$99.00

12-828

EVIDENCE-BASED PRACTICE OF PALLIATIVE MEDICINE

EVIDENCE-BASED PRACTICE OF PALLIATIVE MEDICINE

NATHAN E. GOLDSTEIN, MD

Associate Professor
Director of Research and Quality
Lilian and Benjamin Hertzberg Palliative Care Institute
Brookdale Department of Geriatrics and Palliative Medicine
Mount Sinai School of Medicine
New York, New York;
Physician Investigator
Geriatric Research, Education, and Clinical Center
James J. Peters VA Medical Center
Bronx, New York

R. SEAN MORRISON, MD

Director, National Palliative Care Research Center
Director, Lilian and Benjamin Hertzberg Palliative Care Institute
Hermann Merkin Professor of Palliative Medicine
Brookdale Department of Geriatrics and Palliative Medicine
Mount Sinai School of Medicine
New York, New York;
Physician Investigator
Geriatric Research, Education, and Clinical Center
James J. Peters VA Medical Center
Bronx, New York

ELSEVIER
SAUNDERS

1600 John F. Kennedy Blvd.
Ste 1800
Philadelphia, PA 19103-2899

EVIDENCE-BASED PRACTICE OF PALLIATIVE MEDICINE ISBN: 978-1-4377-3796-7

Notices

Knowledge and best practice in this field are constantly changing. As new research and experience broaden our understanding, changes in research methods, professional practices, or medical treatment may become necessary.

Practitioners and researchers must always rely on their own experience and knowledge in evaluating and using any information, methods, compounds, or experiments described herein. In using such information or methods, they should be mindful of their own safety and the safety of others, including parties for whom they have a professional responsibility.

With respect to any drug or pharmaceutical products identified, readers are advised to check the most current information provided (i) on procedures featured or (ii) by the manufacturer of each product to be administered to verify the recommended dose or formula, the method and duration of administration, and contraindications. It is the responsibility of practitioners, relying on their own experience and knowledge of their patients, to make diagnoses, to determine dosages and the best treatment for each individual patient, and to take all appropriate safety precautions.

To the fullest extent of the law, neither the Publisher nor the authors, contributors, or editors assume any liability for any injury and/or damage to persons or property as a matter of products liability, negligence or otherwise, or from any use or operation of any methods, products, instructions, or ideas contained in the material herein.

The views expressed in this book are those of the authors and/or editors and do not necessarily reflect the position or policy of the Department of Veterans Affairs or the United States government.

Library of Congress Cataloging-in-Publication Data
Evidence-based practice of palliative medicine / [edited by] Nathan E. Goldstein, R. Sean Morrison.
      p. ; cm.
   Includes bibliographical references.
   ISBN 978-1-4377-3796-7 (pbk. : alk. paper)
   I. Goldstein, Nathan E. II. Morrison, R. Sean (Rolfe Sean)
   [DNLM: 1. Palliative Care. 2. Evidence-Based Medicine. WB 310]
   616.02'9–dc23

                                                            2012039834

Content Strategist: Helene Caprari
Senior Content Development Specialist: Jennifer Shreiner
Publishing Services Manager: Anne Altepeter
Senior Project Manager: Doug Turner
Designer: Steve Stave

Printed in the United States of America

Last digit is the print number: 9 8 7 6 5 4 3 2 1

To our patients and their families, who have taught us so much,
And to our partners, Mitchell and Elizabeth, who palliate us in
their own ways

Preface

What Is Palliative Care?

Palliative care is specialized medical care for people with serious illnesses, and the goal is to improve quality of life for both the patient and the family. It is provided by a team of doctors, nurses, social workers, chaplains, and other specialists who work with a patient's other clinicians to provide an added layer of support. Palliative care is appropriate at any age and at any stage in a serious illness, and it can be provided together with curative and disease-directed treatments. Palliative care is different from hospice in that (1) palliative care is given at the same time as life-sustaining or curative treatments whereas hospice is only for patients who have chosen to forego life-sustaining treatments and (2) palliative care is for patients who are at any point in their illness trajectory whereas hospice is for patients who have 6 months or less to live if the disease runs its usual course.

Why Do We Need a New Book About Palliative Care?

Since the early 1990s, the field of palliative medicine has seen exponential growth. In fact, 63% of all hospitals and 85% of mid- to large-size hospitals now report having a palliative care team.[1,2] As the field has grown, so has the evidence base supporting its benefit to patients and their families. Indeed, there is clear evidence that palliative care improves symptom control, helps patients maximize quality of life, and in some cases may help patients live longer.[3-7] As a result of these benefits, palliative care simultaneously reduces costs to hospitals and health care systems.[4,8]

However, many clinicians may not be familiar with the most recent evidence demonstrating the benefits of palliative care. This book provides the most up-to-date evidence (at the time of publication) related to the key, relevant topics encountered during the day-to-day clinical practice of palliative medicine. It is organized in the form of clinical questions, making it more user friendly for the busy practitioner. Each chapter ends with a table that summarizes the key "take-home" points, so the reader can quickly glean the main recommendations or read the entire chapter to get a more in-depth discussion of the topic that includes references to the literature. The chapters are written by clinicians, educators, and researchers across a broad range of disciplines to provide an approach to the practice of palliative medicine from different perspectives.

How Can We Not Thank the Following People?

Publishing a textbook is a daunting task, and we have numerous people to thank. First, thanks to all of our contributors. We are so impressed with their hard work and dedication to our book. Each was given a clinical question and an outline to help organize the material, but it took an incredible amount of work on their part to turn this into the outstanding book that you now hold in your hands. Special thanks go to the team at Elsevier; without our editor, Pam Hetherington, and our amazing developmental editor, Jennifer Shreiner, we would never have been able to complete this book. Thanks to Doug Turner at Elsevier for his work on the proofs, as well. We appreciate the work of Dr. Kathy Foley on the Foreword; we never considered anyone else to author this section and are honored that she would agree to introduce our book in this way. Nate also thanks his partner, Mitchell, and Sean his partner, Elizabeth, and his sons, Kyle and Corey—who help each of us innumerable ways and are always there for us. And last and most important, thanks to our patients and their families, who have taught us so much.

Nathan E. Goldstein and R. Sean Morrison
Mount Sinai School of Medicine

References

1. Voelker R. Hospital palliative care programs raise grade to B in new report card on access. *JAMA.* Dec 7 2011;306(21):2313–2314.
2. Morrison RS, Maroney-Galin C, Kralovec PD, Meier DE. The growth of palliative care programs in United States hospitals. *J Palliat Med.* Dec 2005;8(6):1127–1134.
3. Casarett D, Pickard A, Bailey FA, et al. Do palliative consultations improve patient outcomes? *J Am Geriatr Soc.* Apr 2008;56(4):593–599.
4. Morrison RS, Penrod JD, Cassel JB, et al. Cost savings associated with US hospital palliative care consultation programs. *Arch Intern Med.* Sep 8 2008;168(16):1783–1790.
5. Norton SA, Hogan LA, Holloway RG, Temkin-Greener H, Buckley MJ, Quill TE. Proactive palliative care in the medical intensive care unit: effects on length of stay for selected high-risk patients. *Crit Care Med.* Jun 2007;35(6):1530–1535.
6. Bakitas M, Lyons KD, Hegel MT, et al. Effects of a palliative care intervention on clinical outcomes in patients with advanced cancer: the Project ENABLE II randomized controlled trial. *JAMA.* Aug 19 2009;302(7):741–749.
7. Temel JS, Greer JA, Muzikansky A, et al. Early palliative care for patients with metastatic non-small-cell lung cancer. *N Engl J Med.* Aug 19 2010;363(8):733–742.
8. Morrison RS, Dietrich J, Ladwig S, et al. Palliative care consultation teams cut hospital costs for Medicaid beneficiaries. *Health Aff (Millwood).* Mar 2011;30(3):454–463.

Foreword

The role of palliative medicine has grown and expanded since the early 1990s. The demand for health care professional education and training in this new field of medicine is enormous, which is gratifying to those of us who have advocated for the professionalization of palliative care practice.

We know that educating health care professionals in palliative medicine starts with identifying the common and frequently challenging issues clinicians face as they care for a seriously ill patient. Drs. Goldstein and Morrison, the editors of this new textbook in palliative medicine, have adapted a unique and user-friendly approach that is similar to that of frequently asked questions, and they have assembled a cadre of expert clinicians to provide the evidence-based answers to these common and important questions in palliative medicine.

More than 80 questions define this textbook's domain. They span a diverse range of topics from how to start dosing opioids in an outpatient setting to specific questions about dosing steroids, the use of bisphosphonates, prognostication and difficult conversations, as well as what models of palliative care are appropriate in different settings and what the benefits are of palliative care. In addition to answering a specific question, each chapter provides context, discussion, and pertinent references based on the current available research, coupled with the the authors' clinical expertise and best practices recommendations that give attention to the need for individualized care.

All of the chapters provide substantive information for the busy clinician, and some add a further element to help clinicians advocate for the field of palliative medicine, as evidenced in chapters that address why palliative care is beneficial and needed.

This text's format lends itself to an educational style that is direct, efficient, and practical for busy clinicians and essential for the field. Health care professionals want and need to know the facts quickly and accurately as they contextualize medical information and plan strategies. This text provides a framework to make palliative medicine routinized, prescriptive, evidence based, and integrated. This compendium of questions and answers demonstrates how the field of palliative medicine has advanced and how the practice of improving the quality of life for seriously ill patients and their families has evolved into sophisticated, complex, evidence-based protocols and roadmaps focused on addressing the physical, psychological, and spiritual needs of the sick person and his or her family.

With the increasing demand for palliative care consultations and a limited number of trained specialists to deliver such care, this textbook fills a dual role. It is a powerful teaching tool for nursing and medicial students and trainees, and it is a reliable reference text for senior clinicians who have not been formally trained in palliative medicine but are committed to improving their patients' symptoms and addressing their communication, psychosocial, and spiritual needs.

Clearly, we will succeed in the goal of improving care for those with life-limiting illnesses when health care professionals begin to embrace the answers to the questions raised in this book and integrate them into their daily practice. This textbook will help them achieve this goal.

Kathleen Foley, MD
Professor of Neurology, Neuroscience, and
Clinical Pharmacology
Weill Medical College of Cornell University;
Attending Neurologist
Memorial Sloan-Kettering Cancer Center;
Medical Director
International Palliative Care Initiative
Open Society Foundations

Contributors

Amy P. Abernethy, MD
Associate Professor of Medicine
Division of Medical Oncology
Duke University Medical Center
Durham, North Carolina

Robert M. Arnold, MD
Professor of Medicine
Division of General Internal Medicine
University of Pittsburgh School of Medicine;
Chief, Section of Palliative Care and Medical Ethics
Assistant Director, Institute to Enhance Palliative Care
Director, Institute for Doctor-Patient Communication
Leo H. Criep Chair in Patient Care
UPMC Montefiore Hospital
Pittsburgh, Pennsylvania

Deborah D. Ascheim, MD
Associate Professor
Division of Cardiology
Samuel Bronfman Department of Medicine and
    Department of Health Evidence and Policy
Mount Sinai School of Medicine
New York, New York

Rebecca Aslakson, MD
Assistant Professor
Department of Anesthesiology and Critical Care
    Medicine
The Johns Hopkins University School of Medicine
Baltimore, Maryland

Anthony L. Back, MD
Professor of Medicine
Division of Medical Oncology;
Director, Program in Cancer Communication
Fred Hutchinson Cancer Research Center
University of Washington School of Medicine
Seattle, Washington

Vickie E. Baracos, PhD
Professor of Palliative Care Medicine
Department of Oncology
University of Alberta Faculty of Medicine
    and Dentistry
Edmonton, Alberta, Canada

Susan Block, MD
Chair, Department of Psychosocial Oncology
    and Palliative Care
Dana-Farber Cancer Institute;
Professor of Psychiatry
Department of Medicine
Harvard Medical School;
Co-Director, HMS Center for Palliative Care
Boston, Massachusetts

Barton T. Bobb, MSN, FNP-BC, ACHPN
Advanced Practice Nurse
Thomas Palliative Care Services
Virginia Commonwealth University
Massey Cancer Center
Richmond, Virginia

Jason C. Brookman, MD
Assistant Professor
Department of Anesthesiology and Critical Care
    Medicine
The Johns Hopkins University School of Medicine
Baltimore, Maryland

Melissa D.A. Carlson, PhD, MBA
Assistant Professor
Brookdale Department of Geriatrics and Palliative
    Medicine
Mount Sinai School of Medicine
New York, New York

Thomas Carroll, MD, PhD
Palliative Medicine Fellow
Center for Ethics, Humanities, and Palliative
    Care
University of Rochester School of Medicine
Rochester, New York

Emily J. Chai, MD
Medical Director
Lilian and Benjamin Hertzberg Palliative Care
    Institute
Brookdale Department of Geriatrics and Palliative
    Medicine
Mount Sinai School of Medicine
New York, New York

Harvey M. Chochinov, MD, PhD, OM, FRCPC
Distinguished Professor of Psychiatry
University of Manitoba Faculty of Medicine;
Director, Manitoba Palliative Care Research Unit
CancerCare Manitoba
Winnipeg, Manitoba, Canada

Jessica Cook-Mack, MD
Assistant Professor
Samuel Bronfman Department of Medicine
Mount Sinai School of Medicine
New York, New York

Kenneth E. Covinsky, MD, MPH
Edmund G. Brown, Sr., Professor of Medicine
Division of Geriatrics
University of California, San Francisco
San Francisco, California

Christopher E. Cox, MD, MPH
Assistant Professor of Medicine
Division of Pulmonary, Allergy, and Critical Care
    Medicine
Duke University School of Medicine
Durham, North Carolina

David C. Currow, BMed, MPH, FRACP
Professor of Palliative and Supportive Services
Flinders University
Adelaide, South Australia, Australia

J. Randall Curtis, MD, MPH
Professor of Medicine
Division of Pulmonary and Critical Care
    Medicine
University of Washington School of Medicine
Seattle, Washington

Linda V. DeCherrie, MD
Assistant Professor
Samuel Bronfman Department of Medicine and
    Brookdale Department of Geriatrics and Palliative
    Medicine
Mount Sinai School of Medicine
New York, New York

Ronald M. Epstein, MD
Professor of Family Medicine, Psychiatry, Oncology,
    and Nursing
Director, Center for Communication and Disparities
    Research
University of Rochester Medical Center
Rochester, New York

Mary Ersek, PhD, RN, FAAN
Director
National PROMISE (Performance Reporting and
    Outcomes Measurement to Improve the Standard
    of Care at End-of-Life) Center
Philadelphia Veterans Affairs Medical Center;
Associate Professor
University of Pennsylvania School of Nursing
Philadelphia, Pennsylvania

Kathleen Foley, MD
Professor of Neurology, Neuroscience, and Clinical
    Pharmacology
Weill Medical College of Cornell University;
Attending Neurologist
Memorial Sloan-Kettering Cancer Center;
Medical Director
International Palliative Care Initiative
Open Society Foundations
New York, New York

Laura P. Gelfman, MD
Instructor
Lilian and Benjamin Hertzberg Palliative Care
    Institute
Brookdale Department of Geriatrics and Palliative
    Medicine
Mount Sinai School of Medicine
New York, New York

Eric M. Genden, MD
Professor and Chair
Department of Otolaryngology
Professor of Neurosurgery
Mount Sinai School of Medicine;
Chief, Division of Head and Neck Oncology
Mount Sinai Medical Center
New York, New York

Gabrielle R. Goldberg, MD
Medical Director
The Wiener Family Palliative Care Unit
Assistant Professor
Brookdale Department of Geriatrics and Palliative
    Medicine and Samuel Bronfman Department of
    Medicine
Mount Sinai School of Medicine
New York, New York

Nathan E. Goldstein, MD
Associate Professor
Director of Research and Quality
Lilian and Benjamin Hertzberg Palliative Care
    Institute
Brookdale Department of Geriatrics and Palliative
    Medicine
Mount Sinai School of Medicine
New York, New York;
Physician Investigator
Geriatric Research, Education, and Clinical
    Center
James J. Peters VA Medical Center
Bronx, New York

Rick Goldstein, MD
Attending Physician
Division of Pediatric Palliative Care
Department of Psychosocial Oncology and Palliative
    Care
Dana-Farber Cancer Institute
Children's Hospital Boston
Harvard Medical School
Boston, Massachusetts

Robert Gramling, MD, DSc
Associate Professor
Schools of Medicine and Nursing
Fellowship Director and Co-Director of Research
University of Rochester
Rochester, New York

Corita R. Grudzen, MD, MSHS
Assistant Professor
Department of Emergency Medicine and Brookdale
    Department of Geriatrics and Palliative Medicine
Mount Sinai School of Medicine
New York, New York

The Reverend George Handzo, MA, MDiv, BCC
Senior Consultant
Chaplaincy Care Leadership & Practice
HealthCare Chaplaincy
New York, New York

Paul Hernandez, MDCM, FRCPC
Associate Professor of Medicine
Division of Respirology
Faculty of Medicine
Dalhousie University;
Respirologist
Department of Medicine
Queen Elizabeth II Health Sciences Centre
Halifax, Nova Scotia, Canada

Aluko A. Hope, MD, MSCE
Assistant Professor of Medicine
Division of Critical Care Medicine
Albert Einstein College of Medicine of Yeshiva
    University;
Attending Intensivist
Jay B. Langer Critical Care System
Bronx, New York

Robert Horton, MD
Faculty, Division of Palliative Medicine
Faculty of Medicine
Dalhousie University;
Queen Elizabeth II Health Science Centre
Halifax, Nova Scotia, Canada

Ula Hwang, MD, MPH
Assistant Professor
Department of Emergency Medicine and Brookdale
    Department of Geriatrics and Palliative Medicine
Mount Sinai School of Medicine
New York, New York

Scott A. Irwin, MD, PhD
Chief of Psychiatry
Vice President of Psychosocial Services
San Diego Hospice and the Institute for Palliative
    Medicine
San Diego, California

Vicki A. Jackson, MD, MPH
Assistant Professor of Medicine
Division of Palliative Care
Harvard Medical School;
Chief of Palliative Care
Massachusetts General Hospital
Boston, Massachusetts

Arif Kamal, MD
Assistant Professor of Medicine
Division of Medical Oncology
Department of Medicine
Duke Cancer Institute
Durham, North Carolina

Kenneth L. Kirsh, PhD
Director of Behavioral Medicine and Ancillary
    Services
The Pain Treatment Center of the Bluegrass
Lexington, Kentucky

Kimberly G. Klipstein, MD
Assistant Professor
Department of Psychiatry;
Director, Behavioral Medical and Consultation
    Psychiatry
Mount Sinai Medical Center
New York, New York

Fred C. Ko, MD
Assistant Professor
Brookdale Department of Geriatrics and Palliative
    Medicine
Mount Sinai School of Medicine
New York, New York

Jean S. Kutner, MD, MSPH
Godon Meiklcjohn Endowed
    Professor of Medicine
Division Head, General Internal Medicine
University of Colorado School of Medicine
Denver, Colorado

Alexandra E. Leigh, MD
Assistant Professor of Medicine
Division of Gerontology, Geriatrics, and Palliative
    Care
University of Alabama at Birmingham;
Palliative Care Physician
Birmingham VA Medical Center
Birmingham, Alabama

Stacie K. Levine, MD
Associate Professor
Section of Geriatrics and Palliative Medicine
University of Chicago
Chicago, Illinois

Elizabeth Lindenberger, MD
Program Director
Palliative Medicine Fellowship
Education Director
Lilian and Benjamin Hertzberg Palliative Care
    Institute;
Assistant Professor
Brookdale Department of Geriatrics and Palliative
    Medicine
Mount Sinai School of Medicine
New York, New York

Mara Lugassy, MD
Medical Director
MJHS Hospice and Palliative Care
New York, New York

Jennifer M. Maguire, MD
Clinical Fellow, Pulmonary and Critical Care
    Medicine
Department of Medicine
University of North Carolina
    School of Medicine
Chapel Hill, North Carolina

Deborah B. Marin, MD
Associate Professor
Department of Psychiatry and Brookdale
    Department of Geriatrics and Palliative
    Medicine
Mount Sinai School of Medicine
New York, New York

Diane E. Meier, MD
Director, Center to Advance Palliative Care
Professor and Vice-Chair for Public Policy
Brookdale Department of Geriatrics and Palliative
    Medicine
Gaisman Professor of Medical Ethics
Mount Sinai School of Medicine
New York, New York

Rabbi Edith M. Meyerson, BCC
Palliative Care Chaplain
Lilian and Benjamin Hertzberg Palliative
    Care Institute
Brookdale Department of Geriatrics and Palliative
    Medicine
Mount Sinai School of Medicine
New York, New York

Drew Moghanaki, MD, MPH
Assistant Professor
Department of Radiation Oncology
Virginia Commonwealth University;
Director of Clinical Research
Department of Radiation Oncology
Hunter Holmes McGuire VA Medical Center
Richmond, Virginia

Lori P. Montross, PhD
Director of Psychology and Integrative Medicine
San Diego Hospice and The Institute for Palliative
    Medicine
San Diego, California

R. Sean Morrison, MD
Director, National Palliative Care Research Center
Director, Lilian and Benjamin Hertzberg Palliative
    Care Institute
Hermann Merkin Professor of Palliative Medicine
Brookdale Department of Geriatrics and Palliative
    Medicine
Mount Sinai School of Medicine
New York, New York;
Physician Investigator
Geriatric Research, Education, and Clinical Center
James J. Peters VA Medical Center
Bronx, New York

Alvin H. Moss, MD, FAAHPM
Director
Center for Health Ethics and Law
Professor of Medicine
Medicine, Section of Nephrology
West Virginia University;
Medical Director
Supportive Care Service
West Virginia University Hospital
Morgantown, West Virginia

Ryan R. Nash, MD, MA
Assistant Professor of Medicine
UAB Center for Palliative and Supportive Care
Department of Internal Medicine
University of Alabama, Birmingham
Birmingham, Alabama

Lynn B. O'Neill, MD
Assistant Professor
Department of Medicine
Duke University School of Medicine
Durham, North Carolina

Steve Pantilat, MD
Professor of Clinical Medicine
Department of Medicine;
Director, Palliative Care Program
University of California, San Francisco
San Francisco, California

Steven D. Passik, PhD
Professor
Departments of Psychiatry and Anesthesiology
Vanderbilt University Medical Center
Nashville, Tennessee

Michael W. Rabow, MD, FAAHPM
Professor
Department of Medicine
University of California, San Francisco;
Attending Physician
General Medical Practice and Inpatient Palliative
    Care Service
UCSF Medical Center at Mount Zion;
Director
Symptom Management Service
UCSF Helen Diller Family Comprehensive Cancer
    Care Center
San Francisco, California

Kavitha J. Ramchandran, MD
Clinical Assistant Professor
Department of Medicine
Stanford University School of Medicine
Stanford, California

Aditi Rao, PhD(c), MSN, RN
John A. Hartford Foundation Building Academic
    Geriatric Nursing Capacity Scholar
University of Pennsylvania School of Nursing
Philadelphia, Pennsylvania

Thomas Reid, MD, MA
Assistant Clinical Professor
Department of Medicine
University of California, San Francisco
San Francisco, California

Lynne D. Richardson, MD
Professor
Departments of Emergency Medicine and Health
    Evidence and Policy
Mount Sinai School of Medicine
New York, New York

Christine S. Ritchie, MD, MSPH
Professor of Medicine
Harris Fishbon Distinguished Professor
Department of Medicine
Division of Geriatrics
University of California, San Francisco
San Francisco, California

Graeme Rocker, MD
Professor of Medicine
Head, Division of Respirology
Faculty of Medicine
Dalhousie University;
Queen Elizabeth II Health Science Centre
Halifax, Nova Scotia, Canada

Justine S. Sefcik, MS, RN
National Harford Centers of Gerontological
    Nursing Excellence Patricia G. Archbold
    Scholar
University of Pennsylvania School of Nursing
Philadelphia, Pennsylvania

Joseph W. Shega, MD
Associate Professor of Medicine
Sections of Geriatrics and Palliative Medicine
University of Chicago
Chicago, Illinois

Cardinale B. Smith, MD, MSCR
Assistant Professor
Division of Hematology/Medical Oncology
Tisch Cancer Institute;
Assistant Professor
Lilian and Benjamin Hertzberg Palliative
    Care Institute
Brookdale Department of Geriatrics and Palliative
    Medicine
Mount Sinai School of Medicine
New York, New York

Kristofer L. Smith, MD, MPP
Department of Internal Medicine
Hofstra North Shore-LIJ Medical School
Hofstra University
Hempstead, New York;
Medical Director, Post Acute Care
Department of Internal Medicine
North Shore-LIJ Health System
Manhasset, New York

Lorie N. Smith, MD
Instructor in Medicine
Division of Palliative Care
Harvard Medical School;
Massachusetts General Hospital
Boston, Massachusetts

Thomas J. Smith, MD, FACP
Director of Palliative Medicine
The Johns Hopkins University Medical Institutions;
Professor of Oncology
Sidney Kimmel Comprehensive Cancer Center
Baltimore, Maryland

Theresa A. Soriano, MD
Associate Professor
Department of Medicine
Associate Professor
Brookdale Department of Geriatrics and Palliative
    Medicine
Mount Sinai School of Medicine
New York, New York

Lynn Spragens, MBA
President
Spragens & Associates, LLC
Durham, North Carolina

Knox H. Todd, MD, MPH
Professor and Chair
Department of Emergency Medicine
The University of Texas MD Anderson Cancer Center
Houston, Texas

Rodney O. Tucker, MD, MMM
Associate Professor of Medicine
Division of Gerontology, Geriatrics, and Palliative
    Medicine
University of Alabama at Birmingham
Birmingham, Alabama

Martha L. Twaddle, MD
Associate Professor
Department of Medicine
Rush University Medical Center
Chicago, Illinois;
Chief Medical Officer
Midwest Palliative & Hospice CareCenter
Glenview, Illinois

Jamie H. von Roenn, MD
Professor of Medicine
Division of Medical Oncology
Robert H. Lurie Comprehensive Cancer Center
Northwestern University Feinberg School of Medicine
Chicago, Illinois

Ania Wajnberg, MD
Assistant Professor
Samuel Bronfman Department of Medicine
Mount Sinai School of Medicine
New York, New York

Deborah Waldrop, PhD, MSW
Associate Professor and Associate Dean for Faculty
    Development
School of Social Work
University at Buffalo
Buffalo, New York

Jeremy D. Walston, MD
Raymond and Anna Lublin Professor of Geriatric
    Medicine
Division of Geriatric Medicine and Gerontology
The Johns Hopkins University School of Medicine;
Co-Principal Investigator
Older American Independence Center;
Co-Director
Biology of Healthy Aging Program
Baltimore, Maryland

Monica Wattana, MD
Resident, Department of Emergency Medicine
University of California, Los Angeles
Los Angeles, Californnia

Michelle T. Weckmann, MD
Assistant Professor
Departments of Family Medicine and Psychiatry
University of Iowa
Iowa City, Iowa

Jane L. Wheeler, MS
Medical Instructor
Division of Medical Oncology
Duke University School of Medicine
Durham, North Carolina

Eric Widera, MD
Associate Professor
Division of Geriatrics
University of California, San Francisco;
Director, Hospice and Palliative Care Service
San Francisco VA Medical Center
San Francisco, California

Joanne Wolfe, MD, MPH
Division Chief, Pediatric Palliative Care
Department of Psychosocial Oncology and
    Palliative Care
Dana-Farber Cancer Institute;
Director, Pediatric Palliative Care
Department of Medicine
Children's Hospital Boston;
Associate Professor
Pediatrics
Harvard Medical School
Boston, Massachusetts

Gordon Wood, MD, MSCI
Assistant Professor
Department of Medicine
University of Pittsburgh School of Medicine
Pittsburgh, Pennsylvania

Meng Zhang, MD
Assistant Professor
Samuel Bronfman Department of Medicine
Visiting Doctors Program
Mount Sinai School of Medicine
New York, New York

Contents

Section IV
SPECIAL TOPICS

SYMPTOM MANAGEMENT

PAIN

Chapter 1

How Should Opioids Be Started and Titrated in Routine Outpatient Settings?

GABRIELLE R. GOLDBERG AND CARDINALE B. SMITH

INTRODUCTION AND SCOPE OF THE PROBLEM

Despite recognition of the importance of pain management, availability of effective pain medications in the United States,[1] and multiple published guidelines for the management of pain,[2] the undertreatment of pain in patients with advanced illness continues to be an ongoing and highly prevalent problem.[3] Although numerous organizations such as the World Health Organization (WHO),[4] the American Pain Society,[5] the European Association for Palliative Care, and the American Geriatrics Society[6] have developed guidelines, uncontrolled pain in seriously ill patients persists. The prevalence of undertreatment of cancer pain in particular remains unacceptably high, with nearly half of patients receiving inadequate treatment for their pain.[7] The high prevalence of poorly managed pain is often attributed to barriers to opioid use related to the health care provider, patients and families, and the health care system.[8] Poorly controlled pain has been associated with functional impairment, anxiety, depression, insomnia, and diminished quality of life.[9]

RELEVANT PATHOPHYSIOLOGY

Pain is defined as "an unpleasant sensory and emotional experience associated with actual or potential tissue damage."[10] Pain can be classified as nociceptive, neuropathic, or idiopathic. Nociceptive pain can be further classified as either somatic (resulting from injury to skin and deep tissue) or visceral pain (resulting from injury to internal organs). Visceral pain is often described as dull, vague, or diffuse, whereas somatic pain is more likely to be well localized and described as sharp or intense. The cause of a patient's pain should always be assessed, and disease-specific treatments must be considered[11] and offered where appropriate and consistent with patients' goals of care. The goal of this chapter is to familiarize the reader with an approach to the treatment of pain with opioids; it will not address disease-specific therapies.

End Organ Function

Morphine is metabolized in the liver to morphine-6-glucuronide and morphine-3-glucuronide, both of which are excreted by the kidneys.[12] In the setting of renal failure, these metabolites can accumulate, resulting in a lowering of the seizure threshold. Morphine should therefore be used with caution with mild renal impairment and be avoided in the setting of renal failure.[13] Opioid metabolism is generally impaired in the setting of liver disease, with an increase in oral bioavailability and an increase in elimination half-life.[14] In the setting of severe liver disease, opioids should be used with caution, with a decrease in dose and increased (i.e., longer time between) dosing intervals.[14]

Fentanyl and methadone have few active metabolites and are therefore likely to be safer than other opioids for the treatment of patients with renal or hepatic dysfunction.[13] The most commonly available nonparenteral formulation of fentanyl in the United States is transdermal. As discussed later, transdermal fentanyl should be administered only to a patient who is opioid tolerant, and it should be avoided in patients for whom the opioid dose is being actively titrated. For an in-depth discussion on the use of methadone in treating patients with pain, see Chapters 7 and 8.

Patient Age

Several changes in pharmacokinetics and pharmacodynamics occur with increasing age. Physiological decline in organ function (e.g., decreased glomerular filtration with increased age) and an increased volume of distribution as a result of relative increase in body fat content over skeletal muscle mass can affect the pharmacology of analgesics, and therefore the onset of action, rate of elimination, and half-life of these medications may be altered in older patients.[15] Because of these changes, the prescribing philosophy should be "start low and go slow" (i.e., start at a low dose and increase with caution) when treating older patients with opioids. To be clear, however, older age is not a contraindication to opioid use.

SUMMARY OF EVIDENCE REGARDING TREATMENT RECOMMENDATIONS

Pain Assessment

The experience of pain is subjective, and therefore a patient's report of pain is the gold standard for assessment. The first step in treating a patient is to perform a comprehensive pain assessment. A full pain assessment should take into account the onset, precipitating or alleviating factors, quality, presence or absence of radiation, severity, and timing of the patient's pain. A variety of tools may be used for the assessment of pain severity, including numeric pain intensity rating scales (0 = no pain and 10 = worst possible pain) and the verbal descriptor scales (mild, moderate, or severe). The numeric rating scale offers several advantages, including ease of administration and scoring, multiple response options, and no reported age-related difficulties in its use.[16] For younger patients, the Faces Pain Scale may be more effective than verbal report.[17] (For more information on treating pediatric patients, see Chapter 65.) Clinicians should assess pain intensity regularly, because this helps guide the initial approach to treatment, response to treatment, and need for further titration of medications.

Choosing a Starting Dose

When considering starting a patient on opioids for the treatment of pain in the outpatient setting, several factors must be considered, including the severity of pain, end organ function, patient age, and history of opioid use (Table 1-1). These factors will influence the initial opioid to be used, the starting dose, and the interval of administration. Treatment of pain in the outpatient setting often poses more challenges than pain management in the inpatient setting.

Inpatient settings allow for rapid titration of opioids because the medications can be administered intravenously and may be repeated and increased over minutes to hours. The inpatient setting also allows for controlled dispensing of medication with minimal concern for misuse or diversion. Challenges in the outpatient setting include ensuring that the patient can obtain the prescribed medications (in terms of being able to both afford the medication and find a pharmacy that dispenses opioids[18]), difficulties in monitoring for side effects, and a delay in being able to assess the patient's responses to the medications prescribed (Table 1-2).

Severity of Pain

The WHO developed guidelines for the management of cancer pain in the mid-1990s, and as of 2011 it is currently developing treatment guidelines for the management of acute pain, chronic pain in adults, and chronic pain in children.[4] In the absence of guidelines for pain management in the noncancer population, the WHO Pain Relief Ladder for cancer has been applied to the management of pain in other diseases as well. The WHO recommends a stepwise approach to pain management, with choice of medication based on pain severity, using nonopioids (aspirin and acetaminophen) for mild pain, *mild opioids* (codeine or oxycodone with acetaminophen) for mild to moderate pain, and *strong opioids* such as morphine for moderate to severe pain.[4] The weakness of this approach is that the mild opioids may become limited by the nonopioid component (e.g., in combination medications containing acetaminophen, the total acetaminophen dose for a healthy individual is less than 4 g per 24 hours, and it may be lower in older patients or those with liver disease).[19] Because of concerns about hepatotoxicity with the use of combination opioid agents, the FDA has recommended banning these combination medications.[20] Given these concerns, combination medications will not be further discussed in this chapter. For patients presenting in severe pain, the clinician should consider whether the patient would benefit from inpatient admission to ensure more rapid relief by titrating intravenous opioids as opposed to dose-finding with oral opioids in an outpatient setting.

TABLE 1-1. Issues to Consider When Starting a Patient on an Opioid

- Is the patient opioid naïve?
- What opioids have been effective for the patient in the past?
- What is the patient's age, and does this have an effect on either dose or interval of administration?
- What is the patient's renal function?
- What is the patient's liver function?

TABLE 1-2. Issues to Consider When Prescribing Opioid Medications in the Outpatient Setting

- Does the medication come in the dose you want to prescribe?
- What is the cost of the medication? Does the patient have prescription coverage? Will the patient be able to afford the prescription?
- Where will the patient be filling the prescription?
- Is the medication available at the patient's local pharmacy?
- Did you start the patient on a bowel regimen?
- Have you arranged for a short interval for follow-up with the patient to assess for response to treatment, tolerability, and presence of side effects?

Approach to the Opioid-Naïve Patient

When starting a patient on opioids in the outpatient setting, a short-acting medication that is available orally should be selected; the choices most readily available in the United States are morphine, oxycodone, and hydromorphone. The use of short-acting oral medication allows for active titration. Morphine is generally the opioid of first choice because of its relatively low cost and availability.[2] The recommended starting dose for an opioid-naïve patient is morphine 5 to 10 mg intravenously (IV), which is approximately equivalent to morphine 15 to 30 mg orally (PO) (Table 1-3). The clinician should start at the lower end of this range and reevaluate the patient frequently (either via phone or in subsequent office visits) to determine the optimal starting dose of medication to control the patient's pain. For an older or more debilitated patient, starting at the low end or below this range should be considered.[6] As discussed earlier, oxycodone or hydromorphone would be the preferred oral opioid in patients with a history of renal or liver failure, because their metabolites are not as active as those of morphine. For patients with incident pain that is not constant or that occurs at specific times during the day, the medication should be started on an as-needed basis. For patients with continuous pain, the medication should be prescribed on a standing basis, dosed every 4 hours for patients with normal renal and hepatic function.[21]

In addition to a standing order, patients should also be provided with medications to treat breakthrough pain.[2] Breakthrough pain refers to a transitory increase in pain to greater than moderate intensity that occurs on a baseline or pain of moderate intensity or less in a patient receiving chronic opioid therapy.[22] This pain can be incident (pain is provoked by an event) or may occur spontaneously. The typical dosing recommendations for rescue medications are based largely on anecdotal experience. It has been suggested that the effective dose of breakthrough pain medication is a percentage of the patient's total daily opioid dose, most commonly 10% to 20% of the 24-hour dosage.[2,23] However, current evidence suggests that the dose of opioid for breakthrough pain should be determined by individual titration.[24–26] A useful clinical rule of practice is:

Breakthrough dose = 10% of total 24-hour dosage

The time to peak effect of a short-acting oral opioid is 60 to 90 minutes. Based on the pharmacokinetics of opioids, breakthrough doses of oral opioids can therefore be prescribed every 1 to 2 hours as needed for pain. For example, a patient prescribed morphine 30 mg PO every 4 hours around the clock (a total of 180 mg of morphine in 24 hours) should also receive morphine 18 mg PO every hour as needed for pain. To make administration of this easier, it should be rounded to 15 mg PO every hour as needed.

Approach to the Opioid-Tolerant Patient

Tolerance is defined pharmacologically as loss of drug effect with chronic dosing.[27] Patients currently on opioid therapy or with a prior (or current) history of opioid use will have higher requirements than those who are opioid naïve. Initial dose finding should follow the same guidelines as in the opioid-naïve patient; however, the starting dose will be higher.

Assessment for Response

Assessment for response to an opioid dose should be made at the time of peak effect. Based on the pharmacokinetics of the short-acting oral opioids, if relief has not been obtained in 60 to 90 minutes with an oral opioid, the patient will not receive additional relief despite the fact that the duration of action is 4 hours. Patients should be instructed that if they are requiring the breakthrough doses more frequently than two or three times per day, they should contact their clinician for further titration of the standing medication.

Opioid Titration

Patients should be encouraged to keep a pain journal documenting their use of pain medications and their pain scores. There should be a short time to the next follow-up visit, preferably within 1 week of starting a patient on opioids. This follow-up may occur either in person or by telephone. The clinician should review the patient's use of breakthrough medications, response to the treatment, and presence of side effects (including sedation and constipation). The clinician should also review and calculate the total 24-hour opioid use. Patients with well-controlled pain, requiring no more than 3 breakthrough doses per day, can be started on long-acting opioids, with the total 24-hour opioid dosage divided into 2 daily

TABLE 1-3. Opioid Analgesic Equivalences*

OPIOID AGONISTS	INTRAVENOUS/ SUBCUTANEOUS/ INTRAMUSCULAR (mg)	ORAL/ RECTAL (mg)	DURATION OF EFFECT (hr)
Morphine	10	30	4
Hydrocodone	—	30	4
Oxycodone	—	20	4
Oxymorphone	1	10	4
Hydromorphone	1.5	7.5	4
Fentanyl	†	‡	1-2
Codeine	130	200	4

Modified from Horton JR. Hospital-based opioid analgesia. In: Dunn A, Klotman P, Kathuria N, eds. *Handbook of Hospital Medicine.* Hackensack NJ: World Scientific. In press.

*This table provides a conversion ratio when converting from one opioid medication to another or from one route of administration to another.
†Convert morphine 2 mg PO/24 hr to fentanyl 1 mcg/hr transdermal patch; transdermal fentanyl should never be prescribed for an opioid-naïve patient.
‡Oral fentanyl preparations are available, but their use is complicated and simple conversion ratios do not exist.

doses of long-acting opioid administered every 12 hours. Long-acting opioids will maintain the level of pain control, lessen the pill burden, and decrease the need to wake up at night to take pain medications. Occasionally, patients may report increased pain in the 3 to 4 hours before the next standing dose, requiring the frequent use of breakthrough opioids. This phenomenon is known as end-of-dose failure. In this circumstance, it is reasonable to consider prescribing the long-acting opioid every 8 hours, rather than every 12. The majority of long-acting or sustained-release opioid oral formulations *cannot* be split or crushed, so doses prescribed must be sums or multiples of the available pill sizes. (Crushing or splitting long-acting preparations may counteract the mechanism that ensures delayed, controlled release and thus crushing these medications can potentially result in overdose.) However, select brand-name formulations of long-acting morphine are available in capsules that may be opened and administered via enteral feeding tubes. For example, the patient started on morphine 30 mg PO every 4 hours (180 mg in 24 hours) is taking 1 or 2 breakthrough doses and reports her pain is well controlled. This is a total of 195 to 210 mg of oral morphine daily. Sustained-release morphine tablets are available in 15, 30, 60, 100, and 200 mg. She may be prescribed sustained-release morphine 90 mg PO every 12 hours (180 mg in 24 hours), with continuation of morphine 15 mg PO every 1 to 2 hours as needed for breakthrough pain. A 90-mg long-acting morphine preparation is not available, so the clinician will need to write prescriptions for both sustained-release morphine 60 mg and sustained-release morphine 30 mg to ensure the patient can take the dose of 90 mg every 12 hours.

If the patient requires multiple doses of breakthrough medication in a 24-hour period, her pain is not optimally controlled and the entire 24-hour opioid requirement should be totaled and converted to a long-acting formulation. For example, the patient started on morphine 30 mg PO every 4 hours (180 mg in 24 hours) is requiring 4 breakthrough doses of morphine 15 mg per day (an additional 60 mg in 24 hours) to control her pain. The patient's total 24-hour opioid requirement is 240 mg. She may be prescribed sustained-release morphine 100 mg (note the available formulations reviewed earlier) PO every 12 hours.

Alternatively, if the patient's pain is not well controlled, dose adjustments may be made based on the severity of the pain. Adjustments typically allow for a 25% to 50% dose increase for a patient with mild to moderate pain and a 50% to 100% dose adjustment for a patient with moderate to severe pain. For example, a patient started on morphine 30 mg PO every 4 hours (180 mg in 24 hours) has taken 6 rescue doses of morphine 15 mg per day for the previous 5 days (an additional 90 mg in 24 hours), and she reports her pain is still 10 on a pain scale of 0 to 10. The patient is tolerating a total of 270 mg of morphine in 24 hours; thus her dose can be safely increased by approximately 50% to sustained-release morphine 200 mg PO every 12 hours (400 mg in 24 hours).

Another option for long-acting opioid administration for a patient with well-controlled pain on a stable, standing opioid regimen is the use of transdermal fentanyl. Transdermal administration is particularly useful in patients who are unable to take oral medications or who have enteral feeding tubes. Transdermal fentanyl patches are changed every 72 hours, although some patients may need them changed as frequently as every 48 hours. Because of the longer half-life of transdermal fentanyl, it is not the best choice of opioid for a patient who is still requiring active titration of the analgesic regimen.[2] Transdermal fentanyl is lipophilic and requires a patient to have adequate adipose tissue for effective absorption; it is not recommended for use in patients who are cachectic or very thin. The transdermal absorption can be altered by temperature and moisture, so patients who sweat frequently or live in environments without adequate temperature control may not be good candidates for the transdermal patch. Additionally, the patches should be removed and replaced with an alternative opioid regimen if the patient develops a high fever. Transdermal fentanyl takes 12 to 24 hours to reach peak effect; therefore (1) transdermal fentanyl is *never* an appropriate first-line option for the management of pain in a patient who is opioid naïve and (2) the patient's prior opioid regimen should be continued for the first 12 hours after application of the first fentanyl patch. Each time the clinician evaluates a patient prescribed transdermal fentanyl, the physical examination should verify that the patch has been placed in an area to ensure appropriate absorption.

Opioid Side Effects

Common opioid side effects are listed in Table 1-4. Tolerance develops to all opioid side effects, with the exception of constipation, an expected and predictable consequence of taking opioids. At the time of prescribing opioids, *all* patients should also be started on a prophylactic bowel regimen unless the patient is having diarrhea or has another contraindication to being on a bowel regimen. One of the most commonly used regimens is senna (Senokot) (1 or 2 tablets at bedtime) and docusate (100 mg two or three times per day), although evidence is lacking

TABLE 1-4. Opioid Side Effects

SIDE EFFECT	TIME ON STABLE OPIOID DOSE TO THE DEVELOPMENT OF TOLERANCE
Constipation	Never
Nausea/vomiting	7-10 days
Pruritus	7-10 days
Sedation	36-72 hr
Respiratory depression	Extremely rare when opioids are dosed appropriately

to recommend the addition of docusate to senna as an initial regimen to improve laxation.[28,29] Clinicians should assess for constipation during every follow-up visit after a patient is started on an opioid regimen.

Opioid Rotation

Opioid rotation involves switching from one opioid to another. The clinician should consider opioid rotation when a patient has (1) difficulty tolerating the initial opioid prescribed, because of intolerable side effects (e.g., nausea, pruritus, myoclonus); (2) poor response to pain control with the initial opioid, despite appropriate titration; or (3) worsening of renal or hepatic function.[30,31] When choosing to rotate from morphine to another opioid, oxycodone and hydromorphone are both reasonable alternatives.[32] When rotating opioid medications, the concept of incomplete cross-tolerance, which is the idea that the new drug may be more effective because of differences in potency or drug bioavailability, must be taken into consideration.[9,33] If the patient's pain is well controlled, the equianalgesic dose for the new opioid can be calculated using the Opioid Analgesic Equivalences table (Table 1-3). This dose is then decreased by 25% to 50% to adjust for incomplete cross-tolerance.[31] Clinical judgment should be used in selecting the appropriate dose (e.g., if the pain was not well controlled, the clinician may consider not decreasing the dose or reducing the dose by only 25%). The patient should have close follow-up because the dose initially chosen may require titration.

Opioid Agreements

Written opioid agreements are recommended by consensus guidelines to decrease the risk for opioid misuse.[34] The introduction of an opioid agreement to patients is an opportunity to review potential misperceptions the patient may have about the safety of opioids and their potential side effects and to establish expected treatment outcomes. This discussion has the potential to minimize patient nonadherence with opioid regimens.[35] Agreements may include stipulations such as the patient must obtain opioid prescriptions from only one prescriber, fill the prescription from only one specified pharmacy, and agree to random urine drug screens.[34] Many opioid agreements also clearly state clinical circumstances and behaviors that will lead to discontinuation of opioid prescribing by the clinician or the practice. The limited evidence base for the efficacy of these treatment agreements suggests these agreements may be effective.[36] Opioid agreements should be considered in routine practice because they may provide clinicians with a means of encouraging safer use of opioids through increased compliance with treatment recommendations. They additionally provide a means of consistently and objectively applying ramifications of nonadherence with treatment recommendations.

KEY MESSAGES TO PATIENTS AND FAMILIES

Clinicians should reassure patients and their families that most pain can be effectively treated with available analgesics. Addiction is a common concern for patients and their families, and given the frequency of this concern, clinicians may want to address this proactively. It is important to remind patients that the risk for addiction (defined as persistent use despite harm to self or others) in a patient taking opioids for pain who has no history of abuse is exceedingly low.[19] Likewise, because of misconceptions about opioids, patients and families often have serious concerns about these medications. Clinicians should thus encourage patients and their families to express their concerns about side effects, because these can pose barriers to effective pain management. To engage patients and families in their own care, clinicians may want to encourage the use of a pain journal documenting the timing of administration of standing and breakthrough pain medications and the impact of these medications on pain and function. This information can be very helpful in guiding clinicians in pain management.

CONCLUSION AND SUMMARY

Poor pain management remains a major barrier to high-quality care for patients facing serious illness. Palliative care clinicians have the ability to provide safe and effective pain control for the majority of patients through the appropriate dosing and titration of opioids. Continued research is required to increase the evidence base for the majority of the treatment recommendations provided in this chapter.

SUMMARY RECOMMENDATIONS

- Morphine is the opioid of first choice for the treatment of severe pain.
- Patients on standing opioids should be prescribed rescue medications for breakthrough pain.
- Clinicians should educate patients about the efficacy and side effects of opioids, as well as address any concerns about the use of this class of medication so as to increase patient adherence.
- All patients started on opioids should be started on a bowel regimen unless there is a clear contraindication.
- Opioid treatment agreements should be considered in outpatient practices.

REFERENCES

1. Azevedo Sao Leao Ferreira K, Kimura M, Jacobsen Teixeira M. The WHO analgesic ladder for cancer pain control: twenty years of use. How much pain relief does one get from using it? *Support Care Cancer.* 2006;14(11):1086–1093.
2. Hanks GW, Conno Fd, Cherny N, et al. Morphine and alternative opioids in cancer pain: the EAPC recommendations. *Br J Cancer.* 2001;84(5):587–593.

3. Apolone G, Corli O, Caraceni A, et al. Pattern and quality of care of cancer pain management: results from the Cancer Pain Outcome Research Study Group. *Br J Cancer.* 2009;100(10):1566–1574.

4. Kates M, Perez X, Gribetz J, Swanson SJ, McGinn T, Wisnivesky JP. Validation of a model to predict perioperative mortality from lung cancer resection in the elderly. *Am J Respir Crit Care Med.* 2009;179(5):390–395.

5. *American Pain Society. Principles of Analgesic Use in the Treatment of Acute Pain and Cancer Pain.* 6th ed. Glenview, IL: American Pain Society; 2008.

6. American Geriatrics Society Panel on the Pharmacological Management of Persistent Pain in Older Persons. Pharmacological management of persistent pain in older persons. *J Am Geriatr Soc.* 2009;57(8):1331–1346.

7. Deandrea S, Montanari M, Moja L, Apolone G. Prevalence of undertreatment in cancer pain: a review of published literature. *Ann Oncol.* 2008;19(12):1985–1991.

8. Maltoni M. Opioids, pain, and fear. *Ann Oncol.* 2008;19(1):5–7.

9. Pasero C. *Pain Assessment and Pharmacologic Management.* St. Louis, MO: Mosby; 2011.

10. *International Association for the Study of Pain.* IASP Taxonomy. http://www.iasp-pain.org/AM/Template.cfm?Section=Pain_Definitions. Accessed May 12, 2012.

11. Qaseem A, Snow V, Shekelle P, et al. Evidence-based interventions to improve the palliative care of pain, dyspnea, and depression at the end of life: a clinical practice guideline from the American College of Physicians. *Ann Intern Med.* 2008;148(2):141–146.

12. Coller JK, Christrup LL, Somogyi AA. Role of active metabolites in the use of opioids. *Eur J Clin Pharmacol.* 2009;65(2):121–139.

13. Smith HS. Opioid metabolism. *Mayo Clin Proc.* 2009;84(7):613–624.

14. Hasselstrom J, Eriksson S, Persson A, Rane A, Svensson JO, Sawe J. The metabolism and bioavailability of morphine in patients with severe liver cirrhosis. *Br J Clin Pharmacol.* 1990;29(3):289–297.

15. Rowe JW, Andres R, Tobin JD, Norris AH, Shock NW. The effect of age on creatinine clearance in men: a cross-sectional and longitudinal study. *J Gerontol.* 1976;31(2):155–163.

16. Burton J, Miner J. *Emergency Sedation and Pain Management.* New York, NY: Cambridge University Press; 2007.

17. Wong DL, Baker CM. Pain in children: comparison of assessment scales. *Pediatr. Nurs.* 1988;Jan–Feb;14(1):9–17.

18. Morrison RS, Wallenstein S, Natale DK, et al. "We don't carry that"—failure of pharmacies in predominantly nonwhite neighborhoods to stock opioid analgesics. *N Engl J Med.* 2000;342:1023–1026.

19. Goldstein NE, Morrison RS. Treatment of pain in older adults. *Crit Rev Oncol Hematol.* 2005;54:157–164.

20. Spira A, Ettinger DS. Multidisciplinary management of lung cancer. *N Engl J Med.* 2004;350(4):379–392.

21. American Pain Society. *Principles of Analgesic Use in the Treatment of Acute Pain and Cancer Pain.* 6th ed. Glenview, IL: American Pain Society; 2008.

22. Portenoy RK, Hagen NA. Breakthrough pain: definition, prevalence and characteristics. *Pain.* 1990;41(3):273–281.

23. Gammaitoni AR, Fine P, Alvarez N, McPherson ML, Bergmark S. Clinical application of opioid equianalgesic data. *Clin J Pain.* 2003;19(5):286–297.

24. Christie JM, Simmonds M, Patt R, et al. Dose-titration, multicenter study of oral transmucosal fentanyl citrate for the treatment of breakthrough pain in cancer patients using transdermal fentanyl for persistent pain. *J Clin Oncol.* 1998;16(10):3238–3245.

25. Farrar JT, Cleary J, Rauck R, Busch M, Nordbrock E. Oral transmucosal fentanyl citrate: randomized, double-blinded, placebo-controlled trial for treatment of breakthrough pain in cancer patients. *J Natl Cancer Inst.* 1998;90(8):611–616.

26. Coluzzi PH, Schwartzberg L, Conroy Jr. JD, et al. Breakthrough cancer pain: a randomized trial comparing oral transmucosal fentanyl citrate (OTFC®) and morphine sulfate immediate release (MSIR®). *Pain.* 2001;91(1–2):123–130.

27. Thompson AR, Ray JB. The importance of opioid tolerance: a therapeutic paradox. *J Am Coll Surg.* 2003;196(2):321–324.

28. Hurdon V, Viola R, Schroder C. How useful is docusate in patients at risk for constipation? A systematic review of the evidence in the chronically ill. *J Pain Symptom Manage.* 2000;19(2):130–136.

29. Hawley PH, Byeon JJ. A comparison of sennosides-based bowel protocols with and without docusate in hospitalized patients with cancer. *J Palliat Med.* 2008;11(4):575–581.

30. Manfredi PL, Borsook D, Chandler SW, Payne R. Intravenous methadone for cancer pain unrelieved by morphine and hydromorphone: clinical observations. *Pain.* 1997;70(1):99–101.

31. Fine PG, Portenoy RK. Establishing "best practices" for opioid rotation: conclusions of an expert panel. *J Pain Symptom Manage.* 2009;38(3):418–425.

32. Reid CM, Martin RM, Sterne JA, Davies AN, Hanks GW. Oxycodone for cancer-related pain: meta-analysis of randomized controlled trials. *Arch Intern Med.* 2006;166(8):837–843.

33. Nicholson B. Responsible prescribing of opioids for the management of chronic pain. *Drugs.* 2003;63(1):17–32.

34. Chou R, Fanciullo GJ, Fine PG, et al. Clinical guidelines for the use of chronic opioid therapy in chronic noncancer pain. *J Pain.* 2009;10(2):113–130.

35. Graziottin A, Gardner-Nix J, Stumpf M, Berliner MN. Opioids: how to improve compliance and adherence. *Pain Pract.* 2011;11:574–581.

36. Starrels JL, Becker WC, Alford DP, Kapoor A, Williams AR, Turner BJ. Systematic review: treatment agreements and urine drug testing to reduce opioid misuse in patients with chronic pain. *Ann Intern Med.* 2010;152(11):712–720.

How Should Opioids Be Started and Titrated in Hospital or Inpatient Settings?

CARDINALE B. SMITH AND GABRIELLE R. GOLDBERG

INTRODUCTION AND SCOPE OF THE PROBLEM

Pain is the most common symptom experienced by hospitalized adults.[1] Patients with advanced disease admitted to a hospital setting often have moderate to severe pain and require intravenous opioid therapy.[2] Beginning intravenous opioid therapy in the inpatient setting allows for rapid titration of pain medication, because medication doses may be repeated or the dose escalated over minutes to hours. The inpatient setting also allows for controlled dispensing of opioid medications with little concern for misuse or diversion. Acute severe pain requires rapid application of analgesic strategies and aggressive treatment, which are distinct from chronic management techniques that may be done in the outpatient setting. Numerous adverse outcomes exist to poorly treated pain, including reduced patient satisfaction,[3] depressed mood,[4] decreased quality of life,[5] increased interference with physical functioning,[4] and increased costs resulting from prolongation of hospital stays and delays in return to work.[6,7] In the postoperative setting, complications of poorly controlled pain may include splinting because of chest wall pain, leading to atelectasis and ultimately pneumonia, and deep venous thrombosis[8] resulting from reduced movement because of pain and limiting physical function. Organizations including the World Health Organization (WHO),[9] the American Pain Society,[10] the European Association for Palliative Care,[11] and the American Geriatrics Society[12] have developed guidelines for the treatment of pain, but untreated and poorly controlled pain remains a major problem in hospital settings.

RELEVANT PATHOPHYSIOLOGY

Pain is defined as "an unpleasant sensory and emotional experience associated with actual or potential tissue damage."[13] Pain can be classified as nociceptive, neuropathic, or idiopathic. Nociceptive pain can be further classified as either somatic (resulting from injury to skin and deep tissue) or visceral pain (resulting from injury to internal organs). Visceral pain is often described as dull, vague, or diffuse, whereas somatic pain is more likely to be well-localized and described as sharp or intense.

The cause of a patient's pain should always be assessed and disease-specific treatment offered[14] when appropriate and consistent with patients' goals of care. The focus of this chapter will be on treating pain in the inpatient setting with opioids; a discussion of disease-specific therapies is beyond the scope of this section.

Opioid Pharmacology

It is important to understand the pharmacology of opioids because it dictates the way in which opioids are prescribed and administered. The administration of intravenous opioids is associated with the most rapid onset of analgesia. The time to peak plasma concentration and therefore peak effect of intravenous opioids can vary, although the general range is 5 to 30 minutes. The duration of effect is usually 3 to 4 hours. Opioids are conjugated in the liver and excreted (approximately 90% to 95%) by the kidney.

SUMMARY OF EVIDENCE REGARDING TREATMENT RECOMMENDATIONS

Pain Assessment

The experience of pain is subjective, and therefore a patient's report of pain is the gold standard of assessment. Treatment begins with a comprehensive pain assessment. This includes asking questions to assess time of onset, precipitating or alleviating factors, quality, presence or absence of radiation, severity, and timing of the pain. A variety of tools may be used for the assessment of pain severity, including numeric pain intensity rating scales (0 = no pain and 10 = worst possible pain) and the verbal descriptor scales (mild, moderate, or severe). The numeric rating scale offers several advantages, including ease of administration and scoring, multiple response options, and no reported age-related difficulties in its use.[15] For younger patients and those with cognitive impairments, the Faces Pain Scale may be more effective than verbal report.[16] (For more information on treating pediatric patients, see Chapter 65.) Clinicians should assess pain intensity regularly, because this helps guide the initial approach to treatment, efficacy of current regimen, and need for further titration of medications.

Choosing a Starting Dose

When initiating opioid therapy in the inpatient setting, the severity of pain, end organ function, dose of opioid (if any) currently being taken, the patient's prior experiences with pain, and history of opioid use are all key factors in determining the appropriate regimen. The mu-agonist opioids—morphine, hydromorphone, and fentanyl—are the most commonly used intravenous agents in patients with moderate to severe pain. Methadone is available in an intravenous formulation, but because of its unique pharmacokinetic profile and the complexity relating to its dosing and titration, it should not be used as the initial treatment for pain in the inpatient setting. (For more information on the use of methadone, see Chapters 7 and 8.) In the patient who is opioid naïve, morphine is considered the opioid of choice because of its established effectiveness, availability, familiarity to physicians, simplicity of administration, and relatively lower cost compared to those of other opioids. It is likewise the most appropriate medication for patients on oral morphine who need either titration or escalation of their pain regimen in the inpatient setting.

Opioid Use in Patients With End Organ Dysfunction

Caution should be used with the administration of opioids in patients with renal or hepatic dysfunction. The two major morphine metabolites are morphine-3 glucuronide (M3G) and morphine-6 glucuronide (M6G). M6G appears to contribute to the analgesic activity of morphine.[17,18] M3G does not have analgesic activity and is believed to contribute to the neuroexcitatory side effects. Both M3G and M6G are eliminated by the kidney and, because of a longer half-life than the parent compound, will accumulate faster than morphine itself. The buildup of these metabolites is associated with the most severe toxicities observed with the use of opioids (respiratory depression or obtundation, myoclonus, and seizures).[19] Although evidence regarding the use of opioids in renal and hepatic insufficiency comes from small group pharmacokinetic studies or case reports, which included patients with wide variation in the degree of organ dysfunction, morphine is still not recommended for use in patients with renal

insufficiency.[20] It is also appropriate to consider an alternative opioid for a patient receiving morphine who experiences a decrease in renal function and a concomitant increase in undesirable effects. Fentanyl is considered relatively safe in renal insufficiency because there are no known active metabolites. However, few pharmacokinetic data exist regarding fentanyl in end-stage renal disease.[21] Clinicians should consider starting even the relatively "renal-failure safer" opioids at lower than normal doses to ensure patient safety.[22,23]

In the presence of hepatic impairment, most drugs are subject to significantly impaired clearance, but this has been poorly studied in the clinical setting. The elimination of morphine is greatly reduced in patients with liver disease, and the recommendations have been to decrease the frequency of administration in these patients.[24,25] A paucity of data exist for the use of hydromorphone in patients with hepatic dysfunction, but expert consensus suggests it can be used with caution by increasing (i.e., extending) the dosing interval.[15] In contrast, fentanyl pharmacokinetics do not appear to be altered in patients with cirrhosis and therefore fentanyl may be a reasonable choice in these patients.[25]

Approach to the Opioid-Naïve Patient

The recommended starting dose for an opioid-naïve patient is morphine 5 to 10 mg intravenously (IV), which is approximately equivalent to 15 to 30 mg of oral morphine. An older or more debilitated patient should be started at the lower end of this range. Although this is the dose commonly used, few studies have evaluated the appropriate starting dose for opioid-naïve patients in acute pain. There have been several studies evaluating the utility of beginning various doses and intervals of morphine to achieve appropriate analgesia, particularly in the emergency room setting.[26,27] No one defined standard exists, however, and current practice is based on expert consensus.

Severe pain is considered a medical emergency and should be managed aggressively. Ideally, the starting dose of the opioid should be administered as a bolus or "intravenous push" dose as opposed to a slow infusion over 30 minutes. The peak effect of intravenous opioids is approximately 8 to 15 minutes after administration; therefore the analgesic response can be reevaluated at about 15 minutes after an intravenous push. The dose may then be repeated every 15 minutes if the patient is not sedated and adequate analgesia has not been achieved (see Chapter 1, Table 1-3). A rule of thumb for dose increases is to use 25% to 50% more morphine for mild to moderate pain and 50% to 100% more for moderate to severe pain. A dose increase of less than 25% is likely to have no effect. Repeated intravenous doses are administered in this fashion to titrate to the point of adequate analgesia. Once the adequate dose has been determined, that dose can be prescribed for every 4 hours as a standing order, assuming there is no hepatic or renal dysfunction. Standing scheduled dosing will maintain stable serum drug levels and provide consistent relief.

In addition to a standing order, patients also should be prescribed medications to treat breakthrough pain. Breakthrough pain refers to a transitory increase in pain, to greater than moderate intensity, in a patient receiving chronic opioid therapy.[28] This can be related to incident pain (pain provoked by an event) or pain that occurs spontaneously. Breakthrough pain is treated with rescue medication, which is taken as required (i.e., as needed), rather than on a regular basis.[29] The typical dosing recommendations for rescue medications have been based on anecdotal experience. It has been suggested that the effective dose of breakthrough pain medication is a percentage of the patient's total daily opioid dose (most commonly 10% to 20% of the 24-hour dosing).[30,31] However, current evidence suggests that the dose of opioid for breakthrough pain should be determined by individual titration.[32–34] Future studies on this topic are warranted because the primary objective of previous trials was to evaluate the efficacy of short-acting formulations, not to determine optimal rescue medication dosing. The dosing interval of the rescue medication is based on the pharmacokinetics described earlier. In reality, a rescue dose could be given every 8 to 15 minutes, because this is the time to peak effect of the intravenous opioids. However, in the inpatient setting it is difficult to have a clinician administer a dose that frequently. In clinical practice, these authors suggest calculating the rescue dose as 10% of the total 24-hour dose, given every hour as needed for pain. This interval should be increased to 2 hours for patients with hepatic or renal dysfunction. In a patient requiring frequent administration of rescue doses it is appropriate to consider starting the patient on patient-controlled analgesia (PCA). For example, if a patient is on morphine 4 mg IV every 4 hours (24-hour dose is 24 mg), the rescue medication dose is 2.4 mg IV every hour as needed for pain, although this would be rounded to 2 mg to simplify administration.

Approach to the Opioid-Tolerant Patient

Pharmacologically, tolerance is defined as the loss of drug effect with chronic dosing.[35] Patients on opioid therapy or with a prior history of opioid use will have higher requirements than those who are opioid naïve. Initial dose finding should follow the same guidelines as for the opioid-naïve patient; however, the starting dose will be higher. For example, a patient on long-acting morphine sulfate 45 mg orally (PO) every 12 hours (90 mg in 24 hours) is admitted for progression of disease, with complaints of 10 on a pain scale of 0 to 10 not relieved by the current oral morphine regimen. This is the equivalent of a 24-hour dose of morphine 30 mg IV, or 5 mg IV every 4 hours. Because

the patient has severe pain, the clinician decides to increase the dose by 50% and give a 7.5-mg intravenous morphine bolus dose to treat the acute pain crisis.

Opioid Titration

It is important to ensure accurate and continuous recording of the amount of pain medication necessary to achieve adequate analgesia, because this information will allow safer and more efficient dose titration. After the patient has been started on a regimen of standing opioids and a rescue medication, the total dose of opioids required for effective analgesia is then assessed. In general, the goal is that rescue medications be required no more than two or three times per day. If a patient requires a rescue medication more frequently, the standing dose should be increased. The general practice includes calculating the total opioid doses required in the previous 24-hour period. If the patient's pain is well controlled, this total calculated dose can then be given in divided doses every 4 hours and a new rescue medication dose calculated. If this regimen did not provide adequate relief, the same general rule of thumb applies as described earlier (25% to 50% increase in dose for mild to moderate pain and 50% to 100% increase in dose for moderate to severe pain). For example, a patient is prescribed morphine 4 mg IV every 4 hours and 2 mg IV every hour as needed. The patient has received a total of 5 of the rescue doses (total 24-hour dose is 34 mg). If the pain was well controlled on this regimen, the new dose would be 6 mg IV every 4 hours, with 3 mg IV every hour as needed (doses rounded for ease of administration). If the pain was only moderately controlled, the dose can be increased by 25% to 50%. The new dose would then be 8 mg IV every 4 hours, with 4 mg IV every hour as needed for pain.

Method of Administration

In addition to administering standing opioid doses every 4 hours, the inpatient setting allows for continuous intravenous infusions of pain medications. Depending on the source or severity of pain and the patient's overall health status, continuous intravenous infusions may help achieve better efficacy. This can be achieved either with a continuous "drip" or via a PCA pump. PCA allows a patient to self-administer opioid therapy (according to a clinician's order) to control pain. PCA administration can include a baseline (continuous) infusion, a patient-controlled demand (bolus) dose given at some frequency with a lockout interval, or both; the basal and bolus can each be given alone, or they may be given together. Lockout interval refers to the time between boluses during which the pump will not allow more bolus doses to be administered. Use of PCA has several advantages, the primary being patient convenience. The medication can be administered immediately, removing the delay that often exists when a clinician is required to bring the rescue medication. For a patient with acute severe pain, PCA will allow for more rapid pain relief and faster titration of opioid therapy. Finally, PCA helps to ensure safety; a patient who becomes sedated can no longer press the button for additional doses, thus limiting the risk for respiratory depression. If other individuals press the button to release bolus doses, this can result in administration of potentially unnecessary and unsafe doses of the medication.

Finding the appropriate dose for PCA administration is very similar to the methods described earlier. In general, the majority of patients started on PCA will have been on opioid therapy previously. The first step is to calculate the total opioid doses required in the previous 24-hour period. Expert opinion suggests that 50% to 70% of this dose should be used as the basal (continuous infusion) rate. If the regimen previously used did not provide adequate relief, using the entire 24-hour requirements as the basal dose should be considered. Evidence on the appropriate lockout interval is lacking. Based on the pharmacokinetics of the intravenous opioids the lockout can be between 5 and 30 minutes. In clinical practice the most commonly used intervals are 6, 8, 10, and 15 minutes. In general, the lockout interval should be based on providing adequate analgesic coverage during times when patients need the most coverage (during times when activities or other factors that precipitate pain may occur). The American Pain Society recommends a lockout interval of 5 to 10 minutes for patients with acute pain.[36] The bolus dose given is typically 50% to 150% of the basal dose.[37] In the authors' experience, the general practice is a lockout of 10 minutes with a bolus dose of 50% of the basal amount. The amount of the bolus dose depends on the nature of the pain. Patients who experience severe incident pain may benefit from a relatively higher PCA dose. When intravenous access is not possible, PCA may be administered by the subcutaneous route. Based on risk for local irritation and toxicity, there is a maximum hourly rate that can be given by the subcutaneous route. The maximum rate may be as high as 10 mL per hour, although institutional policies vary.[38] The subcutaneous route may therefore require bags with higher than standard concentrations to keep the hourly maximum volume low. Use of nonstandard concentrations is a potential source of medication error and should be carefully reviewed with the pharmacist and nurse administering the medication. Inappropriate candidates for PCA therapy include patients who are physically or cognitively unable to self-administer demand or breakthrough medication. In other words, patients must be able to interpret their own pain and be able to press the button to administer a bolus dose. Patients, families, and clinicians should be reminded that the PCA bolus should be administered only by the patient. For example, a patient is on morphine 6 mg IV every 4 hours and 4 mg IV every hour as needed (received 10 doses in last the 24 hours). To better control the patient's pain, the clinician decides to start a PCA. The patient received a total of morphine 76 mg IV (6 doses of 6 mg plus 10 doses of 4 mg) in 24 hours. Because the patient rates her current pain as a 5 on a pain rating scale of 0 to 10, it is decided that the basal dose will be 70% of the previous total 24-hour dose. Thus the basal rate should be 2.2 mg per hour (76 mg/24 hr × 70% as basal = 53 mg over 24 hours = 2.2 mg/hr). The orders will be written as follows (note that the doses have been rounded to simplify administration and setting of the pump):

1. Basal rate: Morphine 2.5 mg per hour
2. Bolus dose: Morphine 1.5 mg with a lockout interval of 10 minutes (50% of the basal dose, adjusted for rounding)
3. Maximum hourly dose: 11.5 mg per hour

When starting a basal rate via the PCA it is important to remember that it will take several hours for the dose to reach a steady state. More specifically, it will take 4 to 5 half-lives of a drug to reach a new steady state. Therefore simply starting the basal rate will take 10 to 15 hours for the drug to reach a steady state. In the inpatient setting, this may be an unacceptably long delay to achieve analgesia. It would not be unusual for a patient to use the bolus doses more frequently during this period. A clinician-activated bolus dose ordered in addition to the basal and bolus rate also can be considered. This dose is usually written as 10% of the total 24-hour dose every hour as needed for pain. The clinician-activated bolus is administered by the nurse most commonly by PCA, but can also be given as a separate intravenous dose (bolus or slower infusion). For example, for the patient discussed earlier the orders will now be:

1. Basal rate: Morphine 2.5 mg per hour
2. Bolus dose: Morphine 1.5 mg, with a lockout interval of 10 minutes
3. Maximum hourly dose: 11.5 mg per hour
4. Clinician-administered dose: 6 mg every hour as needed × 4 doses (*Note:* The clinician dose is based on the 24-hour total basal rate, not the maximum hourly dose. The modifier of "×4 doses" is written because if the patient has not achieved appropriate analgesia with the PCA and 4 clinician-administered doses, the patient needs to be reassessed to determine if the entire regimen should be adjusted.)

Opioid Side Effects

Common opioid side effects are listed in Table 2-1. Tolerance develops to all opioid side effects, with the exception of constipation, which is an expected and predictable consequence of taking opioids. At the time of prescribing opioids *all* patients should also be started on a prophylactic bowel regimen, unless the patient has diarrhea or another contraindication to a bowel regimen. One of the most commonly used regimens is senna (Senokot) (1 or 2 tablets at bedtime) and docusate (100 mg two or three times per day), although evidence is lacking to recommend

TABLE 2-1. Opioid Side Effects

SIDE EFFECT	TIME ON STABLE OPIOID DOSE TO THE DEVELOPMENT OF TOLERANCE
Constipation	Never
Nausea/vomiting	7-10 days
Pruritus	7-10 days
Sedation	36-72 hr
Respiratory depression	Extremely rare when opioids are dosed appropriately

the addition of docusate to senna as an initial regimen to improve laxation.[39,40] Clinicians should assess for constipation during every follow-up visit after a patient is started on an opioid regimen. (For further discussion of treating constipation in the setting of opioids, see Chapter 24.)

Opioid Rotation

Opioid rotation involves switching from one opioid to another in an attempt to limit adverse effects or improve analgesia. The clinician should consider opioid rotation when a patient has (1) difficulty with the initial opioid prescribed because of intolerable side effects (e.g., nausea, pruritus, myoclonus), (2) poor response to pain control with the initial opioid despite appropriate titration, or (3) worsening of renal or hepatic function.[41,42] When choosing to rotate from morphine to another opioid, oxycodone and hydromorphone are both reasonable alternatives.[41] If the patient's pain is well controlled, the equianalgesic dose for the new opioid can be calculated using the Opioid Analgesic Equivalences table (see Chapter 1, Table 1-3). When rotating opioid medications, the concept of incomplete cross-tolerance must be taken into consideration, in which the new drug may be more effective because of differences in potency or drug bioavailability. An appropriate dose reduction is to decrease the new opioid dose by 25% to 50% to allow for this incomplete cross-tolerance.[43] Clinical judgment should be used in selecting the appropriate dose (e.g., if the pain is not well controlled, the clinician may consider not decreasing the dose or dose reducing by only 25%). The patient should have close follow-up, because the dose initially chosen may need to be titrated.

KEY MESSAGES TO PATIENTS AND FAMILIES

Clinicians should explain to patients and families that the majority of pain associated with serious illness can be effectively treated with available analgesics. Patients should be empowered to believe that serious pain is a medical emergency and they should expect adequate analgesia in a timely fashion, with particular attention paid to rapid pain control. Addiction and psychological dependence are common concerns for patients and their families, and given the frequency of this concern, clinicians may

want to proactively address this topic. It is important to remind patients that the risk for addiction (defined as persistent use despite harm to self or others) in a patient taking opioids for pain who has no history of abuse is exceedingly low.[44] Likewise, because of misconceptions about opioids, patients and families often have other concerns about these medications. Clinicians should thus encourage patients and their families to express their concerns about side effects, because these can pose barriers to effective pain management.

CONCLUSIONS AND SUMMARY

Pain is a significant symptom experienced by hospitalized patients. Opioids are effective at treating pain in the hospitalized patient and can lead to improved patient outcomes. Palliative care practitioners can provide rapid, effective, and safe pain management for patients in the inpatient setting. The majority of current evidence surrounding the initiation and titration of opioids in the inpatient setting relies on expert opinion and consensus. Further investigative work is needed to improve the evidence base for these treatment recommendations.

SUMMARY RECOMMENDATIONS

- Morphine is the opioid of first choice for the treatment of pain.
- Patients on standing opioids should be prescribed rescue medication for breakthrough pain.
- Patients in severe pain crisis should be given intravenous bolus pain medication until the crisis is resolved.
- Patient-controlled analgesia should be considered for patients with severe pain requiring frequent bolus doses.
- Opioid rotation should be considered for patients with intolerable side effects or poorly managed pain despite adequate titration.

REFERENCES

1. Warfield CA, Kahn CH. Acute pain management: programs in U.S. hospitals and experiences and attitudes among U.S. adults. *Anesthesiology.* 1995;83(5):1090–1094.
2. Desbiens NA, Wu AW. Pain and suffering in seriously ill hospitalized patients. *J Am Geriatr Soc.* 2000;48(5 suppl):S183–S186.
3. Myles PS, Williams DL, Hendrata M, Anderson H, Weeks AM. Patient satisfaction after anaesthesia and surgery: results of a prospective survey of 10,811 patients. *Br J Anaesth.* 2000; 84(1):6–10.
4. Cleeland CS, Gonin R, Hatfield AK, et al. Pain and its treatment in outpatients with metastatic cancer. *N Engl J Med.* 1994;330 (9):592–596.
5. Rustoen T, Moum T, Padilla G, Paul S, Miaskowski C. Predictors of quality of life in oncology outpatients with pain from bone metastasis. *J Pain Symptom Manage.* 2005;30(3):234–242.
6. Stewart WF, Ricci JA, Chee E, Morganstein D, Lipton R. Lost productive time and cost due to common pain conditions in the US workforce. *JAMA.* 2003;290(18):2443–2454.

7. Fortner BV, Demarco G, Irving G, et al. Description and predictors of direct and indirect costs of pain reported by cancer patients. *J Pain Symptom Manage.* 2003;25(1):9–18.
8. Nett MP. Postoperative pain management. *Orthopedics.* 2010;33(9 suppl):23–26.
9. World Health Organization. WHO's pain ladder. http://www.who.int/cancer/palliative/painladder/en/. Accessed May 21, 2012.
10. American Pain Society. *Principles of Analgesic Use in the Treatment of Acute Pain and Cancer Pain.* 6th ed. Glenview, IL: American Pain Society; 2008.
11. Hanks GW, Conno F, Cherny N, et al. Morphine and alternative opioids in cancer pain: the EAPC recommendations. *Br J Cancer.* 2001;84(5):587–593.
12. Society Panel of the Pharmacological Management of Persistent Pain in Older Persons. Pharmacological Management of Persistent Pain in Older Persons. *J Am Geriatr Soc.* 2009;57(8): 1331–1346.
13. *International Association for the Study of Pain.* IASP taxonomy. http://www.iasp-pain.org/Content/NavigationMenu/GeneralResourceLinks/PainDefinitions/default.htm; Accessed October 9, 2012.
14. Qaseem A, Snow V, Shekelle P, et al. Evidence-based interventions to improve the palliative care of pain, dyspnea, and depression at the end of life: a clinical practice guideline from the American College of Physicians. *Ann Intern Med.* 2008;148(2):141–146.
15. Burton J, Miner J. *Emergency Sedation and Pain Management.* New York: Cambridge University Press; 2007.
16. Herr KA, Mobily PR, Kohout FJ, Wagenaar D. Evaluation of the Faces Pain Scale for use with the elderly. *Clin J Pain.* 1998;14(1):29–38.
17. Lotsch J. Opioid metabolites. *J Pain Symptom Manage.* 2005;29 (5 suppl):S10–S24.
18. Portenoy RK, Thaler HT, Inturrisi CE, Friedlander-Klar H, Foley KM. The metabolite morphine-6-glucuronide contributes to the analgesia produced by morphine infusion in patients with pain and normal renal function. *Clin Pharmacol Ther.* 1992;51(4):422–431.
19. Tiseo PJ, Thaler HT, Lapin J, Inturrisi CE, Portenoy RK, Foley KM. Morphine-6-glucuronide concentrations and opioid-related side effects: a survey in cancer patients. *Pain.* 1995; 61(1):47–54.
20. Dean M. Opioids in renal failure and dialysis patients. *J Pain Symptom Manage.* 2004;28(5):497–504.
21. Murphy EJ. Acute pain management pharmacology for the patient with concurrent renal or hepatic disease. *Anaesth Intensive Care.* 2005;33(3):311–322.
22. Pergolizzi J, Boger RH, Budd K, et al. Opioids and the management of chronic severe pain in the elderly: consensus statement of an international expert panel with focus on the six clinically most often used World Health Organization step III opioids (buprenorphine, fentanyl, hydromorphone, methadone, morphine, oxycodone). *Pain Pract.* 2008;8(4):287–313.
23. Rhee C, Broadbent AM. Palliation and chronic renal failure: opioid and other palliative medications—dosage guidelines. *Progr Palliat Care.* 2003;11:183–190.
24. Tegeder I, Lotsch J, Geisslinger G. Pharmacokinetics of opioids in liver disease. *Clin Pharmacokinet.* 1999;37(1):17–40.
25. Rhee C, Broadbent AM. Palliation and liver failure: palliative medications dosage guidelines. *J Palliat Med.* 2007;10(3): 677–685.
26. Mercadante S, Villari P, Ferrera P, Casuccio A, Fulfaro F. Rapid titration with intravenous morphine for severe cancer pain and immediate oral conversion. *Cancer.* 2002;95(1):203–208.
27. Kumar KS, Rajagopal MR, Naseema AM. Intravenous morphine for emergency treatment of cancer pain. *Palliat Med.* 2000;14(3):183–188.
28. Portenoy RK, Hagen NA. Breakthrough pain: definition, prevalence and characteristics. *Pain.* 1990;41(3):273–281.
29. Davies AN, Dickman A, Reid C, Stevens AM, Zeppetella G. The management of cancer-related breakthrough pain: recommendations of a task group of the Science Committee of the Association for Palliative Medicine of Great Britain and Ireland. *Eur J Pain.* 2009;13(4):331–338.
30. Hanks GW, Fd Conno, Cherny N, et al. Morphine and alternative opioids in cancer pain: The EAPC recommendations. *Br J Cancer.* 2001;84(5):587–593.
31. Gammaitoni AR, Fine P, Alvarez N, McPherson ML, Bergmark S. Clinical application of opioid equianalgesic data. *Clin J Pain.* 2003;19(5):286–297.
32. Christie JM, Simmonds M, Patt R, et al. Dose-titration, multicenter study of oral transmucosal fentanyl citrate for the treatment of breakthrough pain in cancer patients using transdermal fentanyl for persistent pain. *J Clin Oncol.* 1998;16(10):3238–3245.
33. Farrar JT, Cleary J, Rauck R, Busch M, Nordbrock E. Oral transmucosal fentanyl citrate: randomized, double-blinded, placebo-controlled trial for treatment of breakthrough pain in cancer patients. *J Natl Cancer Inst.* 1998;90(8):611–616.
34. Coluzzi PH, Schwartzberg L, Conroy Jr JD, et al. Breakthrough cancer pain: a randomized trial comparing oral transmucosal fentanyl citrate (OTFC®) and morphine sulfate immediate release (MSIR®). *Pain.* 2001;91(1–2):123–130.
35. Thompson AR, Ray JB. The importance of opioid tolerance: a therapeutic paradox. *J Am Coll Surg.* 2003;196(2):321–324.
36. Gordon DB, Dahl J, Phillips P, et al. The use of "as-needed" range orders for opiod analgesics in the management of acute pain: a consensus statement of the American Society for Pain Management and the American Pain Society. *Pain Manag Nurs.* 2004;5(52):53–58.
37. Ingram C. *A practical approach to pain management.* Mankato, MN; 2011. http://mnhpc.org/wp-content/uploads/2011/03/1A_Practical_Approach_to_Pain_Mgmt.pdf; Accessed October 9, 2012.
38. Bruera E, Brenneis C, Michaud M, et al. Use of the subcutaneous route for the administration of narcotics in patients with cancer pain. *Cancer.* 1988;62(2):407–411.
39. Hurdon V, Viola R, Schroder C. How useful is docusate in patients at risk for constipation? A systematic review of the evidence in the chronically ill. *J Pain Symptom Manage.* 2000;19(2):130–136.
40. Hawley PH, Byeon JJ. A comparison of sennosides-based bowel protocols with and without docusate in hospitalized patients with cancer. *J Palliat Med.* 2008;11(4):575–581.
41. Manfredi PL, Borsook D, Chandler SW, Payne R. Intravenous methadone for cancer pain unrelieved by morphine and hydromorphone: clinical observations. *Pain.* 1997;70(1):99–101.
42. Fine PG, Portenoy RK. Establishing "best practices" for opioid rotation: conclusions of an expert panel. *J Pain Symptom Manage.* 2009;38(3):418–425.
43. Reid CM, Martin RM, Sterne JA, Davies AN, Hanks GW. Oxycodone for cancer-related pain: meta-analysis of randomized controlled trials. *Arch Intern Med.* 2006;166(8):837–843.
44. Goldstein NE, Morrison RS. Treatment of pain in older adults. *Crit Rev Oncol Hematol.* 2005;54:157–164.

Chapter 3

How Should Patient-Controlled Analgesia Be Used in Patients With Serious Illness and Those Experiencing Postoperative Pain?

Cardinale B. Smith and Gabrielle R. Goldberg

INTRODUCTION AND SCOPE OF THE PROBLEM

Pain is the most common symptom experienced by hospitalized adults. Despite recognition of the importance of effective pain management, undertreatment of pain continues to be widespread.[1] Many patients with serious illness who are admitted to the hospital and those in the postoperative setting will have moderate to severe pain and require opioid therapy. For patients undergoing surgery in the United States, it has been estimated that less than 25% will receive adequate relief of acute pain.[2] Poorly treated pain can result in adverse outcomes, including reduced patient satisfaction,[3] depressed mood,[4] decreased quality of life,[5] worsening of functional status,[4] and increased costs resulting from prolonged hospital stays and delays in return to work.[6,7] In patients undergoing abdominal, thoracic, or cardiac surgery, uncontrolled pain can result in respiratory splinting, increasing the risk for atelectasis, pneumonia, and immobility, with the associated complications of thromboembolic disease and muscular deconditioning.[8] Organizations such as the World Health Organization (WHO),[9] the American Pain Society,[10] the European Association for Palliative Care,[11] and the American Geriatrics Society,[12] have developed guidelines for the treatment of pain, but unfortunately many hospitalized patients continue to have poorly controlled pain.

RELEVANT PATHOPHYSIOLOGY

Types of Pain

Pain is defined as "an unpleasant sensory and emotional experience associated with actual or potential tissue damage."[13] The experience of pain is subjective, and thus a patient's self-report of pain is the gold standard for assessment. Pain can be classified as nociceptive, neuropathic, or idiopathic. Nociceptive pain can be further classified as either somatic (resulting from injury to skin and deep tissue) or visceral pain (resulting from injury to internal organs). Visceral pain is often described as dull, vague, or diffuse, whereas somatic pain is more likely to be well localized and described as sharp or intense.

Opioid Pharmacology

A basic understanding of opioid pharmacology is necessary because it dictates the way opioids are prescribed and administered. The administration of intravenous opioids is associated with the most rapid onset of analgesia but also the shortest duration of action. The time to peak plasma concentration and therefore peak effect of intravenous opioids can vary from approximately 8 to 15 minutes. The time to peak effect of a short-acting oral opioid is 60 to 90 minutes. The duration of effect for both intravenous and oral opioids is usually 3 to 4 hours. Longer-acting oral opioids have varying durations of effect. In general, the duration is 8 to 24 hours, depending on the particular formulation (not including methadone, which has more complex pharmacokinetics and is covered in more detail in Chapters 7 and 8). Opioids are conjugated in the liver and excreted (approximately 90% to 95%) by the kidney. These medications do not have an analgesic efficacy ceiling (i.e., higher doses are associated with greater pain relief), and they can be titrated upward as needed until dose-limiting side effects appear.

SUMMARY OF EVIDENCE REGARDING TREATMENT RECOMMENDATIONS

One of the advantages of intravenous opioid therapy over oral formulations is that the administration of intravenous medications allows for rapid titration because the time to onset is short compared to that of oral medications. This allows for rapid repeat administration and dose escalation to achieve effective pain control. For patients with mild pain the initiation and titration of oral opioid therapy may be appropriate. Conversely, for patients with severe, poorly controlled pain, intravenous administration is the preferred route. Patient–controlled analgesia (PCA) allows patients to self-administer intravenous opioid therapy (according to a clinician's order) with an electronic infusion device to control pain. Typically, PCAs employ intravenous opioids, although the subcutaneous route also can be used. Of note, intravenous and subcutaneous doses are identical. PCA administration can include a baseline (continuous) infusion, a patient-controlled demand (bolus) dose given at some frequency with a lockout interval, or both. The basal and bolus can each be given alone, or they may be given together. The lockout interval is the time between boluses during which the pump will not allow administration of more bolus doses.

PCA offers several advantages. First, PCA therapy reduces the time from the experience of pain to treatment. Specifically, PCA allows medication to be administered immediately, removing the delay that often exists when a nurse is required to bring a rescue intravenous medication. Second, for a patient with acute severe pain, PCA provides faster, individualized titration of opioid therapy than clinician-directed oral or intravenous opioid escalation and thus more rapid pain relief.[14] Finally, PCA helps ensure safety; a patient who becomes sedated can no longer press the button for additional doses, thus limiting the risk for respiratory depression. The following section will discuss the use of PCAs in patients with serious illness and those in the postoperative setting.

The mu-agonist opioids—morphine, hydromorphone, and fentanyl—are the most commonly used intravenous agents in patients with moderate to severe pain. For most opioid-naïve patients, morphine is considered the medication of choice because of its established effectiveness, availability, familiarity to physicians, ease of administration, and relatively low cost. Little evidence exists suggesting major differences in efficacy or side effects between morphine and other commonly used opioids, with the exception of patients with renal insufficiency.[15,16] In the setting of renal insufficiency, the use of a drug with no active metabolites, such as fentanyl, is preferred.[17] Finally, although methadone is available in an intravenous formulation and can be used in PCA, its unusual pharmacokinetic profile and the complexity of its dosing typically relegate its use to situations in which other opioids have not been effective. As a result of its unique properties, methadone should be used only by highly experienced palliative care clinicians. The use of methadone is discussed separately in Chapters 7 and 8.

For patients started on PCA who have previously been receiving opioid therapy, the first step is to calculate the total opioid doses required in the previous 24-hour period. Expert opinion suggests that 50% to 70% of this dose should be used as the basal (continuous infusion) rate (divided over a 24-hour period). If the regimen previously used did not provide adequate relief, using the entire last 24-hour opioid requirement as the basal dose and then calculating the per-hour dose can be considered. In regard to the lockout period, evidence is lacking as to the most appropriate duration. Based on the pharmacokinetics of intravenous opioids, the lockout can be 5 to 30 minutes. In clinical practice the most commonly used intervals are 6, 8, 10, and 15 minutes. In general the lockout interval should be based on providing adequate analgesia during times when activities or factors that precipitate pain are most likely to occur. The American Pain Society recommends a lockout interval of every 5 to 10 minutes for patients with acute pain.[18] The bolus dose is typically 50% to 100% of the basal dose.[19] In the authors' experience, the general practice is a lockout of 10 minutes with a bolus dose of 50% of the basal. The amount of the bolus dose given depends on the nature of the pain. Patients who experience severe incident pain may benefit from a relatively higher PCA bolus dose. When intravenous access is not possible, PCA may be administered by the subcutaneous route. Based on risk for local irritation and toxicity, there is a maximum hourly rate that can be given by the subcutaneous route. The maximum rate may be as high as 10 mL per hour, although institutional policies vary.[20] Inappropriate candidates for PCA therapy include patients who are physically or cognitively unable to safely and effectively self-administer demand or breakthrough medication.[21] Patients, families, and clinicians should be reminded that the PCA bolus should be administered only by the patient. If individuals other than patients press the button to release bolus doses, the inherent safety of the PCA (i.e., the inability of sedated patients to press the button, resulting in overdose) is compromised, resulting in administration of potentially unnecessary and unsafe doses. For example, a patient is on morphine 6 mg intravenously (IV) every 4 hours and 4 mg IV every hour as needed (received 10 doses in last 24 hours). To better control the patient's pain, the clinician decides to start PCA. The patient received a total of morphine 76 mg IV (6 doses of 6 mg + 10 doses of 4 mg) in 24 hours. Because the patient rates her current pain as 5 on a pain scale of 0 to 10, it is decided that the basal dose will be 70% of the previous total 24-hour dose. Thus the basal rate should be 2.2 mg per hour (76 mg/24 hr × 70% as basal = 53 mg over 24 hr = 2.2 mg/hr). The orders will be written as follows (note that the doses have been rounded to make administration and setting of the pump easier):

1. Basal rate: Morphine 2.5 mg/hr
2. Bolus dose: Morphine 1.5 mg with a lockout interval of 10 minutes (50% of the basal dose, adjusted for rounding)
3. Maximum hourly dose: 11.5 mg/hr

When starting a basal rate for PCA it is important to remember that it will take 4 to 5 half-lives, possibly 10 to 15 hours, for the drug to reach a new steady state. This can result in delayed response for patients experiencing severe pain. During this period, it is not unusual for patients to use frequent

TABLE 3-1. Patient-Controlled Anesthesia Dosing for Opioid-Naïve Patients

DRUG	LOADING DOSE	PCA DOSE	LOCKOUT (min)	BASAL RATE*
Morphine	2.5 mg	0.5-2 mg	8	0-0.5 mg/hr
Hydromorphone	0.4 mg	0.1-0.4 mg	6-8	0-0.1 mg/hr
Fentanyl	25 mcg	5-25 mcg	5-6	0-5 mcg/hr

H, Hour; mcg, microgram; mg, milligram.
*Basal rates in opioid-naïve patients should be used with caution.

bolus doses. A clinician-activated bolus dose can be used in addition to the basal and bolus doses and can be administered either by PCA or intravenously as a drip or push. This dose is usually written as 10% of the total 24-hour basal dose every hour as needed for pain. In the previous example, the clinician dose would be 2.5 mg every hour as needed × 4 doses.

For patients who are in the postoperative setting, initial dosing for PCA is different from that for patients with serious, chronic illness. Bolus administration without continuous infusion is the most common method employed for the postoperative patient population. It has been reported that the use of a continuous infusion versus bolus dosing only is associated with no difference in the number of bolus doses given, but the incidence of side effects is increased.[22,23] The routine use of a continuous infusion is not recommended as standard treatment for these patients because postoperative pain is self-limited and the expectation is that the opioid will be tapered quickly. However, a continuous infusion is reasonable in patients who are opioid tolerant and in opioid naïve patients who show high opioid requirements or complain of waking at night in severe pain.[24] Although there is no standard approach to starting PCA administration in opioid-naïve patients, Table 3-1 presents a general consensus starting point.

Data show that PCA versus conventional intravenous opioid analgesia for postoperative pain (e.g., a nurse administering an opioid on patient request) results in improved pain control and greater patient satisfaction with a similar adverse event profile.[25,26] However, few data exist regarding PCA versus oral opioids in this setting. The few studies evaluating oral opioids compared to PCA in the postoperative setting suggest the analgesic outcomes are equivalent.[27–29] However, these studies were conducted in varying types of surgical patients, used different opioids, used novel techniques, and also included the use of adjuvant analgesics. Therefore, no standard technique or guideline is available regarding the most effective approach.

KEY MESSAGES TO PATIENTS AND FAMILIES

Clinicians should help patients and their families understand that pain can inhibit mobility and recovery and effective pain control is critically important to improve both patient comfort and clinical outcomes. The distinction between when pain can be managed with oral agents or with intravenous agents can be confusing for patients, so clarification is helpful. For example, explain that uncomplicated postoperative pain can be managed with oral opioids for many patients, but for those patients who have severe pain, PCA can provide enhanced analgesia and at the same time allow patients more control over administration of their pain medication.

CONCLUSION AND SUMMARY

Pain is a common symptom in hospitalized adults and in the postoperative setting. Many modalities are available to treat these patients. PCA can be a very effective and safe method of pain relief and may allow easier individualization of therapy compared with conventional methods of opioid analgesia. Although oral opioids may be appropriate in some postoperative settings, a longer time is required for titration to adequate relief.

SUMMARY RECOMMENDATIONS

- Morphine is the opioid of first choice for the treatment of severe pain.
- Intravenous patient-controlled analgesia (PCA) provides superior postoperative analgesia and improves patient satisfaction.
- Intravenous PCA allows for more rapid titration of analgesia.

REFERENCES

1. Warfield CA, Kahn CH. Acute pain management: programs in U.S. hospitals and experiences and attitudes among U.S. adults. *Anesthesiology*. 1995;83(5):1090–1094.
2. Phillips DM. JCAHO pain management standards are unveiled: Joint Commission on Accreditation of Healthcare Organizations. *JAMA*. 2000;284(4):428–429.
3. Myles PS, Williams DL, Hendrata M, Anderson H, Weeks AM. Patient satisfaction after anaesthesia and surgery: results of a prospective survey of 10,811 patients. *Br J Anaesth*. 2000;84(1):6–10.
4. Cleeland CS, Gonin R, Hatfield AK, et al. Pain and its treatment in outpatients with metastatic cancer. *N Engl J Med*. 1994;330(9):592–596.
5. Rustoen T, Moum T, Padilla G, Paul S, Miaskowski C. Predictors of quality of life in oncology outpatients with pain from bone metastasis. *J Pain Symptom Manage*. 2005;30(3):234–242.
6. Stewart WF, Ricci JA, Chee E, Morganstein D, Lipton R. Lost productive time and cost due to common pain conditions in the US workforce. *JAMA*. 2003;290(18):2443–2454.

7. Fortner BV, Demarco G, Irving G, et al. Description and predictors of direct and indirect costs of pain reported by cancer patients. *J Pain Symptom Manage.* 2003;25(1):9–18.

8. Nett MP. Postoperative pain management. *Orthopedics.* 2010; 33(9 suppl):23–26.

9. World Health Organization. WHO's pain ladder. http://www.who.int/cancer/palliative/painladder/en/; Accessed May 21, 2012.

10. American Pain Society. *Principles of Analgesic Use in the Treatment of Acute Pain and Cancer Pain.* 6th ed. Glenview, IL: American Pain Society; 2008.

11. Hanks GW, Conno F, Cherny N, et al. Morphine and alternative opioids in cancer pain: the EAPC recommendations. *Br J Cancer.* 2001;84(5):587–593.

12. Pharmacological management of persistent pain in older persons. *J Am Geriatr Soc.* 2009;57(8):1331–1346.

13. *International Association for the Study of Pain.* IASP Taxonomy. http://www.iasp-pain.org/Content/NavigationMenu/GeneralResourceLinks/PainDefinitions/default.htm; Accessed October 9, 2012.

14. Graves DA, Foster TS, Batenhorst RL, Bennett RL, Baumann TJ. Patient-controlled analgesia. *Ann Intern Med.* 1983;99(3):360–366.

15. Rapp SE, Egan KJ, Ross BK, Wild LM, Terman GW, Ching JM. A multidimensional comparison of morphine and hydromorphone patient-controlled analgesia. *Anesth Analg.* 1996;82(5): 1043–1048.

16. Woodhouse A, Hobbes AFT, Mather LE, Gibson M. A comparison of morphine, pethidine and fentanyl in the postsurgical patient-controlled analgesia environment. *Pain.* 1996;64(1):115–121.

17. Smith HS. Opioid metabolism. *Mayo Clin Proc.* 2009;84(7):613–624.

18. Gordon DB, Dahl J, Phillips P, et al. The use of "as-needed" range orders for opiod analgesics in the management of acute pain: a consensus statement of the American Society for Pain Management and the American Pain Society. *Pain Manag Nurs.* 2004;5(52):53–58.

19. Miaskowski C, Burney R, Coyne P, et al. *Guideline for the management of cancer pain in adults and children.* Clinical practice guideline no. 3. Glenview, IL: American Pain Society; 2005.

20. Bruera E, Brenneis C, Michaud M, et al. Use of the subcutaneous route for the administration of narcotics in patients with cancer pain. *Cancer.* 1988;62(2):407–411.

21. Dev R, Del Fabbro E, Bruera E. Patient-controlled analgesia in patients with advanced cancer: should patients be in control? *J Pain Symptom Manage.* 2011;42(2):296–300.

22. Hill HF, Mather LE. Patient-controlled analgesia: pharmacokinetic and therapeutic considerations. *Clin Pharmacokinet.* 1993;24(2):124–140.

23. Etches RC. Patient-controlled analgesia. *Surg Clin North Am.* 1999;79(2):297–312.

24. Macintyre PE. Safety and efficacy of patient controlled analgesia. *Br J Anaesth.* 2001;87(1):36–46.

25. Liu SS, Wu CL. The effect of analgesic technique on postoperative patient-reported outcomes including analgesia: a systematic review. *Anesth Analg.* 2007;105(3):789–808.

26. Hudcova J, McNicol E, Quah C, Lau J, Carr DB. Patient controlled opioid analgesia versus conventional opioid analgesia for postoperative pain. *Cochrane Database Syst Rev.* 2006;(4) CD003348.

27. Striebel HW, Scheitza W, Philippi W, Behrens U, Toussaint S. Quantifying oral analgesic consumption using a novel method and comparison with patient-controlled intravenous analgesic consumption. *Anesth Analg.* 1998;86(5):1051–1053.

28. Ho HS. Patient-controlled analgesia versus oral controlled-release oxycodone: are they interchangeable for acute postoperative pain after laparoscopic colorectal surgeries? *Oncology.* 2008;74(suppl 1):61–65.

29. Rothwell MP, Pearson D, Hunter JD, et al. Oral oxycodone offers equivalent analgesia to intravenous patient-controlled analgesia after total hip replacement: a randomized, single-centre, non-blinded, non-inferiority study. *Br J Anaesth.* 2011;106(6):865–872.

Chapter 4

How Should Opioids Be Used to Manage Pain Emergencies?

GABRIELLE R. GOLDBERG AND CARDINALE B. SMITH

INTRODUCTION AND SCOPE OF THE PROBLEM

A complaint of severe pain should be treated as a medical emergency.[1] Pain emergencies may occur in the setting of *acute pain,* defined as acute "injury to the body…usually due to a definable nociceptive cause."[2] Pain emergencies may also occur in the setting of *breakthrough pain,* defined as "transient flares of severe pain in patients already managed with analgesics."[2] Limited data exist on the prevalence of acute pain crises. In one major cancer center, up to 25% of the consults to the palliative care inpatient service were for assistance in the management of an acute pain crisis.[1] The prevalence of breakthrough pain in patients both with cancer and without cancer receiving treatment for chronic pain is high, ranging from 65% to 85%.[3]

Despite this high prevalence, the management of acute pain in the postoperative and emergency room settings is inadequate.[4] Inadequate management of acute pain has multiple consequences, including reduction in quality of life, poor sleep, impaired physical functioning, and high economic costs because of increased need for hospitalization.[4] Effective pain management results in reducing the incidence of these consequences and the risk for developing chronic pain.[4] Pain can be adequately relieved with opioids in most patients.[5]

RELEVANT PATHOPHYSIOLOGY

Pain is defined as "an unpleasant sensory and emotional experience associated with actual or potential tissue damage."[6] It is a subjective experience, and the gold standard for pain assessment is patient report. Pain can be classified as nociceptive, neuropathic, or idiopathic. Nociceptive pain can be further classified as either somatic (resulting from injury to skin and deep tissue) or visceral (resulting from injury to internal organs). Visceral pain is often described as dull, vague, or diffuse, whereas somatic pain is more likely to be well localized and described as sharp or intense.

The approach to the treatment of acute pain and breakthrough pain emergencies differs because patients experiencing severe breakthrough pain are likely to be on a standing opioid regimen and are therefore opioid tolerant. Opioid-tolerant patients will require higher doses of opioids to achieve therapeutic effect compared with opioid-naïve patients.

Pain emergencies are often associated with progression of the underlying disease. The pain symptom should be urgently treated while the clinician is concurrently considering the underlying cause of the pain and assessing which additional evaluations and interventions would be therapeutic and consistent with the patient's overall goals of care. Thorough evaluation of pain should include a pain history (including onset, prior responses to opioids, quality, radiation, severity, and temporal factors); assessment of the impact of pain on the patient's physical, social, and psychological functioning; and complete physical examination, including neurological evaluation.[1] This comprehensive evaluation is essential because it guides selection of initial opioid type and dose. The assessment must occur rapidly in the setting of an acute pain crisis,[7] although some aspects of this evaluation can be delayed until the patient reaches an acceptable level of pain that will allow patient compliance and tolerability of the evaluation. Disease-specific workup and recommendations are beyond the scope of this chapter.

SUMMARY OF EVIDENCE REGARDING TREATMENT RECOMMENDATIONS

Few prospective controlled trials have been conducted assessing the efficacy of treatment regimens for episodic, breakthrough pain. Therapeutic communication is of utmost importance in treatment of a pain emergency. The palliative care clinician should clearly communicate to the patient that pain control is important, that it will be accomplished in a short time, and that the clinician will remain present with the patient until the crisis is ameliorated. The following discussion is a summary of an approach to the use of opioids for treatment of patients with severe pain (Figure 4-1).

Referral of the Patient to the Appropriate Care Setting

A complaint of severe pain is a pain emergency, and patients should be referred to a care setting that will allow rapid assessment, treatment, and titration of opioids. Given that the route of administration determines the time to peak effect of opioids, severe pain should be treated in a location that allows administration of intravenous or subcutaneous opioid. The time to peak effect of an oral dose of opioid is 60 to 90 minutes and is therefore not appropriate for use in the setting of a pain emergency.[5]

The strongest evidence base for the treatment of acute breakthrough pain indicates administration of oral transmucosal fentanyl.[8] However, given its

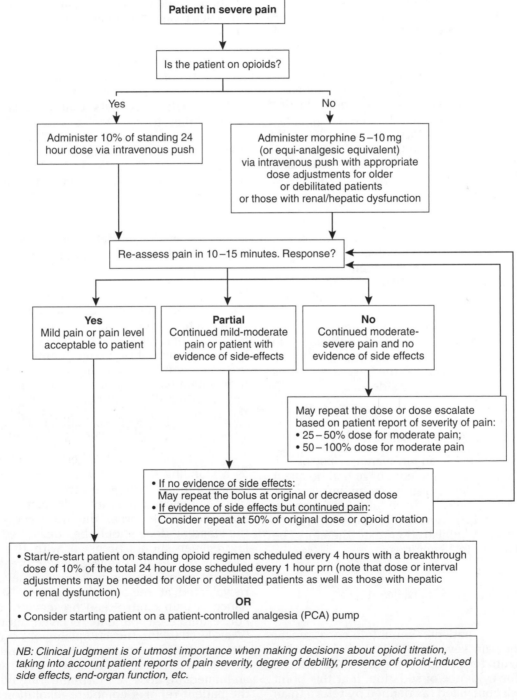

FIGURE 4-1. Approach to treatment of pain emergency.

lower cost and widespread availability, morphine is generally the opioid of first choice.[5,9] In the acute setting of a pain emergency, even in the presence of renal and hepatic dysfunction, morphine can be administered in the short term, with consideration of decreasing the routine starting doses discussed below. (*Note:* Intravenous and subcutaneous opioid dosing for morphine are equivalent; therefore dosing recommendations in the following discussion also may be applied to subcutaneous administration.)

Assessment of Whether Patient Is Opioid-Naive

The initial opioid dose should be based on assessment of whether a patient is opioid naïve or opioid tolerant. A patient on a stable opioid dose for as few as several days is likely to have developed tolerance and will therefore require higher opioid doses to reach the same degree of analgesia as an opioid-naïve patient.

The Opioid-Naïve Patient. The recommended starting dose for an opioid-naïve patient in an acute pain crisis is morphine 5 to 10 mg intravenously (IV) or its equianalgesic equivalent (see Chapter 1, Table 1-3). For older or more debilitated patients, particularly those with renal or hepatic dysfunction, starting at the low end or below this range should be considered. Remember that the duration of action of the opioid is likely to be longer in older patients or in the setting of renal or hepatic dysfunction compared to that in younger or healthier individuals.

The Opioid-Tolerant Patient. The recommended rescue or breakthrough dose for a patient on standing opioids who is in the midst of an acute pain crisis is generally 5% to 20% of the patient's total 24-hour opioid requirement.[10] In the authors' experience, a dose of 10% of the 24-total hour dose is usually sufficient.[11] In the inpatient setting, this dose can be rapidly titrated in a short interval, so dosing at the lower end of this range provides less concern for side effects.

Intravenous Administration of Appropriate Opioid Dose

The time to peak effect of an intravenous dose of opioids is 8 to 15 minutes. If patients have had no effect 15 minutes after administration of an intravenous opioid, they are unlikely to have additional benefit, despite the fact that the duration of effect will be 3 to 4 hours. Repeat administration can therefore be administered after 8 to 15 minutes.

Reassessment for Efficacy and Tolerability at Time to Peak Effect

After 15 minutes, patients should have a repeat assessment of pain severity. Clinicians should also evaluate patients for evidence of opioid side effects, particularly for evidence of sedation. If at this point the pain is well controlled (as defined by return to an acceptable level of pain for the patient), the clinician can consider starting or making adjustments to the standing opioid regimen.

Administration of Additional Opioid for Pain Not Well Controlled

If the patient reports that the pain is partially improved, but continues to be mild to moderate or otherwise unacceptable to the patient and no side effects are evident, the clinician may repeat the opioid dose at the initial dose or a decreased dose. If evidence of side effects is present but the patient reports continued mild to moderate pain, the clinician should consider repeating administration of the opioid, but at 50% of the original dose. When a patient begins to demonstrate side effects, the clinician must closely observe the patient to ensure safety. Another treatment option for inadequate analgesia with evidence of side effects is rotation to another opioid.

If the patient reports that pain is still severe, with minimal to no effect of the initial opioid dose and the clinician determines that no side effects are evident, the patient should be administered a repeat bolus of opioid with a 25% to 50% dose escalation for moderate pain and 50% to 100% dose escalation for severe pain.[7]

Administration of Appropriate Standing Opioid Regimen Based on Opioids Required to Control Pain Emergency

When the patient's pain is controlled, the clinician should determine the total dose of opioid the patient required to get the pain under control and over what length of time the patient received the pain medications. The amount of opioid required to break a pain crisis is often higher than the opioid dose required to maintain patient comfort. The clinician must take into consideration the patient's report of pain and the report or appearance of side effects (particularly the level of sedation). In a patient who reports mild pain with no evidence of side effects, the dose required to break the pain crisis can be prescribed as a standing dose every 4 hours. However, if the patient reports complete resolution of pain or displays evidence of sedation, administering 50% of the dose required to break the crisis every 4 hours as the standing dose should be considered. The standing regimen should be given, with 10% of the total 24-hour opioid dose available for breakthrough or incident pain. The patient's comfort level should be reevaluated at regular, short intervals for maintenance of pain control and presence of side effects. For example, a patient received morphine 4 mg IV at 11:00 AM for the complaint of severe pain. At 11:15 AM the patient was still in moderate to severe pain, with no evidence of side effects, and received an immediate dose of morphine 6 mg IV. At 11:30 AM, the patient reports complete resolution of pain and appears sleepy. The patient received a total of 10 mg of morphine to achieve relief, but is demonstrating some evidence of side effects. The patient can be started on morphine 5 mg IV every 4 hours, with morphine 3 mg IV every 1 hour as needed for breakthrough pain. There should be a plan for frequent follow-up to reassess for pain relief and evidence of side effects.

Administration of Patient-Controlled Analgesia for Appropriate Patient Populations

Patient-controlled analgesia (PCA) should be considered for patients with rapidly accelerating pain requiring ongoing titration and patients with frequent episodes of breakthrough pain.[5] The use of PCA is discussed in Chapters 2 and 3.

KEY MESSAGES TO PATIENTS AND FAMILIES

Patients should understand that their complaint of severe pain will be treated as a medical emergency. It is important that patients be instructed that to provide urgent treatment, their clinician may refer them to a site that will allow intravenous pain medications to be administered. The total amount of medication required to get a pain emergency under control is often higher than the dose of medication required to keep pain under control; therefore patients should be encouraged to take pain medications as prescribed and notify their clinician if pain is not effectively controlled on the prescribed regimen.

CONCLUSION AND SUMMARY

A complaint of severe pain is a medical emergency, and it should be treated as such by clinicians. With effective intravenous titration of opioids, the majority of pain emergencies can be controlled within a short time. While treating a pain emergency with opioids, the clinician should simultaneously be considering the cause of the symptom and appropriate evaluation and nonopioid adjuvant therapies within the context of the patient's overall goals of care. Continued research is required to increase the evidence base for the majority of the treatment recommendations provided in this chapter.

SUMMARY RECOMMENDATIONS

The key steps in responding to a pain emergency are as follows:

- *Step 1:* Refer the patient to the appropriate care setting for administration of intravenous opioids.
- *Step 2:* Determine if patient is receiving opioids.
- *Step 3:* Administer appropriate opioid dose intravenously.
- *Step 4:* Reassess for efficacy at time to peak effect.
- *Step 5:* If pain is not well-controlled, administer additional opioid.
- *Step 6:* Start appropriate standing opioid regimen based on opioids required to control pain emergency.
- *Step 7:* Consider the use of patient-controlled analgesia for the appropriate patient populations.

REFERENCES

1. Moryl N, Coyle N, Foley KM. Managing an acute pain crisis in a patient with advanced cancer: "this is as much of a crisis as a code." *JAMA.* 2008;299(12):1457–1467.
2. Ripamonti C, Bandieri E. Pain therapy. *Crit Rev Oncol Hematol.* 2009;70(2):145–159.
3. Webster LR. Breakthrough pain in the management of chronic persistent pain syndromes. *Am J Manag Care.* 2008;14(5 suppl 1):S116–S122.
4. Sinatra R. Causes and consequences of inadequate management of acute pain. *Pain Med.* 2010;11(12):1859–1871.
5. Hanks GW, Conno Fd, Cherny N, et al. Morphine and alternative opioids in cancer pain: the EAPC recommendations. *Br J Cancer.* 2001;84(5):587–593.
6. *International Association for the Study of Pain.* IASP Taxonomy. http://www.iasp-pain.org/Content/NavigationMenu/GeneralResourceLinks/PainDefinitions/default.htm; Accessed October 9, 2012.
7. Ferrell B, Levy MH, Paice J. Managing pain from advanced cancer in the palliative care setting. *Clin J Oncol Nurs.* 2008;12(4):575–581.
8. Zeppetella G, Ribeiro MD. Opioids for the management of breakthrough (episodic) pain in cancer patients. *Cochrane Database Syst Rev.* 2006;(1):56 CD004311.
9. American Pain Society. *Principles of Analgesic Use in the Treatment of Acute Pain and Cancer Pain.* 6th ed. Glenview, IL: American Pain Society; 2008.
10. Mercadante S, Villari P, Ferrera P, Bianchi M, Casuccio A. Safety and effectiveness of intravenous morphine for episodic (breakthrough) pain using a fixed ratio with the oral daily morphine dose. *J Pain Symptom Manage.* 2004;27(4):352–359.
11. Schrijvers D. Emergencies in palliative care. *Eur J Cancer.* 2011;47(suppl 3):S359–S361.

What Principles Should Guide Oral, Transcutaneous, and Intravenous Opioid Dose Conversions?

LAURA P. GELFMAN AND EMILY J. CHAI

INTRODUCTION AND SCOPE OF THE PROBLEM

Opioids are the foundation of pain management for patients receiving palliative care. They are administered by many different routes, including the oral route for tablets, capsules, or liquids; the parenteral route for intravenous, intramuscular, and subcutaneous means; and the transdermal, transmucosal, and rectal methods of delivery. Insufficient evidence exists that opioids can be effectively and reliably administered by the intranasal or topical route.

The route for opioid administration is selected by a combination of clinical circumstances, including the underlying cause of pain, the need for long-acting pain management, comorbidities, the setting of care (e.g., acute hospital, nursing home, or home), and available opioid formulations.

RELEVANT PATHOPHYSIOLOGY

Whenever feasible and effective, oral administration of opioids is generally preferable. The choice of which oral opioid to use depends on several factors, including the medication's pharmacokinetics and pharmacodynamics, which are discussed in detail in other chapters.

Nevertheless, in some clinical circumstances the parenteral route is desirable, particularly in the setting of escalating pain in which rapid titration of opioids may be necessary. Using the intravenous route may be advantageous in patients who (1) already have an indwelling intravenous line; (2) have generalized edema; (3) develop erythema, soreness, or abscesses; (4) have coagulation disorders; or (5) have poor peripheral circulation.[1] The principal advantage of the intravenous route is that it allows direct administration of the opioid into circulation,

providing a rapid and predictable effect independent of issues relating to absorption.[2] Patients with poorly controlled pain who require rapid escalation because of unstable disease may require aggressive pain treatment by the intravenous route. Practitioners generally favor the intravenous route. However, the subcutaneous route does have advantages, including requiring a smaller needle, providing greater freedom in choosing an injection site, and allowing for less close supervision. Intramuscular injections are both inconvenient and potentially painful.

The care setting may restrict options for administration routes. Although intravenous administration of opioids is feasible in an acute care setting such as a hospital, many other care settings, such as nursing homes or long-term care facilities, may not permit continuous intravenous therapy. Although intravenous regimens are possible at home, they may be logistically difficult to manage. The subcutaneous route is often used in hospice settings, although this route does not always provide sufficiently rapid onset of action. Table 5-1 outlines formulations for each route of administration.

SUMMARY OF EVIDENCE REGARDING TREATMENT OPTIONS

Oral Administration: Pros and Cons

The use of oral medications is predicated on a patient's ability to swallow, which requires appropriate mental status and level of alertness and the physiological ability to both safely swallow and absorb medications. If the patient has difficulty swallowing, nausea, vomiting, or respiratory distress, clinicians should opt for a nonoral administration, including parenteral or transdermal mechanisms.[3] Additionally, patients with gastrointestinal motility disorders, such as malignant bowel obstruction, short gut syndrome, or gastroparesis, may not absorb opioids in a reliable manner.

For those in whom the oral route of administration is feasible, the bioavailability of opioids generally varies, with estimates of oral bioavailability of methadone at nearly 80% compared to approximately 26% for morphine.[4] In spite of the potential variation in opioid bioavailability, the majority of opioids have similar oral absorption, with an onset of action of 30 to 60 minutes and duration of analgesia of about 4 hours. Hydrophilic medications such as morphine,

TABLE 5-1. Potential Routes of Opioid Delivery

| OPIOID | ORAL | | MUCOSAL | | | |
	IMMEDIATE RELEASE (TABLET, CAPSULE, LIQUID)	SUSTAINED RELEASE	ORAL	RECTAL	PARENTERAL	TRANSDERMAL
Morphine	✓	✓	✓	✓	✓	
Oxycodone	✓	✓	✓			
Hydromorphone	✓	✓	✓	✓	✓	
Oxymorphone	✓	✓			✓	
Hydrocodone	✓		✓			
Codeine	✓				✓	
Fentanyl	✓		✓		✓	✓
Methadone	✓		✓	✓	✓	

oxycodone, and hydrocodone all undergo extensive first-pass effect when passing through the liver.[5] If rapid escalation of opioids is needed in an acute care setting, the dose may be titrated intravenously and the patient transitioned back to an oral regimen when a stable effective dose is achieved.

Usually, opioid regimens for chronic pain include a long-acting or continuous analgesic medication, with the addition of a supplemental short-acting opioid for treatment of breakthrough pain. This breakthrough dose is usually a percentage of a patient's total daily opioid dose.[1] A limitation in using oral opioids for breakthrough pain is that oral formulations take longer to relieve pain than the intravenous route. This slow onset of effect makes oral opioids less effective for breakthrough or activity-provoked pain, which may be brief and resolved by the time the oral opioid has reached peak effect.

Routes of Administration for Escalating Pain: Intravenous Versus Subcutaneous

Patients with escalating pain resulting from disease progression generally require a rapid titration of opioid medication. This pain escalation must be distinguished from episodic or breakthrough pain. In patients with cancer, three principal categories of breakthrough pain have been identified: (1) spontaneous pain with no evident precipitating event; (2) incident pain, with an evident precipitating cause or event (e.g., pain with movement or a particular form of activity); and (3) end of dose failure, associated with a reduction in analgesic levels of regularly provided medications below the therapeutic level.[6] The pharmacokinetics of opioids must also be considered when treating breakthrough pain. When patients need a rapid intervention, the intravenous route provides the best drug availability from a pharmacokinetics point of view. When comparing pain relief in the intravenous and oral groups, Elsner and colleagues[7] found that 87% of the patients in the intravenous group reported at least sufficient pain relief after 1 hour, whereas only 26% in the oral group reached similar results after 1 hour. In the same study, they found that intravenous titration is more rapid than oral and subcutaneous titration. Boluses of intravenous and subcutaneous morphine were given every 5 minutes and 30 minutes, respectively. Titration stopped after patients in both groups achieved similar pain intensity, within a mean of 53 minutes for the intravenous group and 77 minutes for the subcutaneous group. The proportion of patients with 30% and 50% pain relief was higher in the intravenous group, despite this group having higher initial scores of pain intensity.

The transition from oral to intravenous opioid requires a stable means of intravenous access. In addition, intravenous delivery is a more costly intervention that requires closer supervision and monitoring, which nearly always necessitates a patient being brought to an inpatient setting. Despite these complexities, rapid control of escalating pain or breakthrough pain is most effectively accomplished using the parenteral route of opioid administration.

The subcutaneous route has many advantages over the intravenous route, principally ease of use, allowing administration of parenteral opioids in lower acuity care settings, such as hospices, nursing homes, or home care. Studies have demonstrated efficacy with both bolus injections and continuous infusion. Simple devices for single-bolus injections show results similar to those achieved with continuous administration.[8] Separately, a gravity-dependent drip method of continuous drug delivery has been found to be a cost-effective, simple technique for ensuring adequate analgesia in resource-scarce environments.[9] The gravity-dependent drip method can be safely administered only by the subcutaneous route for continuous drug delivery because the tissue limits the dose absorbed. A similar gravity-dependent drip administered intravenously may lead to overdose.

In addition, other studies have begun to evaluate the feasibility and efficacy of the subcutaneous route for the management of cancer pain. Cost analyses showed that subcutaneous infusion reduced costs by allowing home discharges or replacing intravenous infusion.[9,10] The subcutaneous route is limited by the amount of fluid that can be delivered at one time. This limit is often set at about 5 mL per hour because most subcutaneous tissue cannot retain more without irritation or damage to surrounding connective tissues. Of note, methadone cannot be administered subcutaneously because of adverse skin reactions.[11]

Unfortunately, few controlled studies have been conducted comparing the subcutaneous and intravenous routes. In a prospective crossover study of inpatients,[12] continuous intravenous and subcutaneous morphine were found to be equianalgesic for most patients when administered as a continuous infusion, showing similar pain-control and adverse-effect profiles. However, patients who needed higher quantities of morphine to achieve adequate analgesia needed higher doses by the subcutaneous route compared to those patients receiving it by the intravenous route. Thus these patients needed higher volumes, suggesting that absorption of high doses may be lower when using the subcutaneous route. In another small study, an intravenous/subcutaneous/oral conversion ratio of 1:2:3 was started by continuous infusion with a simple drip.[9] Intravenous and subcutaneous routes provided similar analgesic effects, although the investigators found the intravenous route to be more potent. Finally, in a randomized clinical trial, subcutaneous morphine titration required more time and higher doses than intravenous titration in patients with exacerbation of cancer pain.[7]

Overall the intravenous route has advantages in higher acuity settings (Table 5-2), where it may be used for purposes other than pain management, such as providing artificial hydration or antibiotics or treatment for emergencies.[13] Patients with cancer may already have a method of permanent venous access (e.g., implanted port for chemotherapy infusions), which allows for easy administration of intravenous pain medications.

Mucosal Route of Delivery: Rectal and Oral

Mucosal delivery routes primarily include the oral and rectal route. In general the rectal route is the choice of last resort given the potential patient discomfort and the fact that this may be a particularly upsetting route of delivery for family caregivers who have to administer the medications. However, when all other means of delivery are not feasible, rectal mucosal delivery offers an alternative. The rate and extent of rectal drug absorption are often lower than with oral absorption; this may be related to the comparatively small surface area available for drug uptake.[14] In addition, the composition of the rectal formulation (solid versus liquid, nature of the suppository base) appears to affect the absorption process because the formulation determines the pattern of drug release. After the opioid is placed in the rectum, it enters systemic circulation through the lower rectal veins.

All opioids can be administered rectally; however, the commercial availability of these medications may vary by country. When not available in suppository form, medications can be compounded by pharmacies using immediate-release tablets in a gelatin capsule. Some authorized pharmacies can prepare suppositories in any strength.

Despite the complexities of administering medications rectally, this route offers distinct advantages over the oral route.[15] The most significant advantage is that the mechanism of absorption is independent of the gastrointestinal tract.[16] Patients with intractable nausea and vomiting, dysphagia, bowel obstruction, or malabsorption are candidates for this alternative route of administration. In addition, this method of delivery offers a substitute for patients who cannot tolerate injections because of bleeding disorders or generalized edema. The rectal route also provides an additional method of opioid delivery in care settings in which intravenous modes of delivery may not be available. Finally, despite family caregiver concerns about the rectal route, the biggest advantage is that unskilled caregivers can easily administer suppositories, even in very sick and frail patients.

In terms of disadvantages of the rectal route, considerable individual variability exists in absorption of rectally administered opioids. This requires careful titration based on individual patient response. Rates of rectal absorption depend on the preparation (differences relate to whether the opioid is dissolved in an aqueous or alcohol-based solution or given as a suppository), the pH of the solutions used, and the amount of feces in the rectum. The rectal route cannot be used in patients with diarrhea, hemorrhoids, anal fissures, or neutropenia, and it is not meant for long-term use. Suppositories can be uncomfortable for patients, and the potential for expulsion of the suppository by a bowel movement further complicates drug absorption. Many patients and caregivers may simply prefer to avoid the rectal route of delivery.

The oral mucosal route of delivery offers several advantages. The oral mucosa is highly permeable—20 times more permeable than the skin—and is highly vascularized. Lipophilic, un-ionized compounds, such as fentanyl, pass through the cellular membranes easily, traveling rapidly through the

---

TABLE 5-2. Advantages and Disadvantages of the Intravenous Route of Opioid Administration[2]

ADVANTAGES	DISADVANTAGES
• Total drug availability and predictable effects • Short onset of action for opioid titration and breakthrough pain • Flexibility modalities: boluses, continuous infusion, patient-controlled analgesia • Unlimited volumes (as opposed to subcutaneous) • Useful for patients unable to take oral route or poor gastrointestinal absorption	• Need to maintain intravenous access • Increased cost • Increased complexity of management for caregivers • Close supervision required • Limited availability of sites for placement of the intravenous catheter (unless permanent access)

oral mucosa into the bloodstream. Moreover, the oral cavity has a relatively uniform temperature and a large surface area, further optimizing this delivery route.[17] Nevertheless, not all drugs are suitable for oral transmucosal administration[17]; in particular, lipophilic drugs are better absorbed than hydrophilic drugs.

Morphine is one of the most commonly used transmucosal opioids, despite evidence that it may not be as effective as other medications.[18] It is poorly absorbed across the oral mucosa because of its low lipid solubility and extensive ionization at the pH level of the mouth. In one study of normal volunteers using sublingual absorption, morphine was only 18% bioavailable, whereas fentanyl was 51% bioavailable.[19] Because clinicians are often not familiar with these data, they may believe that when patients do respond to sublingual morphine, it is because small amounts given sublingually are actually swallowed.

Unlike the pharmacokinetics of most opioids, the short-acting buccal fentanyl tablet[20] (Fentora), offers an onset of pain relief as short as 15 minutes and duration of analgesic effect of approximately 60 minutes. Fentora is absorbed through the buccal mucosa and is 65% bioavailable, reaching blood levels 30% to 50% higher than those of the transmucosal lozenge (see later discussion). This formulation can be effective for management of breakthrough pain in patients who are already receiving opioids, or those who are opioid tolerant, which is defined as those taking the equivalent of at least 60 mg of oral morphine per day.

The oral transmucosal fentanyl citrate lozenge Actiq is another short-acting formulation of fentanyl. The lozenge must be gently rubbed against the buccal mucosa until it has completely dissolved; therefore more active participation is required to correctly use the lozenge.[20,21] Of note, Fentora is not bioequivalent to Actiq and must not be prescribed on a microgram per microgram basis. This may make prescribing difficult, especially for the clinician inexperienced in the use of these formulations. Caution must be used when prescribing these medications because of their rapid onset of action and potential for respiratory depression. Furthermore, because the lozenge has a similar appearance to candy, it must be carefully safeguarded to avoid accidental ingestion by children. In addition, these short-acting formulations of fentanyl are expensive, particularly compared to other opioid preparations.

Transdermal Route of Administration

In the United States, the opioid most commonly used in a transdermal formulation is fentanyl. Compared with oral opioids, the advantages of transdermal fentanyl include a lower incidence of adverse effects (e.g., constipation, nausea and vomiting, and daytime drowsiness), a safety profile allowing it to be used in patients with renal or hepatic impairment,

improved compliance resulting from administration every 72 hours, and decreased use of rescue medication (Table 5-3). It is also associated with a higher degree of patient satisfaction and improved quality of life. Transdermal fentanyl is a useful analgesic for cancer patients who are unable to swallow or have difficulty with absorption resulting from gastrointestinal problems.[22]

Transdermal fentanyl patches produce sustained blood concentrations similar to those of continuous intravenous infusion.[23] The fentanyl patch has a membrane that limits the rate of absorption by a process of passive cutaneous diffusion.[24] The drug forms a depot within the skin before entering microcirculation, resulting in delayed pharmacokinetics.[25] This explains why therapeutic blood levels are attained 12 to 16 hours after initial patch application and why blood levels decrease slowly over 16 to 22 hours after removal.[26,27] As a result of this delayed systemic absorption on application and removal, medication for patients with chronic pain should be titrated to achieve adequate relief with short-acting oral or parenteral opioids before the initiation of transdermal fentanyl. In other words, these patches cannot be used for rapid titration of opioids and this route of administration is not recommended for the treatment of patients with acute, unstable pain syndromes. Instead, transdermal fentanyl should be initiated based on the 24-hour opioid requirement once adequate analgesia has been achieved. During this process, intravenous fentanyl for titration may offer an advantage over other opioids, by avoiding concerns relating to incomplete cross-tolerance because the same opioid is administered intravenously and transdermally.

Transdermal fentanyl may be contraindicated in patients who are cachectic, who are morbidly obese, or who have significant subcutaneous edema because of the mechanism of the cutaneous depot absorption system. Febrile patients should not use transdermal fentanyl, because higher body temperatures may increase the rate of absorption. A pharmacokinetics model[28] suggests that fentanyl blood levels may rise by approximately 33% when body

---

TABLE 5-3. Advantages and Disadvantages of Transdermal Fentanyl

ADVANTAGES	DISADVANTAGES
• Long-acting route of administration and only change every 72 hours • Fentanyl is opioid of choice in patients with renal or hepatic impairment • Easy to use • Useful in patients who cannot take oral medications	• Increased cost • Delayed systemic absorption, unable to use for rapid titration • Unpredictable absorption in cachectic, morbidly obese, or edematous patients • Caution needed when using in febrile or diaphoretic patients

temperature rises to 40°C (104°F) because of a temperature-dependent increase in fentanyl release or changes in the permeability of the membrane as temperature rises. Similarly, this route of administration should be avoided in patients who are particularly diaphoretic as a result of unpredictable absorption and difficulty with the patches adhering to the skin.

The prolonged elimination of transdermal fentanyl can become problematic if patients develop opioid-related adverse effects, especially hypoventilation. Adverse effects do not improve immediately after patch removal and may take many hours to resolve. Patients who experience opioid-related toxicity associated with respiratory depression should be treated immediately with an opioid antagonist such as naloxone and closely monitored for at least 24 hours. Because of the short half-life of naloxone, sequential doses or a continuous infusion of the opioid antagonist may be necessary. For these reasons, transdermal fentanyl should be administered cautiously to patients with preexisting conditions such as emphysema that may predispose them to the development of hypoventilation. Transdermal fentanyl is indicated only for patients who require continuous opioid administration for the treatment of chronic pain that cannot be managed with other medications. Likewise, it is contraindicated in the management of acute postoperative pain, because pain may decrease more rapidly in these circumstances than fentanyl blood levels can be adjusted, leading to the development of life-threatening hypoventilation.[22]

KEY MESSAGES TO PATIENTS AND FAMILIES

Each route of administration has advantages and disadvantages. The most important factor is choosing a route based on the specific clinical circumstances of the patient. Numerous factors related to the patient and the care setting must be considered in this decision, to ensure that medication administration can be accomplished successfully and as conveniently as possible for the patient and the family. By working together with clinicians, the appropriate and most effective route of administration can be selected.

CONCLUSION AND SUMMARY

The primary principles guiding selection of the appropriate route of administration for a specific patient are patient-specific, including comorbidities, ability to use gastrointestinal tract or swallow, ability to absorb medication using different routes of administration, and nature of the pain syndrome. In addition, each route has disadvantages and challenges that must be considered when choosing feasible options based on care settings and available resources.

SUMMARY RECOMMENDATIONS

- The oral route of administration should be used when an effective and stable dose has been achieved.[29]
- The intravenous (parenteral) route of administration should be used for rapid titration for escalating and breakthrough pain.[2,28]
- The subcutaneous route may be a simple, safe, effective, and less expensive parenteral means of opioid administration in select patients.[7,9,10,30]
- Transdermal fentanyl patches are effective for chronic pain regimens and well tolerated; however, these patches cannot be used for titration of opioids and should be used only once a stable dose has been achieved by oral or intravenous administration.[29]
- Mucosal routes of administration can provide an alternative for patients unable to use the gastrointestinal tract, although sublingual morphine has limited efficacy.[5,18]

REFERENCES

1. Hanks GW, Conno F, Cherny N, et al. Morphine and alternative opioids in cancer pain: the EAPC recommendations. *Br J Cancer.* 2001;84(5):587–593.
2. Mercadante S. Intravenous morphine for management of cancer pain. *Lancet Oncol.* 2010;11(5):484–489.
3. Glare P, Walsh D, Groh E, Nelson KA. The efficacy and side effects of continuous infusion intravenous morphine (CIVM) for pain and symptoms due to advanced cancer. *Am J Hosp Palliat Care.* 2002;19(5):343–350.
4. Gourlay GK, Cherry DA, Cousins MJ. A comparative study of the efficacy and pharmacokinetics of oral methadone and morphine in the treatment of severe pain in patients with cancer. *Pain.* 1986;25(3):297–312.
5. Coluzzi PH, Schwartzberg L, Conroy JD, et al. Breakthrough cancer pain: a randomized trial comparing oral transmucosal fentanyl citrate (OTFC) and morphine sulfate immediate release (MSIR). *Pain.* 2001;91(1–2):123–130.
6. Mercadante S. The use of rapid onset opioids for breakthrough cancer pain: the challenge of its dosing. *Crit Rev Oncol Hematol.* 2011;80(3):460–465.
7. Elsner F, Radbruch L, Loick G, Gartner J, Sabatowski R. Intravenous versus subcutaneous morphine titration in patients with persisting exacerbation of cancer pain. *J Palliat Med.* 2005;8(4):743–750.
8. Watanabe S, Pereira J, Tarumi Y, Hanson J, Bruera E. A randomized double-blind crossover comparison of continuous and intermittent subcutaneous administration of opioid for cancer pain. *J Palliat Med.* 2008;11(4):570–574.
9. Koshy RC, Kuriakose R, Sebastian P, Koshy C. Continuous morphine infusions for cancer pain in resource-scarce environments: comparison of the subcutaneous and intravenous routes of administration. *J Pain Palliat Care Pharmacother.* 2005;19(1):27–33.
10. Bruera E, Brenneis C, Michaud M, et al. Use of the subcutaneous route for the administration of narcotics in patients with cancer pain. *Cancer.* 1988;62(2):407–411.
11. Bruera E, Fainsinger R, Moore M, Thibault R, Spoldi E, Ventafridda V. Local toxicity with subcutaneous methadone: experience of two centers. *Pain.* 1991;45(2):141–143.
12. Nelson KA, Glare PA, Walsh D, Groh ES. A prospective, within-patient, crossover study of continuous intravenous and subcutaneous morphine for chronic cancer pain. *J Pain Symptom Manage.* 1997;13(5):262–267.

13. Mercadante S, Intravaia G, Villari P, et al. Clinical and financial analysis of an acute palliative care unit in an oncological department. *Palliat Med.* 2008;22(6):760–767.

14. van Hoogdalem E, de Boer AG, Breimer DD. Pharmacokinetics of rectal drug administration. I. General considerations and clinical applications of centrally acting drugs. *Clin Pharmacokinet.* 1991;21(1):11–26.

15. Davis MP, Walsh D, LeGrand SB, Naughton M. Symptom control in cancer patients: the clinical pharmacology and therapeutic role of suppositories and rectal suspensions. *SCC.* 2002;10(2):117–138.

16. Walsh D, Tropiano PS. Long-term rectal administration of high-dose sustained-release morphine tablets. *SCC.* 2002;10(8):653–655.

17. Zhang H, Zhang J, Streisand JB. Oral mucosal drug delivery: clinical pharmacokinetics and therapeutic applications. *Clin Pharmacokinet.* 2002;41(9):661–680.

18. Coluzzi PH. Sublingual morphine: efficacy reviewed. *J Pain Symptom Manage.* 1998;16(3):184–192.

19. Weinberg DS, Inturrisi CE, Reidenberg B, et al. Sublingual absorption of selected opioid analgesics. *Clin Pharmacol Ther.* 1988;44(3):335–342.

20. Fentanyl buccal tablet (Fentora) for breakthrough pain. *Med Lett Drugs Ther.* 2007;49(1270):78–79.

21. Laverty D. Actiq: an effective oral treatment for cancer-related breakthrough pain. *Br J Community Nurs.* 2007;12(7):311, 313–316.

22. Kornick CA, Santiago-Palma J, Moryl N, Payne R, Obbens EA. Benefit-risk assessment of transdermal fentanyl for the treatment of chronic pain. *Drug Saf.* 2003;26(13):951–973.

23. Grond S, Zech D, Lehmann KA, Radbruch L, Breitenbach H, Hertel D. Transdermal fentanyl in the long-term treatment of cancer pain: a prospective study of 50 patients with advanced cancer of the gastrointestinal tract or the head and neck region. *Pain.* 1997;69(1–2):191–198.

24. Payne R. Transdermal fentanyl: suggested recommendations for clinical use. *J Pain Symptom Manage.* 1992;7(3 suppl): S40–S44.

25. Kornick CA, Santiago-Palma J, Khojainova N, Primavera LH, Payne R, Manfredi PL. A safe and effective method for converting cancer patients from intravenous to transdermal fentanyl. *Cancer.* 2001;92(12):3056–3061.

26. Varvel JR, Shafer SL, Hwang SS, Coen PA, Stanski DR. Absorption characteristics of transdermally administered fentanyl. *Anesthesiology.* 1989;70(6):928–934.

27. Gourlay GK, Kowalski SR, Plummer JL, Cherry DA, Gaukroger P, Cousins MJ. The transdermal administration of fentanyl in the treatment of postoperative pain: pharmacokinetics and pharmacodynamic effects. *Pain.* 1989;37(2):193–202.

28. Southam MA. Transdermal fentanyl therapy: system design, pharmacokinetics and efficacy. *Anticancer Drugs.* 1995;6(suppl 3): 29–34.

29. Mercadante S, Villari P, Ferrera P, Casuccio A, Fulfaro F. Rapid titration with intravenous morphine for severe cancer pain and immediate oral conversion. *Cancer.* 2002;95(1): 203–208.

30. Kumar KS, Rajagopal MR, Naseema AM. Intravenous morphine for emergency treatment of cancer pain. *Palliat Med.* 2000;14(3):183–188.

Which Opioids Are Safest and Most Effective in Renal Failure?

Laura P. Gelfman and Emily J. Chai

INTRODUCTION AND SCOPE OF THE PROBLEM

Most clinicians have experience treating patients with pain who have multiple chronic diseases, many of which may result in renal impairment or renal failure. The cause of pain in patients with a disease primarily of renal origin may be less well understood, despite the fact that many these patients have chronic pain syndromes. More specifically, 37% to 50% of patients on hemodialysis experience chronic pain, with moderate to severe pain in 82%.[1-3] Patients with end-stage renal disease (ESRD) evaluated using a modified version of the Edmonton Symptom Assessment System reported symptoms similar in number and severity to those reported by patients with cancer hospitalized in palliative care settings. Prevalence of pain in patients with renal disease (regardless of cause) persists; even in the last day of life, pain is present in 42% of patients who have stopped dialysis.[4,5] This high prevalence is complicated by the fact that renal failure affects the pharmacokinetics of many drugs, thus limiting the number of treatments available for these patients.

Pain in patients in renal failure may result from numerous causes and is often multifactorial. It may be the result of comorbidities, such as diabetes and vascular disease, with painful sequelae such as ischemic limbs and peripheral neuropathies. Musculoskeletal pain from arthritis in elderly patients with ESRD is one of the most common causes of chronic pain in this patient population. Pain may be a result of the primary renal disease itself (e.g., polycystic kidney disease) or related to the management of the renal failure. Central venous access systems may result in infections that can be painful and subsequent osteomyelitis. Discitis may develop in patients with arteriovenous fistulas, possibly resulting in painful ischemic neuropathies. Recurrent pain from the dialysis itself (e.g., the use of needles to access grafts) and associated muscle cramps and headaches may be perceived as chronic pain by some patients.[6] Numerous painful syndromes that can develop during a patient's time on dialysis are unique to ESRD, such as calciphylaxis, nephrogenic sclerosing fibrosis, dialysis-related amyloidosis, and renal osteodystrophy. Despite these multiple sources of pain and data demonstrating that the vast majority of patients with renal disease experience moderate or severe pain, one study demonstrated that 35% of patients on hemodialysis with chronic pain were not prescribed analgesics and less than 10% were prescribed strong opioids.[7]

Pain management is complicated by altered pharmacokinetics and pharmacodynamics of opioids in patients with renal failure. Other barriers also make pain management in this group particularly challenging; for example, (1) patients with renal disease often have multiple, complex comorbid conditions predisposing them to polypharmacy; (2) renal patients are usually older, which puts them at a higher risk for opioid toxicity and side effects; and (3) clinicians often have difficulties differentiating between opioid side effects and uremic symptoms, which may result in inappropriate withdrawal of opioid treatment.[8]

RELEVANT PATHOPHYSIOLOGY

Regardless of the cause of renal failure, the effect of decreased kidney function may result in variable metabolism of medications and the presence of pharmacologically active metabolites must be considered when prescribing opioids for patients with renal impairment. Palliative care providers need a basic understanding of opioid metabolism to determine which opioids are safest and most effective for patients with renal failure.

Renal impairment or failure affects various aspects of metabolism, including alterations in (1) absorption—resulting from reduced gastric emptying; (2) distribution—from either a decrease in plasma protein-binding resulting from hypoalbuminemia and competitive binding with endogenous substances or an increased volume of distribution caused by volume overload; (3) metabolism—with changes in hepatic drug-metabolizing enzymes; and (4) elimination—resulting from decreases in glomerular filtration, tubular secretion, and reabsorption.[9] The rate of elimination of any drug is proportional to the glomerular filtration rate (GFR).

All opioids are metabolized by the liver to some extent and then excreted by the kidneys. Because opioids are weak organic bases, changes in the urine pH can alter tubular handling and affect the relationship between GFR and renal elimination.[10] Both the choice and dosage of the opioid must be carefully considered in patients with renal failure, with special attention to accumulation of active and toxic metabolites.

Renal Impairment

The following section reviews the pharmacokinetics and pharmacodynamics of each opiate to discuss the safest and most effective opioids in patients with renal impairment.

Morphine. Of all of the opioids, the metabolism of morphine is the most studied. In patients with normal renal function, it is metabolized in the liver to morphine-3-glucuronide (M3G) (55%), morphine-6-glucuronide (M6G) (10%), and normorphine (4%), all of which are excreted by the kidney, along with about 10% of the parent compound.[11,12] Studies have shown that the renal clearance of both morphine and M6G is greater than the creatinine clearance, implying that they are actively secreted by the kidney. Morphine clearance in renal failure is not significantly different from clearance with normal kidney function, but because glucuronide metabolites are renally excreted[11] they will accumulate in renal failure.[13]

The potential accumulation of M6G in patients with reduced renal function has clinical implications.[14] Studies have demonstrated that M6G possesses analgesic effects and depressive effects on the central nervous system, so accumulation in patients with renal disease can result in myoclonus, seizures, and prolonged and profound sedation and respiratory depression.[8] M6G crosses the blood–brain barrier slowly, but once in the central nervous system its effects can be prolonged because it reequilibrates back into the systemic circulation very slowly.[15] This may result in central nervous system effects persisting for some time after discontinuing morphine or dialyzing to remove the M6G because of central nervous system accumulation.[15] The effects of M3G are less clear; however, it is thought to have a low affinity for opioid receptors and has no analgesic activity, although it may antagonize the analgesic effects of both morphine and M6G.[16–18]

Hydromorphone. Like morphine, hydromorphone, a hydrogenated ketone of morphine, is metabolized by the liver to hydromorphone-3-glucuronide (H3G) and its conjugates.[19] All metabolites of hydromorphone are renally excreted. H3G and a small amount of free hydromorphone accumulate in renal failure. Although H3G reportedly has no analgesic activity, it may have a neuroexcitatory effect with accumulation.[20–22] One study investigated hydromorphone pharmacokinetics in volunteers with normal renal function and varying degrees of renal failure. They found that the area under the curve for plasma concentration/time plot increased in a ratio of 1:2:4 for patients with normal renal function, moderate renal failure (creatinine clearance 40-60 mL/min), and severe renal failure (creatinine clearance <30 mL/min), respectively.[23] In a retrospective study, Lee and associates[24] found no significant differences in dose requirements between patients with normal renal function and those with end-stage renal failure when switched from morphine to hydromorphone and adverse effects improved.[24]

Oxycodone. Less is understood about the use of oxycodone in patients with renal failure. Oxycodone undergoes hepatic metabolism principally to oxymorphone and noroxycodone.[25] It is not clear how much of the remaining metabolites exist. The only active metabolite of oxycodone is oxymorphone. In patients with uremia, the elimination half-life of oxycodone is lengthened and the excretion of metabolites is severely impaired. Although oxymorphone does not have a significant pharmacodynamic effect in patients with normal renal function, it is unclear clear how it may affect patients with renal impairment.[26,27] Anecdotal reports suggest oxycodone should be used at reduced doses and increased dosing intervals in this patient population.

Codeine. Codeine is metabolized to codeine-6-glucuronide (81%), norcodeine (2.16%), morphine (0.56%), M3G (2.10%), M6G (0.80%), and normorphine (2.44%). Both codeine and codeine-6-glucuronide are excreted renally.[28] Because codeine and morphine have common metabolites, potential central nervous system affects are a concern. A study by Matzke and colleagues[29] reported significant narcolepsy in three patients with renal failure who were given codeine.

Methadone. Unlike the other opioids, methadone is a synthetic drug. It has both mu-delta opioid agonist activity and N-methyl-D-aspartate (NMDA) receptor antagonism. It is metabolized in the liver into pharmacologically inactive metabolites, with excretion of 10% to 45% in the feces and approximately 20% to 50% in urine as methadone or its metabolites.[30,31] Case studies reported that one oliguric patient excreted 15% of the daily dose in the feces, of which 3% was unchanged methadone, and an anuric patient excreted most of the dose in the feces, again with 3% as unchanged methadone. Methadone is believed to be safe to use in patients with renal disease.[31]

Fentanyl. Fentanyl is a potent, short-acting synthetic opioid with a short half-life of 1.5 to 6 hours. It is metabolized in the liver primarily to norfentanyl (>99%), with smaller amounts of despropionylfentanyl and hydroxyfentanyl. However, no evidence exists that these metabolites are active or toxic.[32] Multiple studies have demonstrated that in patients with renal failure, fentanyl is safe to use, provides good pain control, and has no adverse effects. Although some studies suggest that no dosage adjustment of fentanyl is required for patients with renal failure,[33] others suggest that fentanyl clearance is reduced in patients with moderate to severe uremia, which could result in respiratory depression from gradual drug accumulation.[34,35]

Dialysis

The role of dialysis in the clearance of drugs and their metabolites is complex. Removal of any drug or drug metabolites from the blood by dialysis depends on multiple factors, including the molecular weight of the compound, its solubility, its volume of distribution, the degree to which the drug binds to proteins, and the degree to which it is cleared by nonrenal mechanisms. Drugs or metabolites with a lower molecular weight are more likely to pass through a dialysis filter as free molecules. Drugs or metabolites with greater protein-binding are less likely to be removed by the filter. Molecules with greater water-solubility are more likely to be removed, whereas molecules with a larger volume of distribution are less likely to be removed by unit of time.[10,35]

Additional factors related to the mechanisms of dialysis affect clearance of drugs and their metabolites. The flow rates of the dialysis solution and the patient's blood affect drug removal, influenced by the surface area, pore size, and characteristics of the filter itself. Other dialysis techniques, including continuous renal replacement therapy, the use of more permeable dialysis membranes, and high blood and dialysis flow rates also can affect drug removal. The more efficient dialysis techniques can remove the drug from plasma more effectively (i.e., more rapidly) than the transfer of drug from other tissues, so that after dialysis there can be a "rebound" effect as plasma levels of the active drug rise again.

Unlike hemodialysis, peritoneal dialysis relies on the peritoneum as the filter. The pore size is fixed and the flow rate determined by the volume and frequency of exchanges; thus more frequent exchanges result in more drug removed.[10]

Dialysis and Opioids

Morphine. In patients with uremia, morphine's already low protein-binding is further reduced and its moderate water-solubility increases the likelihood of the drug being removed by dialysis.[36] The slower the flow rate of dialysis, the less morphine that is removed; therefore high-efficiency dialysis techniques are more likely to remove morphine.[37] Although dialysis does remove M6G (the active morphine metabolite), its slow diffusion out of the central nervous system may mean that patients with reduced consciousness resulting from the presence of the metabolite may not immediately improve with dialysis.[15] A study of peritoneal dialysis and morphine determined that approximately 12% of morphine and its glucuronide metabolites are removed with each peritoneal dialysis exchange.[38] These results suggest that the glucuronide metabolites would accumulate with chronic dosing of morphine.

Hydromorphone. Similar to morphine, hydromorphone also has high water-solubility; in addition, it has a low volume of distribution and a low molecular weight. These characteristics suggest that hydromorphone is dialyzable.[39] It does not accumulate in patients on hemodialysis because it is rapidly converted to H3G.

Therefore it is H3G that accumulates between hemodialysis sessions, but it is effectively removed by dialysis.[8] As a result, hydromorphone is safe and effective for use in patients on dialysis, although careful monitoring must be continued.

Oxycodone. Unlike hydromorphone, oxycodone has a greater volume of distribution; the drug is almost 50% protein-bound and is highly water-soluble. No data are available on oxycodone and dialysis, but pharmacodynamics characteristics suggest it is probably dialyzable.[10]

Codeine. Unlike hydromorphone and oxycodone, codeine does not seem to be safe in patients on dialysis. Two of the six patients on dialysis enrolled in a single-dose study of codeine had severe adverse reactions, suggesting that toxic drug accumulation would occur with repeat dosing. This limited evidence suggests that codeine should be avoided in patients on dialysis.[40]

Methadone. Unlike hydromorphone, methadone has high protein-binding and a high volume of distribution, which would suggest it is not well removed by dialysis. However, methadone's moderate water-solubility and low molecular weight make it potentially dialyzable.[41] The more water-soluble metabolite of methadone is readily removed, but this does not have clinical significance because this metabolite is inactive.

Fentanyl. Fentanyl's high protein-binding, low water-solubility, high volume of distribution, and moderately high molecular weight suggest it is not likely to be dialyzed. Limited data support this assumption, however.[36]

SUMMARY OF EVIDENCE REGARDING TREATMENT RECOMMENDATIONS

The degree of renal failure (based on GFR calculations) is an important determinant in selection of appropriate opioid therapy for individual patients. In addition, better data are needed on how dialysis affects opioids. These elements make determining the best medication to use in patients with renal failure difficult. Likewise, it is unclear how treatment recommendations should change for those who develop renal failure while on opioids compared to patients with renal failure who need opioids for pain management. The scarce evidence on the signs and symptoms of opioid overdose in patients with renal impairment compared to patients with normal renal function makes providing treatment recommendations more complicated. More research is needed to determine how to best use opioids other than morphine for patients with renal impairment or on dialysis.

Recommendations

Renal Impairment. In spite of the limitations discussed previously, the literature indicates that morphine should be avoided because of the potential adverse effects of its metabolites. The data are clear that codeine should not be used because active metabolites accumulate in renal failure and are associated with reports of serious adverse effects.[29]

Oxycodone should be used with caution because free oxymorphone, the active metabolite of oxycodone, can accumulate in renal failure and potentially cause toxic and central nervous system–depressant effects in this patient population.

Hydromorphone is thought to be safer for use in patients in renal failure, although the H3G metabolite is neuroexcitatory and can accumulate in renal failure. Methadone appears safe because the metabolites are inactive and both methadone and its metabolites are excreted in the gut. Nevertheless, these data are very limited and may not reflect patient variability.[31] Precautions must be used when prescribing methadone because of its extremely long half-life and complex pharmacokinetics. Some recommend using a dose reduction of methadone for patients with severe renal failure. Fentanyl is also considered safe based on clinical experience. However, some evidence suggests that the parent drug may accumulate in renal failure; therefore its long-term use in patients in renal failure must be carefully monitored.

Dialysis. As discussed earlier, various aspects of dialysis may alter the safety profile of opioid use. Although morphine and the metabolites can be removed by dialysis, they may not be cleared entirely during a dialysis session, leaving a potential reservoir of morphine and metabolites in the central nervous system. This potentially can result in a rebound effect as the medication diffuses out of the central nervous system. Metabolites can accumulate between dialysis sessions; therefore careful dose monitoring is required both during and after dialysis. Given that safer alternatives are available, morphine should be avoided in patients on dialysis.[10] Similarly, codeine should not be used because its metabolites accumulate and have had serious adverse effects in patients on dialysis.[40] Unfortunately, no evidence exists about the effect of dialysis on oxycodone and its metabolites; therefore some have suggested avoiding its use in patients on dialysis.

Hydromorphone is a viable option but should be used with caution. The parent drug can be partially removed by dialysis. However, it is not clear whether its metabolites are cleared with dialysis and accumulation of these metabolites presents a risk. Methadone can be another option for patients on dialysis because its metabolites are inactive and the parent drug is not metabolized. As noted earlier, precautions must be used with methadone given its long half-life.[31] Fentanyl also appears safe for use in the short term for patients on dialysis because its metabolites are inactive. Although concern exists that the parent drug may accumulate in renal failure, no evidence has been reported of its clinical significance. Fentanyl is not dialyzed, so no dose adjustment is necessary. However, fentanyl may adsorb onto the CT 190 dialyzer membrane filter[42]; therefore, if the CT 190 filter used for a patient cannot be changed, rotation to methadone is recommended.

In summary, methadone and fentanyl appear to be the safest opioids because they are not dialyzed. Nevertheless, caution must be used in titrating opioids in patients with renal disease and these patients must be monitored closely.

TABLE 6-1. Opioids in Renal Failure		
PREFERRED	**CONSIDER**	**AVOID**
Methadone	Hydromorphone	Morphine
Fentanyl	Oxycodone	Codeine

KEY MESSAGES TO PATIENTS AND FAMILIES

Pain management is a critical aspect of care for patients with renal impairment or on dialysis. Nevertheless, a limited body of evidence exists to help guide safe and effective opioid choice for this group of patients. In spite of these limitations, some suggested guidelines for opioids selection are available. All opioids should be used with caution and with close monitoring (Table 6-1). Fentanyl and methadone are thought to be the safest opioids for pain management in this patient population. Hydromorphone and oxycodone are to be used with caution. Morphine and codeine are to be avoided. Patients and families should understand that as a patient's renal disease worsens, rotation to safer and more predictable opioid alternatives may be necessary.

CONCLUSION AND SUMMARY

As with all patient populations, the management of pain should be approached in a stepwise manner. By applying the principles behind the World Health Organization's pain ladder to patients with renal impairment or failure, management of pain can be accomplished both safely and effectively[8] (Table 6-2). Given the evidence on metabolism of morphine in patients in renal failure, experts recommend that morphine should be avoided in patients in severe renal failure (GFR <30 mL/min).[10,35,43] In settings in which alternative opioids may not be available, most experts recommend that morphine be given as a single dose to relieve pain until alternative opioids are available. Although anecdotal evidence supports oxycodone as safer than morphine for use in patients in renal failure, oxycodone is recommended only if alternative opioids are not available. Like oxycodone, hydromorphone lacks sufficient evidence to support its use in patients in renal failure, and thus no clear conclusions can be made on its safety and effectiveness in this patient population.

Methadone may be an effective analgesic for use in patients with renal impairment if carefully monitored, although extensive pharmacokinetic and pharmacodynamics are not yet available. Limited evidence supports the use of continuous fentanyl for patients with renal failure. Experts do suggest that, based on its inactive and nontoxic metabolites, fentanyl is safe to use in the last days of life for a patient with advanced chronic kidney disease. The potential for accumulation of the parent drug and an increase in half-life may occur if fentanyl is given as a continuous infusion, and therefore patients should be monitored for signs of opioid toxicity.[25]

TABLE 6-2. Pain Management for Patients With Renal Failure

WHO LADDER	ANALGESIC	RECOMMENDATION	COMMENTS
Step 1	Acetaminophen	Recommended	No dose adjustment necessary.
	Nonsteroidal anti-inflammatories	Use with caution	May have increased bleeding in CKD.
Step 2	Tramadol	Use with caution	Maximum dose of 200 mg daily, associated with lower seizure threshold.
	Codeine	Avoid	Case reports of delayed and unexpected toxicity.
	Dextropropoxyphene	Avoid	Accumulation of parent drug and active metabolites, associated with CNS and cardiac toxicity.
Step 3	Fentanyl	Recommended	
	Methadone	Recommended	Use by experienced clinician.
	Hydromorphone	Recommended	Well tolerated in dialysis patients; toxic metabolites may accumulate in stage 5 CKD, therefore manage conservatively.
	Oxycodone	Insufficient evidence	
	Morphine	Avoid	M6G accumulates and has analgesic and sedating properties.

From Davison SN. The prevalence and management of chronic pain in end-stage renal disease. *J Palliat Med.* 2007;10(6):1277–1287.
CDK, Chronic kidney disease; *CNS,* central nervous system.

SUMMARY RECOMMENDATIONS

- The absorption effect of morphine is unknown. Morphine is glucuronidated to M3G and M6G. Accumulation of M6G leads to increased central nervous system distribution. Morphine is excreted, with accumulation of metabolites. Morphine use should be avoided in renal failure.
- The absorption effect, distribution, and metabolism of codeine are unknown, and it has reduced excretion. Codeine should be avoided in renal failure.
- The absorption effect and distribution of hydromorphone are unknown. No metabolism effects occur, and glucuronidation is preserved. H3G accumulates, possibly resulting in neurotoxicity. Hydromorphone is preferred over morphine because H3G is less neurotoxic than M3G, and patients should be monitored closely.
- The absorption effect, distribution, and metabolism of oxycodone are unknown. Excretion of metabolites is severely metabolized. The metabolites are thought to be less neurotoxic than those of morphine and hydromorphone.
- The absorption effect, distribution, and metabolism of methadone are unknown. Biliary excretion increases as renal excretion decreases. Methadone appears to be safe in renal failure, and no dose recommendations are necessary.
- The absorption effect, distribution, and metabolism of fentanyl are unknown. Case reports suggest that the parent drug may accumulate in the setting of severe renal failure. Fentanyl use appears to be safe in patients with renal failure.
- The absorption effect, distribution, and metabolism of tramadol are unknown. Tramadol and its active metabolites do accumulate. Renal adjustment is required to prevent adverse effects.

REFERENCES

1. Davison SN. Pain in hemodialysis patients: prevalence, cause, severity, and management. *Am J Kidney Dis.* 2003;42(6):1239–1247.
2. Fainsinger RL, Davison SN, Brenneis C. A supportive care model for dialysis patients. *Palliat Med.* 2003;17(1):81–82.
3. Fortina F, Agllata S, Ragazzoni E, et al. Chronic pain during dialysis: pharmacologic therapy and its costs. *Minerva Urol Nefrol.* 1999;51(2):85–87.
4. Chater S, Davison SN, Germain MJ, Cohen LM. Withdrawal from dialysis: a palliative care perspective. *Clin Nephrol.* 2006;66(5):364–372.
5. Cohen LM, Germain M, Poppel DM, Woods A, Kjellstrand CM. Dialysis discontinuation and palliative care. *Am J Kidney Dis.* 2000;36(1):140–144.
6. Davison SN, Jhangri GS. The impact of chronic pain on depression, sleep, and the desire to withdraw from dialysis in hemodialysis patients. *J Pain Symptom Manage.* 2005;30(5):465–473.
7. Davison SN, Jhangri GS, Johnson JA. Cross-sectional validity of a modified Edmonton symptom assessment system in dialysis patients: a simple assessment of symptom burden. *Kidney Int.* 2006;69(9):1621–1625.
8. Davison SN. The prevalence and management of chronic pain in end-stage renal disease. *J Palliat Med.* 2007;10(6):1277–1287.
9. Verbeeck RK, Musuamba FT. Pharmacokinetics and dosage adjustment in patients with renal dysfunction. *Eur J Clin Pharmacol.* 2009;65(8):757–773.
10. Dean M. Opioids in renal failure and dialysis patients. *J Pain Symptom Manage.* 2004;28(5):497–504.
11. Hasselstrom J, Sawe J. Morphine pharmacokinetics and metabolism in humans: enterohepatic cycling and relative contribution of metabolites to active opioid concentrations. *Clin Pharmacokinet.* 1993;24(4):344–354.
12. Andersen G, Christrup L, Sjogren P. Relationships among morphine metabolism, pain and side effects during long-term treatment: an update. *J Pain Symptom Manage.* 2003;25(1):74–91.
13. Sawe J, Odar-Cederlof I. Kinetics of morphine in patients with renal failure. *Eur J Clin Pharmacol.* 1987;32(4):377–382.
14. Wolff J, Bigler D, Christensen CB, Rasmussen SN, Andersen HB, Tonnesen KH. Influence of renal function on the elimination of morphine and morphine glucuronides. *Eur J Clin Pharmacol.* 1988;34(4):353–357.
15. Angst MS, Buhrer M, Lotsch J. Insidious intoxication after morphine treatment in renal failure: delayed onset of morphine-6-glucuronide action. *Anesthesiology.* 2000;92(5):1473–1476.
16. Labella FS, Pinsky C, Havlicek V. Morphine derivatives with diminished opiate receptor potency show enhanced central excitatory activity. *Brain Res.* 1979;174(2):263–271.

17. Lipkowski AW, Carr DB, Langlade A, Osgood PF, Szyfelbein SK. Morphine-3-glucuronide: silent regulator of morphine actions. *Life Sci.* 1994;55(2):149–154.
18. Gong QL, Hedner T, Hedner J, Bjorkman R, Nordberg G. Antinociceptive and ventilatory effects of the morphine metabolites: morphine-6-glucuronide and morphine-3-glucuronide. *Eur J Pharmacol.* 1991;193(1):47–56.
19. Zheng M, McErlane KM, Ong MC. Hydromorphone metabolites: isolation and identification from pooled urine samples of a cancer patient. *Xenobiotica.* 2002;32(5):427–439.
20. Smith MT. Neuroexcitatory effects of morphine and hydromorphone: evidence implicating the 3-glucuronide metabolites. *Clin Exp Pharmacol Physiol.* 2000;27(7):524–528.
21. Babul N, Darke AC, Hagen N. Hydromorphone metabolite accumulation in renal failure. *J Pain Symptom Manage.* 1995;10(3):184–186.
22. Fainsinger R, Schoeller T, Boiskin M, Bruera E. Palliative care round: cognitive failure and coma after renal failure in a patient receiving captopril and hydromorphone. *J Palliat Care.* 1993;9(1):53–55.
23. Durnin C, Hind ID, Wickens MM, Yates DB, Molz KH. Pharmacokinetics of oral immediate-release hydromorphone (Dilaudid IR) in subjects with renal impairment. *Proc West Pharmacol Soc.* 2001;44:81–82.
24. Lee MA, Leng ME, Tiernan EJ. Retrospective study of the use of hydromorphone in palliative care patients with normal and abnormal urea and creatinine. *Palliat Med.* 2001;15(1):26–34.
25. Douglas C, Murtagh FE, Chambers EJ, Howse M, Ellershaw J. Symptom management for the adult patient dying with advanced chronic kidney disease: a review of the literature and development of evidence-based guidelines by a United Kingdom Expert Consensus Group. *Palliat Med.* 2009;23(2):103–110.
26. Fitzgerald J. Narcotic analgesics in renal failure. *Conn Med.* 1991;55(12):701–704.
27. Poyhia R, Seppala T, Olkkola KT, Kalso E. The pharmacokinetics and metabolism of oxycodone after intramuscular and oral administration to healthy subjects. *Br J Clin Pharmacol.* 1992;33(6):617–621.
28. Vree TB, Verwey-van Wissen CP. Pharmacokinetics and metabolism of codeine in humans. *Biopharm Drug Dispos.* 1992;13(6):445–460.
29. Matzke GR, Chan GL, Abraham PA. Codeine dosage in renal failure. *Clin Pharm.* 1986;5(1):15–16.
30. Kreek MJ, Gutjahr CL, Garfield JW, Bowen DV, Field FH. Drug interactions with methadone. *Ann NY Acad Sci.* 1976;281:350–371.
31. Kreek MJ, Schecter AJ, Gutjahr CL, Hecht M. Methadone use in patients with chronic renal disease. *Drug Alcohol Depend.* 1980;5(3):197–205.
32. Labroo RB, Paine MF, Thummel KE, Kharasch ED. Fentanyl metabolism by human hepatic and intestinal cytochrome P450 3A4: implications for interindividual variability in disposition, efficacy, and drug interactions. *Drug Metab Dispos.* 1997;25(9):1072–1080.
33. Fyman PN, Reynolds JR, Moser F, Avitable M, Casthely PA, Butt K. Pharmacokinetics of sufentanil in patients undergoing renal transplantation. *Can J Anaesth.* 1988;35(3 Pt 1):312–315.
34. Koehntop DE, Rodman JH. Fentanyl pharmacokinetics in patients undergoing renal transplantation. *Pharmacotherapy.* 1997;17(4):746–752.
35. Murtagh FE, Chai MO, Donohoe P, Edmonds PM, Higginson IJ. The use of opioid analgesia in end-stage renal disease patients managed without dialysis: recommendations for practice. *J Pain Palliat Care Pharmacother.* 2007;21(2):5–16.
36. Bastani B, Jamal JA. Removal of morphine but not fentanyl during haemodialysis. *Nephrol Dial Transplant.* 1997;12(12):2802–2804.
37. Jamal JA, Joh J, Bastani B. Removal of morphine with the new high-efficiency and high-flux membranes during haemofiltration and haemodialfiltration. *Nephrol Dial Transplant.* 1998;13(6):1535–1537.
38. Pauli-Magnus C, Hofmann U, Mikus G, Kuhlmann U, Mettang T. Pharmacokinetics of morphine and its glucuronides following intravenous administration of morphine in patients undergoing continuous ambulatory peritoneal dialysis. *Nephrol Dial Transplant.* 1999;14(4):903–909.
39. Durnin C, Hind ID, Ghani SP, Yates DB, Cross M. Pharmacokinetics of oral immediate-release hydromorphone (Dilaudid IR) in young and elderly subjects. *Proc West Pharmacol Soc.* 2001;44:79–80.
40. Guay DR, Awni WM, Findlay JW, et al. Pharmacokinetics and pharmacodynamics of codeine in end-stage renal disease. *Clin Pharmacol Ther.* 1988;43(1):63–71.
41. Furlan V, Hafi A, Dessalles MC, Bouchez J, Charpentier B, Taburet AM. Methadone is poorly removed by haemodialysis. *Nephrol Dial Transplant.* 1999;14(1):254–255.
42. Joh J, Sila MK, Bastani B. Nondialyzability of fentanyl with high-efficiency and high-flux membranes [letter]. *Anesth Analg.* 1998;86(2):447.
43. Mercadante S, Arcuri E. Opioids and renal function. *J Pain.* 2004;5(1):2–19.

How Should Methadone Be Started and Titrated in Opioid-Naïve and Opioid-Tolerant Patients?

Laura P. Gelfman and Emily J. Chai

INTRODUCTION AND SCOPE OF THE PROBLEM

Methadone is a unique synthetic opioid agonist with delta receptor affinity, N-methyl-D-aspartate (NMDA) receptor antagonism and monoamine reuptake inhibition. These unique properties make it the opioid of choice for patients with more complex pain syndromes, particularly those with neuropathic pain syndromes. This combination of opioid agonism and NMDA receptor antagonism creates a drug profile that provides effective analgesia with minimal side effects. These benefits have made methadone an increasingly popular second-line opioid for patients whose pain is poorly responsive to other opioids or who develop dose-limiting side effects.[1]

Despite the increasing recognition of the benefits of this medication, methadone is not widely used as a first-line opioid. Its pharmacokinetics and pharmacodynamics, specifically, its multiple drug interactions, long half-life, and highly variable dose conversion from other opioids, limit its use in pain management. Nevertheless, methadone has numerous benefits compared to other opioid medications, including multiple routes for administration, low cost, long half-life, and favorable safety profile for patients with renal failure and those with morphine allergy. Although true of all medications, balancing the risk/benefit ratio is especially important in choosing methadone because of both the potential for serious side-effects and its multiple advantageous properties. These considerations are discussed in detail in Chapter 8. The focus of this chapter is guidelines for safely initiating methadone in opioid-naïve and opioid-tolerant patients. Because of the complexities in using this medication, it is always best for the novice to perform conversions under the guidance of an expert in the use of methadone.

RELEVANT PATHOPHYSIOLOGY

In terms of basic pharmacological principles, the oral bioavailability of methadone is estimated at 80%.[2] Significant variations in methadone's pharmacokinetics exist among individuals, with no clear correlation between methadone plasma levels and analgesic effect.[3]

Methadone's onset of action is similar to that of other opioids—approximately 30 to 60 minutes. At the onset of methadone titration, the duration of analgesia is 4 to 6 hours, again similar to that of other opioids.[4] However, unlike other opioids, the duration of analgesia with long-term dosing may be 8 to 12 hours or longer, with time to peak effect of about 2.5 hours. Because of its longer half-life, steady state will not be reached for several days; for those patients in whom methadone's half-life is closer to 10 days, methadone will not achieve steady state for weeks. Given this variability during the initial titration period, patients are at increased risk for drug accumulation. The concentration of methadone in the blood can rise above the effective analgesic level during this prolonged period before steady state.

Therefore the interval of greatest risk after initiating therapy is days 3 to 5. By initiating therapy with lower doses and longer dosing intervals, there is less risk for accumulation-related side effects, such as excessive sedation and respiratory depression. Typically, when using methadone for analgesia, the dosing is three times per day, although some clinicians have administered it twice daily or four times daily. Once methadone is started, studies have shown that less dose escalation is required compared to that of other opioids.[5]

Because of methadone's unpredictable pharmacodynamics, it is not recommended for use in acute pain management. However, given its long half-life, it is an excellent medication for patients with chronic pain. It can be also be an effective first-line opioid for management of complex pain syndromes in carefully selected patients given that it has advantages over other opioid analgesics, such as acting at multiple receptor sites simultaneously. Still, limited prospective evidence exists for methadone as a first-line opioid for cancer pain management.

The remainder of this chapter focuses on the rotation of other opioids to methadone. Evidence and guidelines are lacking to help clinicians with conversion of methadone back to the other opioids.

This is due in part to the additional pain relieving properties of methadone, including its effect on serotonin and NMDA receptors. Clinicians should rely on individuals with expertise to help them with conversions from methadone to other opioids.

SUMMARY OF EVIDENCE AND TREATMENT RECOMMENDATIONS

Opioid-Naïve Patients

Although methadone is more commonly started after ineffective pain relief with other opioids, in some instances methadone is initiated in opioid-naïve patients. For example, patients with renal failure, morphine allergy, or a need for long-acting pain medication can benefit from methadone as a first-line opioid. This must be done with caution and only in carefully selected patients. Although limited evidence exists on initiation of methadone in this population, practitioners generally recommend starting at a low dose and titrating slowly. One retrospective study demonstrated the safe use of methadone doses starting at 3 mg every 8 hours for opioid-naive patients.[6] Another double-blind study randomly assigned opioid-naïve patients to receive either an oral methadone regimen of 7.5 mg every 12 hours, with 5 mg every 4 hours as needed for breakthrough pain, or slow-release morphine 15 mg every 12 hours, with immediate-release morphine every 4 hours as needed for breakthrough pain.[7] No differences in pain or toxicity were noted at 4 weeks; however, in the methadone group more patients dropped out because of sedation or nausea. Methadone therapy can be initiated with small, fixed doses of 2.5 mg or 5 mg every 12 hours, along with a medication for breakthrough pain. The breakthrough medication may be a different opioid or a smaller dose of methadone prescribed every 3 hours as needed[3] (Table 7-1). Escalation of the methadone dose is stopped once the patient achieves adequate analgesia.

An alternative recommended regimen for starting methadone is 5 mg every 6 to 12 hours, with titration every 3 to 5 days until analgesia is adequate. When steady state is achieved, switch to a dosing schedule of every 8 to 12 hours. For breakthrough pain, methadone or a short-acting opioid may be used, calculated as 10% to 15% of the total 24-hour dose every 2 hours as needed.

Clinicians must carefully titrate methadone in opioid-naïve patients. Because of its long half-life, plasma levels of methadone may take up to 10 days to stabilize.[8] Therefore, during the titration phase, clinicians must balance inadequate analgesia because of insufficient dosing with systemic toxicity resulting from excessive dose.[9] In addition, patients should be warned of methadone's slow onset of action and informed that they should anticipate a gradual improvement in analgesia over time. Methadone doses cannot be titrated frequently even if a patient is not receiving adequate pain relief on the current dose because methadone may take days to reach a steady state. Similarly, if a patient develops the side effect of somnolence and is willing to tolerate this side effect for a few days, the dose can be continued to see if the patient becomes tolerant to this side effect without decreasing the dose. For patients who have inadequate pain relief without significant side effects, the dose can be increased slowly. For patients who report that the pain relief is effective, but not lasting 12 hours, the dose frequency can be increased. Finally, for those patients who do not receive some relief despite dose adjustments or increases, other treatment modalities must be considered, including a slow taper of methadone.[9]

Opioid-Tolerant Patients

The adverse effects of other opioids or poorly controlled pain in spite of appropriate titration typically drive clinicians to provide a trial of methadone. Rotating from one opioid to methadone can be a complex endeavor given the lack of clear evidence about opioid conversion. Although equianalgesic ratios have been published, the majority of the equianalgesic conversion tables from morphine to methadone are based on clinical experience.[10,11] These ratios can underestimate the potency of methadone with repeated doses. Complicating matters further, patients treated previously with high doses of other opioids sometimes paradoxically require less methadone than expected.[12] In addition, large interpatient variability may exist with the equianalgesic conversion ratio, such that a single ratio may not apply to all patients. Particular caution should be used in the case of patients on high but ineffective doses of another opioid; this situation may result in overestimation of the equivalent methadone dose.

When performing opioid rotations, it is necessary to both calculate the initial dose and consider patient characteristics such as age; cognitive, renal, and liver dysfunction; and cardiac and pulmonary comorbidities. For these reasons, conversion to methadone must be done with caution and close monitoring.

Oral Dosing for Opioid-Tolerant Patients

Rotation from oral morphine to oral methadone can be accomplished in several ways. Most conversions recommend that for patients on lower doses of morphine, in the range of a daily dose of 30 to 90 mg

TABLE 7-1. Safe and Effective Starting Doses of Methadone for Opioid-Naïve Patients

WEEK	DOSE	TOTAL DOSE/DAY (mg)
1	2.5 mg PO bid	5
2	5 mg PO bid	10
3	7.5 mg PO bid	15
4	10 mg PO bid	20
5	10 mg PO tid	30
6	20 mg PO bid (or 10 mg PO qid)	40

of oral morphine, the ratio of morphine to methadone should be 4:1. For example, a patient receiving a daily dose of 60 mg of oral morphine should be started on approximately 15 mg of methadone daily. In contrast, in patients on higher doses of morphine, the ratio is 12:1 or greater, such that a patient receiving 400 mg of morphine in a 24-hour period should be started on approximately 35 mg of methadone per day. However, various methadone conversion charts have been developed to account for the variation (Table 7-2). Given the risk for drug accumulation with the long half-life of methadone, the Ayorinde[13] conversion table may be the safest when rotating from other opioids to methadone.

Several approaches are used to rotate from other opioids to methadone. The two primary approaches covered in this chapter are (1) stopping the other opioid completely before initiating therapy with methadone and (2) tapering off the other opioid while gradually increasing the methadone dose over the course of a few days.

A method initially published by Morley and colleagues in 1993[14] and later revised to the Morley and Makin approach[15] involves a protocol of a calculated fixed dose of methadone and the discontinuation of the prior opioid. In this approach, the previous opioid is stopped before the methadone is started, without tapering. For this reason it is often referred to as the "stop and go" methadone conversion regimen. In this scenario, one way to calculate the methadone dose is to use a methadone conversion table. Another way to calculate the fixed dose is to either (1) use a fixed dose of one tenth of the calculated 24-hour oral morphine dose when that dose is less than 300 mg of morphine or (2) when the 24-hour oral morphine dose is greater than 300 mg, the methadone dose should be fixed at 30 mg. Regardless of how the fixed dose is calculated, it should be taken orally *as needed* and not more frequently than every 3 hours because of the risk for tissue accumulation of the drug. Morley and Makin note that methadone requirements usually drop during days 2 to 3 and typically reach steady state on days 4 to 5. Then, on day 6, the amount of methadone taken over the previous 48 hours is calculated and one quarter of this total dose is given in an every-12-hour regimen; this becomes the final stable dose. When the twice-daily steady dose is reached, further adjustments can be made by incrementally increasing the twice-daily dosage by 50% as needed over time. Morley and Makin[15] recommend that the initial use of a fixed ceiling dose of methadone not exceed 30 mg, in combination with as-needed dosing, to prevent the complications of drug accumulation.

Because the conversion is complex and nuanced, what follows is a more concise summary of the stop and go method. First, calculate the methadone dose. If the morphine daily dose is less than 300 mg, calculate the methadone dose to be approximately one tenth of the morphine dose. If the morphine total daily dose is greater than 300, the methadone dose is capped at 30 mg. (In other words, the maximum daily dose of methadone is 30 mg by mouth every 3 hours, or 240 mg in a 24-hour period.) Next, on the first day of the conversion, stop previous opioid therapy and give methadone (as calculated earlier) every 3 to 4 hours as needed (*not* around the clock) for the initial 3 to 5 days. On day 6, divide the total daily dose over the last 48 hours by 4 and give this new fixed dose every 12 hours.

An alternative method is the slower rotation ("reduce and replace") approach, which involves slowly adding methadone while tapering the initial opioid. This approach allows gradual titration of the long-acting methadone and therefore minimizes the risk for toxicity from drug accumulation. With this approach to converting to methadone, the 24-hour methadone dose is first calculated based on the 24-hour oral morphine equivalent using the Ayorinde[13] methadone conversion table (see Table 7-2). On day 1, the total daily dose of morphine is decreased by approximately one third and one third of the total calculated target dose of methadone is started. On day 2, the total daily dose of morphine is decreased by another one third and methadone increased to two thirds of the total target dose. On day 3, morphine is discontinued and methadone increased to 100% of the total calculated target dose.

TABLE 7-2. Equianalgesic Tables for Rotating to Methadone for Opioid-Exposed Patients

FISCH METHOD[21]

OME (mg/day)	CONVERSION RATIO (ORAL MORPHINE/ORAL METHADONE)
<30	2:1
30-99	4:1
100-299	8:1
300-499	12:1
500-999	15:1
≥1000	≥20:1

MERCADANTE METHOD[20]

OME (mg/day)	INITIAL EQUIANALGESIC DOSE RATIO (ORAL MORPHINE/ORAL METHADONE)
<90	4:1
90-300	8:1
>300	12:1

AYONRINDE METHOD[13]

OME (mg/day)	INITIAL EQUIANALGESIC DOSE RATIO (ORAL MORPHINE/ORAL METHADONE)
<100	3:1
101-300	5:1
301-600	10:1
601-800	12:1
801-1000	15:1
>1000	20:1

Data from References 13, 20, and 21.
OME, Oral methadone equivalent.

For example, consider a patient with persistent cancer-related pain despite escalating doses of opioids, for whom the clinical team has made the decision to convert to methadone. The patient is taking oxycodone CR 360 mg with oxycodone IR 160 mg in a 24-hour period—a total of 520 mg per day of oxycodone or an oral morphine equivalent of 780 mg per day. Using the Ayorinde methadone conversion (see Table 7-2), the conversion ratio is 12:1 of oral morphine to methadone because this patient is taking between 600 and 800 oral morphine equivalents per day. This converts to the patient being started on about 66 mg of methadone in a 24-hour period. Next, use the stepwise dosing approach to initiate the reduce and replace method. On day 1, the oxycodone dose would be decreased by one third to approximately 340 mg of oxycodone while adding one third of the target methadone dose (about 22 mg of methadone per day or 8 mg of methadone by mouth every 8 hours). On day 2, the oxycodone dose would be reduced by two thirds of the original dose to approximately 160 mg per day while the methadone dose is increased to two thirds of the target dose (44 mg in 24-hour period or approximately 15 mg by mouth every 8 hours.) Finally, on day 3, the standing oxycodone is discontinued and the full target methadone dose is given (66 mg of methadone as the 24-hour dose or 22 mg by mouth every 8 hours.) On day 4, the as-needed dose of oxycodone could be discontinued and methadone started for breakthrough pain at 10% of the total daily methadone dose (6 mg every 3 hours as needed). By day 4, most patients would reach steady state of methadone. After the calculations are completed, the actual dosing of the medication should be adjusted based on available formulations. For example, 20 mg of methadone every 8 hours will be easier to administer than 22 mg every 8 hours. Similarly, an oral methadone dose of 5 mg for breakthrough pain is easier to administer than a 6-mg dose.

Although many clinicians use variations of the Morley and Makin[15] (stop and go) approach for the conversion to methadone, the gradual transition to methadone allowed by the reduce and replace method is probably a safer approach for clinicians not familiar with methadone. In addition, it may be more reliable in patients who do not understand the concept of taking the medication only as needed or who cannot reliably report pain. Continuation of the short-acting opioid in the stepwise reduce and replace method may also allow for better pain control while the methadone reaches steady state.

Intravenous Dosing of Methadone

Parenteral methadone can be used in patients with pain that is particularly difficult to manage; however, expert consultation is highly recommended because of the complexities in using methadone in this manner. Patient factors for considering use of intravenous methadone include (1) poor tolerance or analgesia with first-line opioids in patients with cancer-related pain; (2) high opioid tolerance (e.g., patients with history of opioid abuse); (3) intense breakthrough pain necessitating intravenous

rescue dosing; (4) patients on an oral methadone regimen with worsening pain who become unable to swallow or who have poor enteral absorption; (5) patients with renal or hepatic failure; and (6) patients needing doses too large to be accommodated by the oral route.

When converting oral methadone to intravenous methadone, the cumulative dose of oral methadone should be reduced by 50% (a 2:1 oral/intravenous ratio). This dose is infused over 24 hours or divided into intermittent dosing and administered every 8 hours.[16] To convert in the opposite direction (i.e., from intravenous to oral), many experts report that the safest approach is to use a 1:1 conversion (i.e., same total daily dose as that given intravenously [IV] over 24 hours). Although methadone has a high oral bioavailability, some patients may need an upward titration close or equal to a 1:2 (intravenous/oral)—that is, twice the intravenous total daily dose.[17] Although limited evidence exists on the conversion from intravenous to oral methadone, a small retrospective study evaluated the ratio of conversion from parenteral to oral methadone and found the ratio to be closer to 1:1.3, meaning the parenteral dose should be multiplied by 1.3 in calculating the appropriate 24-hour oral methadone dose.[18]

Special caution should be taken with intravenous methadone because chlorobutanol, the preservative it contains, independently prolongs the QT interval. Given the risk for QT prolongation with intravenous methadone, guidelines for management suggest that an electrocardiogram (ECG) should be performed (1) before initiation of therapy, (2) after 24 hours of initiation, (3) each time the methadone dose is escalated, and (4) at regular times after titration. Following discharge from the hospital, the ECG should be repeated once after a week of treatment, because of the prolonged half-life in some patients, and again at regular, clinically feasible intervals at subsequent follow-up visits.[19]

Using intravenous methadone creates unique challenges. Unlike oral methadone, the intravenous formulation is expensive and there may be limited availability of the intravenous solution in many settings. In addition, nursing guidelines must be created to ensure patient safety during infusions. Given the often strict regulations of home health agencies regarding the use of intravenous methadone, it may not be possible to discharge patients home on parenteral methadone. For these reasons, intravenous methadone should be administered in close consultation with someone skilled in its use.

KEY MESSAGES TO PATIENTS AND FAMILIES

Families should be reminded that in spite of the stigma and special training required for its use, methadone is a safe and effective treatment for patients with chronic, complex pain syndromes. Although evidence is lacking in support of more precise conversion from other opioids to methadone, significant clinical evidence exists that methadone can be used safely for both opioid-naïve and opioid-exposed patients when used with caution and in the hands of an experienced clinician.

CONCLUSION AND SUMMARY

Methadone should be used with caution and only by clinicians who understand its variable half-life. With appropriate patient selection and careful titration, methadone is an effective, inexpensive, long-acting treatment for complex pain syndromes and for patients with chronic pain from various causes. Under the supervision of appropriate providers, the unique pharmacokinetics of methadone can be used to benefit this patient population. For oral morphine equivalent doses of less than 1200 mg per day, the Ayonride conversion chart and the Morley and Makin method are likely the safest conversion methods. Unfortunately, evidence is lacking for a safe conversion method for an oral morphine equivalent dose of more than 1200 mg per day. Large-scale equianalgesic trials will be necessary to establish a universal morphine-to-methadone conversion method for both low and high doses of morphine.[12] Evidence and guidelines are lacking to help clinicians with conversion of methadone back to the other opioids.

SUMMARY RECOMMENDATIONS

Methadone for Opioid-Naïve Patients

- Methadone is a suitable first-line opioid in select patients when slow onset and long duration of action are advantageous.[17]
- The recommended starting dose in an opioid-naïve patient is 2.5 mg orally every 8 to 12 hours. Frail older patients may need to begin as low as 2.5 mg orally once daily. In the outpatient setting, increases may be made every 5 to 7 days, depending on response.[17]

Methadone for Opioid-Tolerant Patients

- There is no fixed equianalgesic ratio between methadone and other opioids.[13]
- The titration can take several days before reaching steady state.[18]
- Before initiating methadone, the oral morphine equivalent dose must be calculated and then clinicians must choose to either use the Morely and Makin Stop and Go method or the Reduce and Replace method using the Ayonrinde conversion table.[12]

REFERENCES

1. Watanabe S. Methadone: the renaissance. *J Palliat Care.* 2001;17(2):117–120.
2. Davis MP, Walsh D. Methadone for relief of cancer pain: a review of pharmacokinetics, pharmacodynamics, drug interactions and protocols of administration. *SCC.* 2001;9(2):73–83.
3. Bryson J, Tamber A, Seccareccia D, Zimmermann C. Methadone for treatment of cancer pain. *Curr Oncol Rep.* 2006;8(4):282–288.
4. Garrido MJ, Troconiz IF. Methadone: a review of its pharmacokinetic/pharmacodynamic properties. *J Pharmacol Toxicol Methods.* 1999;42(2):61–66.
5. Mercadante S, Casuccio A, Agnello A, Serretta R, Calderone L, Barresi L. Morphine versus methadone in the pain treatment of advanced-cancer patients followed up at home. *J Clin Oncol.* 1998;16(11):3656–3661.
6. De Conno F, Groff L, Brunelli C, Zecca E, Ventafridda V, Ripamonti C. Clinical experience with oral methadone administration in the treatment of pain in 196 advanced cancer patients. *J Clin Oncol.* 1996;14(10):2836–2842.
7. Bruera E, Palmer JL, Bosnjak S, et al. Methadone versus morphine as a first-line strong opioid for cancer pain: a randomized, double-blind study. *J Clin Oncol.* 2004;22(1):185–192.
8. Sawe J. High-dose morphine and methadone in cancer patients: clinical pharmacokinetic considerations of oral treatment. *Clin Pharmacokinet.* 1986;11(2):87–106.
9. Toombs JD. *Oral methadone dosing for chronic pain: a practitioner's guide.* Pain Treat Topics. Updated 2008; http://pain-topics.org/pdf/OralMethadoneDosing.pdf. Accessed April 25, 2012.
10. Ripamonti C, Zecca E, Bruera E. An update on the clinical use of methadone for cancer pain. *Pain.* 1997;70(2–3):109–115.
11. Ripamonti C, Groff L, Brunelli C, Polastri D, Stavrakis A, De Conno F. Switching from morphine to oral methadone in treating cancer pain: what is the equianalgesic dose ratio? *J Clin Oncol.* 1998;16(10):3216–3221.
12. Pollock AB, Tegeler ML, Morgan V, Baumrucker SJ. Morphine to methadone conversion: an interpretation of published data. *Am J Hosp Palliat Care.* 2011;28(2):135–140.
13. Ayonrinde OT, Bridge DT. The rediscovery of methadone for cancer pain management. *Med J Aust.* 2000;173(10):536–540.
14. Morley J, Watt J, Wells J, Miles J, Finnegan M, Leng J. Methadone in pain uncontrolled by morphine. *Lancet.* 1993;342:1243.
15. Morley JS, Makin MK. The use of methadone in cancer pain poorly responsive to other opioids. *Pain Rev.* 1998;5:51–58.
16. Shaiova L, Berger A, Blinderman CD, et al. Consensus guideline on parenteral methadone use in pain and palliative care. *Palliat Support Care.* 2008;6(2):165–176.
17. Manfredi PL, Houde RW. Prescribing methadone, a unique analgesic. *J Support Oncol.* 2003;1(3):216–220.
18. Gonzalez-Barboteo J, Porta-Sales J, Sanchez D, Tuca A, Gomez-Batiste X. Conversion from parenteral to oral methadone. *J Pain Palliat Care Pharmacother.* 2008;22(3):200–205.
19. Shaiova L, Berger A, Blinderman CD, et al. Consensus guideline on parenteral methadone use in pain and palliative care. *Palliat Support Care.* 2008;6(2):165–176.
20. Mercadante S, Casuccio A, Fulfaro F, et al. Switching from morphine to methadone to improve analgesia and tolerability in cancer patients: a prospective study. *J Clin Oncol Oncol.* 2001;19(11):2898–2904.
21. Fisch MJ, Cleeland CS. Managing cancer pain. In: Skeel RT, ed. *Handbook of Cancer Chemotherapy.* Philadelphia: Lippincott Williams & Wilkins; 2003:663.

What Special Considerations Should Guide the Safe Use of Methadone?

Laura P. Gelfman and Emily J. Chai

INTRODUCTION AND SCOPE OF THE PROBLEM

Pain is a debilitating symptom for many people facing serious chronic illness. Most patients can have their pain adequately controlled with the more typical analgesic medications; however, the use of methadone for pain management poses unique challenges. Palliative care clinicians must understand its pharmacology and complex dosing regimens, especially when caring for medically frail or older patients.[1] Methadone was first synthesized in the late 1940s, and its use offers advantages related to its long duration of action and low cost. As an opioid agonist, methadone has cross-tolerance with other opioids, thereby alleviating opioid withdrawal syndrome. This makes it a particularly beneficial agent in those patients with a history of opioid dependence. These same properties make it an ideal medication for management of complex pain syndromes.

Although chemically different from morphine, methadone acts on the opioid receptors, producing a similar analgesic effect. Methadone has also been demonstrated to have antagonist activity at the *N*-methyl-D-aspartate (NMDA) receptor, in addition to antagonist activity at the serotonin and norepinephrine receptors sites, thereby preventing neuronal reuptake at these receptors. This receptor antagonism makes methadone useful for neuropathic pain syndromes. The combination of NMDA receptor antagonism, serotonin and norepinephrine reuptake inhibition, and opioid agonism provides valuable analgesic effects with fewer side effects than other medications in this class.

This chapter will review the special considerations for the safe use of methadone and discuss the patient populations in whom it should be used and those in whom it should be avoided.

RELEVANT PATHOPHYSIOLOGY

Pharmacokinetics

Methadone's unique properties offer benefits different from those of other opioids. Because methadone is a highly lipophilic molecule, it can be administered through a variety of routes, and it has been approved for oral and intramuscular use. It is also available for rectal, intravenous, subcutaneous, epidural, and intrathecal administration.

Oral methadone has a bioavailability nearly 80% of the administered dose compared to 26% for morphine.[2] It is absorbed rapidly from the stomach, and most absorption occurs before transiting beyond the stomach. Following absorption, methadone is widely distributed to the brain, liver, kidneys, muscles, and lungs.[3] Methadone has two phases of distribution: the alpha distribution phase, which occurs in the first 2 to 3 hours, followed by the beta distribution phase, which occurs in the following 8 to 12 hours. The drug binds to tissue more avidly than plasma proteins and can therefore accumulate in tissues with repeated dosing.[4] Methadone also binds to a specific protein called acid glycoprotein (AAG). Because AAG levels fluctuate with physiological changes and this protein interacts with other nonopioid medications such as tricyclic antidepressants, methadone's bioavailability can be altered.

Methadone's onset of action is 30 to 60 minutes after oral administration, which is comparable to those of other immediate-release or short-acting opioids. Plasma concentrations are maintained by the peripheral reservoir. Methadone reabsorption from the tissues may continue for weeks after administration has stopped, thereby sustaining plasma concentrations.

The metabolism of methadone occurs in the liver by the cytochrome P450 (CYP450) enzyme system, primarily CYP3A4. Methadone also inhibits certain CYP450 enzymes, including CYP2D6. The interaction with these enzymes relates to methadone's interaction with numerous medications across a wide array of classes (see later discussion). Unlike other opioids, methadone does not have active metabolites; thus adjusting the dosage of methadone in patients with renal insufficiency is usually not necessary. The duration of analgesia is approximately 3 to 6 hours when methadone therapy is initiated and typically extends to 8 to 12 hours with repeated administration.

Methadone is eliminated primarily by biliary excretion.[3] Although methadone does not accumulate in patients with renal impairment, its elimination can be affected by changes in urinary pH. There is a long and highly variable elimination phase, including the alpha phase, which is 6 to 8 hours in duration, and the beta phase, or second elimination phase, which is 15 to 60 hours in duration. Therefore the half-life of methadone is approximately 24 hours, but it has a very broad range, from 5 to 150 hours, depending on each individual's metabolism.[5] Because of its long half-life, plasma levels of methadone may take 5 to 7 days to reach steady state. It is this variability in duration and time to steady state that pose unique challenges for dosing the medication.

In a study of patients with cancer, an average of 2.4 doses per day was required to maintain adequate pain control.[6] By comparison, oral morphine has a half-life of about 4 hours, so 6 or more doses may be required each day to maintain adequate pain control. For patients with chronic pain who require around-the-clock dosing of opioids, methadone's long duration decreases the frequency of administration, enhances medication compliance, and improves pain control.

Pharmacodynamics

Methadone is a mu-opioid agonist; therefore it possesses both the analgesic properties and the side effects of mu-opioid receptor agonism. Methadone's mu-receptor affinity is similar to that of morphine, but with repeated dosing its analgesic efficacy is greater than that of morphine.[7] There is no clear explanation for the brevity of analgesic effect in view of the long half-life. Methadone's nonopioid actions, including inhibition of the reuptake of monoamines (including serotonin and norepinephrine) and inhibition of NMDA receptors result in additional analgesia.[7] By blocking the activation of the NMDA receptor, which can produce central sensitization, this may help prevent the development of tolerance.[8] This may contribute to methadone's unique ability to attenuate opioid tolerance and reduce hyperalgesia or allodynia. (Of note, some in vitro studies have shown that morphine also will antagonize NMDA receptors, but this occurs at concentrations 8 to 16 times higher than required by methadone.[9]) When methadone is adequately titrated at the time of initiation, frequent or large dosage changes usually are not necessary.

Methadone Side Effects

Side effects associated with methadone are similar to those of other mu-opioid agonists, including pruritus, nausea and vomiting, constipation, dry mouth, somnolence, confusion, sedation, and respiratory depression. Excessive sweating and flushing are common with oral methadone dosing. Sedation is reported less often with methadone than other opioids, but sedation from methadone may lead to more serious consequences because of its long and unpredictable half-life that may lead to accumulation. Toxicities that may occur with initiating therapy or increasing dosage may not become apparent for 2 to 5 days. In a study of patients converted to methadone therapy in an outpatient setting, 20 of 29 participants experienced some degree of toxicity, which was most frequently mild drowsiness during initial titration.[10] In light of the potential for accumulation and toxicity within 2 to 5 days of therapy initiation, the respiratory, cardiac, and central nervous system depression effects of methadone must be closely considered.

Respiratory Depression

Side effects such as sedation and respiratory depression are increased when methadone is combined with alcohol or other drugs. In addition, the respiratory depressant effects of methadone are potentiated when administered concomitantly with other drugs that may affect breathing. An Australian study found benzodiazepines present in 74% of deaths related to methadone and urged particular caution when methadone was prescribed with benzodiazepines.[11] In addition, this effect is exacerbated by the use of methadone in patients with conditions accompanied by hypoxia, hypercapnia, or decreased respiratory reserve.

QT Prolongation

Another serious side effect of methadone is QTc interval prolongation and, ultimately, torsades de pointes. A prolonged QT interval is a proarrhythmic state, associated with an increased risk for ventricular arrhythmia, particularly torsades de pointes, which is a form of polymorphic ventricular tachycardia of varying polarity.[12] Special consideration must be taken in patients with underlying cardiac disease, and careful monitoring of the QTc interval must be conducted during initiation and titration of methadone. The cardiac effects of methadone are also potentiated by concurrent administration of other drugs that prolong the QTc interval or induce torsades de pointes. In addition, clinicians must use particular caution when prescribing methadone to patients with predisposing cardiac risk factors or at risk for development of prolonged QTc interval (Table 8-1).

The risk for drug-induced torsades is increased by coadministration of other medications that prolong the QT interval. This incidence is greatest with antiarrhythmic drugs, particularly those with class III activity.[12] Some medications increase the incident of torsades de pointes through other mechanisms, including intravenous administration, drug–drug interactions (e.g., ketoconazole inhibits the metabolism of methadone), or impaired metabolism. Some individuals may have congenital poor CYP450 2D6 (CYP2D6) metabolizing ability, and therefore these individuals may be exposed to higher plasma concentrations of methadone with the concurrent use of other drugs

TABLE 8-1. Primary Risk Factors for Drug-Induced Torsades de Pointes[12]

Female sex	Cardiac failure
Baseline prolonged QT interval	Recent cardioversion from
Congenital long QT syndrome	atrial fibrillation
Electrolytes imbalance	Hypokalemia
Ventricular arrhythmia	Hypomagnesemia
Bradycardia <50 beats/min	Left ventricular hypertrophy

that are also metabolized by CYP2D6. Some individuals may have an acquired impaired metabolism as a result of hepatic or renal dysfunction. In a small proportion of patients, the use of QT-prolonging drugs will unmask a subclinical congenital long QT syndrome linked to mutations in genes encoding cardiac ion channel proteins.[12] Central sleep apnea may contribute to QT interval prolongation because of the association with bradycardia and QT prolongation and is reported to occur in 30% of patients on methadone maintenance. In summary, the QT interval prolongation associated with methadone may be both dose-related and metabolism-related.

Drug Interactions

Metabolism of methadone may create drug interactions between it and other medications related to methadone's inhibition or induction of CYP450 enzymes (Table 8-2). Specifically, the inhibition of CYP450 enzymes by methadone may cause an increase in toxicity or opioid withdrawal. For example, administration of methadone with a drug that

TABLE 8-2. Medications That Interact With Methadone[17,27]

MEDICATIONS	INCREASE METHADONE CONCENTRATION/EFFECTS	DECREASE METHADONE CONCENTRATION/EFFECTS
Antibiotics	Ciprofloxacin, ketoconazole, fluconazole, macrolide antibiotics (erythromycin, clarithromycin, troleandomycin)	Rifampin
Antiretrovirals	Delavirdine	Amprenavir, efavirenz, nelfinavir, nevirapine, ritonavir
Antidepressants	Fluoxetine, paroxetine, tricyclic antidepressants	
Anticonvulsants	Diazepam	Phenobarbital, phenytoin, carbamazepine
Antacids	Cimetidine, omeprazole	
Cardiac medications	Quinidine, verapamil	
Miscellaneous	Ethanol (acute use) Urinary alkalinizers Grapefruit juice or fruit	Ethanol (chronic use) Urinary acidifiers

inhibits methadone's metabolism or discontinuing a drug that had previously induced methadone's metabolism may result in toxicity related to an increase in the plasma concentration of methadone. In addition, discontinuing a drug that either increases methadone's metabolism or induces the CYP450 enzymes may result in opioid withdrawal.

Some medications can change methadone's absorption, distribution, and metabolism. Methadone's absorption is mediated by gastric pH and P-glycoprotein (Pgp), a transport protein. Changes in gastric pH or the activity of Pgp brought about by certain medications, including verapamil and quinidine, may change methadone absorption.[13,14] Methadone is metabolized principally by the CYP3A4 and CYP2D6 enzymes.[15] Many medications interact with methadone through their effects on these enzymes (see Table 8-2).[15,16] Drugs that inhibit CYP3A4 include fluconazole, fluvoxamine, fluoxetine, paroxetine, human immunodeficiency virus (HIV)–1 protease inhibitors (ritonavir > indinavir > saquinavir), and likely erythromycin and ketoconazole. Selective serotonin reuptake inhibitor (SSRI) antidepressants may inhibit CYP2D6 and therefore can increase methadone plasma levels. Dosing adjustments may be required if these medications are added to or eliminated from a patient's regimen. Analgesics with opioid-antagonist properties, including buprenorphine, butorphanol, dezocine, nalbuphine, nalorphine, and pentazocine, should not be used with methadone because they can displace methadone from mu-opioid receptors. The understanding of these drug interactions of various mechanisms is critical to the safe use of the medication for pain management.[17]

SUMMARY OF EVIDENCE REGARDING TREATMENT RECOMMENDATIONS

Patient Selection for Methadone

Specific factors must be taken into account when considering methadone as a treatment modality for pain management (Table 8-3). Understanding pharmacokinetics, pharmacodynamics, and drug interactions is critical in selection of patients who may be most appropriate to receive methadone. Patients suitable for methadone include those with (1) a true allergy to morphine, (2) significant renal impairment, (3) neuropathic pain, (4) refractory pain, (5) intolerable opioid-related side effects, and (6) a requirement for around-the-clock pain control with a nonoral formulation of an opioid. Relatively low cost is another benefit of methadone (Table 8-4). Methadone is the least expensive long-

TABLE 8-3. Indications for Methadone for Pain Management

Uncontrolled pain	Pain refractory to other
Renal impairment	opioids
Adverse effects of other opioids	Morphine allergy
Lower cost (advantageous in	Neuropathic pain
patients who cannot afford	
more expensive medications)	

TABLE 8-4. Monthly Cost of Methadone Compared to Other Commonly Prescribed Opioids[27]

DRUG AND DOSAGE (QUANTITY)	COST ($)*
Methadone 5 mg PO three times daily (90 pills)	8.00
Sustained-release morphine (generic) 30 mg PO twice daily (60 pills)	101.50
Sustained-release morphine (MS Contin) 30 mg PO twice daily (60 pills)	113.50
Sustained-release oxycodone (OxyContin) 20 mg PO twice daily (60 pills)	176.50
Transdermal fentanyl (Duragesic) 25 mcg per hour (10 patches)	154.00

*Estimated cost to the pharmacist based on average wholesale prices, rounded to the nearest half dollar, in Red Book. Montvale, NJ: Medical Economics Data, 2004. Cost to the patient will be higher, depending on prescription filling fee.

acting opioid available; its cost is a fraction of that of OxyContin (long-acting oxycodone), MS Contin (long-acting morphine), and fentanyl patches.

On the other hand, methadone may not be appropriate for patients (1) with a very short life expectancy (days); (2) prescribed multiple interacting drugs; (3) with a significant cardiac history; (4) with conditions accompanied by a decreased respiratory reserve, hypercapnia, or hypoxia; (5) with significant hepatic impairment; or (6) with a history of or at risk for drug nonadherence.

Patients Receiving Opioid Agonist Therapy

Patients in methadone or buprenorphine maintenance treatment programs who experience acute pain require physicians with specialized training to manage their pain. Clinicians carry many misconceptions about pain management for patients receiving opioid agonist therapy. These misconceptions include (1) the maintenance opioid agonist (methadone or buprenorphine) provides analgesia, (2) use of opioids for analgesia may result in addiction relapse, (3) the additive effects of opioid analgesics and opioid agonist therapy may cause respiratory and central nervous system depression, and (4) reporting pain may be a manipulation to obtain opioid medications or drug-seeking behavior.[18] Patients receiving maintenance therapy with opioids for addiction do not receive sustained analgesia because the duration of action for analgesia for methadone and buprenorphine is 4 to 8 hours; however, the duration of the medication's effect to suppress opioid withdrawal is 24 to 48 hours. In addition, patients receiving maintenance opioids experience cross-tolerance to other opioids and therefore require higher doses of opioid analgesics to achieve adequate pain control.[19]

No evidence has demonstrated that exposure to opioid analgesics in the presence of acute pain increases rates of relapse. Patients receiving opioid agonist therapy typically receive treatment doses that block most euphoric effects of coadministered opioids, theoretically decreasing the likelihood of opioid analgesic abuse.[20] Requests for opioid analgesia from patients receiving opioid agonist therapy may be labeled as drug-seeking behaviors, which are defined as a patient's efforts to obtain opioid medications, including engaging in illegal activities. However, it is important to distinguish between drug-seeking behavior and addiction. This becomes particularly difficult because of a phenomenon known as pseudoaddiction, a state characterized by patients with unrelieved pain who exhibit drug-seeking behaviors and search for alternative sources or increased doses of their analgesic.[21]

Opioid-Induced Hyperalgesia

Patients who experience opioid-induced hyperalgesia may benefit from transitioning to methadone for treatment of pain. Opioid-induced hyperalgesia is the result of a neuroplastic change in pain perception that augments pain sensitivity. Hyperalgesia is described as an enhanced pain response to a noxious stimulus, and opioid induced hyperalgesia occurs after prolonged administration of opioids. It is found more frequently in patients receiving high as opposed to low doses of opioids. Strategies to treat and prevent opioid tolerance and opioid-induced hyperalgesia include using adjuvant drugs for pain treatment (such as anticonvulsants and antidepressants), physical therapy, and opioid rotation. Opioid rotation is a widely used therapeutic technique in which the type of opioid or route of administration is changed to reduce the side effects and improve its analgesic efficacy.[22] The evidence supporting opioid rotation as a means of improving pain control, however, is lacking. The use of buprenorphine (a partial mu-opioid receptor agonist but also a kappa-receptor antagonist) and methadone (a mu-opioid receptor agonist and NMDA receptor antagonist) when coadministered with ketamine (an NMDA receptor antagonist) has been associated with less hyperalgesia.[23]

KEY MESSAGES TO PATIENTS AND FAMILIES

Special care must be taken for the safe use of methadone. Given its historic use for opioid agonist therapy, there is considerable stigma surrounding the use of methadone. Nevertheless, methadone can be used to effectively treat mixed pain syndromes. Data demonstrate that methadone is effective in relieving cancer pain and has analgesic efficacy and a side effect profile similar to those of long-acting morphine. Reports have shown that methadone can be effective at treating neuropathic pain, although evidence is limited supporting this property. Methadone is especially useful for patients with renal impairment, those with morphine allergy, and those in whom a slow onset and long duration of action is beneficial. When prescribed by an experienced clinician, methadone can be administered safely. Nevertheless, considerable caution must be taken for patients who are also taking other medications that cause respiratory or central nervous system depression.

CONCLUSION AND SUMMARY

While methadone has many advantages over other opioids, some special considerations must be taken into account when using it with patients. Methadone can be very effective when treating mixed pain syndromes, including cancer pain and neuropathic pain. It also has properties that make it particularly useful in patients with renal impairment or morphine allergy or in those patients who might benefit from a medication with a slow onset and long duration of action. On the other hand, methadone's long half-life requires that only experienced clinicians oversee its use. Particular caution should be used in patients who are taking other medications that cause respiratory or central nervous system depression, such as benzodiazepines. In the appropriate patient population and under the direction of an experienced clinician, methadone can be used safely and effectively for the management of pain.

SUMMARY RECOMMENDATIONS

- Data suggest that methadone is effective in relieving cancer pain and has an analgesic efficacy and side effect profile similar to that of morphine.[24,25]
- No trial evidence supports the suggestion that methadone is effective at treating neuropathic pain of malignant origin.[24,25]
- Methadone is a suitable first-line opioid in select patients for whom slow onset and long duration of action are beneficial.
- Particular caution is warranted when methadone is prescribed in patients taking benzodiazepines.[26]

REFERENCES

1. Gallagher R. Methadone: an effective, safe drug of first choice for pain management in frail older adults. *Pain Med.* 2009;10(2):319–326.
2. Gourlay GK, Cherry DA, Cousins MJ. A comparative study of the efficacy and pharmacokinetics of oral methadone and morphine in the treatment of severe pain in patients with cancer. *Pain.* 1986;25(3):297–312.
3. Lugo RA, Satterfield KL, Kern SE. Pharmacokinetics of methadone. *J Pain Palliat Care Pharmacother.* 2005;19(4):13–24.
4. Garrido MJ, Troconiz IF. Methadone: a review of its pharmacokinetic/pharmacodynamic properties. *J Pharmacol Toxicol Methods.* 1999;42(2):61–66.
5. Eap CB, Buclin T, Baumann P. Interindividual variability of the clinical pharmacokinetics of methadone: implications for the treatment of opioid dependence. *Clin Pharmacokinet.* 2002;41(14):1153–1193.
6. Mercadante S, Sapio M, Serretta R, Caligara M. Patient-controlled analgesia with oral methadone in cancer pain: preliminary report. *Ann Oncol.* 1996;7(6):613–617.
7. Davis MP, Walsh D. Methadone for relief of cancer pain: a review of pharmacokinetics, pharmacodynamics, drug interactions and protocols of administration. *Support Care Cancer.* 2001;9(2):73–83.
8. Hewitt DJ. The use of NMDA-receptor antagonists in the treatment of chronic pain. *Clin J Pain.* 2000;16(2 suppl):S73–S79.
9. Callahan RJ, Au JD, Paul M, Liu C, Yost CS. Functional inhibition by methadone of N-methyl-D-aspartate receptors expressed in Xenopus oocytes: stereospecific and subunit effects. *Anesth Analg.* 2004;98(3):653–659, table of contents.
10. Hagen NA, Wasylenko E. Methadone: outpatient titration and monitoring strategies in cancer patients. *J Pain Symptom Manage.* 1999;18(5):369–375.
11. Ernst E, Bartu A, Popescu A, Ileutt KF, Hansson R, Plumley N. Methadone-related deaths in Western Australia 1993-99. *Aust N Z J Public Health.* 2002;26(4):364–370.
12. Wilcock A, Beattie JM. Prolonged QT interval and methadone: implications for palliative care. *Curr Opin Support Palliat Care.* 2009;3(4):252–257.
13. de Castro J, Aguirre C, Rodriguez-Sasiain JM, Gomez E, Garrido MJ, Calvo R. The effect of changes in gastric pH induced by omeprazole on the absorption and respiratory depression of methadone. *Biopharm Drug Dispos.* 1996;17(7):551–563.
14. Bouer R, Barthe L, Philibert C, Tournaire C, Woodley J, Houin G. The roles of P-glycoprotein and intracellular metabolism in the intestinal absorption of methadone: in vitro studies using the rat everted intestinal sac. *Fund Clin Pharmacol.* 1999;13(4): 494–500.
15. Eap CB, Buclin T, Baumann P. Interindividual variability of the clinical pharmacokinetics of methadone: implications for the treatment of opioid dependence. *Clin Pharmacokinet.* 2002;41(14):1153–1193.
16. Davis MP, Walsh D. Methadone for relief of cancer pain: a review of pharmacokinetics, pharmacodynamics, drug interactions and protocols of administration. *Support Care Cancer.* 2001;9(2): 73–83.
17. Ripamonti C, Bianchi M. The use of methadone for cancer pain. *Hematol Oncol Clin North Am.* 2002;16(3):543–555.
18. Alford DP, Compton P, Samet JH. Acute pain management for patients receiving maintenance methadone or buprenorphine therapy. *Ann Intern Med.* 2006;144(2):127–134.
19. Doverty M, White JM, Somogyi AA, Bochner F, Ali R, Ling W. Hyperalgesic responses in methadone maintenance patients. *Pain.* 2001;90(1–2):91–96.
20. Jones BE, Prada JA. Drug-seeking behavior during methadone maintenance. *Psychopharmacologia.* 1975;41(1):7–10.
21. Weissman DE, Haddox JD. Opioid pseudoaddiction: an iatrogenic syndrome. *Pain.* 1989;36(3):363–366.
22. Chan BK, Tam LK, Wat CY, Chung YF, Tsui SL, Cheung CW. Opioids in chronic non-cancer pain. *Expert Opin Pharmacother* 2011;12(5):705–720.
23. Silverman SM. Opioid induced hyperalgesia: clinical implications for the pain practitioner. *Pain Physician.* 2009;12(3):679–684.
24. Nicholson AB. Methadone for cancer pain. *Cochrane Database Syst Rev.* 2007;4: CD003971.
25. Mercadante S, Casuccio A, Fulfaro F, et al. Switching from morphine to methadone to improve analgesia and tolerability in cancer patients: a prospective study. *J Clin Oncol.* 2001;19(11):2898–2904.
26. Ernst E, Bartu A, Popescu A, Ileutt KF, Hansson R, Plumley N. Methadone-related deaths in Western Australia 1993-99. *Aust N Z J Public Health.* 2002;26(4):364–370.
27. Toombs JD, Kral LA. Methadone treatment for pain states. *Am Fam Physician.* 2005;71(7):1353–1358.

When Should Corticosteroids Be Used to Manage Pain?

Amy P. Abernethy, Jane L. Wheeler, Arif Kamal, and David C. Currow

INTRODUCTION AND SCOPE OF THE PROBLEM

As a class of drugs, corticosteroid agents comprise several common medications, including hydrocortisone, dexamethasone, prednisone, prednisolone, and methylprednisolone. In the palliative care setting, corticosteroids are used to alleviate various symptoms, including anorexia and cachexia, nausea and vomiting, malignant bowel obstruction, and pain. Their application as a coanalgesic has been described in specific clinical scenarios, such as for relief of symptoms resulting from brain tumors and metastases, spinal cord compression, or superior vena cava syndrome in people with advanced cancer[1] and to treat painful bone metastases.[2] For patients nearing the end of life, physicians often prescribe corticosteroids to help increase appetite, reduce nausea, improve energy and mood, and enhance a person's overall sense of well-being.[3]

Corticosteroids are among the most commonly used medications in palliative care.[4] The prevalence changes by region because corticosteroid prescribing is largely dictated by local norms and concern exists that corticosteroid use is insufficiently monitored in palliative care settings.[5] A survey of German, Swiss, and Austrian palliative care inpatient units revealed that 32% of patients were taking corticosteroids.[6] Similarly, more than 50% of people with cancer in a Swedish palliative care study[7] and 41% of ambulatory people with cancer receiving exclusively supportive care in a Canadian hospital[8] were reported to be on corticosteroids. A study of 100 patients consecutively admitted to a British hospice found that 33% were taking corticosteroids; more than half did not know why they were taking these medications, with few (29%; 8/28) claiming to have benefited and only two with documentation from their referring practice regarding dose and indication.[9]

RELEVANT PATHOPHYSIOLOGY

Corticosteroids are hormonal agents that bind to the glucocorticoid receptor to regulate glucose metabolism. They provide analgesia by (1) inhibiting the synthesis of prostaglandin,[10] which leads to inflammation, and (2) reducing vascular permeability, which results in tissue edema.[11] Corticosteroids also play a role in the nervous system. As lipophilic molecules, they can cross the blood–brain barrier. Steroid receptors in the central and peripheral nervous systems help control neuron growth, differentiation, development, and plasticity.[12] Corticosteroids can reduce neuropathic pain by reducing spontaneous discharge in an injured nerve.[2]

SUMMARY OF EVIDENCE REGARDING TREATMENT RECOMMENDATIONS

The most widely accepted guide to pain management across clinical settings is the World Health Organization (WHO) Three-Step Analgesic Ladder. Although it is frequently suggested that the WHO ladder is too simplistic and inconsistent with contemporary evidence-based practice, it still forms the backbone for most guidelines and provides an overall guide to teaching palliative care pain management, especially in primary care and other non-palliative care settings. Steps two and three of the WHO ladder recommend additional (adjuvant) agents prescribed in conjunction with those initiated in step one to further alleviate pain and potentially address other symptoms. Adjuvant medications, including corticosteroids, are advocated if they directly reduce pain, reduce pain in conjunction with opioid drugs, allow for analgesia at a lower opioid dose, or aid in the management of other concurrent symptoms such as nausea and vomiting, anorexia, and malignant bowel obstruction.[4,13] However, because of their similar mechanisms of action, corticosteroids are unlikely to enhance the analgesic effect of nonsteroidal antiinflammatory drugs (NSAIDs) while predictably adding to risk for toxicity.[2] The combination of these two agents (i.e., NSAIDs and corticosteroids) is not advised, given the resulting increased risk for upper gastrointestinal tract bleeding.

Despite the widespread use of corticosteroids in palliative care, minimal evidence has been presented in the literature to support or refute their use to alleviate pain or other symptoms in this population. A few studies dating to the 1970s demonstrated improvement in symptoms with corticosteroid use. In 1974, dexamethasone was demonstrated to improve appetite in advanced gastrointestinal cancer.[14] However, improvements in appetite did not translate to improvements in cachexia or increases in lean body mass. Since that time, use of corticosteroids to alleviate pain in patients with advanced cancer has been studied, with positive results in several clinical trials,[15–19] although failure to achieve significant impact on pain has also been reported.[20,21] An important randomized trial of adjuvant corticosteroids for patients with advanced cancer who required strong opioids found no additional analgesic benefit, but did report decreased opioid-related gastrointestinal symptoms and improved sense of well-being.[22]

Common evidence-based uses of corticosteroids in cancer pain management include care of patients with brain metastases, in which corticosteroids are used to reduce intracranial pressure and control or prevent cerebral edema,[23,24] and as analgesic adjuvants for patients with spinal metastases.[25] Because of their impact on prostaglandin synthesis, corticosteroids may be most useful in pain syndromes, such as bone pain, that involve prostaglandin release.[2]

Current Recommendations

Currently, the evidence base and expert consensus support consideration of corticosteroids as a coanalgesic for palliative care patients with certain neuropathic pain syndromes (e.g., sympathetic dystrophies); cancer pain including bone pain, infiltration, or nerve compression; headache resulting from intracranial pressure; and pain related to bowel obstruction.[2] Although supporting published literature is less available, other common pain syndromes that may benefit from the introduction of corticosteroids include the pain of stretching of the hepatic capsule as a result of rapidly enlarging liver metastases and acute involution of a necrosing metastatic mass. Existing clinical practice guidelines more generally recommend cautious short-term use of corticosteroids as adjuvant analgesics. The Agency for Healthcare Research and Quality issued guidelines in 1994 recommending the use of corticosteroids as adjuvants at all steps of the WHO Ladder to treat concurrent symptoms that may aggravate the pain syndrome, independently provide pain relief for certain types of pain, and enhance the analgesia provided by opioids.[26,27] Subsequently released, the National Comprehensive Cancer Network Guideline for Adult Cancer Pain recommends a trial of corticosteroids for the acute management of a pain crisis when neural structures or bones are involved, but warns of significant long-term adverse effects.[28] The American Geriatrics Society Panel on the Pharmacological Management of Persistent Pain in Older Persons lists corticosteroids as an option for pain management, but suggests use of the lowest possible dose to prevent side effects, including psychotropic properties, fluid retention, and glycemic effects in the short term and proximal myopathies, changes in body habitus, cardiovascular side effects, and bone demineralization with long-term use.[29]

Current Practice

Dexamethasone is the corticosteroid most commonly prescribed for pain in the palliative care setting. Advantages of dexamethasone over other corticosteroid options, demonstrated at a population level, are that it causes less fluid retention because of its lesser mineralocorticoid effect, has a longer half-life and thus can be taken once daily,[28] and offers higher potency.

Although corticosteroids have excellent oral bioavailability, they may also be administered intravenously or intramuscularly at the same dose. The oral route is preferable.[26] The most appropriate doses of specific corticosteroid drugs have yet to be defined. Dosing of dexamethasone at 2 to 8 mg orally or subcutaneously, from one to three times daily, is generally accepted; others have suggested a starting dose of 10 mg twice daily, tapering thereafter to the minimal effective dose.[2]

Prednisone and prednisolone offer alternatives to dexamethasone; an advantage of prednisolone is lower frequency of myopathy as a side effect. With prednisone, the American Geriatric Society recommends starting at a dose of 5 mg daily, tapering to a lower dose as soon as feasible.[29]

Management of Side Effects

Corticosteroids have many potential side effects that often delimit their usage, for safety reasons, to low-dose, short-term administration or use in patients near the end of life.[29] Because most corticosteroid side effects manifest over the long term, general consensus holds that these drugs are best used for a limited time, at the lowest effective dose, and with frequent monitoring.

Short-term toxicities associated with corticosteroids include hypertension, hyperglycemia, immunosuppression (often manifested by candidiasis), and a wide spectrum of psychiatric complications, including affective disorders, psychotic reactions, and global cognitive impairment.[30] Most patients experience hyperawareness and euphoria with corticosteroids, but up to 20% of patients on high doses report depression, mania, psychosis, or mixed affective state.[31,32] Sleep disturbances and insomnia may require additional medications to resolve. These effects usually appear quickly—most within the first several doses and others within the first few weeks of initiating treatment—and may occur within 1 day of administering the drug. Reduction or discontinuation of the drug generally reverses these short-term toxicities. Long-term adverse effects include Cushing habitus, proximal myopathy (although in some people this may occur relatively early in the course of their use), osteoporosis, and aseptic necrosis of bone (rare).[2]

Because side effects from corticosteroids are diverse and not uncommon, the lowest effective dose should always be used. Side effects accumulate over time; thus corticosteroids are advised for short-term courses of therapy, from 1 to 3 weeks.[33,34] Corticosteroids are used for longer than 3 weeks for palliative care patients who have short- to medium-term prognosis (i.e., <3 months) and in whom side effects are unlikely to develop in the time remaining.

Management of Withdrawal

Symptoms of withdrawal from corticosteroids may include pain, nausea or vomiting, weight loss, depression, fatigue, fever, dizziness, and rebound symptoms that are unmasked on removal of the drug. Addisonian crisis is a life-threatening complication that can cause confusion, coma, cardiovascular shock, and death. It must be considered in all people who have been on corticosteroids and are acutely unwell or facing a systemic stressor such as major surgery. At the end of life, corticosteroid withdrawal is known to exacerbate terminal restlessness. Additionally, fast tapering of corticosteroids may result in a diffuse myalgia/arthralgia withdrawal syndrome requiring a dose increase and slower tapering.[24] The definitions of fast-tapering and the period of exposure to corticosteroids leading to the need for a taper are unclear, and practice varies greatly by discipline. Some clinicians argue that corticosteroid exposure beyond 3 days heralds the need for a taper; others use these agents for up to 6 weeks, arguing that suppression of the pituitary-adrenal axis is likely to take this long. Tapers vary between a few days to a few weeks, depending on chronicity of exposure. In all cases, tapering and ultimate cessation of corticosteroids should be closely monitored for potential side effects.

A clinician might consider continuing corticosteroids for several reasons in a patient with advanced or terminal disease. Continuation of the medication averts the possibility of withdrawal symptoms that may require further medication (e.g., myalgia, arthralgia, abdominal pain, nausea, conjunctivitis, Addisonian crisis) or may be especially problematic in palliative care patients (e.g., exacerbation of terminal restlessness) and avoids causing a rebound of masked symptoms. When prognosis is short, the patient's safety and experience of the remainder of life may be better maintained by continuing rather than discontinuing corticosteroids. A limited prognosis may also mean that the benefits of withdrawing corticosteroids go unrealized and that there is insufficient time for a controlled withdrawal. Additionally, in cases in which patients are unable to communicate distress caused by discontinuation of the corticosteroid, or where withdrawing the medication induces distress in family members, caregivers, or staff, maintenance of the drug may be a legitimate choice. However, this must always be balanced with corticosteroid side effects such as insomnia, hyperglycemia, psychotropic effects, hypertension, and restlessness. Care should always be individualized.

Putting It All Together: A Suggested Evidence-Based Approach

Corticosteroids, properly managed, can play an important role in palliative pain management. To ensure their appropriate and effective usage, the following approach is recommended; these steps are in alignment with expert consensus, existing published evidence, and current clinical practice guidelines. Overall, more evidence is still needed to guide optimal practice.

Because patients in palliative care present with diverse clinical scenarios, including distinct patterns of comorbidity and concurrent symptoms, each patient warrants a brief "n-of-1" trial of the selected corticosteroid; results of this trial should be monitored against specific goals within a defined timeframe. To evaluate progress toward the goal of pain management, a standardized patient-reported measure, such as the Brief Pain Inventory[35] or a simple 0 to 10 numerical rating scale for pain, is best used to evaluate analgesic effect. Concurrent symptoms and potential side effects should be closely and routinely monitored as well; this can be accomplished using a review of systems approach, a comprehensive global symptom assessment such as the Patient Care Monitor,[36] or a palliative care–focused patient-reported instrument such as the Edmonton Symptom Assessment Scale.[37] The corticosteroid should be discontinued if not found to benefit the individual within a week; 3 days may be an adequate trial for many situations (e.g., headache). If effective, the corticosteroid should be maintained at the minimum dose that provides sufficient analgesia without side effects. In general, patients should be maintained on the corticosteroid for less than 3 weeks, but the decision of when and whether to discontinue the corticosteroid should hinge on patient-specific factors, including prognosis, likelihood of side effects from withdrawal, potential to exacerbate other symptoms being masked by the drug, and patient and family experiences and values related to this treatment path. Dexamethasone is currently the corticosteroid best supported by clinical experience, evidence, and guidelines issued by expert panels; dosing is individualized, with a reasonable starting dose totaling 16 mg daily in divided doses, tapering soon after initiation to minimum effective dose.

As with management of other symptoms, pain management using corticosteroids in palliative care warrants a "whole person" orientation. In this "total symptom" framework, modeled after the "total pain" concept introduced by Dame Cecily Saunders in the 1960s,[38] the care plan is carefully designed to minimize the sum total of suffering experienced by the patient and, where possible, the patient's family and caregivers. Pain management is central to optimization of overall quality of life and can work synergistically with the alleviation of other symptoms to enhance patient well-being. In this patient-centered context, factors that will help determine choice of corticosteroid agent, duration of its delivery, and place of corticosteroid treatment within the overall care plan include the individual's prognosis, medical and psychosocial characteristics, and unique circumstances of care. Coanalgesic corticosteroids should be incorporated into the overall pain management plan; whole-person care includes multimodal pain management that optimizes pharmacological and nonpharmacological interventions within the context of the biopsychosocial needs of the patient.

KEY MESSAGES TO PATIENTS AND FAMILIES

Corticosteroids can be useful in alleviating pain, either by their own direct action or in conjunction with other pain medications. These medications may be especially helpful for patients who experience both pain and other simultaneous symptoms that corticosteroids can help alleviate, such as anorexia, nausea and vomiting, and bowel obstruction. They may also sometimes improve mood and reduce anxiety. Because they are associated with various side effects, some of which are serious, corticosteroid use is generally restricted to the short term and at the lowest dose that relieves the patient's symptoms. For these reason, to ensure patient safety, the goal is to taper off corticosteroids as soon as possible, while maintaining relief of the pain and other symptoms.

CONCLUSION AND SUMMARY

Corticosteroids are indicated as adjuvant analgesics for several pain scenarios in palliative care, including bone, visceral, and neuropathic pain in people with advanced cancer and those with spinal cord compression. Because corticosteroids have beneficial effects on other commonly co-occurring symptoms such as anorexia and cachexia, nausea and vomiting, and bowel obstruction, they warrant consideration as a coanalgesic in patients with pain and these concurrent symptoms.[2] The potential side effects of corticosteroids are serious and require that the patient be monitored closely for adverse effects.

SUMMARY RECOMMENDATIONS

- For a patient experiencing pain that is insufficiently relieved by NSAIDs or an opioid, conduct a short (i.e., 3-7 days) n-of-1 trial of the corticosteroid in conjunction with the opioid, monitoring results against specific goals in a defined timeframe.
- If the patient tolerates the corticosteroid well and reports pain relief, continue therapy at a dose of up to 16 mg orally daily in divided doses. Dexamethasone is the current drug of choice; prednisone or prednisolone may be more appropriate for certain patients.
- Discontinue the corticosteroid if it does not achieve the desired pain relief within a predefined timeframe; be sure to communicate this plan to the patient.
- Maintain the patient on the minimum possible corticosteroid dose to achieve the desired effect, for up to 3 weeks.
- If prognosis is longer than 3 weeks, either (1) taper the patient off of the corticosteroid, carefully monitoring for withdrawal symptoms and return of pain, or (2) maintain the patient on the minimum effective dose based on patient-specific considerations.
- Apply this algorithm within a "whole-person," patient-centered context, in which pain is managed using a biopsychosocial approach and corticosteroids are a part of a tailored pharmacological and nonpharmacological analgesic plan.

DISCLOSURE

Dr. Abernethy has research funding from the U.S. National Institutes of Health, U.S. Agency for Healthcare Research and Quality, Robert Wood Johnson Foundation, Pfizer, Eli Lilly, Bristol Meyers Squibb, Helsinn Therapeutics, Amgen, Kanglaite, Alexion, Biovex, DARA Therapuetics, Novartis, and Mi-Co. In the last 2 years she has had nominal consulting agreements (less than $10,000) with Helsinn, Proventys, Amgen, and Novartis.

REFERENCES

1. Wooldridge JE, Anderson CM, Perry MC. Corticosteroids in advanced cancer. *Oncology.* 2001;15(2):225–234.
2. Watanabe S, Bruera E. Corticosteroids as adjuvant analgesics. *J Pain Symptom Manage.* 1994;9(7):442–445.
3. Lundstrom S, Furst CJ. Symptoms in advanced cancer: relationship to endogenous cortisol levels. *Palliat Med.* 2003;17(6):503–508.
4. Vyvey M. Steroids as pain relief adjuvants. *Can Fam Physician.* 2010;56(12):1295–1297.
5. Exton L, Corticosteroids. In: Walsh TD, Caraceni AT, Fainsinger R, et al. eds. *Palliative Medicine.* Philadelphia: Saunders; 797–800.
6. Nauck F, Ostgathe C, Klaschik E, et al. Drugs in palliative care: results from a representative survey in Germany. *Palliat Med.* 2004;18(2):100–107.

7. Lundstrom SH, Furst CJ. The use of corticosteroids in Swedish palliative care. *Acta Oncol.* 2006;45(4):430–437.

8. Riechelmann RP, Krzyzanowska MK, O'Carroll A, Zimmermann C. Symptom and medication profiles among cancer patients attending a palliative care clinic. *Support Care Cancer.* 2007;15(12):1407–1412.

9. Needham PR, Daley AG, Lennard RF. Steroids in advanced cancer: survey of current practice. *BMJ.* 1992;305(6860):24.

10. Haynes JRC. Adrenocortical steroids. In: Goodman EA, ed. *The Pharmacological Basis of Therapeutics.* NewYork: Pergamon; 1990:1436–1458.

11. Yamada K, Ushio Y, Hayakawa T, Arita N, Yamada N, Mogami H. Effects of methylprednisolone on peritumoral brain edema: a quantitative autoradiographic study. *J Neurosurg.* 1983;59(4):612–619.

12. Mensah-Nyagan AG, Meyer L, Schaeffer V, Kibaly C, Patte-Mensah C. Evidence for a key role of steroids in the modulation of pain. *Psychoneuroendocrinology* 2009;34(1).

13. National Comprehensive Cancer Network. *NCCN Guidelines Version 1.2011: Palliative Care.* http://www.nccn.org/professionals/physician_gls/pdf/palliative.pdf; 2011. Accessed May 10, 2012.

14. Moertel CG, Schutt AJ, Reitemeier RJ, Hahn RG. Corticosteroid therapy of preterminal gastrointestinal cancer. *Cancer.* 1974;33(6):1607–1609.

15. Bruera E, Roca E, Cedaro L, Carraro S, Chacon R. Action of oral methylprednisolone in terminal cancer patients: a prospective randomized double-blind study. *Cancer Treat Rep.* 1985;69(7–8):751–754.

16. Della Cuna GR, Pellegrini A, Piazzi M. Effect of methylprednisolone sodium succinate on quality of life in preterminal cancer patients: a placebo-controlled, multicenter study. The Methylprednisolone Preterminal Cancer Study Group. *Eur J Cancer Clin Oncol.* 1989;25(12):1817–1821.

17. Greenberg HS, Kim JH, Posner JB. Epidural spinal cord compression from metastatic tumor: results with a new treatment protocol. *Ann Neurol.* 1980;8(4):361–366.

18. Kozin F, Ryan LM, Carerra GF, Soin JS, Wortmann RL. The reflex sympathetic dystrophy syndrome (RSDS). III. Scintigraphic studies, further evidence for the therapeutic efficacy of systemic corticosteroids, and proposed diagnostic criteria. *Am J Med.* 1981;70(1):23–30.

19. Tannock I, Gospodarowicz M, Meakin W, Panzarella T, Stewart L, Rider W. Treatment of metastatic prostatic cancer with low-dose prednisone: evaluation of pain and quality of life as pragmatic indices of response. *J Clin Oncol.* 1989;7(5):590–597.

20. Popiela T, Lucchi R, Giongo F. Methylprednisolone as palliative therapy for female terminal cancer patients. The Methylprednisolone Female Preterminal Cancer Study Group. *Eur J Cancer Clin Oncol.* 1989;25(12):1823–1829.

21. Vecht CJ, Haaxma-Reiche H, van Putten WL, de Visser M, Vries EP, Twijnstra A. Initial bolus of conventional versus high-dose dexamethasone in metastatic spinal cord compression. *Neurology.* 1989;39(9):1255–1257.

22. Mercadante SL, Berchovich M, Casuccio A, Fulfaro F, Mangione S. A prospective randomized study of corticosteroids as adjuvant drugs to opioids in advanced cancer patients. *Am J Hosp Palliat Med.* 2007;24(1):13–19.

23. Taillibert S, Delattre JY. Palliative care in patients with brain metastases [review]. *Curr Opin Oncol.* 2005;17(6):588–592.

24. Taillibert S, Laigle-Donadey F, Sanson M. Palliative care in patients with primary brain tumors. *Curr Opin Oncol.* 2004;16(6):587–592.

25. Black P. Spinal metastasis: current status and recommended guidelines for management. *Neurosurgery.* 1979;5(6):726–746.

26. Jacox A, Carr DB, Payne R. New clinical-practice guidelines for the management of pain in patients with cancer. *N Engl J Med.* 1994;330(9):651–655.

27. Agency for Healthcare Research, Quality. *Management of cancer pain.* http://www.ncbi.nlm.nih.gov/books/NBK16522/; 1994. Accessed 10.05.12.

28. National Comprehensive Cancer Network. *NCCN Guidelines Version 1.2011: Adult Cancer Pain.* http://www.nccn.org/professionals/physician_gls/pdf/pain.pdf; 2011. Accessed May 5, 2012.

29. American Geriatrics Society Panel on Pharmacological Management of Persistent Pain in Older Persons. Pharmacological Management of Persistent Pain in Older Persons. *J Am Geriatr Soc.* 2009;57(8):1331–1346.

30. Stiefel FC, Breitbart WS, Holland JC. Corticosteroids in cancer: neuropsychiatric complications. *Cancer Invest.* 1989;7(5):479–491.

31. Boston Collaborative Drug Surveillance Program. Acute adverse reactions to prednisone in relation to dosage. *Clin Pharmacol Ther.* 1972;13(5):694–698.

32. Mitchell A, O'Keane V. Steroids and depression. *BMJ.* 1998;316(7127):244–245.

33. Gannon C, McNamara P. A retrospective observation of corticosteroid use at the end of life in a hospice. *J Pain Symptom Manage.* 2002;24(3):328–334.

34. Pereira JL. *The Pallium Palliative Pocketbook: A Peer-Reviewed, Referenced Resource.* Edmonton, Alberta: The Pallium Project; 2008;5.1–5.88.

35. Cleeland CS, Ryan KM. Pain assessment: global use of the Brief Pain Inventory. *Ann Acad Med Singapore.* 1994;23(2):129–138.

36. Abernethy AP, Zafar SY, Uronis H, et al. Validation of the Patient Care Monitor (Version 2.0): a review of system assessment instrument for cancer patients. *J Pain Symptom Manage.* 2010;40(4):545–558.

37. Bruera E, Kuehn N, Miller MJ, Selmser P, Macmillan K. The Edmonton Symptom Assessment System (ESAS): a simple method for the assessment of palliative care patients. *J Palliat Care.* 1991;7(2):6–9.

38. Saunders C. Care of patients suffering from terminal illness at St. Joseph's Hospice, Hackney, London. *Nurs Mirror.* 1964;14:vii–x.

Chapter 10

When Should Nonsteroidal Antiinflammatory Drugs Be Used to Manage Pain?

Amy P. Abernethy, Arif Kamal, and David C. Currow

INTRODUCTION AND SCOPE OF THE PROBLEM

Pain is perhaps the most feared and persistent symptom in palliative care, affecting a major proportion of patients in this setting. In the Study to Understand Prognoses and Preferences for Outcomes and Risks of Treatments (SUPPORT), which was conducted in five teaching hospitals in the United States, family members of the 9105 adults with a life-threatening diagnosis reported moderate to severe pain in these patients at least half of the time.[1] Palliative care populations at elevated risk for insufficiently managed pain include the elderly, those with dementia, and nursing home residents.[2] Studies of U.S. nursing home residents report that 45% to 83% experience some degree of pain.[3-5] This high prevalence of pain led the American Pain Society in the mid-1990s to designate pain as the "fifth vital sign."[6]

Among the most widely used medications in the world, nonsteroidal antiinflammatory drugs (NSAIDs) are frequently used to manage mild to moderate pain or as an adjuvant analgesic for severe pain.[7] As a class of pharmaceutical agents with antipyretic, antiinflammatory, and analgesic effects, the NSAIDs include salicylates, p-amino derivatives, propionic acids, acetic acids, enolic acids, and selective cyclooxygenase-2 (COX-2) inhibitors. They are categorized together to differentiate them from the other major category of antiinflammatory agents, the glucocorticoids (corticosteroids), which operate in a pharmacologically different manner.[8]

RELEVANT PATHOPHYSIOLOGY

Although diverse in their chemical structures, the NSAIDs share a common set of therapeutic properties; principal among these is their ability to reduce edema, erythema, and pain associated with inflammation and to reduce fever. The analgesic effect is attributed to three mechanisms: inhibition of prostaglandin synthesis, inhibition of release of inflammatory mediators from neutrophils, and a central effect that may involve the N-methyl-D-aspartate (NMDA) receptor.[9] A dose-dependent inhibition of prostaglandin formation with NSAIDs was first described in 1971.[8] Since that time, general understanding has held that the effectiveness of NSAIDs is due to inhibition of the COX enzyme; this enzyme has two distinct isoforms: COX-1, which plays an essential role in normal gastrointestinal and platelet function, and COX-2, which is induced in the presence of inflammation[10] and is now understood to play a role in normal renal function.

A summary of commonly used NSAIDs is presented in Table 10-1, divided by class. Traditional "nonselective" NSAIDs inhibit both COX isoforms[11]; a newer class of selective COX-2 inhibitors are more selective for this isoform. Largely, the beneficial antiinflammatory and analgesic actions of NSAIDs have been thought to be associated with COX-2 inhibition and adverse effects (e.g., gastric ulceration, renal toxicity) related to COX-1 inhibition. Although it was attractive to hypothesize that an agent specifically inhibiting COX-2 would provide analgesia without the adverse effects associated with traditional NSAIDs, recent evidence of increased cardiovascular events with selective COX-2 inhibitors demonstrates a more complex picture. To date, the complete pharmacological profile of NSAIDs remains incompletely understood.

SUMMARY OF EVIDENCE REGARDING TREATMENT RECOMMENDATIONS

The World Health Organization (WHO) Three-Step Analgesic Ladder[12] provides the most universally accepted approach to pain management and a starting point for guiding use of NSAIDs in palliative care. The first step of the WHO analgesic ladder addresses the treatment of mild pain, for which the WHO recommends use of a nonopioid with or without an adjuvant analgesic. The guideline suggests that the nonopioid be an NSAID or acetaminophen (i.e., paracetamol). The subsequent two steps of the WHO

TABLE 10-1. Common Nonsteroidal Antiinflammatory Drugs for Mild to Moderate Pain

CLASS	GENERIC NAME	ONSET OF ACTION	DOSING SCHEDULE	RECOMMENDED INITIAL TOTAL DAILY DOSE (mg)	ROUTES OF ADMINISTRATION
Salicylates	Aspirin	2 hr	q4-6 h	2400	PO, PR
	Choline magnesium trisalicylate	2 hr	q8-12 h	1500	PO
	Salsalate	3-4 days	q8-12 h	3000	PO
P-phenol derivatives	Acetaminophen (paracetamol)	10-60 min	q4-6 h	1300	PO, IV
Propionic acids	Ibuprofen	30-60 min	q4-8 h	1200	PO, IV
	Ketoprofen	< 30 min	q6-8 h	200	PO
	Naproxen sodium	1 hr	q6-12 h	1250	PO
Acetic acids	Etodolac	2-4 hr	q6-8 h	600	PO
	Ketorolac	10 min IM, 2-3 hr PO	q4-6 h	120 IV, IM; 40 PO	PO, IV, IM
	Indomethacin	30 min	q8-12 h	100	PO, PR, IV
	Sulindac	3-4 hr	q12 h	400	PO
	Diclofenac	30-60 min	q8 h	150	PO
	Nabumetone	4-6 days	Daily	1000	PO
Enolic acids	Piroxicam	1 hr	Daily	20	PO
	Meloxicam	4-5 hr	Daily	7.5	PO
Selective COX-2–inhibitor	Celecoxib	3 hr	Daily to q12	200	PO

COX, Cyclooxygenase; *IV*, intravenous; *IM*, intramuscular; *PO*, by month; *PR*, rectally; *q*, every.

ladder (mild to moderate pain, moderate to severe pain) require *addition* of an opioid to control pain of increasing severity.

If NSAIDs succeed in achieving the desired pain relief, they have several advantages over opioid and other nonopioid pain medications. These include wide availability, indications for diverse causes of pain, easy administration through oral formulations, relatively lower cost, and additive relief with opioids. Certain disadvantages, however, limit their utility. Unlike opioids, the analgesic effect of NSAIDs has a dose-related ceiling. Therefore alone they are often effective only for mild pain; to treat moderate to severe pain, they generally must be combined with an opioid. NSAIDs carry risk for potentially serious side effects, most notably in the short term, including gastrointestinal bleeding, moderate worsening of hypertension, and acute renal failure. With prolonged use, increased cardiovascular events and chronic renal dysfunction are of serious concern. Additionally, although some NSAIDs are available in parenteral formulations, these are often difficult to obtain because of limited availability.[13]

Despite their widespread use, strong evidence to support the use of NSAIDs for pain management is lacking. A systematic review to assess the safety and efficacy of NSAIDs, alone and in conjunction with opioids, for the treatment of cancer pain included 42 trials that studied NSAIDs versus placebo, compared different NSAIDs to one another, and compared their effect to that of opioids or combination therapy, at various doses. Heterogeneity of study methods and outcomes precluded meta-analyses, and the generally short duration of the included studies inhibited the ability to generalize their results regarding longer-term efficacy and safety. Efficacy was upheld in seven of eight trials, which demonstrated superiority of single doses of an NSAID compared with placebo. Only 4 of 13 studies reported increased efficacy of one

NSAID over another, though frequency of side effects differed between drugs. Of 14 studies, 13 found no or minimal difference between a combination of NSAID plus opioid versus either drug alone; comparisons between various NSAID plus opioid combinations were inconclusive. Four studies demonstrated increased efficacy with increased NSAID dose, without corresponding dose-related increases in side effects. The authors drew a limited conclusion drawn from these data that NSAIDs appear to be more effective than placebo for cancer pain.[14]

Current Recommendations

General principles of best practice for pain management pertain to the use of NSAIDs to manage pain in the palliative care setting. Good pain management in all settings begins with proper assessment of the symptom. Because pain is a highly subjective symptom, patient reporting is accepted as the best assessment method. Many well-recognized, self-reported pain assessment instruments are available, and simple approaches such as a 0 to 10 numeric rating scale or the Wong-Baker FACES Rating Scale, especially for children,[15] are commonly and efficiently used. Patients unable to communicate verbally may indicate the presence of pain through "body language" such as grimacing, restlessness, wincing, clenched fists, body tension, and moaning.[16] In general, an assessment instrument should be chosen in consideration of the individual patient's characteristics and circumstances, and the same instrument should be used over time with that patient to ensure comparability of results in monitoring the patient's experience and results of pain management interventions.[17]

Following assessment, the WHO Three-Step Analgesic Ladder serves as a starting point to guide care under most pain scenarios. If the patient rates pain as mild, from 1 to 3 on a 0 to 10 numeric rating scale, treatment should begin with acetaminophen or an NSAID. The patient should take the chosen pain medication(s) on a scheduled basis rather than contingent on the current pain level. As-needed, or rescue, doses should be available for breakthrough pain or for pain that is insufficiently controlled by the standing regimen.[2] When prescribing as-needed rescue doses in the setting of continuous background NSAID use, the therapeutic ceiling and associated side effects of escalated doses must be carefully considered. For example, ibuprofen dosing that exceeds 2400 mg daily is unlikely to provide additional therapeutic benefit; associated renal insufficiency, exacerbation of hypertension, and tinnitus may occur at higher doses. In the setting of a patient who is currently receiving ibuprofen 800 mg three times daily, additional NSAIDs are likely to offer little benefit. In a case such as this, low-dose opioids would be the most efficacious breakthrough option.

The National Comprehensive Cancer Network (NCCN) provides more detailed, publicly available guidelines for pain management using NSAIDs.[17,18] NCCN guidelines support the use of any NSAID that has proved effective for the patient in the past, and that the patient has tolerated well. If the patient has no such prior history, ibuprofen is suggested as a first choice, administered at a dose of 400 mg three times per day and not to exceed a maximum of 3200 mg per day. An alternative dosing strategy is 800 mg three times daily, although some patients have trouble ingesting this dose. If the patient's pain remains inadequately controlled on the first NSAID, some clinicians switch to an NSAID of a different class (as recommended by the NCCN guidelines). However, in the palliative care setting, if pain is inadequately controlled on an NSAID, addition of an opioid should be considered (especially in light of the systematic review presented earlier and the limited prognoses encountered in palliative care). NSAIDs should be used with caution in patients at high risk for renal, gastrointestinal, or cardiac toxicities, thrombocytopenia, or bleeding disorders. Additionally, in patients with cancer, potential adverse effects associated with chemotherapy (e.g., renal, hepatic, hematological, and cardiovascular toxicities) may be exacerbated by concurrent use of NSAIDs.

Management of Side Effects

Use of NSAIDs must be informed by knowledge of their potentially serious short-term and long-term adverse effects. Primary among these are gastrointestinal side effects ranging from nausea, diarrhea, dyspepsia, and abdominal pain to perforations, ulcerations, and bleeds. A systematic review conducted in 1991 that included 16 studies reported that users of NSAIDs were at threefold greater relative risk for developing serious adverse gastrointestinal events than were nonusers (overall odds ratio [OR] 2.7, 95% confidence interval [CI] 2.5-3.0).[19] Subgroups at elevated risk were patients older than 60 years (OR

5.5, CI 4.6-6.6), patients receiving concomitant glucocorticoids (OR 1.8, CI 1.2-2.8), patients with less than 1 month of NSAID exposure (OR 8.0, CI 6.4-10.1), and patients with 1 to 3 months of exposure (OR 3.3, CI, 2.3-4.8). The last two risk factors indicate that gastrointestinal events tend to occur early and people suffering from these symptoms tend to stop the medication. Women and men appeared to have comparable increased risk for these side effects (OR 2.3, CI 1.9-2.8 and OR 2.4, CI 1.9-3.1, respectively). In subsequent reviews, other risk factors for gastrointestinal bleeding in the setting of NSAIDs included high dose of the NSAID, coadministration of aspirin (also an NSAID) or anticoagulants, coadministration of selective serotonin reuptake inhibitors (SSRIs), history of peptic ulcer disease, history of major organ dysfunction, and significant alcohol use (more than three alcoholic beverages per day).[18,20,21]

The gastrointestinal toxicity of NSAIDs has been attributed to inhibition of COX-1. Selective inhibitors of COX-2 were developed to reduce these effects, but evidence is conflicting regarding whether these drugs actually do reduce incidence of gastrointestinal toxicity.[20] Before the introduction of the COX-2–selective inhibitors, patients at high risk for gastrointestinal effects and taking a conventional NSAID were often also prescribed a gastroprotective agent such as misoprostol or a proton pump–inhibitor.[9] Proton pump–inhibitors reduce gastric acid secretion, whereas agents such as misoprostol reduce prostaglandin synthesis. These approaches have been shown to reduce the risk for gastroduodenal damage by approximately 40%.[22] To avoid gastrointestinal effects, the NCCN advises considering (1) adding an antacid, H_2-receptor antagonist, misoprostol, or a proton pump inhibitor or (2) prescribing a COX-2 inhibitor. The NCCN also advises discontinuing the NSAID if (1) the patient's creatinine or blood urea nitrogen (BUN) doubles or if hypertension develops or worsens, (2) the patient develops peptic ulcer or gastrointestinal hemorrhage, or (3) the patient's liver function tests increase to 1.5 times the upper limit of normal.[18]

Common renal adverse effects of traditional NSAIDs include reductions in glomerular filtration rate (GFR), sodium and potassium excretion, and renal blood flow.[23,24] These effects can lead to fluid and electrolyte disorders, hypertension, acute renal dysfunction, nephrotic syndrome, interstitial nephritis, and renal papillary necrosis. There are differences in renal toxicity among traditional NSAIDs.[25,26] The renal safety profiles of traditional NSAIDs, celecoxib, and rofecoxib have been examined in several large-scale clinical trials, with rofecoxib demonstrating increased renal adverse effects compared to traditional NSAIDs or celecoxib (rofecoxib is now off the market).[27] Factors that place patients at high risk for renal toxicities include age over 60 years, compromised fluid status, multiple myeloma, diabetes, interstitial nephritis, papillary necrosis, and concomitant administration of other nephrotoxic drugs and chemotherapies.[18] If renal toxicities arise, reflected in elevated BUN or creatinine, or newly developed or worsened hypertension, the NSAID should be discontinued immediately.

Liver toxicity is frequently discussed as a risk in the setting of acetaminophen (the other nonopioid alternative to NSAIDs); it is also a major concern with NSAIDs. In fact, given the remarkable prevalence of NSAID use in the general population, NSAIDs are among the most common causes of drug-induced liver injury, with an estimated incidence of up to 20 per 100,000 patient years. Sulindac and diclofenac confer the highest risk, accentuated by use with other hepatotoxic drugs and genetic predisposition.[28] Other toxicities associated with NSAIDs include bleeding and thrombosis. When NSAIDs are prescribed alongside anticoagulants (e.g., warfarin, heparin), the patient may be at considerably increased risk for bleeding complications.

A major point of discussion in the recent past has been the increased risk for vascular events, including myocardial infarction, stroke, and death, in the setting of NSAIDs. Systematic reviews and meta-analyses confirm that (1) COX-2 inhibitors increase the risk for vascular events, especially myocardial infarction; (2) vascular risks with rofecoxib (off the market in the United States) are worse than with celecoxib; (3) naproxen does not have the same vascular risks as COX-2 inhibitors, but traditional NSAIDs other than naproxen also confer some vascular risk, especially diclofenac; and (4) rofecoxib also had substantial risks for arrhythmias and renal effects not seen with celecoxib or traditional NSAIDs.[29,30] When comparing traditional NSAIDs to placebo, the summary rate ratios for vascular events were as follows: 0.92 for naproxen, 1.51 for ibuprofen, and 1.63 for diclofenac.[29] Given current data, it is prudent that patients at high risk for vascular complications, including those with a history of cardiovascular disease, high-risk hypertension, stroke, and transient ischemic attacks, avoid COX-2 inhibitors and likely most nonselective NSAIDs (except perhaps naproxen). If congestive heart failure or hypertension develops or intensifies, the NSAID should be discontinued.[18]

Monitoring for adverse effects of NSAIDs is a vital component of pain management using these agents. NCCN guidelines advise obtaining baseline measures of blood pressure, BUN, creatinine, liver function, complete blood count, and fecal occult blood and repeating these measures every 3 months to check for toxicity.[18] In patients in palliative care with limited prognosis, more frequent monitoring of creatinine and liver function may be warranted given the individual's rapidly changing status.

KEY MESSAGES TO PATIENTS AND FAMILIES

When prescribing NSAIDs, it is important to explain that many options are available. The clinician should reinforce that many patients with mild pain experience relief from use of these drugs and that NSAIDs can be taken orally and, in general, are relatively inexpensive. Patients should be reminded that close monitoring is necessary to ensure that the NSAID is providing sufficient pain relief and ensure safety from side effects. Clinicians should explain that the most common serious side effects of NSAIDs are gastrointestinal toxicities, such as ulcers and bleeding, and compromised kidney or liver function. Sufficient concern exists about heart attack, stroke, and death that people with risk for these events should avoid NSAIDs, especially the COX-2 inhibitors (though naproxen may be adequately safe in this setting). Patients and their families should be told in advance that if these or other toxicities appear, the NSAID should be discontinued and a different drug category will be tried until pain relief is achieved without toxicity.

CONCLUSION AND SUMMARY

NSAIDs have a useful role in pain management for patients in palliative care. In patients for whom they provide sufficient analgesia, NSAIDs possess several advantages, including widespread availability, ease of administration through oral formulation, acceptance by patients and families, and low relative cost. However, potentially serious adverse effects of NSAIDs require that they be not be administered to patients at high risk for their various toxicities and that patients be closely monitored for the possible emergence of adverse reactions.

SUMMARY RECOMMENDATIONS

- Assess the individual's pain using a well-established, patient-reported (where possible) assessment instrument that is well-matched to the individual patient. Use the same instrument over time to monitor the impact of pain management.
- Communicate with patients and family members or caregivers, where appropriate, regarding pain relief that can be achieved by NSAIDs, potential side effects, and how the patient will be monitored to detect side effects early and avoid serious adverse effects.
- Toxicities differ among NSAIDs; therefore, if an NSAID achieves analgesia but its use is limited by side effects, it may be prudent to try the patient on a different NSAID (one with a different toxicity profile). However, after trying two NSAIDs, if pain relief is insufficient or side effects occur, implement a different approach to pain management (e.g., use of opioids).
- Continue use of the NSAID if sufficient pain relief is achieved, as indicated by the patient's self-report in regular pain assessments.
- Monitor for potential adverse effects by regular measurement of blood pressure, blood urea nitrogen, creatinine, liver function, complete blood count, and fecal occult blood. Monitor for bleeding and vascular events.

REFERENCES

1. The SUPPORT Principal Investigators. A controlled trial to improve care for seriously ill hospitalized patients. The Study to Understand Prognoses and Preferences for Outcomes and Risks of Treatments (SUPPORT). *JAMA* 1995;274(20):1591–1598.
2. Morrison LJ, Morrison RS. Palliative care and pain management. *Med Clin North Am.* 2006;90(5):983–1004.
3. Ferrell BA. Pain evaluation and management in the nursing home. *Ann Intern Med.* 1995;123(9):681–687.
4. Ferrell BA, Ferrell BR, Rivera L. Pain in cognitively impaired nursing home patients. *J Pain Symptom Manage.* 1995;10(8):591–598.
5. Parmelee PA, Smith B, Katz IR. Pain complaints and cognitive status among elderly institution residents. *J Am Geriatr Soc.* 1993;41(5):517–522.
6. Molony SL, Kobayashi M, Holleran EA, Mezey M. Assessing pain as a fifth vital sign in long-term care facilities: recommendations from the field. *J Gerontol Nurs.* 2005;31(3):16–24.
7. Mills JA. Nonsteroidal anti-inflammatory drugs (first of two parts). *N Engl J Med.* 1974;290(14):781–784.
8. Vane JR. Inhibition of prostaglandin synthesis as a mechanism of action for aspirin-like drugs. *Nat New Biol.* 1971;231(25):232–235.
9. Dickman A, Ellershaw J. NSAIDs: gastroprotection or selective COX-2 inhibitor? *Palliat Med.* 2004;18(4):275–286.
10. Vane JR, Botting RM. Mechanism of action of nonsteroidal anti-inflammatory drugs. *Am J Med* 1998;104(3A):30.
11. Komhoff M, Grone HJ, Klein T, Seyberth HW, Nusing RM. Localization of cyclooxygenase-1 and -2 in adult and fetal human kidney: implication for renal function. *Am J Physiol* 1997;272(4 Pt 2):F460–F468.
12. World Health Organization. *WHO's Three-Step Pain Relief Ladder.* http://www.who.int/cancer/palliative/painladder/en/; 2011. Accessed January 9, 2012.
13. Jacox A, Carr DB, Payne R, et al. *Management of Cancer Pain: Clinical Practice Guideline No. 9.* AHCPR Publication 94–0592 Rockville, MD: Agency for Health Care Policy and Research; 1994.
14. McNicol E, Strassels S, Goudas L, Lau J, Carr D. Nonsteroidal anti-inflammatory drugs, alone or combined with opioids, for cancer pain: a systematic review. *J Clin Oncol.* 2004;22(10):1975–1992.
15. Wong DL, Hockenberry-Eaton M, et al. *Whaley and Wong's Nursing Care of Infants and Children.* 6th ed St. Louis: Mosby; 1999:1756–1757.
16. Puntillo KA, White C, Morris AB, et al. Patients' perceptions and responses to procedural pain: results from Thunder Project II. *Am J Crit Care.* 2001;10(4):238–251.
17. National Comprehensive Cancer Network. *NCCN Clinical Practice Guidelines in Oncology: Palliative Care, Version 2.2011.* http://www.nccn.org/professionals/physician_gls/pdf/palliative.pdf; 2011. Accessed January 9, 2012.
18. National Comprehensive Cancer Network. *NCCN Clinical Practice Guidelines in Oncology: Adult Cancer Pain, Version 2.2011.* http://www.nccn.org/professionals/physician_gls/pdf/pain.pdf; 2011. Accessed January 9, 2012.
19. Gabriel SE, Jaakkimainen L, Bombardier C. Risk for serious gastrointestinal complications related to use of nonsteroidal anti-inflammatory drugs: a meta-analysis. *Ann Intern Med.* 1991;115(10):787–796.
20. Shah S, Thomas B. Nonsteroidal anti-inflammatory analgesics and gastrointestinal protection in palliative care patients. *Palliat Med.* 2004;18(8):739–740.
21. Dalton SO, Johansen C, Mellemkjaer L, Norgard B, Sorensen HT, Olsen JH. Use of selective serotonin reuptake inhibitors and risk of upper gastrointestinal tract bleeding: a population-based cohort study. *Arch Intern Med.* 2003;163(1):59–64.
22. Raskin JB, White RH, Jaszewski R, Korsten MA, Schubert TT, Fort JG. Misoprostol and ranitidine in the prevention of NSAID-induced ulcers: a prospective, double-blind, multicenter study. *Am J Gastroenterol.* 1996;91(2):223–227.
23. Palmer BF. Renal complications associated with use of nonsteroidal anti-inflammatory agents. *J Investig Med.* 1995;43(6):516–533.
24. Murray MD, Brater DC. Renal toxicity of the nonsteroidal anti-inflammatory drugs [review]. *Annu Rev Pharmacol Toxicol.* 1993;33:435–465.
25. Levy RA, Smith DL. Clinical differences among nonsteroidal antiinflammatory drugs: implications for therapeutic substitution in ambulatory patients. *DICP.* 1989;23(1):76–85.
26. Day RO, Graham GG, Williams KM, Champion GD, de Jager J. Clinical pharmacology of non-steroidal anti-inflammatory drugs. *Pharmacol Ther.* 1987;33(2–3):383–433.
27. Zhao SZ, Reynolds MW, Lejkowith J, Whelton A, Arellano FM. A comparison of renal-related adverse drug reactions between rofecoxib and celecoxib, based on the World Health Organization/Uppsala Monitoring Centre safety database. *Clin Ther.* 2001;23(9):1478–1491.
28. Aithal GP, Day CP. Nonsteroidal anti-inflammatory drug-induced hepatotoxicity. *Clin Liver Dis.* 2007;11(3):563–575, vi–vii.
29. McGettigan P, Henry D. Cardiovascular risk and inhibition of cyclooxygenase: a systematic review of the observational studies of selective and nonselective inhibitors of cyclooxygenase 2. *JAMA.* 2006;296(13):1633–1644.
30. Zhang J, Ding EL, Song Y. Adverse effects of cyclooxygenase 2 inhibitors on renal and arrhythmia events: meta-analysis of randomized trials. *JAMA.* 2006;296(13):1619–1632.

What Is Neuropathic Pain? How Do Opioids and Nonopioids Compare for Neuropathic Pain Management?

Ula Hwang, Monica Wattana, and Knox H. Todd

INTRODUCTION AND SCOPE OF THE PROBLEM

As defined by the 2008 International Association for the Study of Pain (IASP), neuropathic pain is "pain caused by a lesion or disease of the somatosensory system."[1] Worldwide estimates of the prevalence of neuropathic pain range from 3% to 8% in the genral population.[2–4] Common disease-related neuropathic conditions include diabetes, postherpetic neuralgia (PHN), peripheral nerve injury, human immunodeficiency virus (HIV) neuropathy, and trigeminal neuralgia.[5] The prevalence of neuropathic pain among patients with cancer, however, is much higher, with estimates ranging from 19 to 39%.[6] Older adults are at greater risk for neuropathic pain because they have fewer inhibitory nerves, lower endorphin levels, and a slowed capacity to reverse nerve sensitization.

Pain associated with nerve injury or dysfunction is clinically characterized by negative somatosensory signs (abnormal or sensory deficits, paresthesias [e.g., tingling sensation]), positive signs (e.g., spontaneous shooting or electric shocklike symptoms), and evoked symptoms (e.g., thermal hypersensitivity to heat and cold, mechanical allodynia, and pain in response to a nonnociceptive stimulus such as light touch).

RELEVANT PATHOPHYSIOLOGY

The pathophysiology of neuropathic pain fundamentally differs from that of other painful conditions. Neuropathic pain symptoms result from focal disruptions in normal afferent neuronal signaling pathways in the peripheral and central nervous systems; other painful conditions rely on these pathways being intact.[7–9] The underlying causal mechanism responsible for altered somatosensory signaling can be classified as peripheral or central. Understanding these mechanisms may allow more focused therapies and increase the likelihood of treatment success.

After peripheral nerve injury, inflammatory mediators initiate signaling cascades calling for increased expression of sodium channels on cell membranes of injured and surrounding neurons.[7,10] Upregulation of these sodium channels lowers the threshold of activation, leading to ectopic activity within individual nociceptors comprising Aδ and C fibers within the afferent pain pathway. Clinically, this aberrant activity correlates with sensations of paroxysmal shooting pain or continuous pain that occurs in the presence or absence of a stimulus.[11] These chemical mediators also create "ephaptic conduction," in which ectopic activity is seen in uninjured fibers resulting from cross-talk with nearby injured fibers.[7] Spontaneous activity also occurs via upregulation of aberrant forms of receptor proteins in cell membranes of peripheral nociceptors. The normal forms of these receptor proteins are only minimally expressed under normal conditions.[8] An example of aberrant receptor upregulation is the heat activation protein TRPV1. In normal nociceptors, the TRPV1 receptor is activated by noxious heat stimuli above 41° C. In injured nociceptors, receptor activation occurs at 38° C; thus spontaneous activity can occur at normal body temperature. Another hallmark of neuropathic pain is that patients experience abnormal sensation with areas of hypersensitivity adjacent to or mixed with areas of sensory deficit.[8,12] This peripheral sensitization may be caused by the sprouting of collateral fibers from intact adjacent sensory axons into the skin of denervated areas.

Central sensitization causes alterations in communication from peripheral afferent fibers to higher order neurons within the dorsal root ganglion of the spinal cord and brain. Two proposed mechanisms are hyperexcitability and disinhibition. Mechanical allodynia, the sensation of pain on light touch, is a common feature of neuropathic pain.[8] Hyperexcitablity may cause mechanical allodynia through activation of second-order pain pathway neurons by intact non–pain conducting peripheral afferent fibers. This activation occurs by phosphorylation of N-methyl-D-aspartate (NMDA) and α-amino-3-hydroxy-5-methyl-4-isoxazolepropionic acid (AMPA) receptors and expression of voltage-gated sodium channels within postsynaptic membranes.[8] Disinhibition occurs at many levels within the central nervous system. Peripheral nerve lesions cause loss of inhibitory regulation through chemical cascades, resulting in apoptosis of inhibitory γ-aminobutyric acid (GABA) ergic interneurons in the spinal cord. Lesions within the central nervous system may also cause neuropathic pain symptoms via the release of chemical modulators.

SUMMARY OF EVIDENCE REGARDING TREATMENT RECOMMENDATIONS

Neuropathic pain treatment begins with an initial pain assessment. Differentiating neuropathic from nociceptive pain will guide appropriate treatment. Nociceptive pain is caused by acute illness (from injury or inflammatory processes) that results in actual or potential tissue damage that activates pain receptors to warn or protect individuals. Neuropathic pain results from lesions or malfunction of the nervous system and serves no purpose. Clinical examination of patients with chronic neuropathic pain may reveal autonomic abnormalities such as tropic skin changes, motor weakness, tremors, and dystonia. More commonly, however, the clinical examination is completely normal. Unfortunately, there is often overlap of neuropathic and nociceptive pain mechanisms (mixed pain). Neurophysiological testing for peripheral nerve conduction disorders is not as effective for small Aδ and C fibers; thus these tests are of limited utility. Some value has been found in autonomic function testing using the quantitative sudomotor axon reflex test (QSART)[13] and nerve biopsies to determine the extent of neuropathy.[8] Many of these tests, however, are not specific for neuropathic pain and are also abnormal in peripheral neuropathies not associated with pain.[14]

Several tools have been developed and validated to differentiate neuropathic from nociceptive pain and generally consist of a combination of self-report and physical findings that can be conducted at the bedside.[15] The Neuropathic Pain Diagnostic Questionnaire (DN4) has high sensitivity and specificity and is easy to use (Table 11-1).[16,17]

In a recent systematic review of treatment options for neuropathic pain, pharmacological options are the mainstay. In randomized controlled clinical trials, meta-analyses, and consensus statements, five classes of medications are reported to be effective[5,8,18–22]: (1) antidepressants with reuptake-blocking effects; (2) anticonvulsants with calcium-modulating actions; (3) opioids; (4) topical agents; and (5) combination therapy. In part, because underlying pain-generating mechanisms and causes of neuropathic pain are often heterogeneous or unknown, many patients experience suboptimal pain relief from these therapies. To increase patient compliance, realistic treatment goals should be established early in the course of therapy.

TABLE 11-1. Neuropathic Pain Diagnostic Questionnaire to Distinguish Nociceptive From Neuropathic Pain

SIGN/SYMPTOM	YES = 1	NO = 0
Does the pain have one or more of the following characteristics?		
• Burning	1	0
• Painful cold	1	0
• Electric shocks	1	0
Does the area of pain also have one or more of the following?		
• Tingling	1	0
• Pins and needles	1	0
• Numbness	1	0
• Itching	1	0
Examination		
• Decrease in touch sensation (soft brush)	1	0
• Decrease in prick sensation (von Frey hair no. 13)	1	0
• Movement of a soft brush in the area causes or increases pain	1	0
TOTAL:		

Score each item. Score: 0-3 = likely nociceptive pain; ≥4 = likely neuropathic pain

Modified from Arnstein P. Best practices in nursing care to older adults: try this. *Specialty Practice Series*. 2010; SP1; and Bouhassira D, Attal N, Alchaar H, et al. Comparison of pain syndromes associated with nervous or somatic lesions and development of a new neuropathic pain diagnostic questionnaire (DN4). *Pain*. 2005;114(1-2):29-46, Appendix B.

A stepwise process is best to identify which drug or drug combination provides the greatest pain relief with the fewest side effects, especially in older adults with multiple comorbidities.[8,23] Given multiple neuropathic causes for pain, combination therapies generally produce greater pain relief and fewer side effects than an escalating monotherapeutic approach.[24]

Antidepressants

Tricyclic antidepressants (TCAs) and selective serotonin and norepinephrine reuptake inhibitors (SSNRIs) block cholinergic, adrenergic, histaminergic, and sodium channels or inhibit serotonin and norepinephrine reuptake. Because of their ability to relieve pain independent of their antidepressant effects, these drugs should be first-line agents in patients with coexisting depression. TCAs (nortriptyline, imipramine, desipramine) are the most effective of the antidepressants, followed by SSNRIs (venlafaxine, duloxetine), in relieving neuropathic pain, particularly in the setting of diabetic neuropathy, nerve injury, PHN, and central poststroke pain.[20,23,25] These agents also have major side effects, including cardiac conduction abnormalities, dry mouth, urine retention, sedation, dizziness, nausea, and orthostatic hypotension. Patients should be cautioned about these and have baseline electrocardiograms before initiating therapy. Careful titration during dose escalation is essential, particularly with

TCAs. Of note, selective serotonin reuptake inhibitors (SSRIs) (citalopram, paroxetine) provide little to no analgesic effect and are not recommended. For TCAs, doses should be titrated to effect over 6 to 8 weeks, with at least 2 weeks at the maximum tolerated dose. For SSNRIs, 4 to 5 weeks is sufficient.

Anticonvulsants

The calcium channel α2-δ ligands agents gabapentin and pregabalin are effective in treating painful diabetic polyneuropathy, PHN, and mixed neuropathic conditions. These drugs mimic GABA and bind the α2-δ subunit of calcium channels, effectively reducing the influx of calcium into neuronal cells that have a wide distribution of calcium channels. This in turn decreases the release of glutamate, norepinephrine, and substance P at the synapses. Side effects include dizziness, sedation, dry mouth, difficulty concentrating, and weight gain. Trial durations of 4 weeks are recommended.

Opioids

Commonly used opioids and opioid-analogs found effective in neuropathic pain include morphine, oxycodone, and tramadol. These drugs function as mu-receptor agonists and also inhibit norepinephrine and serotonin reuptake. Side effects include sedation, constipation, dizziness, and nausea. Compared to placebo, tramadol is highly effective in reducing neuropathic pain and no more or less effective than other opioids. Tramadol trials should last up to 4 weeks.

Topical Agents

Topical agents such as 5% lidocaine patches block sodium channels and are indicated for certain conditions, such as postherpetic neuralgia. The benefit of these agents is their minimal side effects, which are generally limited to rash or erythema localized to the site of application. Trial durations of 2 weeks are recommended.

Combination Therapy

Combination therapy is often needed to achieve satisfactory neuropathic pain relief. Although recent studies have found the addition of oxycodone ineffective when enhancing pregabalin effects,[26] other studies have found the addition of oxycodone to gabapentin,[27] morphine to gabapentin,[28] nortriptyline to gabapentin,[29] and topical lidocaine to pregabalin[30] more effective at lower combined doses than for each drug as single agents. For a summary of these agents and their mode of action and duration of treatment, see Table 11-2.

KEY MESSAGES TO PATIENTS AND FAMILIES

Those with neuropathic pain may find their symptoms difficult to describe, and the failure to accurately diagnose neuropathic pain may decrease the likelihood of successful treatment. These painful conditions often cause significant interference with activities of daily living, such as sleeping, working, or concentrating, and may be difficult to treat. Although primary care and palliative care clinicians can treat many with neuropathic pain, specialized treatment by pain physicians or neurologists may be necessary for those with resistant symptoms. Nonpharmacological therapies, such as exercise, stress management, and relaxation therapies are often advised, and a variety of pharmacological interventions are available. Those with neuropathic pain should realize that there is much yet to be learned about the condition and that their doctors may be unable to answer all of their questions. It is important to find a physician who pays adequate attention to the patient's concerns and is available for questions. Although for many neuropathic pain conditions there is no absolute cure, treatment options can minimize symptoms and maximize quality of life.

CONCLUSION AND SUMMARY

Neuropathic pain is caused by a lesion or disease of the somatosensory system. It encompasses a diverse group of conditions that share common underlying mechanisms.[11] Neuropathic pain symptoms result from disruptions in normal nerve signaling pathways in the peripheral and central nervous system. Rational therapies targeted to specific underlying pathological processes may yield more efficient symptom control than nonspecific therapies; therefore, a basic understanding of these mechanisms is important to those who treat pain.[8] The mainstays of neuropathic treatment are pharmacological therapies, including antidepressants, anticonvulsants, opioids, and topical agents. These medications may each be given alone or in combination. Many recent studies demonstrate successful reduction of pain with combination therapy. Jointly, these agents are effective at lower doses than when used alone.

Critical steps in successful treatment of neuropathic pain are appropriate assessment for the presence of neuropathic pain, counseling about treatment options, understanding that these agents may require weeks of gradual titration, education regarding side effects associated with treatment, and establishing clear patient and caregiver expectations. Although complete pain relief may not always be feasible, functional recovery and improved quality of life are realistic goals.

TABLE 11-2. Pharmacological Treatment Agents for Neuropathic Pain

AGENT	MODE OF ACTION	NEGATIVE SIDE EFFECTS	POSITIVE SIDE EFFECTS	STARTING DOSE/MAXIMUM DOSE	TITRATION	DURATION OF ADEQUATE TRIAL
Antidepressants Tricyclic antidepressants: nortriptyline, desipramine	Inhibition of serotonin/norepinephrine reuptake, sodium channel blocking, anticholinergic	Sedation, anticholinergic effects, cardiac arrhythmias	Concurrent treatment of depression	25 mg/150 mg daily	Increase by 25 mg every 3-7 days as tolerated	6-8 wk (at last 2 wk maximum tolerated dose)
Selective serotonin and norepinephrine reuptake inhibitors (SSNRIs): duloxetine, venlafaxine	Inhibition of serotonin/norepinephrine reuptake	Nausea	Concurrent treatment of depression	*Duloxetine:* 30 mg daily/60 mg 2 × daily *Venlafaxine:* 37.5 mg daily or twice daily/225 mg daily	*Duloxetine:* Increase by 60 mg after 1 week as tolerated *Venlafaxine:* Increase by 37.5-75 mg each week as tolerated	4 wk 4-6 wk
Anticonvulsants Gabapentin, pregabalin	Decreased release of glutamate, norepinephrine, substance P, affecting calcium channels	Sedation, dizziness	No major drug–drug interaction	*Gabapentin:* 100-300 mg 1-3 × day/1200 mg 3 × day *Pregabalin:* 50 mg 3 × day/200 mg 3 × day	*Gabapentin:* Increase by 100-300 mg 3 × day every 1-7 days *Pregabalin:* Increase by 300 mg daily after 3-7 days, then 150 mg daily every 3-7 days	4 wk 4 wk
Opioids Morphine, tramadol	μ-Receptor agonists	Sedation, nausea, vomiting, constipation	Rapid onset analgesic effect	*Morphine:* 10-15 mg every 4 hours, no max *Tramadol:* 50 mg 1-2 × daily/400 mg daily	*Morphine:* Convert to long-acting or fentanyl transdermal patches *Tramadol:* Increase by 50-100 mg every 3-7 days	4-6 wk 4 wk
Topical Agent 5% Lidocaine patch	Sodium channel blocking	Rash, local erythema	No systemic effects	1-3 patches/3 patches daily	Must remove patch every 12 hours (i.e., 12 hours on, 12 hours off)	2 wk
Combination Therapy Gabapentin-morphine[28]	Above-listed mechanisms; synergistic mode of action	Sedation, nausea, constipation, dizziness	Synergistic effect in pain relief; drug combination requires lower doses than each drug alone	*Gabapentin:* 300 mg total daily/2400 mg total daily *Morphine:* 15 mg total daily/60 mg total daily	*Gabapentin and morphine:* Increase to maximum tolerated or ceiling dose every 3-7 days	3-4 wk
Gabapentin-oxycodone[27]				*Gabapentin:* Maximum dose tolerated by patient *Oxycodone:* 5 mg prolonged release every 12 hours	*Gabapentin:* Already at maximum tolerated *Oxycodone:* Titrate by one dose level every 3-7 days	Up to 12 wk
Gabapentin-nortriptyline[29]				*Gabapentin:* 400 mg 3 × day/3600 mg total daily *Nortriptyline:* 10 mg 3 × day/100 mg total daily	*Gabapentin:* Increase to maximum tolerated or ceiling dose every 3-7 days *Nortriptyline:* Increase by 10 mg every 3-7 days as tolerated to ceiling dose	6 wk

Data from References 5, 8, 21, 22, 27-29.

SUMMARY RECOMMENDATIONS

- Assessment for neuropathic pain (i.e., differentiating neuropathic versus nociceptive pain) should be conducted with validated screening tools (e.g., the Neuropathic Pain Diagnostic Questionnaire).
- Patients should be educated about neuropathic pain, treatment options, side-effects, and realistic goals and expectations of pain relief.
- Therapy is initiated based on the disease causing neuropathic pain (if applicable). Pharmacological options include tricyclic antidepressants (nortriptyline, desipramine, imipramine), selective serotonin and norepinephrine reuptake inhibitors (duloxetine, venlafaxine), anticonvulsants (gabapentin, pregabalin), topical agents, and opioids or tramadol.
- Pain and health-related quality of life should be reassessed and therapies titrated accordingly, as follows:
  - Substantial pain relief (pain score of 3 or less on a pain scale of 0 to 10) and tolerable side effects: Continue treatment.
  - Partial pain relief (pain score of 4 or greater on a pain scale of 0 to 10): Consider addition of other first-line agents for combination therapy.
  - Inadequate or no pain relief and target dose achieved: Switch to another first-line agent.

For more information on this stepwise approach, see Dworkin RH, O'Connor AB, Backonja M, et al. Pharmacologic management of neuropathic pain: evidence-based recommendations. *Pain*. 2007;132:237-251.

REFERENCES

1. Jensen TS, Baron R, Haanpaa M, et al. A new definition of neuropathic pain. *Pain*. 2011;152:2204-2205.
2. Torrance N, Smith BH, Bennett MI, Lee AJ. The epidemiology of chronic pain of predominantly neuropathic origin: results from a general population survey. *J Pain*. 2006;7:281-289.
3. Gustorff B, Dorner T, Likar R, et al. Prevalence of self-reported neuropathic pain and impact on quality of life: a prospective representative survey. *Acta Anaesthesiol Scand*. 2008;52:132-136.
4. Toth C, Lander J, Weibe S. The prevalence and impact of chronic pain with neuropathic pain symptoms in the general population. *Pain Med*. 2009;10(5):918-929.
5. Finnerup NB, Sindrup SH, Jensen TS. The evidence for pharmacological treatment of neuropathic pain. *Pain*. 2010;150:573-581.
6. Bennett GJ, Rayment C, Hjermstad M, Aass N, Caraceni A, Kaasa S. Prevalence and aetiology of neuropathic pain in cancer patients: a systematic review. *Pain*. 2012;153:359-365.
7. Pasero C. Pathophysiology of neuropathic pain. *Pain Manag Nurs*. 2004;5(4 suppl 1):3-8.
8. Baron R, Binder A, Wasner G. Neuropathic pain: diagnosis, pathophysiological mechanisms, and treatment. *Lancet Neurol*. 2010;9:807-819.
9. Beydoun A, Backonja MM. Mechanistic stratification of antineuralgic agents. *J Pain Symptom Manage*. 2003;25:s18-s30.
10. Baron R. Mechanisms of disease: neuropathic pain—a clinical perspective. *Nat Clin Pract*. 2006;2(2):95-106.
11. Dworkin RH. An overview of neuropathic pain: syndromes, symptoms, signs, and several mechanisms. *Clin J Pain*. 2002;18:343-349.
12. Vranken JH. Mechanisms and treatment of neuropathic pain. *Cent Nerv Syst Agents Med Chem*. 2009;9(1):71-78.
13. Low VA, Sandroni P, Fealy RD, et al. Detection of small-fiber neuropathy by sudomotor testing. *Muscle Nerve*. 2006;34:57-61.
14. Horowitz SH. The diagnostic workup of patients with neuropathic pain. *Med Clin North Am*. 2007;91:21-30.
15. Bennett MI, Attal N, Backonja M, et al. Using screening tools to identify neuropathic pain. *Pain*. 2007;127(3):199-203.
16. Arnstein P. Best practices in nursing care to older adults: try this. *Specialty Practice Series*. 2010; SP1.
17. Bouhassira D, Attal N, Alchaar H, et al. Comparison of pain syndromes associated with nervous or somatic lesions and development of a new neuropathic pain diagnostic questionnaire (DN4). *Pain*. 2005;114(1-2):29-46 Appendix B.
18. Moulin DE, Clark AG, Gilron I, et al. Pharmacological management of chronic neuropathic pain: conseusus statement and guidelines from the Canadian Pain Society. *Pain Res Manag*. 2007;12:13-21.
19. Finnerup NB, Otto M, Jensen TS, Sindrup SH. An evidence-based algorithm for the treatment of neuropathic pain. *Med Gen Med*. 2007;15:36.
20. Jensen TS, Madsen CS, Finnerup NB. Pharmacology and treatment of neuropathic pains. *Curr Opin Neurol*. 2009;22:467-474.
21. Dworkin RH, O'Connor AB, Audette J, et al. Recommendations for the pharmacological management of neuropathic pain: an overview and literature update. *Mayo Clin Proc*. 2010;85(suppl 3):s3-s14.
22. Attal N, Crucco G, Baron R, et al. EFNS guidelines on the pharmacological treatment of neuropathic pain: 2010 revision. *Eur J Neurol*. 2010;17:1113-1123.
23. Dworkin RH, O'Connor AB, Backonja M, et al. Pharmacologic management of neuropathic pain: evidence-based recommendations. *Pain*. 2007;132:237-251.
24. Baron R. Neuropathic pain: a clinical perspective. *Handb Exp Pharmacol*. 2009;(194):3-30.
25. Finnerup NB, Otto M, McQuay HJ, Jensen TS, Sindrup SH. Algorithm for neuropathic pain treatment: an evidence based proposal. *Pain*. 2005;118:289-305.
26. Zin CS, Nissen LM, O'Callaghan JP, Duffull SB, Smith MT, Moore BJ. A randomized, controlled trial of oxycodone versus placebo in patients with postherpetic neuralgia and painful diabetic neuropathy treated with pregabalin. *J Pain*. 2010;11:462-471.
27. Hanna M, O'Brien C, Wilson MC. Prolonged-release oxycodone enhances the effects of exisitng gabapentin therapy in painful diabetic neurpathy patients. *Eur J Pain*. 2008;12:804-813.
28. Gilron I, Bailey JM, Holden RR, Weaver DF, Houlden RL. Morphine, gabapentin, or their combination for neuropathic pain. *N Engl J Med*. 2005;352:1324-1334.
29. Gilron I, Bailey JM, Tu D, Holden RR, Jackson AC, Houlden RL. Nortriptyline and gabapentin, alone and in combination for neuropathic pain: a double-blind, randomised controlled crossover trial. *Lancet*. 2009;374(9697):1252-1261.
30. Baron R, Mayoral V, Leijon G, Binder A, Stiegerwald I, Serpell M. Efficacy and safety of combination therapy with 5% lidocaine medicated plaster and pregabalin in post-herpetic neueralgia and diabetic polyneuropathy. *Curr Med Res Opin*. 2009;25:1677-1687.

Chapter 12

Should Bisphosphonates Be Used Routinely to Manage Pain and Skeletal Complications in Cancer?

Arif Kamal, Jennifer M. Maguire, David C. Currow, and Amy P. Abernethy

INTRODUCTION AND SCOPE OF THE PROBLEM

Bone is a common site of metastatic disease in advanced malignancies such as breast, lung, prostate, thyroid, and kidney cancers and multiple myeloma. Approximately 70% of patients with advanced prostate or breast cancer and up to 40% of patients with other advanced cancers will develop bone metastases.[1] Bone metastases may be the lone site of distant disease in up to 20% of women with advanced breast cancer and 50% of men with advanced prostate cancer, often translating into a more favorable prognostic category.[2]

Bone metastases portend a significant risk for future skeletal complications and associated morbidity while also often becoming a source of pain and restricted activity. Additionally, early bone loss and increased risk for skeletal-related events can result from medications such as antihormonal treatments given to patients with breast and prostate cancer, long-term heparin anticoagulants used for venous thromboembolism or prophylaxis, and cumulative glucocorticoid exposure (e.g., as an antineoplastic, antiemetic, or adjuvant pain medication).

Pain may be a presenting symptom in up to 80% of patients with bone metastases[3] and often requires a multimodality approach for evaluation and treatment. Uncontrolled incident pain may limit mobility and activity, ultimately leading to deconditioning, decreased functional status, and poor quality of life. This highlights the importance of preventing skeletal-related events and considering bone-directed agents as adjuvant pain options in nonfracture bone pain.

Without bone-targeted therapies, many patients with bone metastases would eventually experience a skeletal-related event. These events include pathological fractures, spinal cord compression, need for surgery or radiotherapy to the bone, and hypercalcemia of malignancy.[4] Untreated bone metastases present a significant fracture risk of 20% to 40% annually and the potential for significant skeletal complications every 3 to 6 months in the absence of bone-targeted therapies.[1] Remarkably, in a placebo-controlled bisphosphonate trial in multiple myeloma, more than 40% of patients who did not receive bisphosphonate suffered from a skeletal event within 36 weeks.[5] The potential morbidity and mortality effects of these events are significant and range from hospitalization to emergent surgery to death. Evidence demonstrates that skeletal-related events can affect survival, reduce quality of life,[6] or result in performance status declines that may preclude future disease-directed therapy.[7]

Standardized management that addresses bone-related pain and prevention of skeletal-related events is essential to prevent complications, suffering, and premature death. This includes the early implementation and regular use of bisphosphonates, which were approved by the U.S. Food and Drug Administration (FDA) in the 1990s for use in advanced cancer. Bisphosphonates can be prescribed as adjuvant with other pain therapies, including opioids and radiotherapy, as the primary bone-directed treatment for metastatic bone involvement or as an adjuvant to other ongoing cancer-directed therapies.

RELEVANT PATHOPHYSIOLOGY AND PHARMACOLOGY

Osteoblastic and Osteolytic Bone Metastases

Advanced cancer disrupts the normal homeostasis between bone production by osteoblasts and bone resorption by osteoclasts through disruption of the receptor activator of nuclear factor κ-B ligand (RANKL) loop. A key factor for osteoclast differentiation and activation, RANKL can be either inhibited, producing osteoblastic bone metastases (e.g., in prostate cancer) when osteoclast activity is attenuated[8] or cleaved into its more active form, thus increasing osteoclast activity[9] and creating osteolytic bone metastases (e.g., in breast and lung cancer).

Additionally, as growth factors are released from the bone matrix through increased resorption, a positive feedback loop is created inducing local tumor cells to increase osteoclast-promoting cytokine secretion. Through this mechanism, others have described the creation of a "vicious cycle" in which osteolysis perpetuates indefinitely until osteoclast activity is inhibited.[10]

Bisphosphonate Mechanism of Action

Bisphosphonates are structural analogs of pyrophosphates, a naturally occurring component of bone crystal deposition, and are composed of two phosphate groups (thus the name "bis"phosphonates). Various side chain modifications of the basic pyrophosphate structure gives rise to the multiple generations of bisphosphonates with differing levels of activity. Bisphosphonates generally work in several ways: absorbing calcium phosphate to provide physicochemical protection, suppressing the normal functioning of mature osteoclasts, and preventing osteoclast precursors from maturing. The two classes of bisphosphonates are nonnitrogenous (e.g., etidronate, clodronate) and nitrogenous (pamidronate, zoledronate [zoledronic acid]). Bone resorption is the primary process implicated in pain from bone metastases and decreased bone integrity, making the osteoclast the key therapeutic target for skeletal metastases. Nonnitrogenous bisphosphonates are ingested and metabolized by osteoclasts, which leads to osteoclast apoptosis and death. Nitrogenous bisphosphonates bind and block the enzyme farnesyl diphosphate synthase in the 3-hydroxy-3-methylglutaryl coenzyme A (HMG-CoA) reductase pathway, effecting osteoclastogenesis, cell survival, and cytoskeletal integrity.

SUMMARY OF EVIDENCE REGARDING TREATMENT RECOMMENDATIONS

Evidence for the use of bisphosphonates for pain from bone metastases were recently reviewed in a Cochrane meta-analysis.[11] The endpoints studied included the proportion of patients with pain relief, reduction in analgesic consumption, and quality of life. The proportion of patients with pain relief was reported in six placebo-controlled and two open-controlled studies. At week 4, the cumulative odds ratio (OR) for pain relief was 2.21 (95% CI 1.19-4.12) and at week 12 the OR was 2.49 (95% CI 1.38-4.48). The number needed to treat (NNT) was 11 after 4 weeks and improved to 7 at week 12. The best pain relief response was seen within 12 weeks for tumor sites except prostate cancer; the OR ranged from 1.83 (95% CI 1.11-3.04) to 8.47 (95% CI 2.69-27) for any primary site. A trend toward improved pain control with bisphosphonates was observed in patients with prostate cancer (OR 1.54, 95% CI 0.97-2.44, $p = .07$).[12]

The mean analgesic consumption as an endpoint was reported in a subgroup of studies. There was a decrease of 6.4 mg of morphine equivalents with use of intravenous clodronate; in this crossover trial with 60 patients with osseous metastases and pain, patients and providers who chose therapies blindly reliably chose the bisphosphonate as the agent that improved pain more than placebo ($p = .03$).[13] A similar study reported an average change in morphine equivalents of +10 mg for the treatment arm and +62 mg for the placebo arm ($p = .096$).[14] Three other studies did not show such a benefit. Pooled results showed an OR in favor of the treatment group, with week 4 OR 2.81 (95% CI 1.24-6.38) and week 12 OR 2.37 (95% CI 1.1-5.12). Some studies have also reported less decrease in QOL after at least 9 months of therapy with bisphosphonates.[15,16]

Despite the fact that these studies and the systematic review demonstrate the role of bisphosphonates in reducing pain in the setting of bone metastases, it should be noted that these data are for adjuvant management as a part of an overall pain management regimen. These data do not support bisphosphonates as the primary analgesic (first-line analgesic) but rather as a coanalgesic in the setting of opioid and nonopioid pain medications. The role of bisphosphonates as a primary analgesic is unclear.

Data supporting the role of bisphosphonates in managing skeletal-related events are explicit. Results of large trials from previous decades demonstrate the role of bisphosphonates in prevention and treatment of skeletal-related events in breast cancer and myeloma[17]; more recent results demonstrate a decreased proportion of patients experiencing a skeletal-related event in prostate cancer[18] and other solid tumors.[19] In a study of patients with solid tumors other than breast or prostate cancer, zoledronate 4 mg significantly reduced skeletal-related events from 47% to 38% ($p = .039$), with a delay in median time to first event from 163 days to 230 days ($p = .023$).[19] A recent systematic review also concluded that both the decreased risk for fractures (OR 0.65 [95% CI 0.55-0.78], $p < .0001$) and increased time to first skeletal-related event support the use of bisphosphonates.[20] These study results have translated into clinical effectiveness; regular use of modern bisphosphonates has reduced the number of patients suffering from skeletal-related events by 30% to 50%, resulting in improvements in quality of life and better preservation of function.[21]

Current Recommendations

Consensus guidelines recommend the regular use of bisphosphonates with osteolytic bone metastases from breast cancer,[22] other solid tumors, and multiple myeloma from the time of diagnosis and continued indefinitely.[21,23] Additionally, bisphosphonates are recommended for treatment of hypercalcemia of malignancy.[24]

Guidance regarding treatment of therapy-related bone loss in cancer has also been published. Because aromatase-inhibitors cause bone loss at more than twice the rate of physiological postmenopausal bone loss,[25] resulting in an increased fracture risk for women,[26] current recommendations from several consensus groups, including the American Society of Clinical Oncology (ASCO) and the St. Gallen Panel, endorse the routine use of bisphosphonates in women with aromatase-inhibitor–induced bone loss.[27] Androgen deprivation therapy is a common treatment for men with locally advanced or metastatic prostate cancer that increases the potential risk for fractures.[28] The National Comprehensive Cancer Network Clinical Practice Guidelines recommend screening in men on androgen-deprivation therapy and all men aged 70 and older.[29]

Current screening guidelines also support routine evaluation in patients with high risk for decreased bone mineral density. ASCO[30] and the U.S. Preventive Services Task Force[31] recommend bone mineral density screening for all women age 65 years and older and for women aged 60 to 64 who are at high risk for bone loss. ASCO guidelines go further to suggest bone mineral density screening for women with breast cancer who have risk factors such as family history of fractures or body weight less than 70 kg, and prior nontraumatic fracture in all postmenopausal women receiving aromatase-inhibitor therapy or premenopausal women with therapy-induced ovarian failure.

Many cancer pain management guidelines mention bisphosphonates as an adjuvant strategy when bone metastases are present, but discussions of the role of bisphosphonates are scant.

Current Practice: Choosing an Agent

Table 12-1 lists the bisphosphonate agents and their availability and relative potency. As a result of the abundance of data on patients with cancer in the United States, zoledronate and pamidronate have emerged as the bisphosphonates of choice for use in these patients. These remain the only two FDA-approved bisphosphonates for treatment of pain from bone metastases and prevention of skeletal-related events. Zoledronate has been directly compared with pamidronate and clodronate to reduce skeletal-related events in head-to-head fashion; clodronate, ibandronate, and pamidronate have never been compared directly. Zoledronate was shown not inferior to pamidronate in regard to time to first skeletal-related event, cumulative risk for skeletal-related events, and reductions in bone pain in patients with breast cancer and multiple myeloma.[32] In the recently published Myeloma XI trial, zoledronate 4 mg intravenously every 3 to 4 weeks significantly reduced the proportion of patients with skeletal-related events compared with clodronate.[33]

Currently, no oral bisphosphonate has FDA approval or is routinely used for skeletal metastases in the United States. Bisphosphonate infusions can be given through peripheral or central venous access; pamidronate infusions can be over as short as 60 minutes, and zoledronate is often given over 15 minutes. For renal insufficiency, slowing pamidronate infusions is recommended and the dose for zoledronate must be adjusted for creatinine clearance of 60 mL per minute or less. Both agents require regular monitoring of serum creatinine and calcium; oral calcium and vitamin D supplementation are recommended during treatment.

Possible Harms

Table 12-2 lists the potential side effects of bisphosphonate medications. Types of reactions include fever, flulike reactions, nausea, allergic reactions, hypocalcemia, and osteonecrosis of the jaw. The recent Cochrane review of bisphosphonates for skeletal pain calculated the number needed to harm at 16 (95% CI 12-27) for discontinuation because of adverse effects.[11] The most feared adverse event in the regular use of

TABLE 12-2. Possible Adverse Events: Monitoring, and Treatment Approach

ADVERSE EVENT	MONITORING AND TREATMENT APPROACH
Osteonecrosis of the jaw	Dental evaluation before treatment, with delay between dental extraction and other major dental procedures and initiation Physician assessment of oral and dental hygiene at baseline Regular oropharyngeal examination before administration
Hypocalcemia	Routine calcium and albumin monitoring before administration
Renal dysfunction	Routine creatinine clearance monitoring before administration; dose adjustment and change of infusion rate as necessary
Fever	Prophylactic or adjuvant use of antipyretic medications
Nausea	Use of antiemetics before initiation

TABLE 12-1. Bisphosphonates Studied in Cancer: Route, Dosing, and Potency

AGENT	ROUTE	COMMON DOSE	AVAILABLE	RELATIVE POTENCY
Etidronate	PO	20 mg/kg daily	Europe	1
	IV	7.5 mg/kg IV daily × 3 days		
Clodronate	PO	1600 mg/day	Europe	10
	IV	300 mg/day for up to 10 days		
Pamidronate	IV	60-90 mg over 90-120 min	United States, Europe	100
Zoledronate	IV	4 mg over 15 min infusion	United States, Europe	10,000

IV, Intravenous; *PO*, By mouth.

bisphosphonates is the development of osteonecrosis of the jaw. This condition, characterized by exposed bone in the oral cavity that does not resolve within 6 weeks with appropriate dental care in the absence of osteoradionecrosis or malignant bone disease of the jaw, has an incidence in patients with metastatic cancer of approximately 1%[34] or less[35] in those exposed to bisphosphonates. Longer follow-up in a recent clinical trial of zoledronate versus denosumab, a novel RANKL inhibitor, has an incidence of osteonecrosis of the jaw of 1% at 2 to 3 years,[36] suggesting the risk is higher when patients have longer exposure; because people with metastatic cancer live longer, the cumulative risk is generally unknown. The major risk factor for development of osteonecrosis of the jaw is length of exposure; the median number of treatment cycles was 35 infusions for patients developing the condition versus 15 infusions for those who did not ($p < 0.001$).[37] In another multivariate analysis, use of dentures and history of dental extraction were associated with increased risk for development of osteonecrosis of the jaw whereas other dental disease such as periodontitis and root canal treatment were not associated.[38] In an Italian study of 154 patients, a significant reduction in the incidence of osteonecrosis of the jaw from 3.2% to 1.3% was observed after the implementation of baseline mouth assessments by a dental team, with all appropriate dental care completed before the first infusion.[39]

Putting It All Together: An Evidence-Based Approach

Based on the results of large, randomized controlled trials conducted since the 1990s, bisphosphonates have become the standard of care for the prevention and treatment of skeletal-related events. It remains critically important to identify and treat skeletal metastases with bisphosphonates to prevent future events. An analysis of four major placebo-controlled bisphosphonate trials demonstrated the prevalence of pathologic fractures as high as 52% at 2 years, need for radiation therapy as high as 43% in breast cancer, and spinal cord compression approaching 10% in prostate cancer patients.[40]

For management or prevention of skeletal-related events, the standard regimen is either pamidronate or zoledronate given on a regular basis on 3-week or 4-week cycles. Oral agents do not have approval in the United States or evidence for use in cancer settings. The optimal type, route, and duration for administration remain uncertain because of lack of head-to-head comparisons and long-term follow-up with less frequent dosing. Many providers will administer bisphosphonates monthly for up to 2 years in solid tumors and then consider less frequent dosing in the absence of new skeletal lesions or skeletal-related events. For either of these, returning to a monthly regimen is recommended. In multiple myeloma, despite advancing antimyeloma treatments with immunological agents and proteosome-inhibitors, bone lesions do not heal, even in patients who have been in remission for several years. Therefore response to antimyeloma treatment does not necessarily reduce or eliminate the risk for future skeletal morbidity alone[41] and necessitates indefinite, regular administration. Ongoing studies accounting for the long half-life of bisphosphonates are examining the optimal frequency and duration.

Despite more than 50 randomized studies in the topic area, heterogeneity among trial designs for bone pain control preclude the ability to make robust conclusions. Insufficient evidence exists to use bisphosphonates in the first-line setting as the predominant pain control strategy for bony metastases. They may be considered adjunct to both opioid and nonopioid analgesics and other interventions such as radiotherapy or radiopharmaceuticals therapy. For example, McQuay and colleagues[42] reviewed the efficacy of radiotherapy for at least 50% pain relief, showing an NNT 3.6 (95% CI 3.2-3.9), with a median duration of pain relief of 12 weeks. This is lower than the NNT of 7 for bisphosphonates.

The development of a skeletal-related event is not a sign of bisphosphonate treatment failure; rather, treatment should still be considered indefinitely to delay further events. Many clinicians extend time intervals once 1 to 2 years of consecutive bisphosphonate has been delivered. Despite the lack of evidence, this approach may be reasonable during periods of disease control when bone resorption may be more controlled with cytotoxic therapies. If the disease progresses or a new skeletal-related event occurs, the standard dose and schedule should be resumed.

KEY MESSAGES TO PATIENTS AND FAMILIES

Clinicians should explain to patients and their families that bisphosphonates are the primary bone-directed therapy used to prevent skeletal-related events in solid tumors with metastatic bone disease and multiple myeloma. They should clarify that these medications have also been proved to reduce pain and analgesic use in most advanced solid tumors. When discussing the medications, it is important to stress that although generally safe, bisphosphonates may cause immediate reactions (e.g., fever, flulike symptoms) or, rarely, serious complications such as renal failure or osteonecrosis of the jaw. Patients should follow up with their clinicians so they can be monitored closely.

CONCLUSION AND SUMMARY

Bisphosphonates are the standard of care for prevention of skeletal-related events in advanced solid tumors with bone involvement and multiple myeloma. Through inhibiting osteoclast activity, bisphosphonates have been proved to reduce fractures, treat hypercalcemia, and reduce pain. Currently, the role of bisphosphonates in pain control is as an adjuvant modality to analgesics and radiotherapy. Most serious adverse reactions are rare and preventable by baseline screening for risk factors, close follow-up, and prompt discontinuation and supportive measures when present; nonetheless, osteonecrosis of the jaw is a major complication of bisphosphonate therapy that warrants close monitoring.

SUMMARY RECOMMENDATIONS

- Bisphosphonates should be considered the standard of care for prevention of skeletal-related events in all patients with metastatic cancer affecting the bones.
- Bisphosphonate therapy should be continued and changed to a bisphosphonate with increased potency if a skeletal-related event occurs during regular administration.
- Bisphosphonates reduce pain and analgesic use but lack the data to be used as the main pain management strategy for metastatic bone pain; they should be considered as adjunctive therapy.
- Bisphosphonates should be continued for 12 weeks during a trial for pain control to fully assess efficacy.
- The optimal frequency of bisphosphonates after 1 to 2 years of stable bone disease is unknown; some clinicians reduce the frequency for patient time and cost considerations.
- Close vigilance of oral and dental health can prevent chronic complications of osteonecrosis of the jaw, which typically resolves with supportive measures only.

REFERENCES

1. Coleman RE. Clinical features of metastatic bone disease and risk of skeletal morbidity. *Clin Cancer Res.* 2006;12:6243s–6249s.
2. Plunkett TA, Smith P, Rubens RD. Risk of complications from bone metastases in breast cancer: implications for management. *Eur J Cancer.* 2000;36:476–482.
3. Janjan NA, Payne R, Gillis T, et al. Presenting symptoms in patients referred to a multidisciplinary clinic for bone metastases. *J Pain Symptom Manage.* 1998;16:171–178.
4. Coleman RE. Bisphosphonates: clinical experience. *Oncologist.* 2004;9(suppl 4):14–27.
5. Berenson JR, Lichtenstein A, Porter L, et al. Efficacy of pamidronate in reducing skeletal events in patients with advanced multiple myeloma. Myeloma Aredia Study Group. *N Engl J Med.* 1996;334:488–493.
6. Saad F. New research findings on zoledronic acid: survival, pain, and anti-tumour effects. *Cancer Treat Rev.* 2008;34:183–192.
7. Patel N, Adatia R, Mellemgaard A, et al. Variation in the use of chemotherapy in lung cancer. *Br J Cancer.* 2007;96:886–890.
8. Logothetis CJ, Lin SH. Osteoblasts in prostate cancer metastasis to bone. *Nat Rev Cancer.* 2005;5:21–28.
9. Lynch CC, Hikosaka A, Acuff HB, et al. MMP-7 promotes prostate cancer-induced osteolysis via the solubilization of RANKL. *Cancer Cell.* 2005;7:485–496.
10. Santini D, Galluzzo S, Zoccoli A, et al. New molecular targets in bone metastases. *Cancer Treat Rev.* 2010;36(suppl 3):S6–S10.
11. Wong R, Wiffen PJ. Bisphosphonates for the relief of pain secondary to bone metastases. *Cochrane Database Syst Rev* 2002; CD002068.
12. Yuen KK, Shelley M, Sze WM, et al. Bisphosphonates for advanced prostate cancer. *Cochrane Database Syst Rev.* 2006; CD006250.
13. Ernst DS, Brasher P, Hagen N, et al. A randomized, controlled trial of intravenous clodronate in patients with metastatic bone disease and pain. *J Pain Symptom Manage.* 1997;13:319–326.
14. Ernst DS, MacDonald RN, Paterson AH, et al. A double-blind, crossover trial of intravenous clodronate in metastatic bone pain. *J Pain Symptom Manage.* 1992;7:4–11.
15. Harvey HA, Lipton A. The role of bisphosphonates in the treatment of bone metastases: the U.S. experience. *Support Care Cancer.* 1996;4:213–217.
16. Hortobagyi GN, Theriault RL, Porter L, et al. Efficacy of pamidronate in reducing skeletal complications in patients with breast cancer and lytic bone metastases. Protocol 19 Aredia Breast Cancer Study Group. *N Engl J Med.* 1996;335:1785–1791.
17. Coleman RE. Risks and benefits of bisphosphonates. *Br J Cancer.* 2008;98:1736–1740.
18. Saad F. Zoledronic acid significantly reduces pathologic fractures in patients with advanced-stage prostate cancer metastatic to bone. *Clin Prostate Cancer.* 2002;1:145–152.
19. Rosen LS, Gordon D, Tchekmedyian S, et al. Zoledronic acid versus placebo in the treatment of skeletal metastases in patients with lung cancer and other solid tumors: a phase III, double-blind, randomized trial. The Zoledronic Acid Lung Cancer and Other Solid Tumors Study Group. *J Clin Oncol.* 2003;21:3150–3157.
20. Ross JR, Saunders Y, Edmonds PM, et al. A systematic review of the role of bisphosphonates in metastatic disease. *Health Technol Assess.* 2004;8:1–176.
21. Aapro M, Abrahamsson PA, Body JJ, et al. Guidance on the use of bisphosphonates in solid tumours: recommendations of an international expert panel. *Ann Oncol.* 2008;19:420–432.
22. Hillner BE, Ingle JN, Berenson JR, et al. American Society of Clinical Oncology guideline on the role of bisphosphonates in breast cancer. American Society of Clinical Oncology Bisphosphonates Expert Panel. *J Clin Oncol.* 2000;18:1378–1391.
23. Cuzick J, Decensi A, Arun B, et al. Preventive therapy for breast cancer: a consensus statement. *Lancet Oncol.* 2011;12:496–503.
24. Russell RG. Bisphosphonates: the first 40 years. *Bone.* 2011; 49:2–19.
25. Hadji P. Aromatase inhibitor-associated bone loss in breast cancer patients is distinct from postmenopausal osteoporosis. *Crit Rev Oncol Hematol.* 2009;69:73–82.
26. Coleman RE, Banks LM, Girgis SI, et al. Skeletal effects of exemestane on bone-mineral density, bone biomarkers, and fracture incidence in postmenopausal women with early breast cancer participating in the Intergroup Exemestane Study (IES): a randomised controlled study. *Lancet Oncol.* 2007;8:119–127.
27. Hadji P, Aapro MS, Body JJ, et al. Management of aromatase inhibitor-associated bone loss in postmenopausal women with breast cancer: practical guidance for prevention and treatment. *Ann Oncol.* 2011;22:2546–2555.
28. Oefelein MG, Ricchuiti V, Conrad W, et al. Skeletal fracture associated with androgen suppression induced osteoporosis: the clinical incidence and risk factors for patients with prostate cancer. *J Urol.* 2001;166:1724–1728.
29. Mohler JL. The 2010 NCCN clinical practice guidelines in oncology on prostate cancer. *J Natl Compr Canc Netw.* 2010;8:145.
30. Hillner BE, Ingle JN, Chlebowski RT, et al. American Society of Clinical Oncology 2003 update on the role of bisphosphonates and bone health issues in women with breast cancer. *J Clin Oncol.* 2003;21:4042–4057.
31. Nelson HD, Helfand M, Woolf SH, et al. Screening for postmenopausal osteoporosis: a review of the evidence for the U.S. Preventive Services Task Force. *Ann Intern Med.* 2002;137: 529–541.
32. Rosen LS, Gordon D, Kaminski M, et al. Zoledronic acid versus pamidronate in the treatment of skeletal metastases in patients with breast cancer or osteolytic lesions of multiple myeloma: a phase III, double-blind, comparative trial. *Cancer J.* 2001;7:377–387.
33. Morgan GJ, Davies FE, Gregory WM, et al. First-line treatment with zoledronic acid as compared with clodronic acid in multiple myeloma (MRC Myeloma IX): a randomised controlled trial. *Lancet.* 2010;376:1989–1999.

34. Khosla S, Burr D, Cauley J, et al. Bisphosphonate-associated osteonecrosis of the jaw: report of a task force of the American Society for Bone and Mineral Research. *J Bone Miner Res.* 2007;22:1479–1491.
35. Coleman R, Woodward E, Brown J, et al. Safety of zoledronic acid and incidence of osteonecrosis of the jaw (ONJ) during adjuvant therapy in a randomised phase III trial (AZURE: BIG 01–04) for women with stage II/III breast cancer. *Breast Cancer Res Treat.* 2011;127(2):429–438.
36. Henry DH, Costa L, Goldwasser F, et al. Randomized, double-blind study of denosumab versus zoledronic acid in the treatment of bone metastases in patients with advanced cancer (excluding breast and prostate cancer) or multiple myeloma. *J Clin Oncol.* 2011;29:1125–1132.
37. Bamias A, Kastritis E, Bamia C, et al. Osteonecrosis of the jaw in cancer after treatment with bisphosphonates: incidence and risk factors. *J Clin Oncol.* 2005;23:8580–8587.
38. Vahtsevanos K, Kyrgidis A, Verrou E, et al. Longitudinal cohort study of risk factors in cancer patients of bisphosphonate-related osteonecrosis of the jaw. *J Clin Oncol.* 2009;27:5356.
39. Ripamonti CI, Maniezzo M, Campa T, et al. Decreased occurrence of osteonecrosis of the jaw after implementation of dental preventive measures in solid tumour patients with bone metastases treated with bisphosphonates: the experience of the National Cancer Institute of Milan. *Ann Oncol.* 2009;20:137–145.
40. Gralow JR, Biermann JS, Farooki A, et al. NCCN Task Force Report: Bone Health in Cancer Care. *J Natl Compr Canc Netw.* 2009;7(suppl 3):S1–S32; quiz S33–S35.
41. Epstein J, Walker R. Myeloma and bone disease: "the dangerous tango". *Clin Adv Hematol Oncol.* 2006;4:300–306.
42. McQuay HJ, Carroll D, Moore RA. Radiotherapy for painful bone metastases: a systematic review. *Clin Oncol (R Coll Radiol).* 1997;9:150–154.

Chapter 13

Should Bisphosphonates Be Used Routinely to Manage Pain and Skeletal Complications in Other Conditions?

JENNIFER M. MAGUIRE, ARIF KAMAL, DAVID C. CURROW, AND AMY P. ABERNETHY

INTRODUCTION AND SCOPE OF THE PROBLEM

Bone loss not related to age, referred to as secondary osteoporosis, presents a significant potential for morbidity and mortality in patients with chronic or life-threatening illnesses. Increasingly, as palliative care aims to evaluate and treat patients with serious illness earlier in the course of their illness, when disease-directed therapies are still ongoing, palliative medicine professionals may encounter patients who are potential candidates for bone-directed therapies. The goal remains prevention; dramatic consequences of untreated bone loss are often fracture, pain, accelerated and ultimately irreversible debility, hospitalization, rehabilitation, and sometimes death.

Secondary osteoporosis accounts for almost half of all cases of bone loss in the United States.[1] Bone loss may result from chronic medications, diseases that directly impair bone integrity or cause an imbalance between bone production and resorption, or a combination of both. Medications used long term that may cause bone loss include corticosteroids (technically glucocorticoids), heparin, anticonvulsants, and immunosuppressants. Medical conditions that may cause decreased bone density include endocrine dysfunction (e.g., hyperparathyroidism, hypogonadism), gastrointestinal malabsorption syndromes (e.g., gastric bypass, celiac disease), rheumatoid arthritis, cystic fibrosis, posttransplantation states, severe liver disease, and long-term immobility. A comprehensive list of medical conditions involving loss of bone density is presented in Table 13-1.

Although a multitude of medications and diseases result in secondary osteoporosis, the leading cause for all patients—and certainly relevant to palliative medicine—is long-term glucocorticoid use.

Patients on long-term therapy should be assessed for secondary bone loss and considered for prevention and treatment strategies. Further, the ease of glucocorticoid prescription and duration of intervention can increase the prevalence, morbidity, and mortality from selected dermatological, pulmonary, renal, and rheumatological disorders.

Do bisphosphonates have a clear role in the prevention and management of fractures in secondary osteoporosis? In primary osteoporosis, bisphosphonates have been shown to effectively reduce the risk for primary osteoporotic vertebral fractures by approximately 50%.[2] For secondary osteoporosis, the greatest evidence base supporting the role of bisphosphonates is in glucocorticoid-induced osteoporosis. Although it is important to acknowledge that other conditions, such as posttransplantation states[3] and cystic fibrosis,[4] have high rates of fractures and sporadic evidence for bisphosphonates, the majority of this chapter will address bone loss secondary to chronic glucocorticoid use.

RELEVANT PATHOPHYSIOLOGY

Glucocorticoid-induced osteoporosis is the result of diverse medication effects on several types of bone cells. These include stimulating osteoclastogenesis, thus increasing the number of cells responsible for bone resorption; decreasing osteoblast function and life span; increasing osteoblast apoptosis; impairing preosteoblast formation; and increasing osteocyte apoptosis, thereby interfering with the normal management process of the osteocyte in directing bone repair.[5,6] Overall, this creates an imbalance among bone formation, maintenance, and resorption that may result in decreased bone quality and increased fracture risk even before measurable decrements in bone mineral density are observed.[7]

Other direct molecular effects of glucocorticoids include blocking the stimulatory effect of insulin-like growth factor 1 (IGF-1) on bone formation[8] (similar to the deficiency seen in insulin-dependent diabetes mellitus [IDDM]), increasing levels of receptor activator of nuclear factor κ B ligand (RANKL), resulting in increased bone resorption[9] and decreasing estrogen, testosterone, and androgen levels,[10] which stimulates bone production.

TABLE 13-1. Causes of Non–Malignancy-Associated Secondary Osteoporosis

MEDICATIONS	DISEASES OR DISORDERS
Glucocorticoids	Hypogonadism
Antiseizure medications	Excessive alcohol consumption
Heparins	Renal insufficiency
Antihormonal agents	Chronic respiratory disorders
Immunosuppressants	Rheumatoid arthritis
• Cyclosporin A	Hyperthyroidism
• Tacrolimus	Hyperparathyroidism
• Mycophenolate mofetil	Smoking
	Immobility
	Diabetes mellitus type 1
	Solid organ transplant
	Cushing syndrome
	Human immunodeficiency virus
	Hemochromatosis
	Inflammatory bowel disease
	Severe liver disease

TABLE 13-2. Data for World Health Organization Fracture Risk Assessment Tool (FRAX) Calculation

Patient age (or date of birth)
Sex
Weight (kg)
Height (cm)
History of previous fracture
History of parent fracturing hip
Current smoking status
Current glucocorticoid use
Medical history of rheumatoid arthritis
Presence of disorder strongly associated with osteoporosis*
Consumption of 3 or more units of alcohol per day[†]
Femoral neck bone mineral density values (optional)

*Includes type 1 diabetes mellitus, osteogenesis imperfecta in adults, untreated long-standing hyperthyroidism, hypogonadism or premature (<45 years) menopause, chronic malnutrition or malabsorption, and chronic liver disease.
[†]In the United States a unit of alcohol is defined as one glass of beer, a single measure of spirits, or a medium-sized glass of wine.

SUMMARY OF EVIDENCE REGARDING TREATMENT RECOMMENDATIONS

Current Guidelines

Recommendations for screening for bone loss come from the Bone Mass Measurement Act of 1997.[11] Bone mass measurement is reimbursed by Medicare for five categories, two of which address secondary osteoporosis. These include patients receiving long-term glucocorticoids at doses of prednisone greater than or equal to 7.5 mg per day (or equivalent) and patients with known hyperparathyroidism. Longitudinal measurement may be repeated as often as every 6 months for monitoring glucocorticoid-treated patients to detect bone loss and during treatment with a bisphosphonate. When making decisions, absolute fracture risk incorporating comorbidities, patient age, and family history is more appropriate than defining a specific T-score cutoff from the bone mineral density examination alone. In fact, the absolute threshold for which interventions should be considered has no consensus, and depending on the guidelines followed, may range from a T score of –1.0 to –1.5. The World Health Organization (WHO) Fracture Risk Assessment (FRAX) tool is an example of a tool that does not rely on a T score from bone mineral density testing. The calculator for the FRAX scale can be found at http://www.shef.ac.uk/FRAX/.

The FRAX combines demographics, family history, social history, and medical history with optional bone mineral density values to calculate a 10-year probability of fracture. Current Medicare guidelines recommend therapeutic interventions, which may include bisphosphonates in addition to calcium and vitamin D supplementation, for patients with a 10-year FRAX risk of 3% for hip fractures and 20% for all major fractures.[12] For example, consider a 70-year-old obese white woman (weight 70 kg, height 135 cm, body mass index 38.4) with a parental history of hip fracture who is a current smoker and taking chronic glucocorticoids; she has a major osteoporotic fracture risk of 21% and hip fracture risk of 7.4% at 10 years. Current guidelines suggest medical intervention in this patient. Information necessary to complete a FRAX is listed in Table 13-2.

Guidelines for the prevention and treatment of glucocorticoid-induced bone loss have been published. The American College of Rheumatology (ACR)[11] and Royal College of Physicians[13] endorse the use of bisphosphonates to prevent and treat bone loss in patients receiving glucocorticoids. The ACR recommends bisphosphonates for all patients starting long-term glucocorticoid treatments, regardless of bone mineral density values, relying more on clinical data than radiological criteria. In premenopausal women, because of the potential teratogenic effects to a fetus, they recommend patients be counseled and educated on the risks before initiating bisphosphonate therapy.

Clinical Practice

Primary osteoporosis from age-related bone loss is a diagnosis made either clinically or radiographically, with outlined diagnostic thresholds for bone mineral density scans or medical history. No clear-cut recommendations are available for evaluation of secondary osteoporosis outside of glucocorticoid-induced bone loss.[1] Because as little as 5 mg per day of prednisone (or equivalent) reduces bone mineral density and increases the risk for vertebral and nonvertebral fractures as early as 3 to 6 months after initiating therapy,[14] early recognition of prolonged glucocorticoid use and risk factors for bone loss are necessary even in patients who may be receiving low or temporary doses of glucocorticoids. Based on clinical trials, these patients are candidates for bisphosphonates for the prevention of fracture.

Stoch and colleagues[15] conducted a placebo-controlled clinical trial of once-weekly oral alendronate in patients receiving glucocorticoid therapy. The study showed an increase in bone density in the axial skeleton and decreased biochemical markers of bone turnover in the alendronate group. Both a Cochrane Database review and a meta-analysis concluded that in more than 800 patients across 13 trials, bisphosphonates were effective at preventing and treating glucocorticoid-related osteoporosis. Because of the overwhelming evidence, risedronate, zoledronic acid, and alendronate are approved by the U.S. Food and Drug Administration (FDA) for prevention and treatment of glucocorticoid-induced osteoporosis. Comparative studies assessing fracture risk among alendronate, risedronate, and zoledronic acid have not been performed.

Conflicting data exist regarding the decrease in bone mineral density in patients using inhaled glucocorticoids. Wong and associates[16] studied 196 adults with asthma who used inhaled glucocorticoids for a median duration of 6 years. They found a dose-response effect with a negative correlation between total inhaled glucocorticoid and bone mineral density. Another retrospective study found an increase in all nonvertebral and specifically hip fractures among people with chronic obstructive pulmonary disease using inhaled medications. No difference was found between inhaled glucocorticoids and inhaled bronchodilators, suggesting the risk may be related more to the underlying respiratory disease.[17]

If glucocorticoids are discontinued because of an acute event, such as fracture, the optimal duration of bisphosphonate therapy after the fracture is unknown. Some evidence suggests that fracture risk with the use of oral glucocorticoids does not return to baseline until 2 years after discontinuation.[14] If the underlying disease and its associated independent risks for secondary osteoporosis (e.g., rheumatoid arthritis) continue despite stopping glucocorticoids, this should be considered in determining the total bisphosphonate duration.

Putting It All Together

Because of the significant prevalence of fractures and their associated morbidity and potential mortality, it is of utmost importance to develop a screening strategy for patients at risk for secondary osteoporosis. Usually these are patients taking glucocorticoids for more than 3 months who require preventive strategies with regular bisphosphonates independent of bone mineral density. Also, these are patients who are at high risk because of medications, diseases, or lifestyle choices, which along with demographic and family history information, may place them at high risk for future fracture-related complications without bone-directed therapy (a list of reversible risk factors is listed in Table 13-3). Regular implementation of the WHO FRAX into clinical decision making is valuable. Although not necessary but often helpful to monitor bone integrity changes while on therapy, bone mineral density testing may be performed as often as every 6 months.

In palliative care, key considerations are the risk for fracture and its sequelae, duration of time a patient will be exposed to that risk, and challenge of

TABLE 13-3. Suggested Lifestyle Measures for Prevention of Secondary Osteoporosis
Smoking cessation
Regular weight-bearing exercise
Calcium intake of at least 1200 mg/day
Vitamin D of at least 800 international units/day
Reducing alcohol intake to <2 units/day*

*In the United States a unit of alcohol is defined as one glass of beer, a single measure of spirits, or a medium-sized glass of wine.

balancing appropriate pharmaceutical-based prevention strategies with the accumulating polypharmacy encountered as life closes. Clearly, the palliative care practitioner must take prognosis, quality of life, and comorbidities into consideration as decisions are made about whether to prescribe bisphosphonates for secondary osteoporosis. Bisphosphonates prescribed for preventive purposes should be routinely reevaluated at predetermined assessment times (e.g., every 3 or 6 months) to determine whether the intervention should be continued given the updated overall clinical status of the patient. Communication with the patient and family about intent, planned duration of therapy, and precautions is critical.

Lack of head-to-head comparisons among FDA-approved bisphosphonates for glucocorticoid-induced osteoporosis emphasizes the importance of considering patient costs and potential compliance (with daily versus monthly regimens) when selecting an agent. Additionally, close monitoring of renal function and for possible adverse events such as osteonecrosis of the jaw requires regular patient and provider interactions and, rarely, dose adjustments, supportive measures, or discontinuation.

Despite overwhelming evidence, the importance of patient and provider education cannot be overstated. Evidence shows that most patients are not being adequately educated on the importance of bone-directed therapies (including calcium, vitamin D, and bisphosphonates) to prevent glucocorticoid-induced bone loss.[18] A systematic review of 24 studies reported the prevalence of evidence-based compliance with bone density testing or bone-protective agents to be only 23% and 42%, respectively. This highlights the greater need for both patient and provider understanding of the importance of evaluation and prevention strategies.

KEY MESSAGES TO PATIENTS AND FAMILIES

Clinicians should screen all patients on long-term, high-risk medications (e.g., glucocorticoids) or who have high-risk medical conditions (cystic fibrosis, solid organ transplantation) for secondary osteoporosis. As part of this screening, the patient and family can be educated as to the fact that up to half of all osteoporosis is from non–age-related sources. Early recognition is key to prevention of fractures, pain, immobility, and possible death. In terms of explaining risk factors, the clinician should inform the patient and family that age, weight, height, medical history, family history, and alcohol and smoking history are considered when assessing for fracture risk. High-risk patients should be counseled and receive a bisphosphonate. It is important to remind patients on even small doses of glucocorticoids that they are at risk for bone loss and thus they should be considered for bisphosphonate treatment. Patients should understand that bisphosphonates have been proven in clinical trials and are FDA-approved for prevention and treatment of glucocorticoid-induced osteoporosis. Finally, a discussion with patients or families about the use of bisphosphonates in the palliative care setting should address the balance of risks, anticipated prognosis, intended benefit, and competing concerns such as polypharmacy.

CONCLUSION AND SUMMARY

Fracture prevention from secondary osteoporosis requires early recognition of high-risk patients; lifestyle, medication, and medical factors; regular screening for formal risk assessment; and prompt treatment. Bisphosphonates have been FDA-approved for prevention and treatment of secondary osteoporosis from long-term glucocorticoid use, independent of current bone density deficit. They have also been used in other high-risk medical conditions; guidelines and evidence for use have been extrapolated from glucocorticoid experience and are not as robust. Patients and providers should be mindful of the cumulative doses of glucocorticoids taken over the course of several intermittent disease exacerbations or when taken continuously over 3 months or more. Bisphosphonates, once started, should be monitored for efficacy with regular bone mineral density testing and ought to be continued until the causative factor is reversed, radiographic evidence of bone fragility is reversed, or, in cases of normal bone density, up to 2 years after the cause is eliminated. In addition to early recognition and treatment, compliance remains of utmost importance to prevent a very real risk for fracture and significant morbidity.

SUMMARY RECOMMENDATIONS

- Lifestyle, medications, and medical history may all contribute to an increased risk for secondary osteoporosis and fracture.
- All patients receiving long-term glucocorticoids should have regular fracture risk assessment, which includes a directed medical history and physical examination and may include a radiographic bone density evaluation, at baseline and routinely every 6 months to 1 year.
- The World Health Organization Fracture Risk Assessment Tool (FRAX) should be an integral part of risk assessment; it does not require formal bone density testing.
- Bisphosphonates are the standard of care for prevention of secondary osteoporosis in all persons taking (or predicted to take) prednisone 5 mg (or equivalent glucocorticosteroid) for 3 months or longer.
- Bisphosphonates should be continued indefinitely while chronic glucocorticoids are prescribed and up to 2 years after they are discontinued.
- Recognizing patient and provider undercompliance in taking and prescribing bisphosphonates for high-risk patients is essential to preventing significant morbidity and mortality related to fractures.
- When a fracture occurs in the setting of secondary osteoporosis and the patient is not on bisphosphonates, the offending cause should be minimized or removed if possible (e.g., discontinue or decrease glucocorticoids) and bisphosphonate therapy initiated.
- Decisions to prescribe bisphosphonates in the palliative care setting should balance risk, anticipated prognosis, intended benefit, and competing concerns such as polypharmacy.

REFERENCES

1. National Institutes of Health Consensus Development Panel on Osteoporosis Prevention, Diagnosis, and Therapy. Highlights of the conference. March 7-29, 2000. *South Med J.* 2001;94: 569–573.
2. Bianchi G, Sambrook P. Oral nitrogen-containing bisphosphonates: a systematic review of randomized clinical trials and vertebral fractures. *Curr Med Res Opin.* 2008;24:2669–2677.
3. Crawford BA, Kam C, Pavlovic J, et al. Zoledronic acid prevents bone loss after liver transplantation: a randomized, double-blind, placebo-controlled trial. *Ann Intern Med.* 2006;144: 239–248.
4. Conwell LS, Chang AB. Bisphosphonates for osteoporosis in people with cystic fibrosis. *Cochrane Database Syst Rev.* 2009; CD002010.
5. Yao W, Cheng Z, Busse C, et al. Glucocorticoid excess in mice results in early activation of osteoclastogenesis and adipogenesis and prolonged suppression of osteogenesis: a longitudinal study of gene expression in bone tissue from glucocorticoid-treated mice. *Arthritis Rheum.* 2008;58:1674–1686.
6. Manolagas SC. Corticosteroids and fractures: a close encounter of the third cell kind. *J Bone Miner Res.* 2000;15:1001–1005.
7. Manolagas SC, Weinstein RS. New developments in the pathogenesis and treatment of steroid-induced osteoporosis. *J Bone Miner Res.* 1999;14:1061–1066.
8. Canalis E, Bilezikian JP, Angeli A, et al. Perspectives on glucocorticoid-induced osteoporosis. *Bone.* 2004;34:593–598.
9. Deal C. Potential new drug targets for osteoporosis. *Nat Clin Pract Rheumatol.* 2009;5:20–27.
10. Lane NE, Lukert B. The science and therapy of glucocorticoid-induced bone loss. *Endocrinol Metab Clin North Am.* 1998;27: 465–483.
11. American College of Rheumatology Ad Hoc Committee on Glucocorticoid-Induced Osteoporosis. Recommendations for the prevention and treatment of glucocorticoid-induced osteoporosis: 2001 update. *Arthritis Rheum.* 2001;44:1496–1503.
12. Gralow JR, Biermann JS, Farooki A, et al. NCCN Task Force Report: bone health in cancer care. *J Natl Compr Canc Netw.* 2009;3(suppl 7):S1–S32; quiz S33–S35.

13. Compston J. US and UK guidelines for glucocorticoid-induced osteoporosis: similarities and differences. *Curr Rheumatol Rep.* 2004;6:66–69.

14. van Staa TP, Leufkens HG, Cooper C. The epidemiology of corticosteroid-induced osteoporosis: a meta-analysis. *Osteoporos Int.* 2002;13:777–787.

15. Stoch SA, Saag KG, Greenwald M, et al. Once-weekly oral alendronate 70 mg in patients with glucocorticoid-induced bone loss: a 12-month randomized, placebo-controlled clinical trial. *J Rheumatol.* 2009;36:1705–1714.

16. Wong CA, Walsh LJ, Smith CJ, et al. Inhaled corticosteroid use and bone-mineral density in patients with asthma. *Lancet.* 2000;355:1399–1403.

17. van Staa TP, Leufkens HG, Cooper C. Use of inhaled corticosteroids and risk of fractures. *J Bone Miner Res.* 2001;16:581–588.

18. Blalock SJ, Norton LL, Patel RA, et al. Patient knowledge, beliefs, and behavior concerning the prevention and treatment of glucocorticoid-induced osteoporosis. *Arthritis Rheum.* 2005;53:732–739.

When Should Radiotherapy Be Considered for Pain Management and What Principles Should Guide the Consideration of Limited-Fraction Versus Full-Dose Radiotherapy?

DREW MOGHANAKI AND THOMAS J. SMITH

INTRODUCTION AND SCOPE OF THE PROBLEM

Pain is a symptom frequently experienced by patients with metastatic cancer. Pain can be related to treatment effects, including prior surgical intervention, radiotherapy, and chemotherapy, or to tumor growth when systemic chemotherapies can no longer halt disease progression. Mass effect, nerve impingement, or destruction of soft or bony tissue are often the cause of a patient's pain. In these latter circumstances, palliative radiotherapy can provide effective treatments with an 80% to 90% response rate to specific anatomic targets with minimal side effects. Unfortunately, palliative radiotherapy is often unnecessarily delayed and underused[1] and indeed is often considered an alternative strategy to standard opioid therapy when it may actually be the better initial strategy.[2,3] For example, consider the case of a 60-year-old man with an obstructing prostate cancer and osseous metastases. He began to complain of intense bony pain secondary to destructive lesions in his right humerus, left ribs, and bilateral hips. He remained hospitalized for poorly controlled pain, despite appropriate medical management, because he was deemed a poor candidate for orthopedic intervention. The managing medical oncologist promptly ordered an inpatient radiation oncology consultation, which led to recommendation for single 8-Gy fraction radiotherapy to each of the three painful sites (Figure 14-1). With prophylactic ondansetron 8 mg given orally 1 hour before radiotherapy, the patient tolerated treatment without side effects. Pain relief was noticed within a few days, and the patient was soon discharged. Twenty-two months later, the patient was ambulating without assistance, remained off analgesics, and his pain relief remained durable while on androgen-deprivation therapy. No associated long-term toxicities were noted.

The utility of therapeutic radiation to shrink tumors and provide pain relief was noted within weeks of the discovery of x-rays in 1896. With modern advancements making treatment safer than before, currently more than two thirds of all patients with cancer receive radiation at some point during their treatment, and approximately one fourth of all radiation treatments delivered are for palliative intent.[4] Nevertheless, referrals for palliative radiotherapy, like those for hospice, are often made late—near death—when palliative radiotherapy becomes less effective as symptomatic tumors continue to destroy normal tissue. This chapter presents the rationale for the importance of frequent and early referrals to radiation oncology for pain management in the palliative setting. Furthermore, this chapter briefly outlines how radiation therapy works, summarizes the benefits of a comprehensive radiation oncology evaluation, and provides an update on modern techniques that enable the safe delivery of radiation therapy with fewer side effects than ever before. It also provides a practical overview of when physicians can refer to radiation oncology and what patients can expect.

RELEVANT PATHOPHYSIOLOGY AND PROCESSES

Radiation therapy kills tumor cells through a combination of direct and indirect DNA damage. Whereas naturally occurring DNA repair proteins often effectively repair this damage in normal cells, malignant cells are less equipped and thus secondarily pushed into interphase death, mitotic catastrophe, or cell-mediated apoptosis. The pain relief associated with radiation therapy results from rapid tumor shrinkage.

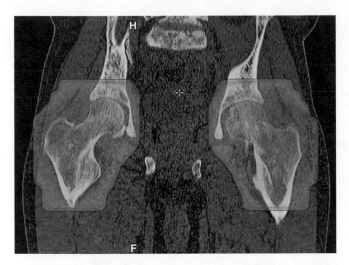

Figure 14-1. Bilateral hip irradiation. Using CT-based treatment planning, a three-dimensional conformal plan was developed within 1 hour. Note effective sparing of bowel and bladder while providing full coverage of areas at risk for fracture, including the acetabulum and femoral neck. *F*, Direction of feet placed back; *H*, direction of head. Please visit our website at www.expertconsult.com to view this image in color.

TABLE 14-1. Issues to Consider When Assessing Whether Patients With Cancer-Related Pain Should Receive Radiation Therapy

1. Is the pain related to the malignancy? If not, what is the cause?
2. If considering palliative radiotherapy, do we have confirmation the patient is incurable? (That is, avoid missing an opportunity for prescribing curative radiotherapy.)
3. Might there be a more effective alternative approach to relieving pain without radiation therapy?
4. Does the pain signal a potentially impending complication that may not be completely prevented with radiotherapy alone?
5. How long does the patient have to live? (It is important to remember when answering this question that physicians often overestimate prognosis.)
6. Can the tumor be identified on imaging to facilitate targeting?
7. How large of a volume would need to be treated and what normal structures might be exposed?
8. If previously irradiated, can the current target safely receive repeat irradiation?
9. Are the logistics of treatment possible (e.g., transportation, caregiver support to facilitate treatment, and payment)? (For patients in hospice care, a discussion with the hospice medical director may be required.)

Although the early benefits of radiation therapy may be related to damage of localized cells, producing pain modulators (e.g., lymphocytes), the durable benefits are related to long-term tumor shrinkage or even eradication, which facilitates restoration of normal osseous and soft tissue structures.

With numerous ongoing technological advancements, modern linear accelerators can currently deliver effective doses of therapeutic radiation to highly specific anatomic targets while minimizing exposure of adjacent normal tissues. This involves utilization advancements in three-dimensional imaging and treatment-planning computer programs that help design conformal "dose clouds" specific to targets of interest. A typical course of palliative radiotherapy can range from 1 to 15 treatments and often can be designed in a single day. Various dosing schedules are used, and the dose is measured in units of gray (Gy) or centigray (cGy). The total prescription dose depends on the size of each daily treatment and traditionally is 8 to 37.5 Gy. It is helpful to remind patients that pain may begin to dissipate within several days, but is rarely noticed immediately and may take up to 2 weeks to show benefit.

Consultation With a Radiation Oncologist

Radiation oncologists can be helpful in determining which patients are appropriate for radiotherapy, and it is useful to include them early in the clinical decision-making process.[5] Table 14-1 outlines key elements the radiation oncologist addresses during the evaluative workup of a patient for radiation therapy. Given that tumors can involve any anatomic site, the radiation oncologist is particularly adept at evaluating radiographic images to correlate with the patient's presenting symptoms to assess whether palliative radiotherapy can be of benefit.[6] The expertise provided by the radiation oncologist can help clarify the differential diagnosis for a patient's symptoms, including ensuring that radiation therapy is not being considered for a nonmalignant process (e.g., ensuring that a cardiac origin of chest pain has been considered for a patient with known rib metastases).

In many cases, the radiation oncologist may be helpful in determining when other specialties should be consulted to determine the best treatment for a patient. For example, when evaluating a patient with bone metastases, evaluation of structural integrity is critical. In weight-bearing bones, orthopedic stabilization may be indicated, particularly if there is more than 50% cortical bone destruction. Table 14-2 outlines many factors that should be considered when evaluating a patient for radiation therapy, some to be determined by the primary team and others by the radiation oncologist.

Particular considerations apply to patients with vertebral disease, in whom surgical stabilization of the spine may be preferred before radiotherapy. For patients whose tumors in the spine are radioresistant, such as melanoma or renal cell carcinoma, surgical debulking can help provide a more durable benefit. The American Society for Radiation Oncology (ASTRO) provides guidelines for identifying patients

TABLE 14-2. Issues for the Team to Consider in Decision Making on the Utility of Radiation Therapy

CLINICAL SCENARIO	CONSIDERATION
Treatment goals	1. Establish medically appropriate goals for patient comfort. 2. Recognize the high therapeutic ratio of radiation therapy. 3. Get radiation oncologist involved early, as the expert in managing this treatment modality in patients with cancer.
Back pain in the patient with cancer	Back pain: Consider initial MRI (CT delays diagnosis). Cord compression is an emergency—begin corticosteroids, consider immediate evaluation by spine surgeon. Vertebroplasty to be considered if no cord compression; shown to improve pain relief in a recently published international phase III trial.[12] (The patient will still need radiation therapy, and the surgical service performing the vertebroplasty procedure may not make a referral in the postoperative period. A member of the oncological team caring for the patient may need to be responsible for ensuring the patient receives consultation with a radiation oncologist.)
Weight-bearing bone	Make non–weight bearing, consider orthopedic stabilization before radiotherapy.
Other pain in the patient with cancer	Refer whenever pain is localized (may reduce need for systemic treatment). Neuropathic pain and incident pain may be effectively treated when other modalities have failed.
Concurrent chemotherapy and radiation	May be able to give palliative radiation concurrently, though discouraged if visceral organs may be irradiated. The radiation oncologist should be involved in the decision to use concurrent chemoradiotherapy if the goal is purely palliative, because there is no evidence for or against this practice.
Prior radiation	Engage radiation oncologist to determine if a repeat course is feasible. (Withholding additional radiotherapy may ultimately be worse for patient.) SABR/SBRT may an option, although myelopathy is a known risk, depending on the experience at the radiation center. Remember that repeat irradiation is an acceptable alternative and can improve the patient's quality of life, especially if the goal of the radiation treatment is palliative. Overestimation of life-expectancy can sometimes preclude an opportunity to provide effective pain relief.

CT, Computed tomography; *MRI,* magnetic resonance imaging; *SABR,* stereotactic ablative radiation therapy (also known as stereotactic body radiation therapy [SBRT].

TABLE 14-3. Characteristics of Patients With Spinal Cord or Brain Metastases for Whom Surgical Intervention Should Be Considered Before Radiotherapy Offered

CHARACTERISTIC	CONSIDERATION
Patient	<65 yr old and medically fit for surgery ECOG 0 or 1; able to walk or impaired for <48 hr Realistic survival >3 mo Slow progression (days to weeks) of symptoms
Cancer	Radioresistant cancer that will not improve with radiation (e.g., melanoma, sarcoma) Rest of the disease controlled Previous spinal cord radiation
Radiographic	Solitary site No visceral metastases, slowly growing cancer Spinal instability can be ameliorated with surgery, or brain lesion amenable to surgery

Modified from Lutz S, Berk L, Chang E, et al. Palliative radiotherapy for bone metastases: an ASTRO evidence-based guideline. *Int J Radiat Oncol Biol Phys.* 2011;79:965-976.

ECOG, Eastern Cooperative Oncology Group.

who may benefit from surgical decompression[7]; the guidelines are presented in Table 14-3 and expanded to include decisions about patients with brain metastases. These guidelines consider factors such as age, performance status, and overall prognosis. Other questions to consider when evaluating patients for potential surgical decompression of the spinal cord include the following:

- Will radiotherapy reverse all associated symptoms, such as neurological impairment?
- What is the risk of fracture after radiotherapy?
- Does the patient's prognosis justify a prolonged postoperative recovery period?

For the latter concern, vertebroplasty has emerged as a less invasive alternative to improve structural integrity in the spine, which at times may even provide immediate relief of pain before radiotherapy is delivered to eradicate the local tumor.[8] The radiation oncologist must consider all of these factors when considering whether to refer the patient to a spine surgeon while at the same time recognizing the risks inherent in delaying treatment of lesions that have the potential for damaging the spinal cord or other central nervous system structures.

Simulation

When a patient has been determined to be appropriate for palliative radiation and the decision has been made that this treatment is in line with the patient's goals of care, the treatment planning begins. The first step is a simulation, a process that begins by setting patients in an anatomic position that can be reproduced for each treatment. A treatment-planning computed tomography (CT) scan then provides the radiation oncologist with a three-dimensional rendition of the patient's internal anatomy. Using planning software, the grossly

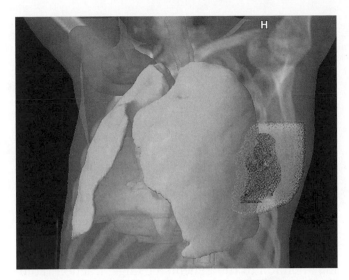

Figure 14-2. Example three-dimensional conformal treatment planning to target two separate painful metastatic lesions involving the right humerus and left ribs. The blue cloud around the right humerus denotes the volume to be targeted. Dose coverage is displayed for the left rib lesion, providing assurance of where the dose is being delivered, which in this case minimizes incidental exposure of the heart and lungs. *H*, Direction of head placed back. Please visit our website at www.expertconsult.com to view this image in color.

visible tumor is contoured on axial slices, and the target volume is delineated by including an expanded margin to ensure coverage of subclinical extension, depending on natural routes of spread. Next, conformal radiation beams are oriented from various angles to develop the most effective treatment plan with the goal of maximizing target coverage while minimizing normal tissue exposure from entrance and exit beams. Developing three-dimensional conformal plans was highly time-consuming only a few years ago; however, they can now be designed in the same day in centers with adequate resources. An example of a palliative three-dimensional conformal treatment plan is illustrated in Figure 14-2, demonstrating coverage of a large, painful, metastatic lesion of the ribs while ensuring minimal incidental exposure of the lungs.

An older treatment-planning technique consisting of traditional fluoroscopic simulation is often still used. Also known as two-dimensional planning, this strategy relies on bony landmarks to define treatment volumes and may not necessarily take less time to design. Treatment planning is not as precise, and differences in clinical outcomes may be hard to measure, particularly for patients in palliative care who do not survive long enough to experience normal tissue radiation toxicity. Many centers in the United States no longer have fluoroscopic simulators and have moved exclusively to CT-based treatment-planning.

Additional technologies include intensity modulated radiation therapy (IMRT), which can be delivered with most modern linear accelerator treatment machines and tomotherapy machines. The main advantage of this resource-intensive and more expensive technology relates to increased ability to develop more conformal treatment plans. For patients treated with curative intent, the time-consuming process of designing an IMRT plan, which may take up to 2 weeks, justifies its use. However, for patients with metastatic disease and active pain, the gains in sparing of normal tissue are often negligible and difficult to measure, and thus this mode of planning is rarely used for palliation.

Stereotactic ablative radiation therapy (SABR), also known as stereotactic body radiation therapy (SBRT), is an emerging technology available only in limited centers. Using image guidance, highly conformal focused beams of high-dose radiation can be delivered with the intent to provide ablative treatment. This technique is highly resource-intensive and expensive, and it has the pitfall of a highly conformal therapy with potential for incomplete tumor coverage. Given the effectiveness of conventional external beam radiotherapy techniques, it is difficult to justify SABR/SBRT. However, given its increased tumoricidal efficacy, palliative investigators have begun to evaluate its role for vertebral metastases. Initial experience has demonstrated severe toxicities, including myelopathy, vertebral body fractures, bronchial stenosis, and fatal esophageal necrosis. Therefore its use is currently cautioned in the initial setting and reserved for consideration only on a protocol or in the setting of repeat irradiation at a highly experienced center.[7]

SUMMARY OF EVIDENCE REGARDING TREATMENT RECOMMENDATIONS

The benefits of palliative radiotherapy can be seen with only minor tumor shrinkage and are usually noticed within the first 2 weeks, but may take up to 6 weeks for maximum effect. Overall reported success rates range from 50% to 100%.[9-12] This variability in effectiveness likely relates to the degree of pain from local tissue destruction, which may include soft tissue, bony tissue, and nerves. It is important to remember that uncontrolled tissue destruction may lead to permanent organ dysfunction; however, this can be avoided with palliative radiotherapy earlier in the disease process. Although opioid therapy can temporarily relieve patient discomfort, uncontrolled tumor progression can cause irreversible pain syndromes that are particularly difficult to manage when involving the brachial, celiac, and sacral plexus. When tumors become refractory to chemotherapy, prompt referral for radiation oncology evaluation is encouraged.

Short courses of radiation can increase the speed of pain relief and decrease the patient's burden of having to travel to the radiation center. In the 1920s, Claude Regaud established the principle of fractionated radiotherapy to maintain tumoricidal efficacy while minimizing normal tissue injury.[13] Subsequent studies demonstrated improved tumor control with multiple radiation treatments and confirmed the reduced risk for late side effects with longer courses.[14] These principles set the premise for protracted courses of radiotherapy. However, the need for complete sterilization of tumors and concern for minimizing late effects is less of an issue in patients undergoing palliative treatment. In fact, numerous prospective randomized clinical trials have failed to show increased rates of long-term toxicities with single versus longer courses of radiotherapy.[7] More than 100 reported palliative fractionation schemes are available, ranging from 1 to 20 treatments.[15] Results from 25 randomized clinical trials, 20 prospective single-arm studies, and 4 meta-analyses firmly established equivalent pain relief with treatment schedules ranging from 1 to 20 treatments.[12,15] The three largest randomized trials, each enrolling 700 to 1100 patients, confirm equivalent pain relief and freedom from opioid use and failed to demonstrate difference in toxicity (Table 14-4).[16–19] Shorter courses offer several benefits, including increased patient convenience; decreased caregiver burden; reduced number of medical appointments at the end of life; fewer challenges associated with transportation (e.g., having to travel a distance in the setting of a patient with reduced mobility); reduced clinical resource usage; and improved cost-effectiveness.[20–22] Data also suggest decreased side effects with shorter courses.[19] Given the shorter time associated with treatment regimens, single-fraction radiotherapy may facilitate more rapid turnaround time to address other issues with terminally ill patients.

Despite equivalent clinical benefits, many radiation oncologists remain reluctant to adopt single-fraction radiotherapy.[23–25] Reasons for variations in prescription patterns include lack of experience with large fraction sizes, (unfounded) concerns regarding efficacy and side effects, departmental policy, and reimbursement.[25,26] Studies have demonstrated shorter courses are most commonly used in countries where reimbursement does not depend on the number of fractions.[27,28] Adoption of single-fraction radiotherapy, as well as current practices, in the United States have lagged behind those in other countries.[20,29] An ASTRO panel assembled to address this issue concluded there has been a delay in incorporating evidence and that further randomized trials are unnecessary.[1] This practice pattern has been largely attributed to financial influences, in which the difference between a course of single versus 10 fractions may be $1381 versus $3493 based on 2008 Medicare reimbursement. This does not include direct medical costs, such as additional visits, and nonmedical costs, such as time away from home, travel, lost productivity, or caregiver sacrifice.[22,30]

An additional concern about single fraction radiotherapy is the documented two-fold increased incidence of repeat treatments. However, exploratory analyses have demonstrated this may not necessarily be secondary to an increased risk for progression, but instead may be an artifact of practitioner bias associated with earlier repeat treatment at lower pain scores. This may also be influenced by the increased safety margin related to repeat irradiation after single fraction treatment.[31,32] In a 2011 report from ASTRO, a task force of experts to develop a guideline regarding the care of patients with bone metastases stated no further clinical trials were necessary to confirm the benefit of single-fraction radiotherapy, even in critical structures such as the spine.[7] With increasing attention to the benefits of single fraction radiotherapy, ASTRO continues to work with international organizations to develop more uniform guidelines.

When widespread disease leads to diffuse pain refractory to chemotherapy, larger volumes of radiation therapy may be considered. Hemibody radiotherapy is a less commonly used strategy to sequentially treat both upper and lower halves of the body, with a planned break in between.[33] All tumor types respond to such wide-field radiotherapy techniques, and pain relief with single-dose hemibody radiotherapy is roughly 60% within first 48 hours and 80% by 1 week, with a plateau of benefit by 2 weeks. In the clinical trial RTOG 8206, 73% of patients had some relief, 66% had 50% relief, and 19% had a complete response with no need for additional analgesics.[34] The mean duration of pain relief lasted 15 weeks. Approximately 50% to 66% of patients maintained relief for the remainder of their lives, and an exploratory subset analysis of patients with prostate cancer actually suggested prolonged survival at 1 year. Lack of response was associated with irreversible normal tissue destruction. Of note, all patients were pretreated with intravenous fluids, corticosteroids, and antiemetics. Side effects included nausea lasting several hours (50% patients) and diarrhea lasting up to a week (16% of patients). Almost 50% had marrow suppression requiring 6 weeks for recovery; therefore selection of patients with adequate marrow reserve is encouraged.

TABLE 14-4. Evidence for Short-Course Versus Long-Course Radiation

STUDY	NO. OF SUBJECTS	FRACTIONS (GRAY × NUMBER OF TREATMENTS)	PATIENTS WHO HAD AT LEAST SOME RELIEF OF PAIN (%)	PATIENTS WHO HAD COMPLETE RESOLUTION OF PAIN (%)	PATIENTS WHO DEVELOPED ACUTE TOXICITY (%)	PATIENTS WHO DEVELOPED LATE TOXICITY (%)	REPEAT RADIATION TREATMENT NEEDED (%)
BPTWP[17]	775	8 Gy × 1	78	57	30	2	23
		4 Gy × 5 or 3 Gy × 10	78	58	32	1	10
RTOG 9714[19]	898	8 Gy × 1	66	15	10	4	18
		3 Gy × 10	66	18	17	4	9
Dutch[16]	1171	8 Gy × 1	72	37	Equivalent	4	25
		4 Gy × 6	69	33	Equivalent	2	7

BPTWP, Bone Pain Trial Working Party; *Gy,* gray; *RTOG,* Radiation Therapy Oncology Group.

Cost-Effectiveness

One argument often cited against the use of radiotherapy is its high cost. However, compared to pharmacotherapy, palliative radiotherapy can actually be cost-effective, as demonstrated in a Cleveland Clinic study published in 1998. In this study, patients receiving palliative radiotherapy on average had a 5-point decrease in pain (on a pain rating scale of 0 to 10). The cost of palliative radiotherapy was $1200 to $2500, compared to an estimated annual opioid cost of $9000 to $36,000.[22]

In general, short-course radiation compared to longer course radiation gives equal relief from pain, similar life expectancy and quality-adjusted life expectancy, and lower costs. The largest trial in the Netherlands showed equal results with less cost to society for short-course radiation to bone metastases.[35] In palliative treatment of non–small cell lung cancer, better survival justified the use of the longer, 10-fraction treatment rather than 2-fraction treatment.[36] In the United States, single fraction treatment of bone metastases was the preferred treatment in the largest clinical trial, RTOG 97-14.[19] It was found to cost less than 10 treatments, and the cost-effectiveness analysis showed that if repeat treatment costs were included, the incremental cost-effectiveness ratio of the 10-fraction plan was only an additional $6973 per quality-adjusted life year (considered an acceptable use of societal resources).[37]

Possibility of Repeat Irradiation

In patients who previously received radiation, a repeat course of treatment is traditionally discouraged. Radiation therapy prescriptions often expose adjacent normal tissues to their tolerance doses, which can lead to significant cellular and vascular atrophy. The long-term effects of radiation therapy are cumulative, and normal tissue breakdown is of concern. However, in highly selected cases, a repeat course of radiation can be considered and often provides significant pain relief in 46% to 87% of patients.[7] The evaluation for repeat irradiation involves a technical reconstruction of recommended current treatment volumes in relation to previous treatment plans. In the repeat irradiation setting, safety margin expansion can be altered to minimize repeated exposure to normal tissue. To get the external beam radiotherapy to the target area, treatment planning can aim to spread the dose to previously untreated tissues. In patients with good performance status but uncontrolled pain, IMRT or SABR/SBRT also can be considered to improve dose conformality.

Some patients with well-controlled metastatic disease but local recurrences are being studied prospectively using proton repeat irradiation. Definitive doses may be safely delivered using this modality when control is desired in the face of previous treatment for patients with masses too large for stereotactic methods. The expense of treatment—$50,000 or more—makes this prohibitive in most cases.

Although not as effective as an initial course of palliative radiotherapy, repeat irradiation (regardless of technique) often can provide meaningful pain relief, particularly when tumors have become refractory to chemotherapy. Given that issues of late radiation toxicity related to cumulative doses are less of an issue in patients with a poor prognosis, repeat irradiation is a reasonable option to pursue in patients with residual disease.

Side Effect Recognition and Management

The side effects of radiation are typically limited to the structures exposed and thus can be predicted (Table 14-5). For example, a patient's hair should never fall out with radiation therapy unless the scalp is exposed. Most acute effects are self-limited and resolve within several weeks with supportive care. Nutritional counseling is encouraged to ensure patients have the best opportunity to heal from these temporary normal tissue reactions.

Acute reactions are often easily managed. The more concerning side effects, consequences of cellular and vascular atrophy that may lead to decreased normal tissue function and perfusion and ultimately organ dysfunction, may develop months to years later. The treatment planning process uses established tolerance

TABLE 14-5. Acute Toxicities Related to Radiation Therapy and Suggested Supportive Care

ORGAN EXPOSED	ACUTE TOXICITY	ONSET	RESOLUTION	SUPPORTIVE CARE
Oral cavity	Mucositis	1-2 wk	2 wk after finish	Analgesics, IVF prn
Larynx	Hoarseness, dysphagia, odynophagia	1-2 wk	2-4 wk after finish	Analgesics, IVF prn
Esophagus	Dysphagia, odynophagia	1-2 wk	2-4 wk after finish	Analgesics, IVF prn
Bowel	Nausea, diarrhea	1-2 wk	2-4 wk after finish	Antiemetics, Antidiarrheal agents
Bladder	Urinary urgency, frequency, dysuria	1-2 wk	2-4 wk after finish	Antispasmodic agents, NSAIDs
Liver	Nausea, fever, chills (chemical hepatitis)	1-3 days	5-7 days after finish	Antiemetics
Hair loss after whole-brain radiation	Not applicable	14-21 days	Months	Ensure iron, thyroid stores are repleted

IVF prn, Intravenous fluids as needed; *NSAIDs,* nonsteroidal antiinflammatory drugs.

doses to avoid irreversible damage of critical structures, such as the spinal cord, lung, kidney, and liver. Although these issues are most important in curable patients, the consideration may be different in the dying patient. For example, repeat treatment of the spinal cord that causes degeneration and paralysis in 3 months may be acceptable for someone with terrible pain whose life-expectancy may be shorter than the time required for side effects to manifest.

KEY MESSAGES TO PATIENTS AND FAMILIES

Radiotherapy is a highly effective therapy with minimal side effects for patients with cancer whose pain is due to the tumor itself. Patients and families often have concerns about radiation therapy; many of these are addressed in Table 14-6. For patients in whom a longer (≥10 fraction) course is recommended, the clinician should encourage the patient and family to speak with the radiation oncologist about a shorter course of only 1 to 5 treatments to increase the speed of relief as well as maximize convenience for the patient and family.

CONCLUSION AND SUMMARY

Radiation therapy is very effective in palliating symptoms of cancer. Most patients can expect pain or symptom relief within days and maintain that relief until the end of their life. Despite the effectiveness of radiation, it is given too infrequently and often too late. Some of the barriers to effective radiation use include lack of knowledge about modern short-course techniques, concerns about availability, and the perception that radiation is expensive or not covered under the Medicare hospice benefit. Indeed, most patients can be treated with short courses (1 to 5 fractions, not ≥10), and radiation therapy is within the geographic reach of most patients in the United States. Radiation therapy can be cost-effective and can be used within the Medicare hospice benefit. Increased adoption of short courses of radiation will likely become more prevalent in the United States in the near future as a result of health care reform and efforts by organizations such as American Society of Radiation Oncology and the American College of Radiology.

The physician involved in care of the patient with incurable cancer has many options when patients develop pain, and it is important that early referral to radiation therapy be a key element in the treatment plan of these patients.

SUMMARY RECOMMENDATIONS

- Radiation therapy is an effective anticancer therapy, with an 80% to 90% response rate.
- It can provide prompt, effective, and durable pain relief, but is underused because of current clinical practices that administer chemotherapy as first-line treatment for symptom control until symptoms become severe.
- Radiation therapy is most effective before tumors cause significant tissue damage; thus clinicians should refer patients for radiation therapy early in their disease course.
- A preponderance of evidence exists demonstrating equivalency with shorter courses, and a prescription of 1 to 5 treatments may soon become the standard of care worldwide for patients with advanced disease.

TABLE 14-6. Key Messages to Patients and Families About Radiation Therapy

1. Do not conceal pain or other symptoms related to concerns about your cancer, because effective treatment is available. A course of radiation therapy will not detract from long-term goals.
2. Radiation therapy is not limited to care for patients at the end of life; it can be used for a potentially curable tumor while awaiting response to systemic treatment.
3. Radiation therapy is highly effective and safe; normal tissues are easily avoided with modern techniques.
4. Early consultation with a radiation oncologist is essential, because it may increase the efficacy of treatment.
5. Each patient and cancer is unique, and the location of the cancer determines the best course of treatment.
6. Single or short-course treatments are excellent options. If necessary because of pain recurrence, repeat treatment is an option.
7. Toxicity can be minimized with the use of medications, such as antiemetics for nausea and nonsteroidal antiinflammatory drugs for increased pain related to large, bony-lesion flare posttreatment.
8. Multiple precautions are taken to ensure symptom relief while maintaining safety, such as dose calculations, avoiding normal tissue, and calibration measurements.
9. Radiation for pain or shortness of breath can be effective within a few days.

REFERENCES

1. Janjan N, Lutz ST, Bedwinek JM, et al. Therapeutic guidelines for the treatment of bone metastasis: a report from the American College of Radiology Appropriateness Criteria Expert Panel on Radiation Oncology. *J Palliat Med.* 2009;12:417–426.
2. Lutz S, Lupu D, Johnstone P, et al. The influence of the newly formed hospice and palliative medicine subspecialty on radiation oncology and end-of-life care. *J Am Coll Radiol.* 2008;5:1102–1105.
3. Khatcheressian J, Harrington SB, Lyckholm LJ, et al. 'Futile care': what to do when your patient insists on chemotherapy that likely won't help. *Oncology (Williston Park).* 2008;22: 881–888; discussion 893, 896, 898.
4. Janjan NA. An emerging respect for palliative care in radiation oncology. *J Palliat Med.* 1998;1:83–88.
5. Lutz S, Spence C, Chow E, et al. Survey on use of palliative radiotherapy in hospice care. *J Clin Oncol.* 2004;22:3581–3586.
6. Abrams HL, Spiro R, Goldstein N. Metastases in carcinoma: analysis of 1000 autopsied cases. *Cancer.* 1950;3:74–85.
7. Lutz S, Berk L, Chang E, et al. Palliative radiotherapy for bone metastases: an ASTRO evidence-based guideline. *Int J Radiat Oncol Biol Phys.* 2011;79:965–976.
8. Berenson J, Pflugmacher R, Jarzem P, et al. Balloon kyphoplasty versus non-surgical fracture management for treatment of painful vertebral body compression fractures in patients with cancer: a multicentre, randomised controlled trial. *Lancet Oncol.* 2011;12:225–235.

9. Bartelink H, Battermann J, Hart G. Half body irradiation. *Int J Radiat Oncol Biol Phys.* 1980;6:87–90.
10. Kuban DA, Delbridge T, el-Mahdi AM, et al. Half-body irradiation for treatment of widely metastatic adenocarcinoma of the prostate. *J Urol.* 1989;141:572–574.
11. Nag S, Shah V. Once-a-week lower hemibody irradiation (HBI) for metastatic cancers. *Int J Radiat Oncol Biol Phys.* 1986;12:1003–1005.
12. Chow E, Harris K, Fan G, et al. Palliative radiotherapy trials for bone metastases: a systematic review. *J Clin Oncol.* 2007;25:1423–1436.
13. Regaud C. The influence of the duration of irradiation on the changes produced in the testicle by radium. *Int J Radiat Oncol Biol Phys.* 1977;2:565–567.
14. Thames Jr HD, Withers HR, Peters LJ, et al. Changes in early and late radiation responses with altered dose fractionation: implications for dose-survival relationships. *Int J Radiat Oncol Biol Phys.* 1982;8:219–226.
15. Fairchild A, Barnes E, Ghosh S, et al. International patterns of practice in palliative radiotherapy for painful bone metastases: evidence-based practice? *Int J Radiat Oncol Biol Phys.* 2009;75:1501–1510.
16. Steenland E, Leer JW, van Houwelingen H, et al. The effect of a single fraction compared to multiple fractions on painful bone metastases: a global analysis of the Dutch Bone Metastasis Study. *Radiother Oncol.* 1999;52:101–109.
17. Bone Pain Trial Working Party. 8 Gy single fraction radiotherapy for the treatment of metastatic skeletal pain: randomised comparison with a multifraction schedule over 12 months of patient follow-up. *Radiother Oncol.* 1999;52:111–121.
18. Tong D, Gillick L, Hendrickson FR. The palliation of symptomatic osseous metastases: final results of the Study by the Radiation Therapy Oncology Group. *Cancer.* 1982;50:893–899.
19. Hartsell WF, Scott CB, Bruner DW, et al. Randomized trial of short- versus long-course radiotherapy for palliation of painful bone metastases. *J Natl Cancer Inst.* 2005;97:798–804.
20. Bradley NM, Husted J, Sey MS, et al. Review of patterns of practice and patients' preferences in the treatment of bone metastases with palliative radiotherapy. *Support Care Cancer.* 2007;15:373–385.
21. Kirkbride P, Barton R. Palliative radiation therapy. *J Palliat Med.* 1999;2:87–97.
22. Macklis RM, Cornelli H, Lasher J. Brief courses of palliative radiotherapy for metastatic bone pain: a pilot cost-minimization comparison with narcotic analgesics. *Am J Clin Oncol.* 1998;21:617–622.
23. Kachnic L, Berk L. Palliative single-fraction radiation therapy: how much more evidence is needed? *J Natl Cancer Inst.* 2005;97:786–788.
24. Booth M, Summers J, Williams MV. Audit reduces the reluctance to use single fractions for painful bone metastases. *Clin Oncol (R Coll Radiol).* 1993;5:15–18.
25. Ben-Josef E, Shamsa F, Williams AO, et al. Radiotherapeutic management of osseous metastases: a survey of current patterns of care. *Int J Radiat Oncol Biol Phys.* 1998;40:915–921.
26. van der Linden YM, Steenland E, van Houwelingen HC, et al. Patients with a favourable prognosis are equally palliated with single and multiple fraction radiotherapy: results on survival in the Dutch Bone Metastasis Study. *Radiother Oncol.* 2006;78:245–253.
27. Lievens Y, Kesteloot K, Rijnders A, et al. Differences in palliative radiotherapy for bone metastases within Western European countries. *Radiother Oncol.* 2000;56:297–303.
28. Lievens Y, Van den Bogaert W, Rijnders A, et al. Palliative radiotherapy practice within Western European countries: impact of the radiotherapy financing system? *Radiother Oncol.* 2000;56:289–295.
29. Maher EJ, Coia L, Duncan G, et al. Treatment strategies in advanced and metastatic cancer: differences in attitude between the USA, Canada and Europe. *Int J Radiat Oncol Biol Phys.* 1992;23:239–244.
30. Konski A, James J, Hartsell W, et al. Economic analysis of radiation therapy oncology group 97–14: multiple versus single fraction radiation treatment of patients with bone metastases. *Am J Clin Oncol.* 2009;32:423–428.
31. Roos DE, Turner SL, O'Brien PC, et al. Randomized trial of 8 Gy in 1 versus 20 Gy in 5 fractions of radiotherapy for neuropathic pain due to bone metastases (Trans-Tasman Radiation Oncology Group, TROG 96.05). *Radiother Oncol.* 2005;75:54–63.
32. van der Linden YM, Lok JJ, Steenland E, et al. Single fraction radiotherapy is efficacious: a further analysis of the Dutch Bone Metastasis Study controlling for the influence of retreatment. *Int J Radiat Oncol Biol Phys.* 2004;59:528–537.
33. Perez CA. *Principles and Practice of Radiation Oncology.* 4th ed. Philadelphia: Lippincott Williams & Wilkins; 2004:2397.
34. Poulter CA, Cosmatos D, Rubin P, et al. A report of RTOG 8206: a phase III study of whether the addition of single dose hemibody irradiation to standard fractionated local field irradiation is more effective than local field irradiation alone in the treatment of symptomatic osseous metastases. *Int J Radiat Oncol Biol Phys.* 1992;23(1):207–214.
35. van den Hout WB, van der Linden YM, Steenland E, et al. Single- versus multiple-fraction radiotherapy in patients with painful bone metastases: cost-utility analysis based on a randomized trial. *J Natl Cancer Inst.* 2003;95:222–229.
36. van den Hout WB, Kramer GW, Noordijk EM, et al. Cost-utility analysis of short- versus long-course palliative radiotherapy in patients with non-small-cell lung cancer. *J Natl Cancer Inst.* 2006;98:1786–1794.
37. Hillner BE, Smith TJ. Efficacy does not necessarily translate to cost effectiveness: a case study in the challenges associated with 21st-century cancer drug pricing. *J Clin Oncol.* 2009;27:2111–2113.

When Should Radiopharmaceuticals Be Considered for Pain Management?

Drew Moghanaki and Thomas J. Smith

INTRODUCTION AND SCOPE OF THE PROBLEM

Most patients with cancer achieve control of pain with conventional opioids; however, as many as 10% to 20% will not experience adequate analgesia or will have significant side effects from pain medications.[1] Additionally, in some clinical scenarios bone pain is particularly difficult to control (e.g., diffuse bony disease in the setting of breast or prostate cancer) or patients with bone pain have been treated with maximum doses of external beam radiation therapy. In these types of patients, radiopharmaceuticals such as radioactive strontium or samarium can play an important role in long-term palliation.

RELEVANT PATHOPHYSIOLOGY

Bone pain and bone destruction are caused by hematogenous spread of cancer to the bone marrow, explaining why the vertebrae, long bones, and weight-bearing bones are most commonly affected and why joints, filled with compact hard bone, are almost never involved. The process of bone metastasis has been understood at the molecular level for some years. This bone formation is regulated by the activation of the receptor for the nuclear factor B (RANK)/RANK ligand (RANKL)/osteoprotegerin system.[2] Calcium homeostasis is normally mediated by parathyroid hormone, but epithelial cancers such as lung or breast cancer often produce an embryonic form of this protein, parathyroid hormone-related protein (PTHrP). This mimics parathyroid hormone in stimulating distal renal tubule (but not gastrointestinal tract) absorption of calcium and stimulates osteoclasts to reabsorb bone. Both of these mechanisms increase serum calcium levels. Solid tumors also produce other activating hormones, including interleukin (IL)-1, IL-6, tumor growth factor (TGF), tumor necrosis factor (TNF), and granulocyte-colony stimulating factor (G-CSF).[2] Hematological malignancies most commonly have excess PTHrP, but produce a number of other locally bone-active cytokines such as IL-6, IL-1, and lymphotoxin (TNF-β), as well as extrarenal production of calcitriol (1,25-[OH]$_2$D$_3$).[2]

Pain is a common accompaniment of bone metastases regardless of the type of cancer or underlying hormonal mechanisms. Some pain, especially movement or incident pain, may be a direct consequence of bone movement irritating nerves. The dull, deep, aching pain often experienced by cancer patients has been attributed to osteoclasts generating protons, which then produces local acidosis. This in turn stimulates nociceptors in the bone.[3]

The activity of radionuclides results from their rapid absorption into the bone matrix. They deliver small particles with very short path lengths and irradiate anything within the radius of the path length. (Table 15-1 outlines the properties of the most commonly used radiopharmaceuticals.) This mechanism explains both their analgesic effect and the side effect of pancytopenia by irradiation of normal bone marrow. To combat bone pain produced by osteoclast-activated bone destruction and direct bone invasion by cancer, an effective treatment must destroy the cancer cells, osteoclasts, and osteoblasts.

SUMMARY OF EVIDENCE REGARDING TREATMENT RECOMMENDATIONS

In diffuse skeletal involvement, radiopharmaceuticals can provide high rates of pain relief.[4-14] ^{32}P was one of the first radionuclides to be used, and it was rapidly adopted and used for decades after reports of its effectiveness were published as early as 1939.[15,16] The advantages of this systemic agent included its availability in both oral and injectable forms and its specificity for the rapidly turning-over bone, with the phosphorous element binding directly to the hydroxyapatite molecules of bone. The overall response rates were 80% for breast and prostate cancer bone pain, and palliation was often seen within 2 weeks. Surprisingly, no dose-dependent response was identified. The main drawback was the frequency of pancytopenia, because ^{32}P has a propensity for bone marrow destruction. When secondary

TABLE 15-1. Properties of Available Compounds

ISOTOPE	HALF-LIFE (DAYS)	TYPE OF RADIOACTIVE PARTICLE	PENETRATION OF THE RADIOACTIVE PARTICLE (mm)
Strontium-89 (^{89}Sr)	50.5	β- (electron)	2.4
Samarium-153 (^{153}Sm)	1.9	β- (electron)	0.6
Phosphorus-32 (^{32}P)	14.3	β- (electron)	3 to 8

acute myeloid leukemia and myelodysplastic syndromes were reported, use of ^{32}P declined rapidly, although some have argued that the transformation to leukemia may have been due to subsequent chemotherapy agents and not necessarily ^{32}P.[17,18]

Radionuclides in more common use today are strontium-89 and samarium-153, with radium-223 under investigation (NCT00699751). These compounds target osteoblastic activity, which is ideal for breast and prostate cancers that produce PTHrP. Strontium mimics calcium, so it is rapidly absorbed into the bony matrix. As noted in Table 15-1, the half-life of ^{89}Sr is 14 days and in diseased bone 51 days. ^{89}Sr may take 7 to 20 days after administration to provide relief. Conversely, ^{153}Sm has a very short half-life of 1.9 days and releases its radiation much more quickly, which translates into more rapid pain relief. See Table 15-2 for a comparison of these agents.

Excellent reviews comparing the use and efficacy of ^{89}Sr and ^{153}Sm are available in the 2011 American Society for Radiation Oncology consensus paper.[19] For both agents, pain relief has been correlated with a reduction in alkaline phosphatase levels and decreased technetium-99 m uptake[20] on bone scan. Reports show its use does not obviate need for external beam radiation therapy.[20]

Pretreatment Evaluation

In practice, radionuclides are used most for patients with epithelial cancers such as breast and prostate cancer, rather than for hematological malignancies or other solid tumors. One reason for this is because the cancer has to be sufficiently "bone-seeking" to primarily involve bony structures. Patients must also have an appropriately long prognosis for the treatments to be effective. Although lung cancers may be bone-avid, they spread to other organs so aggressively that bone disease is rarely the limiting symptom. Hematological malignancies such as myeloma or lymphoma can respond well to radionuclides, but the associated bone marrow suppression makes the disease more difficult to treat with systemic radiopharmaceuticals. Table 15-3 provides a clinical checklist to aid in identifying patients who may benefit from radiopharmaceuticals.

Administering the Radionuclide

Each department of nuclear medicine has its own method for administering the radionuclide, but all follow standard safety checklists.[21] One typically should

TABLE 15-3. Criteria for Identifying Patients Appropriate for Radiopharmaceuticals

Indications
Recent bone scan showing sites of osteoblastic metastatic disease
Diffuse painful skeletal involvement
Cancer refractory to other systemic therapies
Poorly controlled pain (despite appropriate analgesics) or analgesic intolerance

When to Consider Other Therapies
Asymptomatic metastatic disease
Osteolytic disease
Limited metastatic sites, more amenable to external beam radiation therapy
Disease sensitive to systemic agents
Analgesia medications are well tolerated by the patients
Life expectancy <3 mo

Contraindications
Pregnancy
Renal failure (glomerular filtration rate <30 mL/min)
Spinal cord compression
Present or impending pathological fracture
Hemoglobin <9, white blood cell count <3.5, or platelets <60

TABLE 15-2. Clinical Comparison of Available Radionuclides

AGENT	ROUTE	RESPONSE RATE (%)	TIME TO ONSET; DURATION OF ACTION	MECHANISM OF ACTION	COMMENTS
Strontium-89 (^{89}Sr)	IV	70	1-2 wk; 6 mo	Mimics calcium	May cause transient early flare; associated with good pain response
Samarium-153 (^{153}Sm)	IV	70	1 wk; 4 mo	Phosphonate complex co-localizes with osteoblastic activity	Distribution similar to that of bone scan technetium-99 m

wait at least 4 to 6 weeks after the last chemotherapy treatment so bone marrow is spared the combined suppressive effects of the chemotherapy and radionuclide. The actual administration is much like that of the technetium-99m given for a bone scan—the nuclear medicine physician gives the intravenous injection followed by a saline flush. The radiation safety officer or appointee will oversee the process and instruct the patient on disposal of radioactive urine.

Costs and Cost-Effectiveness

Radiopharmaceuticals are expensive. At our institution, the reimbursement paid by Medicare for strontium is $3499.76 (trade name Metastron, Current Procedural Technology [CPT]/Healthcare Common Procedure Coding System [HCPCS] code A9600) and for samarium is $7454.58 (trade name Quadramet, CPT/HCPCS code A9604); insurance typically reimburses all or most of the cost. The professional fee for administration is $324.59 (CPT Code 79101, treatment of painful bone metastases). In general, these medications are considered cost-effective because the associated reduced analgesic and hospital use offset the cost the of radionuclide.[22] One report recommends that treatment be given to patients with prostate cancer who are in hospice and have good performance status (Karnofsky 60 or higher, Eastern Cooperative Oncology Group [ECOG] 0 to 1, or up and ambulatory), because they are most likely to benefit and live long enough to justify the cost.[23] Given the large initial expense, it is unlikely that any hospice in the United States could afford to give these medications under their capitated payment system. However, given the reduction in need for analgesic medications in the 3 to 6 months after treatment, it may be appropriate to give them immediately before a patient is enrolled in hospice.

KEY MESSAGES TO PATIENTS AND FAMILIES

Radionuclide injection is an underused and very effective method to treat bone pain in patients with diffusely metastatic cancer. It only works on the bone disease to relieve pain, and thus external beam radiation is usually needed to prevent fractures. Both radioactive strontium and samarium can reduce blood counts, but this side effect is easily managed. Patients with breast and prostate cancer are most likely to benefit from radiopharmaceutical therapies, because metastatic disease primarily involves bone in these two conditions.

CONCLUSION AND SUMMARY

Radionuclide injections are effective in 70% or more of patients with breast and prostate cancer to relieve pain from bone metastases. For the treatment to work, a recent positive bone scan must show the metastases and the bones must be the primary area of metastases. Pain relief typically starts within days and may last months. The major side effect is bone marrow suppression. The American Society for Radiation Oncology has called for future studies to examine an earlier prophylactic role for radiopharmaceuticals in patients with limited bone metastases, with or without combination chemotherapy, bisphosphonates, or denosumab. The optimal mode of delivery (external beam radiation versus radiopharmaceuticals versus a combination of the two) and optimum dosing are the subject of future research.

SUMMARY RECOMMENDATIONS

- Radionuclides such as radioactive strontium and samarium are highly effective in the control of bone pain in selected patients.
- The most appropriate patients for radiopharmaceuticals are those with: epithelial cancers such as prostate and breast cancer, multiple sites of disease but predominantly in the bone, a positive technetium-99m bone scan, a life-expectancy longer than 3 months, and good bone marrow reserve.
- Most patients have bone pain relief within days and maintenance of pain relief for months. The main side effect is bone marrow suppression 4 to 6 weeks after treatment.

REFERENCES

1. Meuser T, Pietruck C, Radbruch L, Stute P, Lehmann KL, Grond S. Symptoms during cancer pain treatment following WHO-guidelines: a longitudinal follow-up study of symptom prevalence, severity and etiology. *Pain.* 2001;93:247–257.
2. Clines GA, Guise TA. Hypercalcaemia of malignancy and basic research on mechanisms responsible for osteolytic and osteoblastic metastasis to bone. *Endocr Relat Cancer.* 2005;12:549–583.
3. Julius D, Basbaum AI. Molecular mechanisms of nociception. *Nature.* 2001;413:203–210.
4. Lubitz JD, Riley GF. Trends in Medicare payments in the last year of life. *N Engl J Med.* 1993;328:1092–1096.
5. Alberts AS, Smit BJ, Louw WK, et al. Dose response relationship and multiple dose efficacy and toxicity of samarium-153-EDTMP in metastatic cancer to bone. *Radiother Oncol.* 1997;43:175–179.
6. Anderson PM, Wiseman GA, Dispenzieri A, et al. High-dose samarium-153 ethylene diamine tetramethylene phosphonate: low toxicity of skeletal irradiation in patients with osteosarcoma and bone metastases. *J Clin Oncol.* 2002;20:189–196.
7. Bolger JJ, Dearnaley DP, Kirk D, et al. Strontium-89 (Metastron) versus external beam radiotherapy in patients with painful bone metastases secondary to prostatic cancer: preliminary report of a multicenter trial. UK Metastron Investigators Group. *Semin Oncol.* 1993;20:32–33.
8. Franzius C, Schuck A, Bielack SS. High-dose samarium-153 ethylene diamine tetramethylene phosphonate: low toxicity of skeletal irradiation in patients with osteosarcoma and bone metastases. *J Clin Oncol.* 2002;20:1953–1954.
9. McEwan AJ, Amyotte GA, McGowan DG, et al. A retrospective analysis of the cost effectiveness of treatment with Metastron in patients with prostate cancer metastatic to bone. *Eur Urol.* 1994;26(suppl 1):26–31.
10. Porter AT, McEwan AJ. Strontium-89 as an adjuvant to external beam radiation improves pain relief and delays disease progression in advanced prostate cancer: results of a randomized controlled trial. *Semin Oncol.* 1993;20:38–43.

11. Porter AT, McEwan AJ, Powe JE, et al. Results of a randomized phase-III trial to evaluate the efficacy of strontium-89 adjuvant to local field external beam irradiation in the management of endocrine resistant metastatic prostate cancer. *Int J Radiat Oncol Biol Phys.* 1993;25:805–813.

12. Robinson RG, Preston DF, Schiefelbein M, et al. Strontium 89 therapy for the palliation of pain due to osseous metastases. *JAMA.* 1995;274:420–424.

13. Serafini AN, Houston SJ, Resche I, et al. Palliation of pain associated with metastatic bone cancer using samarium-153 lexidronam: a double-blind placebo-controlled clinical trial. *J Clin Oncol.* 1998;16:1574–1581.

14. Windsor PM. Predictors of response to strontium-89 (Metastron) in skeletal metastases from prostate cancer: report of a single centre's 10-year experience. *Clin Oncol (R Coll Radiol).* 2001;13:219–227.

15. Friedell HL, Storaasli JP. The use of radioactive phosphorus in the treatment of carcinoma of the breast with widespread metastases to bone. *Am J Roentgenol Radium Ther.* 1950;64:559–575.

16. Erf LA, Lawrence JH. Clinical studies with the aid of radioactive phosphorus. I. The absorption and distribution of radiophosphorus in the blood and its excretion by normal individuals and patients with leukemia. *J Clin Invest.* 1941;20:567–575.

17. Finazzi G, Caruso V, Marchioli R, et al. Acute leukemia in polycythemia vera: an analysis of 1638 patients enrolled in a prospective observational study. *Blood.* 2005;105:2664–2670.

18. Berlin NI. Treatment of the myeloproliferative disorders with 32P. *Eur J Haematol.* 2000;65:1–7.

19. Lutz S, Berk L, Chang E, et al. Palliative radiotherapy for bone metastases: an ASTRO evidence-based guideline. *Int J Radiat Oncol Biol Phys.* 2011;79:965–976.

20. Janjan N, Lutz ST, Bedwinek JM, et al. Therapeutic guidelines for the treatment of bone metastasis: a report from the American College of Radiology Appropriateness Criteria Expert Panel on Radiation Oncology. *J Palliat Med.* 2009;12:417–426.

21. Pandit-Taskar N, Batraki M, Divgi CR. Radiopharmaceutical therapy for palliation of bone pain from osseous metastases. *J Nucl Med.* 2004;45:1358–1365.

22. McEwan AJ, Amyotte GA, McGowan DG, MacGillivray JA, Porter AT. A retrospective analysis of the cost effectiveness of treatment with Metastron in patients with prostate cancer metastatic to bone. *Eur Urol.* 1994;26(suppl 1):26–31.

23. Schmeler K, Bastin K. Strontium-89 for symptomatic metastatic prostate cancer to bone: recommendations for hospice patients. *Hosp J.* 1996;11(2):1–10.

What Principles Should Guide the Prescribing of Opioids for Non–Cancer-Related Pain?

Steven D. Passik and Kenneth L. Kirsh

INTRODUCTION AND SCOPE OF PROBLEM

Few issues in medicine have generated heated debate like the topic of whether to use opioid medications in the treatment of non–cancer-related pain. Although opioids have no inherent moral value, issues of abuse, diversion, and addiction related to this class of medications are a serious social issue. The views of many in health care concerning the use of opioids tend to be steeped in myth and misconception, with physicians making pronouncements that are typically based on social conventions as opposed to scientific evidence.[1] However, in the appropriately selected patient, these medications can provide relief to considerable suffering. Unfortunately, these types of negative attitudes can result in substandard treatment for patients with chronic pain who might benefit from long-term opioid therapy.

In more recent years, high-profile legal cases and arrests of physicians for inappropriate prescribing of opioid medications have been theorized to have a chilling effect on physicians' treatment of chronic pain.[2] Further regulatory scrutiny of opioid prescribing, in some states, has resulted in the loss of licensure for some physicians, usually accompanied by frenzied negative media coverage. The lack of long-term efficacy, the problem of opioid-induced hyperalgesia, and adverse side effects have been described as major problems when opioids are used.[3] These and other issues created a suspicious and controversial environment for the use of opioids in the treatment of chronic pain. This suspicion and inertia may lead to patient suffering, and thus these issues are not academic but rather immediate and critical. However, the misuse of this class of medications can lead to considerable suffering and social cost.

The problem of treating pain has become a serious concern. Seventy-five million Americans suffer with chronic, persistent pain,[4] resulting in an estimated 60 billion dollars of lost work productivity and over 100 billion in health care costs.[5–8] The U.S. Senate voted the decade 2000 to 2010 to be the "Decade of Pain Control and Research" and pledged to support research and education in this critically important area.[9] Unfortunately, the amount of money funneled into research on pain has been woefully small and represented only a small fraction of available research monies.[10] It is no wonder, then, that empirically based evidence in the realm of pain management tends to be lacking.

In addition to a lack of research in the pain field generally, many barriers prevent the appropriate treatment of non–cancer-related pain. Societal, patient, and physician barriers still plague treatment of the patient with chronic pain. Numerous studies and surveys have shown that pain continues to be poorly treated. A list of some potential barriers culled from the extant literature is shown in Table 16-1.[11–19] Critics of these barriers suggest that they do not account for the continued poor treatment this class of patients receives and the tendency for patients with non–cancer-related pain to be marginalized.[20–22]

Risks in pain medicine can be understood to affect three areas: risks to the patient, risks to the prescriber, and risks to society.[21] Risks to the patient frequently entail risks to the prescriber and society as well (e.g., medication side effects, the costs of side effects, interactions, liability issues). The prescriber and the patient are both placed at risk when they operate from ignorance concerning pain syndromes, diagnosis, physiology, pharmacology, and treatment. Therefore risks to the pain medicine specialist can come through both omission and commission. It is therefore a responsibility of the individual pain prescriber to understand the risks involved in the medical management of pain, to reduce those risks as much as possible, and to keep a current knowledge base. The following are a set of suggestions to keep in mind when considering the prescription of opioid medications for patients with non–cancer-related pain.

Principles for Prescribing Opioids in Non–Cancer-Related Pain

The treatment of patients with chronic non–cancer-related pain with opioid therapy requires attentiveness to the risks to the prescriber, the patient, and society. To achieve successful outcomes, five categories are proposed to ensure quality care. These are assessment of the pain complaint, patient

TABLE 16-1. Barriers to the Appropriate Treatment of Non–Cancer-Related Pain

Fear of addiction when using opioids
Legal obstacles and fear of regulatory agency sanctions (especially when using opioids)
Fear of side effects of medications
Ignorance of proper assessment of pain
Lack of appropriate education in pain management
Beliefs in how "proper" patients should respond (i.e., the "good patient")
Ignorance of pain physiology
Failure to identify pain relief as a priority
Failure of the health care system to hold clinicians, physicians, and others accountable for pain relief
Cost constraints and inadequate insurance coverage
Patient reluctance to take medications

Data from References 11-19.

evaluation for comorbidities, treatment initiation, scheduled medication management, and prescriber improvement.

As a first step in considering opioid therapy for patients with non–cancer-related pain, a complete history should be obtained and comprehensive physical examination performed focused on the pain complaint.[23,24] This full patient assessment and evaluation must be completed on the first visit because it sets the stage for everything that follows. The history should establish the most consistent diagnosis for pain generation, and the physical examination helps support that diagnosis. It is recommended that a prescriber use a diagram of the body, front and back, head to toe, to diagram the pain complaints and number them. This provides a logical approach to each of the problems. Although this first evaluation is time-intensive, the time spent will be more than recovered in future visits.

Before leaving the issue of patient assessment, it is important to remember that simply conducting an evaluation is not enough. Documentation of the assessment is crucial. Indeed, documentation is one of the major weaknesses of prescribers who have problems with regulatory boards or federal agencies.[25] The prescriber who is interested in treating chronic pain should document in detail all correspondence with the patient and patient visits. Also, obtaining a record of previous treatments and treating prescribers is critical. Although old records may be difficult to obtain, reasonable attempts should be made. These records can establish patterns of treatment, suggest potential problems with and for the patient, and suggest previous successful strategies. Additionally, they can identify patterns of behavior that may or may not suggest risks. Patients may bring in old records; frequently this is done in an effort to help the prescriber. However, this should not be the only set of records to be obtained. Efforts to get original records can be useful, because comparison of these two sets of records can be illustrative of the trustworthiness of the patient.

The second principle to keep in mind when considering opioid therapy is to perform a patient evaluation for comorbidities. Patients with chronic pain frequently have multiple comorbidities. Obstructive sleep apnea may be more common, especially in patients on long-term opioid therapy.[26] In addition, insomnia and sleep disturbance are common and endocrinopathy patterns, such as thyroid dysfunction, are being identified that can play a role in exacerbating or initiating chronic pain.

The third principle concerns the initiation of treatment with an opioid analgesic. As a first step, we must remember that informed consent is necessary because it is the foundation by which we engage in any therapy. Patients need to know the risks and potential benefits, and this is no less true with scheduled medications. Also, when starting a controlled substance, patients should be strongly encouraged to obtain their scheduled medications from a single pharmacy.[27] Communication with a local pharmacist is a critical component in monitoring patients and opioid usage, especially if the state does not have a prescription monitoring program in place. When deciding on an opioid agent for a patient, long-acting opioids should be considered when possible. Although data to support this notion are conflicting, the use of short-acting agents in animals has been shown to create micro-withdrawal events at the trough of their serum levels, which might increase pain in humans.[28] Finally, before initiation of opioid therapy, a risk assessment should be performed. Various screening tools have appeared in the literature in the past few years to aid in risk stratification. Choosing which tools to use can be daunting; however, a recent review conducted a thorough comparison of the tools.[29] Many clinicians find the Opioid Risk Tool to be useful when brevity is needed and the Screener and Opioid Assessment for Patients with Pain (SOAPP) to be good a choice for a slightly longer tool to implement in clinical practice.[30–32]

The fourth principle involves treatment maintenance. It is recommended that the 4 A's— analgesia, activities of daily living, adverse side effects, and potentially aberrant behaviors—should be assessed at every visit.[33] A charting tool has been created to help in this regard, but simple documentation around these areas will suffice.[34] In addition, patient goals should be identified and followed. What does the patient want to achieve? All patients with chronic pain want "less pain," but pain patients are also expected to become more functional. Although other patients (e.g., a patient with diabetes) are not held to a similar need to show improved function, this is a laudable and important goal. Further, if a patient is placed on a scheduled medication and there is no improvement in the patient's pain levels, quality of life, or function, the treatment should be modified or even discontinued. Finally, patients should be seen regularly for follow-up, which, although a provision of many states regulatory boards, is never defined well.[35] New patients should likely be seen on a monthly basis, whereas more established patients with minimal risk factors can be seen every 2 to 3 months.

Additional safeguards should be employed at various times during treatment maintenance, although not required at every visit. The first is the implementation of urine drug screens. Urine drug screen results are important because they may offer information that the patient is positive for illicit substances or negative for prescribed opioids (a potential sign of diversion). Studies have shown that approximately 29% of urine drug tests are positive in patients who show no visible physical signs of abuse or aberrant behaviors.[36] Pill or patch counts should also be used because they give an estimate of patient compliance and should always be done in front of the patient and with a witness. The pills should be counted twice and the patient, physician, and witness should sign a form indicating how many pills were present. This documentation should be in the permanent patient record. Also, if available, prescription monitoring program reports should be used to review whether the patient has been engaging in doctor shopping activities (i.e., obtaining multiple prescriptions for controlled substances from multiples providers). It is still not clear if prescription monitoring programs have a significant impact on diversion, but they do represent a standard of care in states where they exist and therefore should be used.

As a final principle, it is necessary that all prescribers consider engaging in ongoing efforts to improve their knowledge base and familiarity with opioid medications. Prescribers should not be afraid to get a second opinion on a patient. This helps to establish due diligence in prescribing, and the outside consultation helps document the treatment regimen and goals of therapy. Prescribers should also consider obtaining specific pain education and certifications. Training in the treatment of chronic pain is easy to obtain and should be part of a primary care physician's continuing education. Prescribers should also be familiar with the pain literature and continue to read journals in this specialty. Keeping up with the knowledge base is critical in proper diagnosis and treatment.

RELEVANT PATHOPHYSIOLOGY

When thinking about whether opioid analgesics should be considered for use in non–cancer-related pain, it is important to ask a more fundamental question regarding what differences actually exist in the generation of pain complaints. To this end, if the pain generator is different or works through a different mechanism, perhaps the opioid class simply would not be an appropriate choice in regard to pathways and targets for treatments and intervention. The short answer to this query, however, is that there is "nothing inherently unique about the mechanisms involved in the production of the nociception."[37] Therefore we are left with a distinction that is largely dependent on other factors, such as psychosocial issues and our own personalization of issues as more or less worthy of clinical intervention attention.

SUMMARY OF EVIDENCE REGARDING TREATMENT RECOMMENDATIONS

Although many recommendations have been made in regard to how long-term management for non–cancer-related pain should be conducted, the reality is that much of the extant evidence is either at a rather low level of complexity or altogether lacking. For example, it has often been recommended that management of chronic non–cancer-related pain include treatment contingencies for failures on medication trials, that multimodal therapy be used, that longer acting medications be used for an around-the-clock strategy, and that clinicians always have an exit strategy for reevaluating and discontinuing medication trials that have suboptimal results.[38] However, when looking at the evidence base for these recommendations, we have rarely gone past the "good idea" level of evidence.

It has been postulated that we should obtain informed consent for pain management efforts. This should include a discussion about long-term goals and risks involved in opioid therapy. In recent reviews, this notion has been rated as having a strong recommendation but rather low-quality evidence. Similarly, going past informed consent to include a written agreement (formerly discussed as "contracts") to define the expectations and responsibilities of both the patient and the provider has been rated with a weak recommendation and overall low-quality evidence.[38,39]

When it comes to treating high-risk patients with non–cancer-related pain with opioids, a good deal of common wisdom exists. For example, it is often stated that high-risk patients (e.g., a history of drug abuse, psychiatric issues, other aberrant drug-taking behaviors) can be treated with opioid medications only if they can be monitored more frequently and in a stringent fashion. This would include, for example, use of frequent urine drug screens, pill and patch counts, more frequent patient contact, and referral to a mental health professional. Further, common wisdom dictates that patients engaging in ongoing aberrant behaviors or otherwise showing themselves to have intractable behaviors or no apparent benefit from opioids should be tapered or weaned from their medication trial. Although this all seems appropriate, the fact remains that reviews have given these ideas a strong recommendation while acknowledging that currently we only have low-quality evidence. Other ideas, such as rotating a patient's opioid medication as the dose escalates, have been proposed to carry a weak recommendation and low-quality evidence.[38,39]

KEY MESSAGES TO PATIENTS AND FAMILIES

Over the course of 15 to 20 years a dramatic expansion has occurred in the prescribing of opioids that began in cancer pain management and has been applied to the much more diverse population of those with non–cancer-related pain. This has generally been a positive development, with those in pain having unprecedented access to opioids and other controlled substances. However, along with the growing public health problem of poorly treated chronic pain, a dramatic upsurge in abuse, addiction, diversion, and overdose has occurred. Therefore a major paradigm shift in opioid therapy for non–cancer-related pain has occurred. The field has moved from an essentially "all low risk model," in which patients are given latitude to self-titrate much like those with cancer, to an approach that begins with risk stratification and then matches the management to risk level. The risk transcends the patients, to include those in their environment that might seek access to their medications for abuse and diversion (see the discussion of diversion in Chapter 17). Therefore highly structured management includes maneuvers foreign to many patients, such as agreements, monitoring techniques, and an insistence on agreeing to multimodal therapies, which is now the rule rather than the exception. Patient messaging then has to prepare patients for this paradigm, anticipate their concerns, and find ways to help them understand the empowerment and protection this affords the compliant patient and the early detection of problems of nonadherence in those who may have (anticipated or unanticipated) problems in this domain. The latter is particularly important; in the setting of incorrect media messages about the addiction liability of mere exposure to pain medications, the careful practitioner can reassure concerned patients with appropriate techniques for early detection of problems.

CONCLUSION AND SUMMARY

The treatment of non–cancer-related pain with opioid therapy is likely to remain a controversial topic for some time. The answer is not to forgo prescribing opioids for chronic pain but rather to be educated in the use of these medications while not hindering the moral imperative to alleviate suffering. The current science and evidence base have a great deal of room for improvement, but in the meantime it is important to ameliorate patient suffering. To this end, although we "lack good data... we cannot delay treatment until the answers are in."[40]

SUMMARY RECOMMENDATIONS

- All opioid therapy should begin with risk assessment and stratification without making assumptions about risk on the part of the practitioner.
- When the decision to embark an opioid trial has been made, the next decision is equally important—how should opioid therapy be delivered to this patient to ensure safety and compliance?
- The opioid trial management often necessitates maneuvers that are foreign to many patients; therefore efforts to inform, educate, empower, and not infantilize patients should be a priority.

REFERENCES

1. Loeser JD. Opiophobia and opiophilia. In: Meldrum ML, ed. *Opioids and Pain Relief: A Historical Perspective—Progress in Pain Research and Management*, vol. 25. Seattle, WA: IASP Press; 2003:1–4.
2. Fishman SM, Papazian JS, Gonzalez S, Riches PS, Gilson A. Regulating opioid prescribing through prescription monitoring programs: balancing drug diversion and treatment of pain. *Pain Med*. 2004;5:309–324.
3. Chu LF, Angst MS, Clark D. Opioid-induced hyperalgesia in humans. *Clin J Pain*. 2008;24:479–496.
4. Gureje O, Von Korff M, Simon GE, Gater R. Persistent pain and well-being: A World Health Organization study in primary care. *JAMA*. 1998;280:147–151.
5. Stewart WF, Ricci JA, Chee E, Lipton R. Work-related cost of pain in the United States: results from the American Productivity Audit-Abstracts from the tenth World Congress of Pain. 2002. Seattle, WA: IASP Press; 2002:224.
6. Stewart WF, Ricci JA, Chee E, Morganstein D, Lipton R. Lost productive time and cost due to common pain conditions in the US workforce. *JAMA*. 2003;290:2443–2545.
7. Ferrell BR. The cost of comfort: economics of pain management in oncology. *Oncol Econ*. 2000;1:56–61.
8. Portenoy RK. Issues in the economic analysis of therapies for cancer pain. *Oncology*. 1995;9(suppl):71–78.
9. Nelson R. Decade of pain control and research gets into gear in USA. *Lancet*. 2003;362:1129.
10. Max MB. How to move pain and symptom research from the margin to the mainstream. *J Pain*. 2003;4:355–360.
11. Ferrell BR, Cronin Nash C, Warfield C. The role of patient-controlled analgesia in the management of cancer pain. *J Pain Symptom Manage*. 1992;7:149–154.
12. Hoffmann DE. Pain management and palliative care in the era of managed care: issues for health insurers. *J Law Med Ethics*. 1998;26:267–289.
13. Cleeland CS, Gonin R, Hatfield AK, et al. Pain and its treatment in outpatients with metastatic cancer. *N Engl J Med*. 1994;330:592–596.
14. Grossman SA, Sheidler VR, Swedeen K, Mucenski J, Piantadosi S. Correlation of patient and caregiver ratings of cancer pain. *J Pain Symptom Manage*. 1991;6:53–57.
15. Hoffmann DE. Pain management and palliative care in the era of managed care: issues for health insurers. *J Law Med Ethics*. 1998;26:267–289.
16. Proulx K, Jacelon C. Dying with dignity: the good patient versus the good death. *Am J Hosp Palliat Care*. 2004;21:116–120.
17. Moseley L. Unraveling the barriers to reconceptualization of the problem in chronic pain: the actual and perceived ability of patients and health professionals to understand the neurophysiology. *J Pain*. 2003;4:184–189.
18. Ferrell BR. The role of ethics committees in responding to the moral outrage of unrelieved pain. *Bioethics Forum*. 1997;13:11–16.
19. Dar R, Beach CM, Barden PL, Cleeland CS. Cancer pain in the marital system: a study of patients and their spouses. *J Pain Symptom Manage*. 1992;7:87–93.
20. Rich BA. An ethical analysis of the barriers to effective pain management. *Camb Q Healthc Ethics*. 2000;9:54–70.
21. Peppin JF. Bioethics and Pain. In: Boswell MV, Cole BE, eds. *Weiner's Pain Management: A Practical Guide for Clinicians*. 7th ed. Boca Raton, FL: CRC Press; 2005:1377–1392.
22. Peppin JF. The marginalization of chronic pain patients on chronic opioid therapy. *Pain Physician*. 2009;12:493–498.
23. Gourlay DL, Heit HA, Almahrezi A. Universal precautions in pain medicine: a rational approach to the treatment of chronic pain. *Pain Med*. 2005;6:107–112.
24. Gourlay D, Heit H. Universal precautions: a matter of mutual trust and responsibility. *Pain Med*. 2006;7:210–211.
25. Bovbjerg RR, Aliago P, Gittler J, et al. *State Discipline of Physicians: Assessing State Medical Boards Through Case Studies*. Washington, DC: U.S. Department of Health and Human Services; February, 2006.
26. Webster LR, Choi Y, Desai H, et al. Sleep-disordered breathing and chronic opioid therapy. *Pain Med*. 2008;9(4):425–432.
27. Strickland JM, Huskey A, Brushwood DB. Pharmacist-physician collaboration in pain management practice. *J Opioid Manag*. 2007;3:295–301.

28. Cooper ZD, Truong YN, Shi YG, Woods JH. Morphine depriva-tion increases self-administration of the fast- and short-acting mu-opioid receptor agonist remifentanil in the rat. *J Pharmacol Exp Ther.* 2008;326:920–929.
29. Passik SD, Kirsh KL, Casper D. Addiction-related assess-ment tools and pain management: Instruments for screening, treatment planning, and monitoring compliance. *Pain Med.* 2008;99(suppl 2):S145–S166.
30. Akbik H, Butler SF, Budman SH, Fernandez K, Katz NP, Jamison RN. Validation and clinical application of the Screener and Opioid Assessment for Patients with Pain (SOAPP). *J Pain Symptom Manage.* 2006;32:287–293.
31. Butler SF, Budman SH, Fernandez K, Jamison RN. Validation of a screener and opioid assessment measure for patients with chronic pain. *Pain.* 2004;112:65–75.
32. Webster LR, Webster RM. Predicting aberrant behaviors in opioid-treated patients: preliminary validation of the Opioid Risk Tool. *Pain Med.* 2005;6:432–442.
33. Passik SD, Kirsh KL, Whitcomb L, et al. A new tool to assess and document pain outcomes in chronic pain patients receiv-ing opioid therapy. *Clin Ther.* 2004;26:552–561.
34. Passik SD, Kirsh KL, Whitcomb L, et al. Monitoring outcomes during long-term opioid therapy for noncancer pain: results with the Pain Assessment and Documentation Tool. *J Opioid Manag.* 2005;1:257–266.
35. Gilson AM, Maurer MA, Joranson DE. State medical board mem-bers' beliefs about pain, addiction and diversion and abuse: a changing regulatory environment. *J Pain.* 2007;8:682–691.
36. Katz NP, Sherburne S, Beach M, et al. Behavioral monitoring and urine toxicology testing in patients receiving long-term opioid therapy. *Anesth Analg.* 2003;97:1097–1102.
37. Turk DC. Remember the distinction between malignant and benign pain? Well, forget it. *Clin J Pain.* 2002;18(2):75–76.
38. Chou R, Fanciullo GJ, Fine PG, et al. Clinical guidelines for the use of chronic opioid therapy in chronic noncancer pain. *J Pain.* 2009;10(2):113–130.
39. Fine PG, Finnegan T, Portenoy RK. Protect your patients, pro-tect your practice: practical risk assessment in the structur-ing of opioid therapy in chronic pain. *J Fam Pract.* 2010;59(9): (suppl 2) S1–S16 .
40. Covington EC. Opioiphobia, opiophilia, opioagnosia. *Pain Med.* 2000;1:217–223.

What Approaches Should Be Used to Minimize Opioid Diversion and Abuse in Palliative Care?

STEVEN D. PASSIK AND KENNETH L. KIRSH

INTRODUCTION AND SCOPE OF THE PROBLEM

The abuse of prescription medications, particularly opioids, has increased over the last decade to a level that some have described as epidemic.[1,2] At the same time, chronic pain has remained a serious public health concern whose treatment may be hampered by prescribers' fear of diversion and abuse of scheduled medications and the regulatory scrutiny that may follow.[3–6] Further, a growing illicit market operates in the diversion and sale of these drugs and misuse of these medications has led to overdose and death. Deaths from the nonmedical use of prescription opioid medications have increased dramatically over the last decade,[7] and as opioid-related overdose deaths have increased, so too has public outcry.

What do these issues mean with regard to patients in palliative care settings? Unfortunately, there is still a problem of undertreating pain in these patients.[8] In one advanced disease type, cancer, it has been reported that approximately 40% to 50% of patients with metastatic disease and 90% of patients with terminal cancer or other advanced diseases experience unrelieved pain.[9–11] Furthermore, inadequate treatment of cancer pain is an even greater possibility if the patient is a member of an ethnic minority, female, elderly, a child, or a substance abuser.[12]

Home Hospice and Palliative Care

Hospice and palliative care is as important part of many communities and can bring great comfort to patients with serious illness and their families and loved ones. This is also a cost-effective option for reducing health care disparities in medically underserved areas. Although not specific to rural and underserved areas, the study by Serra-Prat and colleagues[13] examined the effects of home-based palliative care service on patients. In their study, patients treated using the services of the home-based palliative care model were compared to patients receiving standard of care. They found that patients receiving home-based care had fewer emergency department and outpatient visits and had shorter length of hospital stays. This resulted in a net savings of 71% compared to costs in the patients receiving standard of care only. Similarly, Brumley and colleagues[14] documented a total cost savings of 45% for palliative care as opposed to patients receiving standard of care. DiCosimo and colleagues[15] realized similar savings in a study of an Italian-based patient population of patients and Burke[16] in patients in England. Even when more expensive home technologies are employed (e.g., in-home infusion therapies), Witteveen and colleagues[17] demonstrated savings of $8000 per patient compared to a similar length hospital stay.

Pain management is an essential aspect of care in the dying patient.[18] Across the United States, hospice organizations have taken an active role in reducing pain and improving the quality of life of dying people. For most patients receiving hospice care, pain management proceeds in an uneventful fashion where issues of drug addiction or diversion are concerned. However, in some cases, when patients or their family members have preexisting substance abuse problems, management becomes more difficult and complex. Hospice and palliative care professionals struggle disproportionately with this small percentage of patients. Given the high prevalence of addiction in our society in general and the rising tide of prescription drug abuse and diversion in particular, palliative care professionals responsible for case management must be attentive to signs indicating problems with substance abuse or drug diversion and develop case management strategies for coping with these challenges.

Substance Abuse in Hospice and Palliative Care

Aggressive treatment of pain in patients in hospice care is sometimes hampered by misplaced fears of addiction. These fears on the part of patients and families are often the primary barriers to pain management.[19] Although most fears of addiction are misplaced, in some patients and families, a history of drug or alcohol abuse makes these concerns a reality. Addiction is a common problem in our society, and prescription drug abuse has been on the rise.[20] Aggressive pain management in hospice can sometimes be complicated by the presence of addiction in the patient or family members, and although these cases represent a minority, they are labor-intensive and emotionally draining, raising difficult clinical and ethical dilemmas.[21] Very little empirical study has been done on this issue, although clinical experience suggests it is no less common than might be expected based on the norms of drug abuse in the population at large.

In the small number of empirical studies related to this issue, substance abuse and misuse among patients admitted to hospice units is not uncommon and is often missed in both initial assessments and longer term follow-up. A survey conducted by Bruera and colleagues[22] found that more than 25% of patients with cancer admitted to a palliative care unit had a problem with alcohol abuse. However, only one third of the patients with alcohol abuse had a documented diagnosis of alcoholism in their charts, even though all of these patients had undergone numerous hospital admissions and medical interventions. Other patients in hospice and palliative care settings may develop psychiatric conditions related to end-of-life issues, with still others having preexisting psychiatric disorders. These patients also may be at increased risk for abusing and misusing prescribed medication. Such patients have been referred to as "chemical copers,"[22,23] and their patterns of drug use are problematic at times, leading to overmedication and poor outcomes.

Little doubt exists that substance abuse–related issues make case management more difficult. Adequate pain control is more difficult to obtain and maintain when patients are abusing substances.[24] In addition, families with substance abuse problems tend to have poorer coping skills and more chaotic home environments than families without these problems.[25,26] To further complicate the situation, hospice and palliative care involve more than the identified patient. Friends and family members are also intimately involved in end-of-life care, and they also have the opportunity to engage in misuse or diversion of the patient's prescribed medication. Because hospice and palliative care occur within the context of the family and community, chaotic, dysfunctional family behavior can have a serious impact on patient management. Some dying patients will have family members who are substance abusers, who are psychiatrically ill, or who have criminal histories.

Unchecked substance abuse perpetuates a dying patient's suffering, while complicating symptom management, impeding diagnosis and treatment of psychiatric problems, and creating tension for an already fragile social support network of family and caregivers.[27]

Counseling, medication, and pain and symptom management techniques that are not beyond the scope of routine clinical practice can be used to successfully provide supportive care that patients and their caregivers need to allow for desired outcomes in end-of-life care.

Some clinicians and nurses fail to appreciate the deleterious impact of addiction on palliative care efforts, whereas others view addiction as an intractable problem for which interventions are likely to fail in any case. Furthermore, some of these clinicians may not only believe that is it impossible to successfully decrease a patient's use of alcohol or illicit substance while in palliative care but may also erroneously believe that such a decrease is tantamount to depriving a dying patient of a source of pleasure.[27] In fact, chemically dependent patients spend very little of their time high or euphoric, even when engaging in substance use. Instead, the majority of their time is spent feeling depressed, isolated, and withdrawn or engaging in behaviors they consider demeaning or degrading, particularly those related to drug procurement. Indeed, what is so mystifying about addiction is the tenacity of behaviors that are so infrequently and inconsistently rewarded. The typical mental state of the chemically dependent individual is rarely one of euphoria; instead, it is more often a global state of unpleasantness, boredom, and loneliness. This suffering is no less a legitimate target of hospice and palliative care intervention than any other form simply because it is at the patient's (or family's) own hand. The nihilism that sometimes characterizes the approach to this problem may simply lead to more unchecked abuse-related behavior and perpetuation of suffering.

Drug Diversion in Hospice and Palliative Care

Anecdotal evidence suggests that diversion occurs in at least some hospice and palliative care cases,[28,29] but there are no empirical studies on this issue. Pain medications can be diverted for several reasons. Some family members may have a preexisting substance abuse disorder and may abuse the medication prescribed to the patient for pain relief. Some anecdotal evidence suggests that family members or caregivers may use the patient's pain medication to deal with the stress of coping with the illness. In other situations, the patient or the patient's family may divert the drugs by selling them or allowing them to be sold on the street to provide funds for basic needs. Until basic data on drug diversion associated with hospice patients is gathered, the severity and the scope of the problem remain unknown.

The relative monetary value of prescription drugs is also an unavoidable issue. Diversion of prescription drugs can provide patients and their families extra funds at a stressful time. Monies obtained through illicit sales of prescription drugs can improve patient quality of life by providing needed goods and services that might be otherwise unavailable or by allowing the patient or the family access to luxuries typically inaccessible to them. Unfortunately, because of the widespread problem of addiction and prescription drug abuse, pain medications typically prescribed to hospice patients are easily converted to cash in most communities in the United States. Pain medications may represent unexpected resources some patients and families are unable to resist exploiting. The phenomenon of the "patient dealer," new in drug abuse and diversion circles over the past few years, is noted to have begun in Maine with a woman with advanced cancer selling her medications.[30]

Establishing Definitions of Abuse and Addiction for Advanced Illness

Identification of recommendations for managing abuse and diversion necessitates defining these key terms in the context of palliative care. An appropriate definition of addiction exemplifies that it is a chronic disorder characterized by "the compulsive use of a substance resulting in physical, psychological, or social harm to the user and continued use despite the harm."[31] Although this definition is not without fault, it emphasizes that addiction is essentially a psychological and behavioral syndrome.[32,33]

A differential diagnosis should also be considered if questionable behaviors occur during pain treatment. A true addiction (substance dependence) is only one of many possible interpretations. A diagnosis of pseudoaddiction should also be taken into account if the patient reports distress associated with unrelieved symptoms.[34] Impulsive drug use may also be indicative of another psychiatric disorder, diagnosis of which may have therapeutic implications. On occasion, aberrant drug-related behaviors appear to be causally remotely related to a mild encephalopathy, with perplexity concerning the appropriate therapeutic regimen. On rare occasions, questionable behaviors imply criminal intent. These diagnoses are not mutually exclusive.[32,33]

Varied and repeated observations over time may be necessary to categorize questionable behaviors properly. Perceptive psychiatric assessment is crucial and may require evaluation by consultants who can elucidate the complex interactions among personality factors and psychiatric illness. Some patients may be self-medicating symptoms of anxiety or depression, insomnia, or problems of adjustment (e.g., boredom resulting from decreased ability to engage in usual activities and hobbies). Yet others may have character pathology that may be the more prominent determinant of drug-taking behavior. Patients with borderline personality disorders, for example, may use prescription medications in an impulsive manner that regulates inner tension; expresses anger at physicians, friends, or family; or improves the chronic emptiness of boredom. Psychiatric assessment is vitally important for both the population without a prior history of substance abuse and the popula-

tion of known substance abusers who have a high incidence of psychiatric comorbidity.[35]

General Guidelines

Recommendations for long-term administration of potential medications of abuse, such as opioids, to patients at risk for substance abuse or diversion are based exclusively on clinical experience. Research is needed to ascertain the most effective strategies and to empirically identify patient subgroups that may be most responsive to different approaches. Pain and symptom management is often complicated by various medical, psychosocial, and administrative issues in the population of patients with a substance use disorder. The most effective team may include a physician with expertise in pain or palliative care, nurses, social workers, and, when possible, a mental health care provider with expertise in the area of addiction medicine.[32,36]

As a first step, it is important to conduct a good substance use history. In an effort to not offend, threaten, or anger patients, clinicians many times avoid asking patients about drug abuse. There is also often the expectation that patients will not answer truthfully. However, obtaining a detailed history of duration, frequency, and desired effect of drug use is vital. Adopting a nonjudgmental position and communicating in an empathetic and truthful manner is the best strategy when taking a patient substance use history.[33,36]

A gradual approach and style for the interview can be beneficial in slowly introducing the assessment of drug abuse. This approach begins with broad and general inquires regarding the role of drugs in the patient's life, such as caffeine and nicotine, and gradually proceeds to more specific questions regarding illicit drugs. This interview style can also assist in discerning any coexisting psychiatric disorders, which can significantly contribute to aberrant drug-taking behavior. When identified, treatment of comorbid psychiatric disorders can greatly enhance management strategies and decrease the risk for relapse.[33,36]

When deciding on a pain regimen for a patient in palliative care who has pain and is at risk for abuse issues, long-acting opioid medications should be considered. The use of long-acting analgesics in sufficient amounts may assist in minimizing the number of rescue doses needed, theoretically lessen cravings, and decrease the risk for abuse of prescribed medications, given the possible difficulty in using short-acting formulations in patients with substance use histories. Rather than being overly concerned regarding the choice of drug or route of administration, the prescribing of opioids and other drugs of potential abuse should be done in a setting of limits and guidelines.[33,36]

As an ongoing monitoring technique, frequent visits and regular assessments of significant others who can contribute information regarding the patient's drug use may be required. It may also be necessary to have patients who have been actively abusing drugs in the recent past to submit urine specimens for regular screening of illicit or licit but unprescribed drugs to promote early recognition of aberrant drug-related behaviors. In informing the patient of this approach, it should be explained as a method of monitoring that can reassure the clinician and provide a foundation for aggressive symptom-oriented treatment, thus enhancing the therapeutic alliance with the patient.[33,36]

Many nondrug approaches can be used to assist patients in coping with chronic pain in advanced illness. Such educational interventions may include relaxation techniques, ways of thinking and describing the experience of pain, and methods of communicating physical and emotional distress to staff members. Although nondrug interventions may be helpful adjuvants to management, they should not be perceived as substitutes for drugs targeted at treating pain or other physical or psychological symptoms.[33,36]

Written agreements that clearly state the roles of the team members and the rules and expectations for the patient are helpful when structuring outpatient treatment. While using the patient's behaviors as the basis for the level of restrictions, graded agreements should be enforced that clearly state the consequences of aberrant drug use.[33,36] In addition to adding a written agreement to the treatment plan, it may be advisable for at-risk patients to be seen more frequently. Frequent visits allow the opportunity of prescribing small quantities of drugs, which may decrease the temptation to divert and provide a motive for keeping appointments.[33,36]

As a final note, the clinician should involve family members and friends in the treatment plan. These meetings will not only allow the clinician and other team members to become familiar with the family but will also assist the team to identify family members who are using illicit drugs. Referral of these identified family members to drug treatment can be offered and portrayed as a manner of gathering support for the patient. The patient should also be prepared to cope with family members or friends who may attempt to buy or sell the patient's medications. These meetings will also assist the team to identify dependable individuals who can serve as a source of strength and support for the patient during treatment.[33,36]

RELEVANT PATHOPHYSIOLOGY

Substance use disorders are a consistent phenomenon in the United States, with estimated base rates of 6% to 15%.[37–40] The prevalence of drug abuse certainly touches medically ill patients and can negatively influence the manner in which pain is treated. Given the relative paucity of data specific to palliative care, the base rates can be assumed to be at least close to the national average. Therefore this is a significant problem worthy of consideration in palliative care treatment efforts.

SUMMARY OF EVIDENCE REGARDING TREATMENT RECOMMENDATIONS

Given that few data are available on the incidence and prevalence of diversion and abuse in patients in palliative care, many of the treatment recommendations for managing these issues are minimal or nonexistent. In the field of non–cancer-related pain, which has a greater awareness of these issues, a relative lack of data exists, as well as a general acknowledgment that risk management efforts may have strong recommendations but almost all of them have weak levels of evidence.[41,42]

KEY MESSAGES TO PATIENTS AND FAMILIES

Nonmedical use of opioids often seems innocent enough. Well-intentioned sharing of medications of every variety is generally thought to be a benevolent act by patients and families. Someone having a stressful day or having just learned of bad news might be the recipient of a benzodiazepine by a concerned family member or friend; someone traveling on a long flight might borrow a sleep aid; a student facing finals might share a friend's stimulant medications to get through an "all-nighter"; or someone with a new or even simply temporarily worsened pain, might be offered an opioid. For some, these actions might be innocent and helpful, but patients and families must realize that for other, more vulnerable recipients it could the beginning of a long and slippery decent into addiction. Are those sharing medications aware of the risks to the recipient despite their good intentions? It seems as though most are not, and this necessitates a more absolute message of never sharing these medications.

Furthermore, patients are not always aware of the street value and other attractions of their medications to their relatives, their friends, and even people servicing their homes. Thus it is the responsibility of every patient to secure the controlled substances in their home. If individuals in society are unable to each take responsibility for their pain medications and stem the tide of abuse and diversion, the entire future of the availability of pain medications to people who need them is in jeopardy. Patients must secure their controlled substances, understand their responsibility for them differs from that for noncontrolled pain medications (e.g., people generally leave ibuprofen on a countertop), and inventory them so that they will know if any are taken.

In some instances, for example, with low-risk patients, messaging might end with these admonitions against sharing and cautions regarding storage. However, for those with histories of drug abuse or who maintain contact with people who might want to borrow, buy, or trade for their medications, the role of urine screening and other forms of monitoring are essential and must be explained to patients. In the authors' practices, cases of elder abuse have been uncovered in which the older patient tested negative for prescribed pain medications, only to then reluctantly admit that they were being stolen by family and that the patient had been threatened to keep reporting pain to maintain the supply. Other patients with drug abuse might test negative for their prescribed medication and positive for cocaine, having traded the former for the latter. Thus patients should be alerted to the fact that monitoring for adherence is a safeguard for them and that problems in this arena that might reflect diversion will be discovered, discussed, and managed.

CONCLUSION AND SUMMARY

Treating patients who are experiencing chronic pain from advanced illness and a substance use disorder or who may be diverting medications is challenging because these issues can significantly complicate each other. Using a treatment plan that involves a team approach that recognizes and responds to these complex needs is the optimum strategy to facilitate treatment. Although pain management may continue to be challenging, even when all treatment plan procedures are implemented, the health care team's goal should be the highest level of pain management for all patients in the palliative care setting.

SUMMARY RECOMMENDATIONS

- Clinicians should never ignore the potential for drug diversion in any setting in which pain management with controlled substances is being practiced.
- A range of monitoring and management techniques can limit diversion and should be applied appropriately in response to risk stratification and assessment.
- All patients should be educated about the importance of not sharing medications, maintaining safe storage techniques for controlled substances, and monitoring inventory of medications.

REFERENCES

1. Manchikanti L. Prescription drug abuse: what is being done to address this new drug epidemic? Testimony before the Subcommittee on Criminal Justice, Drug Policy and Human Resources. *Pain Physician.* 2006;9:287–321.
2. National Center on Addiction and Substance Abuse. Controlled prescription drug abuse at epidemic level. *J Pain Palliat Care Pharmacother.* 2006;20:61–64.
3. Passik SD, Heit H, Kirsh KL. Reality and responsibility: a commentary on the treatment of pain and suffering in a drug-using society. *J Opioid Manag.* 2006;2:123–127.
4. Hertz JA, Knight JR. Prescription drug misuse: a growing national problem. *Adolesc Med Clin.* 2006;17:751–769.
5. Passik SD. Issues in long-term opioid therapy: unmet needs, risks, and solutions. *Mayo Clin Proc.* 2009;84:593–601.
6. Wunsch MJ, Cropsey KL, Campbell ED, Knisely JS. OxyContin use and misuse in three populations: substance abuse patients, pain patients, and criminal justice participants. *J Opioid Manag.* 2008;4:73–79.
7. Wysowski DK. Surveillance of prescription drug-related mortality using death certificate data. *Drug Saf.* 2007;30:533–540.
8. Crane RA, Wilson PC, Behrens G. Pain control in hospice home care: management guidelines. *Am J Hosp Palliat Care.* 1990;7:39–42.
9. Glajchen M, Fitzmartin RD, Blum D, Swanton R. Psychosocial barriers to cancer pain relief. *Cancer Pract.* 1995;3(2):76–82.
10. Ramer L, Richardson JL, Cohen MZ, Bedney C, Danley KL, Judge EA. Multimeasure pain assessment in an ethnically diverse group of patients with cancer. *J Transcult Nurs.* 1999;10(2):94–101.
11. Ward SE, Goldberg N, Miller-McCauley V, et al. Patient-related barriers to management of cancer pain. *Pain.* 1993;52:319–324.
12. Joranson DE, Gilson AM. Policy issues and imperatives in the use of opioids to treat pain in substance abusers. *J Law Med Ethics.* 1994;22(3):215–223.
13. Serra-Prat M, Gallo P, Picaza JM. Home palliative care as a cost-saving alternative: evidence from Catalonia. *Palliat Med.* 2001;15(4):271–278.
14. Brumley RD, Enguidanos S, Cherin DA. Effectiveness of a home-based palliative care program for end-of-life. *J Palliat Med.* 2003;6(5):715–724.
15. Di Cosimo S, Pistillucci G, Ferretti G, et al. Palliative home care and cost savings: encouraging results from Italy. *N Z Med J.* 2003;116(1170):U370.
16. Burke K. Palliative care at home to get further funds if it saves money. *BMJ.* 2004;328:544.
17. Witteveen PO, van Groenestijn MA, Blijham GH, Schrijvers AJ. Use of resources and costs of palliative care with parenteral fluids and analgesics in the home setting for patients with end-stage cancer. *Ann Oncol.* 1999;10(3):161–165.
18. Whitecar PS, Jonas AP, Clasen ME. Managing pain in the dying patient. *Am Fam Physician.* 2000;61(3):755–764.
19. Ward SE, Goldberg N, Miller-McCauley V. Patient-related barriers to management of cancer pain. *Pain.* 1993;52:319–324.
20. U.S. Substance Abuse and Mental Health Administration. *National Household Survey on Drug Abuse.* Baltimore, MD: U.S. Substance Abuse and Mental Health Administration; 2001.
21. Bruera E. Ethical issues in palliative care research. *J Palliat Care.* 1994;10(3):7–9.
22. Bruera E, Moyano J, Seifert L, Fainsinger RL, Hanson J, Suarez-Almazor M. The frequency of alcoholism among patients with pain due to terminal cancer. *J Pain Symptom Manage.* 1995;10:599–604.
23. Kirsh KL, Jass C, Bennett DS, Hagen JE, Passik SD. Initial development of a survey tool to detect issues of chemical coping in chronic pain patients. *Palliat Support Care.* 2007;5:219–226.
24. McCorquodale S, De Faye B, Bruera E. Palliative care rounds: case report: pain control in an alcoholic cancer patient. *J Pain Symptom Manage.* 1993;8:177–180.
25. Cook B, Winokur G. Alcoholism as a family dysfunction. *Psychiatr Ann.* 1993;23:508–512.
26. Mansky P. Reminiscence of an addictionologist: thought of a researcher and clinician. *Psychiatr Q.* 1993;64:81–106.
27. Passik SD, Theobald DE. Managing addiction in advanced cancer patients: why bother? *J Pain Symptom Manage.* 2000;19:229–234.
28. Schaum M, Schaum A. Hospices: medical and legal considerations. *Leg Med.* 1985;297–322.
29. Thornton ES. Possible diversion of pain medication occurs in home hospice setting. *Oncol Nurs Forum.* 1996;23:118.
30. Hancock CM. OxyContin use and abuse. *Clin J Oncol Nurs.* 2002;6(2):109.
31. Rinaldi RC, Steindler EM, Wilford BB. Clarification and standardization of substance abuse terminology. *JAMA.* 1988;259:555–557.
32. Passik SD, Portenoy RK, Ricketts PL. Substance abuse issues in cancer patients. I. Prevalence and diagnosis. *Oncology.* 1998;12(4):517–521.
33. Passik SD, Portenoy RK. Substance abuse issues in palliative care. In: Berger A, Portenoy R, Weissman D, eds. *Principles and Practice of Supportive Oncology.* Philadelphia: Lippincott-Raven Publishers; 1998:513–524.

34. Passik SD, Webster L, Kirsh KL. Pseudoaddiction revisited: a commentary on clinical and historical considerations. *Pain Manage*. 2011;1:239–248.

35. Khantzian EJ, Treece C. DSM-III psychiatric diagnosis of narcotic addicts. *Arch Gen Psychiatry*. 1985;42:1067–1071.

36. Passik SD, Portenoy RK, Ricketts PL. Substance abuse issues in cancer patients. II, Evaluation and treatment. *Oncology*. 1998;12(5):729–734.

37. Muirhead G. Cultural issues in substance abuse treatment. *Patient Care*. 2000;5:151–159.

38. Gfroerer J, Brodsky M. The incidence of illicit drug use in the United States 1962–1989. *Br J Addict*. 1992;87:1345–1351.

39. Colliver JD, Kopstein AN. Trends in cocaine abuse reflected in emergency room episodes reported to DAWN. *Public Health Rep*. 1991;106:59–68.

40. Regier DA, Myers JK, Kramer M, et al. The NIMH epidemiology catchment area program. *Arch Gen Psychiatry*. 1984;41:934–941.

41. Chou R, Fanciullo GJ, Fine PG, et al. Clinical guidelines for the use of chronic opioid therapy in chronic noncancer pain. *J Pain*. 2009;10(2):113–130.

42. Fine PG, Finnegan T, Portenoy RK. Protect your patients, protect your practice: Practical risk assessment in the structuring of opioid therapy in chronic pain. *J Fam Pract*. 2010;59(9) (suppl 2): S1–S16.

Chapter 18

When Should Epidural or Intrathecal Opioid Infusions and Pumps Be Considered for Pain Management?

Barton T. Bobb and Thomas J. Smith

INTRODUCTION AND SCOPE OF THE PROBLEM

Most patients can achieve satisfactory pain control and tolerable side effects with the standard World Health Organization (WHO) Three-Step Analgesic Pain Ladder. However, some patients simply cannot tolerate pain medications regardless of route, because of sedation or other side effects, or never achieve adequate pain control. The number of patients who do not achieve satisfactory pain control varies from 10% to 20%[1] and is likely to depend on who inquires about the patients' pain, the patients' expectations, and the level of attention paid to side effects.[2]

The use of epidural (alongside the epidural sac, with diffusion into the spinal fluid) and intrathecal (intraspinal, or delivery of the medications directly to the spinal fluid) therapy can be a significant help to patients with unrelieved pain, unsatisfactory side effects, or both.[2] Consider the following case that illustrates the benefit of these systems. L.G. was a 48-year-old woman with progressively worsening pain in her lower back and left pelvis resulting from metastatic adenocarcinoma of unknown primary that was growing in the left psoas muscle. Sustained-release oxycodone 360 mg per day plus ketamine 50 mg by mouth every 6 hours did not control the pain but did induce somnolence. A trial of methadone 120 mg daily plus oxycodone 140 mg every 4 hours also failed to produce adequate analgesia, especially in terms of pain with movement. An epidural trial (placing an epidural for testing of medication effect) was successful (at least 50% reduction in pain scores), with 7 mg per hour of preservative-free morphine and 7 mL per hour of 0.25% bupivacaine. The patient's functional ability also improved. An intrathecal pump was placed with morphine, bupivacaine, and baclofen. After several weeks, clonidine

(α_2-adrenergic agonist) was added to the intrathecal pump in place of the bupivacaine, with excellent pain relief, and an epidural pump with 0.25% bupivacaine was added to target her new specific vertebral erosion pain. Her pain remained well controlled and she died a few weeks later comfortably at home with hospice.

This chapter reviews the indications and data on the effectiveness of epidural and intrathecal therapy; however, discussion of the implantation or management of these pumps is beyond the scope of this text.

RELEVANT PATHOPHYSIOLOGY

Epidural and intrathecal pain medications target nerve conduction pathways in the spinal cord. Intrathecal opioids reduce the release of presynaptic neurotransmitters and inhibit pain impulse transmission by making the nerve membranes in the postsynaptic neurons in the dorsal horn more negative, thus preventing depolarization.[1]

Two main reasons account for the success of this treatment compared to oral, intravenous, or transdermal treatments: the ability to give different classes of drugs for which there is no oral equivalent and the ability to escalate drugs with fewer side effects. The ability to give different and more effective drugs is one of the key advantages of intrathecal treatment, and this delivery system is likely to become even more effective in the future as new analgesic medications are discovered. The local anesthetics are the best example of this therapy; their primary mechanism of action is to prevent nerve conduction (achieve neuronal blockade) by blocking sodium channels, and no effective oral equivalent exists. Table 18-1 lists the main differences between conventional treatments and epidural and intraspinal treatments.

The other main advantage of epidural and intrathecal drug delivery is the ability to escalate doses of opioids, often with the patient having few or no side effects.[3] These opioids can act directly on opioid receptors in the spinal cord without affecting the brain, so 1 mg of intrathecal morphine is equivalent to about 300 mg oral morphine. Conversion ratios of medications from oral or intravenous routes to epidural and intraspinal doses have been recommended by consensus[4]; the commonly accepted conversion ratios are listed in Table 18-2. Of note, no clinical trials

TABLE 18-1. Differences Between Conventional and Epidural and Intraspinal Delivery Routes for Analgesic Medications

DRUG CLASS	CONVENTIONAL	EPIDURAL/INTRASPINAL
Opioids	Available, limited by side effects.	Many available.
α-Adrenergic agonists	Only one drug available, dexmedetomidine; limited by intravenous infusion and cost.[25]	Clonidine is effective and inexpensive.
Local anesthetics	Mexiletine is the only oral agent available; limited[26] or no efficacy[27] in randomized trials.	Bupivacaine and lidocaine-type drugs commonly used.
Calcium channel blockers (e.g., ziconotide)	Oral drugs ineffective for pain relief.	Ziconotide effective.
Muscle relaxants (e.g., baclofen)	Available, limited by side effects and efficacy.	Intrathecal baclofen as third-line option or for spasms.

TABLE 18-2. Conversion Between Conventional and Epidural and Intraspinal Opioid Doses

DOSE	MORPHINE (mg)	HYDROMORPHONE (mg)	SUFENTANIL (mcg)
Oral dose	300	60	Not available
Intravenous dose	100	20	1
Epidural dose	10	2	0.01
Intraspinal dose	1	0.25	0.001

Modified from Krames ES: Intraspinal opioid therapy for chronic nonmalignant pain: current practice and clinical guidelines. *J Pain Symptom Manage.* 1996;11:333-e52; and Kedlaya D, Reynolds L, Waldman S. Epidural and intrathecal analgesia for cancer pain. *Best Pract Res Clin Anaesthesiol.* 2002;16:651-665.

have been conducted comparing the effectiveness of conversion ratios for infused versus oral, intrathecal, and epidural medications, so the ratios currently in use are based on expert consensus. Therefore the clinician should proceed cautiously when converting oral to intrathecal doses and the reverse, because the ratio in some individuals has been demonstrated to be as low as 12:1 as opposed to the more commonly accepted consensus ratio of 300:1.[5]

Placement of Catheters

In epidural delivery of medications, the skin between the 3rd and 4th vertebrae is cleansed and sterilely prepared; then the usual approach is for the anesthesiologist to use a hollow-bore needle to thread a small catheter alongside the epidural sac. Anesthesiologists may "tunnel" the epidural catheter by starting the approach 3 to 4 cm laterally and then taking the epidural catheter out away from the midline; this better anchors the catheter and appears to have a lower incidence of infection.[6] These catheters are connected to external pumps and are suitable for use for weeks or months. The incidence of infection is surprisingly low, although it has been reported in up to 10% patients.[7] Infection is often related to the length of time the patient has had the infusion,[8] and in the authors' experience it has not been a dose-limiting factor.

Intraspinal catheters are placed by neurosurgery under fluoroscopy at most institutions, although they can be placed at the bedside. These catheters tend to be more securely placed than a tunneled epidural catheter and are therefore less likely to fall out, but infection in the intrathecal space is more serious than skin or epidural infection. The amount of opioid required is generally only 10% of the epidural requirement, that is, 1% of systemic requirement if converted directly from systemic use. Finally, several medications (including baclofen and ziconotide) can be given only intrathecally.

Programmable Intrathecal Pump Placement

Should an epidural or intrathecal catheter trial be successful and the patient has a realistic life expectancy of more than 3 months,[9] a programmable pump is an appropriate next step.[10] These pumps usually are placed by neurosurgeons or other trained physicians, with policy varying by institution. The surgery is generally fairly short (approximately 1.5 hours); an incision is made in the spine, where the catheter is inserted; another incision is made in the abdomen, where the pump is placed and secured; and a track for the catheter to run from the back to the abdomen is made with a trocar. Although complications related to intrathecal pump surgery are overall quite rare (<1% of patients), the more serious potential postoperative complications include wound infection, wound hematoma or seroma, meningitis, and cerebrospinal fluid leak, which is often accompanied by a post–dural puncture headache.

A clinical pearl that may be useful is to evaluate the success of the epidural trial by sending the patient home for several days to ensure that the pain is relived with this more invasive delivery system. This allows the clinician to titrate the medications to ensure the best analgesia, rather than only being able to try a single injection of intrathecal morphine. The epidural can be removed at the time the intraspinal drug delivery system is placed. Others use a single injection of preservative-free opioid or local anesthetic and, if pain is relieved, proceed to full treatment, because this is simpler to do in the outpatient setting and has a lower infection risk. A second pearl is to establish a team for the evaluation and management of these patients. This should include clinicians who together can perform the outpatient evaluation, inpatient management, pharmacy conversions and prescriptions, and home health care. Diagramming and planning each step of the process helps ensure success.

Epidural Medications

The following section presents the most commonly used medications and the expected side effects. Of note, all of these medications must be preservative-free.

Opioids. Side effects of epidural opioids may routinely include urinary retention, nausea and vomiting, and pruritus, but respiratory depression, sedation, and constipation also may occur. The starting dose is generally based on a patient's prior daily opioid use and given as a continuous infusion at a dose that is 10% of the patient's prior systemic opioid use per hour (e.g., a patient using 120 mg of intravenous morphine equivalent per day, or 5 mg per hour, could be started on 0.5 mg per hour of epidural morphine). Fentanyl, primarily because of its lipophilic nature, does not act spinally when administered via continuous epidural infusion and is therefore not usually given epidurally for chronic cancer pain[11]; sufentanil can be substituted[1] but is very expensive.

Local Anesthetics. Ropivacaine and bupivacaine are used primarily for continuous infusion. A starting dose is usually 4 mL per hour of low-concentration ropivacaine or bupivacaine. Side effects for all local anesthetics include hypotension, bradycardia and arrhythmia, loss of sensation (potentially even motor blockade, although any nerve damage is usually temporary), seizures, and other central nervous system side effects such as dizziness and altered mental status. Ropivacaine has less incidence of motor block and fewer cardiovascular side effects, but it is significantly more expensive and therefore not used routinely for home epidural or intrathecal purposes.

Clonidine. Clonidine acts as an α_2-receptor adrenergic agonist and can have a synergistic effect if given with opioids. The starting dose is usually around 30 mcg per hour. The most common potential side effects are hypotension, sedation, and bradycardia.

Intrathecal Medications

Although morphine and ziconotide are technically the only Food and Drug Administration–approved medications for intrathecal pain management, a variety of other medications are usually safe, have demonstrated efficacy, are used routinely, and are covered by insurance.[1] All medications used should be preservative-free.

Opioids. Intrathecal opioids are 10 times more potent than opioids administered by the epidural route, and starting doses are adjusted accordingly (e.g., a patient receiving morphine 100 mg per day epidurally would get 10 mg per day by intrathecal delivery). The most common side effects include nausea and vomiting, peripheral edema, sedation, pruritus, and decreasing testosterone levels over time.[12,13] Higher concentrations of morphine and hydromorphone in particular have been associated with increased long-term risk for developing an inflammatory catheter tip mass, called a granuloma.[14] For patients expected to survive longer than a year, it is recommended to try to limit the maximum concentration of morphine to 20 mg per mL and hydromorphone to 10 mg per mL.[14] For patients expected to live less than a year, the concentration of morphine can be compounded up to 50 mg per mL and hydromorphone up to 100 mg per mL.[15]

Bupivacaine. The usual intrathecal starting dose of bupivacaine is 3 to 5 mg per day.[3] This medication is particularly useful for neuropathic pain, either as a single agent or as a second-line agent added to an opioid. The most common side effects include perineal or lower extremity loss of sensation (and potentially even function, which can result in urinary or fecal retention or incontinence and lower extremity weakness) and postural hypotension.

Clonidine. The usual starting dose of intrathecal clonidine is 50 mcg per day; it is usually not given as a single agent in cancer pain.[3] Instead, it is used primarily as a second-line or third-line agent added to help treat refractory nociceptive and neuropathic pain. The most common potential side effects are primarily hypotension, sedation, and edema.

Ziconotide. A novel calcium channel blocker derived from the neurotoxin of the conus magnus sea snail, ziconotide is effective in refractory pain[16]; however, its use is limited by the fairly narrow therapeutic window, short period of stability when mixed with most other drugs, and frequent occurrence of central nervous system side effects.[17] Significant side effects include a variety of nervous system and psychiatric symptoms such as dizziness, altered mental status, depression, hallucinations, abnormal gait, slurred speech, and sedation, but ziconotide can also cause symptoms such as nausea and elevated creatine kinase levels.[14]

Baclofen. Although primarily useful if spasms are a significant symptom, baclofen can help relieve pain through its action as a γ-aminobutyric acid (GABA) agonist. The starting dose is 25 to 50 mcg per day. Side effects include nausea, sedation, and headache. It must also be noted that high-dose baclofen should never be stopped abruptly to avoid potentially severe withdrawal symptoms that can lead to severe injury, seizures, and even death.[14]

Intrathecal Pump Filling and Titration

The refilling process involves accessing the programmable intrathecal pump aseptically using a special refill kit, with a second provider holding the noncoring needle in place to ensure it does not slip out during this process (this would be a potentially cata-strophic scenario that could result in patient death if enough medication was accidentally administered subcutaneously).[18] After removing the remaining fluid from the pump, the pump is slowly filled with the medication from the new syringe that has been prepared in advance (all the while ensuring that all of the medication is actually going into the pump). Most programmable intrathecal pumps have a 40-mL capacity, but some are made to hold only 20 mL of fluid. Most patients with 40-mL pumps usually return for pump refill every 3 to 6 months, depending on the concentration of the medications in the pump.

The next step of the process involves programming the pump, which includes the ability to deliver a differ-ent dose of medication (if requested by the patient), and then printing the old and new pump settings. In the inpatient setting, intrathecal pump increases are sometimes made as often as every 12 hours (versus every 24 hours in an outpatient setting), and the rate routinely can be conservatively increased up to 15% if nonopioids are in the pump and up to 20% if the pump contains only opioids.[3] If the patient has been given a patient therapy manager,[19] the pump can be programmed to deliver an extra dose of medication (i.e., a bolus) at the specific rate and frequency pro-grammed. A general guideline is to give 5% to 10% of the patient's daily dose every 4 to 8 hours as needed (as rapidly as over 10 to 15 minutes with opioid only in the pump and over 40 or more minutes if the pump contains multiple drugs). The sophisticated nature of the pump also enables providers to program varying rates of infusion throughout the day to match fluc-tuating patterns of pain as necessary. A side port on the programmable pump can be accessed to not only withdraw the medication that is in the catheter in the patient's spine but also withdraw cerebrospinal fluid to test for infection.

General contraindications to using intraspinal or intrathecal pumps include patients on anticoagu-lants (because of a concern for spinal hematoma), active infection, and obstruction of cerebrospi-nal fluid flow by metastasis or anatomy. A relative contraindication is not having a team or physician willing to manage the pump after placement.[20]

In terms of system-based issues relating to the use of these pumps, not all hospices will accept patients with epidural pumps. In general, placement of a cath-eter is outside of acceptable hospice per-diem pay-ments, but once the catheter is placed, the drugs are all generic (except ziconotide), are cost-effective, and could be covered by the hospice benefit. These treat-ments may thus require negotiation with the home care provider.

SUMMARY OF EVIDENCE REGARDING TREATMENT RECOMMENDATIONS

Good Level I evidence exists for the use of epidural and intrathecal treatments in the care of selected patients.[21] This evidence is listed in Table 18-3. At least five studies from single institutions document efficacy and safety, but all are uncontrolled. The assessments of pain relief vary from the clinician's opinion to formal testing and are not standardized. No reports of harm to a series of patients have been published.

Smith and colleagues[22] performed a randomized clinical trial of comprehensive medical management versus comprehensive medical management plus intraspinal drug delivery systems. They random-ized 202 patients in five countries to the best guide-line–based treatment by an experienced team to the same management plus a Medtronic Synchromed pump. The primary outcome was pain relief without excess toxicity. The primary outcomes are shown in Table 18-4. More patients achieved pain relief with-out toxicity. The average pain relief was 60% with intrathecal management and 37% with conventional management. Drug toxicity scores were dramatically better, and survival was better at 6 months if patients were either randomized to receive a pump or received one in crossover ($p = .06$).[23] Even the patients with the most refractory pain achieved substantial relief of both pain and drug side effects if they crossed over

TABLE 18-3. Evidence for the Effectiveness of Implantable Drug Delivery Systems From Nonrandomized Clinical Trials

STUDY, YEAR OF PUBLICATION	PATIENTS	RESULTS
Devulder,[7] 1994	33 over 5 yr	25 with "good" (<5) pain relief; 3 developed meningitis.
Hassenbusch,[28] 1990	69 over 6 yr	41 with decrease in pain on visual analog scale from 8.6 to 3.8 at 1 month.
Onofrio,[29] 1990	53 over 7 yr	34/51 (67%) had good quality of life as determined by neurosurgeon.
Penn,[30] 1987	35 over 5 yr	28/35 patients had satisfactory results.
Gestin,[31] 1997	50 over 4 yr	Authors conclude that long-term intrathecal morphine provided satisfactory pain relief, few side effects, and a high degree of patient autonomy.

Modified from Smith TJ, Coyne P. What is the evidence for implantable drug delivery systems for refractory cancer pain? *Support Cancer Ther.* 2004;1:185-189.
Note: All trials were single-site and were retrospective. None had control groups.

TABLE 18-4. Impact of Implantable Drug Delivery Systems on Clinical Success, Pain Visual Analog Scale Scores, and Drug Toxicity as Treated in a Randomized Controlled Trial

	BY 4 WK		BY 12 WK	
CLINICAL SUCCESS	IDDS	Non-IDDS	IDDS	Non-IDDS
≥20% relief of pain or toxicity	46/52 (88.5%) $p = 0.02$	65/91 (71.4%)	47/57 (82.5%) $p = 0.55$	35/45 (77.8%)
≥20% relief of both pain and toxicity	35/52 (67.3%) $p = 0.0003$	33/91 (36.3%)	33/57 (57.9%) $p = 0.01$	15/45 (33.3%)
Average pain relief (% changes from adjusted regression model)	7.49-3.19 (60%) $p = 0.002$	7.81-4.81 (37%)	7.81-3.89 (47%) $p = 0.23$	7.21-4.53 (42%)
Comprehensive toxicity score (% changes from adjusted regression model)	7.41-2.7 (55%) $p = 0.0003$	6.43-5.44 (20%)	6.68-2.30 (66%) $p = 0.01$	6.73-4.13 (37%)
Survival at 6 mo (%)	IDDS/no implant: 59.2 IDDS/implant: 54.3 CMM/implant: 51.8 CMM/no implant: 31.5			

Modified from Smith TJ, Coyne P. What is the evidence for implantable drug delivery systems for refractory cancer pain? *Support Cancer Ther.* 2004;1:185-189.
CMM, Comprehensive medical management; *IDDS,* implantable drug delivery system.

to receive a pump, and these patients lived 3 months past the point at which intraspinal therapy is likely to be cost-effective.[24] A replication trial was planned by the North Center Cancer Treatment Group, but the steering committee and pain specialists determined that the evidence was sufficient for recommendation without another trial. No randomized trials have been conducted on different ways of testing whether epidural or intraspinal therapy will be effective.

KEY MESSAGES TO PATIENTS AND FAMILIES

Clinicians should explain that patients are appropriate for these types of procedures when they are receiving 100 to 200 mg daily of oral morphine or its equivalent without pain relief or when they have intolerable side effects. Clinicians should first explore the risks and benefits of the procedure with the patient and family. It may be necessary to have a discussion about life expectancy and how this relates to which device may be appropriate for a patient. Clinicians should explore discharge options, including whether a local hospice provider will accept patients with an implanted pump, with the patient and family when creating a plan of care.

CONCLUSION AND SUMMARY

Most patients achieve acceptable pain relief with oral medications, but some have intractable pain or side effects despite appropriate therapy. For this group of patients, epidural, intrathecal, or intraspinal therapy is an important proven option that provides superior analgesia, fewer drug toxicities, and possibly longer survival. The first step to advanced therapy is recognition of appropriate candidates; this usually includes those with intractable pain

or with intolerable side effects from their analgesics. Patients with a limited life expectancy (e.g., <3 months) may benefit from a tunneled epidural catheter and external pump. Patients with a longer time to live may benefit from in implantable drug delivery system.

SUMMARY RECOMMENDATIONS

- Epidural and intraspinal therapy have been proven effective to manage refractory pain in many settings.
- Patients are appropriate for these therapies if they are on 100 mg or more of oral morphine daily and continue to have refractory pain or intolerable side effects.
- These systems offer the advantages of better pain relief, fewer systemic side effects, and the ability to use different classes of medications, such as local anesthetics, for which there is no oral equivalent.

REFERENCES

1. Tay W, Ho KY. The role of interventional therapies in cancer pain management. *Ann Acad Med Singapore.* 2009;38(11):989–997.
2. Krames E. Implantable devices for pain control: spinal cord stimulation and intrathecal therapies. *Best Pract Res Clin Anaesthesiol.* 2002;16(4):619–649.
3. Coyne PJ, Smith T, Laird J, et al. Effectively starting and titrating intrathecal analgesic therapy in patients with refractory cancer pain. *Clin J Oncol Nurs.* 2005;9(5):581–583.
4. Krames ES. Intraspinal opioid therapy for chronic nonmalignant pain: current practice and clinical guidelines. *J Pain Symptom Manage.* 1996;11(6):333–352.
5. Sylvester RK, Lindsay SM, Schauer C. The conversion challenge: from intrathecal to oral morphine. *Am J Hosp Palliat Care.* 2004;21(2):143–147.

6. Iksilara MC, Diccini S, Barbosa DA. Infection incidence in patients with tunneled peridural catheter. *Rev Bras Enferm.* 2005;58(2):152–155.

7. Devulder J, Ghys L, Dhondt W, Rolly G. Spinal analgesia in terminal care: risk versus benefit. *J Pain Symptom Manage.* 1994;9(2):75–81.

8. Smitt PS, Tsafka A, Teng-van de Zande F, et al. Outcome and complications of epidural analgesia in patients with chronic cancer pain. *Cancer.* 1998;83(9):2015–2022.

9. Christakis NA, Lamont EB. Extent and determinants of error in doctors' prognoses in terminally ill patients: prospective cohort study. *BMJ.* 2000;320(7233):469–472.

10. Coyne PJ, Smith TJ, Bobb B, Lyckholm LJ. Epidural screening before intrathecal analgesia. *J Pain Palliat Care Pharmacother.* 2008;22(1):69–70.

11. Ginosar Y, Riley ET, Angst MS. The site of action of epidural fentanyl in humans: the difference between infusion and bolus administration. *Anesth Analg.* 2003;97(5):1428–1438.

12. Elliott JA, Horton E, Fibuch EE. The endocrine effects of long-term oral opioid therapy: a case report and review of the literature. *J Opioid Manag.* 2011;7(2):145–154.

13. Katz N, Mazer NA. The impact of opioids on the endocrine system. *Clin J Pain.* 2009;25(2):170–175.

14. Deer T, Krames ES, Hassenbusch S, et al. Management of intrathecal catheter-tip inflammatory masses: an updated 2007 consensus statement from an expert panel. *Neuromodulation.* 2007;11(2):77–91.

15. Stearns L, Boortz-Marx R, Du Pen S, et al. Intrathecal drug delivery for the management of cancer pain: a multidisciplinary consensus of best clinical practices. *J Support Oncol.* 2005;3(6):399–408.

16. Staats PS, Yearwood T, Charapata SG, et al. Intrathecal ziconotide in the treatment of refractory pain in patients with cancer or AIDS: a randomized controlled trial. *JAMA.* 2004;291(1):63–70.

17. Osenbach RK. Intrathecal drug delivery in the management of pain. In: Fishman SM, Ballantyne JC, Rathmell JP, eds. *Bonica's Management of Pain.* 4th ed.Philadelphia: Wolters Kluwer/Lippincott Williams and Wilkins; 2010:1437–1458.

18. Coyne PJ, Hansen LA, Laird J, et al. Massive hydromorphone dose delivered subcutaneously instead of intrathecally: guidelines for prevention and management of opioid, local anesthetic, and clonidine overdose. *J Pain Symptom Manage.* 2004;28(3):273–276.

19. Rauck RL, Cherry D, Boyer MF, et al. Long-term intrathecal opioid therapy with a patient-activated, implanted delivery system for the treatment of refractory cancer pain. *J Pain.* 2003;4(8):441–447.

20. British Pain Society. *Intrathecal drug delivery for the management of pain and spasticity in adults: recommendations for best clinical practice.* Available at http://www.britishpainsociety.org/book_ittd_main.pdf; 2008. Accessed November 15, 2011.

21. Smith TJ, Coyne P. What is the evidence for implantable drug delivery systems for refractory cancer pain? *Support Cancer Ther.* 2004;1(3):185–189.

22. Smith TJ, Staats PS, Deer T, et al. Randomized clinical trial of an implantable drug delivery system compared with comprehensive medical management for refractory cancer pain: impact on pain, drug-related toxicity, and survival. *J Clin Oncol.* 2002;20:4040–4049.

23. Smith TJ, Coyne PJ, Staats PS, et al. An implantable drug delivery system (IDDS) for refractory cancer pain provides sustained pain control, less drug-related toxicity, and possibly better survival compared with comprehensive medical management (CMM). *Ann Oncol.* 2005;16:825–833.

24. Smith TJ, Coyne PJ. Implantable drug delivery systems (IDDS) after failure of comprehensive medical management (CMM) can palliate symptoms in the most refractory cancer pain patients. *J Palliat Med.* 2005;8(4):736–742.

25. Roberts SB, Wozencraft CP, Coyne PJ, Smith TJ. Dexmedetomidine as an adjuvant analgesic for intractable cancer pain. *J Palliat Med.* 2011;14(3):371–373.

26. O'Connor AB, Dworkin RH. Treatment of neuropathic pain: an overview of recent guidelines [review]. *Am J Med.* 2009;122 (suppl 10):S22–S32.

27. Wallace MS, Magnuson S, Ridgeway B. Efficacy of oral mexiletine for neuropathic pain with allodynia: a double-blind, placebo-controlled, crossover study. *Reg Anesth Pain Med.* 2000;25(5):459–467.

28. Hassenbusch SJ, Pillay PK, Magdinec M, et al. Constant infusion of morphine for intractable cancer pain using an implanted pump. *J Neurosurg.* 1990;73:405–409.

29. Onofrio BM, Yaksh TL. Long-term pain relief produced by intrathecal morphine infusion in 53 patients. *J Neurosurg.* 1990;2:200–209.

30. Penn RD, Paice JA. Chronic intrathecal morphine for intractable pain. *J Neurosurg.* 1987;67:182–186.

31. Gestin Y, Vainio A, Pegurier AM. Long-term intrathecal infusion of morphine in the home care of patients with advanced cancer. *Acta Anaesthesiol Scand.* 1997;41:12–17.

Chapter 19

When Should Nerve Blocks Be Used for Pain Management?

Rebecca Aslakson, Jason C. Brookman, and Thomas J. Smith

INTRODUCTION AND SCOPE OF THE PROBLEM

Pain is the most feared problem in patients with advanced illness; it is highly prevalent in cancer and in many other advanced diseases such as human immunodeficiency virus and acquired immunodeficiency syndrome, congestive heart failure, and renal failure. Most patients achieve satisfactory relief of their pain with the World Health Organization (WHO) Three-Step Analgesic Ladder,[1] but 10% to 20% do not.[2] These patients are living substantially longer than in the past and have more complicated symptoms and expectations.[3] Consequently, an extension of the ladder has been proposed that includes interventional pain management and nerve blocks.[4]

This chapter discusses diagnostic nerve blocks, which are used to establish a diagnosis or do a trial of treatment, and therapeutic nerve blocks, which are used to treat active pain. There are two types of therapeutic blocks: nonneurolytic nerve blocks, usually with a local anesthetic and corticosteroid, and neurolytic nerve blocks, with a nerve-killing agent such as absolute ethanol.

Any nerve that can be reached by a needle is a candidate for a local nerve block. This includes not only the commonly known spinal nerve root injections and celiac plexus and splanchnic nerve blocks but also the less commonly used blocks such as brachial plexus and peroneal nerve blocks. Blocks may be one-time immediate injections or the placement of a catheter for several days to help "reset" a nerve with long-lasting relief. (For more information on the use of implantable systems for the delivery of pain medications, see Chapter 18.)

The most important knowledge about nerve blocks for the noninterventional pain professional is to use blocks early. Given their effectiveness, they should be common practice but unfortunately are too often withheld "until things get bad." One of the most common responses after a patient has had a nerve block is "I wish I had done this months ago."

RELEVANT PATHOPHYSIOLOGY

Pain is a complicated phenomenon with multiple sites of origination of pain impulses, propagation, reinforcement or inhibition, central nervous system and spinal cord "wind up," and psychological responses.[5] Nerves blocks, on the other hand, are relatively simple, local procedures designed to interrupt the pain impulse temporarily or permanently, allowing both immediate relief of pain and remodeling of the nerve or its response to pain.

Several classes of drugs are used in nerve blocks, all common and familiar. The most frequently used are local anesthetics such as short-acting lidocaine and longer-acting bupivacaine. Corticosteroids administered in a local-release depot form are familiar to most health care professionals and have mainly local reaction. However, prolonged use can lead to systemic absorption and long-term side effects such as osteoporosis and cataracts, but these reactions are rare. The drug with the most permanent effect is absolute (100%) ethanol, which directly kills nerve fibers and the blood supply to local nerves.

Local nerve blocks have several mechanisms of action, which are, as in all pain relief measures, complicated. The "unwinding" of a pain impulse is always multifactorial, with components of local nerve pain impulse relief, relief of inflammation, reduction in propagation of the impulse, and even remodeling of the nerve itself. Other mechanisms include disruption of vascular supply, alterations in gene expression and protein production, and secondary messengers. The interested reader is referred to other works that explore these common mechanisms of pain relief.[6,7] Sympathetic nerve blocks are localized to the sympathetic ganglion area and have some effect on vascular supply, but are thought to work primarily by interruption of nociceptive afferent fibers from the areas involved with the cancer.[8] Knowing anatomy and neurophysiology is critical to ensure that the ganglion to be blocked is separated anatomically from the somatic nerves; potential complications include sensory and motor dysfunction in important areas such as the ganglion impar in front of the sacral-coccyx junction and the celiac plexus.

Techniques for Blocks

The contraindications for blocks are similar to those for any invasive procedure, and providers must always weigh the benefits of immediate and thorough pain relief versus the risks of the procedure. Common contraindications include a bleeding diathesis caused by anticoagulation or antiplatelet agents. The risk for bleeding is proportionally the same as with other procedures, but the adverse consequences of a large hemorrhage into the retroperitoneal space or even a small hemorrhage near the spinal cord or a nerve facet may be severe.

Routine care before and after the block is similar to that in other procedures. Most centers require the patient to be observed for several hours afterward to ensure pain relief and absence of allergic reactions, hypotension, or significant diarrhea.

The earliest blocks, such as a celiac plexus block from the posterior approach, were done with knowledge of anatomy only. Modern practitioners typically use radiological tools to directly visualize the nerve or surrounding anatomy. Types of imaging used include fluoroscopy, computed tomography, magnetic resonance imaging visualization, and ultrasound localization. Furthermore, with the advent of safe and effective endoscopy, more blocks are being done through real-time endoscopic interventions. A comparison of the block types is presented in Table 19-1.

Ultrasound allows direct visualization of the nerve to give safer and more effective access to the region for the block. Previous studies demonstrated that ultrasound increases the likelihood and quality of a successful block and decreases time to onset of analgesia.[9] Ultrasound is also particularly helpful when the anatomy has been changed by scar, prior therapy, or metastases. Newer ultrasound capability permits direct visualization of the nerve, blood vessels, and distribution of the injection.[10]

SUMMARY OF EVIDENCE REGARDING TREATMENT RECOMMENDATIONS

Effect on Pain

In general, nerve blocks are successful in relieving pain. The number of randomized clinical trials comparing "sham" to real nerve blocks is limited because of the multitude of problems conducting randomized trials.[11] Consequently, some placebo effect may occur, but the preponderance of evidence is overwhelmingly positive. A summary of typical results is listed in Table 19-2.

Effect on Survival

A landmark study done in the 1990s established that pain relief might have an impact on patient survival (Table 19-3). In pancreatic cancer, deep visceral pain is highly prevalent, with 78% to 82% of patients even having this pain as a presenting symptom.[12] In this study, patients who were to undergo a Whipple procedure were randomized before surgery to a celiac plexus block with saline or with 100% alcohol. For the whole group, pain was improved but there was no difference in survival. However, for the 34 patients who had typical pancreatic cancer–related visceral pain before surgery, improvement occurred in survival as well as pain control.[13] This led to the supposition that if pain were controlled, patients would live longer as well as better. This trial was repeated 10 years later; the results are shown in Table 19-3. Pain control was somewhat better, but overall survival was unchanged.[14] One of the explanations given for these lesser effects was that pain management improved substantially from 1990 to 2000, such that the later study patients were not subjected to unrelenting pain. Further research has shown that only one block (0.75% bupivacaine 20 mL and 98% alcohol 10 mL) is needed, instead of two, with similar results.[15]

Underuse of Nerve Blocks

Given the positive evidence, why are nerve blocks not used more frequently and earlier? A multitude of reasons likely exist for delaying patient referral for a nerve block. The first is lack of knowledge of nerve blocks by noninterventional pain physicians. The second is lack of a good referral network or the perception that the results of local nerve block are not as good as reported. In general, for any interventional procedure, a strong relationship exists among higher patient volume, provider experience, and medical

TABLE 19-1. Approaches to Blocks

APPROACH	ADVANTAGES AND DISADVANTAGES
Anatomic	Universally available without equipment using traditional anatomic landmarks and elicitation of paresthesias.
Fluoroscopic guided	Requires inexpensive equipment; enables direct visualization of both anatomic landmarks and needle position.
Nerve stimulation guided	Nerve stimulator attached to 22-gauge needle is advanced to area to be blocked. Motor nerves are stimulated first, causing a contraction visible to the operator, before any pain is felt. The nerve can then be blocked.* If not successful, second attempts are less apt to work because the nerve will be anesthetized already, preventing twitches.
CAT guided	Requires expensive equipment, but allows for direct visualization of anatomic landmarks, position of needle, and distribution of the anesthetic fluid.
Ultrasound guided	Localizes the exact area and surrounding blood vessels, allowing visualization of the block liquid.
ERCP or endoscopic guided	Has the theoretical advantage of being concurrently diagnostic (brushing and biopsy) and therapeutic (stent placement or nerve block to control pain).

CAT, Computer axial tomograph; *ERCP,* endoscopic retrograde cholangiopancreatographic.
*Franco CD, Vieira ZE. 1,001 subclavian perivascular brachial plexus blocks: success with a nerve stimulator. *Reg Anesth Pain Med.* 2000;25:41-46.

TABLE 19-2. Evidence Summary for Nerve Blocks

TYPE OF BLOCK	INDICATION	EFFECT ON PAIN	SIDE EFFECTS TO NOTE
Intraabdominal and Ganglion Blocks			
Celiac plexus*	Deep visceral pain, especially from the pancreas or nearby organs	70%-96% success in pancreas cancer often lasting months[a] May be very successful in pancreatitis[b]	Hypotension, diarrhea
Superior hypogastric plexus block*	Pelvic pain from recurrent rectal, bladder, uterine, cervical cancer	If diagnostic block is successful, long-lasting pain relief in 72% of patients,[c] whether done early or late in the course[d]	Hypotension, diarrhea
Splanchnic nerve block*	Deep visceral pain for more diffuse metastases or sites of disease	Good to excellent success[e]	
Stellate ganglion block	Menopausal hot flashes Upper extremity pain PHN Angina Raynaud disease Angina pectoris Phantom limb pain CRPS	Safe, with 64% reduction in hot flashes[f] Safe and effective but few randomized or large trials[f]	Paresthesias, anesthesias
Ganglion impar block, anterior to the sacrococcygeal junction	Perineal pain	Good to excellent relief for perineal and coccyx pain, 90% response with >50% reduction in pain[g]	
Plexopathy Pain			
Brachial plexus	Chronic pain from cancer, scar, radiation, accidents	Few large series but small reports detail excellent pain relief[h]	Thoracic ganglion blocks may be highly effective in similar patients[i]
Lumbar sympathetic block	Lower extremity cancer pain, phantom pain, CRPS, PHN, or pelvic/urogenic pain Vertebral fracture pain	Few large series Recent randomized trial, L2 block for osteoporosis/fracture pain helped for 2 wk but not beyond[j]	
Peroneal or popliteal nerve	Chronic ischemia-related or cancer-related pain	Good results in chronic ischemia with local anesthetic or combined with morphine[k]	Few to no trials in chronic pain

[a]*Eisenberg* E, Carr DB, Chalmers TC. Neurolytic celiac plexus block for treatment of cancer pain: a meta-analysis. *Anesth Analg.* 1995;80:290-295.
[b]Wong GY, Sakorafas GH, Tsiotos GG, Sarr MG. Palliation of pain in chronic pancreatitis: use of neural blocks and neurotomy. *Surg Clin North Am.* 1999;79:873-893.
[c]Eisenberg E, Carr DB, Chalmers TC. Neurolytic celiac plexus block for treatment of cancer pain: a meta-analysis. Anesth Analg. 1995;80:290-295.
[d]de Oliveira R, dos Reis MP, Prado WA. The effects of early or late neurolytic sympathetic plexus block on the management of abdominal or pelvic cancer pain. *Pain.* 2004;110:400-408.
[e]Erdine S. Celiac ganglion block. *Agri.* 2005;17:14-22.
[f]Haest K, Kumar A, Van Calster B, et al. Stellate ganglion block for the management of hot flashes and sleep disturbances in breast cancer survivors: an uncontrolled experimental study with 24 weeks of follow-up. *Ann Oncol.* 2012;23(6):1449-1454.
[g]Agarwal-Kozlowski K, Lorke DE, Habermann CR, Am Esch JS, Beck H. CT-guided blocks and neuroablation of the ganglion impar (Walther) in perineal pain: anatomy, technique, safety, and efficacy. *Clin J Pain.* 2009;25:570-576.
[h]Mukherji SK, Wagle A, Armao DM, Dogra S. Brachial plexus nerve block with CT guidance for regional pain management: initial results. *Radiology.* 2000;216:886-890.
[i]Yoo HS, Nahm FS, Lee PB, Lee CJ. Early thoracic sympathetic block improves the treatment effect for upper extremity neuropathic pain. *Anesth Analg.* 2011;113:605-609.
[j]Ohtori S, Yamashita M, Inoue G, et al. L2 spinal nerve-block effects on acute low back pain from osteoporotic vertebral fracture. *J Pain.* 2009;10:870-875.
[k]Keskinbora K, Aydinli I. Perineural morphine in patients with chronic ischemic lower extremity pain: efficacy and long-term results. *J Anesth.* 2009;23:11-18.
*Only visceral pain responds, not bone or muscle pain from the same region.

CRPS, Complex regional pain syndrome; *PHN,* postherpetic neuralgia.

TABLE 19-3. Effect of Celiac Plexus Block in Pancreatic Cancer

STUDY, YEAR	EFFECT ON PAIN	EFFECT ON SURVIVAL
Lillimoe,[13] 1993	Pain significantly better in the alcohol group compared to saline block ($p < .05$)	~6 mo in alcohol vs. 2-3 mo for saline block ($p < .001$)
Wong,[14] 2004	Mean pain at week 1 was reduced by 53% compared to 27% with standard treatment ($p < .001$) 14% of patients with NCPB reported moderate or severe pain in the first 6 weeks compared to 40% of opioid only ($p = .005$)	Not statistically different, but at 1 year 16% of patients with NCPB were alive compared to 6% of opioid-only ($p = .26$)

NCPB, Neurolytic celiac plexus block.

outcomes; this has not been well studied, however, with regard to nerve blocks.[16] It does appear that visual guidance, such as ultrasound, allows for easier learning than with nerve stimulators.[17]

KEY MESSAGES TO PATIENTS AND FAMILIES

Most patients have their pain satisfactorily controlled by the usual pain medications, but some require nerve blocks or other, more invasive pain procedures. Some common situations in which nerve blocks may significantly improve pain management include the abdominal pain of pancreatic cancer and localized "plexopathy" pain from damage to a group of nerves such as the brachial plexus under the shoulder.

The advantage of nerve blocks is that the effect is immediate. Depending on both injection technique and the cause of the pain, relief may be permanent or may require repeat injections in a few months. If the pain is relieved with a local anesthetic, corticosteroids can be injected to give longer-lasting pain relief by reducing local swelling and inflammation. An injection of 100% absolute alcohol may permanently kill the nerve that is causing the pain.

Other types of blocks involve placing a small catheter along the nerve and giving local anesthetics or pain medicines as a constant infusion. It is even possible to "reset" a damaged nerve such that pain relief continues even when the pain medication is stopped.

Patients and families should explore whether a nerve block is right for them either when they have unrelieved pain, particularly if related to an abdominal malignancy such as pancreatic cancer, or when they have significant side effects from the common pain medications.

CONCLUSION AND SUMMARY

Nerve blocks have a strong clinical record of pain relief, allowing better pain management and reduction in drug side effects. The evidence for most types of nerve blocks is not from large randomized, controlled trials but rather observational or single-arm studies. In general, 50% to 90% of patients have substantial relief of pain from a nerve block that is evident immediately, with no major side effects. Nerve blocks are underused in the management of pain in patients with serious illness, so consultation with specialists skilled in their use should occur early in the course of a patient's disease.

SUMMARY RECOMMENDATIONS

- Nerve blocks have an excellent track record of effectiveness and safety in routine clinical practice. The evidence is nearly all from single-arm and single-center trials, with few randomized trials, but the evidence is consistent. In general, nerve blocks are used too little and too late by most practitioners. Health care professionals who manage pain should develop a close working relationship with interventional pain specialists who can assist with these procedures.
- Nerve blocks are particularly useful for deep somatic pain, for example, from intraabdominal malignancies such as pancreatic cancer or liver metastases. Blocks are also useful for localized plexopathy-related pain.
- Immediate side effects after intraabdominal blocks for which the clinician should monitor include transient worsening of pain, hypotension, and diarrhea. Serious side effects are unusual.

REFERENCES

1. Zeppetella G. The WHO analgesic ladder: 25 years on. *Br J Nurs.* 2011;20:S4–S6.
2. Meuser T, Pietruck C, Radbruch L, Stute P, Lehmann KL, Grond S. Symptoms during cancer pain treatment following WHO-guidelines: a longitudinal follow-up study of symptom prevalence, severity and etiology. *Pain.* 2001;93:247–257.
3. Raphael J, Hester J, Ahmedzai S, et al. Cancer pain. I. Physical, interventional and complimentary therapies; management in the community; acute, treatment-related and complex cancer pain—a perspective from the British Pain Society endorsed by the UK Association of Palliative Medicine and the Royal College of General Practitioners. *Pain Med.* 2010;11:872–896.
4. Christo PJ, Mazloomdoost D. Interventional pain treatments for cancer pain. *Ann N Y Acad Sci.* 2008;1138:299–328.
5. Jensen MP. A neuropsychological model of pain: research and clinical implications. *J Pain.* 2010;11:2–12.
6. Campbell JN, Meyer RA. Mechanisms of neuropathic pain [review]. *Neuron.* 2006;52:77–92.
7. Jarvis MF, Boyce-Rustay JM. Neuropathic pain: models and mechanisms. *Curr Pharm Des.* 2009;15:1711–1716.
8. Kaplan R, Portenoy RK. *Cancer pain management: interventional therapies.* Up To Date, Version 19.3 2011.
9. Walker KJ, McGrattan K, Aas-Eng K, Smith AF. Ultrasound guidance for peripheral nerve blockade. *Cochrane Database Syst Rev* 2009;(4) CD006459.
10. Jeng CL, Rosenblatt MA. *Overview of peripheral nerve blocks.* Up To Date, Version 19.3 2011.
11. Dworkin RH, Turk DC, Peirce-Sandner S, et al. Research design considerations for confirmatory chronic pain clinical trials: IMMPACT recommendations. *Pain.* 2010;149:177–193.
12. Sharma C, Eltawil KM, Renfrew PD, Walsh MJ, Molinari M. Advances in diagnosis, treatment and palliation of pancreatic carcinoma: 1990-2010. *World J Gastroenterol.* 2011;17:867–897.
13. Lillemoe KD, Cameron JL, Kaufman HS, et al. Chemical splanchicectomy in patients with unresectable pancreatic cancer: a prospective randomized trial. *Ann Surg.* 1993;217:447–457.
14. Wong GY, Schroeder DR, Carns PE, et al. Effect of neurolytic celiac plexus block on pain relief, quality of life, and survival in patients with unresectable pancreatic cancer: a randomized controlled trial. *JAMA.* 2004;291:1092–1099.
15. Leblanc JK, Al-Haddad M, McHenry L, et al. A prospective, randomized study of EUS-guided celiac plexus neurolysis for pancreatic cancer: one injection or two? *Gastrointest Endosc.* 2011;74(6):1300–1307.
16. Konrad C, Schüpfer G, Wietlisbach M, Gerber H. Learning manual skills in anesthesiology: is there a recommended number of cases for anesthetic procedures? *Anesth Analg.* 1998;86:635–639.
17. Luyet C, Schüpfer G, Wipfli M, Greif R, Luginbühl M, Eichenberger U. Different learning curves for axillary brachial plexus block: ultrasound guidance versus nerve stimulation. *Anesthesiol Res Pract.* 2010:309462. Epub 2011 Jan 20.

DYSPNEA

Chapter 20

What Interventions Are Effective for Managing Dyspnea in Cancer?

Amy P. Abernethy, Arif Kamal, Jennifer M. Maguire, and David C. Currow

INTRODUCTION AND SCOPE OF THE PROBLEM

Dyspnea, as defined by a consensus panel of the American Thoracic Society, is "a subjective experience of breathing discomfort that consists of qualitatively distinct sensations that vary in intensity.[1]" Often termed "shortness of breath" or "breathlessness," dyspnea is one of the most common symptoms experienced by patients with advanced disease. The majority of patients with advanced cancer report dyspnea at some point,[2] as do most imminently dying patients.[3] The incidence of dyspnea increases significantly in the 1 to 3 months before death.[4,5] The symptom afflicts nearly half of all patients receiving end-of-life care, and half of those afflicted report severe dyspnea.[6]

The particularly subjective nature of dyspnea makes clinical management challenging.[7] The American Thoracic Society explains that the experience of dyspnea "derives from interactions among multiple physiological, psychological, social, and environmental factors and may induce secondary physiological and behavioral responses."[1] The way in which dyspnea manifests and its reported nature and severity are thus determined by patient perception,[1] with patient descriptions of dyspnea varying based on an array of factors such as the individual's underlying disease, ethnic or racial background, previous experiences, and emotional state. To incorporate the various aspects of dyspnea into a conceptual framework, "total dyspnea" has been described.[8] As a symptom description, total dyspnea involves the interaction of four domains of suffering—physical, psychological, interpersonal, and existential—in an attempt to fully capture patients' experience of this disabling and distressing symptom.

RELEVANT PATHOPHYSIOLOGY

Dyspnea results from three main physiological abnormalities: (1) increased load requiring greater respiratory effort, such as from airway obstruction; (2) increase in the proportion of respiratory muscle required to maintain a normal workload, which may be due to weakening of the relevant muscles; and (3) increase in ventilation requirements resulting from conditions such as fever or anemia. In patients with cancer, the cause of dyspnea may be identified in a specific anatomic condition and associated comorbidity such as pulmonary obstruction (chronic obstructive pulmonary disease [COPD], reactive airways, cough and secretions, mass lesions), pulmonary restriction (fibrosis or other interstitial disease, effusions, fibrosis, infections, kyphosis, obesity), mismatch between perfusion and oxygenation (anemia, pulmonary hypertension, heart failure, pulmonary embolism), and fatigue and weakness (cancer-associated, anorexia/cachexia syndrome, cancer-associated fatigue and muscle wasting, chemotherapy effect, multiple sclerosis, amyotrophic lateral sclerosis). These specific abnormalities can usually be measured, imaged, or inferred from the patient's underlying disease to provide clues to the cause of the dyspnea.

Dyspnea often results from systemic effects of illness, instead of or in addition to identifiable localized causes. In a national study, 24% of patients in hospice care with no known cardiopulmonary involvement (e.g., local cancer involvement, pleural effusions, pulmonary infections) reported experiencing dyspnea[2]; likewise, in patients in hospice care with no known cardiopulmonary disorder, both prevalence and severity of dyspnea increases significantly as death approaches.[5] Systemic changes such as asthenia and cachexia, both of which affect more than 80% of patients with advanced cancer, are suggested as causes in many of these cases.[9]

In addition to anatomic causes, emotional, spiritual, and existential distress can induce or worsen dyspnea in the patient with cancer. Anxiety and panic both factor importantly in the development of dyspnea and, in turn, are exacerbated by its presence—setting up a pernicious spiral of cause and symptom. The association between symptoms of breathlessness and anxiety is well-documented.[10] This association bears notice given the high prevalence of anxiety in palliative care populations. Compared to control patients, patients with underlying anxiety or panic disorders have an exaggerated experience of dyspnea.[11] Additionally, the effect of spiritual distress on dyspnea has been described.[12]

In the accepted neurophysiological model, dyspnea is thought to begin with the activation of sensory receptors involved with respiration; this sends an afferent impulse to the central nervous system, which then directs an efferent impulse toward the respiratory muscles. Mismatch between these signals and modulation of systems may contribute to the perception of dyspnea.[13]

Endogenous opioids (i.e., endorphins) have been thought to attenuate the sensation of dyspnea at the central nervous system level since 1985.[14] A recent important investigation conducted in opioid-naïve volunteers has added to the understanding of the mechanisms of efficacy of exogenous opioids, which remain the mainstay of global therapy for dyspnea.[15] In this double-blind, cross-over study, levels of β-endorphin were measured at rest and after exercise in 17 patients with COPD undergoing a 10-minute treadmill exercise test. Patients received either intravenous saline or naloxone, an opioid antagonist. A three-fold increase in serum β-endorphin levels was observed from rest to postexercise. Mean self-reported dyspnea scores throughout exercise were significantly higher in patients when they received naloxone, suggesting a need for further studies to identify ways of accentuating the effect of endogenous opioids on dyspnea.

Investigations with positron emission tomography[16–18] and functional magnetic resonance imaging have added to the knowledge of how dyspnea activates cortical and cerebellar systems.[19]

SUMMARY OF EVIDENCE REGARDING TREATMENT RECOMMENDATIONS

Because of the complex biopsychosocial causes of dyspnea, effective management requires a multidimensional and individualized approach. The clinician's first step is to establish the goals of care, in conjunction with the patient and other relevant individuals such as family members and informal caregivers. If dyspnea in a patient with cancer is caused by a modifiable anatomic condition or treatable disease, the initial aim is to reduce the dyspnea by targeting this cause. If the cancer has been maximally treated, no alterable physiological cause is identified, and the patient's dyspnea persists, the clinical approach shifts to one focused on global symptom management, targeting the breathlessness rather than the disease.[20] Treatment options for managing dyspnea in the patient with cancer include pharmacological, surgical, and other nonpharmacological interventions; regardless of treatment choice, outcomes will be optimized if the clinician addresses as many as possible of the individual-specific contributing factors, including anxiety; other symptoms; nonmedical stressors, such as interpersonal, relational, and financial concerns; and spiritual or existential distress.

Pharmacological Management

Opioids. Opioids are the mainstay of pharmacological management for dyspnea and have been more studied and commonly employed than any other class of pharmacological agents for relieving this symptom.[21] In addition to their direct ventilator and vasodilatory effects,[22] opioids appear to relieve dyspnea indirectly by ameliorating anxiety and pain, both of which often contribute to the dyspnea cycle; the positive effects of opioids on anxiety and pain have been extensively reviewed.[23] A study of endogenous opioids during dyspnea (discussed earlier)[15] showed that dyspnea was attenuated by endogenous, circulatory opioids during treadmill exercise in opioid-naïve dyspneic patients; this effect was reversed by the administration of an opioid antagonist, naloxone. The threefold increase in endogenous opioids from rest to end of exercise suggested a mechanism by which exogenous opioids may also benefit the patient experiencing dyspnea.

Randomized controlled trials have studied opioids, particularly morphine, in oral, parenteral, and nebulized forms. A systematic review and meta-analysis of placebo-controlled trials in dyspnea showed a statistically significant effect for oral or parenteral opioids only; study populations spanned various diseases.[24] Subgroup analysis did not reveal a positive effect of nebulized opioids, but conclusions should be cautiously drawn because available studies were small and of poor quality. Two subsequent systematic reviews[25,26] in patients with cancer examined various modalities of opioid administration and reached similar conclusions about the efficacy of both oral and parenteral opioids. Although one small study by Bruera and colleagues[27] showed comparable dyspnea relief with nebulized morphine and subcutaneous morphine, seven other placebo-controlled trials did not replicate these results.

Recommendations for opioid dosing and titration rest on the results of two important clinical trials. A double-blind, controlled trial assigned 48 opioid-naïve dyspneic patients to sustained-release oral morphine 20 mg once daily or placebo for 4 days, followed by 4 days of the alternative.[28] Participants in the morphine arm reported significant benefits with respect to dyspnea and insomnia. Another study in patients with prior opioid exposure found that titrating to significantly higher doses (50% above baseline) conferred no additional dyspnea relief compared to increasing the dose in smaller increments (25% above baseline).[29] Subsequently, a phase 2 dose increment study has helped to determine a minimum effective daily dose for opioids for dyspnea improvement; a secondary purpose was to evaluate whether the clinical benefit is maintained over time.[30] Participants (n = 85) received escalating doses of sustained-release oral morphine, starting at 10 mg per day and increasing in increments of 10 mg to a maximum 30 mg per day if patients experienced less than a 10% reduction in dyspnea over their own baseline. In 65% of participants, opioids reduced dyspnea by at least 10% and 53% sustained the benefit for 3 months. For 70% of participants, 10 mg per day was the beneficial dose. This study was the first to demonstrate that low doses of sustained opioids provide significant and enduring relief of dyspnea. Based on these two studies, the recommended starting dose in opioid-naïve dyspneic patients is sustained-release morphine 10 to 20 mg daily in divided doses, with active evaluation and gradual titration to desired effect.

Although most trials of opioids for dyspnea have studied morphine, a few studies have investigated common nonmorphine opioids. A small study of oral hydromorphone (n = 14) showed significant dyspnea relief at a mean dose of 2.5 mg.[31] A pilot trial of nebulized or systemic hydromorphone versus saline demonstrated dyspnea improvement in all groups, suggesting the importance of a possible placebo effect for any dyspnea intervention.[32] A small case series showed promising results using the oral, transmucosal form of fentanyl.[33,34]

Safety is a limiting concern when clinicians consider the use of opioids to treat dyspnea; the feared risks are respiratory depression and accelerated death. The application of opioids to alleviate dyspnea dates back to the late nineteenth century; they were used for this purpose until the 1950s, when concerns were raised about respiratory depression and carbon dioxide retention with opioid use.[35] Discrediting this fear, subsequent studies[36,37] demonstrated a decrease in respiratory rate and improvement in dyspnea with morphine or hydromorphone titration, but no significant changes in other respiratory parameters (i.e., no opioid-induced respiratory depression). These results and the lack of evidence of accelerated death led the American College of Chest Physicians to recommend, in its 2010 Consensus Statement on the Management of Dyspnea in Patients with Advanced Lung or Heart Disease, that physicians titrate oral and parenteral opioids for the relief of dyspnea.[38]

Anxiolytics. Because patients with anxiety disorders frequently report a cluster of symptoms (e.g., dyspnea, anxiety, depression), benzodiazepans and selective seretonin reuptake inhibitors (SSRIs) are sometimes used to relieve dyspnea indirectly by treating their anxiety disorder. SSRIs may also exert a direct effect on neural centers that control the perception of breathlessness.

Benzodiazepines have been studied both alone and in conjunction with opioids. An early (1980) exploratory study reported diazepam efficacy in four patients with severe obstructive airway disease and without severe hypoxia at rest.[39] Subsequent trials of clorazepate,[40] alprazolam,[41] and diazepam[42] failed to show any dyspnea benefit for patients compared to placebo.

Midazolam has been most studied by the Navigante group in Brazil. Their first trial enrolled patients with advanced cancer who were opioid- and benzodiazepine-naïve with a life expectancy of less than 1 week and compared three arms: morphine alone, midazolam alone, and morphine plus midazolam.[43] Modest benefit was achieved with the addition of the benzodiazepine to morphine, leading to reduction in dyspnea intensity and decreased breakthrough dyspnea. A 2010 study by the same group demonstrated both equal efficacy and overall safety of oral midazolam versus oral opioid.[44] The investigators randomized outpatient participants (n = 63) who had severe dyspnea (mean dyspnea >8.5 on a numeric rating scale of 0-10) to oral morphine or oral midazolam at starting doses of 3 mg and 2 mg, respectively. Doses were increased to an effective dose using a fast-titration schedule over 2 hours; patients were then followed daily for 5 days. At least 50% of both patient groups had dyspnea alleviated during the 2-hour titrating phase, with no significant difference between agents. During the 5-day follow-up phase, midazolam proved superior to morphine in controlling both baseline and breakthrough dyspnea. The most common adverse effect was mild somnolence that did not interfere with further medical workup and that did not differ significantly between the two agents. However, the role of midazolam remains controversial because of the short duration of studies and the severely dyspneic nature of the included populations, whose disease was causing acute rather than chronic dyspnea. Safety and efficacy results may not be generalizable[45] and the compatibility of doses of opioids and benzodiazepine has not been demonstrated. Clinical trials of SSRIs are underway.

Inhaled Furosemide. Furosemide may reduce dyspnea because of its inhibitory effect on the cough reflex, preventive effect on bronchoconstriction in asthma, and possible indirect actions on sensory nerve endings in the airway epithelium. Inhaled furosemide has been studied in patients with cancer.[46,47] Placebo-controlled studies of inhaled furosemide delivered to patients with COPD have shown a significant improvement in dyspnea scores with exercise.[48,49] A recent double-blind study of 15 patients with cancer (primarily lung cancer) randomized participants to receive either nebulized furosemide 40 mg, nebulized 0.9% saline, or no treatment in random order over 3 consecutive days.[46] Of the 15 participants, 6 reported dyspnea relief with any nebulized treatment; neither saline nor furosemide proved statistically superior. This small study confirmed findings from another study in patients with cancer (n = 7) that investigated a 20-mg furosemide dose.[50] Otherwise, most reports of inhaled furosemide benefits in patients with cancer are case reports and case series.

Oxygen. Patients frequently request supplemental oxygen to relieve dyspnea,[51,52] and this therapy is commonly prescribed in hospitals.[53] Long-term oxygen therapy is indicated and generally reimbursable for patients with severe hypoxemia (i.e., $Pao_2 \leq 55$ mm Hg at rest). Data to support use of oxygen therapy come mainly from studies in COPD. In clinical trials in which patients with COPD with significant hypoxemia received oxygen therapy, patients experienced improvement in both survival and quality of life. Two early landmark trials demonstrated a clear survival advantage with continuous or nocturnal oxygen in patients with hypoxemia and COPD whose measured Pao_2 was less than 55 mm Hg or less than <60 mm Hg with cor pulmonale or other evidence of end-organ damage resulting from hypoxia.[54,55]

Palliative oxygen is used when patients experience persistent dyspnea but do not meet criteria for long-term oxygen therapy, that is, when Pao_2 is above 55 mm Hg. A Cochrane review of studies of palliative oxygen therapy in adult patients with chronic terminal illness in nonacute settings included eight randomized, controlled trials measuring dyspnea in patients with cancer, heart failure, and kyphoscoliosis.[56] Individually, all of the included studies had small study populations and most were underpowered to detect a 25% difference in dyspnea. Conflicting findings made the overall results inconclusive. The included studies that focused on cancer-related dyspnea studied palliative oxygen therapy use both at rest and with activity; differing results were reported. The authors of the systematic review concluded that the available studies failed to demonstrate a consistent effect of palliative oxygen for dyspnea, although certain populations of patients may significantly benefit from this intervention. Other systematic reviews in cancer dyspnea[25,57] suggest that oxygen benefit may be seen only in patients with severe hypoxemia.

A recent large international double-blind, randomized, controlled trial of palliative oxygen versus medical air (i.e., room air with ambient partial pressure of oxygen) for patients without hypoxemia ($Pao_2 > 55$ mm Hg) sought to clarify whether this intervention benefits patients with persistent dyspnea.[58] Participants received gas (oxygen or medical air) by concentrator through nasal cannulae at 2 L per minute and were instructed to use it for at least 15 hours per day for 7 days. Neither gas demonstrated superiority in improving quality of life or relieving the sensation of breathlessness, but both dyspnea and quality of life improved over the study period in both arms. These results suggest that patients may benefit from the motion of any gas over the face or nasal passages, rather than from the properties of a specific gas such as oxygen. Further analysis suggested that patients with higher baseline dyspnea derived more benefit preferentially from palliative oxygen than did patients with lower baseline dyspnea and that most benefit from the intervention occurred in the first 48 hours; nearly all symptomatic and functional improvements occurred in the first 3 days. The underlying illness and cause did not predict therapeutic benefit; similar effects were observed in patients with cancer and those without cancer. This study calls into question the common practice of prescribing oxygen therapy for refractory dyspnea; if oxygen is prescribed, patients should be monitored closely and the intervention discontinued if no benefit is realized after 3 days. Because some patients who might benefit from oxygen therapy may not want to receive it[59] and because the data on treatment preferences of patients with dyspnea are not conclusive, palliative oxygen should be delivered only with careful consideration of the intervention's potential benefit versus patient burden and costs; this conversation should include the patient and caregiver whenever possible. An "N of 1" trial can help guide treatment choice.[60]

Further qualification of the role and relative benefit of palliative oxygen comes from a German study comparing opioids versus oxygen therapy for patients receiving palliative care.[61] The study enrolled 46 terminally ill patients with baseline hypoxemia (<90% Sao_2) or normoxemia but without uncontrolled symptoms. For symptom relief, patients received either 4 L of supplemental oxygen by nasal cannula or titrated basal opioids with the option for breakthrough opioids. Outcomes were respiratory rate, dyspnea intensity, and Sao_2 and $Paco_2$ values. Patients receiving opioids were more likely to have dyspnea intensity reduced, and the opioid group experienced no increased hypercarbia compared to the oxygen group. Oxygen provided no benefit at rest in either hypoxemic or normoxemic patients.

Nonpharmacological Management

Consistent with the results of the palliative oxygen trial described earlier, simple interventions based on the movement of air may safely and inexpensively relieve dyspnea for certain patients. In a randomized crossover trial, use of a handheld electric fan directed toward the face was compared to use of the same fan directed toward the leg.[62] Participants (n = 50), all of whom had advanced disease, used the fan for 5 minutes; they reported significant decrease in dyspnea when the moving air was directed toward the face but not toward the leg. Some participants experienced continued benefit and some experienced new benefit during the 10-minute washout period after cessation of the fan intervention.

Used to treat the sensation of breathlessness, pulmonary rehabilitation is usually provided in the United States as a multidisciplinary, hospital-based, outpatient program, although it is sometimes available in home, community, or inpatient settings. The intervention is intensive; a typical regimen consists of supervised low- or high-intensity aerobic exercise sessions lasting 3 to 4 hours per session, scheduled three times per week for 6 to 12 weeks. The benefits of pulmonary rehabilitation, demonstrated in many clinical trials, include improvement in exercise capacity and health-related quality of life and reduction in dyspnea severity. Pulmonary rehabilitation may be especially beneficial for patients with severe dyspnea whose symptoms seem out of proportion to the severity of their disease.[63] These data were derived in the setting of COPD, and therefore the effects in patients with advanced cancer are largely unknown.

Other nonpharmacological approaches to management of dyspnea include vibration of the patient's chest wall, electrical stimulation of leg muscles to help with exercise tolerance, walking aids, relaxation and breathing training, music, case management, and psychotherapy. A comprehensive review, entitled "Non-pharmacological Interventions for Breathlessness in Advanced Stages of Malignant and Non-malignant Diseases," is available through the Cochrane series of systematic reviews.[64] Of note, studies support vibration of patient's chest wall, electrical stimulation of leg muscles, walking aids, and breathing training as effective interventions for dyspnea relief.

Surgical and Other Procedural Interventions for Dyspnea. In patients with lung cancer, dyspnea can result from obstruction either in the airways, caused by mass lesions, or in the lung parenchyma, resulting from pleural effusions. Pleural effusions can be addressed by many surgical and procedural approaches, including mechanical and chemical pleurodesis, placement of tunneled pleural catheters, and open or video-assisted thoracoscopic pleurectomy. Advantages of tunneled pleural catheters are their ease of placement, low complication rate, and potential to improve quality of life, symptoms, and general comfort in patients with end-stage malignancies.[65] A decision analysis that compared the cost-effectiveness of a commonly used brand of tunneled pleural catheter to that of talc pleurodesis for malignant pleural effusion found similar effectiveness of the two interventions, although the pleurodesis proved more cost-effective by 0.006 quality-adjusted life year at an $840 lower cost.[66] The cost-effectiveness of catheters increased (reducing cost to $100,000 per quality-adjusted life year) when patients had a prognosis of less than 6 weeks.

A prospective study of interventional bronchoscopy to relieve dyspnea and improve quality of life in patients with malignant central respiratory obstructions showed dyspnea improvement in 85% of patients; approximately half reported an improvement in overall quality of life.[67]

Lung volume reduction surgery (LVRS) is considered in patients with severe COPD who are symptomatic despite maximal medical therapy and pulmonary rehabilitation. In patients with predominantly upper lobe emphysema and low exercise capacity, LVRS improves dyspnea and exercise tolerance and confers a survival advantage.[68] Furthermore, LVRS has been shown to be superior in reducing need for supplemental oxygen up to 2 years after surgery[69] and decreasing frequency of COPD exacerbations.[70] However, the procedure has limitations: the 90-day postoperative mortality rate is approximately 5%, and major pulmonary and cardiac postoperative morbidity can exceed 20%.[71] This procedure may be of interest in a small number of cases for patients with cancer who have comorbid COPD.

Emerging and Complementary Therapies for Dyspnea. Several emerging and complementary therapies may be effective in alleviating dyspnea in patients with cancer. Heliox, a mixture of oxygen and helium (20% to 28% and 72% to 80%, respectively), increases SaO_2, improves exercise tolerance, and decreases dyspnea scores in patients with lung cancer compared to oxygen alone.[72] However, it is limited by expense, cumbersome logistics (use requires a nonrebreathing mask; gas is delivered in large tanks), lack of routine availability, and lack of guidelines for patient selection.[73]

Acupuncture offers a nonpharmaceutical, minimally invasive approach to dyspnea. A prospective study of 20 patients with cancer-related dyspnea at rest treated with acupuncture reported that 70% of participants experienced significant dyspnea improvement; benefit peaked at 90 minutes and lasted up to 6 hours.[74] However, a 2008 systematic review[25] and Cochrane Database review[64] found inadequate evidence to recommend acupuncture, or the related intervention acupressure, as a routine intervention for dyspnea control in patients with cancer.

KEY MESSAGES TO PATIENTS AND FAMILIES

The key first step in working with patients and families is to explain that dyspnea is a complex symptom that varies substantially from one patient to another; in addition to physical causes, other factors such as anxiety and subjective interpretation contribute to creating the dyspnea experience and determining how much suffering it entails. Patients and families should understand that if aspects of the cancer itself are causing the patient's dyspnea, dyspnea treatment first focuses on these anatomic and physiological causes; that is, the clinician targets the cancer and its physical effects to eliminate the resulting symptoms. If this fails, the next step is to explain to the patient and the family that when the patient's disease is being fully treated or when treatment has concluded but dyspnea persists, the clinician will apply a more global treatment strategy to manage the symptom. Overall, opioids are the mainstay of these global approaches to dyspnea, and patients should understand that these medications are effective and safe. A range of options for the treatment of dyspnea are available, and the clinician should walk the patient and family through these. The first is oxygen delivered from canisters or concentrators, which may be effective for patients with severe dyspnea. In patients who do not qualify for reimbursable long-term oxygen therapy, simple moving air such as that generated by the use of a small fan can provide similar relief. The next step is to explain that other therapies are possible in light of the individual patient's circumstances and needs, and these may include pulmonary rehabilitation, benzodiazepines, SSRIs, and acupuncture. Finally, the clinician needs to explain the importance of paying proper attention to anxiety, fear, and other psychological stressors, because these are important given that the related emotional states can fuel a spiral of worsening dyspnea. The clinician may recommend that the patient try psychotherapy, relaxation techniques, music, visualization, or other methods of interrupting the dyspnea spiral.

CONCLUSION AND SUMMARY

Dyspnea is a common and disabling symptom experienced by a majority of patients with cancer, especially as disease advances and they approach the end of life. Strategies aimed at reversing anatomic and physiological causes may relieve dyspnea and represent a first target of intervention. When underlying causes cannot be modified, global therapies focused on symptom relief should be enlisted; these also can be employed in conjunction with disease-targeted approaches. Opioids, preferably in oral formulation, are the standard first-line pharmacological treatment. Emerging data are providing evidence to position the role of anxiolytics (e.g., benzodiazepines, SSRIs) and inhaled furosemide as pharmacological adjuncts. Although oxygen is often prescribed to alleviate dyspnea in people who are not hypoxemic, it may be no more effective than less burdensome approaches and its use should be discontinued if patients do not experience meaningful relief within 3 days of initiation. Nonpharmacological options warranting consideration include vibration of patient's chest wall, electrical stimulation of leg muscles, walking aids, and breathing training; further data may support the use of pulmonary rehabilitation and acupuncture. Regardless of the treatment selected, a multidisciplinary approach should address the psychosocial, spiritual, and existential components contributing to the individual's "total dyspnea" experience, because suffering from this symptom transcends its physical impact.

SUMMARY RECOMMENDATIONS

- Identify disease-related and other anatomic or physiological causes of the dyspnea and treat these to directly relieve the symptom.
- In conjunction with treatment options, or if the disease has been maximally treated, initiate global therapies targeting the symptom itself rather than underlying disease.
- Use opioids as a first-line treatment option. Sustained-release oral morphine 10 mg per day is a reasonable starting point and may provide sufficient symptom relief.
- Use oxygen therapy for patients with severe hypoxemia ($Pao_2 \leq 55$ mm Hg at rest); for patients with mild to moderate hypoxemia ($Pao_2 > 55$ mm Hg), a brief N-of-1 trial should be conducted and the therapy discontinued if the patient does not report meaningful benefit within 3 days.
- Consider other nonpharmacological approaches where available and as appropriate to the individual patient; options include a fan, pulmonary rehabilitation, and acupuncture. For certain patients, surgical intervention may be warranted and effective.
- Provide care for this biopsychosocial symptom in a "whole person," patient-centered context, in which dyspnea management addresses the psychological, interpersonal, social, spiritual, and existential aspects of the symptom.

REFERENCES

1. American Thoracic Society. Dyspnea. Mechanisms, assessment, and management: a consensus statement. American Thoracic Society. *Am J Respir Crit Care Med.* 1999;159(1):321–340.
2. Reuben DB, Mor V. Dyspnea in terminally ill cancer patients. *Chest.* 1986;89(2):234–236.
3. Lynn J, Teno JM, Phillips RS, et al. Perceptions by family members of the dying experience of older and seriously ill patients. SUPPORT Investigators: Study to Understand Prognoses and Preferences for Outcomes and Risks of Treatments. *Ann Intern Med.* 1997;126(2):97–106.
4. Elmqvist MA, Jordhoy MS, Bjordal K, Kaasa S, Jannert M. Health-related quality of life during the last three months of life in patients with advanced cancer. *Support Care Cancer.* 2009;17(2):191–198.
5. Currow DC, Smith J, Davidson PM, Newton PJ, Agar MR, Abernethy AP. Do the trajectories of dyspnea differ in prevalence and intensity by diagnosis at the end of life? A consecutive cohort study. *J Pain Symptom Manage.* 2010;39(4):680–690.
6. Kutner JS, Kassner CT, Nowels DE. Symptom burden at the end of life: hospice providers' perceptions. *J Pain Symptom Manage.* 2001;21(6):473–480.
7. Currow DC, Ward AM, Abernethy AP. Advances in the pharmacological management of breathlessness. *Curr Opin Support Palliat Care.* 2009;3(2):103–106.
8. Abernethy AP, Wheeler JL. Total dyspnoea. *Curr Opin Support Palliat Care.* 2008;2(2):110–113.
9. Bruera EF, Fainsinger RL. Clinical management of cachexia and anorexia. In: Doyle D, ed. *Oxford Textbook of Palliative Medicine.* Oxford: Oxford Medical; 1993:330–337.
10. Bruera E, Schmitz B, Pither J, Neumann CM, Hanson J. The frequency and correlates of dyspnea in patients with advanced cancer. *J Pain Symptom Manage.* 2000;19(5):357–362.
11. Nardi AE, Freire RC, Zin WA. Panic disorder and control of breathing. *Respir Physiol Neurobiol.* 2009;167(1):133–143.
12. Edmonds P, Higginson I, Altmann D, Sen-Gupta G, McDonnell M. Is the presence of dyspnea a risk factor for morbidity in cancer patients? *J Pain Symptom Manage.* 2000;19(1):15–22.
13. O'Donnell DE, Banzett RB, Carrieri-Kohlman V, et al. Pathophysiology of dyspnea in chronic obstructive pulmonary disease: a roundtable. *Proc Am Thorac Soc.* 2007;4(2):145–168.
14. Santiago TV, Edelman NH. Opioids and breathing. *J Appl Physiol.* 1985;59(6):1675–1685.
15. Mahler DA, Murray JA, Waterman LA, et al. Endogenous opioids modify dyspnoea during treadmill exercise in patients with COPD. *Eur Respir J.* 2009;33(4):771–777.
16. Banzett RB, Mulnier HE, Murphy K, Rosen SD, Wise RJ, Adams L. Breathlessness in humans activates insular cortex. *NeuroReport.* 2000;11(10):2117–2120.
17. Parsons LM, Egan G, Liotti M, et al. Neuroimaging evidence implicating cerebellum in the experience of hypercapnia and hunger for air. *Proc Natl Acad Sci U S A.* 2001;98(4):2041–2046.
18. Liotti M, Brannan S, Egan G, et al. Brain responses associated with consciousness of breathlessness (air hunger). *Proc Natl Acad Sci USA.* 2001;98(4):2035–2040.
19. Evans KC, Banzett RB, Adams L, McKay L, Frackowiak RS, Corfield DR. BOLD fMRI identifies limbic, paralimbic, and cerebellar activation during air hunger. *J Neurophysiol.* 2002;88(3):1500–1511.
20. Abernethy AP, Currow DC. Need for mechanistically focused research of global systemic interventions in palliative care. *J Pain Symptom Manage.* 2010;40(3):e5–e8.
21. Kamal AH, Maguire JM, Wheeler JL, Currow DC, Abernethy AP. Dyspnea review for the palliative care professional: treatment goals and therapeutic options. *J Palliat Med.* 2012;15:106–114.
22. Kaye AD, Hoover JM, Ibrahim IN, et al. Analysis of the effects of fentanyl in the feline pulmonary vascular bed. *Am J Ther.* 2006;13(6):478–484.
23. Tenore PL. Psychotherapeutic benefits of opioid agonist therapy. *J Addict Dis.* 2008;27(3):49–65.
24. Jennings AL, Davies AN, Higgins JP, Gibbs JS, Broadley KE. A systematic review of the use of opioids in the management of dyspnoea. *Thorax.* 2002;57(11):939–944.

25. Ben-Aharon I, Gafter-Gvili A, Paul M, Leibovici L, Stemmer SM. Interventions for alleviating cancer-related dyspnea: a systematic review. *J Clin Oncol.* 2008;26(14):2396–2404.

26. Viola R, Kiteley C, Lloyd NS, Mackay JA, Wilson J, Wong RK. The management of dyspnea in cancer patients: a systematic review. *Support Care Cancer.* 2008;16(4):329–337.

27. Bruera E, Sala R, Spruyt O, Palmer JL, Zhang T, Willey J. Nebulized versus subcutaneous morphine for patients with cancer dyspnea: a preliminary study. *J Pain Symptom Manage.* 2005;29(6):613–618.

28. Abernethy AP, Currow DC, Frith P, Fazekas BS, McHugh A, Bui C. Randomised, double blind, placebo controlled crossover trial of sustained release morphine for the management of refractory dyspnoea. *BMJ.* 2003;327(7414):523–528.

29. Allard P, Lamontagne C, Bernard P, Tremblay C. How effective are supplementary doses of opioids for dyspnea in terminally ill cancer patients? A randomized continuous sequential clinical trial. *J Pain Symptom Manage.* 1999;17(4):256–265.

30. Currow DC, McDonald C, Oaten S, et al. Once-daily opioids for chronic dyspnea: a dose increment and pharmacovigilance study. *J Pain Symptom Manage.* 2011;42(3):388–399.

31. Clemens KE, Klaschik E. Effect of hydromorphone on ventilation in palliative care patients with dyspnea. *Support Care Cancer.* 2008;16(1):93–99.

32. Charles MA, Reymond L, Israel F. Relief of incident dyspnea in palliative cancer patients: a pilot, randomized, controlled trial comparing nebulized hydromorphone, systemic hydromorphone, and nebulized saline. *J Pain Symptom Manage.* 2008;36(1):29–38.

33. Benitez-Rosario MA, Martin AS, Feria M. Oral transmucosal fentanyl citrate in the management of dyspnea crises in cancer patients. *J Pain Symptom Manage.* 2005;30(5):395–397.

34. Gauna AA, Kang SK, Triano ML, Swatko ER, Vanston VJ. Oral transmucosal fentanyl citrate for dyspnea in terminally ill patients: an observational case series. *J Palliat Med.* 2008;11(4):643–648.

35. Wilson RH, Hoseth W, Dempsey ME. Respiratory acidosis. I. Effects of decreasing respiratory minute volume in patients with severe chronic pulmonary emphysema, with specific reference to oxygen, morphine and barbiturates. *Am J Med.* 1954;17(4):464–470.

36. Clemens KE, Quednau I, Klaschik E. Is there a higher risk of respiratory depression in opioid-naive palliative care patients during symptomatic therapy of dyspnea with strong opioids? *J Palliat Med.* 2008;11(2):204–216.

37. Clemens KE, Klaschik E. Symptomatic therapy of dyspnea with strong opioids and its effect on ventilation in palliative care patients. *J Pain Symptom Manage.* 2007;33(4):473–481.

38. Mahler DA, Selecky PA, Harrod CG, et al. American College of Chest Physicians consensus statement on the management of dyspnea in patients with advanced lung or heart disease. *Chest.* 2010;137(3):674–691.

39. Mitchell-Heggs P, Murphy K, Minty K, et al. Diazepam in the treatment of dyspnoea in the 'Pink Puffer' syndrome. *Q J Med.* 1980;49(193):9–20.

40. Eimer M, Cable T, Gal P, Rothenberger LA, McCue JD. Effects of clorazepate on breathlessness and exercise tolerance in patients with chronic airflow obstruction. *J Fam Pract.* 1985;21(5):359–362.

41. Man GC, Hsu K, Sproule BJ. Effect of alprazolam on exercise and dyspnea in patients with chronic obstructive pulmonary disease. *Chest.* 1986;90(6):832–836.

42. Woodcock AA, Gross ER, Geddes DM. Drug treatment of breathlessness: contrasting effects of diazepam and promethazine in pink puffers. *Br Med J (Clin Res Ed).* 1981;283(6287):343–346.

43. Navigante AH, Cerchietti LC, Castro MA, Lutteral MA, Cabalar ME. Midazolam as adjunct therapy to morphine in the alleviation of severe dyspnea perception in patients with advanced cancer. *J Pain Symptom Manage.* 2006;31(1):38–47.

44. Navigante AH, Castro MA, Cerchietti LC. Morphine versus midazolam as upfront therapy to control dyspnea perception in cancer patients while its underlying cause is sought or treated. *J Pain Symptom Manage.* 2010;39(5):820–830.

45. Currow DC, Abernethy AP. Potential opioid-sparing effect of regular benzodiazepines in dyspnea: longer duration of studies needed. *J Pain Symptom Manage.* 2010;40(5):e1–e2; author reply e2–e4.

46. Wilcock A, Walton A, Manderson C, et al. Randomised, placebo controlled trial of nebulised furosemide for breathlessness in patients with cancer. *Thorax.* 2008;63(10):872–875.

47. Kohara H, Ueoka H, Aoe K, et al. Effect of nebulized furosemide in terminally ill cancer patients with dyspnea. *J Pain Symptom Manage.* 2003;26(4):962–967.

48. Ong KC, Kor AC, Chong WF, Earnest A, Wang YT. Effects of inhaled furosemide on exertional dyspnea in chronic obstructive pulmonary disease. *Am J Respir Crit Care Med.* 2004;169(9):1028–1033.

49. Jensen D, Amjadi K, Harris-McAllister V, Webb KA, O'Donnell DE. Mechanisms of dyspnoea relief and improved exercise endurance after furosemide inhalation in COPD. *Thorax.* 2008;63(7):606–613.

50. Stone P, Rix, Kurowska A, Tookman. Re: nebulized furosemide for dyspnea in terminal cancer patients. *J Pain Symptom Manage.* 2002;24(3):274–275 author reply 275–276.

51. Abernethy AP, Currow DC, Frith P, Fazekas B. Prescribing palliative oxygen: a clinician survey of expected benefit and patterns of use. *Palliat Med.* 2005;19(2):168–170.

52. Roberts CM. Short burst oxygen therapy for relief of breathlessness in COPD. *Thorax.* 2004;59(8):638–640.

53. Escalante CP, Martin CG, Elting LS, et al. Dyspnea in cancer patients: etiology, resource utilization, and survival-implications in a managed care world. *Cancer.* 1996;78(6):1314–1319.

54. Nocturnal Oxygen Therapy Trial Group. Continuous or nocturnal oxygen therapy in hypoxemic chronic obstructive lung disease: a clinical trial. *Ann Intern Med.* 1980;93(3):391–398.

55. Report of the Medical Research Council Working Party. Long term domiciliary oxygen therapy in chronic hypoxic cor pulmonale complicating chronic bronchitis and emphysema. *Lancet.* 1981;1(8222):681–686.

56. Cranston JM, Crockett A, Currow DC. Oxygen therapy for dyspnea in adults. *Cochrane Database Syst Rev.* 2008;Jul 16;(3):CD004769.

57. Uronis HE, Currow DC, McCrory DC, Samsa GP, Abernethy AP. Oxygen for relief of dyspnoea in mildly- or non-hypoxaemic patients with cancer: a systematic review and meta-analysis. *Br J Cancer.* 2008;98(2):294–299.

58. Abernethy AP, McDonald CF, Frith PA, et al. Effect of palliative oxygen versus room air in relief of breathlessness in patients with refractory dyspnoea: a double-blind, randomised controlled trial. *Lancet.* 2010;376(2):784–793.

59. Currow DC, Fazekas B, Abernethy AP. Oxygen use: patients define symptomatic benefit discerningly. *J Pain Symptom Manage.* 2007;34:113–114.

60. Nonoyama ML, Brooks D, Guyatt GH, Goldstein RS. Effect of oxygen on health quality of life in patients with chronic obstructive pulmonary disease with transient exertional hypoxemia. *Am J Respir Crit Care Med.* 2007;176:343–349.

61. Clemens KE, Quednau I, Klaschik E. Use of oxygen and opioids in the palliation of dyspnoea in hypoxic and non-hypoxic palliative care patients: a prospective study. *Support Care Cancer.* 2009;17(4):367–377.

62. Galbraith S, Fagan P, Perkins P, Lynch A, Booth S. Does the use of a handheld fan improve chronic dyspnea? A randomized, controlled, crossover trial. *J Pain Symptom Manage.* 2010;39(5):831–838.

63. Casaburi R, ZuWallack R. Pulmonary rehabilitation for management of chronic obstructive pulmonary disease. *N Engl J Med.* 2009;360(13):1329–1335.

64. Bausewein C, Booth S, Gysels M, Higginson I. Non-pharmacological interventions for breathlessness in advanced stages of malignant and non-malignant diseases. *Cochrane Database Syst Rev.* 2008;(2) CD005623.

65. Monsky WL, Yoneda KY, MacMillan J, et al. Peritoneal and pleural ports for management of refractory ascites and pleural effusions: assessment of impact on patient quality of life and hospice/home nursing care. *J Palliat Med.* 2009;12(5):811–817.

66. Olden AM, Holloway R. Treatment of malignant pleural effusion: PleuRx catheter or talc pleurodesis? A cost-effectiveness analysis. *J Palliat Med.* 2010;13(1):59–65.

67. Amjadi K, Voduc N, Cruysberghs Y, et al. Impact of interventional bronchoscopy on quality of life in malignant airway obstruction. *Respiration.* 2008;76(4):421–428.

68. Naunheim KS, Wood DE, Mohsenifar Z, et al. Long-term follow-up of patients receiving lung-volume-reduction surgery versus medical therapy for severe emphysema by the National Emphysema Treatment Trial Research Group. *Ann Thorac Surg.* 2006;82:431–443.

69. Snyder ML, Goss CH, Neradilek B, et al. Changes in arterial oxygenation and self-reported oxygen use after lung volume reduction surgery. *Am J Respir Crit Care Med.* 2008;178(4):339–345.
70. Washko GR, Fan VS, Ramsey SD, et al. The effect of lung volume reduction surgery on chronic obstructive pulmonary disease exacerbations. *Am J Respir Crit Care Med.* 2008;177(2):164–169.
71. Naunheim KS, Wood DE, Krasna MJ, et al. Predictors of operative mortality and cardiopulmonary morbidity in the National Emphysema Treatment Trial. *J Thorac Cardiovasc Surg.* 2006; 131(1):43–53.

72. Ahmedzai SH, Laude E, Robertson A, Troy G, Vora V. A double-blind, randomised, controlled Phase II trial of Heliox28 gas mixture in lung cancer patients with dyspnoea on exertion. *Br J Cancer.* 2004;90(2):366–371.
73. Mathous C, Morgan SM, Hall JB, et al. Heliox in the treatment of airflow obstruction: a critical review of the literature. *Respir Care.* 1997;42:1034–1042.
74. Filshie J, Penn K, Ashley S, Davis CL. Acupuncture for the relief of cancer-related breathlessness. *Palliat Med.* 1996;10(2): 145–150.

What Is the Role of Opioids in Treatment of Refractory Dyspnea in Advanced Chronic Obstructive Pulmonary Disease?

ROBERT HORTON AND GRAEME ROCKER

INTRODUCTION AND SCOPE OF THE PROBLEM

This chapter outlines a supporting rationale and approach to the use of opioids in management of refractory dyspnea in the patient with advanced chronic obstructive pulmonary disease (COPD). Incapacitating dyspnea in the latter stages of COPD is a significant source of suffering that profoundly affects quality of life. Despite a range of potential interventions, dyspnea is a symptom that remains inadequately relieved for approximately half of all patients who continue to live and die with debilitating breathlessness.[1]

Palliative care services that initially focused on addressing the needs of patients with advanced cancer have evolved to focus more broadly on addressing unmet needs and symptoms in patients with a multitude of chronic, progressive illnesses.[2-4] Models of care and treatment regimens developed for patients with advanced malignancy may not transfer well to patients with other chronic illnesses. In COPD it is particularly prudent to consider an individualized approach to management of refractory dyspnea with the understanding that specific management strategies may differ significantly from standardized approaches to management of persistent dyspnea in the later stages of advanced malignancy.

Although this chapter focuses specifically on the use of opioids, it must be stressed that nonpharmacological and behavioral interventions as well as the potential of other medications in the management of refractory dyspnea remain of paramount importance and have been discussed extensively elsewhere.[5-9]

A small but growing body of evidence supports the effectiveness of opioids for treatment of refractory dyspnea in patients with advanced COPD.[10-12] Yet, many physicians are reluctant to prescribe opioids in this setting. Reluctance to consider opioids for treatment of refractory dyspnea earlier in the disease trajectory is reenforced in part by a dearth of evidence describing long-term use and a lack of consensus on opioid use among professional societies and practice guidelines.

Despite a limited body of evidence, it is increasingly accepted that a therapeutic trial of opioids should be considered not only in end-of-life situations but also for stable patients with COPD whenever breathlessness is severe and continues at intolerable levels despite optimal conventional therapy.[9,14,15] The role of opioids in this setting is the subject of ongoing studies to address many outstanding questions. In the absence of a comprehensive evidence base, this chapter reviews the current state of thinking on this issue and outlines an approach to using opioids in COPD that is supported by current evidence as well as expert-based consensus.

RELEVANT PATHOPHYSIOLOGY

Total Dyspnea

In the most simplistic terms, dyspnea has been defined as the uncomfortable awareness of breathing. More nuanced definitions acknowledge that dyspnea arises from a complex interaction between physical symptoms that contribute to dyspnea intensity and an emotional response to those symptoms that contributes to dyspnea-related distress. Thus dyspnea is a complex symptom resulting from signals originating from multiple sources in the central nervous system, upper airways, lungs, and chest wall. These signals are processed in higher brain centers, where they are interpreted along with associated behavioral, cognitive, emotional, contextual, and environmental cues, resulting in an individualized perception of dyspnea. This complexity of interaction can result in a wide range of symptoms affecting physical, emotional, social, and spiritual well-being. Just as the interaction among these factors contributes to the conceptual framework of "total pain," it is recognized that this interaction contributes similarly to shape the experience of total dyspnea.[16] The degree to which these various factors influence the final symptom of dyspnea is likely highly individualized and may have a profound impact on the individual's experience and response to various interventions and treatments. Recent advances in neural imaging are beginning to shed light on the extent of limbic and paralimbic activation in dyspnea,[17-20] supporting a multifaceted approach to management that addresses both underlying physical causes while simultaneously addressing the significant contribution of anxiety, fear, and other emotions.

How Do Opioids Influence Dyspnea?

Although exact mechanisms are not clearly understood, traditionally opioids are thought to modulate the perception of dyspnea through several pathways and mechanisms of action resulting in a reduction in total ventilation, an increase in ventilatory efficiency with exercise, a reduction in responses to hypoxia and hypercapnia, a reduction in the drive to breathe, and effects on bronchoconstriction. Exercise performance–related dyspnea in COPD was recognized many years ago to be improved by exogenous opioids[21] and more recently affected by endogenous opioids.[22]

Advances in neural imaging have provided additional insights into the role of the limbic system[23] and the ability of opioids to alter the central perception of dyspnea.[24] The ability of opioids to attenuate limbic responses associated with dyspnea may be at the root of their therapeutic potential.

Dyspnea Intensity Versus Dyspnea Distress

Patients with COPD make clear distinctions between physical descriptors related to dyspnea intensity and dyspnea-related affective distress, qualities of which appear to be specific and measurable.[25-27] This distinction is further supported by comparative analysis of the linguistic terms used by patients with COPD to describe their dyspnea, revealing that despite comparable descriptors of dyspnea intensity to age-matched controls, typically only patients with COPD choose affective descriptors such as "frightening," "worried," "helpless," "depressed," and "awful" to characterize their breathing.[28] Opioids have been shown to be effective in reducing dyspnea intensity,[10-12] but the essence of their therapeutic value may be in their potential to reduce the accompanying distress and suffering experienced as dyspnea intensity worsens. The challenge is to identify which of these variable factors contributing to the construct of total dyspnea are affected by opioids and to distinguish between them when making decisions about initiating treatment.

SUMMARY OF EVIDENCE REGARDING TREATMENT RECOMMENDATIONS

What Evidence Supports the Use of Opioids?

Experience with opioid use in advanced COPD is limited, even though it has been more than two decades since morphine was first reported to be associated with a reduction in dyspnea symptoms.[29] Until recently, the use of opioids over longer periods (weeks and months or beyond) has received little attention or support, and the research has mostly focused on short-term effects over hours or days.[10]

The use of opioids for dyspnea is the subject of a Cochrane review in which 11 of 18 studies reported only patients with COPD (range 7-19 patients). This review confirmed overall beneficial effects of both oral and parenteral opioids on dyspnea ($p = .001$) and, from a meta-regression, that both were more effective than placebo,[12] a conclusion supported by a subsequent report in 2004.[30] By contrast, nebulized opioids did not appear to have any effect on dyspnea. It is noteworthy that 14 of the 18 randomized, controlled trials reviewed involved single dosing of opioids. Four multiple-dosing studies over a week or more involving patients with COPD used oral diamorphine,[31] dihydrocodeine,[21] or morphine.[32] Table 21-1 summarizes evidence on opioid efficacy and side effects accrued from these studies.

Subsequent to the 2002 systematic review, Abernethy and colleagues[10] published the results of a placebo-controlled crossover trial of 48 patients (mostly with COPD) in which daily use of a sustained-release morphine formulation had predominantly beneficial effects. In this 4-day crossover study, using sustained-release morphine 20 mg per 24 hours, the effects were positive, with patients reporting improvements in their refractory dyspnea and better sleep. The effect on dyspnea was more evident later in the day. Constipation was a problem for some patients. Of the original cohort of 48, 10 withdrew from the study; only 5 withdrew for likely morphine-related side effects. Despite some adverse effects, this study was the first adequately powered randomized, controlled trial that supported the use of opioids for the symptomatic relief of dyspnea. Secondary analyses of the study data failed to demonstrate a relation between severity of dyspnea and subsequent response to opioids.[34]

A recent open-label dose increment and pharmacovigilance study evaluated once-daily sustained-release morphine in doses ranging from 10 to 30 mg in 83 patients with chronic dyspnea, 54% of whom had COPD.[11] Sixty-two percent of patients experienced a minimum 10% improvement in dyspnea over baseline (average 30%), yielding a number needed to treat of 1.6 and number needed to harm of 4.6. Dyspnea was controlled in 70% of patients on 10 mg per day, and benefit was sustained for 3 months for one third of patients. Constipation, drowsiness, and nausea and vomiting were the most commonly encountered side effects; there were no reported cases of hospitalization for respiratory depression or decreased

TABLE 21-1. Multiple Dosing Studies of Opioids for Dyspnea Among Patients With Chronic Obstructive Pulmonary Disease

STUDY, YEAR	NUMBER OF PATIENTS	OPIOID PREPARATION	STUDY DESIGN	STUDY DURATION	DYSPNEA MEASUREMENT	RESULTS	SIDE EFFECTS
Currow,[11] 2011	N = 83, 45 with COPD	Morphine SR 10, 20, 30 mg OD	Open label, dose increment study	3 mo, 30 patient-years of data	VAS for dyspnea 2 × daily	62% of patients had minimum 10% reduction in dyspnea, NNT = 1.6 NNH = 4.6; 70% of patients controlled on 10 mg per day	Constipation was the most common. No hospitalizations for respiratory depression, reduced LOC, or delirium.
Abernethy,[10] 2003	N = 48 (COPD n = 42)	Morphine SR 20 mg 4-day crossover vs. placebo	Clinical study in the community	4 days	VAS for dyspnea at day 4	Better dyspnea scores both mornings ($p = 0.01$) and evening ($p < 0.05$)	More constipation with morphine; other side effects not significant.
Poole,[32] 1998	N = 16 (FEV$_1$ <1.5 l)	Morphine SR 10-20 mg OD or bid	Preregimen and 6-wk exercise testing in study center	6 wk × 2, plus 2-wk washout	CRQ for quality of life, 6-min walk	NS overall, but mastery scale favored placebo; 6-min walk test worse with morphine	Opioid withdrawal syndrome: 4/16; patients on morphine more likely to report nausea, anorexia, constipation, or drowsiness ($p = 0.004$).
Eiser et al,[31] 1991	N = 18 (pink puffer, mean FEV$_1$ 36%)	Diamorphine 2.5 or 5 mg PO qid	Preregimen and 2-wk exercise testing in study center	2 wk × 3, crossover, no washout	VAS for dyspnea; 6-min walk	NS	4 withdrew (chest infection, itching, constipation, headache); mild nausea: "several" with constipation or vomiting (3/14)
Johnson,[35] 1983	N = 19 FEV$_1$ <1.2 MRC ≥3	Dihydrocodeine 15 mg PO 30 min preexercise, up to tid	Preregimen and 1 wk pedometer testing in the home	weekly, crossover × 3 (third wk alternate-day codeine)	VAS for dyspnea; pedometer distance	Dyspnea reduced by 18%, walk distance up 17%	Similar among placebo and treated groups
Woodcock,[21] 1981	N = 12 MRC >3	Dihydrocodeine 1 mg/kg PO OD, vs. oxygen, alcohol, or caffeine 45 min preexercise	Exercise testing (treadmill, in hospital)	4 days	VAS for dyspnea	20% reduction in dyspnea, 18% increase in exercise tolerance 45 min after codeine	Nausea and vomiting (5/16); constipated/ drowsy (2/16)

COPD, Chronic obstructive pulmonary disease; *CRQ*, Chronic Respiratory Disease Questionnaire; *FEV$_1$*, forced expiratory volume in 1 second; *LOC*, level of consciousness, *Morphine SR*, sustained-release morphine; *MRC*, Medical Research Council Dyspnea Scale; *NNH*, number needed to harm; *NNT*, number needed to treat; *NS*, not significant; *OD*, once daily; *VAS*, visual analog scale.

level of consciousness. Qualitative data published in abstract form confirm that both patients and their families find opioids helpful in advanced COPD.[13]

Barriers to Use of Opioids

For physicians, barriers to opioid use in COPD include discomfort and inexperience with managing potential side effects, fears about respiratory depression, and concerns about addiction and dependence. In addition, clinicians have a lack of knowledge regarding opioid pharmacokinetics, which may result in discomfort with appropriate initiation, dose titration, and monitoring of clinical response and side effects.

Advice from professional societies and clinical practice guidelines has often been unclear and at times contradictory. Until recently, there has been a lack of explicit expert guidance on this issue and considerable variation in recommendations. A 2004 position paper from the European Respiratory Society and the American Thoracic Society made no recommendations.[36] Previous Canadian, Australian, and American guidelines and policy statements on COPD included guarded or nonspecific recommendations for considering opioids for severe dyspnea.[37–40]

A 1999 position paper from the American Thoracic Society specifically counseled against the use of opioids in COPD except in terminal stages,[41] and the Global Initiative for Chronic Obstructive Lung Disease made passing, cautious reference regarding the use of opioids suggesting that their use may cause serious adverse effects and that benefits may be limited to a few sensitive individuals.[42]

Evidence amassed to date regarding the use of opioids in patients with COPD has raised questions about the veracity of these assertions. There have been no reported cases of clinically significant respiratory depression in the medical literature resulting from carefully initiated and appropriately titrated oral opioids. Several studies within the systematic review by Jennings and colleagues[12] attest to the lack of adverse short-term effect on blood gases. More recent studies have also confirmed that appropriate initiation and monitoring of opioids over the longer term in stable patients with COPD is safe and well tolerated.[11,43] In 2010 the American College of Chest Physicians published a consensus statement on the management of dyspnea in advanced heart and lung disease supporting the role of oral and parenteral opioids in providing relief of dyspnea and recommending individualized dose titration.[15] Most recently the Canadian Thoracic Society offered specific recommendations on initiation and dose titration of oral opioids as an adjunctive treatment to reduce dyspnea and improve quality of life in the setting of refractory dyspnea in COPD.[14]

Fears of using potentially powerful medications with side effects or of implications of using a controlled substance or having them in the house often underpins initial reluctance by patients and families to consider opioids.[13] Case reports indicate that any initial reluctance may be supplanted by the reduction in dyspnea distress that opioids induce and that for some, the improvements in quality of life have been profound.[32,44–46]

Refractory Versus Acceptable, Manageable, or Tolerable Dyspnea

Dyspnea is considered refractory when individual symptoms persist at an intolerable level despite optimal conventional treatment.[47] Complete relief from all manifestations of dyspnea in the latter stages of COPD is not a realistic goal for the vast majority of patients. Interventions aimed at palliating dyspnea need to be clearly focused on alleviating the most distressing aspects of the total dyspnea complex, striking a reasonable balance between achieving acceptable or tolerable levels of dyspnea related distress and avoiding medication related side-effects. Reduction in dyspnea-related distress in the advanced stages of disease in response to opioids might occur in the absence of accompanying improvement in functional status or exercise tolerance. An individualized approach to choice of agent, route of delivery, and meticulous titration targeted to achieving individually defined acceptable, manageable, or tolerable levels of dyspnea in return for minimized opioid-related side effects is most likely to be successful within the paradigm of COPD. This approach is similar to that endorsed by patients prescribed opioids for the management of cancer pain[48] and is supported by recent Canadian Thoracic Society guidelines on treatment of refractory dyspnea in COPD.[14]

The Concept of Dyspnea and Opioid Responsiveness

Opioid responsiveness in the context of refractory dyspnea has been defined as the attainment of acceptable, manageable, or tolerable levels of dyspnea-related distress in response to initiation and titration of opioid therapy that may or may not be accompanied by an associated reduction in dyspnea intensity.[49]

Variability in degree of opioid responsiveness in pain is well described.[50–53] More recently it has been proposed that dyspnea as a symptom may show variation in response to opioids based on several potential factors.[34,49] Identification of the most relevant factors may allow us to predict with more accuracy which patients with refractory dyspnea are most likely to respond to opioids, allowing clinicians to target therapies to those most likely to benefit and avoid adverse outcomes in those less likely to respond.

Although definitive evidence regarding opioid responsiveness in dyspnea is lacking and the subject of ongoing research,[47] it has been proposed that dyspnea is most likely to be responsive to opioid therapy in the following situations[49]:
- Dyspnea is strongly associated with the presence of fear, anxiety, or panic.
- The patient perceives dyspnea intensity is steadily worsening over time.

- The patient perceives an inability to control dyspnea by pacing, reduction in activity, or practicing cognitive or behavioral interventions.
- Dyspnea is unpredictable in onset.

Dyspnea Crisis

Although the potential exists for opioids to reduce dyspnea intensity in the setting of more chronic dyspnea, the proposal has been made that the magnitude of opioid response may increase as patients' dyspnea experience approaches crisis proportions and beneficial effects may wane or side effects may predominate in situations in which dyspnea, although disabling, is more chronic, stable, and predictable.[49] Dyspnea crisis in the setting of COPD has been defined as an acute onset or escalation of dyspnea that may or may not be predictable and is strongly associated with the following[49]:

- Fear, anxiety, or panic (limbic activation)
- Sense of loss of control (inability to reverse by pacing activity or breathing techniques)
- Experience of dyspnea as a distinct departure from background or baseline dyspnea

Although likely more prevalent in the advanced stages of disease, dyspnea crisis may occur earlier in the disease trajectory secondary to potentially reversible underlying causes such as an acute COPD exacerbation or pneumonia. Opioids are widely used to manage dyspnea crisis toward the end of life; however, their use as adjunctive treatment for dyspnea crisis earlier in the trajectory of COPD has not been evaluated.

Initiation and Titration of Opioids for Refractory Dyspnea

Opioid therapy is one of several potential approaches to the management of severe dyspnea that includes both conventional pharmacological and nonpharmacological interventions that should be optimized first (Figure 21-1). Nevertheless, given that a high proportion of patients with advanced COPD continue to experience intolerable dyspnea despite conventional interventions, people struggling with dyspnea related to COPD should not be denied an appropriately initiated and monitored trial of opioids, balancing benefits and any adverse effects as in any other clinical encounter. Of note, unlike almost all other medications in the pharmacopoeia, opioids can be titrated effectively and safely over a wide range of doses to therapeutic effect. A "start low, go slow" approach is important for several reasons, but gaining patients' and families' confidence is key. Gaining the confidence of the "opioid-naïve physician" unaccustomed to prescribing opioids in this situation is also important.

Initiation of treatment with a single, once-daily oral long-acting preparation of morphine at a starting dose of 10 mg, though not without side effects, has been shown to be effective, safe, and tolerable for a majority of patients with refractory dyspnea in COPD.[11] Although potentially more costly than more frequent dosing with immediate-release morphine, this approach offers obvious benefits in terms of convenience and compliance.

Although longer-term data evaluating efficacy and tolerability of oral morphine equivalent of less than 10 mg and greater than 30 mg per day have yet to be reported, preliminary unpublished data from a mixed methods study evaluating initiation of an atypically small starting dose (0.5 mg) of oral immediate-release morphine every 4 hours gradually titrated to effect indicate that this approach is not only safe and well tolerated but also contributes to profound improvements in quality of life for select individuals.[13,47]

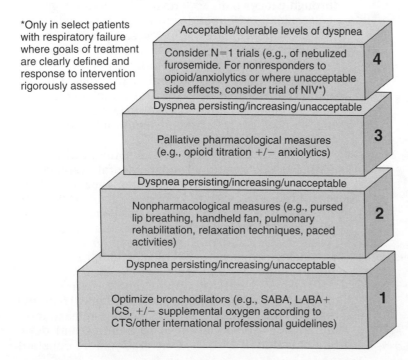

*Only in select patients with respiratory failure where goals of treatment are clearly defined and response to intervention rigorously assessed

Acceptable/tolerable levels of dyspnea

4 — Consider N=1 trials (e.g., of nebulized furosemide. For nonresponders to opioid/anxiolytics or where unacceptable side effects, consider trial of NIV*)

Dyspnea persisting/increasing/unacceptable

3 — Palliative pharmacological measures (e.g., opioid titration +/− anxiolytics)

Dyspnea persisting/increasing/unacceptable

2 — Nonpharmacological measures (e.g., pursed lip breathing, handheld fan, pulmonary rehabilitation, relaxation techniques, paced activities)

Dyspnea persisting/increasing/unacceptable

1 — Optimize bronchodilators (e.g., SABA, LABA+ ICS, +/− supplemental oxygen according to CTS/other international professional guidelines)

FIGURE 21-1. The dyspnea ladder in chronic obstructive pulmonary disease. The ladder describes a stepwise approach to the management of severe dyspnea in patients with advanced COPD. *CTS,* Canadian Thoracic Society; *ICS,* inhaled corticosteroids; *LABA,* long-acting β-agonists; *NIV,* noninvasive ventilation; *SABA,* short-acting β-agonists. *(Modified from Marciniuk DD, Goodridge D, Hernandez P, et al. Managing dyspnea in patients with advanced chronic obstructive pulmonary disease: a Canadian Thoracic Society clinical practice guideline. Can Respir J. 2011;18(2):69-78; and Rocker GM, Sinuff T, Horton R, Hernandez P. Advanced chronic obstructive pulmonary disease: innovative approaches to palliation. J Palliat Med. 2007;10(3):783-797.)*

Table 21-2 outlines this more cautious consensus-based approach to opioid initiation and titration in the setting of advanced COPD supported by the Canadian Thoracic Society.[14]

In contrast to patients with cancer, patients with COPD usually have lived with slowly progressive breathlessness for years. Commonly encountered opioid-related side effects (constipation, nausea, sedation, and impaired cognition) may significantly impair quality of life for some patients who may prefer to live with some degree of breathlessness rather than experience persistent opioid side effects. Education of patients and family members and an anticipatory management plan that meticulously addresses side effects is crucial. Patients who experience delirium or unexpected sedation related to progressive or rapid dose escalation on a regimen that might be considered routine when treating pain may be extremely reluctant to revisit opioid use in the future. Thus, in a stable patient, it may be preferable to initiate treatment with a low starting dose and ensure gradual dose escalation is tailored to individual response and tolerability. If confidence with opioids is lost through a "forced pace" regimen, patients will have lost an important and rare therapeutic intervention for dyspnea. This approach may seem overly cautious, but it is aimed at minimizing noncompliance resulting from opioid-related side effects, accepting the tradeoff that it may take time to see a therapeutic response.

Nebulized Opioids

A 2002 Cochrane review of opioids in the treatment of dyspnea concluded that in contrast to oral and parenteral opioids, there was insufficient evidence to support use of nebulized opioids.[12] Nevertheless, some case series and uncontrolled studies support a possible role for nebulized opioids in the treatment of refractory dyspnea.[54,55] More recently it has become clear that the way nebulized opioids are administered may play a role in determining their efficacy.[56] It is also probable that the individual pharmacokinetic properties of the administered opioid are a key factor. Nebulized fentanyl, for example, is lipophilic and rapidly absorbed, achieving similar serum levels to parenteral administration within 5 minutes,[57] making it potentially well suited to treatment of acute episodic dyspnea. At present, evidence supporting beneficial effects of nebulized fentanyl is limited to uncontrolled case series in cancer-related dyspnea.[55,58]

A 2009 article highlights recruitment difficulties (two patients over 18 months) in a randomized cross-over trial (nebulized fentanyl versus placebo). Both patients demonstrated marked reduction in dyspnea intensity measured by visual analog scale in response to nebulized fentanyl in comparison to placebo.[59] These results underscore the potential value of N-of-1 trials in evaluation of novel agents in clinical situations in which options are limited and evidence from randomized, controlled trials is lacking or difficult to obtain.[60] Canadian investigators are currently conducting a randomized placebo-controlled trial of the effect of inhaled fentanyl on dyspnea and exercise tolerance in patients with moderate to severe COPD.[61] Given that patients with COPD are often familiar with and have access to nebulized delivery of bronchodilators, delivery of opioids by this route, if effective, could offer a valuable means of providing rapid relief for refractory episodic dyspnea.

Advances in Opioid Delivery

Recently available sublingual, buccal, and nasal formulations of fentanyl aimed at the treatment of breakthrough cancer pain[55,62-66] resulted in some degree of reclassification of opioids (Table 21-3) and expanded treatment possibilities, offering easily administered formulations with rapid onset and shorter duration of action without active metabolites. These preparations are potentially suited to treating brief but severe episodes of incidental or spontaneous dyspnea that plague patients in the latter stages of COPD and often lead to repeated presentations to the emergency department.[67]

It may be crucial to make a clear distinction between resting versus exertional and incidental dyspnea and acute versus chronic dyspnea when considering the role of therapeutic options in general, in addition to the specific issue of opioid responsiveness and opioid pharmacokinetics that might influence therapeutic choices. Episodic severe dyspnea that comes on quickly and lasts an average of 30 minutes every morning after dressing is likely to be more appropriately managed with a lipophilic rapidly acting, short-duration opioid such as intranasal or buccal fentanyl than an oral formulation of immediate-release morphine with a peak action of 60 minutes and duration of action of 4 hours. Conversely, more constant

---

TABLE 21-2.   Suggested Protocol for Managing Refractory Dyspnea With Opioid Therapy in Chronic Obstructive Pulmonary Disease

Initiate opioid therapy with oral immediate-release morphine syrup—titrate slowly at weekly intervals over a 4- to 6-week period.

Start therapy with morphine 0.5 mg PO q24h for 2 days, then increase to 0.5 mg PO q4h while awake for remainder of week 1.

If tolerated and indicated, increase to morphine 1 mg PO q4h while awake in week 2, increasing by 1 mg/wk or 25% dosage increments/wk until the lowest effective dose that appropriately manages the dyspnea is achieved.

When a stable dosage is achieved (i.e., no significant dose change for 2 weeks and dyspnea managed), a sustained-release preparation at a comparable daily dose could be considered for substitution.

If patients experience significant opioid-related side effects such as nausea or confusion, substitution of an equipotent dose of oral hydromorphone could be considered.

Stool softeners and laxatives should be routinely offered to prevent opioid-associated constipation.

From Marciniuk D, Goodridge D, Hernandez P, et al. Managing dyspnea in patients with advanced chronic obstructive pulmonary disease: a Canadian Thoracic Society clinical practice guideline. *Can Respir J.* 2011;18(2):69–78.

TABLE 21-3. Commonly Available Opioids by Onset and Duration of Action

CLASSIFICATION	PREPARATION	ONSET	DURATION OF ACTION
Short acting	Morphine	30-60 min	3-4 hr
	Hydromorphone	30-60 min	3-4 hr
	Oxycodone	30-60 min	3-4 hr
Long acting	Morphine SR	3-4 hr	8-12 hr
	Oxycodone SR	3-4 hr	8-12 hr
	Fentanyl transdermal patch	12-24 hr	48-72 hr
Rapid onset	Fentanyl oral transmucosal	15 min	1-3 hr
	Fentanyl buccal tablet	10-15 min	1-3 hr
	Fentanyl sublingual tablet	10-15 min	1-3 hr
	Fentanyl intranasal spray	10-15 min	1-3 hr

unrelieved or poorly controlled background dyspnea that is present most of the day may be more appropriately treated with a longer-acting, slower-onset, orally administered opioid such as sustained-release morphine. To date, the current literature supporting the potential for rapidly acting opioids to alleviate refractory incident dyspnea is limited to case reports.[54,55,68]

KEY MESSAGES TO PATIENTS AND FAMILIES

The key message for patients with COPD and their families is that the use of opioids to control dyspnea is both safe and effective. Concerns about these medications, including those relating to fear of addiction, side effects, and that the medications will induce respiratory depression, are common and should be addressed preemptively when prescribing opioids. If this is not done, it is likely that the patient will avoid taking the medications and continue to suffer needlessly. Clinicians should also discuss the relationship of shortness of breath with anxiety and panic and help patients and families understand that each can worsen the other. Thus the critical elements in working with patients with COPD and their families is to both prescribe the appropriate medications and provide education about the disease and the ways opioids can effectively treat symptoms.

CONCLUSION AND SUMMARY

In the setting of refractory dyspnea in advanced COPD, it appears that opioids are neither panacea nor poison. Research that aims to clarify their role and efficacy is in its infancy. Many unanswered questions remain:

- What is the most effective initiation dose, dosing interval, titration schedule, and delivery route? How are these affected by the opioid pharmacokinetic profile?
- How do beneficial and adverse effects of opioids change over time?
- What factors influence response to opioids in COPD?
- What factors influence compliance with opioid therapy? How does compliance change over time?

- Do patients with COPD experience incidence of opioid-induced complications similar to those of other patients with refractory dyspnea?
- What is the relative risk/benefit of using opioids in patients with refractory dyspnea and chronic hypercapnia?

Ongoing initiatives address these and other questions to provide further insight and allow clinicians to refine their individual approach to using opioids in this setting.

SUMMARY RECOMMENDATIONS

- Conventional therapy should be optimized for chronic obstructive pulmonary disease.
- Therapy should be initiated with either a single, once-daily oral dose of 24-hour sustained-release morphine 10 mg or immediate-release morphine 0.5 to 1 mg of every 4 hours while awake.
- Side effects, especially constipation, should be anticipated and preemptively managed.
- Opioids should be titrated gradually to achieve acceptable balance between side effects and individualized target for acceptable, manageable, or tolerable dyspnea.

REFERENCES

1. Elkington H, White P, Addington-Hall J, Higgs R, Edmonds P. The healthcare needs of chronic obstructive pulmonary disease patients in the last year of life. *Palliat Med.* 2005;19(6):485–491.
2. Twaddle ML. The trend to move palliative care upstream. *J Palliat Med.* 2003;6(2):193–194.
3. Murtagh FE, Preston M, Higginson I. Patterns of dying: palliative care for non-malignant disease. *Clin Med.* 2004;4(1): 39–44.
4. Murray SA, Boyd K, Kendall M, Worth A, Benton TF, Clausen H. Dying of lung cancer or cardiac failure: prospective qualitative interview study of patients and their carers in the community. *Br Med J.* 2002;325(7370):929.
5. Booth S, Bausewein C, Higginson I, Moosavi SH. Pharmacological treatment of refractory breathlessness. *Expert Rev Respir Med.* 2009;3(1):21–36.
6. Bausewein C, Booth S, Gysels M, Higginsin I. Non-pharmacological interventions for breathlessness in advanced stages of malignant and non-malignant diseases. *Cochrane Database Syst Rev.* 2008;(2):CD005623.

7. Currow DC, Abernethy AP. Pharmacological management of dyspnoea. *Curr Opin Support Palliat Care.* 2007;1(2):96–101.

8. Currow DC, Ward AM, Abernethy AP. Advances in the pharmacological management of breathlessness. *Curr Opin Support Palliat Care.* 2009;3(2):103–106.

9. Rocker G, Horton R, Currow DC, Goodridge D, Young J, Booth S. Palliation of dyspnoea in advanced COPD: revisiting a role for opioids. *Thorax.* 2009;64(10):910–915.

10. Abernethy AP, Currow DC, Frith P, Fazekas BS, McHugh A, Bui C. Randomised, double blind, placebo controlled crossover trial of sustained release morphine for the management of refractory dyspnoea. *Br Med J.* 2003;327(7414):523–528.

11. Currow DC, McDonald C, Oaten S, et al. Once-daily opioids for chronic dyspnea: a dose increment and pharmacovigilance study. *J Pain Symptom Manage.* 2011;42:386–389.

12. Jennings AL, Davies AN, Higgins JP, Gibbs JS, Broadley KE. A systematic review of the use of opioids in the management of dyspnoea. *Thorax.* 2002;57(11):939–944.

13. Rocker G, Young J, Donahue M, et al. Perspectives of patients, family caregivers and physicians about the use of opioids for refractory dyspnea in advanced chronic obstructive pulmonary disease. *CMAJ,* 2012;18(9):E497–E504.

14. Marciniuk D, Goodridge D, Hernandez P, et al. Managing dyspnea in patients with advanced chronic obstructive pulmonary disease: a Canadian Thoracic Society clinical practice guideline. *Can Respir J.* 2011;18(2):69–78.

15. Mahler DA, Murray JA, Waterman LA, et al. Endogenous opioids modify dyspnoea during treadmill exercise in patients with COPD. *Eur Respir J.* 2009;33(4):771–777.

16. Abernethy AP, Wheeler JL. Total dyspnoea. *Curr Opin Support Palliat Care.* 2008;2(2):110–113.

17. von Leupoldt A, Sommer T, Kegat S, et al. The unpleasantness of perceived dyspnea is processed in the anterior insula and amygdala. *Am J Respir Crit Care Med.* 2008;177(9):1026–1032.

18. von Leupoldt A, Sommer T, Kegat S, et al. Dyspnea and pain share emotion-related brain network. *Neuroimage.* 2009;48(1):200–206.

19. Peiffer C. Dyspnea and emotion: what can we learn from functional brain imaging? *Am J Respir Crit Care Med.* 2008;177(9):937–939.

20. Peiffer C, Costes N, Hervé P, Garcia-Larrea L. Relief of dyspnea involves a characteristic brain activation and a specific quality of sensation. *Am J Respir Crit Care Med.* 2008;177(4):440–449.

21. Woodcock AA, Gross ER, Gellert A, Shah S, Johnson M, Geddes DM. Effects of dihydrocodeine, alcohol, and caffeine on breathlessness and exercise tolerance in patients with chronic obstructive lung disease and normal blood gases. *N Engl J Med.* 1981;305(27):1611–1616.

22. Mahler DA, Murray JA, Waterman LA, et al. Endogenous opioids modify dyspnoea during treadmill exercise in patients with COPD. *Eur Respir J.* 2009;33(4):771–777.

23. Herigstad M, Haven A, Wiech K, Pattinson KT. Dyspnoea and the brain. *Respir Med.* 2011;105(6):809–817.

24. Pattinson KT, Governo RJ, MacIntosh BJ, et al. Opioids depress cortical centers responsible for the volitional control of respiration. *J Neurosci.* 2009;29(25):8177–8186.

25. Smith J, Albert P, Bertella E, Lester J, Jack S, Calverly P. Qualitative aspects of breathlessness in health and disease. *Thorax.* 2009;64(8):713–718.

26. Carrieri-Kohlman V, Donescy-Cuenco D, Park SK, Mackin L, Nguyen HQ, Paul SM. Additional evidence for the affective dimension of dyspnea in patients with COPD. *Res Nurs Health.* 2010;33(1):4–19.

27. Lansing RW, Gracely RH, Banzett RB. The multiple dimensions of dyspnea: review and hypotheses. *Respir Physiol Neurobiol.* 2009;67(1):53–60.

28. Williams M, Cafarella P, Olds T, Petkov J, Frith P. The language of breathlessness differentiates between patients with COPD and age-matched adults. *Chest.* 2008;134(3):489–496.

29. Light RW, Muro JR, Sato RI, Stansbury DW, Fischer CE, Brown SE. Effects of oral morphine on breathlessness and exercise tolerance in patients with chronic obstructive pulmonary disease. *Am Rev Respir Dis.* 1989;139(1):126–133.

30. Foral PA, Malesker MA, Huerta G, Hilleman DE. Nebulized opioids use in COPD. *Chest.* 2004;125(2):691–694.

31. Eiser N, Denman WT, West C, Luce P. Oral diamorphine: lack of effect on dyspnoea and exercise tolerance in the "pink puffer" syndrome. *Eur Respir J.* 1991;4(8):926–931.

32. Poole PJ, Veale AG, Black PN. The effect of sustained-release morphine on breathlessness and quality of life in severe chronic obstructive pulmonary disease. *Am J Respir Crit Care Med.* 1998;157(6 Pt 1):1877–1880.

33. Johnson MA, Woodcock AA, Geddes DM. Dihydrocodeine for breathlessness in "pink puffers." *Br Med J.* 1983;286(6366): 675–677.

34. Currow DC, Plummer J, Frith P, Abernethy AP. Can we predict which patients with refractory dyspnea will respond to opioids? *J Palliat Med.* 2007;10(5):1031–1036.

35. Johnson MA, Woodcock AA, Rehahn M, Geddes DM. Are "pink puffers" more breathless than "blue bloaters"? *Br Med J.* 1983;286(6360):179–182.

36. Celli BR, MacNee W. Standards for the diagnosis and treatment of patients with COPD: a summary of the ATS/ERS position paper. *Eur Respir J.* 2004;23(6):932–946.

37. Abramson MJ, Crockett AJ, Frith PA, McDonald CF. COPDX: an update of guidelines for the management of chronic obstructive pulmonary disease with a review of recent evidence. *Med J Aust.* 2006;184(7):342–345.

38. O'Donnell DE, Aaron S, Bourbeau J, et al. State of the Art Compendium: Canadian Thoracic Society recommendations for the management of chronic obstructive pulmonary disease. *Can Respir J.* 2004;11(suppl B):7B–59B.

39. Selecky PA, Eliasson CA, Hall RI, et al. Palliative and end-of-life care for patients with cardiopulmonary diseases: American College of Chest Physicians position statement. *Chest.* 2005;128(5):3599–3610.

40. Lanken PN, Terry PB, Delisser HM, et al. An official American Thoracic Society clinical policy statement: palliative care for patients with respiratory diseases and critical illnesses. *Am J Respir Crit Care Med.* 2008;177(8):912–927.

41. American Thoracic Society. Dyspnea: mechanisms, assessment, and management—a consensus statement. *Am J Respir Crit Care Med.* 1999;159(1):321–340.

42. Rabe KF, Hurd S, Anzueto A, et al. Global strategy for the diagnosis, management, and prevention of chronic obstructive pulmonary disease: GOLD executive summary. *Am J Respir Crit Care Med.* 2007;176(6):532–555.

43. Currow DC, Kenny B, McDonald C, et al. Multisite open label dose ranging study to determine the minimum effective dose of sustained release morphine (SRM) for reducing refractory breathlessness. *Eur J Palliat Care.* 1991;4:926–931.

44. Rocker GM, Sinuff T, Horton R, Hernandez P. Advanced chronic obstructive pulmonary disease: innovative approaches to palliation. *J Palliat Med.* 2007;10(3):783–797.

45. Markowitz AJ, Rabow M. Management of dyspnea in patients with far-advanced lung disease. *JAMA.* 2001;285(10):1331–1337.

46. Robin ED, Burke CM. Single-patient randomized clinical trial: opiates for intractable dyspnea. *Chest.* 1986;90(6):888–892.

47. Rocker GM, Demmons J, Donahue M, Young J, Simpson AC, Horton R, Hernandez P. Using opioids to treat refractory dyspnea in advanced COPD: early insights from a clinical trial. *Chest.* 2011;140(4):543A.

48. Zelman DC, Smith MY, Hoffman D, et al. Acceptable, manageable, and tolerable days: patient daily goals for medication management of persistent pain. *J Pain Symptom Manage.* 2004;28(5):474–487.

49. Horton R, Rocker G, Currow D. The dyspnea target: can we zero in on opioid responsiveness in advanced chronic obstructive pulmonary disease? *Curr Opin Support Palliat Care.* 2010;4(2):92–96.

50. Mercadante S. Predictive factors and opioid responsiveness in cancer pain. *Eur J Cancer.* 1998;34(5):627–631.

51. Mercadante S, Portenoy RK. Opioid poorly-responsive cancer pain. III. Clinical strategies to improve opioid responsiveness. *J Pain Symptom Manage.* 2001;21(4):338–354.

52. Mercadante S, Portenoy RK. Opioid poorly-responsive cancer pain. II. Basic mechanisms that could shift dose response for analgesia. *J Pain Symptom Manage.* 2001;21(3):255–264.

53. Mercadante S, Portenoy RK. Opioid poorly-responsive cancer pain. I. Clinical considerations. *J Pain Symptom Manage.* 2001;21(2):144–150.

54. Sitte T, Bausewein C. Intranasal fentanyl for episodic breathlessness. *J Pain Symptom Manage.* 2008;36(6):e3–e6.

55. Coyne PJ, Viswanathan R, Smith TJ. Nebulized fentanyl citrate improves patients' perception of breathing, respiratory rate, and oxygen saturation in dyspnea. *J Pain Symptom Manage.* 2002;23(2):157–160.

56. Krajnik M, Podolec Z, Siekierka M, et al. Morphine inhalation by cancer patients: a comparison of different nebulization techniques using pharmacokinetic, spirometric, and gasometric parameters. *J Pain Symptom Manage.* 2009;38(5):747–757.

57. Mather LE, Woodhouse A, Ward ME, Farr SJ, Rubsamen RA, Eltherington LG. Pulmonary administration of aerosolised fentanyl: pharmacokinetic analysis of systemic delivery. *Br J Clin Pharmacol.* 1998;46(1):37–43.

58. Schultheis CP. Nebulized fentanyl provides subjective improvements for patients with dyspnea. *Oncol Nurs Forum.* 2005;32(1):15.

59. Smith TJ, Coyne P, French W, Ramakrishnan V, Corrigan P. Failure to accrue to a study of nebulized fentanyl for dyspnea: lessons learned. *J Palliat Med.* 2009;12(9):771–772.

60. Guyatt GH, Heyting A, Jaeschke R, Keller J, Adaci JD, Roberts RS. N of 1 randomized trials for investigating new drugs. *Control Clin Trials.* 1990;11(2):88–100.

61. Jensen D, Alsuhall A, Viola R, Dudgeon DJ, O'Donnell DE. Inhaled fentanyl citrate improves dynamic airway function, exertional dyspnea and exercise endurance in COPD. *Am J Respir Crit Care Med.* 2011;183:A5627.

62. de Leon-Casasola OA. Current developments in opioid therapy for management of cancer pain. *Clin J Pain.* 2008;24 (suppl 10):S3–S7.

63. Rauck RL, Tark M, Reves E, et al. Efficacy and long-term tolerability of sublingual fentanyl orally disintegrating tablet in the treatment of breakthrough cancer pain. *Curr Med Res Opin.* 2009;25(12):2877–2885.

64. Mercadante S, Radbruch L, Davies A, et al. A comparison of intranasal fentanyl spray with oral transmucosal fentanyl citrate for the treatment of breakthrough cancer pain: an open-label, randomised, crossover trial. *Curr Med Res Opin.* 2009;25(11):2805–2815.

65. Fentanyl buccal tablet (Fentora) for breakthrough pain. *Med Lett Drugs Ther.* 2007;49(1270):78–79.

66. Hill L, Schug SA. Recent advances in the pharmaceutical management of pain. *Expert Rev Clin Pharmacol.* 2009;2(5): 543–557.

67. Bailey PH. The dyspnea-anxiety-dyspnea cycle: COPD patients' stories of breathlessness "it's scary when you can't breathe". *Qual Health Res.* 2004;14(6):760–778.

68. Benitez-Rosario MA, Martin AS, Feria M. Oral transmucosal fentanyl citrate in the management of dyspnea crises in cancer patients. *J Pain Symptom Manage.* 2005;30(5):395–397.

What Nonopioid Treatments Should Be Used to Manage Dyspnea Associated With Chronic Obstructive Pulmonary Disease?

PAUL HERNANDEZ

INTRODUCTION AND SCOPE OF THE PROBLEM

Dyspnea is a key symptom that has a negative impact on functional status and quality of life in individuals living with chronic obstructive pulmonary disease (COPD). Prevalence and intensity of dyspnea tend to increase as COPD disease severity increases. Effective strategies to manage dyspnea require a basic understanding of the mechanisms of this cardinal symptom. This chapter reviews the pathophysiology and management of dyspnea in COPD, including clinical measurement and conventional pharmacological and nonpharmacological treatments. Palliative use of opioids to treat refractory dyspnea in advanced COPD is discussed in Chapter 21.

RELEVANT PATHOPHYSIOLOGY

Mechanisms of Dyspnea

Current understanding of the pathophysiology of dyspnea in COPD has grown considerably in recent years. Dyspnea is a complex and individualized symptom that can be defined as a "subjective experience of breathing discomfort."[1] Numerous peripheral and central neural receptors and pathways contribute to the experience of dyspnea. Like pain, dyspnea is a multidimensional symptom; two main components have been proposed—one related to sensory aspects (e.g., intensity, spatial, temporal awareness) and one related to affective aspects. On the basis of recent functional neuroimaging studies, the affective component of dyspnea (similar to pain) is thought to be processed in central limbic structures, the insular cortex, cingulate gyrus, and amygdale.[2]

Individuals are normally unaware of the act of breathing. Respiratory drive, generated at the level of the brainstem, produces the motor output that results in ventilation. Ventilation is monitored and automatically adjusted in response to many afferent sensory inputs integrated centrally, including those coming from receptors in chest wall, lung parenchyma, upper and lower airways, and chemoreceptors.[3] It has long been hypothesized that conscious awareness of breathing and dyspnea occurs when an imbalance exists between the level of neural respiratory drive and resultant ventilation (i.e., neuromechanical dissociation).[4] Individuals can voluntarily focus attention on their breathing. Respiratory sensation is further modulated by affective state (e.g., anxiety, depression), endogenous opioids, and activity of other sensory modalities (e.g., distractive stimuli).

The mechanisms of dyspnea in COPD are multiple and complex. Neuromechanical factors likely predominate over chemoreceptor stimulation, except during acute events resulting in worsened hypoxemia or hypercapnia. COPD is caused by inhalation of noxious stimuli (e.g., cigarette smoke) triggering persistent inflammation and remodeling of airways, lung parenchyma, and vasculature.[5] The pathophysiology of COPD is characterized by partially reversible expiratory airflow limitation and lung hyperinflation.[3] This is due to small airway collapse during expiration from loss of tethering parenchymal lung attachments (emphysema) and small airway obstruction from excess mucus, airway inflammation, and remodeling (chronic bronchitis) combined with reduced driving pressure for expiratory airflow from a loss of elastic recoil (emphysema). As a result, lung emptying is incomplete; end-expiratory lung volume is usually increased at rest and further dynamically increases with increased ventilation, such as during exertion, anxiety, or panic attacks. Hyperinflation (increased end-expiratory lung volume) increases work and oxygen costs of breathing (increased threshold and elastic loads) while causing functional inspiratory muscle weakness (resulting from abnormal chest geometry and respiratory muscle shortening) and possibly negatively affecting cardiac performance. Emphysema is also associated with increased physiological dead space (e.g., wasted) ventilation. Ultimately, neuromechanical dissociation and associated dyspnea occur as a result of increased respiratory neuromuscular output and effort in the face of reduced respiratory response (e.g., tidal volume, level of carbon dioxide).

COPD is not only a lung disease; it is also associated with important systemic manifestations that can further contribute to exercise intolerance and dyspnea, particularly at advanced stages of the disease. Systemic inflammation, malnutrition, inactivity, inadequate levels of anabolic hormones, and medication side effects are all factors that can lead to skeletal muscle wasting and reduced aerobic capacity.[6] During exertion, excess carbon dioxide production results from early-onset anaerobic metabolism and lactic acid production by exercising skeletal muscles requiring buffering with bicarbonate. The outcome is an increase in ventilatory drive and dyspnea. Patients also may have difficulty differentiating between symptoms causing exercise intolerance related to peripheral muscle fatigue and dyspnea.

SUMMARY OF EVIDENCE REGARDING TREATMENT RECOMMENDATIONS

Clinical Measurement of Dyspnea

Individuals with COPD use a variety of qualitative descriptors of their dyspnea experience that may reflect not only increased effort or work of breathing (e.g., "difficult breathing") but also neuromechanical dissociation (e.g., "cannot get a deep breath in," "unsatisfied breath"), air hunger (e.g., "out of breath," "suffocating"), and emotional consequences of this distressing symptom (e.g., "frightening," "awful").[7] Descriptors of dyspnea are also influenced by gender, language, and cultural factors. Proper clinical assessment requires that the health care professional and patient speak the same "language of dyspnea"; otherwise, dyspnea may go unrecognized or underappreciated.

The ability to accurately quantify the intensity of the sensation of dyspnea in response to a given stimulus and its impact on disability and health-related quality of life is critical to guide treatment decisions. Instruments and scales, with their own psychometric properties, are available to measure dyspnea in clinical and research settings.[8] Instrument choice should be guided by the purpose of the measurement; *discriminative* scales are used to compare level of dyspnea among individuals, whereas *evaluative* scales are responsive to change in dyspnea within an individual over time (both acutely and chronically) or in response to an intervention. Example instruments are briefly described in the following section.

For the assessment of levels of acute dyspnea in response to a stimulus such as exercise, several validated instruments are available. The two most commonly used are the visual analog scale (VAS) and the 0 to 10 category-ratio scale (CR-10).[8] Both scales provide descriptors at the ends of the scales as anchors (although a modified CR-10 exists without a ceiling). Use of the VAS requires patients to position their level of dyspnea on a line drawn between two descriptive anchors (e.g., "no shortness of breath" and "maximal shortness of breath"). The CR-10 provides numeric choices with corresponding verbal descriptors non-linearly spaced between 0 and 10.

In terms of measuring chronic level of dyspnea, discriminative and evaluative instruments are available. The Medical Research Council Questionnaire (MRC scale) is a discriminative 5-point scale of dyspnea (1-5 originally, 0-4 in the modified version) that assesses level of disability (e.g., activity limitation) related to dyspnea. The MRC dyspnea scale, particularly when incorporated into a multidimensional index of COPD disease severity such as BODE (a composite index that includes *b*ody mass index, airway *o*bstruction, *d*yspnea, and *e*xercise tolerance) has been demonstrated to better predict mortality and better correlate with health-related quality of life than the standard spirometry measurement of lung function impairment, forced expired volume in 1 second (FEV_1), alone.[9–11]

Two multidimensional dyspnea scales, the Baseline Dyspnea Index (BDI) and the Transition Dyspnea Index (TDI), are interviewer-administered questionnaires that rate initial level of dyspnea (BDI, discriminative) and change in dyspnea over time since baseline (TDI, evaluative).[12] These two scales rate dyspnea in relation to functional impairment, magnitude of difficulty, and magnitude of effort performing daily activities.

The dyspnea domain of the Chronic Respiratory Disease Questionnaire (CRQ, a disease-specific, health-related quality of life instrument) is another well-validated scale that can be used as a discriminative and evaluative instrument to measure chronic levels of dyspnea during activities of daily living. Longer, interviewer-administered (e.g., patients select 5 daily activities from a menu of 25 choices that are most important to them) and standardized, short-form (e.g., activities are prechosen for patients) versions are available.[13,14] Dyspnea is rated on a 7-point Likert scale for each of the 5 activities. This instrument has been shown to be responsive to change in level of dyspnea following treatment with medications and nonpharmacological interventions, such as pulmonary rehabilitation.

Management of Dyspnea

The comprehensive goals of COPD management include slowing disease progression, relieving symptoms (notably dyspnea), improving exercise tolerance, improving health-related quality of life, preventing and treating complications (including exacerbations), and reducing mortality.[15] National and international clinical practice guidelines have been produced over the past decade that provide clinicians with recommendations in the comprehensive management of COPD.[5,15,16] To specifically address dyspnea, the most prevalent and distressing symptom experienced by most patients with COPD, the Canadian Thoracic Society (CTS) recently proposed an evidence-based, stepwise approach to dyspnea management.[17] This guideline added evidence to the concept of a "dyspnea ladder" (Figure 22-1) proposed by Rocker

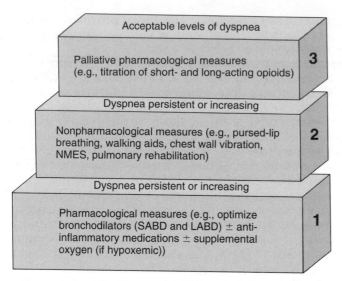

FIGURE 22-1. The dyspnea ladder in chronic obstructive pulmonary disease. *LABD,* Long-acting bronchodilators; *NMES,* neuromuscular electrical muscle stimulation; *SABD,* short-acting bronchodilators. *(Modified from Marciniuk DD, Goodridge D, Hernandez P, et al. Managing dyspnea in patients with advanced chronic obstructive pulmonary disease: a Canadian Thoracic Society clinical practice guideline.* Can Respir J. *2011;18(2): 69-78; and Rocker GM, Sinuff T, Horton R, Hernandez P. Advanced chronic obstructive pulmonary disease: innovative approaches to palliation.* J Palliat Med. *2007;10(3):783-797.)*

and colleagues,[18] itself an adaptation of the "pain ladder" familiar to palliative care clinicians. It was recommended in the CTS guidelines that patients initially be managed with pharmacological therapies, primarily bronchodilators. If dyspnea persists despite optimal pharmacotherapy, nonpharmacological therapies should be introduced. Ultimately, for refractory dyspnea, particularly in patients with advanced COPD, opioid therapy may be initiated and titrated to achieve tolerable levels of dyspnea balanced with acceptable side effects.

Optimizing Pharmacotherapy

Bronchodilators are the mainstay for symptomatic treatment of dyspnea and exercise intolerance in COPD.[5,15] Two main classes of bronchodilator medications are used in COPD: β_2-agonists and anticholinergics. Both drug classes are preferably delivered by inhalation and are available in short-acting (4-8 hours) and long-acting (12-24 hours) forms. Bronchodilators reduce airway smooth muscle tone, increasing airway diameter and decreasing airway resistance. As a result, expiratory airflow increases, enhancing lung emptying and thereby reducing both static and dynamic hyperinflation. It has been postulated that dyspnea relief following bronchodilation relates to improved neuromechanical coupling (i.e., reduced central motor output or effort in the face of decreased work of breathing; decreased threshold and elastic loads) and improved respiratory muscle function (improved geometry, length-tension relationship).[3]

Short-acting bronchodilators are usually initiated on an as-needed basis for relief of dyspnea. The need for regular short-acting bronchodilators for persistent or more severe dyspnea leads to the addition of a regular long-acting bronchodilator for convenience, improved compliance, and improved efficacy. Combining the two classes of bronchodilators has been shown to further improve lung function compared to either class alone.[5] Individual symptomatic response and adverse effects need to be closely monitored.

A growing number of handheld inhaler devices are available, including pressurized metered-dose inhalers that can be used with or without a spacer and breath-actuated, dry powder inhalers. Inhaler technique must be assessed and corrected at regular visits. With proper instruction, given the widely available choices of handheld devices, it is rare for a patient with COPD to require the use of a nebulized bronchodilator to achieve effective inhaled drug delivery.

Two classes of antiinflammatory medications are available for treatment of COPD: inhaled corticosteroids and phosphodiesterase-4 (PDE4) inhibitors. The exact mechanisms by which antiinflammatory mechanisms relieve dyspnea in COPD are unclear. It has been postulated that by reducing leukocyte infiltration of airways and lung parenchyma, these medications modulate vagally mediated sensory receptors and their afferent signals transmitted for central processing.[19]

Although inhaled corticosteroids are first-line antiinflammatory medications in asthma, their role is limited in COPD, except when used in combination with long-acting β_2-agonist bronchodilators. In COPD, inhaled corticosteroid and long-acting β_2-agonist combination inhalers have been shown to reduce the number of key inflammatory cells and mediators, reduce exacerbations, and improve lung function, exercise tolerance, and health-related quality of life.[5] In light of the lack of evidence for efficacy and concern for serious adverse effects, long-term use of systemic corticosteroids in stable COPD is not recommended.[15]

PDE4 inhibitors have also been shown to reduce the number of key inflammatory cells and mediators, as well as reduce the number of exacerbations in COPD; however, because they are not bronchodilators their effect on improving lung function and dyspnea is modest.[15] Only one PDE4 inhibitor (roflumilast) is currently approved in some countries for use in COPD as a once-daily, oral medication. Adverse effects include gastrointestinal upset and weight loss, but this medication class is generally better tolerated with fewer drug–drug interactions than methylxanthines, which are older, nonselective phosphodiesterase inhibitors with weak bronchodilator and debatable antiinflammatory properties in COPD.

Dyspnea intensity and perception can be amplified by the presence of anxiety, panic, and depression. These psychological disturbances are common in COPD and should be sought and appropriately treated when identified.[18] However, despite the relationship between mood disturbances and dyspnea, limited evidence exists that anxiolytic medications (e.g., benzodiazepines, serotonergics) or antidepressant medications (e.g., tricyclic antidepressants, selective serotonin-reuptake inhibitors) benefit patients with COPD specifically in terms of reducing dyspnea.[17]

Supplemental oxygen may reduce dyspnea during exertion through changes in breathing pattern (e.g., decreased respiratory frequency and minute ventilation), resulting in reduced levels of dynamic hyperinflation.[20] The benefit of long-term oxygen therapy in the management of patients with COPD complicated by chronic, severe hypoxemia is well established.[21,22] Whether supplemental oxygen also improves chronic dyspnea in this setting is less clear.[18] Short-term use of oxygen during activity may improve exercise capacity, exercise training during pulmonary rehabilitation, and dyspnea.[18] The routine long-term use of supplemental oxygen in patients with COPD without severe hypoxemia for dyspnea management is not recommended.

Table 22-1 provides a summary of medications used in treatment of COPD. Typical doses and routes of administration are shown; however, available doses, formulations, and approved indications will vary among countries.[15]

Optimizing Nonpharmacotherapy

Through self-management education, patients with COPD can acquire disease-specific knowledge and skills to better self-manage acute exacerbations and their day-to-day symptoms, such as dyspnea.[23] One such self-management program (Living Well With COPD) was evaluated in a multicenter randomized, controlled trial involving patients with severe COPD.[24] Compared to patients receiving usual care, patients in the intervention group had reduced acute health care resource use and improved health-related quality of life. Patients were taught by a COPD educator nonpharmacological strategies that may have been helpful in reducing dyspnea. These skills included proper inhaler technique for medication delivery, breathing training techniques, energy conservation, and relaxation techniques.

TABLE 22-1. Pharmacotherapy for Chronic Obstructive Pulmonary Disease

MEDICATION	ROUTE(S) OF ADMINISTRATION*	DURATION OF ACTION (hr)	TYPICAL DOSES* (mcg)
Bronchodilators			
β_2-Agonists, short-acting			
Fenoterol	pMPI	4-6	100-200
Salbutamol	pMDI	4-6	100-200
Salbutamol	Neb	4-6	5000
Terbutaline	DPI	4-6	400-500
β_2-Agonists, long-acting (LABA)			
Formoterol	DPI, pMDI	12	4.5-12
Indacaterol	DPI	24	75-300
Salmeterol	DPI, pMDI	12	25-50
Anticholinergics, short-acting			
Ipratropium bromide	pMDI	6-8	20-40
Ipratropium bromide	Neb	6-8	500
Oxitropium bromide	pMDI	6-8	100
Oxitropium bromide	Neb	6-8	1500
Anticholinergics, long-acting			
Tiotropium bromide	DPI	24	18
Methylxanthines			
Aminophylline	Oral	Up to 24	
Theophylline	Oral	Up to 24	
Antiinflammatories			
Inhaled corticosteroids (ICS)			
Beclomethasone	DPI, pMDI	12	50-400
Budesonide	DPI	12	100-400
Budesonide	Neb	12	200-500
Fluticasone propionate	DPI, pMDI	12	50-500
Phosphodiesterase-4 inhibitors			
Roflumilast	Oral	24	500
Antiinflammatory and Bronchodilator Combined			
Combination ICS/LABA in a Single Inhaler			
Budesonide/Formoterol	DPI	12	200-400/4.5-12
Fluticasone/Salmeterol	DPI, pMDI	12	50-500/25-50

Modified from Global Initiative for Chronic Obstructive Pulmonary Disease. *Global strategy for the diagnosis, management, and prevention of chronic obstructive pulmonary disease.* Updated 2010. Available at www.goldcopd.org; Accessed October 10, 2012.
DPI, Dry powdered inhaler; *pMDI,* pressurized metered-dose inhaler.
*Not all doses and formulations are available or have an approved indication for use in COPD in all countries.

Breathing training techniques include pursed-lip breathing and diaphragmatic breathing.[25] Pursed-lip breathing involves expiring through the increased resistance of partially closed lips. It promotes slower and deeper breathing at rest and during exertion. Patients with COPD may do pursed-lip breathing spontaneously or can be taught to use this breathing technique when experiencing dyspnea. Improvements in dyspnea with pursed-lip breathing correlate with reductions in end-expiratory lung volume and greater reserves in inspiratory muscle pressure-generating capacity.[26] In contrast, although the deep breathing associated with diaphragmatic breathing may improve arterial blood gases in individuals with severe COPD, it is at the expense of increased work of breathing and increased dyspnea.[27]

Simple walking aids, such as a rollator, have been investigated in individuals with COPD.[28] Dyspnea improves during exercise in association with increased walking distances and decreased need for rest stops compared to walking without a walking aid. Translating the acute benefits of a walking aid into improved activity levels and quality of life at home requires proper instruction and support to individuals regarding how to make best use of these devices.[29]

In-phase, chest wall vibration is another technique that has been studied in individuals with COPD, at rest, with hypercapnia, and during lower-extremity and upper-extremity exercise.[30,31] In this technique, external high-frequency vibrations are applied to intercostal muscles in phase with the respiratory cycle (e.g., to inspiratory muscles during inspiration). Acute application of this techniques results in decreased respiratory frequency, increased tidal volume, stable minute ventilation, improved gas exchange, and reduced dyspnea. This acute effect on dyspnea suggests that respiratory sensation may be mediated by afferent information from chest wall respiratory muscles being integrated centrally.

Relatively strong evidence exists for the benefit of neuromuscular electrical muscle stimulation (NMES) in improving muscle strength and reducing dyspnea in COPD.[17,25,32,33] NMES involves application of surface patch electrodes over specific muscle groups (e.g., quadriceps) to electrically induce contractions of that muscle, according to individual tolerance, for a defined period (e.g., 20-30 minutes) and frequency (e.g., 3-5 times per week). Passive training of peripheral muscles with NMES can be employed alone or as an adjunct to an active exercise training program.[32,33] However, one limitation to widespread access to some nonpharmacological measures (e.g., chest wall vibration and NMES) to manage dyspnea is the requirement for expertise from knowledgeable health care professionals and specialized equipment.

Pulmonary rehabilitation has become an established standard of care means to alleviate symptoms, particularly dyspnea, in COPD.[34–36] Pulmonary rehabilitation is defined as a "multidisciplinary, and comprehensive intervention…designed to reduce symptoms, optimize functional status, increase participation, and reduce health-care costs through stabilizing or reversing systemic manifestations of the disease. Comprehensive pulmonary rehabilitation programs include patient assessment, exercise training, education, and psychosocial support."[35] Pulmonary rehabilitation programs typically last from 6 to 12 weeks, with individuals attending two to five sessions per week; exercise training is considered a mandatory component. Programs can be effectively delivered in the ambulatory care, inpatient hospital, community, and home-based settings.

Two systematic reviews concluded insufficient evidence exists to support the use of other nonpharmacological measures, such as handheld fan, distractive auditory stimuli (e.g., music), acupuncture, acupressure, relaxation training, psychotherapy, and counseling and support programs, to reduce dyspnea in COPD.[17,25]

KEY MESSAGES TO PATIENTS AND FAMILIES

Clinicians should help patients and families understand that there are a multitude of therapies that have been shown to improve symptoms, quality of life, and mortality in patients with COPD. In particular, these modalities can improve the sensation of breathlessness that is familiar to patients with advanced lung disease. Whereas some of these treatments, such as oxygen or inhaled β-agonists, may be familiar to patients, others are relatively new. The palliative care clinician may not necessarily be prescribing all of these therapies, but it is essential to understand their mechanisms of action to better educate patients and families about their use and benefits.

CONCLUSION AND SUMMARY

Treatment of dyspnea is a key management goal for clinicians providing care to individuals with COPD. An effective management strategy includes the choice of appropriate clinical measurement instruments, pharmacological treatments, and nonpharmacological therapies. Through such an approach, individuals with COPD can anticipate relief from this common and distressing symptom.

SUMMARY RECOMMENDATIONS

- Dyspnea is a common, distressing, multidimensional symptom that should be assessed using validated measurement tools at baseline and in response to treatment in all individuals living with COPD.
- Evidence-based dyspnea management in COPD should be approached in a stepwise fashion. Initial pharmacological management of dyspnea requires optimization of bronchodilators. For persistent dyspnea, other pharmacological and nonpharmacological therapies may be effective adjuncts.

REFERENCES

1. American Thoracic Society. Dyspnea: mechanisms, assessment, and management—a consensus statement. *Am J Respir Crit Care Med.* 1999;159(1):321–340.
2. Von Leupoldt A, Sommer T, Kegat S, et al. The unpleasantness of perceived dyspnea is processed in the anterior insula and amygdale. *Am J Respir Crit Care Med.* 2008;177:1026–1032.
3. O'Donnell DE, Banzett RB, Carrieri-Kohlman V, et al. Pathophysiology of dyspnea in chronic obstructive pulmonary disease. *Proc Am Thorac Soc.* 2007;4:145–168.
4. Campbell EJ, Howell JB. The sensation of breathlessness. *Br Med Bull.* 1963;19:36–40.
5. O'Donnell DE, Aaron S, Bourbeau J, et al. Canadian Thoracic Society recommendations for management of chronic obstructive pulmonary disease: 2007 update. *Can Respir J.* 2007;14(suppl B): 5B–32B.
6. American Thoracic Society, European Respiratory Society. Statement on skeletal muscle dysfunction in chronic obstructive pulmonary disease. *Am J Respir Crit Care Med.* 1999;159(1):S1–S40.
7. Williams M, Cafarella P, Olds T, et al. The language of breathlessness differentiates between patients with COPD and age-matched adults. *Chest.* 2008;134(3):489–496.
8. Mahler DA, Guyatt GH, Jones PW. Clinical measurement of dyspnea. In: Mahler DA, ed. *Dyspnea.* New York: Marcel Dekker; 1998:149–198.
9. Nishimura K, Izumi T, Tsukino M, Oga T, on behalf of the Kansai COPD Registry and Research Group in Japan. Dyspnea is a better predictor of 5-year survival than airway obstruction in patients with COPD. *Chest.* 2002;121:1434–1440.
10. Hajiro T, Nishimura K, Tsukino M, et al. A comparison of the level of dyspnea vs. disease severity in indicating the health-related quality of life of patients with COPD. *Chest.* 1999;116:1632–1637.
11. Celli BR, Cote CG, Marin JM, et al. The body-mass index, airflow obstruction, dyspnea, and exercise capacity index in chronic obstructive pulmonary disease. *N Engl J Med.* 2004;350:1005–1012.
12. Mahler DA, Weinberg DH, Wells CK, Feinstein AR. The measurement of dyspnea: contents, interobserver agreement, and physiologic correlates of two new clinical indexes. *Chest.* 1984;85:751–758.
13. Guyatt GH, Berman LB, Townsend M, et al. A measure of quality of life for clinical trials in chronic lung disease. *Thorax.* 1987;47:773–778.
14. Schunemann HJ, Griffith L, Jaeschke R, et al. A comparison of the original Chronic Respiratory Questionnaire with a standardized version. *Chest.* 2003;124:1421–1429.
15. Global Initiative for Chronic Obstructive Pulmonary Disease. *Global strategy for the diagnosis, management, and prevention of chronic obstructive pulmonary disease.* Updated 2010. www.goldcopd.org. Accessed October 10, 2012.
16. Celli BR, MacNee W, Agusti A, et al. Standards for the diagnosis and treatment of patients with COPD: a summary of the ATS/ERS position paper. *Eur Respir J.* 2004;23:932–946.
17. Marciniuk DD, Goodridge D, Hernandez P, et al. Managing dyspnea in patients with advanced chronic obstructive pulmonary disease: a Canadian Thoracic Society clinical practice guideline. *Can Respir J.* 2011;18(2):69–78.
18. Rocker GM, Sinuff T, Horton R, Hernandez P. Advanced chronic obstructive pulmonary disease: innovative approaches to palliation. *J Palliat Med.* 2007;10(3):783–797.
19. Mahler DA. Understanding mechanisms and documenting plausibility of palliative interventions for dyspnea. *Curr Opin Support Palliat Care.* 2011;5:71–76.
20. O'Donnell DE, D'Arsigny C, Webb KA. Effects of hyperoxia on ventilatory limitation during exercise in advanced chronic obstructive pulmonary disease. *Am J Respir Crit Care Med.* 2001;163:892–898.
21. Medical Research Council Working Party. Long term domiciliary oxygen in chronic hypoxic cor pulmonale complicating chronic bronchitis and emphysema. *Lancet.* 1981;1: 681–686.
22. Nocturnal Oxygen Therapy Group. Continuous or nocturnal oxygen therapy in chronic obstructive pulmonary disease. *Ann Intern Med.* 1980;93:391–398.
23. Bourbeau J, Nault D. Self-management strategies in chronic obstructive pulmonary disease. *Clin Chest Med.* 2007;28:617–628.
24. Bourbeau J, Julien M, Maltais F, et al. Reduction of hospital utilization in patients with chronic obstructive pulmonary disease: a disease-specific management intervention. *Arch Intern Med.* 2003;163:585–591.
25. Bausewein C, Booth S, Gysels M, Higginson I. Non-pharmacological interventions for breathlessness in advanced stages of malignant and non-malignant diseases. *Cochrane Database Syst Rev.* 2008;16(2):CD005623.
26. Spahija J, de Marchie M, Grassino A. Effects of imposed pursed-lips breathing on respiratory mechanics and dyspnea at rest and during exercise in COPD. *Chest.* 2005;128(2):640–650.
27. Vitacca M, Clini E, Bianchi L, Ambrosino N. Acute effects of deep diaphragmatic breathing in COPD patients with chronic respiratory insufficiency. *Eur Respir J.* 1998;11(2):408–415.
28. Gupta R, Goldstein R, Brooks D. The acute effects of a rollator in individuals with COPD. *J Cardiopulm Rehabil.* 2006;26(2):107–111.
29. Gupta R, Brooks D, Lacasse Y, Goldstein R. Effect of rollator use on health-related quality of life in individuals with COPD. *Chest.* 2006;130(4):1089–1095.
30. Nakayama H, Sibuya M, Yamada M, et al. In-phase chest wall vibration decreases dyspnea during arm elevation in chronic obstructive pulmonary disease. *Intern Med.* 1998;37:831–835.
31. Sibuya M, Yamada M, Kanamaru A, et al. Effect of chest wall vibration on dyspnea in patients with chronic respiratory disease. *Am J Respir Crit Care Med.* 1994;149(5):1235–1240.
32. Neder JA, Sword D, Ward SA, et al. Home based neuromuscular electrical stimulation as a new rehabilitative strategy for severely disabled patients with chronic obstructive pulmonary disease. *Thorax.* 2002;57(4):333–337.
33. Vivodtzev I, Pepin J-L, Vottero G, et al. Improvement in quadriceps strength and dyspnea in daily tasks after 1 month of electrical stimulation in severely deconditioned and malnourished COPD. *Chest.* 2006;129(6):1540–1548.
34. Ries AL, Bauldoff GS, Carlin BW, et al. Pulmonary Rehabilitation. Joint ACCP/AACVPR evidence-based clinical practice guidelines. *Chest.* 2007;131(5):4S–42S.
35. Nici L, Donner C, Wouters E, et al. American Thoracic Society/European Respiratory Society statement on pulmonary rehabilitation. *Am J Respir Crit Care Med.* 2006;173:1390–1413.
36. Lacasse Y, Martin S, Lasserson TJ, Goldstein RS. Meta-analysis of respiratory rehabilitation in chronic obstructive pulmonary disease: a Cochrane systematic review. *Eura Medicophys.* 2007;43(4):475–485.

What Interventions Are Effective for Managing Dyspnea in Heart Failure?

NATHAN E. GOLDSTEIN AND DEBORAH D. ASCHEIM

INTRODUCTION AND SCOPE OF THE PROBLEM
RELEVANT PATHOPHYSIOLOGY
SUMMARY OF EVIDENCE REGARDING TREATMENT
  RECOMMENDATIONS
KEY MESSAGES TO PATIENTS AND FAMILIES
CONCLUSION AND SUMMARY

INTRODUCTION AND SCOPE OF THE PROBLEM

Heart failure is a chronic and progressive illness typically associated with multiple comorbidities. It is a leading cause of death in the United States. Patients with heart failure have a multitude of symptoms, including fatigue, cachexia, anorexia, and pain.[1] The most common symptom in patients with heart failure, however, is dyspnea. Numerous studies have attempted to determine the prevalence of dyspnea for patients with heart failure, with a wide range of results. For example, in the Study to Understand Prognoses and Preferences for Outcomes and Risks of Treatments (SUPPORT), a prospective cohort study of more than 9000 patients at five academic medical centers across the United States, the rate of dyspnea for patients with advanced heart failure near the end of life was 60%.[2] One study of outpatients with heart failure who were earlier in the course of their disease found a rate of dyspnea of 55%,[3] and another demonstrated a prevalence of rate of 65%.[1] However, in a study in Sweden, review of the charts for 80 patients with heart failure determined the prevalence of shortness of breath was between 85% and 90%.[4]

RELEVANT PATHOPHYSIOLOGY

The mechanisms of dyspnea in patients with heart failure are complex and not well understood.[5] In general, dyspnea may have three sources: (1) an increase in respiratory effort needed to overcome a particular pathological condition (e.g., heart failure–related pulmonary congestion), (2) an increase in the proportion of muscle needed to maintain the work of breathing (which may be particularly applicable in patients with end-stage heart failure who have muscle wasting and thus need to recruit additional muscle mass to breathe), and (3) an increase in ventilatory requirements such as in hypercapnia.[6] Others have postulated that the sensation of dyspnea may be due to neurochemical derangements that are detected in various pathways.[7] However, physiological studies of patients with heart failure indicate that the mechanism may be even more complex. For example, although decreased cardiac output could result in increased dead space ventilation (i.e., alveoli that are ventilated but not perfused), patients with chronic heart failure actually have decreased $Paco_2$. Perfusion in the apical portions of the lung in patients with heart failure is not reduced, and this does not seem to change with exertion.[8] These findings make it clear that the sensation of dyspnea is most likely multifactorial and cannot be explained by any one mechanism.

From a neurological perspective, the sensation of dyspnea may be due to interaction among afferent signals in the central nervous system (e.g., chemoreceptors, pulmonary vagal afferent nerves, peripheral mechanoreceptors), the brainstem, and the cerebral cortex. The interaction of these afferent systems results in signals to respiratory muscles to increase breathing.[7] Although this is still not well understood, it does help elucidate the relationship between dyspnea and symptoms such as anxiety, because these fibers may synapse in the limbic system and thereby trigger emotional reactions.[6,7] The interplay between dyspnea and the central nervous system may also explain some of the effects of morphine in terms of relieving dyspnea, particularly given the presence of mu receptors in the brain and spinal cord. The dyspnea-relieving effects of morphine may also be due to binding to peripheral mu receptors in the lungs and alveoli.[7] Ongoing exploration of the pathophysiological mechanism of dyspnea in heart failure promises to provide additional clarity with regard to the cause of this highly prevalent symptom.[8]

The sensation of dyspnea is subjective and may not correlate to oxygen saturation, respiratory rate, or partial pressures of oxygen or carbon dioxide in the blood. This is reinforced by the fact that dyspnea is often related to not only underlying pathophysiology but also psychological, social, and environmental factors that can result in both worsening and amelioration of the symptom.[6] Measurement of dyspnea should include evaluating its severity during activities of daily living and exercise and its overall impact on the patient's health status.[5] Assessment can be performed using standard scales, such as the Memorial Symptom Assessment Scale[9] or the Edmonton Symptoms Assessment Scale.[10] One instrument that is often used to measure dyspnea is the Borg scale, which relates the sensation of shortness of breath to activity level.[6] Scales specifically designed for assessing dyspnea in patients with heart failure are in development.[6,11]

SUMMARY OF EVIDENCE REGARDING TREATMENT RECOMMENDATIONS

A useful approach to treating dyspnea in patients with heart failure is to divide the treatments into two categories: those that treat the underlying disease and those that treat the symptom (Table 23-1).[6] Indeed, the best treatment for dyspnea is treatment of the patient's underlying heart failure. Although a complete review of the treatment for heart failure is well beyond the scope of this chapter, a few key therapies can be outlined. Diuretics continue to be the mainstay of treatment for patients with heart failure, because they not only treat the patient's dyspnea but have also been shown to improve survival and physical functioning. Over time, patients become progressively resistant to escalating doses of diuretics; thus adding additional diuretics or other therapies may become necessary. This may include aquapheresis (e.g., hemofiltration), or for patients with concomitant renal failure, which is often a result of heart failure, hemodialysis may be indicated.[12] Patients with recurrent pleural effusion may occasionally benefit from thoracentesis.[13] These mechanisms of removing fluid are on the more invasive end of the spectrum, and their use depends somewhat on the patient's overall goals of care.

In terms of other treatments for heart failure that may relieve dyspnea, afterload reduction with long-acting nitrates can be effective. Data have also demonstrated that angiotensin-converting enzyme inhibitors reduce dyspnea.[14] Likewise, intravenous inotropes and vasodilators provide effective relief of dyspnea in patients with advanced chronic heart failure and those with an acute exacerbation.[12] Peptide agonists (e.g., nesiritide) have also been shown to reduce dyspnea in patients with decompensated heart failure, although some recent data have demonstrated conflicting evidence.[15]

In terms of symptomatic treatment of dyspnea in patients with advanced, end-stage heart failure, morphine is commonly used. Doses used for the treatment of dyspnea in patients with heart failure are often much lower than those used for patients with pain; a starting dose of oral morphine 2 to 3 mg may be effective in relieving symptoms.[12,13,16] For patients with renal failure resulting from their heart failure, using equivalent doses of medications with fewer active metabolites (e.g., hydromorphone) can be considered. Studies on the use of nebulized morphine for the treatment of dyspnea in heart failure have not shown it to be beneficial.[17] Conversely, studies of nebulized fentanyl in cancer-related dyspnea are more promising.[18] Because of the strong relationship between dyspnea and anxiety, low-dose benzodiazepines are often used in patients with dyspnea, although there is little evidence for their use as front-line therapies without opioids.[7] Numerous studies have examined the use of oxygen for patients with dyspnea who do not have hypoxia. Results of these trials are mixed overall, and it has been suggested that the benefit may be related to the moving of gas past the nares and stimulation of the trigeminal nerve as opposed to correcting a disturbance in ventilation.[12,19–21] Use of a fan may stimulate this reflex as well. (Patients with hypoxia, however, should be given oxygen.) Exercise and strength training, acupuncture, and meditation and relaxation have all been suggested to relive dyspnea in patients with advanced heart failure, although the data to support these interventions is generally of poor quality.[12,22]

KEY MESSAGES TO PATIENTS AND FAMILIES

Clinicians should help patients and families understand that dyspnea is a common symptom in patients with advanced heart failure. There are multiple modalities that can be used to treat shortness of breath, some of which are the same therapies used to treat the underlying disease. Family members often can be taught to administer symptomatic treatment such as opioids or benzodiazepines, so proper education on the use of these medications and their side effects is important. When prescribing opioids, extra education may be required to distinguish this use from that of treating pain, both to ensure the medication is used appropriately and to assuage patient and caregiver fears about the side effects of this class of medications.

CONCLUSION AND SUMMARY

Dyspnea in patients with advanced heart failure is a highly prevalent symptom. The pathophysiology related to this symptom is not well understood, although it is thought to be due to a complex interaction between peripheral and central receptors that results in the sensation of breathlessness. The interaction of these neurological pathways in the brain may explain some of the anxiety that often accompanies dyspnea. Treatment of shortness of breath should target the underlying heart failure and address symptoms directly. Education of patients and families is important so they understand the treatments being used and how to appropriately dose medications. Further research is needed to better understand the pathophysiology behind dyspnea and expand available treatment options.[23]

TABLE 23-1. Treatments for Heart Failure Patients With Dyspnea[12]

Therapies targeted at heart failure
    Diuretics
    Vasodilators (e.g., nitrates)
    Inotropes
    Aquapheresis (e.g., ultrafiltration, dialysis)
Therapies targeted at symptom
    Opioids
    Benzodiazepines
    Oxygen
    Exercise therapy
    Relaxation therapy
    Acupuncture

Data from Adler ED, Goldfinger JZ, Kalman J, Park ME, Meier DE. Palliative care in the treatment of advanced heart failure. *Circulation.* 2009;120(25):2597-2606.

SUMMARY RECOMMENDATIONS

- Because the best symptomatic treatment for patients with heart failure is to maximize the treatment of the disease itself, ensure that the patient's treatment regimen is optimal. Consultation with a cardiologist or heart failure specialist may be beneficial.
- Low dose opioids – with doses lower than those used for pain – may be beneficial. Because many patients with heart failure also have renal insufficiency, consider using opioids with less active metabolites.
- Dyspnea is often associated with anxiety, so treatment of anxiety may be beneficial for these patients.
- In addition to opioids and benzodiazepines, other therapies that may be effective for heart failure patients with dyspnea include oxygen, use of a fan, exercise therapy, relaxation therapy, and acupuncture.

REFERENCES

1. Bekelman DB, Rumsfeld JS, Havranek EP, et al. Symptom burden, depression, and spiritual well-being: a comparison of heart failure and advanced cancer patients. *J Gen Intern Med.* 2009;24(5):592–598.
2. Lynn J, Teno JM, Phillips RS, et al. Perceptions by family members of the dying experience of older and seriously ill patients. *Ann Intern Med.* 1997;126(2):97–106.
3. Blinderman CD, Homel P, Billings JA, Portenoy RK, Tennstedt SL. Symptom distress and quality of life in patients with advanced congestive heart failure. *J Pain Symptom Manage.* 2008;35(6):594–603.
4. Nordgren L, Sorensen S. Symptoms experienced in the last six months of life in patients with end-stage heart failure. *Eur J Cardiovasc Nurs.* 2003;2(3):213–217.
5. West RL, Hernandez AF, O'Connor CM, Starling RC, Califf RM. A review of dyspnea in acute heart failure syndromes. *Am Heart J.* 2010;160(2):209–214.
6. Martin DE. Palliation of dyspnea in patients with heart failure. *Dimens Crit Care Nurs.* 2011;30(3):144–149.
7. Elia G, Thomas J. The symptomatic relief of dyspnea. *Curr Oncol Rep.* 2008;10(4):319–325.
8. Clark AL. Origin of symptoms in chronic heart failure. *Heart.* 2006;92(1):12–16.
9. Portenoy RK, Thaler HT, Kornblith AB, et al. The Memorial Symptom Assessment Scale: an instrument for the evaluation of symptom prevalence, characteristics and distress. *Eur J Cancer.* 1994;30A(9):1326–1336.
10. Chang VT, Hwang SS, Feuerman M. Validation of the Edmonton Symptom Assessment Scale. *Cancer.* 2000;88(9):2164–2171.
11. Goodlin SJ. Palliative care in congestive heart failure. *J Am Coll Cardiol.* 2009;54(5):386–396.
12. Adler ED, Goldfinger JZ, Kalman J, Park ME, Meier DE. Palliative care in the treatment of advanced heart failure. *Circulation.* 2009;120(25):2597–2606.
13. Pantilat SZ, Steimle AE. Palliative care for patients with heart failure. *JAMA.* 2004;291(20):2476–2482.
14. Johnson MJ, Oxberry SG. The management of dyspnoea in chronic heart failure. *Curr Opin Support Palliat Care.* 2010;4(2):63–68.
15. Intravenous nesiritide vs nitroglycerin for treatment of decompensated congestive heart failure: a randomized controlled trial. *JAMA.* 2002;287(12):1531–1540.
16. Goldfinger JZ, Adler ED. End-of-life options for patients with advanced heart failure. *Curr Heart Fail Rep.* 2010;7(3):140–147.
17. Jennings AL, Davies AN, Higgins JP, Gibbs JS, Broadley KE. A systematic review of the use of opioids in the management of dyspnoea. *Thorax.* 2002;57(11):939–944.
18. Coyne PJ, Viswanathan R, Smith TJ. Nebulized fentanyl citrate improves patients' perception of breathing, respiratory rate, and oxygen saturation in dyspnea. *J Pain Symptom Manage.* 2002;23(2):157–160.
19. Abernethy AP, McDonald CF, Frith PA, et al. Effect of palliative oxygen versus room air in relief of breathlessness in patients with refractory dyspnoea: a double-blind, randomised controlled trial. *Lancet.* 2010;376(9743):784–793.
20. Booth S, Wade R, Johnson M, Kite S, Swannick M, Anderson H. The use of oxygen in the palliation of breathlessness: a report of the expert working group of the Scientific Committee of the Association of Palliative Medicine. *Respir Med.* 2004;98(1):66–77.
21. Russell SD, Koshkarian GM, Medinger AE, Carson PE, Higginbotham MB. Lack of effect of increased inspired oxygen concentrations on maximal exercise capacity or ventilation in stable heart failure. *Am J Cardiol.* 1999;84(12):1412–1416.
22. Pozehl B, Duncan K, Hertzog M. The effects of exercise training on fatigue and dyspnea in heart failure. *Eur J Cardiovasc Nurs.* 2008;7(2):127–132.
23. Goodlin SJ, Hauptman PJ, Arnold R, et al. Consensus statement: palliative and supportive care in advanced heart failure. *J Card Fail.* 2004;10(3):200–209.

GASTROINTESTINAL

Chapter 24

What Medications Are Effective in Preventing and Relieving Constipation in the Setting of Opioid Use?

STACIE K. LEVINE AND JOSEPH W. SHEGA

INTRODUCTION AND SCOPE OF THE PROBLEM

Constipation resulting from opioid use, commonly referred to as opioid-related constipation, opioid-induced bowel dysfunction, and opioid-induced constipation, is one of the most distressing symptoms experienced by patients, especially those with advanced illness. The prevalence of constipation from all causes, including opioid-induced constipation, in hospitalized patients with cancer ranges from 10% to 70%, with more than 50% of persons reporting constipation on admission to hospice.[1,2] It is estimated that among patients on long-term opioid therapy for pain management, 15% to 90% will develop constipation.[3,4] Moreover, studies suggest fewer than half of patients find effective relief from current treatment options, including prescription and over-the-counter laxatives and stool softeners.[3] Inadequately managed constipation can lead to decline in functional performance, nutritional intake, socialization, and quality of life.[5] Health care usage increases as dissatisfied patients seek treatment in office settings and hospital emergency departments. Unlike other side effects of opioid medications, such as nausea and sedation, tolerance to the constipation-related side effects of opioid medication develops very slowly or not at all. Patients with opioid-induced constipation may present with a range of symptoms, such as hard, dry stools; straining; incomplete evacuation; abdominal distention; anorexia; nausea; and vomiting. This may lead to complications such as fecal impaction with obstipation, overflow incontinence, and life-threatening bowel obstruction[6,7] (Table 24-1). Patients may elect to forgo opioid therapy to avoid these adverse effects.[3] Expert opinion supports prevention as the cornerstone of the management of opioid-induced constipation, so starting laxative medications at the same time a patient is started on opioids is advisable.

RELEVANT PATHOPHYSIOLOGY

Opioid receptors are located throughout the peripheral and central nervous systems. Of the three subtypes—mu, delta, and kappa—the mu receptors are most involved in opioid-induced constipation. Opioids induce constipation through peripheral and central mechanisms. Exogenous opioids bind to mu receptors located in the small intestine and inhibit the release of neurotransmitters such as acetylcholine, which in turn interrupts peristalsis and delays transit through the small bowel. At the same time, opioids reduce intestinal secretions normally induced by prostaglandins and vasoactive intestinal polypeptides by binding to receptors in the submucosal plexus. This in turn leads to an increase in fluid and electrolyte absorption from the small and large intestine, resulting in dry, hard stools that are difficult to pass.[3] Opioids also increase anal sphincter tone, reducing the urge to defecate by central effects[8] (Table 24-2).

SUMMARY EVIDENCE REGARDING TREATMENT RECOMMENDATIONS

Evaluation

Considerable variability exists in the meaning of the word *constipation* to patients and health care practitioners. One consideration is stool frequency, which normally varies from once per week to several times a day. Other symptoms include too much straining with bowel movements, passage of small hard stools, or a sense that the bowels have not emptied completely. To better characterize constipation, consensus groups have made attempts to create a standard definition. The Rome criteria were developed to better define functional constipation and take into account bowel movement frequency with associated discomfort.[9] The Bowel Function Index is a reliable and valid measure that evaluates the impact and severity of opioid-induced constipation among

TABLE 24-1. Manifestations of Opioid-Induced Constipation

PRIMARY SYMPTOMS	SECONDARY SYMPTOMS
Dry, hard stool	Gastroesophageal reflux
Small bowel movements	Anorexia
Decrease in stool frequency	Nausea and vomiting
Change in flatus	Urinary retention
Straining	Interference with drug absorption and digestion
Incomplete defecation	Fecal impaction
Abdominal distention	Anal fissures
Abdominal bloating	Overflow incontinence
	Obstruction

TABLE 24-2. Pathophysiology of Opioid-Induced Constipation

PHYSIOLOGICAL CHANGE	RESULT
Inhibition of release of acetylcholine from myenteric plexus	Relaxation of longitudinal muscles in small intestine and colon
	Increased intestinal smooth muscle tone
	Decrease in peristalsis
Increase in segmental contraction	Prolonged transit of intestinal contents and increase in time for reabsorption of water and electrolytes from the bowel
Decrease in gastric, intestinal, biliary, and pancreatic secretions	Reduction in digestion and absorption of micronutrients and macronutrients
Increase tone at ileocecal valve and decrease in defecation reflex	
Decreased sensitivity to rectal sensation	Impaired distal evacuation

TABLE 24-3. Contributors to Constipation in Patients in Palliative Care

Gastrointestinal Disorders
Tumors
Rectal prolapse
Anal fissure
Stricture
Hemorrhoids

Drugs
Analgesics (e.g., opioids, tramadol)
Anticholinergics (e.g., tricyclic antidepressants, antihistamines, antispasmodics)
Antihypertensives (e.g., calcium channel antagonists, β-adrenergic antagonists)
Antiarrhythmics (e.g., amiodarone)
5-Hydroxytryptamine (5-HT3) antiemetics (e.g., ondansetron)
Anticonvulsants (e.g., carbamazepine)
Chemotherapeutic agents (e.g., vinca alkaloids, alkylating agents)
Antidepressants
Diuretics (loop, thiazides)
Neuroleptics
Antiparkinsonian drugs (e.g., benztropine, dopamine agonists)
Bile acid sequestrants
Antacids (aluminum or calcium-containing)
Iron supplementation
Calcium supplementation

Neurological Disorders
Peripheral neuropathies
Spinal cord lesions
Parkinson disease
Cerebrovascular disease
Multiple sclerosis

Metabolic and Electrolyte Abnormalities
Hypercalcemia
Hypokalemia
Uremia
Hypothyroidism
Diabetes mellitus
Hypoparathyroidism

Other
Decreased mobility
Poor fluid intake
Inadequate dietary fiber
Emotional stress

patient populations with and without cancer.[10–12] When considering opioid-induced constipation, any recent change in bowel habits, if persistent, warrants further investigation.

Taking an adequate history and performing a physical examination are essential first steps in evaluating a patient with constipation, including opioid-induced constipation. The history should detail frequency and consistency of stools (both current and baseline before opioid use); associated factors such as nausea, vomiting, and obstipation; history of laxative use; activity level; diet; prescription and over-the-counter medications; comorbid conditions; and any other related symptoms, such as pain with defecation. Clinicians should also consider and mitigate other contributors to opioid-induced constipation whenever possible (e.g., discontinuation of calcium supplements) (Table 24-3).

Physical examination should focus on abdominal distention, presence or absence of bowel sounds, evaluation for masses, tenderness to palpation, and, when indicated, rectal examination for fecal impaction, perianal fissures, and ulcerations. The rectum may be empty if hard or impacted stool is higher up in the bowel. In addition, patients presenting with fecal impaction may pass loose stools or develop fecal seepage and stool incontinence that may be mistaken for normal bowel movements (often referred to as overflow fecal incontinence). Constipation may be the first sign of spinal cord compression, and patients who are at risk should undergo a complete neurological assessment, including evaluation for saddle anesthesia and rectal tone.[13] Some patients may benefit from radiological imaging, such as abdominal radiography, computed tomography scans, and spinal magnetic resonance imaging, depending on the clinical presentation of symptoms of constipation and goals of care.

Prevention

The goal of laxative therapy is to achieve comfortable defecation, with most patients benefiting from one nonforced bowel movement every 1 to 2 days. Because tolerance does not develop to constipating effects of opioids, prophylactic treatment with stool softeners and laxatives is considered the standard of care for as long as opioids are prescribed. Other preventive measures such as increasing fluid intake and dietary fiber, scheduled toileting, and regular physical activity should be considered, but may not be feasible or appropriate in persons with advanced illness.

Pharmacological Treatment

No studies have been reported indicating superiority of one conventional laxative versus another in the management of opioid-induced constipation.[14] Current recommendations are largely based on a few case reports, anecdotal experience, and clinical observations. A consensus group recently published a best practices document that combines expert opinion with existing limited evidence.[15] Selection of laxative depends on the nature of the stools, causes of constipation, and acceptability to the patient. Treatment must be individualized because each agent has considerable side effects that can limit tolerability. Because rectal interventions may be uncomfortable and embarrassing for a patient, oral therapies are usually considered first-line treatment.[13] Expert opinion supports prevention as the cornerstone of the management of opioid-induced constipation, which starts with a scheduled combination of stool softener plus a stimulant. An escalation of laxatives is recommended every 2 days if constipation persists, using a stepwise approach as depicted in Figure 24-1. Current evidence does not identify a linear relationship between opioid dose and amount of laxative required; however, as opioid doses are increased additional laxatives are usually necessary to manage opioid-induced constipation. The following is a description of commonly used classes of medications for management of opioid-induced constipation (Table 24-4).

Bulk-Forming Agents. Fiber bulking agents are organic polymers that absorb and maintain water in the stool, leading to increased frequency of bowel movements in persons with functional constipation. Examples of agents in this category include psyllium seed, bran, and methylcellulose. Without concomitant fluid intake, stools become hard and difficult to pass, potentially worsening constipation. Therefore these agents are not recommended for use in persons with advanced illness or in older adults, and they have shown no benefit in persons with opioid-induced constipation.[16]

Surfactant Laxatives. Stool softeners, such as docusate sodium, act as detergents by allowing water into the stool, making it softer and more voluminous. These agents are generally well tolerated but ineffective if fluid intake is inadequate. Efficacy as a standalone agent in opioid-induced constipation is poor; therefore it is common practice to provide an additional laxative in combination with stool softeners.[17]

Osmotic Laxatives. The hyperosmolar osmotic laxatives enhance laxation by causing secretion of water into the intestinal lumen, leading to softer

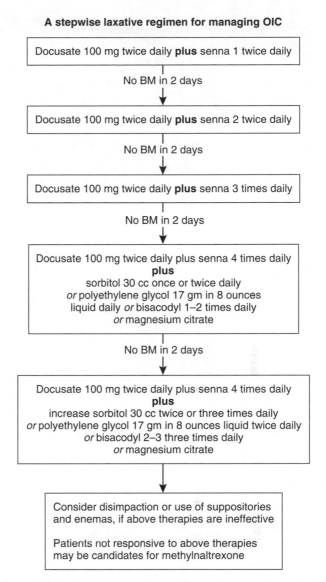

A stepwise laxative regimen for managing OIC

Docusate 100 mg twice daily **plus** senna 1 twice daily

No BM in 2 days

Docusate 100 mg twice daily **plus** senna 2 twice daily

No BM in 2 days

Docusate 100 mg twice daily **plus** senna 3 times daily

No BM in 2 days

Docusate 100 mg twice daily plus senna 4 times daily
plus
sorbitol 30 cc once or twice daily
or polyethylene glycol 17 gm in 8 ounces
liquid daily *or* bisacodyl 1–2 times daily
or magnesium citrate

No BM in 2 days

Docusate 100 mg twice daily plus senna 4 times daily
plus
increase sorbitol 30 cc twice or three times daily
or polyethylene glycol 17 gm in 8 ounces liquid twice daily
or bisacodyl 2–3 three times daily
or magnesium citrate

Consider disimpaction or use of suppositories and enemas, if above therapies are ineffective

Patients not responsive to above therapies may be candidates for methylnaltrexone

FIGURE 24-1. Stepwise laxative regimen for managing opioid-induced constipation.

stools and enhanced propulsion.[17,18] They may be composed of sugars, such as lactulose or sorbitol; magnesium salts, such as magnesium citrate; or inert substances, such as polyethylene glycol. The individual compounds differ in their efficacy and tolerability largely because of variability in digestion by colonic bacteria.[18]

Lactulose is a nonabsorbable synthetic disaccharide composed of galactose and fructose. In the colon it is fermented by bacteria into acetic, formic, and lactic acid, hydrogen, and carbon dioxide. This process lowers intraluminal pH, stimulating peristalsis, and also leads to an influx of water into the lumen through its osmotic effects.[6] Although less expensive, it often requires multiple daily doses to produce laxation and tends to be less well tolerated than other osmotic laxatives.

Sorbitol is a nonabsorbable sugar alcohol that exerts its osmotic effects within the colon. It is less expensive and may produce less nausea and gas than lactulose.[16]

TABLE 24-4. Commonly Used Laxatives for Opioid-Induced Constipation

GROUP	ACTION	AGENTS	LATENCY	SIDE EFFECTS/CAUTIONS
Bulking agents	Increase fecal bulk, retain fluid in gut lumen	Psyllium seed, bran, methylcellulose	Days	Bloating, flatulence, abdominal pain Risk of exacerbating constipation if inadequate fluid intake Generally not recommended in patients with advanced illness
Osmotics	Draw and maintain water within gut lumen, increase fluid secretion in small bowel	Magnesium sulfate (e.g., Milk of Magnesia, Magnesium citrate, epsom salt)	1-3 hr	Abdominal cramping, watery stools, dehydration, hypermagnesemia, hypocalcemia, hyperphosphatemia Not recommended in patient with cardiac and renal disease
		Lactulose	24-48 hr	Bloating, flatulence, colic, sweet taste, hypokalemia, hypernatremia, lactic acidosis, acid–base disturbance
		Sorbitol	24-48 hr	Abdominal cramping, bloating, flatulence, sweet taste
		Polyethylene glycol (e.g., MiraLax)	0.5-1 hr	Nausea, abdominal cramping, bloating, diarrhea, flatulence, fecal incontinence Aspiration into lungs can result in pulmonary edema
Stimulants	Alter intestinal permeability, stimulates myenteric plexus to induce peristalsis	Anthroquinones: senna, cascara	6-12 hr	Abdominal cramping, colic, melanosis coli with chronic use
		Bisacodyl	6-12 hr	Abdominal cramping, electrolyte imbalance
Surfactants	Detergents, lubricate and soften stools	Docusate sodium	12-72 hr	Limited efficacy, not recommended as solo agent
Suppositories	Reflex evacuation through direct stimulation	Glycerin	0.25-1 hr	Rectal irritation, ineffective if feces located higher in colon
		Bisacodyl	0.25-1 hr	Rectal irritation, ineffective if feces located higher in colon
Enemas	Draw water into lumen	Saline, sodium phosphate	0.5-1 hr	Dehydration, hypocalcemia, hyperphosphatemia Not recommended in patients with renal disease
	Distention, facilitating peristalsis	Tap water, soapsuds, mineral oil	0.5-1 hr	Repeated tap water enemas may lead to fluid and electrolyte abnormalities Soapsuds have been associated with chemical colitis
Opioid receptor antagonists	Competitive opioid antagonist	Naloxone	0.5-4 hr	Opioid withdrawal; not indicated in most patients
	Selective peripheral opioid antagonist	Methylnaltrexone	0.5-4 hr	Abdominal cramps, nausea, soft stools, diarrhea, flatulence, nausea Contraindicated in setting of bowel obstruction

Polyethylene glycol is an isoosmotic laxative that is nonabsorbable and binds water molecules to increase volume and soften stools, resulting in enhanced peristalsis.[18] Although limited data exist comparing agents for opioid-induced constipation, a recent Cochrane review favored polyethylene glycol over lactulose in outcomes of stool frequency and consistency, relief of abdominal pain, and need for additional products for chronic constipation.[19]

Stimulant Laxatives. Stimulant laxatives increase peristalsis and intestinal secretions by stimulating the myenteric plexus and altering fluid and electrolyte transport.[15,18] At low doses they inhibit the reabsorption of sodium and water from the gut and at higher doses stimulate sodium and water influx into the intestinal lumen.[18] Senna and bisacodyl are prodrugs that are activated in the gastrointestinal tract by bacterial action in the colon and small intestinal enzymes, respectively. Both can result in abdominal cramping and bloating during activation.[15,17]

Lubricant Laxatives. Lubricant laxatives are used to soften the fecal mass. They are used primarily for fecal impaction but have otherwise limited value in opioid-induced constipation. If used orally, mineral oil may interfere with the absorption of fat-soluble vitamins and increase bleeding risk through prolonged prothrombin time.[6] These medications may be contraindicated in patients with difficulty swallowing because of concerns about aspiration.

Rectal Laxatives. Suppositories and enemas are alternatives to oral therapies in patients in palliative care but are often reserved for refractory constipation because of patient-related discomfort, inconvenience, and embarrassment. They may be contraindicated in patients with myelosuppression because of an increased risk for bleeding and infection, and their use should be carefully aligned with the patient's goals of care. Soft stools in the rectum may be evacuated by a bisacodyl suppository; however, this may be ineffective if feces are located more proximal in the intestines.[16] Hard stools in the rectum may be softened with a glycerin suppository or mineral oil retention enemas overnight and, if necessary, followed by manual disimpaction. Large-scale manual disimpactions may require premedication with opioids or benzodiazepines to lessen patient discomfort. A variety of enemas exist, with no evidence supporting one agent over another. Most types of enemas work directly as mechanical stimulants through the insertion of tap water alone or tap water mixed with baking soda or mild hand soap into the rectum. Enemas can also be buffered with a sodium phosphate solution to draw additional water into the intestinal lumen, which may lead to intense cramping from colonic irritation. The use of any enema should be limited to an as-needed basis because of patient discomfort and propensity toward mucosal inflammation and fluid and electrolyte disturbances when used repeatedly.[13,16,18]

Other Agents. Several other agents, including colchicine, lubiprostone, and misoprostol, have been studied in chronic functional constipation. However, their efficacy and role in the management of opioid-induced constipation remains unknown.[17] Metoclopramide is a prokinetic agent that inhibits the action of dopamine and augments acetylcholine release at the muscarinic receptors in gastrointestinal smooth muscle.[20] To date, it has only been studied in disorders of the upper gastrointestinal tract and has unknown benefit in opioid-induced constipation.[21] Prucalopride, a selective 5-hydroxytryptamine receptor 4 (5-HT4) receptor agonist, has shown benefit in persons with chronic severe functional constipation; however, it has not been studied in persons with opioid-induced constipation.[22]

Opioid Rotation. All opioids are associated with increased risk for constipation, and an aggressive bowel regimen should be implemented whenever initiating opioid therapy. Little evidence exists that switching route of administration from oral to intravenous formulation decreases risk.[16,23] However, a few published studies have demonstrated a reduced tendency toward constipation for transdermal fentanyl compared to other sustained-release oral opioids in patients with noncancer and cancer pain.[4,24–26]

Opioid Antagonists. Because opioid analgesia is primarily mediated through opioid receptors in the central and peripheral nervous systems, a rational approach to management of opioid-induced constipation is to combine opioid analgesics with opioid receptor antagonists that do not cross the blood–brain barrier.

Naloxone is a nonselective opioid receptor antagonist that, when given intravenously, reverses all peripheral and centrally acting opioid mechanisms when it rapidly crosses the blood–brain barrier. When given orally there is extensive elimination through hepatic first-pass metabolism, resulting in less than 2% systemic bioavailability.[27] Oral naloxone can improve opioid-induced constipation; however, it has a narrow therapeutic window and increasing doses may result in opioid withdrawal.[28] Several published and ongoing studies evaluate the efficacy and tolerability of extended-release naloxone given in combination with extended-release opioid agonists such as oxycodone.[27] Because of inconsistent dosing regimens and need for vigilant clinical monitoring, naloxone is not indicated for opioid-induced constipation.

Methylnaltrexone and alvimopan are quaternary opioid antagonists. These agents are 200 times more potent at selectively blocking peripheral mu receptors over central mu receptors. The quaternary functional group on these compounds increases polarity of the compound and decreases lipid solubility, limiting their ability to cross the blood–brain barrier. When given in combination with opioid analgesics, these agents prevent or reverse the peripheral pathways involved in opioid-induced constipation without interfering with analgesia. Alvimopan is currently approved only for in-hospital treatment of postoperative ileus in adult patients after bowel resection. It is dosed as 12 mg orally before surgery and daily postoperatively for a maximum of 7 days. The drug is generally well tolerated, with reported adverse events of nausea, vomiting, and abdominal discomfort. Long-term safety studies are ongoing.[27] Methylnaltrexone is a methylated derivative of naltrexone with low oral bioavailability. In 2008 it was approved for the management of opioid-induced constipation in patients in palliative care and hospice who do not respond to other laxative therapies. It is given subcutaneously and dosed by weight (0.15 mg/kg), with most patients falling into the 8-mg or 12-mg dose range. Studies show that 30% of patients treated successfully achieve laxation within 30 minutes of the first subcutaneous dose, with up to 80% responding by 4 hours.[29–31] The recommended dosing interval is every 2 days, with no more than one dose given in a 24-hour period. Dosage should be reduced by 50% if creatinine clearance is less than 30 mL per minute. Methylnaltrexone is generally well-tolerated, with adverse effects such as abdominal cramps, diarrhea, flatulence, and nausea being reported. Rare cases of bowel perforation after methylnaltrexone have been reported in persons predisposed to changes in the underlying structural integrity of the GI mucosa (e.g., malignancy, Ogilvie syndrome, peptic ulcer disease). As with alvimopan, long-term safety and efficacy studies for methylnaltrexone are ongoing.[14,27]

KEY MESSAGES TO PATIENTS AND FAMILIES

Constipation from opioid medications is very common and, if undertreated, may lead to further discomfort and complications. The best first step is prevention; when able, patients should incorporate a steady intake of fluids and fiber and increase their level of activity. Bowel evacuation should be timed for after meals, and patients should not prolong defecation when the urge arises. The addition of stool softeners and stimulants are an essential first step for prophylaxis of constipation and should be consistently taken when on chronic opioid therapies. If ineffective, adjustments in bowel regimen are necessary. Any change in bowel habits should be reported to a clinician to facilitate a timely evaluation and treatment of underlying causes.

CONCLUSION

The use of opioid medications to treat pain and nonpain symptoms in patients in palliative care is common. Side effects, such as opioid-induced constipation, if untreated may add to the discomfort if not appropriately anticipated and treated. A thorough evaluation and comprehensive treatment plan to prevent opioid-induced constipation should be implemented at the start of opioid therapy. Patients requiring regular use of opioids should be started on a combination of stool softeners and laxatives, with medications titrated to achieve a soft bowel movement every 1 to 2 days. When possible, eliminating other contributors to constipation, such as medications, should occur. Severe constipation should be evaluated by digital rectal examination, with consideration given to radiological imaging to rule out obstruction. Patients with constipation that does not improve with conventional therapy may be candidates for selective peripheral antagonists.

SUMMARY RECOMMENDATIONS

- Opioid-induced constipation is common in patients in palliative care, and clinicians should consider starting a laxative regimen at the same time a patient is started on opioids.
- Stool softeners and oral laxatives are an appropriate starting regimen, and the medications can be gradually increased or others added based on the severity of the patient's constipation.
- Severe constipation should be evaluated by digital rectal examination, with consideration given to radiological imaging to rule out obstruction.
- Patients with constipation that does not improve with conventional therapy may be candidates for selective peripheral antagonists.

REFERENCES

1. McMillan S. Assessing and managing opiate-induced constipation in adults with cancer. *Cancer Control.* 2004;11(suppl 1):3–9.
2. Sykes N. Constipation and diarrhea. In: Hanks G, Cherny NI, Christakis NA, et al, eds. *Oxford textbook of Palliative Medicine.* 4th ed. Oxford: Oxford University Press; 2010: 833–842.
3. Panchal SJ, Muller-Schwefe P, Wurzelmann JI. Opioid-induced bowel dysfunction: prevalence, pathophysiology and burden. *Int J Clin Pract.* 2007;61(7):1181–1187.
4. Cherny N, Ripamonti C, Pereira J, et al. Strategies to manage the adverse effects of oral morphine: an evidence-based report. *J Clin Oncol.* 2001;19:2542–2554.
5. Annunziata K, Bell T. Impact of opioid-induced constipation on patients and healthcare resource use. *Eur J Pain.* 2006;10 (suppl 1):S172.
6. Clemens KE, Klaschik E. Management of constipation in palliative care patients. *Curr Opin Support Palliat Care.* 2008;2:22–27.
7. Kurz A, Sessler DI. Opioid-induced bowel dysfunction: pathophysiology and potential new therapies. *Drugs.* 2003;63(7):649–671.
8. Branch RL, Butt TF. Drug-induced constipation. *Adverse Drug React Bull.* 2009;(257): 987–990.
9. Longstretch GF, Thompson WG, Chey WD, et al. Functional bowel disorders. *Gastroenterology.* 2006;130:1480–1491.
10. Slappendel R, Simpson K, Dubois D, Keininger DL. Validation of the PAC-SYM questionnaire for opioid-induced constipation in patients with chronic low back pain. *Eur J Pain.* 2006; 10:209–217.
11. Marquis P, De La Loge C, Dubois D, et al. Development and validation of the Patient Assessment of Constipation Quality of Life questionnaire. *Scand J Gastroenterol.* 2005;40:540–551.
12. Rentz AM, Yu R, Muller-Lissner S, Leyendecker P. Validation of the bowel function index to detect clinically meaningful changes in opioid-induced constipation. *J Med Econ.* 2009;12:371–383.
13. Gevirtz C. Update on the management of opioid-induced constipation. *Top Pain Manage.* 2007;23(3):1–12.
14. Candy B, Jones L, Goodman ML, et al. Laxatives or methylnaltrexone for the management of constipation in palliative care patients. *Cochrane Database Syst Rev.* 2011;(1): CD003448.
15. Librach SL, Bouvette M, De Angelis C, Pereira JL. Consensus recommendations for the management of constipation in patients with advanced, progressive illness. *J Pain Symptom Manage.* 2010;40(5):761–773.
16. Herndon CM, Jackson KC, Hallin PA. Management of opioid-induced gastrointestinal effects in patient receiving palliative care. *Pharmacotherapy.* 2002;22(2):240–250.
17. Thomas J. Opioid-induced bowel dysfunction. *J Pain Symptom Manage.* 2008;35:103–113.
18. Gallagher PF, O'Mahony D, Quigley EM. Management of chronic constipation in the elderly. *Drugs Aging.* 2008;25(10):807–821.
19. Lee-Robichaud H, Thomas K, Morgan J, Nelson RL. Lactulose versus polyethylene glycol for chronic constipation. *Cochrane Database Syst Rev.* 2010;(7): CD007570.
20. Longo WE, Vernava AM. Prokinetic agents for lower gastrointestinal motility disorders. *Dis Colon Rectum.* 1993;36:696–708.
21. Boyle G, Mounsey A, Crowell K. What is the role of prokinetic agents for constipation? *J Fam Pract.* 2009;58(4):220d–220f.
22. Camillieri M, Kerstens R, Rykx A, Vandeplassche L. A placebo-controlled trial of prucalopride for severe chronic constipation. *N Engl J Med.* 2008;358:2344–2354.
23. Muzumdar A, Mishra S, Bhatnagar S, Gupta D. Intravenous morphine can avoid distressing constipation associated with oral morphine. *Am J Hosp Palliat Med.* 2008;25(4):282–284.
24. Staats PS, Markowitz J, Schein J. Incidence of constipation associated with long-acting opioid therapy: a comparative study. *South Med J.* 2004;97(2):129–134.
25. Allan L, Richarz U, Simpson K, Slappendel R. Transdermal fentanyl versus sustained release oral morphine in strong-opioid naïve patients with chronic low back pain. *Spine.* 2005;30:2484–2490.
26. Allan L, Hays H, Jensen NH, et al. Randomised crossover trial of transdermal fentanyl and sustained release oral morphine for treating chronic non-cancer pain. *BMJ.* 2001;322:1154–1158.
27. Holzer P. Opioid antagonists for prevention and treatment of opioid-induced gastrointestinal effects. *Curr Opin Anaesthesiol.* 2010;23:616–622.
28. Harris JD. Management of expected and unexpected opioid-related side effects. *Clin J Pain.* 2008;24(4):S8–S13.
29. Thomas J, Karver S, Cooney GA, et al. Methylnaltrexone for opioid-induced constipation in advanced illness. *N Engl J Med.* 2008;358(22):2332–2343.
30. Chamberlain BH, Cross K, Winston JL, et al. Methylnaltrexone treatment of opioid-induced constipation in patients with advanced illness. *J Pain Symptom Manage.* 2009;38(5):683–690.
31. Slatkin N, Thomas J, Lipman AG, et al. Methylnaltrexone for treatment of opioid-induced constipation in advanced illness patients. *J Support Oncol.* 2009;7:39–46.

Chapter 25

How Should Medications Be Initiated and Titrated to Reduce Acute and Delayed Nausea and Vomiting in the Setting of Chemotherapy?

STACIE K. LEVINE AND JOSEPH W. SHEGA

INTRODUCTION AND SCOPE OF THE PROBLEM

Chemotherapy-induced nausea and vomiting (CINV) remains one of the most unpleasant, distressing, and feared symptoms of cancer patients, afflicting 70% to 80% of those undergoing treatment,[1] with 10% to 44% experiencing anticipatory symptoms.[2,3] The incidence and severity vary based on the chemotherapeutic agent, dose, schedule, and concomitant therapies along with individual patient characteristics. When poorly controlled, CINV leads to dehydration, anorexia, weight loss, electrolyte disturbances, and diminished quality of life. Fear surrounding CINV may result in administration delays, dose reductions, or discontinuation of treatment altogether, mitigating the symptomatic control and life prolongation benefits resulting from antitumor therapy. The advent of 5-HT3 and NK_1 antagonists that specifically target neuroreceptors implicated in CINV has dramatically improved the prevention and acute control of symptoms. However, delayed CINV remains difficult to control and poses a substantial burden for patients.[4]

RELEVANT PATHOPHYSIOLOGY

Chemotherapy is postulated to induce nausea and vomiting through several neurophysiological pathways. The most common mechanism is direct stimulation of the chemoreceptor trigger zone within the area postrema of the brain, which can be reached by emetogenic chemicals via blood or cerebrospinal fluid. Activation of receptors in the area postrema leads to stimulation of the vomiting center, resulting in nausea and emesis. Other mechanisms implicated in CINV include activation of peripheral pathways through stimulation of receptors within the gastrointestinal mucosa, the cortical pathway (psychogenic causes or abnormal tastes and smells), and the vestibular apparatus. Neurotransmitters such as dopamine, serotonin, histamine, vasopressin, and substance P, located within central and peripheral pathways, induce emesis when binding to their corresponding receptors.[5] The current strategy in the management of CINV is to target multiple implicated receptors simultaneously to facilitate synergy and achieve optimal symptom control.

CINV is categorized by symptom timing—anticipatory, acute, and delayed. Table 25-1 describes the timeframe for each category and recognized risk factors. Timing of symptoms is an important determinant for treatment strategies.[6,7]

SUMMARY OF EVIDENCE REGARDING TREATMENT RECOMMENDATIONS

The prophylactic use of antiemetics has dramatically reduced the frequency of CINV. For example, in patients who receive cisplatin, a highly emetogenic agent, CINV has decreased in prevalence from almost 100% to 25% or less.[8] Based on the success of this strategy, The American Society of Clinical Oncology (ASCO),[9] National Comprehensive Cancer Network (NCCN),[10] and Multinational Association of Supportive Care in Cancer (MASCC)[11] published clinical practice guidelines on antiemetic choice based on emetic risk (ASCO and NCCN guidelines reported in Tables 25-2 and 25-3). Although evidence-based tools to assess emetic risk for an individual patient are lacking, it is recommended that providers evaluate the emetic potential of each regimen and target medium-risk and high-risk agents for prevention. Several patient-related factors are also known to increase the risk for CINV (see Table 25-1); however, the role of these factors in the selection of antiemetic prophylaxis remains limited.[12]

TABLE 25-1. Categories of Chemotherapy-Induced Nausea and Vomiting

CATEGORY	TIMING	RISK FACTORS
Anticipatory	A conditioned response that may occur before, during, or after chemotherapy and is triggered by factors associated with chemotherapy administration such as smells, tastes, sights, and anxiety	Poor control of acute or delayed CINV, younger age, history of motion sickness
Acute	Within 24 hr of chemotherapy	Advanced age, female, history of motion sickness, low alcohol intake, emesis during pregnancy
Delayed	>24 hr after chemotherapy, may last several days	Carboplatin, doxorubicin, cyclophosphamide, dose of chemotherapy, prior history acute or delayed CINV

CINV, Chemotherapy-induced nausea and vomiting.

TABLE 25-2. Estimated Emetogenic Risk of Intravenous Chemotherapeutic Agents

EMETOGENIC RISK (INCIDENCE OF EMESIS WITHOUT ANTIEMETICS)	CHEMOTHERAPEUTIC AGENT	
High (>90%)	Carmustine	Dactinomycin
	Cisplatin	Lomustine
	Cyclophosphamide (>1500 mg/m^2)	Mechlorethamine
	Dacarbazine	Pentostatin
		Streptozotocin
Moderate (30%-90%)	Altretamine	Ifosfamide
	Carboplatin	Irinotecan
	Cyclophosphamide (<1500 mg/m^2)	Melphalan
	Cytarabine (>1000 mg/m^2)	Mitoxantrone (>12 mg/m^2)
	Daunorubicin	Oxaliplatin
	Doxorubicin	Temozolomide
	Epirubicin	Trabectedin
	Idarubicin	Treosulfan
Low (10%-30%)	Asparaginase	Mitomycin
	Bortezomib	Mitoxantrone (<12 mg/m^2)
	Cetuximab	Paclitaxel
	Cytarabine (<1000 mg/m^2)	Peg-asparaginase
	Docetaxel	Pemetrexed
	Etoposide	Teniposide
	5-Fluorouracil	Thiotepa
	Gemcitabine	Topotecan
	Methotrexate (>100 mg/m^2)	Trastuzumab
Minimal (<10%)	Bevacizumab	Hormone
	Bleomycin	Interferon
	Busulfan	Mercaptopurine
	Chlorambucil	Methotrexate (<100 mg/m^2)
	2-Chlorodeoxyadenosine	Rituximab
	Cladribine	Thioguanine
	Cytarabine (<100 mg/m^2)	Vinblastine
	Fludarabine	Vincristine
	Hydroxyurea	Vinorelbine

Data from References 10 and 23.

High Emetogenic Potential

Before 2003 the standard antiemetic therapy for high-risk chemotherapy was a combination of 5-hydroxy-tryptamine (5-HT3) receptor antagonist and dexamethasone. Since then, the addition of aprepitant, a neurokinin-1 receptor antagonist, to this regimen has further reduced the incidence of CINV. Comparison studies of two-drug (5-HT3 plus dexamethasone) versus three-drug (5-HT3, dexamethasone, and aprepitant) therapies for cisplatin-based chemotherapy showed superiority in acute emesis (7%-17% three-drug arm versus 19%-33% two-drug arm [*p*<.001]).[8,13,14] Patients receiving aprepitant were also 15% less likely to have delayed emesis and reported a higher improvement in quality of life.[15] Studies evaluating the effect of aprepitant on delayed emesis with use of highly emetogenic agents also showed superiority of aprepitant plus dexamethasone versus dexamethasone alone (24%-32% two-drug arm versus 45%-53% dexamethasone [*p*<.001]).[14,16] Suggested ASCO and NCCN regimens for prevention of acute and delayed CINV are listed in Table 25-3.

TABLE 25-3. Recommended Regimens for Prevention of Chemotherapy-Induced Nausea and Vomiting Based on Category of Emetic Risk

EMETIC RISK CATEGORY	ASCO GUIDELINES	NCCN GUIDELINES
High (>90%)	*Acute:* Day 1: 5-HT3 RA + dexamethasone + aprepitant *Delayed:* Days 2-4: dexamethasone + aprepitant	*Acute:* Day 1: 5-HT3 RA + dexamethasone + aprepitant +/– lorazepam *Delayed:* Days 2-4: dexamethasone + aprepitant (days 2 and 3), +/– lorazepam (days 2-4)
Moderate (30%-90%)	Anthracycline/cyclophosphamide: *Acute:* Day 1: 5-HT3 RA + dexamethasone + aprepitant *Delayed:* Days 2 and 3: aprepitant Other chemotherapies: *Acute:* Day 1: 5-HT3 RA + dexamethasone *Delayed:* Days 2 and 3: 5-HT3 RA *or* dexamethasone	Anthracycline/cyclophosphamide and select others: *Acute:* Day 1: 5-HT3 RA + dexamethasone + aprepitant +/– lorazepam *Delayed:* Days 2 and 3: aprepitant +/– dexamethasone (days 2-4) +/– lorazepam (days 2-4) Other chemotherapies: *Acute:* Day 1: 5-HT3 RA + dexamethasone +/– lorazepam *Delayed:* Days 2-4: 5-HT3 RA *or* dexamethasone, +/– lorazepam
Low (10%-30%)	*Acute:* Day 1: Dexamethasone *Delayed:* No routine prophylaxis	Dexamethasone +/– lorazepam *or* metoclopramide +/– lorazepam *or* prochlorperazine +/– lorazepam *Delayed:* No routine prophylaxis
Minimal (<10%)	No routine prophylaxis	No routine prophylaxis

Data from Basch E, Prestrud AA, Hesketh PJ, et al: *Antiemetics: American Society of Clinical Oncology clinical practice guideline update.* Alexandria, VA: American Society of Clinical Oncology; 2011; and *NCCN clinical practice guidelines in oncology for antiemesis. v.1.2012,* National Comprehensive Cancer Network; 2011.
ASCO, American Society of Clinical Oncology; *NCCN,* National Comprehensive Cancer Network;
5-HT3 RA, 5-HT3 receptor antagonist.

Moderate Emetogenic Potential

Multiple double-blind randomized, controlled trials have demonstrated superiority of 5-HT3 receptor antagonists compared to placebo in the prevention of nausea and emesis in patients receiving moderately emetic chemotherapy. A meta-analysis of 11 trials demonstrated a decreased risk for acute emesis with an odds ratio of 0.47 (confidence interval [CI] 0.39-0.58).[17] This class contains five drugs (Table 25-4), and multiple studies have demonstrated equivalency in antiemetic efficacy and safety.[15] Current guidelines do not recommend one agent over another. Both ASCO and NCCN recommend a triple combination (5-HT3, dexamethasone, and aprepitant) in persons receiving anthracycline- and cyclophosphamide-based regimens and differ in their recommendations for prevention of delayed CINV in persons receiving moderately emetogenic chemotherapy (see Table 25-3).

Low Emetogenic Potential

ASCO guidelines recommend the use of corticosteroids alone for the first 24 hours of chemotherapy and no prophylaxis beyond 24 hours for acute CINV in agents with low emetic potential. The NCCN guidelines recommend prochlorperazine or metoclopramide as alternatives to dexamethasone, all with or without the addition of lorazepam (see Table 25-3). Neither guideline recommends routine prophylaxis for delayed CINV.

Minimally Emetogenic Potential

All guidelines agree that for acute or delayed CINV no antiemetic therapies need to be administered prophylactically in patients receiving agents with low emetic risk.

Anticipatory Nausea and Vomiting

The most effective method for preventing anticipatory nausea and vomiting is to prescribe an effective antiemetic regimen before chemotherapy. Other suggested nonpharmacological methods include relaxation, systematic desensitization, hypnosis, guided imagery, music therapy, acupuncture, and acupressure.[18-20] Because of their anxiolytic and amnestic effects, short-acting benzodiazepines such as alprazolam and lorazepam have been used to prevent anticipatory symptoms. However, no prospective trials have been conducted to determine their efficacy in this setting.[21]

Management of Breakthrough and Refractory Nausea and Vomiting

The use of prophylactic regimens with high-risk and moderate-risk emetogenic chemotherapies has greatly reduced the incidence of CINV. Despite these interventions, some patients continue to experience breakthrough or refractory symptoms. To date, few prospective randomized trials of therapeutic

TABLE 25-4. Antiemetic Agents for Chemotherapy-Induced Nausea and Vomiting

CLASS	DRUG NAME	DOSING	MECHANISM OF ACTION	SIDE EFFECTS/PRECAUTIONS
5-HT3 receptor antagonist	Dolasetron (Anzemet)	*Oral:* 100 mg *IV:* 100 mg or 1.8 mg/kg	Antagonism of 5-HT3 receptors located in vagal afferents, solitary tract nucleus of the vagus nerve, and chemoreceptor trigger zone of area postrema	Headache, constipation, transient elevation aminotransferases. Equivalent in efficacy and toxicity at recommended doses. Palonosetron has longer half-life and binding activity than others.
	Granisetron (Kytril)	*Oral:* 2 mg *IV:* 1 mg or 0.01 mg/kg *Transdermal patch:* 3.1 mg q24h, max 7 days		
	Ondansetron (Zofran)	High risk—*Oral:* 24 mg Moderate risk—*Oral:* 16 mg *IV:* 8 mg or 0.15 mg/kg Available generic, ODT, and mucous membrane film		
	Palonosetron (Aloxi)	High risk—*IV:* 0.25 mg Moderate risk—*Oral:* 5 mg		
	Tropisetron	*IV/Oral:* 5 mg Not available in United States		
NK$_1$ receptor antagonist	Aprepitant (Emend)	High risk and those receiving combination anthracycline and cyclophosphamide—*Oral:* 125 mg day 1, then 80 mg days 2-4 Moderate risk—*Oral:* 125 mg day 1, then 80 mg days 2 and 3	Antagonism of NK$_1$ receptors in the GI tract and vomiting center, the binding sites of tachykinin substance P	Fatigue, hiccups, constipation, anorexia, headache
Corticosteroids	Dexamethasone	High risk—*Oral:* 12 mg day 1, 8 mg days 2-4 Moderate risk: Without aprepitant—*IV:* 8 mg, then oral 8 mg days 2 and 3 With aprepitant—*Oral:* 12 mg day 1, then 8 mg days 2 and 3	Reduction of peritumoral inflammation and prostaglandin production	Numerous, but especially: hyperglycemia, epigastric burning, sleep disturbances
Benzamine analogs	Metoclopramide (Reglan)	Prophylaxis—*IV:* 1.2 mg/kg over 15 min, give 30 min before chemotherapy, then every 2 hr for 2 doses, then every 3 hr for 3 doses	Antagonizes central and peripheral dopamine receptors At high doses acts as 5-HT3 receptor antagonist	Sedation, extrapyramidal reactions at high doses
Antipsychotics	Haloperidol (Haldol)	*Oral/IV:* 0.5-2 mg q6-8 hr	Antagonizes central and peripheral dopamine receptors	Sedation, extrapyramidal reactions, QT prolongation
	Olanzapine (Zyprexa)	*Oral:* 2.5-10 mg daily	Blocks dopaminergic, serotoninergic, adrenergic, histaminic, and muscarinic receptors	Sedation, akathisia, dizziness, tremor, hyperglycemia
Benzodiazepines	Lorazepam	Prophylaxis—*IV:* Single dose 0.025-0.005 mg/kg, max 4 mg, slowly 30 min before chemotherapy, may supplement with 1-2 mg/hr oral as needed	Adjunctive therapy for antianxiety effects, may be useful given 1 or more days before chemotherapy for anticipatory emesis	Sedation, dizziness, asthenia, falls
Cannabinoids	Dronabinol	Initial—*Oral:* 5 mg/m^2 2 hr before chemotherapy and every 4 hr after, max 4-6 doses/day Titrate up by 2.5 mg/m^2 to a per-dose max 15 mg/m^2	Adjunctive therapy for patients intolerant or refractory to 5-HT3, corticosteroids, or aprepitant	Sedation, euphoria, dizziness, hallucinations, dry mouth
	Nabilone	Initial—*Oral:* 1 mg q12h starting 3 hr before chemotherapy; titrate by 2 mg/dose to max 6 mg/day in 3 divided doses		

GI, Gastrointestinal; *ODT,* oral dissolving tablets.

agents have been conducted in this population.[22] Breakthrough symptoms may respond to the addition of a benzodiazepine or antipsychotic, or substituting high-dose metoclopramide for the 5-HT3 antagonist.[21,23] Cannabinoids such as dronabinol and nabilone are approved by the U.S. Food and Drug Administration for patients with CINV who have failed to respond to conventional antiemetics. However, their use is limited by potent side effects and a narrow therapeutic index.[24] Although antihistamines are often used, studies with agents such as hydroxyzine or diphenhydramine have not demonstrated antiemetic activity for CINV.[12] Olanzapine, an atypical antipsychotic, has potential antiemetic properties because of its effect on multiple receptor sites implicated in the nausea and vomiting pathway. Prospective trials of olanzapine in combination with the 5-HT3 antagonist dexamethasone have demonstrated high prevention rates for acute and delayed CINV in patients receiving high and moderate emetic chemotherapies.[25–27] The dosing for agents and their side effects are listed in Table 25-4.

KEY MESSAGES TO PATIENTS AND FAMILIES

Patients receiving chemotherapy for cancer are often faced with distressing side effects such as nausea and vomiting. The advent of less toxic cancer therapies and targeted antiemetic therapies have led to a significant decline in the incidence of nausea and vomiting. Patients and families should discuss with their clinician potential emetic risk when reviewing cancer treatments.

CONCLUSION AND SUMMARY

Considerable progress has been made over the past few decades in reduction of the incidence of acute and delayed CINV, although there is still work to do. The goal of therapy is to prevent nausea and vomiting throughout the entire period of emetic risk using the lowest maximally effective dose of antiemetic before chemotherapy. Choice of antiemetic should be based on the emetic risk of chemotherapeutic agents, and toxicity and side effects of antiemetics should also be considered.

SUMMARY RECOMMENDATIONS

- Chemotherapy-induced nausea and vomiting is a frequent side effect in patients with cancer, and its potential should be discussed with patients when reviewing treatment options.
- Antiemetics should be considered to prevent acute and delayed nausea and vomiting in the setting of chemotherapy.
- Choice of antiemetics and timing of dosing should be approached in a systematic manner, and the clinician should consider patient risk factors as well as the potential of the chemotherapeutic agent to induce nausea and vomiting.

REFERENCES

1. Morran C, Smith DC, Anderson DA, McArdle CS. Incidence of nausea and vomiting with cytotoxic chemotherapy: a prospective randomized trial of antiemetics. *Br Med J.* 1979;1:1323–1324.
2. Vainio A, Auvinen A. Prevalence of symptoms among patients with advanced cancer: an international collaborative study. Symptom Prevalence Group. *J Pain Symptom Manage.* 1996;12:3–10.
3. Abernethy AP, Wheeler JL, Zafar SY. Detailing of gastrointestinal symptoms in cancer patients with advanced disease: new methodologies, new insights, and a proposed approach. *Curr Opin Support Palliat Care.* 2009;3:41–49.
4. Nevidjon B, Chaudhary R. Controlling emesis: evolving challenges, novel strategies. *J Support Oncol.* 2010;8(2):1–10.
5. Hsu ES. A review of granisetron, 5-hydrotryptamine receptor antagonists, and other antiemetics. *Am J Therapeut.* 2010;17:476–486.
6. Markman M. Progress in preventing chemotherapy-induced nausea and vomiting. *Cleve Clin J Med.* 2002;69:609–617.
7. Gralla RJ, Osoba D, Kris MG, et al. Recommendations for the use of antiemetics: evidence-based, clinical practice guidelines. American Society of Clinical Oncology. *J Clin Oncol.* 1999;17:2971–2994.
8. Hesketh PJ, Grunberg SM, Gralla RJ, et al. The oral neurokinin-1 antagonist aprepitant for the prevention of chemotherapy-induced nausea and vomiting: a multinational, randomized, double-blind, placebo-controlled trial in patients receiving high-dose cisplatin. The Aprepitant Protocol 052 Study Group. *J Clin Oncol.* 2003;21:4112–4119.
9. Prevention of chemotherapy and radiotherapy-induced emesis: results of Perugia Consensus Conference. Antiemetic Subcommittee of the Multinational Association of Supportive Care in Cancer (MASCC). *Ann Oncol.* 1998;9:811–819.
10. National Comprehensive Cancer Network. NCCN clinical practice guidelines in oncology. v.1 2007. Antiemesis. Available at http://www.nccn.org; Accessed 26.10.11.
11. Kris MG, Hesketh PJ, Somerfield MR, et al. American Society of Clinical Oncology guideline for antiemetics in oncology: update 2006. *J Clin Oncol.* 24(18):2932–2947.
12. Jordan K, Sippel C, Schmoll HJ. Guidelines for antiemetic treatment of chemotherapy-induced nausea and vomiting: past, present, and future recommendations. *Oncologist.* 2007;12: 1143–1150.
13. Navari RM, Reinhardt RR, Gralla RJ, et al. Reduction of cisplatin-induced emesis by a selective neurokinin-1 receptor antagonist: L-754,030. Antiemetics Trials Group. *N Engl J Med.* 1999;340:190–195.
14. Warr DG, Grunberg SM, Gralla RJ, et al. The oral NK(1) antagonist aprepitant for the prevention of acute and delayed chemotherapy-induced nausea and vomiting: pooled data from two randomised, double-blind, placebo controlled trials. *Eur J Cancer.* 2005;41:1278–1285.
15. Naeim A, Sydney M, Lorenz KA, et al. Evidence-based recommendations for cancer nausea and vomiting. *J Clin Oncol.* 2008;26(23):3903–3910.
16. De Wit R, Herrstedt J, Rapoport B, et al. The oral NK(1) antagonist, aprepitant, given with standard antiemetics provides protection against nausea and vomiting over multiple cycles of cisplatin-based chemotherapy: a combined analysis of two randomized, placebo-controlled phase III clinical trials. *Eur J Cancer.* 2004;40:403–410.
17. Jantunen IT, Kataja W, Muhonen TT, et al. An overview of randomised studies comparing 5HT3 receptor antagonists to

conventional anti-emetics in the prophylaxis of acute chemotherapy-induced vomiting. *Eur J Cancer.* 1997;33:66–74.

18. Morrow GR, Morrell C. Behavioral treatment for the anticipatory nausea and vomiting induced by cancer chemotherapy. *N Engl J Med.* 1982;307:1476–1480.

19. Ezzo J, Vickers A, Richardson MA, et al. Acupuncture-point stimulation for chemotherapy-induced nausea and vomiting. *J Clin Oncol.* 2005;23:7188–7198.

20. Redd WH, Andrykowski MA. Behavioral intervention in cancer treatment: controlling aversion reactions to chemotherapy. *J Consult Clin Psych.* 1982;50(6):1018–1029.

21. Navari RM. Overview of the updated antiemetic guidelines for chemotherapy-induced nausea and vomiting. *Comm Oncol.* 2007;4(4):3–11.

22. Jones JM, Qin R, Bardia A, et al. Antiemetics for chemotherapy-induced nausea and vomiting occurring despite prophylactic antiemetic therapy. *J Pall Med.* 2011;14(7):810–814.

23. Roila F, Herrstedt J, Aapro M, et al. Guideline update for MASCC and ESMO in the prevention of chemotherapy and radiation-therapy-induced nausea and vomiting: results of the Perugia consensus conference. *Ann Oncol.* 2010;21(S5):v232–v243.

24. Tramer MR, Carroll D, Campbell FA, et al. Cannabinoids for control of chemotherapy-induced nausea and vomiting: a quantitative systematic review. *BMJ.* 2001;323:16–21.

25. Navari RM, Einhorn LH, Loehrer Sr. PJ, et al. A phase II trial of olanzapine, dexamethasone, and palonosetron for the prevention of chemotherapy-induced nausea and vomiting. A Hooiser Oncology Group study. *Support Care Cancer.* 2007;15:1285–1291.

26. Aapro MS, Grunberg SM, Manikhas GM, et al. A phase III, double-blind, randomized trial of palonosetron compared with ondansetron in preventing chemotherapy-induced nausea and vomiting following emetogenic chemotherapy. *Ann Oncol.* 2006;17:1441–1449.

27. Schmoll HJ, Aapro MS, Poli-Bigelli S, et al. Comparison of an aprepitant regimen with a multiple day ondansetron regimen, both with dexamethasone, for antiemetic efficacy in high-dose cisplatin treatment. *Ann Oncol.* 2006;17:1000–1006.

Chapter 26

How Should Medications Be Initiated and Titrated to Prevent and Treat Nausea and Vomiting in Clinical Situations Unrelated to Chemotherapy?

STACIE K. LEVINE AND JOSEPH W. SHEGA

INTRODUCTION AND SCOPE OF THE PROBLEM

Nausea, vomiting, and retching are common and distressing symptoms encountered in patients with advanced illness.[1] These symptoms have been reported in up to 70% of patients with cancer, and they also occur frequently in noncancer diagnoses such as congestive heart failure, acquired immunodeficiency virus (AIDS), and hepatic and renal failure.[2,3] Nausea, especially when accompanied by emesis, can result in serious complications such as electrolyte imbalances, dehydration, aspiration, Mallory-Weiss tears, and malnutrition. Numerous factors can contribute to nausea and vomiting in persons with advanced illness, including metabolic derangements (e.g., hyponatremia, hypercalcemia, uremia), medications (e.g., opioids, antidepressants, cholinesterase inhibitors), changes in gastric and bowel motility, central nervous system disorders (e.g., increased intracranial pressure, anxiety), and autonomic dysfunction resulting from malnutrition and poor performance status.[4] Interventions to reduce nausea and vomiting involve awareness of the mechanism of emetogenic pathways, careful patient assessment, and prescribing of medications tailored to the suspected cause.

RELEVANT PATHOPHYSIOLOGY

The emetic response involves coordination of various pathways and associated receptors through the physiological control center called the vomiting center (Figure 26-1). The vomiting center is located in the lateral reticular formation of the medulla and receives central and peripheral input. Central afferents to the vomiting center include the cerebral cortex, higher brainstem, thalamus, hypothalamus, and vestibular system. Peripheral afferents arrive by the vagus and splanchnic nerves from mechanoreceptors and chemoreceptors in the gastrointestinal tract and serosa (see Figure 26-1). Neuroreceptors within each pathway exist and may include dopamine, serotonin, histamine, opioid, cannabanoid, and neurokinin receptors. The pathogenesis of nausea and vomiting involves the trigger of release of neurotransmitters specific to these receptors by emetogenic stimuli. For example, the chemoreceptor trigger zone (CTZ) is located in the area postrema of the fourth ventricle of the brain, where there is effectively no blood–brain barrier, allowing noxious stimuli such as certain medications, bacterial toxins, and metabolic products to stimulate dopamine (D_2) receptors in the CTZ to induce nausea and emesis. It is important to recognize that one or more of these pathways may contribute to nausea and vomiting (Table 26-1), and assessment and treatment should be targeted to suspected causes.[5]

Symptoms and Evaluation

Many assessment tools are available to measure nausea and vomiting, including unidimensional, multidimensional, and global quality of life scales.[1] When caring for persons with advanced illness, respondent burden and the patient's cognitive and emotional state may help guide measure selection, with a general preference for tools that are convenient and easy to use. Selection of the measure reflects the clinical situation, cultural and social factors, and how the information will be used. Unidimensional scales such as the visual analog scale are of benefit because of rapid assessment, ease of use, and low patient burden, but they evaluate only the presence and severity of the symptom and may not identify other related symptoms as are seen in clusters. Multidimensional tools such as the Edmonton Symptom Assessment Scale (ESAS) provide additional information on other symptoms as well as nausea, such as pain, drowsiness, and appetite.[6] Global measures such as the McMaster Quality of Life Scale evaluate the impact of physical symptoms on patients' psychological distress and functional status.[7]

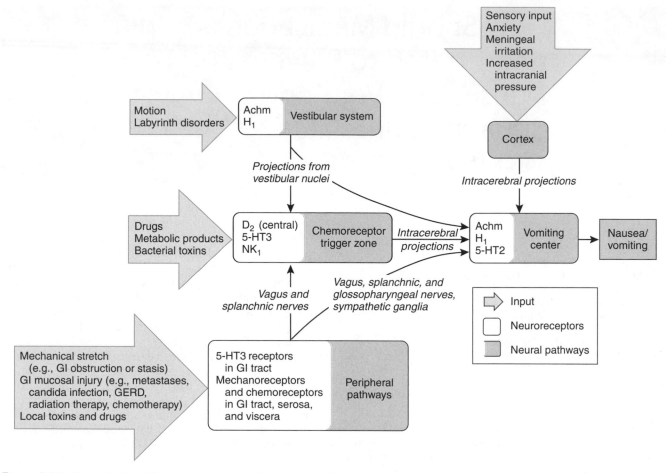

Figure 26-1. Interrelationships between neural pathways that mediate nausea and vomiting. *Achm,* Muscarinic acetylcholine receptor; *D₂,* dopamine type 2 receptor; *GERD,* gastroesophageal reflux; *GI,* gastrointestinal; *H₁,* histamine type 1 receptor; *NK1,* neurokinin type 1 receptor; *5-HT2,* 5-hydroxytryptamine type 2 receptor; *5-HT3,* 5-hydroxytryptamine type 3 receptor. *(From Wood GJ, Shega JW, Lynch B, Von Roenn JH: Management of intractable nausea and vomiting in patients at the end of life.* JAMA. *2007;298:1196-1207, 2007. ©2007 American Medical Association. All rights reserved.)*

A thorough history and physical examination are essential first steps in determining the underlying cause(s) of nausea and vomiting. Attention should be given to frequency, onset, duration, associated exacerbating and relieving factors, and consistency and volume of emesis. Large-volume, feculent emesis may suggest a partial or complete bowel obstruction. Small-volume emesis after meals may be due to gastric stasis. Associated symptoms such as pain, vertigo, headaches, and fever may provide additional information leading to diagnosis. A history of syncope or early satiety should raise the possibility of autonomic insufficiency. Medication history is also essential because many prescription and over-the-counter drugs may contribute to nausea and vomiting (see Table 26-1). Suspect medications include recently initiated therapies and those that have been taken for longer durations, because disease progression may precipitate medication-related adverse effects. Comorbid medical conditions such as gastroesophageal reflux disease, peptic ulcer disease, diabetes, autoimmune disorders, and alcoholism may also increase the risk of emesis.

Physical examination may provide additional clues to the cause, such as papilledema (increased intracranial pressure), thrush (esophageal irritation), abdominal distention and reduced bowel sounds (bowel obstruction), and fecal impaction (constipation). In appropriate patients, laboratory values may reveal renal or hepatic failure, hypercalcemia, ketoacidosis, or drug toxicity. Upright abdominal films may reveal air–fluid levels consistent with bowel obstruction or fecal matter indicating impaction. Neuroimaging may be indicated when brain metastases or other pathology are suspected.

SUMMARY OF EVIDENCE REGARDING TREATMENT RECOMMENDATIONS

Before initiation of pharmacologic therapy, environmental stimuli should be identified and eliminated. This may include avoiding strong cooking smells and fragrances. Also, necrotic or infected tissue from wounds can produce unpleasant odors that trigger

TABLE 26-1. Cause-Based Classification of Nausea and Vomiting

CLINICAL SYNDROME	GENERAL CAUSE	FEATURES	RECEPTOR PATHWAYS	TREATMENT
Chemical	*Medications:* Opioids, digoxin, anticonvulsants, antibiotics, antifungals, cytotoxics, SSRIs, iron *Toxins:* Ischemic bowel, infection, tumor products *Metabolic:* Renal failure, liver failure, hypercalcemia, hyponatremia, ketoacidosis	Drug toxicity, associated underlying disease, constant nausea, variable vomiting	Stimulation of D_2 +/− 5-HT3 in CTZ Chemotherapy stimulates serotonin release in GI tract, 5-HT3 on vagus Chemotherapy stimulates NK_1 receptors in brain	Check drug levels, stop offending drug Treat underlying cause Haloperidol or phenothiazine 5-HT3 antagonists for CINV and radiation-related NK_1 for CINV
Impaired gastric emptying	*Medications:* Opioids, tricyclic antidepressants, phenothiazines, anticholinergics Ascites Hepatosplenomegaly Autonomic dysfunction Tumor infiltration	Epigastric fullness or pain, early satiety, flatulence, reflux, hiccups, large-volume emesis	Gastric mechanoreceptors stimulate vagal afferents to the VC Additional receptors: H_1, Achm	Treat underlying cause(s) Prokinetics (metoclopramide) Large-volume paracentesis
Visceral causes	Peritoneal carcinomatosis Bowel obstruction Gastroenteritis, gastritis Constipation, fecal impaction Mesenteric metastases Stretched liver capsule Ureteral distention	Diffuse, dull aching or crampy abdominal pain that may radiate to shoulder, back, other parts of abdomen	Gut/serosal mechanoreceptors stimulate vagal afferents to the VC	Aggressive bowel regimen Reduce acid secretions with H_2-blocker or proton pump inhibitor Medical or surgical management of obstruction Corticosteroids may reduce tumor mass
Cortical	Increased intracranial pressure: Intracranial tumor, cerebral infarct, infection, bleed Meningeal irritation Leptomeningeal carcinomatosis Anxiety, pain	Headache, visual changes, focal neurological deficits, altered sensorium	Direct stimulation of receptors in vomiting center (5-HT2, Achm, H_1) via intracerebral projections	Treat reversible cause Benzodiazepines Corticosteroids may reduce tumor mass
Vestibular	Medications Motion sickness Labyrinthine disorders	Symptoms correspond to position change, vertigo	Stimulation of Achm and histamine in the vestibular apparatus	Stop offending drug Meclizine Antihistamines

Modified from Glare P, Pereira G, Kristjanson LJ, Stockler M, et al. Systemic review of the efficacy of antiemetics in the treatment of nausea in patients with far-advanced cancer. *Support Care Cancer.* 2004;12:432-440.
Achm, Anticholinergic muscarinic; *CINV,* chemotherapy induced nausea and vomiting; *SSRI,* selective serotonin reuptake inhibitor; *VC,* vomiting center.

symptoms. The sense of taste and smell may be altered in advanced disease, and previously innocuous food and drink may suddenly become nauseating.

The next step is to prioritize the differential diagnosis of conditions contributing to nausea and vomiting and treat underlying conditions consistent within the goals of care (e.g., an infection or cancer progression). At the same time, an antiemetic that blocks the most likely implicated receptors in the physiological pathway should be chosen. With the lack of well-designed studies, the evidence base to support antiemetic regimens is limited and current management is largely based on anecdotal experience and expert opinion. A recent systematic review of antiemetics for emesis in cancer unrelated to chemotherapy and radiation therapy found weak evidence supporting antiemetic choices, except for studies involving the treatment of bowel obstruction[8] (see Chapter 27). Uncontrolled studies report a higher response rate compared to standard regimens (75%-93% for both nausea and vomiting), with randomized,

controlled trials reporting a much lower response rate to these agents (nausea 23%-36%, vomiting 18%-52%).[9] Two approaches, cause-based and empirical, used to manage nausea and emesis in patients in palliative care are described in the literature.[9] The empirical approach involves trying various antiemetics without regard to the underlying cause of nausea and vomiting and may be effective.[10,11] The cause-based approach has been more widely adopted by the palliative care community and deemed moderately effective, but limited evidence supports its use in clinical practice.[12] This approach involves matching knowledge of emetogenic pathways and the supposed emetogenic stimulus to the drug, or combination of drugs, most likely to block that stimulus. The following section describes antiemetics commonly used in nausea and vomiting unrelated to chemotherapy (Table 26-2). Discussion of the agents used for chemotherapy-induced nausea and vomiting and bowel obstruction may be found in Chapters 25 and 27, respectively.

TABLE 26-2. Common Receptor-Specific Therapies for Nausea and Emesis Not Related to Chemotherapy

CLASS	DRUG	RECEPTOR	SITE	DOSING	SIDE EFFECTS
Dopamine antagonists	Promethazine	D_2, Achm, H_1	CTZ	*PO/IV:* 12.5-25 mg q6h *Rectally:* 25 mg q6h	Sedation, orthostatic hypotension, extrapyramidal side effects
	Prochlorperazine	D_2	CTZ	*PO/IV:* 5-10 mg q6h *Rectally:* 25 mg q6h	
	Chlorpromazine	D_2	CTZ	*PO:* 10-25 mg q4h *IV:* 25-50 mg q4h *Rectally:* 50-100 mg q4h	
	Haloperidol	D_2	CTZ	*PO/subcutaneously:* 0.5-5 mg q8-12h	
Prokinetic	Metoclopramide	D_2, 5-HT3, Achm	CTZ, GI tract	*PO/IV/subcutaneously:* 10-20 mg q6h	Avoid in complete GI obstruction
Serotonin antagonist	Ondansetron	5-HT3	GI tract, CTZ, VC	*PO/ODT/IV:* 4-8 mg q4-8h	Constipation, diarrhea, fatigue, headache, possible QTc prolongation
Antihistamines	Diphenhydramine	H_1	Vestibular	*PO/IV/subcutaneously:* 25-50 mg q6h	Dry mouth, drowsiness, confusion, urinary retention
	Meclizine	H_1	Vestibular	*PO:* 12.5-50 mg q6h	Dry mouth, drowsiness, blurred vision
Anticholinergics	Hyoscyamine	Achm	Vestibular	*PO/SL:* 0.125-0.25 mg q4h *IV/subcutaneously:* 0.25-0.5 mg q4h	Dry mouth, blurred vision, urinary retention, constipation, confusion
	Scopolamine	Achm	Vestibular	*Transdermal patch:* 1-3 applied q72h *Gel:* 0.25% applied topically q4-6h	
Antidepressant	Mirtazapine	5-HT3	GI tract, CTZ, VC	*PO:* 15-45 mg at night	Dizziness, blurred vision, sedation, somnolence, malaise, increased appetite, weight gain, dry mouth, constipation, vivid dreams
Atypical antipsychotic	Olanzapine	D_2, Achm, 5-HT3, H_1	GI tract, CTZ, VC	*PO:* 2.5-10 mg q24h	Increased appetite, weight gain, hyperglycemia, sedation, reduced seizure threshold, increased serum lipids

Achm, Anticholinergic muscarinic; *CTZ,* chemoreceptor trigger zone; *D1, D2,* dopamine receptors; *GI,* gastrointestinal; *ODT,* oral dissolving tablet; *SL,* sublingual; *VC,* vomiting center.

Pharmacological Treatments

Dopamine Antagonists. Of the D_2 antagonists, haloperidol has the most potent effect at the CTZ, minimizing the effect of dopamine at the D_2 receptor in the CTZ, thereby reducing input into the vomiting center.[13] Ondansetron is also a dopamine antagonist and, at higher doses, a 5-HT3 antagonist. Metoclopramide is a benzamide derivative with both antiemetic and prokinetic properties. The antiemetic action is due to its antagonist activity at the D_2 receptors and, at higher doses, 5-HT3 receptors in the area postrema of the CTZ. This gastroprokinetic activity is thought to be mediated by muscarinic activity, D_2 antagonism, and 5-HT4 agonist activity in the periphery. The efficacy of orally administered metoclopramide has been well documented in treating delayed gastric emptying in patients with cancer and opioid-related nausea and vomiting.[4] Sustained plasma concentrations are required to suppress nausea and emesis, resulting in the need to administer short-acting oral or parenteral medication frequently. Patients requiring subcutaneous infusions to treat chronic nausea have been reported.[14]

5-HT3 Antagonists. The discovery of 5-HT3–selective receptor antagonists has revolutionized the treatment of chemotherapy-induced nausea and vomiting.[15] Although they are commonly used in the management of nausea and emesis from other causes, they do not reverse nausea mediated by dopaminergic pathways (e.g., opioids) and have not been tested in populations without cancer, such as patients with AIDS. Thus their current indications are for chemotherapy and radiation therapy–induced or postoperative nausea and vomiting.

Antihistamines and Anticholinergics. The antihistamine and anticholinergic medications are thought to exert their antiemetic effects in the vestibular pathway by blocking acetylcholine and histamine receptors in the vestibulocochlear nerve. They are most commonly used in motion-related nausea and vomiting.[16]

Corticosteroids. The mechanism of action of corticosteroids in treatment of nausea and vomiting is not well understood but has been postulated to be due to reduction in release of serotonin or activation of corticosteroid receptors in the central nervous system.[17] Although few data support efficacy for symptoms unrelated to chemotherapy,[18] anecdotal experience has found corticosteroids to be effective in reducing symptoms in patients with intractable nausea and vomiting,[19] particularly when scheduled around the clock.

Mirtazapine. Mirtazapine is a tetracyclic antidepressant that antagonizes the 5-HT3 receptor and is often tried as an antiemetic in patients with refractory symptoms. Evidence to support its use is limited to case reports and small studies in patients with cancer.[20,21]

Olanzapine. Olanzapine is an atypical antipsychotic known to block several receptors implicated in the emesis pathway. Its efficacy has been demonstrated in small case reports; however, larger controlled studies are warranted.[22,23]

Cannabanoids. Cannabanoids, such as dronabinol and nabilone, can be effective antiemetics in persons with cancer and AIDS[24,25]; however, their use may be limited by adverse effects such as delirium and sedation, especially in older adults.

Other Drugs. Lorazepam, diphenhydramine, haloperidol, and metoclopramide (ABHR) and diphenhydramine, dexamethasone, and metoclopramide (BDR) suppositories and topical gels are compounded, combination preparations often used in home hospice in patients who are not able to swallow medication. Although they are easy to use and generally well-tolerated, there is no evidence to support their efficacy.[19]

Nonpharmacological Measures

Acupressure, acupuncture, transcutaneous electrical nerve stimulation, and guided imagery are examples of nonpharmacological measures used to treat nausea and vomiting. Although limited evidence exists to support their efficacy, a recent Cochrane review showed superiority of P6 acupuncture point stimulation over sham treatment in pooled data from 26 trials of more than 3000 patients. The majority of these studies were in postoperative sickness, chemotherapy-induced, and pregnancy-related nausea and vomiting.[26]

Role of Palliative Sedation

If symptoms remain intractable despite multimodal interventions, palliative sedation may be considered in patients with limited life expectancy. No standard regimen exists for sedation of patients with intractable nausea; however, propofol has been considered to be the ideal agent because of its sedative effects and antiemetic effects on the 5-HT3 receptors.[27]

KEY MESSAGES TO PATIENTS AND FAMILIES

Patients and families should understand that nausea and vomiting are common, distressing symptoms experienced by patients living with advanced illness. The best initial step in treatment is to identify and treat potential precipitants, including environmental factors such as strong odors and aversive foods. A thoughtful history and physical examination often identifies causes, allowing clinicians to choose the best treatment. In most cases, these symptoms can be controlled with medications targeting the potential cause(s).

CONCLUSION AND SUMMARY

Control of nausea and vomiting involves identifying and removing potential triggers, consideration of potentially involved emetogenic pathways and neurotransmitters, and selecting medications that antagonize the corresponding receptors. Clinicians should choose a route of administration that ensures maximal absorption, in this setting often excluding the oral route. The dose should be titrated carefully, with special attention paid to potential side effects and drug interactions. If symptoms persist, reassess the patient to search for overlooked cause(s) and consider an additional or alternative treatment. Terminally ill patients who continue to have refractory symptoms despite aggressive treatment may be candidates for palliative sedation.

SUMMARY RECOMMENDATIONS

- Controlling nausea and vomiting involves identifying and removing potential triggers, consideration of potentially involved emetogenic pathways and neurotransmitters, and selecting medications that antagonize the corresponding receptors.
- Before initiation of pharmacologic therapy, environmental stimuli that may be triggering the nausea or vomiting should be identified and eliminated.
- If symptoms persist, reassess the patient to search for overlooked cause(s) and consider an additional or alternative treatment.

REFERENCES

1. Saxby C, Ackroyd R, Callin S, et al. How should we measure emesis in palliative care? *Palliat Med.* 2007;21:369–383.
2. Barnes S, Gott M, Payne S, et al. Prevalence of symptoms in a community-based sample of heart failure patients. *J Pain Symptom Manage.* 2006;32(3):208–216.
3. Norval DA. Symptoms and sites of pain experienced by AIDS patients. *S Afr Med J.* 2004;94(6):450–454.

4. Kumar G, Hayes KA, Clark R. Efficacy of a scheduled IV cocktail of antiemetics for the palliation of nausea and vomiting in a hospice population. *A J Palliat Med.* 2008;25(3):184–189.

5. Hanks G, Cherny NI, Christakis NA, Fallon M, Kaasa S, Portenoy RK, eds. Gastrointestinal symptoms. In: *Oxford Textbook of Palliative Medicine.* 4th ed. Oxford: Oxford University Press; 2010:801–811.

6. Bruera E, Kuehn N, Miller M. The Edmonton Symptom Assessment System (ESAS): a simple method for the assessment of palliative care patients. *J Palliat Care.* 1991;7(2):6–9.

7. Sterkenburg C, King B, Woodward C. A reliability and validity study of the McMaster Quality of Life Scale (MQLS) for a palliative population. *J Palliat Care.* 1996;12:18–25.

8. Davis MP, Hallerberg G. A systematic review of the treatment of nausea and/or vomiting in cancer unrelated to chemotherapy or radiation. *J Pain Symptom Manage.* 2010;39(4):756–767.

9. Glare P, Pereira G, Kristjanson LJ, et al. Systemic review of the efficacy of antiemetics in the treatment of nausea in patients with far-advanced cancer. *Support Care Cancer.* 2004;12:432–440.

10. Bruera E, Belzile M, Neumann C, et al. A double blind crossover study of controlled release metoclopramide and placebo for the chronic nausea and dyspepsia of advanced cancer. *J Pain Symptom Manage.* 2000;19:427–435.

11. Hardy J, Daly S, McQuade B, et al. A double blind, randomized parallel group, multinational, multicentre study comparing single dose ondansetron 24 mg po with placebo and metoclopramide 10 mg po in the treatment of opioid induced nausea and emesis in cancer patients. *Support Care Cancer.* 2002;10:231–236.

12. Stephenson J, Davies A. An assessment of aetiology-based guidelines for the management of nausea and vomiting in patients with advanced cancer. *Support Care Cancer.* 2006;14:348–353.

13. Critchley P, Plach N, Grantham M, et al. Efficacy of haloperidol in the treatment of nausea and vomiting in the palliative patient: a systematic review. *J Pain Symptom Manage.* 2001;22(2):631–634.

14. Bruera E, Seifert L, Watanabe S, et al. Chronic nausea in advanced cancer patients: a retrospective assessment of a metoclopramide-based antiemetic regimen. *J Pain Symptom Manage.* 1996;11:147–153.

15. Jordan K, Schmoll HJ, Aapro MS. Comparative activity of antiemetic drugs. *Crit Rev Oncol Hematol.* 2007;61(2):162–175.

16. Cranwell-Bruce L. Antiemetic drugs. *MEDSURG Nurs.* 2009;18(5):309–313.

17. Lohr L. Chemotherapy-induced nausea and vomiting. *Cancer J.* 2008;14(2):85–93.

18. Bruera E, Moyano JR, Sala R, et al. Dexamethasone in addition to metoclopramide for chronic nausea in patients with advanced cancer: a randomized control trial. *J Pain Symptom Manage.* 2004;28(4):381–388.

19. Wood G, Shega J, Lynch B, Von Roenn J. Management of intractable nausea and vomiting in patients at the end of life. *JAMA.* 2007;298(10):1196–1207.

20. Theobald DE, Kirsh KL, Holtsclaw E, et al. An open-label, crossover trial of mirtazapine (15 mg and 30 mg) in cancer patients with pain and other distressing symptoms. *J Pain Symptom Manage.* 2002;23(5):442–447.

21. Thompson DS. Mirtazapine for the treatment of depression and nausea in breast and gynecological oncology. *Psychosomatics.* 2000;41(4):356–359.

22. Jackson WC, Tavernier L. Olanzapine for intractable nausea in palliative care patients. *J Palliat Med.* 2003;6:251–255.

23. Passik SD, Lundberg J, Kirsh KL, et al. A pilot exploration of the antiemetic activity of olanzapine for the relief of nausea in patients with advanced cancer and pain. *J Pain Symptom Manage.* 2002;23:526–532.

24. Flynn J, Hanif N. Nabilone for the management of intractable nausea and vomiting in terminally staged AIDS. *J Palliat Care.* 1992;8(2):46–47.

25. Hall W, Christie M, Currow D. Cannabanoids and cancer: causation, remediation, and palliation. *Lancet Oncol.* 2005;6(1):35–42.

26. Ezzo J, Streitberger K, Schneider A. Cochrane systematic reviews examine P6 acupuncture-point stimulation for nausea and vomiting. *J Altern Complement Med.* 2006;12(5):489–495.

27. Lundstrom S, Zachrisson U, Furst CJ. When nothing helps: propofol as sedative and antiemetic in palliative cancer care. *J Pain Symptom Manage.* 2005;30(6):570–577.

What Interventions Are Effective for Relieving Acute Bowel Obstruction in Cancer and Other Conditions?

STACIE K. LEVINE AND JOSEPH W. SHEGA

INTRODUCTION AND SCOPE OF THE PROBLEM

Malignant bowel obstruction is a common complication of gastrointestinal and ovarian cancers, usually occurring in the advanced stage of illness, with a recent prospective study reporting an average life expectancy of 80 days at the time of presentation.[1] Retrospective studies report a wide range in incidence, with malignant bowel obstruction occurring in 5% to 51% of ovarian and 10% to 28% of gastrointestinal cancers.[2] Bowel obstruction less commonly occurs in gastric and pancreatic cancer and malignancies that frequently metastasize to the abdomen, such as breast and lung cancer. The pathogenesis of obstruction may be the direct effect of the malignancy, as a secondary effect from cancer-related treatments, or from nonmalignant causes[3] (Table 27-1). The acuity and severity of associated symptoms (pain, nausea, vomiting), along with the issues that arise surrounding nutrition, often lead to substantial patient and family distress that can be ameliorated by an experienced and skilled treatment team.

RELEVANT PATHOPHYSIOLOGY

In the early phase of obstruction, luminal contents accumulate proximally, damaging the epithelium. This triggers an inflammatory response with subsequent release of prostaglandins, vasoactive peptide, and other secretagogues.[4] These inflammatory mediators stimulate a large influx of fluid into the gut lumen with concomitant decreased reabsorption of water, sodium, and other electrolytes. Bowel dilation and wall edema ensue, leading to colicky pain, nausea, and vomiting. Despite little movement of intestinal contents, the bowel continues to contract, leading to a self-perpetuating, cyclic sequence of events (distention-secretion-distention) with further influx of fluid and worsening distention and symptoms[5,6] (Figure 27-1). Without early intervention, patients become quickly dehydrated, develop electrolyte disturbances, and experience a substantial symptom burden. The natural history of partial to complete mechanical bowel obstruction usually progresses over several days, with the timing and severity of progression depending largely on cause and location (Table 27-2). For example, obstructions from ovarian tumors are more likely to occur in the small bowel or sigmoid colon.[3] Tumors in the jejunum and those that infiltrate the small bowel are less likely to have the degree of distention as seen in the large bowel.[6]

Symptoms and Evaluation

Symptoms of bowel obstruction may vary and depend somewhat on the site of obstruction and the cause. Nausea is a frequent complaint triggered by local distention and stimulation of mechanoreceptors, leading to direct stimulation of the chemoreceptor trigger zone by the vagus and splanchnic nerves. Nausea can often lead to vomiting, although vomiting may occur without any preceding symptoms. Patients with proximal obstruction in the stomach or small bowel may present with intermittent or continuous bilious vomiting within 45 minutes of a meal. Vomiting from colonic obstruction generally occurs later and may present with foul-smelling, fecaloid material. Abdominal pain is typically characterized as periumbilical, colicky, and traveling in waves; pain that is well localized or increases with palpation may signal peritoneal irritation or perforation. Absence of feces or flatus suggests a complete obstruction. Patients with incomplete obstruction may present with overflow incontinence as a result of liquefaction of fecal material by intestinal bacteria.[5]

The physical examination can provide additional clues as to whether an obstruction is present. Classic findings include a distended, tender abdomen with high-pitched hyperactive bowel sounds. However, it is not uncommon for patients to have a nontender abdomen and hypoactive bowel sounds.[7]

The evaluation for bowel obstruction depends on the goals of care. A review of medications may identify potential contributors to stasis, such as opioids or anticholinergics. However, the benefits of these therapies typically outweigh potential harms, particularly in the

TABLE 27-1. Causes of Mechanical Bowel Obstruction

Malignant: Direct
Gynecological (ovarian) and gastrointestinal
 Direct tumor invasion
 Extrinsic compression
 Altered motility from dissemination of tumor
 Postradiation fibrosis
Lung, breast, melanoma
 Direct spread to abdomen
Peritoneal carcinomatosis

Malignant: Indirect
Radiation enteritis
Surgical adhesions
Intraperitoneal chemotherapy

Nonmalignant
Complications of diverticulitis
Anastomotic strictures after previous surgery
Fecal impaction (e.g., secondary to medications)
Hernia
Pseudoobstruction from altered extrinsic neural control of
 gut (e.g., neurological disorders, diabetes, gastric surgery)
Medications (e.g., anticholinergics)

↑ Stasis of gut contents, epithelial damage

↑ Inflammation and release of prostaglandins, vasoactive peptide, and secretagogues

↑ Bowel contraction **Obstruction** ↑ Intestinal, pancreatic, and biliary secretions

↑ Influx of sodium and water into gut lumen

↑ Abdominal cramping, colicky pain, nausea, vomiting

↓ Reabsorption of water and electrolytes

↑ Intestinal hyperemia, bowel edema, distention

FIGURE 27-1. Distention-secretion-distention cycle in bowel obstruction.

TABLE 27-2. Types of Obstruction From Malignancy

LOCATION	RESULT
Intraluminal	Intussusception, occlusion of lumen
Intramural	Impaired peristalsis, occlusion of lumen
Mesenteric, omental masses, adhesions	Extramural obstruction
Infiltration of enteric or celiac plexus	Dysmotility

TABLE 27-3. Contraindications for Surgery in Patients With Bowel Obstruction

Previous laparotomy with adhesions
Diffuse intraabdominal tumors
Peritoneal carcinomatosis
Multiple obstruction sites
Limited life expectancy
Poor nutritional status
Multiple comorbidities
Presence of large volume of ascites
Poor performance status
Patient preference for more conservative (i.e., nonsurgical) therapies

palliative care setting.[4,5] A laboratory evaluation may identify abnormalities that exacerbate an obstruction (e.g., hypokalemia, hypercalcemia) and can be readily treatable. Confirmatory diagnosis is usually achieved through abdominal radiographs revealing air–fluid levels and distended loops of bowel. Contrast radiographs may be helpful in identifying the site or extent of the obstruction. Gastrograffin is preferred over barium because gastrograffin is not absorbed or retained and therefore will not interfere with future endoscopic procedures. Abdominal computed tomography may provide more detailed information regarding extent of disease to allow for therapeutic decisions regarding possibility of intervention procedures.[4,5]

SUMMARY OF EVIDENCE REGARDING TREATMENT RECOMMENDATIONS

Interventional Management

Surgical Resection. Treatment of bowel obstruction depends largely on the cause, condition of the patient, goals of care, and predicted prognosis. Before the mid-1980s the mainstay treatment for patients with bowel obstruction due to malignancy was either palliative surgery or, if patients were not surgical candidates, nasogastric suction with intravenous hydration. Operative approaches include intestinal resection or bypass, debulking, and diversion (e.g., colostomy). Although surgery remains the treatment of choice and should be considered in all cases of bowel obstruction, several potential contraindications must be considered (Table 27-3). Also, surgery is not always a viable option in patients with advanced disease given the limited life expectancy. Surgical intervention carries significant perioperative morbidity and mortality. A series of studies evaluating persons with advanced gynecological malignancies found an operative mortality of 9% to 40%, with a complication rate of 9% to 90%.[5] Postoperative morbidities include fistula formation, incision dehiscence, local and systemic infections, bleeding, and thrombosis. Based on previous studies showing a high morbidity and mortality associated with surgical management, a general rule of thumb is that persons with a life expectancy of 2 months or less or poor performance status should forgo surgery and focus on medical management.[5] Taken together, surgical management of malignant bowel obstruction necessitates a thoughtful discussion among providers with patients and families.

Venting Procedures. In certain patients with a reasonable life expectancy, placement of percutaneous endoscopic gastrostomies may be indicated to provide symptom relief from nausea and vomiting and as a means of providing nutrition once the obstruction resolves.

Stenting. Self-expanding metallic stents (SEMS) are possible alternatives for persons with esophageal, gastric outlet, proximal small-bowel, and large-bowel obstructions. Use of SEMS for large-bowel obstructions was first reported in 1991[8] and has been gaining popularity as an alternative or bridge to surgery. Endoscopic treatment of malignancy is less invasive than surgery, allows shorter length of stay, and may avert surgical emergencies that are associated with high morbidity.[9] Although no randomized, controlled studies have compared clinical outcomes, prospective studies have found SEMS to be cost-effective, with a reduced need for permanent colostomy[10] and reduced use of intensive care unit resources.[9] Comprehensive systematic reviews for malignant bowel obstruction have found initial technical success rates approaching 92%, with mortality less than 1%.[11] SEMS placement for obstruction caused by gynecological malignancies has demonstrated results similar to those in patients with colorectal cancer.[12] Outcomes for their use in treatment of benign strictures have been mixed.[9,13,14] A large systematic review examining incidence of early complications in 1198 patients found a perforation rate of 3.8 %, (associated with predilation of the stenosis), stent migration 11.8%, and reobstruction 7.3%.[15] However, the decision to pursue stent placement should be carefully considered because late complications (migration, obstruction, perforation, tenesmus) may occur in 50% of patients. Use of palliative chemotherapy may worsen complication rate.[16] Also, there are no available studies examining long-term survival or quality of life measures.[17] Authors conclude that for patients with potentially curable lesions, stenting should be considered only if surgery is scheduled shortly after stent placement. Those with

incurable obstructing colorectal cancer eligible for chemotherapy and with a long life expectancy should consider palliative treatments other than SEMS.[16,18] Contraindications to SEMS include diffuse peritoneal carcinomatosis, multiple areas of obstruction, and perforation. Stenting of rectal obstruction that is too close to the anal verge may lead to pain, tenesmus, and fecal incontinence.[3]

Pharmacological Management

Baines and colleagues[19] published the first report on using medications for the treatment of malignant bowel obstruction in 1985. Since then, numerous studies have been published examining the efficacy of pharmacological agents for malignant bowel obstruction not amenable to surgical intervention. Several classes of therapies have been found effective and target the underlying pathophysiology of obstruction[4,20,21] (Table 27-4). Through synergistic action these agents reduce intestinal secretions and intraluminal hypertension to interrupt the cycle of distention-secretion-distention (see Figure 27-1). Pharmacological strategies for management of bowel obstruction include decompression and hydration along with a combination of analgesics, antispasmodics, antiemetics, and drugs to control bowel secretions. Multiple studies have found that patients treated with this strategy demonstrated improvement in nausea, vomiting, colic, and abdominal pain.[4,22,23] Establishing early treatment increases the possibility of return of bowel function, permitting eating, improvement in quality of life, and possibly survival.[4,21] The oral route is often not possible in

TABLE 27-4. Medication Management for Malignant Bowel Obstruction

AGENT	ACTION	DOSE	SIDE EFFECTS/CAUTION
Octreotide	Antispasmodic, decreases intestinal secretions	*Subcutaneous bolus:* 50-100 mcg q8h *Infusion:* Start at 10-20 mcg/hr, titrate every 24 hr to achieve symptom relief	Expense, pain at injection site, localized skin reaction Long-term use has been associated with biliary sludging and hyperglycemia Warming the vial in hands before injection may reduce pain at injection site
Haloperidol	Antiemetic	*IV/subcutaneous:* 0.5-1 mg q6-8 h	Extrapyramidal reactions, QT prolongation
Metoclopramide	Antidopaminergic, antiemetic, and prokinetic	*IV/subcutaneous bolus:* 10-20 mg q6h *Subcutaneous infusion:* 2-4 mg/hr *Rectal:* 10 mg q8h	Extrapyramidal reactions, dry mouth Contraindicated in complete bowel obstruction
Scopolamine hydrobromide	Decreases peristalsis, decreases intestinal secretions	*Subcutaneous bolus:* 0.1-0.4 mg q6h *IV/subcutaneous infusion:* 0.1 mg/hr *Topical:* 1.5-mg patch q72h	Dry mouth, urinary retention, dry mouth, blurry vision, confusion
Glycopyrrolate	Antisecretory	*Subcutaneous bolus:* 0.2-0.4 mg q2-4 h *IV/subcutaneous infusion:* 0.02 mg/hr	Fewer CNS side effects than scopolamine
Corticosteroids	Reduces inflammatory edema, decreases secretion of water and sodium into lumen	Dexamethasone—*IV/subcutaneous:* 4 mg q8h	Numerous side-effects, including oral candidiasis, gastric hemorrhage, muscle atrophy, euphoria, elevated blood glucose, adrenal insufficiency Limited data on oral, rectal, or topical use Unpleasant perianal sensation (IV formulation)

CNS, Central nervous system.

patients, and alternative routes such as intravenous or subcutaneous should be considered. Subcutaneous therapies with hypodermoclysis have the advantages of ease of use, minimal discomfort, and easy maintenance at home. Several of the therapies used for the medical management of malignant bowel obstruction can be administered through nontraditional routes, including rectal, buccal, sublingual, and transdermal.

Octreotide. Octreotide, a somatostatin analog, is a potent antisecretagogue with a complex mechanism of action. Through its direct effect on intestinal smooth muscle, influx of gastric and intestinal secretions into the lumen is decreased, thus reducing intestinal distention.[24–26] Octreotide also directly inhibits neurotransmission in peripheral nerves of the gastrointestinal tract, thereby decreasing peristalsis and splanchnic blood flow.[26] When the vicious cycle of distention-secretion-distention is interrupted, bowel wall edema and ischemia decrease, reducing painful intestinal cramping and the risk for intestinal necrosis and perforation. Early use of octreotide in malignant bowel obstruction aids in the restoration and maintenance of bowel function and control of gastrointestinal symptoms.[27,28] Peak plasma concentrations are achieved at 0.5 to 2 hours in most patients, with a duration of effect of approximately 12 hours.[21] Studies have shown a reduction in placement of, and output from, nasogastric tubes with the use of octreotide in patients with malignant bowel obstruction.[4,21] Moreover, patients undergoing bowel resection who received octreotide perioperatively had a greater success rate of intestinal anastomosis,[29] with some able to avoid surgery altogether.[30,31] Octreotide is generally well-tolerated in patients in palliative care, but administration remains burdensome with subcutaneous injections every 8 hours or intravenous or subcutaneous continuous infusions. Also, these therapies are relatively expensive, which may limit their use, particularly in the hospice setting.[32] The development of newer, long-acting somatostatin analogues is currently being evaluated in the palliative management of malignant bowel obstruction. Initial studies have found octreotide LAR (octreotide acetate for injectable suspension) to be well-tolerated, with an acceptable safety profile.[24,25] Expense remains a significant issue, although the use of long-acting compounds may decrease the time spent in the hospital without the need for frequent injections or continuous infusions.

Corticosteroids. The evidence-base surrounding the use of corticosteroids for malignant bowel obstruction continues to be evaluated, but theoretically these agents have the potential to improve symptoms and alter the natural course of the disease. Specifically, the corticosteroid's antiinflammatory activity diminishes bowel wall edema and the resultant decrease in gut transit. In addition, corticosteroids may function as antisecretory agents by reducing salt and water secretion into the gut lumen. The consequence of these actions includes analgesia and antinausea effects, along with potential relief of the obstruction.[33,34]

Usual practice is for corticosteroids to be administered for 3 to 5 days at the time of presentation and titrated downward depending on the patient's symptoms. Several routes of administration are available, including oral, intravenous, subcutaneous, and rectal. A Cochrane review, originally published in 1999 and updated in 2009 found a trend for evidence that dexamethasone given intravenously at a range of 6 to 16 mg per day may enhance resolution of bowel obstruction with a number needed to treat of 6. The number of side effects in the studies was low, and the use of corticosteroids did not appear to affect short-term survival.[2] Common side effects of corticosteroids include delirium, hyperglycemia, fungal infections, gastrointestinal upset and bleeding, hypertension, and muscle weakness.

Anticholinergics. Anticholinergics are often provided in combination with analgesics and antiemetics to reduce gastrointestinal secretions. Their mechanism of action is to competitively inhibit muscarinic receptors in the smooth muscle of the gastrointestinal wall, thereby impairing ganglionic neural transmission.[22] In addition to decreasing secretions, this blockade can decrease the colicky pain frequently associated with malignant bowel obstruction, thereby providing a coanalgesic effect. Hyoscine bromide (scopolamine) is available in the United States only as a hydrobromide salt, which can penetrate the central nervous system, leading to delirium. Glycopyrrolate is a quaternary amine with antimuscarinic activity that has similar clinical efficacy to scopolamine but because of structural differences has markedly decreased central nervous system side effects. A handful of studies found octreotide to be superior to hyoscine bromide in reducing intestinal secretions, number of vomiting episodes, amount of fatigue, and appetite improvement. Octreotide was also found to be superior in improving chances of nasogastric tube removal.[32,35,36] Because it has a different mechanism of action than octreotide, expert opinion recommends the addition of anticholinergic agents to further reduce secretions in persons with severe inoperable obstruction who are already on octreotide.[6]

Antiemetic Agents. Prokinetic drugs such as metoclopramide may be effective in the setting of a partial bowel obstruction. They work by binding to the 5-hydroxytryptophan 4 (5-HT4) receptor and releasing acetylcholine, which binds to cholinergic receptors to increase gut motility.[4,5] The resultant increase in motility decreases stasis and mitigates the feeling of nausea. In the setting of complete obstruction, metoclopramide should be discontinued because it may worsen cramping.[20,21] If metoclopramide is not an option or if nausea persists, therapies that target the chemoreceptor trigger zone can often be helpful. These include agents that block dopaminergic (haloperidol or other antipsychotic) and serotoninergic receptors and are usually scheduled around the clock.

Hydration. The value of hydration in the management of malignant bowel obstruction continues to be debated. Anecdotal experience has led to concern that parenteral hydration may further fuel an increase in secretions, thereby worsening symptoms.[35] At the same time, the metabolic derangements that accompany dehydration may further nausea and vomiting. One small study of 17 patients with inoperable bowel obstruction found that the administration of parenteral hydration over 500 mL per day significantly reduced symptoms of nausea and drowsiness.[36] Further studies are needed to delineate the role of hydration in this patient population. Despite the lack of consensus, many experts recommend limiting intravenous hydration to less than 50 mL per hour until gastrointestinal symptoms improve.[36]

KEY MESSAGES TO PATIENTS AND FAMILIES

Malignant bowel obstruction is an emergent condition that requires early assessment and intervention. Patients with a history of colorectal and gynecological cancers are at increased risk, especially during the advanced stage of illness. Patients presenting with worsening nausea and vomiting, abdominal distention, colicky abdominal pain, and constipation should be evaluated for bowel obstruction. The management of bowel obstruction varies, depending on the underlying cause, number and sites of obstruction, physical condition of the patient, life expectancy, and goals of care. Some patients may benefit from interventions such as a nasogastric tube, gastrostomy tube, stenting, or surgical resection. For others, medical management may represent the best treatment option, with a combination of therapies that help alleviate the obstruction, provide analgesia, and relieve nausea and vomiting.

CONCLUSION AND SUMMARY

Despite limited evidence from randomized, controlled trials, common practice in the medical management of malignant bowel obstruction is a multimodal approach, combining drugs with relatively low toxicities and different mechanisms of action to improve gastrointestinal symptoms. Patients with a reasonable life expectancy who do not have contraindications should also be considered for endoscopic or surgical interventions in addition to ongoing medical management.

SUMMARY RECOMMENDATIONS

- Bowel obstruction is a common complication of gastrointestinal and ovarian cancers, usually occurring in the advanced stage of illness. A thorough history and physical examination should be conducted in persons presenting with nausea and vomiting who have bowel obstruction.
- The management of bowel obstruction varies depending on the underlying cause, number and sites of obstruction, physical condition of the patient, life expectancy, and goals of care.
- Treatment options include interventions such as a nasogastric tube, a gastrostomy tube, stenting, or surgical resection. For others, medical management may represent the best treatment option, with a combination of therapies that help alleviate the obstruction, provide analgesia, and relieve nausea and vomiting.

REFERENCES

1. Chakraborty A, Selby D, Gardiner K, et al. Malignant bowel obstruction: natural history of a heterogeneous patient population followed prospectively over two years. *J Pain Symptom Manage.* 2011;41(2):412–420.
2. Feuer DDJ, Broadley KE. Corticosteroids for the resolution of malignant bowel obstruction in advanced gynecological and gastrointestinal cancer. *Cochrane Database Syst Rev.* 1999;(3): CD001219.
3. Dekovich AA. Endoscopic treatment of colonic obstruction. *Curr Opin Gastroenterol.* 2008;25:50–54.
4. Mercadante S, Ferrera P, Villari P, Marrazzo A. Aggressive pharmacological treatment for reversing malignant bowel obstruction. *J Pain Symptom Manage.* 2004;28:412–416.
5. Ripamonti C, Bruera E. Palliative management of malignant bowel obstruction. *Int J Gynecol Cancer.* 2002;12:135–143.
6. Ripamonti C, Mercadante S. How to use octreotide for malignant bowel obstruction. *J Support Oncol.* 2004;2:357–364.
7. Schrijvers D, Van Fraeyenhove F. Emergencies in palliative care. *Cancer J.* 2010;16(5):514–520.
8. Dohmoto M. New method: endoscopic implantation of rectal stent in palliative treatment of malignant stenosis. *Endosc Digest.* 1991;3:1507–1512.
9. Meisner S, Hensler M, Knop FK, et al. Self-expanding metal stents for colonic obstruction: experiences from 104 procedures in a single center. *Dis Colon Rectum.* 2004;47:444–450.
10. Osman H, Rashid HI, Sathananthan M, Parker MC. The cost effectiveness of self-expanding metal stents in the management of malignant left sided large bowel obstruction. *Colorectal Dis.* 2000;2:233–237.
11. Khot UP, Wenk Lang A, Murali K, Parker MC. Systematic review of the efficacy and safety of colorectal stents. *Br J Surg.* 2002;89:1096–1102.
12. Caceres A, Zhou Q, Iasonos A, et al. Colorectal stents for palliation of large bowel obstructions in recurrent gynecological cancer: an updated series. *Gynecol Oncol.* 2008;108:482–485.
13. Law WL, Choi HK, Chu KW, Tung HM. Radiation stricture of rectosigmoid treated with self-expanding metallic stent. *Surg Endosc.* 2002;16:1106–1107.
14. Dormann AJ, Deppe H, Wigginghaus B. Self-expanding metallic stents for continuous dilatation of benign stenoses in gastrointestinal tract – first results of long-term follow-up in interim stent application in pyloric and colonic obstructions. *Z Gastroenterol.* 2001;39:957–960.
15. Sebastian S, Johnston S, Geoghegan T, et al. Pooled analysis of the efficacy and safety of self-expanding metal stenting in malignant colorectal obstruction. *Am J Gastroenterol.* 2004;99:2051–2057.
16. Fernandez-Esparrach G, Bordas JM, Giraldez MD, et al. Severe complications limit long-term clinical success of self-expanding metal stents in patients with obstructive colorectal cancer. *Am J Gastroenterol.* 2010;105:1087–1093.
17. Tilney HS, Lovegrove RE, Purkayastha S, et al. Comparison of colonic stenting and open surgery for malignant large bowel obstruction. *Surg Endosc.* 2007;21:225–233.
18. Dronamraju SS, Ramamurthy S, Kelly SB, Hyat M. Role of self-expanding metallic stents in the management of malignant obstruction of the proximal colon. *Dis Colon Rectum.* 2009;52(9):1657–1661.
19. Baines M, Oliver DJ, Carter RL. Medical management of intestinal obstruction in patients with advanced malignant disease. *Lancet.* 1985;2:990–993.
20. Abernathy AP, Wheeler JL, Zafar SY. Detailing of gastrointestinal symptoms in cancer patients with advanced disease: new methodologies, new insights, and a proposed approach. *Curr Opin Support Palliat Care.* 2009;3:41–49.
21. Weber C, Zuilian GB. Malignant irreversible intestinal obstruction: the powerful association of octreotide to corticosteroids, antiemetics, and analgesics. *Am J Hosp Palliat Med.* 2009;26(2):84–88.
22. Mercadante S, Casuccio A, Mangione S. Medical treatment for inoperable malignant bowel obstruction: a qualitative systematic review. *J Pain Symptom Manage.* 2007;33:217–223.
23. Fainsinger RL, Spachynski K, Hanson J, Bruera E. Symptom control in terminally ill patients with malignant bowel obstruction. *J Pain Symptom Manage.* 1994;9:12–18.

24. Matulonis UA, Seiden MV, Roche M, et al. Long-acting octreotide for the treatment and symptomatic relief of bowel obstruction in advanced ovarian cancer. *J Pain Symptom Manage.* 2005;30:563–569.

25. Massacesi C, Galeazzi G. Sustained release octreotide may have a role in the treatment of malignant bowel obstruction. *Palliat Med.* 2006;20:715–716.

26. Kvols LK, Wolterinf EA. Role of somatostatin analogs in the clinical management of non-neuroendocrine solid tumors. *Anticancer Drugs.* 2006;17:601–608.

27. Mercadante S, Spoldi E, Carceni A, et al. Octreotide in relieving gastrointestinal symptoms due to bowel obstruction. *Palliat Med.* 1993;7:295–299.

28. Mercadante S, Kargar J, Nicolosi G. Octreotide may prevent definitive intestinal obstruction. *J Pain Symptom Manage.* 1997;13:352–355.

29. Mercadante S, Avola G, Maddaloni S, et al. Octreotide prevents the pathological alterations of bowel obstruction in cancer patients. *Support Care Cancer.* 1996;4:393–394.

30. Sun X, Li X, Li H. Management of intestinal obstruction in advanced ovarian cancer: an analysis of 57 cases. *Zhonghua Zhong Liu Za Zhi.* 1995;17:39–42.

31. Hisanaga T, Shinjo T, Morita T, et al. Multicenter prospective study on efficacy and safety of octreotide for inoperable malignant bowel obstruction. *Jpn J Clin Oncol.* 2010;40(8):739–745.

32. Mystakidou K, Tsilka E, Kalaidopoulou O, et al. Comparison of octreotide administration vs. conservative treatment in the management of inoperable bowel obstruction in patients with far advanced cancer: a randomized, double-blind, controlled clinical trial. *Anticancer Res* 2002;22:1187–1192.

33. Laval G, Girarder J, Lassauniere J, et al. The use of steroids in the management of inoperable intestinal obstruction in terminal cancer patients: do they remove the obstruction? *Palliat Med.* 2000;14:3–10.

34. Hardy J, Ling J, Mansi J, et al. Pitfalls in placebo-controlled trials in palliative care: dexamethasone for the palliation of malignant bowel obstruction. *Palliat Med.* 1998;12:437–442.

35. Mercadante S, Ripamonti C, Casuccio A, Zecca E, Groff L. Comparison of octreotide and hyoscine butylbromide in controlling gastrointestinal symptoms due to malignant inoperable bowel obstruction. *Support Care Cancer.* 2000;8:188–191.

36. Ripamonti C, Mercadante S, Groff L, et al. Role of octreotide, scopolamine butylbromide, and hydration in symptom control of patients with inoperable bowel obstruction and nasogastric tubes: a prospective randomized trial. *J Pain Symptom Manage.* 2000;19(1):23–34.

ANOREXIA, CACHEXIA, AND FEEDING DIFFICULTIES

Chapter 28

What Medications Are Effective in Improving Anorexia and Weight Loss in Cancer?

VICKIE E. BARACOS

INTRODUCTION AND SCOPE OF THE PROBLEM

The onset of involuntary weight loss is often the first clinical sign of the presence of malignant disease, and in cancers that are incurable by currently available therapies, weight loss of large magnitude, culminating in emaciation, can be seen in any palliative care setting.

The estimated prevalence of cancer cachexia is variously reported. Cachexia prevalence will depend on the demographics of body weight in specific geographic regions. Given the prevalence of obesity in westernized countries,[1] the marked shift in body weight renders the definition of clinically significant weight loss in patients with cancer a moving target. In the United States, it has been estimated that cancer cachexia may affect approximately 1.3 million people.[2] The prevalence of cancer cachexia varies depending on the type of malignancy, with the greatest frequency of weight loss (approximately 50%-85% of patients) observed in gastrointestinal, pancreatic, lung, and colorectal cancers at diagnosis and before initiation of chemotherapy.[3,4] Weight loss is an acknowledged feature of the disease trajectory of all incurable malignancies, which contribute to an estimated 7.4 million deaths per year worldwide.[5]

Cachexia has been recognized since ancient times as an adverse effect of cancer. It is associated with reduced physical function,[6] reduced tolerance to anticancer therapy,[7,8] and reduced survival.[4,9] The evident physical wasting and loss of appetite that patients commonly experience, particularly in advanced stages of cancer, coupled with the poor efficacy of nutritional supplementation to reverse cachexia, impart a substantial burden of distress on the patient and family. Often family members hold a strong belief that increased caloric intake can enhance patient quality of life and prolong survival, and patients often feel significant distress when family members insist on offering food.[10,11] Thus the progression of cancer cachexia and associated physical wasting can have profound effects on the family environment, including distress, frustration, and heightened anxiety regarding outcomes of the disease.[12–14]

RELEVANT PATHOPHYSIOLOGY

Cancer cachexia is a complex multidimensional problem for which there has been no generally agreed classification system or treatment algorithm. Recently, several international consensus groups have worked to develop a conceptual framework for the cause-based diagnosis of cancer-associated malnutrition[15] and cachexia.[16] The motivation for these efforts was concern that multiple, often discordant, definitions for these terms are found in the literature and that lack of uniformly accepted definition, diagnostic criteria, and classification has impeded advancement in both clinical trials and clinical practice.

The efforts of the consensus groups create a jumping-off point for the diagnosis, staging, and intervention for cancer cachexia, with agreement on the following key points:

1. The specific erosion of skeletal muscle (i.e., lean tissue) is the physiologically and nutritionally important element of weight loss. Connected with this point is the important finding that many cancer patients whose body weight is normal, overweight, or even obese, may harbor very significant muscle wasting. This severe muscle wasting (also known as sarcopenia) is an occult condition, and while hidden behind a mantle of adipose tissue, is related to reduced survival[17] and increased toxicity of systemic antineoplastic therapy.[8,18]

The presence of occult muscle wasting brings into view the need of objective measures of skeletal muscle mass in the clinical assessment of patients with cancer.[16]

2. Pathophysiology is characterized by a negative protein and energy balance driven by a variable combination of reduced food intake and abnormal metabolism. The degree to which food intake is decreased and metabolism is increased is a characteristic of a given patient, disease type, and stage. Quantification of protein and calorie intake is useful.

3. Reduced food intake is attributable to primary anorexia, as well as other symptoms affecting oral intake. A clinical distinction is to be made between alterations occurring in the brain, such as decreased central drive to eat, and secondary causes of impaired food intake (e.g., stomatitis, constipation, decreased upper gastrointestinal motility [causing early satiety and nausea], dyspnea, pain, and poor dietary habits), which should be recognized early because they might prove readily reversible.

4. Hypercatabolism aggravates weight loss. This is provoked by tumor burden, systemic inflammation, and other catabolic factors. The tumor and its metastases may reach a mass sufficient to result in a quantitatively significant energy expenditure[19]; however, changes may occur in host tissue, such as increased sensitivity to lipolytic factors[20] or resistance to the normal anabolic actions of insulin[21] that underlie weight loss. A known feature of cancer cachexia is the tumor-induced activation of the host immune system involving proinflammatory cytokines.[22] Increased production of interleukin (IL)-1β, IL-6, interferon-γ, and tumor necrosis factor (TNF)-α, may be the primary catabolic triggers of skeletal muscle loss.[22–25] These metabolic changes define the reason that cachexia, unlike simple malnutrition, cannot be fully reversed by conventional nutritional support, although some of these metabolic changes are potentially reversible with suitable antiinflammatory therapy. Finally, new findings of potentially great importance relate to antineoplastic agents as specific catabolic effectors. In particular, several targeted therapies promote weight loss and skeletal muscle catabolism.[26,27] This is suggested to occur because pathways of muscle anabolism and of tumor cell proliferation share common elements.

5. Clinical progression of malnutrition and wasting occurs over time. A staging system to what is essentially a progressive and cumulative problem of depletion should be applied. This is an exceedingly important point in relation to therapy and in recognition of cancer cachexia as a continuum. Fearon and colleagues[16] proposed three stages of clinical relevance: precachexia, cachexia, and refractory cachexia. Because the underlying metabolic abnormalities responsible for the eventual clinical manifestations of cachexia are likely present before overt weight loss, it seems reasonable to identify cachexia in its earliest stages (precachexia) with a view to delay or prevent the onset of cachexia. On the other end of the spectrum, cachexia can be clinically refractory as a result of very advanced disease (the presence of rapidly progressive cancer unresponsive to anticancer therapy). This stage is associated with profound anorexia and active catabolism or the presence of factors that render active management of weight loss no longer possible or appropriate. Refractory cachexia is characterized by a low performance status (World Health Organization score 3 or 4) and a life expectancy of less than 3 months. Thus cachexia may be viewed as an end-of-life condition that is managed primarily through palliative approaches in the refractory phase, whereas cachexia may be present early in the progression of cancer and approachable by nutritional and pharmacological treatment.

SUMMARY OF EVIDENCE REGARDING TREATMENT RECOMMENDATIONS

Treatment recommendations for cancer cachexia must be based on its stage and cause. Management of precachexia is based on early identification, preventive intervention, and monitoring for progression to cachexia. Cachexia requires multimodal management based on its specific phenotype, with priority also given to the reversal of symptoms contributing to low dietary intake. In the instance of refractory cachexia, palliation of symptoms and psychosocial support come to the forefront. Historically, cancer cachexia was viewed as an end-of-life condition and managed primarily through palliative approaches. Randomized clinical trials of therapies for cancer cachexia have largely been conducted in populations well within the last 3 months preceding death and hence within the refractory stage. Of note, the most extensively studied therapies to date are compounds that palliate the profound anorexia in advanced cancer, progestins and corticosteroids (see later discussion).

A useful systematic review of pharmacological therapies for cancer-associated anorexia and weight loss in adult patients with nonhematological malignancies was published in 2005.[28] The review encompassed articles in MEDLINE, EMBASE, CINAHL, and Cochrane Control Trials Register. At that time only 55 studies met inclusion criteria, and the largest number of studies involved progestins (29 trials conducted in 4139 patients) and corticosteroids (6 studies conducted in 637 patients). Only two classes of drugs (progestins and corticosteroids) were found to have sufficient evidence to support their use in cancer cachexia. Few studies have examined other agents, with at most two or three trials on any given agent. A general paucity of clinical trials exists on cancer cachexia; approximately 10 trials with a randomized design are currently listed as recruiting patients on www.ClinicalTrials.gov, an international registry of clinical research.

Precachexia

Precachexia is a concept that first appeared in the literature in 2010, and currently diagnostic criteria for precachexia remain under discussion. Because earlier diagnosis may be important for the prevention and treatment of cachexia, diagnostic criteria specific for precachexia have been proposed.[29] These criteria include the presence of an underlying chronic disease such as cancer, unintentional weight loss of low grade (≤5% within 6 months), a chronic or recurrent systemic inflammatory response, and disease-associated anorexia. Because the underlying metabolic abnormalities responsible for the eventual clinical manifestations of cachexia are likely present before overt weight loss, it seems reasonable to employ nutritional and pharmacological strategies to delay or prevent the onset of cachexia; however, this approach requires clinical validation. Several randomized clinical trials currently in progress adopt the approach of initiation of cachexia therapy immediately on diagnosis and concurrently with planned therapy such as radiation and chemotherapy. Such studies challenge current paradigms and will determine the efficacy of early intervention.

Cachexia

Cachexia requires multimodal management based on its specific phenotype, with priority also given to the reversal of symptoms contributing to low dietary intake. Macdonald and associates[30] detailed a list of potentially correctable problems likely to interfere with food intake or assimilation and emphasized the need to screen for and meticulously manage all of them. Specific issues included treatable psychological factors (anxiety, depression, family distress, spiritual distress), eating problems (poor appetite, disturbed taste or smell, dental issues, mouth sores, thrush, dry mouth, dysphagia, regurgitation, early satiety, nausea and vomiting, bowel obstruction, constipation, malabsorption, fistulas, fatigue, inability to sleep, pain) and metabolic disorders (diabetes, adrenal insufficiency, hypogonadism, thyroid insufficiency).

At the point that each patient's underlying primary disease, comorbidities, and the foregoing potentially correctable problems are being managed optimally, treatment of cachexia may be undertaken. Consideration should be given to the following specific domains:

1. *Oral intake.* In general it is important to emphasize the need for a broad balanced diet and to explain the importance of maintaining food intake, to undergo cancer therapy or optimize quality of life. It is important to explore what patients consider to be a normal diet and to identify the principal daily source of protein in the diet. On average, weight-losing cancer patients are in energy deficit on the order of 250 to 400 kilocalories (Kcal) per day, and because protein requirements are not decreased, it is necessary to increase the fraction of protein in the diet to gain or maintain diminished skeletal muscle mass. The exact protein intake required has not been defined, but it is important to note that the majority of healthy adults over 65 years of age cannot maintain nitrogen balance at less than 1g of protein per kilogram of body weight per day. Red or white meat, fish, dairy products, and protein–enriched supplements are possible sources. Patients will often benefit from specialist dietary assessment and advice from a dietitian.

2. *Exercise.* The average physical activity levels of patients with advanced cancer still attending the outpatient clinic is reduced by approximately 40% to 50%.[31] Patients with advanced cancer are generally elderly and have significant musculoskeletal, cardiopulmonary, or other comorbidity, making many forms of exercise beyond their capacity. The consequences of inactivity in healthy older adults are significant, with rapid reduction of protein biosynthesis and loss of muscle mass and muscle function.[32] It is vital to explain to patients the value of exercise to counteract muscle wasting. Simply maintaining mobility and walking are reasonable goals to set. Motivated patients may benefit from a program of training developed by a physiotherapist.

3. *Antiinflammatory.* The amount of evidence is growing concerning the role of systemic inflammation in most forms of cachexia. Inflammatory mediators contribute to both reduced food intake and uncontrolled catabolism. No antiinflammatory strategy has been proven to be of benefit in cachexia. However, two common approaches are nonsteroidal antiinflammatory drugs (NSAIDs)[33] and fish oil (eicosapentaenoic acid). NSAIDs with a low incidence of gastrointestinal side effects, such as ibuprofen, can be taken long term with or without gastric mucosal protection. Fish oil is an alternative and may be perceived as more natural to some patients. A dose of 1.5 to 2g per day of eicosapentaenoic acid is recommended and can be taken as fish oil capsules or a fish oil–enriched oral nutritional supplement. Several studies have shown preliminary evidence suggesting benefits for the retention of lean body mass and overall survival.[34–38]

Additional specific pharmacological agents for cancer cachexia have been subjected to limited investigation (i.e., cannabinoids, anabolic steroids); however, their efficacy remains unproved. Investigational new drugs are appearing in Phase I and II clinical trials, targeting stimulation of appetite in the hypothalamus (i.e., the gastric appetite-stimulating hormone ghrelin) and skeletal muscle anabolism (i.e., selective androgen receptor modulators, antagonists to myostatin).

Refractory Cachexia

Refractory cachexia is characterized by severe anorexia, intense catabolism, and often substantial frustration and distress in patients and family in regard to this highly visible manifestation of progressive disease. The benefits of nutritional supplementation may be impaired because of underlying catabolic processes and impairment of anabolism. Overall, randomized trials of nutritional intervention have shown minimal clinical efficacy.[39]

Appetite stimulants, including corticosteroids and progestational agents, are effective in increasing food intake and weight, but these effects are generally short lived and, similar to nutritional supplementation, have limited long-term benefits on patient quality of life.[28] Due to their well-known adverse effects, particularly with longer duration of use, corticosteroids may be more suitable for patients with a short life expectancy, especially if they have other symptoms that may be simultaneously alleviated (i.e., pain or nausea). Megestrol acetate (Megace *ES*, Par Pharmaceutical Companies, Inc., Spring Valley, NY) is a synthetic progestational agent approved for treatment of weight loss, severe malnutrition, and suppressed appetite in patients with acquired immunodeficiency syndrome.[40] Progestogens can stimulate appetite in some patients with cancer cachexia; however, fat mass and water retention are the primary components of any increase in weight, with no effects on muscle mass and no clear improvement in patient quality of life or prolongation of survival.

Several authors have emphasized the need for assessment of patients for distress related to eating, altered body image and feelings of pressure, guilt, and relational stress and the corresponding need psychosocial support for patients and families during the refractory stage of cachexia.[16,41] Physical wasting is highly evident, and anorexia and other symptoms disrupt the rhythm of meal preparation and sharing of food in the family. Family members may hold a strong belief that increased caloric intake can enhance patient quality of life and prolong survival. Patients often feel significant distress when family members focus on offering food[42] or apply pressure to eat. Health care providers may assist in this context by providing clarification of the causes and outcomes of the disorder and in doing so may relieve some of the burden on patients and caregivers and dissipate conflict over food intake.

KEY MESSAGES TO PATIENTS AND FAMILIES

Unplanned weight loss is frequently one of the earliest signs of the presence of cancer, and for cancers which are not curable, weight loss is expected to develop hand-in-hand with the progression of the disease. Patients, family members, and health care professionals all struggle with this weight loss, which can be large and is usually associated with a loss of appetite and enjoyment of food. Clinicians should work to help patients and families understand that treatment of cancer-associated weight loss is possible, involving the combined efforts of patient and family, physician, dietitian, and physical therapist. However the expectation of weight gain must be moderated, because body weight often does not increase in response to nutritional supplementation in the

same degree that it does in healthy people. In addition to maintaining food intake, especially protein, exercise may help gain muscle and maintain physical function. Clinicians may prescribe medications to increase appetite and assist in weight gain, as well as to manage symptoms that interfere with eating. It is important to emphasize that cancer causes loss of pleasurable sensations from food and the desire to eat. In this situation, it is helpful for family members to avoid pressuring the cancer patient to eat, because this is likely to cause distress and frustration.

CONCLUSION AND SUMMARY

Cancer cachexia is a complex multidimensional problem for which there has been no generally agreed on classification system or treatment algorithm. Cancer cachexia thus remains a significant medical problem with few therapeutic options. Recently, international consensus has been achieved on a conceptual framework for the definition and classification of cancer cachexia. This crucial set of concepts will assist in advancement in both in clinical trials and clinical practice and provide a means to develop cachexia therapy specific to its stage and specific cause.

SUMMARY RECOMMENDATIONS

- Involuntary weight loss should be assessed at the time of cancer diagnosis and over the disease course to detect the onset of cachexia.
- Key elements to be included in clinical assessment of the cachexia syndrome include the loss of skeletal muscle mass, dietary intake, symptoms which impair oral intake, and inflammation.
- A multimodal approach to treating cachexia includes the combined efforts of patient and family, physician, dietitian, and physical therapist.
- Clinicians should emphasize that cancer causes loss of pleasurable sensations from food and the desire to eat. Family members should avoid pressuring the cancer patient to eat, because this is likely to cause distress and frustration.

REFERENCES

1. Flegal KM, Carroll MD, Ogden CL, Curtin LR. Prevalence and trends in obesity among US adults, 1999–2008. *JAMA.* 2010;303(3):235–241.
2. Morley JE, Thomas DR, Wilson MM. Cachexia: pathophysiology and clinical relevance. *Am J Clin Nutr.* 2006;83(4):735–743.
3. Bruera E. ABC of palliative care: anorexia, cachexia, and nutrition. *BMJ.* 1997;315:1219–1222.
4. Dewys WD, Begg C, Lavin PT, et al. Prognostic effect of weight loss prior to chemotherapy in cancer patients. Eastern Cooperative Oncology Group. *Am J Med.* 1980;69(4):491–497.
5. World Health Organization. *2009 Cancer Key facts.* http://www.who.int/mediacentre/factsheets/fs297/en/. Accessed September 3, 2012.
6. Moses AWG, Slater C, Preston T, et al. Reduced total energy expenditure and physical activity in cachectic patients with pancreatic cancer can be modulated by an energy and protein dense oral supplement enriched with n-3 fatty acids. *Br J Cancer.* 2004;90(5):996–1002.

7. Bachmann J, Heiligensetzer M, Krakowski-Roosen H, et al. Cachexia worsens prognosis in patients with resectable pancreatic cancer. *J Gastrointest Surg.* 2008;12(7):1193–1201.

8. Prado CM, Antoun S, Sawyer MB, Baracos VE. Two faces of drug therapy in cancer: drug-related lean tissue loss and its adverse consequences to survival and toxicity. *Curr Opin Clin Nutr Metab Care.* 2011;14(3):250–254.

9. Fearon KCH, Voss AC, Hustead DS. Cancer Cachexia Study Group. Definition of cancer cachexia: effect of weight loss, reduced food intake and systemic inflammation on functional status and prognosis. *Am J Clin Nutr.* 2006;83(6):1345–1350.

10. Reid J, McKenna H, Fitzsimons D, McCance T. The experience of cancer cachexia: a qualitative study of advanced cancer patients and their family members. *Int J Nurs Stud.* 2009; 46(5):606–616.

11. McClement S. Cancer anorexia-cachexia syndrome: psychological effect on the patient and family. *J Wound Ostomy Continence Nurs.* 2005;32(4):264–268.

12. Strasser F, Palmer JL, Schover LR, et al. The impact of hypogonadism and autonomic dysfunction on fatigue, emotional function, and sexual desire in male patients with advanced cancer: a pilot study. *Cancer.* 2006;107(12): 2949–2957.

13. Tchekmedyian NS, Cella D. Clinical usefulness of quality-of-life evaluations: the case of anorexia. *Contemp Oncol.* 1995; 20:30–33.

14. Cella D, Bonomi AE, Leslie WT, et al. Quality of life and nutritional well-being: measurement and relationship. *Oncology.* 1993;7:105–111.

15. Jensen GL, Mirtallo J, Compher C, et al. for the International Consensus Guideline Committee. Adult starvation and disease-related malnutrition: a proposal for etiology-based diagnosis in the clinical practice setting from the International Consensus Guideline Committee. *JPEN-Parenter Enter.* 2010;34:156–159.

16. Fearon K, Strasser F, Anker SD, et al. Definition and classification of cancer cachexia: an international consensus. *Lancet Oncol.* 2011;12(5):489–495.

17. Prado CM, Lieffers JR, McCargar LJ, et al. Prevalence and clinical implications of sarcopenic obesity in patients with solid tumours of the respiratory and gastrointestinal tracts: a population-based study. *Lancet Oncol.* 2008;9(7):629–635.

18. Prado CM, Baracos VE, McCargar LJ, et al. Sarcopenia as a determinant of chemotherapy toxicity and time to tumor progression in metastatic breast cancer patients receiving capecitabine treatment. *Clin Cancer Res.* 2009;15(8):2920–2926.

19. Lieffers JR, Mourtzakis M, Hall KD, et al. A viscerally driven cachexia syndrome in patients with advanced colorectal cancer: contributions of organ and tumor mass to whole-body energy demands. *Am J Clin Nutr.* 2009;89(4):1173–1179.

20. Agustsson T, Rydén M, Hoffstedt J, et al. Mechanism of increased lipolysis in cancer cachexia. *Cancer Res.* 2007;67(11): 5531–5537.

21. Asp ML, Tian M, Wendel AA, Belury MA. Evidence for the contribution of insulin resistance to the development of cachexia in tumor-bearing mice. *Int J Cancer.* 2010;126(3):756–763.

22. Baracos VE. Cancer-associated cachexia and underlying biological mechanisms. *Ann Rev Nutr.* 2006;26:435–461.

23. Argiles JM, Busquets S, Felipe A, Lopez-Soriano FJ. Molecular mechanisms involved in muscle wasting in cancer and ageing: cachexia versus sarcopenia. *Int J Biochem Cell Biol.* 2005;37(5): 1084–1104.

24. Gullett N, Rossi P, Kucuk O, Johnstone PA. Cancer-induced cachexia: a guide for the oncologist. *J Soc Integr Oncol.* 2009;7(4):155–169.

25. Mantovani G, Maccio A, Madeddu C, et al. Phase II nonrandomized study of the efficacy and safety of COX-2 inhibitor celecoxib on patients with cancer cachexia. *J Mol Med.* 2010; 88(1):85–92.

26. Desar IM, Thijs AM, Mulder SF, et al. Weight loss induced by tyrosine kinase inhibitors of the vascular endothelial growth factor pathway. *Anticancer Drugs.* 2012;23(2):149–154.

27. Antoun S, Birdsell L, Sawyer MB, et al. Association of skeletal muscle wasting with treatment with sorafenib in patients with advanced renal cell carcinoma: results from a placebo-controlled study. *J Clin Oncol.* 2010;28(6):1054–1060.

28. Yavuzsen T, Davis MP, Walsh D, et al. Systematic review of the treatment of cancer-associated anorexia and weight loss. *J Clin Oncol.* 2005;23(33):8500–8511.

29. Muscaritoli M, Anker SD, Argiles J, et al. Consensus definition of sarcopenia, cachexia and precachexia: joint document elaborated by Special Interest Groups (SIG) "cachexia-anorexia in chronic wasting diseases" and "nutrition in geriatrics". *Clin Nutr.* 2010;29(2):154–159.

30. MacDonald N, Easson AM, Mazurak VC, et al. Understanding and managing cancer cachexia. *J Am Coll Surg.* 2003;197:143–161.

31. Dahele M, Skipworth R, Wall L, et al. Objective physical activity and self-reported quality of life in patients receiving palliative chemotherapy. *J Pain Symptom Manage.* 2007;33(6):676–685.

32. Kortebein P, Ferrando A, Lombeida J, et al. Effect of 10 days of bed rest on skeletal muscle in healthy older adults. *JAMA.* 2007;297(18):1772–1774.

33. Preston T, Fearon KCH, McMillan DC, et al. Effect of ibuprofen on the acute phase response and protein metabolism in weight-losing cancer patients. *Br J Surg.* 1995;82(2):229–234.

34. Murphy RA, Yeung E, Mazurak VC, Mourtzakis M. Influence of eicosapentaenoic acid supplementation on lean body mass in cancer cachexia. *Br J Cancer.* 2011;105(10):1469–1473.

35. Ries A, Trottenberg P, Elsner F, et al. A systematic review on the role of fish oil for the treatment of cachexia in advanced cancer: an EPCRC cachexia guidelines project. *Palliat Med.* 2012;26(4) 294–304.

36. Weed HG, Ferguson ML, Gaff RL, et al. Lean body mass gain in patients with head and neck squamous cell cancer treated perioperatively with a protein- and energy-dense nutritional supplement containing eicosapentaenoic acid. *Head Neck.* 2011;33(7):1027–1033.

37. Fearon KC, Barber MD, Moses AG, et al. Double-blind, placebo-controlled, randomized study of eicosapentaenoic acid diester in patients with cancer cachexia. *J Clin Oncol.* 2006;24(21):3401–3407.

38. Murphy RA, Mourtzakis M, Chu QS, et al. Nutritional intervention with fish oil provides a benefit over standard of care for weight and skeletal muscle mass in patients with nonsmall cell lung cancer receiving chemotherapy. *Cancer.* 2011;117:1775–1782.

39. Fearon KC, Von Meyenfeldt MF, Moses AG, et al. Effect of a protein and energy dense N-3 fatty acid enriched oral supplement on loss of weight and lean tissue in cancer cachexia: a randomised double blind trial. *Gut.* 2003;52(10):1479–1486.

40. Megace ES. (megestrol acetate oral suspension) *Full prescribing information.* Spring Valley, NY: Par Pharmaceutical Companies, Inc; 2008. Available at http://www.megacees.com/PDF/Megace_ES_Portrait_PI.pdf. Accessed September 3, 2012.

41. Dodson S, Baracos VE, Jatoi A, et al. Muscle wasting in cancer cachexia: clinical implications, diagnosis, and emerging treatment strategies. *Annu Rev Med.* 2011;62:265–279.

42. McClement S. Cancer anorexia-cachexia syndrome: psychological effect on the patient and family. *J Wound Ostomy Continence Nurs.* 2005;32(4):264–268.

29

What Therapeutic Strategies Are Effective in Improving Anorexia and Weight Loss in Nonmalignant Disease?

VICKIE E. BARACOS

INTRODUCTION AND SCOPE OF THE PROBLEM

Cachexia is a term commonly understood by health care professionals. It describes a condition characterized by the presence of involuntary weight loss and culminating in a state of emaciation. This was described aptly by Hippocrates: "a sharp nose, hollow eyes, sunken temples...."

Until recently, no agreement had been reached on an operational definition of and diagnostic criteria for cachexia; this lack of definition motivated international groups of experts to develop a uniformly accepted definition, diagnostic criteria, and classification to advance clinical practice. Clearly defined diagnostic criteria are also essential for development and approval of potential therapeutic agents. The definition provided by an international consensus group chaired by Evans and colleagues[1] is as follows:

Cachexia is a complex metabolic syndrome associated with underlying illness and characterized by loss of muscle with or without loss of fat mass. The prominent clinical feature of cachexia is weight loss in adults (corrected for fluid retention) or growth failure in children (excluding endocrine disorders). Anorexia, inflammation, insulin resistance and increased muscle protein breakdown are frequently associated with cachexia. Cachexia is distinct from starvation, age-related loss of muscle mass, primary depression, malabsorption and hyperthyroidism and is associated with increased morbidity. (p. 793)

This definition makes several key distinctions. Although cachexia is often associated with reduced food intake, it differs from simple malnutrition by the presence of underlying disease[1,2]; involuntary weight loss does not occur in healthy individuals and conversely is associated with a host of chronic conditions, including cancer, diabetes, untreated acquired immunodeficiency syndrome (AIDS), chronic obstructive pulmonary disease (COPD), chronic heart failure, chronic renal failure, and rheumatoid arthritis. Chapter 28 discusses cancer cachexia, the most well studied cachexia in chronic diseases. It should be noted that several acute conditions, such as trauma, burn, and sepsis, are associated with acute and sometimes severe weight loss related to the cachexia of chronic disease. In all of these conditions the underlying disease or injury variously adds to the development of weight loss through inflammation, insulin resistance, increased catabolism of skeletal muscle, and increased overall energy expenditure.

Von Haehling and Anker[3] described cachexia as a major underestimated and unmet medical need. According to the estimated prevalence of cachexia in patients affected by chronic diseases, this ranges from a low of 5% to 15% in advanced COPD or chronic heart failure to as much as 60% to 80% in advanced cancer. Those authors calculated the population prevalence of cachexia, concluding that the most frequent cachexia subtypes are, in order of frequency, COPD cachexia, cardiac cachexia, cancer cachexia, and cachexia of chronic renal failure. In industrialized countries (North America, Europe, Japan), the overall prevalence of cachexia (resulting from any disease) is thought to be growing and currently about 1%, that is, affecting about 9 million patients. It is of relevance that older people develop multiple comorbid conditions, and it is not unusual for a person over 70 years of age to have more than one condition associated with cachexia. For example, atherosclerotic disease, depression, chronic kidney disease, cognitive impairment, obstructive sleep apnea syndrome, lung cancer, osteoporosis, diabetes, heart failure, sarcopenia, aortic aneurysm, arrhythmias, and pulmonary embolism are all highly prevalent among older COPD patients.[4]

Cachexia is associated with mortality. Large degrees of weight loss and low body mass index are poor prognostic factors in chronic heart failure.[5] Perhaps not surprisingly, having been obese or overweight in the first place is protective and longer survival has been documented in patients with initially heavy body weights across a range of cachexia-associated conditions.[6-8]

Cachexia is a source of psychological distress. The evident physical wasting and loss of appetite that patients commonly experience, particularly in advanced stages of the progression of cachexia impart a substantial burden of distress on patient and family. Psychological distress associated with cachexia has been most studied in malignant disease. Often family members hold a strong belief that increased caloric intake can enhance patient quality of life and prolong survival, and patients often feel significant distress when family members insist on offering food.[9,10] Thus the progression of cancer cachexia and its associated physical wasting can have profound effects on the family environment, including distress and frustration and heightened anxiety regarding outcomes of the disease.[11,12]

RELEVANT PATHOPHYSIOLOGY

Cachexia is a complex multidimensional problem, and several points of its pathophysiology are important for the diagnosis and treatment of the condition. The following five key points are agreed upon:

1. *The specific erosion of skeletal muscle (i.e., lean tissue) is the physiologically and nutritionally important element of weight loss.* As described earlier, cachexia is "characterized by loss of muscle with or without loss of fat mass."[1] Connected with this point is the important finding that many patients whose body weight is normal, overweight, or even obese may harbor very significant muscle wasting. This severe muscle wasting (also known as sarcopenia) is an occult condition, and while hidden behind a mantle of adipose tissue, is related to reduced physical function and survival.[13] The presence of occult muscle wasting brings into view the need for objective measures of skeletal muscle mass in clinical assessment, and this is accessible simply by anthropometry[14] or image–based technologies such as dual energy x-ray.[15–17] The perceived importance of muscle explains the emphasis on therapeutic approaches with essential amino acid supplementation[16,18] and anabolic agents.[17]

2. *The pathophysiology is characterized by a negative protein and energy balance driven by a variable combination of reduced food intake and abnormal metabolism.* The degree to which food intake is decreased and metabolism increased is a characteristic of a given patient, disease type, and stage. Quantification of protein and calorie intake is useful. Several micronutrients that are essential in the diet for humans, such as n-3 polyunsaturated fatty acids and vitamin D, have been proposed to contribute to the wasting of skeletal muscle and loss of physical function in cachexia.[19,20]

3. *Reduced food intake is attributable to primary anorexia and other symptoms affecting oral intake.* A clinical distinction is to be made between alterations occurring in the brain, such as decreased central drive to eat, and secondary causes of impaired food intake, such as constipation, decreased upper gastrointestinal motility (causing early satiety and nausea), dyspnea, pain, and poor dietary habits. These secondary causes should be recognized early because they might prove readily reversible.

4. *Hypercatabolism aggravates weight loss.* This is provoked by disease, systemic inflammation, and other catabolic factors. Increased resting energy expenditure per kilogram of fat-free (lean) body mass has been characterized in COPD, chronic heart failure, and chronic renal failure[13,21–23]; however, changes may occur in host tissue, such as increased lipolysis and proteolysis or resistance to the normal anabolic actions of insulin,[24] that underlie weight loss. A feature of cachexia is the activation of the host immune system, involving proinflammatory cytokines.[24] Increased production of interleukin (IL)-1β, IL-6, interferon-γ, and tumor necrosis factor (TNF)-α, may be the primary catabolic triggers of skeletal muscle loss in addition to anorexia.[25] Of importance, these metabolic changes define the reason that cachexia, unlike simple malnutrition, cannot be fully reversed by conventional nutritional support. Some of these metabolic changes are potentially reversible with suitable antiinflammatory therapy.

5. *The clinical progression of malnutrition and wasting occurs over time.* The need exists to apply a staging system to what is essentially a progressive and cumulative problem of depletion. This is an important point in relation to therapy and in recognition of cachexia as a continuum. Fearon and colleagues[26] proposed three stages of clinical relevance: precachexia, cachexia, and refractory cachexia. Because the underlying metabolic abnormalities responsible for the eventual clinical manifestations of cachexia are likely present before overt weight loss, it seems reasonable to identify cachexia in its earliest stages (precachexia) with a view to delay or prevent its onset. Compared with the relatively rapid course of metastatic cancer and cancer cachexia, the evolution of cachexia in some chronic diseases is slower, giving much opportunity for preemptive treatments. The concept of refractory cachexia is relatively new and has arisen in discussion of cancer cachexia and the lack of efficacy of cachexia therapy in the end stages of disease. It can be clinically refractory as a result of advanced disease that is unresponsive to treatment, such as in end-stage renal failure. This stage is associated with profound anorexia and active catabolism or the presence of factors that render active management of weight-loss no longer possible or appropriate. Refractory cachexia is characterized by a low performance status and life expectancy of less than 3 months. Thus cachexia may be viewed as an end-of-life condition that is managed primarily through palliative approaches in the refractory phase, whereas cachexia may be present early in the progression of disease and approachable by nutritional and pharmacological treatment.

SUMMARY OF EVIDENCE REGARDING TREATMENT RECOMMENDATIONS

Treatment recommendations for cachexia must be based on its stage and cause. Management of pre-cachexia is based on early identification, preventive intervention, and monitoring for progression to cachexia. Cachexia requires multimodal management based on its specific phenotype, with priority also given to the reversal of symptoms contributing to low dietary intake. Potentially correctable problems likely to interfere with food intake or assimilation require meticulous management. Specific issues include treatable psychological factors (anxiety, depression, family distress, spiritual distress), eating problems (poor appetite, disturbed taste or smell, dental issues, mouth sores, thrush, dry mouth, dysphagia, regurgitation, early satiety, nausea and vomiting, constipation, malabsorption, fistulas, fatigue, inability to sleep, pain), and metabolic disorders (diabetes, adrenal insufficiency, hypogonadism, thyroid insufficiency).

Treatment of cachexia in nonmalignant disease is not particularly well informed by clinical trials. A general paucity of clinical trials on cachexia persists, and the majority of those done pertain to cancer cachexia. A recent search revealed only 99 studies including the term *cachexia* listed on www.ClinicalTrials.gov, an international registry of clinical research. Of these, 75% are on cancer cachexia, with the remaining 25% concerning cachexia of human immunodeficiency virus (HIV) infection, COPD, chronic heart failure, or chronic renal failure. Trials on nonmalignant disease include interventions on n-3 polyunsaturated fatty acids for cachexia in COPD and chronic heart failure, enteral nutrition formulas, infliximab for COPD cachexia, and three studies of megestrol acetate for HIV-associated cachexia.

Currently no drugs are approved for either cachexia or anorexia in most conditions. However, some recent reviews are useful to develop a clinical decision-making strategy for cachexia therapy. Some of these are specific to a given disease and therapy, such as the review by Aaronson and colleagues[27] on the safety of anabolic testosterone therapy in cardiac disease. Hypogonadism has been considered a problem contributing to muscle wasting in elderly men for some time, and a more recent development is consideration of this therapy in elderly men affected by chronic diseases.[28] A related topic is the use of anabolic steroids to promote muscle anabolism.[29] Some authors discuss the chronic diseases in a broader context; for example, Vogelmeier and Wouters[28] discuss a constellation of systemic effects of COPD, including cachexia, osteoporosis, vitamin D deficiency, and physical inactivity. These are considered comorbidities of COPD, may have an impact on morbidity and mortality, and are interrelated. Muscle wasting is an outcome of cachexia and vitamin D deficiency and is potentiated by physical inactivity; therefore a rational approach to patient management cannot consider any of these in isolation. Cogent discussions of the pathophysiology that is common to cachexia and spans multiple chronic diseases have been published. Maddocks and colleagues[30] discuss the rationale for exercise to attenuate the effects of cachexia by modulating muscle metabolism, insulin sensitivity, and levels of inflammation, as well as the challenges in its clinical application. McHugh and Miller-Saultz[31] provide an overview of the assessment and management of gastrointestinal symptoms across the spectrum of advanced incurable illness, including anorexia, cachexia, nausea, vomiting, and constipation. Thomas[32] and Braun and Marks[25] consider the application of orexigenic medications to improve appetite in the elderly and in cachexia. Of these, ghrelin or small molecules that mimic its action are attracting current interest.[33] Ghrelin is a growth hormone–releasing peptide that is mainly secreted by the stomach and participates in a variety of physiological processes. Ghrelin stimulates food intake by hypothalamic neurons and causes a positive energy balance and body weight gain by decreasing fat usage and promoting adipogenesis. Preliminary trials suggest that it may prove valuable in the management of disease-induced cachexia. Several nutritional recommendations are seen to span the range of cachexias, including nutritional therapy for muscle wasting[34] and n-3 polyunsaturated fatty acids as nondrug anti-inflammatory therapy.[35]

At the point at which each patient's underlying primary disease, comorbidities, and potentially correctable problems are being managed optimally, treatment of cachexia may be undertaken. Consideration should be given to the following three domains:

1. *Oral intake.* In general, it is important to emphasize the need for a broad, balanced diet and to explain the importance of maintaining food intake, to undergo disease-directed therapies or to optimize quality of life. It is important to explore what patients consider to be a normal diet and identify the principal daily source of protein in the diet. It is necessary to increase the fraction of protein in the diet to either gain or maintain diminished skeletal muscle mass.[16,18] The exact protein intake required has not been defined for most chronic diseases, but it is important to note that the majority of healthy adults over 65 years of age cannot maintain nitrogen balance at less than 1 g of protein per kilogram body weight per day. Red or white meat, fish, dairy products, and protein-enriched supplements are possible sources. Patients often benefit from specialist dietary assessment and advice from a dietician.

2. *Exercise.* The average physical activity levels of patients with chronic diseases are minimal. Patients are generally elderly and have significant musculoskeletal, cardiopulmonary, or other comorbidity making many forms of exercise beyond their capacity. The consequences of inactivity in healthy older adults are impressive, with rapid reduction of protein biosynthesis and loss of muscle mass and function.[36] It is vital to explain to patients the value of exercise to counteract muscle

wasting. Simply maintaining mobility and walking are reasonable goals to set. Motivated patients may benefit from a program of training developed by a physiotherapist.

3. *Antiinflammatory.* A growing body of evidence demonstrates the role of systemic inflammation in most forms of cachexia. Inflammatory mediators contribute to both reduced food intake and uncontrolled catabolism. No ideal antiinflammatory strategy has been proved of benefit in cachexia. However, two common approaches are nonsteroidal antiinflammatory drugs (NSAIDs)[37] and fish oil (eicosapentaenoic acid). NSAIDs with a low incidence of gastrointestinal side effects such as ibuprofen can be taken long term with or without gastric mucosal protection. Fish oil is an alternative that may be perceived as more natural to some patients. Eicosapentaenoic acid 1.5 to 2 g per day is recommended and can be taken either as fish oil capsules or a fish oil–enriched oral nutritional supplement.

Several authors emphasize the need for assessment of patients for distress related to eating, including altered body image; feelings of pressure, guilt, and relational stress; and the corresponding need for psychosocial support for patients and families during the refractory stage of cachexia.[26,38] Physical wasting is highly evident, and anorexia and other symptoms disrupt the rhythm of meal preparation and sharing of food in the family. Family members may hold a strong belief that increased caloric intake can enhance patient quality of life and prolong survival. Patients often feel significant distress when family members focus on offering food or apply pressure to eat.[9,10] Health care providers may assist in this context by providing clarification of the causes and outcomes of the disorder and in doing so may relieve some of the burden on patients and caregivers and dissipate conflict over food intake.

KEY MESSAGES TO PATIENTS AND FAMILIES

Clinicians should help patients and families understand that unplanned weight loss is frequently one of the earliest signs of the presence of chronic disease. For patients with conditions that are not curable, weight loss is expected to develop hand-in-hand with disease progression. Patients, family members, and health care professionals all struggle with this weight loss, which can be large and is usually associated with a loss of appetite and enjoyment of food.

It is important to explain that treatment of weight loss is possible, involving the combined efforts of patient and family, physicians, nurses, dietitians, and physical therapists. However, the expectation of weight gain must be moderated, because body weight often does not increase in response to nutritional supplementation in the same degree that it does in healthy people. In addition to maintaining food intake, especially protein, exercise may help gain muscle and maintain physical function. Clinicians

should explain that treatments are available that may increase appetite, assist in weight gain, and manage symptoms that interfere with eating.

In working with patients and families, clinicians may want to acknowledge that illness causes loss of pleasurable sensations from food and the desire to eat. In this situation, it is helpful for family members to avoid pressuring the patient to eat, because this is likely to cause distress and frustration.

CONCLUSION AND SUMMARY

Cachexia is a complex multidimensional problem with no generally agreed upon classification system or treatment algorithm. It thus remains a significant medical problem with limited therapeutic options. Recently, international consensus was achieved on a conceptual framework for the definition and classification of cachexia. This crucial set of concepts will assist in the advancement of both clinical trials and clinical practice, and they provide a means to develop cachexia therapy specific to its stage and cause.

SUMMARY RECOMMENDATIONS

- Patients with chronic illnesses should be monitored for involuntary weight loss and loss of lean body mass.
- Key elements to be included in the clinical assessment of cachexia include age-related changes, specific comorbidities, level of physical functioning, the presence of symptoms effecting oral intake, and the presence of inflammation.
- A multimodal approach to treating cachexia should include the combined efforts of patient and family, physician, nurse, dietitian, and physical therapist.
- Clinicians should emphasize that cachexia causes loss of pleasurable sensations from food and the desire to eat. Family members should avoid pressuring the patient to eat, because this is likely to cause distress and frustration.

REFERENCES

1. Evans WJ, Morley JE, Argilés J, et al. Cachexia: a new definition. *Clin Nutr.* 2008;27(6):793–799.
2. Jensen GL, Mirtallo J, Compher C, et al for the International Consensus Guideline Committee. Adult starvation and disease-related malnutrition: a proposal for etiology-based diagnosis in the clinical practice setting from the International Consensus Guideline Committee. *JPEN J Parenter Enteral Nutr.* 2010;34:156–159.
3. von Haehling S, Anker SD. Cachexia as a major underestimated and unmet medical need: facts and numbers. *J Cachexia Sarcopenia Muscle.* 2010;1(1):1–5.

4. Corsonello A, Antonelli Incalzi R, Pistelli R, et al. Comorbidities of chronic obstructive pulmonary disease. *Curr Opin Pulm Med.* 2011;17(suppl 1):S21–S28.

5. Anker SD, Ponikowski P, Varney S, et al. Wasting as independent risk factor for mortality in chronic heart failure. *Lancet.* 1997;349(9058):1050–1053.

6. Davos CH, Doehner W, Rauchhaus M, et al. Body mass and survival in patients with chronic heart failure without cachexia: the importance of obesity. *J Card Fail.* 2003;9(1):29–35.

7. Kalantar-Zadeh K, Kopple JD. Obesity paradox in patients on maintenance dialysis. *Contrib Nephrol.* 2006;151:57–69.

8. Horwich TB, Fonarow GC. Reverse epidemiology beyond dialysis patients: chronic heart failure, geriatrics, rheumatoid arthritis, COPD, and AIDS. *Semin Dial.* 2007;20(6):549–553.

9. Reid J, McKenna H, Fitzsimons D, McCance T. The experience of cancer cachexia: a qualitative study of advanced cancer patients and their family members. *Int J Nurs Stud.* 2009;46(5):606–616.

10. McClement S. Cancer anorexia-cachexia syndrome: psychological effect on the patient and family. *J Wound Ostomy Continence Nurs.* 2005;32(4):264–268.

11. Tchekmedyian NS, Cella D. Clinical usefulness of quality-of-life evaluations: the case of anorexia. *Contemp Oncol.* 1995;20:30–33.

12. Cella D, Bonomi AE, Leslie WT, et al. Quality of life and nutritional well-being: measurement and relationship. *Oncology.* 1993;7:105–111.

13. Sergi G, Coin A, Marin S, et al. Body composition and resting energy expenditure in elderly male patients with chronic obstructive pulmonary disease. *Respir Med.* 2006;100(11):1918–1924.

14. Noori N, Kopple JD, Kovesdy CP, et al. Mid-arm muscle circumference and quality of life and survival in maintenance hemodialysis patients. *Clin J Am Soc Nephrol.* 2010;5(12):2258–2268.

15. Thibault R, Cano N, Pichard C. Quantification of lean tissue losses during cancer and HIV infection/AIDS. *Curr Opin Clin Nutr Metab Care.* 2011;14(3):261–267.

16. Solerte SB, Gazzaruso C, Bonacasa R, et al. Nutritional supplements with oral amino acid mixtures increases whole-body lean mass and insulin sensitivity in elderly subjects with sarcopenia. *Am J Cardiol.* 2008;101(11A):69E–77E.

17. Storer TW, Woodhouse LJ, Sattler F, et al. A randomized, placebo-controlled trial of nandrolone decanoate in human immunodeficiency virus-infected men with mild to moderate weight loss with recombinant human growth hormone as active reference treatment. *J Clin Endocrinol Metab.* 2005;90(8):4474–4482.

18. Dal Negro RW, Aquilani R, Bertacco S, et al. Comprehensive effects of supplemented essential amino acids in patients with severe COPD and sarcopenia. *Monaldi Arch Chest Dis.* 2010;73(1):25–33.

19. Gordon PL, Doyle JW, Johansen KL. Association of 1,25-dihydroxyvitamin D levels with physical performance and thigh muscle cross-sectional area in chronic kidney disease stage 3 and 4. *J Ren Nutr.* 2012;22(4):423–433.

20. Dawson-Hughes B. Serum 25-hydroxyvitamin D and muscle atrophy in the elderly. *Proc Nutr Soc.* 2012;71(1):46–49.

21. Kao CC, Hsu JW, Bandi V, et al. Resting energy expenditure and protein turnover are increased in patients with severe chronic obstructive pulmonary disease. *Metabolism.* 2011;60(10):1449–1455.

22. Wang AY, Sea MM, Tang N, et al. Energy intake and expenditure profile in chronic peritoneal dialysis patients complicated with circulatory congestion. *Am J Clin Nutr.* 2009;90(5):1179–1184.

23. Fragasso G, Salerno A, Lattuada G, et al. Effect of partial inhibition of fatty acid oxidation by trimetazidine on whole body energy metabolism in patients with chronic heart failure. *Heart.* 2011;97(18):1495–1500.

24. Skyba P, Ukropec J, Pobeha P, et al. Metabolic phenotype and adipose tissue inflammation in patients with chronic obstructive pulmonary disease. *Mediators Inflamm.* 2010:173498; 2010, (doi:10.1155/2010/173498).

25. Braun TP, Marks DL. Pathophysiology and treatment of inflammatory anorexia in chronic disease. *J Cachexia Sarcopenia Muscle.* 2010;1(2):135–145.

26. Fearon K, Strasser F, Anker SD, et al. Definition and classification of cancer cachexia: an international consensus. *Lancet Oncol.* 2011;12(5):489–495.

27. Aaronson AJ, Morrissey RP, Nguyen CT, Willix R, Schwarz ER. Update on the safety of testosterone therapy in cardiac disease. *Expert Opin Drug Saf.* 2011;10:697–704.

28. Vogelmeier CF, Wouters EF. Treating the systemic effects of chronic obstructive pulmonary disease. *Proc Am Thorac Soc.* 2011;8(40):376–379.

29. Gullett NP, Hebbar G, Ziegler TR. Update on clinical trials of growth factors and anabolic steroids in cachexia and wasting. *Am J Clin Nutr.* 2010;91(4):1143S–1147S.

30. Maddocks M, Murton AJ, Wilcock A. Improving muscle mass and function in cachexia: non-drug approaches. *Curr Opin Support Palliat Care.* 2011;5(4):361–364.

31. McHugh ME, Miller-Saultz D. Assessment and management of gastrointestinal symptoms in advanced illness. *Prim Care.* 2011;38(2):225–246.

32. Thomas DR. Use of orexigenic medications in geriatric patients. *Am J Geriatr Pharmacother.* 2011;9(2):97–108.

33. Angelidis G, Valotassiou V, Georgoulias P. Current and potential roles of ghrelin in clinical practice. *J Endocrinol Invest.* 2010;33(11):823–838.

34. Morley JE, Argiles JM, Evans WJ, et al for the Society for Sarcopenia, Cachexia, and Wasting Disease. Nutritional recommendations for the management of sarcopenia. *J Am Med Dir Assoc.* 2010;11(6):391–396.

35. Fasano E, Serini S, Piccioni E, Innocenti I, Calviello G. Chemoprevention of lung pathologies by dietary n-3 polyunsaturated fatty acids. *Curr Med Chem.* 2010;17(29):3358–3376.

36. Kortebein P, Ferrando A, Lombeida J, et al. Effect of 10 days of bed rest on skeletal muscle in healthy older adults. *JAMA.* 2007;297(16):1772–1774.

37. Preston T, Fearon KCH, McMillan DC, et al. Effect of ibuprofen on the acute phase response and protein metabolism in weight-losing cancer patients. *Br J Surg.* 1995;82:229–234.

38. Dodson S, Baracos VE, Jatoi A, et al. Muscle wasting in cancer cachexia: clinical implications, diagnosis, and emerging treatment strategies. *Annu Rev Med.* 2011;62:265–279.

Chapter 30

When Should Enteral Feeding by Percutaneous Tube Be Used in Patients With Cancer and in Patients With Non–Cancer-Related Conditions?

Thomas Reid and Steve Pantilat

INTRODUCTION AND SCOPE OF THE PROBLEM

Artificial nutrition by means of a feeding tube—enteral nutrition—can provide needed calories and nutrients for patients who are unable to eat. Such tubes can pass transnasally or percutaneously and terminate in either the stomach or the small intestine. If the problem preventing a patient from eating is temporary, as is often the case in the intensive care unit during acute illness and after some operations, this intervention can be lifesaving. Whereas nasogastric tube feeding tubes may be used for short-term enteral nutrition, use for more than a few weeks generally requires percutaneous tube placement. This chapter focuses on these latter interventions.

In the United States, more than 200,000 gastrostomy tubes are placed annually in patients with Medicare coverage[1] and prevalence rates for gastrostomy tubes in nursing homes ranges from 7.5% to 40%.[2] In the palliative care setting, gastrostomy tubes are considered most commonly for patients with neurological disorders (especially dementia and stroke) and oropharyngeal and esophageal obstruction (usually resulting from cancer), as well as for patients with any advanced illness who are losing weight.[3] They may also be placed to facilitate medication administration or to relieve a permanent bowel obstruction (venting gastrostomy). Near the end of life, questions often arise about the effectiveness and appropriateness of gastrostomy. Does it prolong life? Does it promote comfort or detract from it? How should clinicians navigate the complex cultural, family, and personal meanings attached to feeding?

Gastrostomy: What Is It and How Is It Done?

Percutaneous endoscopic gastrostomy (PEG) and percutaneous endoscopic jejunostomy (PEJ), defined by where the tube terminates, are endoscopic procedures to insert a plastic tube through the abdominal wall into the gastrointestinal tract. In the case of PEG placement, an endoscope is introduced into the stomach, where a light identifies its position through the abdominal wall.[3] A guidewire is inserted through the abdominal wall into the stomach, grasped by the endoscope, and pulled back up through the esophagus. The wire is attached to the gastrostomy tube, which is then pulled back into the stomach and out through the skin. Other surgical and radiological approaches exist, all of which also require sedation and incision in the abdominal wall. When the procedure is complete, a balloon or internal bumper remains inside the lumen of the stomach to seal the entry point and prevent the tube from being inadvertently removed, and an external bumper is attached just over the skin to prevent further movement into the body. Feeding via the tube is usually started 24 hours after placement, although a recent meta-analysis supports starting as soon as 3 hours.[4]

Contraindications to gastrostomy include active coagulopathy, thrombocytopenia, abdominal wall abnormalities, organomegaly, large ascites, varices, recent myocardial infarction, hemodynamic instability, and sepsis.[5]

Risks and Complications Associated With Percutaneous Endoscopic Gastrostomy. Complications with PEG are associated with upper endoscopy, PEG placement, and the presence of the tube in the body.[5] Although serious complications are rare, overall long-term complications are common, with estimates ranging from 32% to 70%.[6] In healthy outpatients, mortality related to upper endoscopy is very low (<0.01%).[5] The risk for aspiration (0.3%-1%), severe hemorrhage (0.02%-0.06%), and perforation (0.008%-0.04%) are also low. Complications related to the PEG procedure itself include pneumoperitoneum (approximately 50%, generally benign), bowel injury, fistula formation, liver or spleen injury, and hemorrhage into various areas. Postprocedural complications include peptic ulcer disease (15%), diarrhea, tube dislodgement (1.6%-4.4%), infection (3% with prophylactic antibiotics), gastrointestinal bleeding (2.5%), ileus or gastroparesis (1%-2%), peristomal leakage (1%-2%), peristomal pain, gastric outlet obstruction, volvulus, and buried bumper syndrome (1.5%-1.9%), in which the internal bumper is pulled too tight against the stomach wall and gradually erodes into the extragastric tissue.

Percutaneous Endoscopic Gastrostomy Versus Nasogastric Tube. A recent Cochrane review found that complications in the first month and incidence of pneumonia at 6 months are no different between PEG and nasogastric tube for enteral nutrition.[7] Lower-quality evidence finds that PEG is associated with a lower prevalence of recurrent displacements and treatment interruptions but no difference in mortality, suggesting that PEG should be used if enteral access is needed for more than 30 days.[8] Separate Cochrane reviews favored PEG for stroke but found no difference for head and neck cancer.[9,10] Patients and families often prefer a gastrostomy for social reasons, comfort, and convenience.

Expectations of Benefit of Gastrostomy

Health care provider expectations for feeding tubes include improved nutrition (93%), hydration (60%), and survival (58%; predict 1-2 months with versus 1-3 years without placement); providing medications (55%); preventing aspiration (49%); facilitating nursing home placement (22%); diminishing pain (14%); and decreasing obstruction (12%).[11]

Surrogate expectations of benefit from PEG placement include improved nutrition (96%), health (93%), survival (90%), quality of life (87%), and comfort (79%); fewer problems eating (83%); fewer choking episodes (79%); and providing nutrition in absence of hunger or thirst (70%).[12] Surrogates report understanding the benefits of gastrostomy more than the risks. Of note, only 40% believed that the gastrostomy tube improved the patient's quality of life when surveyed 2 or more months after placement.[13]

RELEVANT PATHOPHYSIOLOGY

Two key issues driving the use of gastrostomy tubes in patients with advanced illness are the often mistaken beliefs that a patient is dying from lack of nutrition and that better nutrition will improve outcomes. However, in the terminal phase of disease it is common for patients to develop cachexia, defined as "a complex metabolic syndrome associated with underlying illness and characterized by loss of muscle with or without loss of fat mass."[14] Tissue wasting occurs with or without adequate nutritional intake and is usually accompanied by anorexia (loss of the desire to eat), early satiety, anemia, edema, weakness, and fatigue.[15] In patients with cancer, these symptoms are referred to as the cancer anorexia-cachexia syndrome (CACS) and eventually occur in up to 80% of cases.[14] The pathophysiology of CACS is only partially understood but appears to be driven by complex host–cancer cytokine interactions that induce the body to favor catabolism over anabolism. Patients with other advanced diseases such as heart failure, chronic obstructive pulmonary disease (COPD), human immunodeficiency virus (HIV) infection, acquired immunodeficiency syndrome (AIDS), and renal failure also can develop cachexia. In all cases, cachexia is a poor prognostic sign. Of importance, because cachexia is a metabolic disorder, it does not respond to additional nutritional support. A more detailed discussion of cachexia may be found in Chapter 28.

SUMMARY OF EVIDENCE REGARDING TREATMENT RECOMMENDATIONS

In the palliative care setting, strong supporting evidence does not exist in regard to any specific disease for which tube feeding is commonly recommended.[16] A recent Cochrane review sought to evaluate the effect of artificial nutrition on the quality and length of life of patients in palliative care, but no studies were sufficiently rigorous to meet the inclusion criteria.[17] Several prospective observational studies that examined mortality after placement of feeding tubes in mixed-disease populations in a variety of settings found high mortality after PEG placement (12%-22% at 1 month, 30% at 6 months, 50%-63% at 1 year, and 81% at 3 years).[6,12,18–20]

For patients who will receive gastrostomy, a mortality benefit may be associated with deferring placement until after hospital discharge. In one retrospective case-control study, compared with inpatients in whom a PEG was placed, the risk for death within 30 days was sevenfold lower for patients in community nursing homes (4% versus 29%) and half as great for matched inpatient controls who did not receive a PEG (13% versus 29%).[21] None of the patients in nursing homes and very few (6%) of the inpatients had their tubes placed for temporary nutritional support. Dementia or other serious cognitive dysfunction was present in 85% of the patients in nursing homes, 52% of the inpatients receiving PEGs, and 19% of the matched controls and was the most common indication for tube placement in the first two groups.

A second study by the same authors followed two groups of patients who received PEGs for any reason. For the first 2 years, all consecutive patients had their tubes placed in the hospital as close to the request as possible.[22] During the subsequent 2 years, patients were required to wait 30 days after discharge before placement. Both groups had a high proportion of cognitively impaired patients (80%-85%). Thirty-day mortality rates were identical from the time of admission but 40% lower from the time of the request for PEG and 87.5% lower from the time of PEG insertion in the patients in whom the procedure was postponed. Given the high baseline 30-day mortality, these differences may result from preventing tubes being placed in patients with very limited prognoses. It may also be possible that deferring the decision to the less-pressured outpatient setting results in better decision making. Regardless of the underlying cause, these and other data have led some to propose nasogastric tube feeding for a 30-day waiting period before PEG insertion.

Cancer

Nutrition support in surgical oncology is generally beneficial, short-term, and provided by nasogastric tube. Except in patients with head and neck cancer (discussed later), for nonsurgical cancer patients the benefit of enteral nutrition depends almost entirely on the patient's functional and nutritional status. In patients with limited prognoses and poor quality of life, no data support improved survival and patients with cancer who receive PEGs generally report poorer quality of life. Guidelines also recommend against enteral nutrition for patients undergoing routine radiation, chemotherapy, or stem cell transplant.[23] In contrast, enteral feeding is recommended for patients with good functional status and quality of life if they are losing weight from insufficient nutritional intake or are expected to consume less than 60% of their estimated energy expenditure for more than 10 days.[23]

Head and Neck Cancers. Patients with head and neck cancers are at high risk for nutritional deficiency from CACS, anatomic obstruction, and side effects of chemoradiation treatments, including dysphagia, odynophagia, dysgeusia, xerostomia, tissue necrosis, and infections.[24] Between 60% and 100% of treated patients with head and neck cancers receive enteral feeding for a median of 21 to 29 weeks, with 10% to 30% of tubes still in place after 1 year.[24,25] No evidence indicates that placing a tube prophylactically improves any clinically important outcome, and tube placement may be associated with worse quality of life.[24] For those who do receive enteral nutrition, insufficient evidence exists to recommend any one type of tube.[10]

Patients Without Cancer

Dementia. Dementia is perhaps the most controversial indication for gastrostomy. In the United States, dementia accounts for 30% of gastrostomy placements[6] and 34% of patients with dementia in nursing homes have gastrostomy tubes.[20,26] Hopes for gastrostomy in this population include prolonging survival, improving quality of life, preventing or healing pressure ulcers, increasing functional capacity, and reducing aspiration. A Cochrane review of both nasogastric and PEG feeding for older people with advanced dementia found no randomized trials but did summarize seven prospective cohort studies.[27] Unfortunately, the best available evidence

(summarized in the following section) is not of sufficient quality to draw definitive conclusions regarding causality for any outcome. Based on the best available data, for patients with advanced dementia, tube feeding does not affect survival, quality of life, pressure ulcers formation or healing, or functional capacity.

Mortality. Only one study in the Cochrane review showed increased survival with tube feeding compared to oral feeding, and that finding became insignificant after controlling for factors including functional impairment and age.[28] Two studies showed increased mortality with tube feeding.[29,30] In the remaining four studies no differences occurred in mortality. In two studies published since the Cochrane review, approximately half of patients with dementia lived longer than 1 year and 25% longer than 3 years after PEG, with no difference in mortality rates compared with patients without dementia receiving PEGs.[31,32]

Quality of Life. Improved quality of life is a challenging outcome to measure in patients with dementia, and no study in the Cochrane review assessed it. Surrogates of patients in nursing home who have advanced dementia reported greater satisfaction with end-of-life care when feeding tubes were not present.[33]

Aspiration. Many observational studies show that enteral nutrition with nasogastric, PEG, or PEJ tubes does not reduce the risk for aspiration or pneumonia and in patients with dementia may even increase it.[27,34,35] Aspiration pneumonia rates in the only study in the Cochrane review to report them were significantly higher for those fed by gastrostomy tube rather than orally (67% versus 17%).[36] This finding is not surprising because gastrostomy tubes do not prevent aspiration of oral secretions. In these patients, careful hand feeding has been advocated as an alternative to gastrostomy. Although oral feeding may lead to weight gain (0.5 to 2.0 kg over 16 months) in moderately to severely demented patients, it does not affect function, cognition, or mortality.[37]

Pressure Ulcer Healing and Prevention. Two of the trials included in the Cochrane review showed an insignificant trend toward a lower prevalence and smaller number of pressure ulcers. Most other data suggest that enteral nutrition has no effect on ulcer formation or healing.[35]

Stroke. Up to half of patients who experience strokes have dysphagia, difficulty with self-feeding, or severe cognitive impairment, with half of these either dying or recovering function within the first 2 weeks.[9] The remainder will require artificial nutrition and hydration to survive. Strong data show no benefit to tube feeding in first week after stroke, allowing clinicians time to assess whether function will return.[16] If nutrition support is required after that time, placing a PEG tube instead of a nasogastric tube is associated with lower mortality (odds ratio [OR] 0.28), fewer treatment failures (OR 0.10), and improved nutrition (measured by albumin, +0.7 g/dL).[9] Of those patients with stroke who receive PEG tubes, a quarter die within a month and another quarter regain enough swallowing ability to have the tube removed within 2 to 3 years.[38] In the remaining half of patients, enteral feeding is withdrawn or becomes essentially permanent.

For patients with stroke who otherwise have what they would consider an adequate quality of life, starting artificial nutrition with a PEG tube is a reasonable option. However, the decision to withdraw this intervention may be more difficult as the likelihood for functional improvement dims.

Amyotrophic Lateral Sclerosis. Evidence-based practice guidelines from the American Academy of Neurology (AAN) recommend that PEG placement should be considered to stabilize weight and to prolong survival in patients with amyotrophic lateral sclerosis (ALS).[39] A recent Cochrane review evaluated enteral feeding for patients with ALS.[40] No randomized clinical trials were found. The three prospective and eight retrospective trials that met the inclusion criteria weakly supported the AAN recommendations.

Poor Prognostic Factors. Low albumin (OR 2.1 to 3), age older than 80 years (OR 1.8), comorbid congestive heart failure (OR 1.5), previous subtotal gastrectomy (OR 2.6), receiving a PEG in the hospital, poor functional status (bedridden), and disorientation are independent risk factors for increased mortality after gastrostomy.[22,29-31,41]

Important Considerations

Hunger and Starvation. A major concern of surrogates and family members is whether a patient who is not eating or receiving enteral feeding will be hungry or "starve to death." Although it is impossible to know if severely cognitively impaired patients suffer because of their decreased intake at the end of life, available evidence suggests they do not and may even be more comfortable without artificial nutrition and hydration.

With only small amounts of food and water given at the request of the patient, 63% of terminally ill, mentally aware patients admitted to a comfort care unit never experienced hunger and initial hunger in nearly all of the others (34%) eventually disappeared.[42] Patients who do not eat develop a ketogenic state that is associated with reduced hunger, and carbohydrate loads in this setting may stimulate hunger.[43] Fasting causes endorphin release and slows metabolism through reduced cortisol secretion and increased inactivation of thyroxine. Finally, not providing artificial nutrition and hydration at the end of life is associated with decreased respiratory secretions, coughing, nausea, vomiting, and diarrhea.

The issue of starving to death conjures up distressing images of famine-stricken people that anyone would want to avoid. Explaining that the weight loss, anorexia, cachexia, and decreased oral intake associated with terminal illnesses is different from starvation and typically is a consequence of the dying process rather than its cause can alleviate worry.

Comfort Feeding. In the palliative care setting, comfort feeding, in which the primary focus of eating is pleasure and quality of life, can achieve many patient and surrogate goals and obviate the need for gastrostomy. Comfort feeding allows the patient to enjoy the taste and texture of food and drink and also encourages human contact and interaction.[44]

Legal and Ethical Issues

Law. Although the Supreme Court has ruled that artificial nutrition and hydration is a medical treatment that patients and surrogates may refuse, the evidence a surrogate must provide regarding a patient's preference varies among states.[45] In 20 states and the District of Colombia, where the evidentiary threshold for discontinuing tube feeds is higher than for other interventions, it is especially important to ask patients to document their preferences in advance and surrogates to thoroughly consider patients' goals before artificial nutrition and hydration is initiated.[46]

Ethics. A strong consensus supports withholding or withdrawing any life-sustaining intervention in the service of a patient's wishes. Although no ethical distinction exists between the two practices, clinicians and surrogate decision-makers may find it more difficult to withdraw an intervention such as enteral feeding than to withhold it in the first place. In most cases the argument for withdrawing artificial nutrition is actually stronger than that for withholding it, because experience has usually provided evidence of its specific failure to achieve the patient's goals.[47]

Religion, Culture, Language, and Psychology. Differences in religious and cultural norms affect how clinicians, patients, and families make decisions regarding enteral nutrition. Groups and families that have experienced hunger or deprivation may have especially strong concerns about withholding nutritional support.[45] The symbolic power of food and the act of eating cannot be overstated. Surrogates may insist on enteral feeding because it demonstrates their love and dedication to the patient. Decreased intake can also be an emotionally powerful sign of failure—of the patient for not eating and of the caregiver for not providing food.

KEY MESSAGES TO PATIENTS AND FAMILIES

Although all potentially difficult conversations with patients and families benefit from excellent communication skills and family meeting structure, specific issues should be considered when discussing enteral feeding for patients with advanced disease. Helpful phrases for achieving key communication goals are provided in Table 30-1. Common emotional concerns such as starvation and the meaning of food may be the most important factors driving a decision and should be explored early in any conversation about gastrostomy, even if the patient or family does not raise them. Finally, because decisions about enteral nutrition often arise in patients who lack capacity, it is especially important to discuss preferences directly with patients while they are still able to participate in the decision.

TABLE 30-1. Suggestions for Language to Use in Discussing Gastrostomy and Enteral Feeding With Patients and Surrogates

GOAL	SUGGESTED LANGUAGE
Determine patient/surrogate understanding using open-ended questions	"How have things been going for you/your loved one?" "What is your understanding of your/your loved one's medical situation?"
Elicit values	"When you think about the future what do you hope for?" "When you think about what lies ahead, what worries you the most?"
Choose language carefully	Use "artificial nutrition" or "nutrition by a tube." Do not use words such as "feeding" or "eating."
Elicit understanding of gastrostomy tube	"How were you hoping the gastrostomy tube would help?"
Correct misconceptions	"I wish that the artificial nutrition would make her stronger/more alert/gain weight/fight the cancer/more comfortable/prevent infections or pneumonia, but unfortunately it can't do that for her."
Address potential harms of gastrostomy	"Unfortunately, extra formula and water doesn't help her body get better. It tends to go to the wrong places like her belly or lungs, and may actually make her less comfortable." "This is the body's way of shutting down. It's part of how we die."
Address starvation and hunger directly	"I can see that you would worry about starvation. It's terrible to think of that. What we know, however, is that for people like your mother, who have dementia/cancer and cannot eat, dementia/cancer leads to their death, not starvation."
Make a recommendation as appropriate	"Given what you have told me about your mother and my understanding of her condition, I recommend that we not start the artificial nutrition."
Validate the emotions a family is feeling	"I can see that your father has really benefitted from everything you've done. You must care for him very much. He's lucky to have you looking out for him."
Suggest a time-limited trial	"It sounds like you hope putting in a tube will help you/your mother be stronger/more alert and interactive. We'll probably be able to tell if that's working within a month. Let's plan to revisit the decision at that time to discuss if artificial nutrition is still the right decision for her."

Emphasize Artificiality

Though jargon usually impedes communication with patients and families, discussions of gastrostomy placement and artificial nutrition and hydration may be exceptions. Use of the phrases "artificial nutrition" or "nutrition by a tube" instead of "eating" helps to emphasize that a gastrostomy tube is a medical intervention that is qualitatively different from the familiar act of eating.

Provide Information

Elicit patient and surrogate assumptions about the perceived benefits of artificial nutrition and hydration and respectfully correct misperceptions. Explain that in advanced illness the body cannot benefit from and may even be harmed by artificial nutrition and hydration. Discuss the psychosocial impact of the actions that may be necessary to prevent the tube from becoming dislodged, such as using restraints or limiting mobility, social activity, and physical intimacy.

Set Limits at the Outset (Time-Limited Trials)

Gastrostomy tubes are frequently placed when clinical outcomes are uncertain and the benefits of a tube are unclear, yet once in place the tubes and

artificial nutrition and hydration are often psychologically, socially, or legally difficult to withdraw. When patients or families choose to have a gastrostomy under such circumstances, it may be helpful to propose a time-limited trial. Discuss a timeframe after which the patient and/or surrogate will reassess whether artifical nutrition and hydration is meeting the goals and expectations (benefits and risks) they previously described. Depending on the likelihood of success, present this date as a default stopping point or an opportunity to reevaluate. If possible, try to make explicit the conditions under which they would want to stop artificial nutrition and hydration, recognizing that survival as the outcome may become de facto evidence of efficacy.

Consider a Waiting Period

No difference exists in 30-day complications between nasogastric and PEG tubes, and some evidence suggests increased mortality associated with urgent PEG procedures; therefore consider suggesting a 30-day waiting period before PEG tube placement, especially for inpatients. A delay allows decision-makers time to adjust to what may be a new medical situation, provides patients time to recover function or try comfort feeding, and removes the environmental pressure to "get things done" that often exists in the hospital setting.

CONCLUSION AND SUMMARY

Although clinicians, patients, and families often believe that gastrostomy and enteral feeding can be beneficial, in the palliative care setting they rarely are. The catabolic state resulting from CACS that affects up to 80% of patients with cancer means that enteral nutrition has no role in the care of patients with advanced cancer who are losing weight. However, in patients with cancer who have good functional status and quality of life and those with head and neck cancers who are unable to consume sufficient calories, gastrostomy may be beneficial. Unfortunately, enteral feeding likely does not provide any benefit for patients with advanced dementia and may even increase aspiration. Careful hand feeding and comfort feeding are reasonable options for addressing goals of providing care and nutrition to these patients. In the last weeks and months of life, careful and compassionate communication about gastrostomy that acknowledges both the emotional and cultural significance of food and the data showing that enteral nutrition is not beneficial can lead to better decisions.

SUMMARY RECOMMENDATIONS

- In patients with limited prognoses and poor quality of life (terminal phase of disease) no data support improved survival or quality of life with enteral nutrition, and patients with cancer who receive PEGs generally report poorer quality of life.
- No role exists for routine enteral nutrition for patients undergoing radiation, chemotherapy, or stem cell transplant.
- Enteral feeding is recommended for cancer patients with good functional status and quality of life if they are losing weight because of insufficient nutritional intake or are expected to consume less than 60% of their estimated energy expenditure for longer than 10 days.
- Even though most patients with head and neck cancers will receive enteral feeding for many months or even years, there is no evidence that prophylactic gastrostomy improves any clinically important outcome.
- For patients with severe dementia, gastrostomy very likely does not increase survival, improve quality of life or functional capacity, prevent aspiration pneumonia or pressure ulcer formation, or promote the healing of pressure ulcers.
- Enteral nutrition should be avoided in the first week after stroke.
- For dysphagic stroke survivors who require enteral nutrition, a PEG is better than a nasogastric tube.
- Cachexia in advanced illness and near the end of life is a natural process that is not reversed by providing artificial nutrition and hydration.

- The need for enteral feeding often portends a poor prognosis with high mortality after PEG placement.
- When gastrostomy is chosen, consider a time-limited trial or a 30-day waiting period.
- Choose words carefully when discussing the emotionally charged issues of gastrostomy and enteral nutrition.

REFERENCES

1. Duszak R, Mabry MR. National trends in gastrointestinal access procedures: an analysis of Medicare services provided by radiologists and other specialists. *J Vasc Interv Radiol.* 2003;14(8):1031–1036.
2. Lin L-C, Li M-H, Watson R. A survey of the reasons patients do not chose percutaneous endoscopic gastrostomy/jejunostomy (PEG/PEJ) as a route for long-term feeding. *J Clin Nurs.* 2011;20(5–6):802–810.
3. Kurien M, McAlindon ME, Westaby D, Sanders DS. Percutaneous endoscopic gastrostomy (PEG) feeding. *BMJ.* 2010;340:c2414.
4. Szary NM, Arif M, Matteson ML, et al. Enteral feeding within three hours after percutaneous endoscopic gastrostomy placement: a meta-analysis. *J Clin Gastroenterol.* 2011;45(4):e34–e38.
5. Schrag SP, Sharma R, Jaik NP, et al. Complications related to percutaneous endoscopic gastrostomy (PEG) tubes: a comprehensive clinical review. *J Gastrointestin Liver Dis.* 2007;16(4):407–418.
6. Cervo FA, Bryan L, Farber S. To PEG or not to PEG: a review of evidence for placing feeding tubes in advanced dementia and the decision-making process. *Geriatrics.* 2006;61(6):30–35.
7. Gomes CA, Lustosa SAS, Matos D, et al. Percutaneous endoscopic gastrostomy versus nasogastric tube feeding for adults with swallowing disturbances. *Cochrane Database Syst Rev.* 2010;(11):CD008096.
8. American Gastroenterological Association. Medical position statement: guidelines for the use of enteral nutrition. *Gastroenterology.* 1995;108(4):1280–1281.
9. Bath PM, Bath FJ, Smithard DG. Interventions for dysphagia in acute stroke. *Cochrane Database Syst Rev.* 2000;(2):CD000323.
10. Nugent B, Lewis S, O'Sullivan JM. Enteral feeding methods for nutritional management in patients with head and neck cancers being treated with radiotherapy and/or chemotherapy. *Cochrane Database Syst Rev.* 2010;(3):CD007904.
11. Hanson LC, Garrett JM, Lewis C, et al. Physicians' expectations of benefit from tube feeding. *J Palliat Med.* 2008;11(8):1130–1134.
12. Carey T, Hanson L, Garrett J, et al. Expectations and outcomes of gastric feeding tubes. *Am J Med.* 2006;119(6):527 e11–527.e16.
13. Mitchell SL, Berkowitz RE, Lawson FM, Lipsitz LA. A cross-national survey of tube-feeding decisions in cognitively impaired older persons. *J Am Geriatr Soc.* 2000;48(4):391–397.
14. Evans WJ, Morley JE, Argilés J, et al. Cachexia: a new definition. *Clin Nutr.* 2008;27(6):793–799.
15. Bennani-Baiti N, Davis MP. Cytokines and cancer anorexia cachexia syndrome. *Am J Hosp Palliat Med.* 2008;25(5):407–411.
16. Koretz RL, Avenell A, Lipman TO, Braunschweig CL, Milne AC. Does enteral nutrition affect clinical outcome? A systematic review of the randomized trials. *Am J Gastroenterol.* 2007;102(2):412–429.
17. Good P, Cavenagh J, Mather M, Ravenscroft P. Medically assisted nutrition for palliative care in adult patients. *Cochrane Database Syst Rev.* 2008;(4):CD006274.
18. Callahan CM, Haag KM, Weinberger M, et al. Outcomes of percutaneous endoscopic gastrostomy among older adults in a community setting. *J Am Geriatr Soc.* 2000;48(9):1048–1054.
19. Pruthi D, Duerksen DR, Singh H. The practice of gastrostomy tube placement across a Canadian regional health authority. *Am J Gastroenterol.* 2010;105(7):1541–1550.
20. Teno JM, Mitchell SL, Skinner J, et al. Churning: the association between health care transitions and feeding tube insertion for nursing home residents with advanced cognitive impairment. *J Palliat Med.* 2009;12(4):359–362.

21. Abuksis G, Mor M, Segal N, et al. Percutaneous endoscopic gastrostomy: high mortality rates in hospitalized patients. *Am J Gastroenterol.* 2000;95(1):128–132.

22. Abuksis G. Outcome of percutaneous endoscopic gastrostomy (PEG): comparison of two policies in a 4-year experience. *Clin Nutr.* 2004;23(3):341–346.

23. Bozzetti F, Arends J, Lundholm K, et al. ESPEN Guidelines on Parenteral Nutrition: non-surgical oncology. *Clin Nutr.* 2009;28(4):445–454.

24. Locher JL, Bonner JA, Carroll WR, et al. Prophylactic percutaneous endoscopic gastrostomy tube placement in treatment of head and neck cancer: a comprehensive review and call for evidence-based medicine. *JPEN-J Parenter Enteral Nutr.* 2011;35(3):365–374.

25. Paleri V, Patterson J. Use of gastrostomy in head and neck cancer: a systematic review to identify areas for future research. *Clin Otolaryngol.* 2010;35(3):177–189.

26. Mitchell SL, Teno JM, Roy J, Kabumoto G, Mor V. Clinical and organizational factors associated with feeding tube use among nursing home residents with advanced cognitive impairment. *JAMA.* 2003;290(1):73–80.

27. Sampson E, Candy B, Jones L. Enteral tube feeding for older people with advanced dementia. *Cochrane Database Syst Rev.* 2009;(2):CD007209.

28. Jaul E, Singer P, Calderon-Margalit R. Tube feeding in the demented elderly with severe disabilities. *Isr Med Assoc J.* 2006;8(12):870–874.

29. Nair S, Hertan H, Pitchumoni CS. Hypoalbuminemia is a poor predictor of survival after percutaneous endoscopic gastrostomy in elderly patients with dementia. *Am J Gastroenterol.* 2000;95(1):133–136.

30. Alvarez-Fernández B, García-Ordoñez MA, Martínez-Manzanares C, Gómez-Huelgas R. Survival of a cohort of elderly patients with advanced dementia: nasogastric tube feeding as a risk factor for mortality. *Int J Geriatr Psychiatry.* 2005;20(4):363–370.

31. Higaki F, Yokota O, Ohishi M. Factors predictive of survival after percutaneous endoscopic gastrostomy in the elderly: is dementia really a risk factor? *Am J Gastroenterol.* 2008;103(4):1011–1016.

32. Gaines DI, Durkalski V, Patel A, DeLegge MH. Dementia and cognitive impairment are not associated with earlier mortality after percutaneous endoscopic gastrostomy. *JPEN-J Parenter Enteral Nutr.* 2008;33(1):62–66.

33. Engel SE, Kiely DK, Mitchell SL. Satisfaction with end-of-life care for nursing home residents with advanced dementia. *J Am Geriatr Soc.* 2006;54(10):1567–1572.

34. Finucane TE, Bynum JP. Use of tube feeding to prevent aspiration pneumonia. *Lancet.* 1996;348(9039):1421–1424.

35. Finucane TE, Christmas C, Travis K. Tube feeding in patients with advanced dementia: a review of the evidence. *JAMA.* 1999;282(14):1365–1370.

36. Peck A, Cohen CE, Mulvihill MN. Long-term enteral feeding of aged demented nursing home patients. *J Am Geriatr Soc.* 1990;38(11):1195–1198.

37. Hanson LC, Ersek M, Gilliam R, Carey TS. Oral feeding options for people with dementia: a systematic review. *J Am Geriatr Soc.* 2011;59(3):463–472.

38. Skelly RH. Are we using percutaneous endoscopic gastrostomy appropriately in the elderly? *Curr Opin Clin Nutr Metab Care.* 2002;5(1):35–42.

39. Miller RG, Jackson CE, Kasarskis EJ, et al. Practice parameter update: the care of the patient with amyotrophic lateral sclerosis—drug, nutritional, and respiratory therapies (an evidence-based review). Report of the Quality Standards Subcommittee of the American Academy of Neurology. *Neurology.* 2009;73(15):1218–1226.

40. Katzberg HD, Benatar M. Enteral tube feeding for amyotrophic lateral sclerosis/motor neuron disease. *Cochrane Database Syst Rev.* 2011;(1):CD004030.

41. Friedenberg F, Jensen G, Gujral N, Braitman LE, Levine GM. Serum albumin is predictive of 30-day survival after percutaneous endoscopic gastrostomy. *JPEN J Parenter Enteral Nutr.* 1997;21(2):72–74.

42. McCann RM, Hall WJ, Groth-Juncker A. Comfort care for terminally ill patients: the appropriate use of nutrition and hydration. *JAMA.* 1994;272(16):1263–1266.

43. Winter SM. Terminal nutrition: framing the debate for the withdrawal of nutritional support in terminally ill patients. *Am J Med.* 2000;109(9):723–726.

44. Palecek EJ, Teno JM, Casarett DJ, et al. Comfort feeding only: a proposal to bring clarity to decision-making regarding difficulty with eating for persons with advanced dementia. *J Am Geriatr Soc.* 2010;58(3):580–584.

45. Heuberger R. Artificial nutrition and hydration at the end of life. *J Nutr Elder.* 2010;29(4):347–385.

46. Sieger CE, Arnold JF, Ahronheim JC. Refusing artificial nutrition and hydration: does statutory law send the wrong message? *J Am Geriatr Soc.* 2002;50(3):544–550.

47. Casarett D, Kapo J, Caplan A. Appropriate use of artificial nutrition and hydration: fundamental principles and recommendations. *N Engl J Med.* 2005;353(24):2607–2612.

When Should Parenteral Feeding Be Considered for Patients With Cancer and for Patients With Non–Cancer-Related Conditions?

Thomas Reid and Steve Pantilat

INTRODUCTION AND SCOPE OF THE PROBLEM

Artificial nutrition and hydration given intravenously, termed parenteral nutrition (PN), can provide needed calories and nutrients for patients who are unable to eat. For patients with a functioning gut who need artificial nutrition and hydration, enteral nutrition (EN) is generally preferred (see Chapter 30).[1] When gut function is interrupted temporarily, PN can be lifesaving. Longer-term PN, most notably at home, is more controversial in the palliative care setting because it is associated with high rates of complications, high cost, and potentially reduced quality of life.

Parenteral Nutrition: What Is It and How Is It Done?

PN provides macronutrients and essential micronutrients directly into the venous system. The parenteral route may be used to provide all required nutrition, known as total parenteral nutrition (TPN), or to supplement oral or tube feeding. PN may be delivered through a peripheral or central intravenous catheter. Peripheral delivery can accommodate only lower osmolarity solutions (usually achieved with decreased dextrose concentrations), is shorter term (<2 weeks), and may not be feasible in patients with poor peripheral access, high nutritional requirements, or fluid restrictions.[2] For short-term to medium-term administration, a directly inserted central line or peripherally inserted central catheter (PICC) may be used. If PN is likely to be needed for months or longer, a tunneled line or subcutaneous infusion port is preferred to reduce the risk for infection.[3] PN formulas consist of dextrose, amino acids, electrolytes, and some vitamins and trace mineral supplements. Chloride and acetate are titrated to create a physiological pH level. Lipid emulsions are commonly provided in a separate delivery bag. As with all nutritional supplementation, analysis of needs and current intake determines the composition of the formula for a particular patient. When PN is started, it requires close clinical monitoring of electrolytes, blood glucose, and markers of nutritional status, such as prealbumin. With longer-term use, intermittent monitoring of trace elements (zinc, copper, selenium) and vitamins (B_{12}, folate, D) is also necessary.

Risks and Complications

Although no absolute contraindications to providing PN exist, the significant risks must be considered whenever it is started. The major risks in PN may be divided into three categories: mechanical, infective, and metabolic.[1-3] Mechanical risks are primarily those associated with placing an intravenous line, including bleeding, pneumothorax, misplacement, pain, air embolism, and arrhythmias. Once the line is in place, mechanical risks include thrombosis, line failure requiring replacement, phlebitis, and infiltration. The prevalence of most of these complications depends on the location of the line and the technique used to place it but generally are significant in only 1% to 4% of patients.

Despite recent advances in infection prevention, central venous catheters still carry a significant risk for infection, with resultant spread of organisms to the bloodstream and possible sepsis. Compared with those whose lines are used for other purposes, patients receiving PN are 4 times more likely (5 per 1000 catheter days) to develop line infections and are at particular risk for fungemia.[3] Mortality for each infection is high, estimated to be 12% to 25%. Finally, even with close monitoring, metabolic complications can occur, including hyperglycemia, liver function abnormalities, refeeding syndrome (hypophosphatemia, hypomagnesemia, and hypokalemia), steatosis, cholestasis, and cholecystitis (4% after 3 months). Long-term use over years is also associated with end-stage liver disease (approximately 50%) and metabolic bone disease (40%-100%).

RELEVANT PATHOPHYSIOLOGY

Cachexia

A 2007 consensus conference defined cachexia as "a complex metabolic syndrome associated with underlying illness and characterized by loss of muscle with or without loss of fat mass."[4] Cachexia is a pathological process and is distinct from starvation and age-related loss of muscle mass. Some definitions also exclude primary depression, malabsorption, and hyperthyroidism. Diseases that are commonly associated with cachexia include cancer (see later discussion); heart failure; chronic obstructive pulmonary disease (COPD); human immunodeficiency virus (HIV); malabsorptive diseases, including various forms of inflammatory bowel disease; chronic kidney disease; chronic infection; and sepsis.

Clinically, cachexia results in weight loss and may be associated with anorexia, inflammation, insulin resistance, and increased muscle protein breakdown. These factors often manifest as weakness and fatigue. To diagnose cachexia a patient should demonstrate either a body mass index less than 20 or weight loss of at least 5% over fewer than 12 months plus three of five additional criteria: decreased muscle strength, fatigue, anorexia, low fat-free mass index, and abnormal biochemistry (albumin <3.2, hemoglobin <12, C-reactive protein >5 mg/L). Of importance, because cachexia is a metabolic disorder, it usually does not respond to nutritional support.

Cancer and the Anorexia-Cachexia Syndrome

More than 80% of patients with advanced cancer develop cachexia, usually accompanied by anorexia, early satiety, anemia, and edema—often despite seemingly adequate nutritional intake.[5] Together, these symptoms are referred to as the cancer anorexia-cachexia syndrome (CACS). As with other forms of cachexia, the pathophysiology of this disorder is only partially understood but is probably related to complex host–cancer cytokine interactions that induce the body to favor catabolism over anabolism.

Key to any discussion of PN in CACS is the observation that nutritional support generally does not restore lean body mass because protein catabolism is rate-limiting. Studies of the potential for certain medications and nutritional supplements and formulas to reverse this process are ongoing.

SUMMARY OF EVIDENCE REGARDING TREATMENT RECOMMENDATIONS

Parenteral Versus Enteral Nutrition

In nearly all cases in which the gut is functional, EN is preferred over PN because it is more physiological, is associated with fewer complications, and costs much less. Physiologically, EN helps improve gut function and stimulate gut immunity, maintaining the mucosal barrier and gut-associated lymphoid tissue.[1] The higher rate of infections seen with PN is likely due in part to its immunosuppressive effect relative to EN. Data pertaining to particular diseases and settings are discussed in the following section.

Conditions Commonly Appropriate for Parenteral Nutrition

PN is generally considered when nutrition has been inadequate and oral or enteral feeding or supplementation efforts have either failed or are impractical. If the patient has a functioning gut, oral or enteral nutrition is nearly always preferred over PN. In the palliative care setting, PN is typically considered for patients with malignant bowel obstruction or head and neck cancer, but it may be requested in other situations. Of importance, PN does not have to be total and should usually be supplemented by and eventually replaced with EN as soon as possible.

Concern for Nonrecommended Use

Given the high cost and serious complications associated with PN, significant concern exists for its use outside of guidelines in the United States. The American Society for Parenteral and Enteral Nutrition (ASPEN) and the European Society for Clinical Nutrition and Metabolism (ESPEN) published evidence-based guidelines for the appropriate use of PN.[6–18] Even hospitals that have made previous efforts to control the ordering of inappropriate PN have recently been found to follow guidelines only 32% of the time.[1] Use of PN outside of guideline recommendations results in longer hospital stays and higher overall costs (approximately $4000 per patient) without changes in outcome.[1,19] In the United States, it is estimated that moving 10% of patients on PN to EN would save $92 million annually from reduced adverse events and shorter hospital stays. There is some evidence that using a specialized nutrition support team may reduce rates of inappropriate PN use.[1]

Guidelines for the Use of Parenteral Nutrition

Evidence for PN from the ASPEN and ESPEN guidelines is reviewed in the following section, supplemented by information from meta-analyses and randomized clinical trials published since the guidelines. Where research has explored the potential benefits of avoiding EN, comparisons with PN are discussed. Except as specified, all other sections assume that EN is not feasible and generally focus on when in an illness it is appropriate to begin PN. They also assume that PN is otherwise consistent with the patient's goals of care, which for permanent enteral failure—when PN itself becomes a life-sustaining intervention—is often the single most important consideration. In all cases, initiating PN use during a proinflammatory phase of illness (e.g., early in sepsis treatment) or when the patient is hemodynamically unstable is associated with increased risk for complications. This discussion is limited to the use of PN in the palliative care setting.

Palliative Care. A Cochrane review examining the effect of medically assisted nutrition on the length and quality of life of patients receiving primarily palliative care found no randomized clinical trials or prospective controlled trials and concluded that insufficient data were available to make recommendations.[20] Three less rigorous prospective studies included in the review that examined home PN, mostly in cancer patients, showed average survival of 3 to 4 months. No quantitative data on quality of life were available, but positive features of home PN identified in one qualitative study were assurance that nutrition needs were being met and a shift in the focus of eating from nutrition to comfort. Negative features were nausea, vomiting, drowsiness, headache, and restriction on family life and social involvement. Complications in this population were catheter sepsis (0.67 cases per year of treatment), deep vein thrombosis (0.16), and metabolic instability (0.50).

Cancer. As with other forms of nutrition support, although PN may stimulate tumor growth in many cancers, there is no evidence that this stimulation has any clinical effect.[16]

Nonsurgical Oncology. For short-term treatment of patients with cancer who have severe mucositis or severe radiation enteritis and cannot tolerate nasoenteric tubes, PN is generally accepted but not proved to be of benefit.[16,21] In patients who have undergone bone marrow transplant, routine PN is associated with increased infections and longer hospital stays.[21] Absent other indications for its use (e.g., gastrointestinal failure) PN is otherwise ineffective and probably harmful (increased morbidity and mortality) for most well-nourished patients with cancer, especially during chemotherapy or radiation. In the inpatient setting, PN is generally considered for malnourished patients with cancer who cannot tolerate EN, although no data support this practice.

For patients with incurable cancer and permanent gastrointestinal failure (e.g., malignant bowel obstruction) the benefit of PN depends almost entirely on their functional and nutritional status. If prognosis and quality of life are initially poor (terminal phase of disease) PN is unlikely to help. For patients with a good quality of life who are more likely to die of malnutrition than their disease (generally with prognoses greater than 2-3 months) and who cannot tolerate oral intake or EN, PN may be reasonable if it is otherwise consistent with their goals of care.[16] Retrospective data when these patients receive PN show a median survival of 6.5 months, suggesting a survival benefit

over the days to weeks expected without any supplementation or the 2 to 3 months likely with fluids alone and without additional nutrition.[22] Data examining the effect of PN on quality of life in these patients are generally mixed and largely retrospective. A less challenging and more cost-effective alternative for some of these patients may be intravenous fluids alone (see later discussion).

Although most data do not support PN for patients with a functioning gut, a single randomized clinical trial examining patients receiving noncurative chemotherapy for advanced colorectal cancer who were still able to eat did show positive results.[23] When these patients received supplemental PN in addition to baseline intense oral nutrition therapy they reported improved quality of life by week 18, decreased overall gastrointestinal symptoms, and increased survival (16.7 versus 10.2 months). EN supplementation was not studied, so it is unclear whether these results could be achieved less invasively.

Surgical Oncology. As with most other major surgeries, if EN is not feasible, PN starting a week preoperatively decreases complications and mortality in malnourished patients with cancer who are undergoing surgery.

Non–Cancer-Related Conditions

Liver Disease. Compared with EN, PN has been associated with increased infection rates and more metabolic complications in most liver diseases and after liver transplant.[24] Expert consensus is that long-term PN should generally be avoided because it may worsen existing cirrhosis and liver failure, promote cholestasis, and increase risks for sepsis, coagulopathy, and death.

Renal Failure. Guidelines diverge on the utility of PN given as a supplement during outpatient hemodialysis sessions (intradialytic PN or IDPN), with ASPEN opposing its use and ESPEN in favor of offering it if nutritional counseling and oral nutritional supplements are unsuccessful. Overall, IDPN does not appear to affect quality of life, although it may reduce hospitalizations, increase weight, and raise albumin levels.[10,15] Mortality data in retrospective studies are mixed. The sole randomized clinical trial performed to date showed no difference in 2-year mortality for patients receiving a year of IDPN in addition to oral nutritional supplements, although patients whose prealbumin rose more than 30 mg per liter over 3 months were 54% less likely to die in the same period.[25]

Heart and Lung Disease. No outcome data exist regarding the effect of PN on advanced cardiopulmonary diseases, although the volume load may be expected to worsen the condition of patients with heart failure.

HIV and AIDS. A Cochrane review showed that home TPN had no significant impact on overall survival or rate of rehospitalization for patients with advanced HIV or AIDS.[26]

Cognitive Impairment and Stroke. No data specifically address the use of PN in stroke, dementia, or other advanced cognitive impairment. Although data do not support the use of EN in dementia and cognitive impairment, appropriate patients with stroke who are dysphagic may benefit from EN. Given the additional burdens and costs associated with PN, it seems reasonable to conclude that it is unlikely to be of benefit in the former group.

Important Considerations

Hunger and Starvation. The common and quite significant concern of patients, surrogates, and family members that a patient who is not eating or receiving nutrition will be hungry or "starve to death" is discussed in detail in Chapter 30. Although it is not possible to know whether severely cognitively impaired patients suffer because of their decreased intake at the end of life, the available evidence suggests that they do not and may even be more comfortable without artificial nutrition and hydration.

Weaning From Parenteral Nutrition. Abrupt discontinuation of PN (as opposed to tapering) does not seem to produce clinically significant hypoglycemia.[12]

Alternatives to Parenteral Nutrition When Enteral Nutrition Is Not Feasible. Patients may survive for weeks to months without nutrition; however, without fluid intake they will generally die within weeks. When EN is not feasible, artificial hydration alone may be a reasonable alternative to PN in patients with otherwise good quality of life and prognoses limited by their disease rather than their nutritional status (generally <2-3 months). Hydration may be delivered intravenously, subcutaneously (hypodermoclysis), or per rectum (proctoclysis).[27] Insufficient data are available to directly evaluate the mortality and quality of life effects of these interventions. For patients with prognoses of days to weeks, the burdens of artificial hydration (especially with dextrose-containing fluids, which may reverse the palliative effects of ketosis) are similar to those of PN (e.g., increased secretions, urination, bladder distension, third spacing) and usually outweigh any potential benefits.[28]

Legal and Ethical Issues. The important legal, ethical, religious, cultural, linguistic, and psychological factors that often have a strong impact on the decision to use, withhold, or withdraw PN are generally very similar to those for EN. The chief difference is that, consciously or unconsciously, patients, families, and providers tend to view PN as more obviously a medical intervention ("unnatural") than gastrostomy with EN. As a result, decisions to withhold or withdraw PN may be less controversial.

KEY MESSAGES TO PATIENTS AND FAMILIES

All potentially difficult conversations with patients and families benefit from excellent communication skills and careful family meeting structure. The specific issues and phrasing to consider when discussing PN for patients with advanced disease are similar to those for gastrostomy (see Chapter 30).

Emphasize Artificiality

Although medical terminology usually impedes communication with patients and families, PN may be an exception. Use the phrases "artificial nutrition" or "nutrition by vein" instead of "eating" or "feeding" to emphasize that PN is a medical intervention that is qualitatively different from the familiar act of eating.

Provide Information

Provide as much data as the patient or family is willing to hear. Where relevant to the disease process or stage of illness, explain how the body may not benefit from (or may even be harmed by) PN and discuss CACS. Encourage decision-makers to consider the burden of laboratory testing and the psychosocial impact of limitations imposed by the duration of daily therapy and the need to protect the catheter, such as decreased mobility, social activity, and physical intimacy.

Anticipate and Explore Assumptions About Eating and Food

If not made explicit, emotional, psychological, and cultural assumptions will still drive decision-making, can impede communication, and may evoke defensiveness if the patient or family is inadvertently challenged. Ask about the meanings of food, eating, and other important related topics, such as hunger and starvation early in any conversation about PN.

Avoid "Care" Versus "No Care"

A narrow focus on the procedure may be perceived by patients and families as a stark choice between "feeding" and "not feeding" or more profoundly between "care" and "no care." This dynamic can be prevented in several ways. First, always discuss artificial nutrition as one of several options. Second, if issues of duty or demonstrating caring are paramount, validate the emotions a family is feeling and the sacrifices they have already made in the care of their loved one. In addition, it may be helpful to discuss other ways to show love or fulfill responsibility. Finally, focus on what *will* be done, rather than what will *not* be done. A detailed description of palliative measures and ways that a family can stay involved may help the family and the patient feel confident that the family will still be able to care for their loved one without PN.

Discuss Direct Requests for Parenteral Nutrition

Help families to place direct requests for PN in the broader context of artificial nutrition and hydration as it relates to a patient's goals of care. As in other circumstances, if artificial nutrition and hydration seems reasonable for a patient with advanced illness, the least burdensome delivery method is the one the clinician should offer. PN would be indicated only if EN were indicated but not feasible.

Set Limits at the Outset (Time-Limited Trials)

PN may be started when clinical outcomes are uncertain and its benefits are unclear, yet once started it may be psychologically, socially, or legally difficult to withdraw. When patients or families choose PN under such circumstances, it may be helpful to propose a time-limited trial. Discuss a timeframe after which the patient and/or surrogate will reassess whether PN is meeting the goals and expectations (benefits and risks). Depending on the likelihood of success, present this date as a default stopping point or an opportunity to reevaluate. If possible, try to make explicit the conditions under which they would want to stop PN.

CONCLUSION AND SUMMARY

Although clinicians, patients, and families often hope that PN may extend and improve life when EN is not feasible, in the palliative care setting this is probably only true when quality of life is already adequate and prognosis is limited by nutritional deficiency rather than underlying disease. The increased cost, complications, and immunosuppression associated with PN compared with EN mean that if artificial nutrition and hydration is indicated, the enteral route should always be used if possible. As with all forms of nutrition support, the catabolic state resulting from CACS that affects up to 80% of cancer patients means that PN has no role in the care of patients with advanced cancer who are losing weight. In the last weeks and months of life, careful and compassionate communication about artifical nutrition and hydration that acknowledges both the emotional and cultural significance of food and the absence of data supporting a beneficial effect from PN can lead to better decisions.

SUMMARY RECOMMENDATIONS

- In all cases, PN should be used only when EN is not feasible.
- Cachexia at the end of life is a natural process that is not reversed by providing artificial nutrition and hydration as either PN or EN.
- In the palliative care setting, long-term use of PN should be considered only in patients with good functional status who have a prognosis longer than 2 to 3 months and in whom EN is not feasible.
- Consider intravenous hydration as an alternative to PN in patients with limited prognosis who are unable to take fluids by mouth or tube, but who otherwise have a prognosis of weeks to months.
- PN should not be given routinely during cancer treatment, but may be helpful in patients experiencing severe treatment-related mucositis or enteritis in whom oral or enteral nutrition is not possible.
- Consider proposing a time-limited trial if a patient or surrogate requests PN when its benefits are uncertain.

REFERENCES

1. Martin K, DeLegge M, Nichols M, et al. Assessing appropriate parenteral nutrition ordering practices in tertiary care medical centers. *JPEN J Parenter Enteral Nutr.* 2011;35(1):122–130.
2. Ghosh D, Neild P. Parenteral nutrition. *Clin Med.* 2010;10(6): 620–623.
3. Kulick D, Deen D. Specialized nutrition support. *Am Fam Physician.* 2011;83(2):173–183.
4. Evans WJ, Morley JE, Argilés J, et al. Cachexia: a new definition. *Clin Nutr.* 2008;27(6):793–799.
5. Bennani-Baiti N, Davis MP. Cytokines and cancer anorexia cachexia syndrome. *Am J Hosp Palliat Med.* 2008;25(5):407–411.
6. McClave SA, Martindale RG, Vanek VW, et al. Guidelines for the provision and assessment of nutrition support therapy in the adult critically ill patient: Society of Critical Care Medicine (SCCM) and American Society for Parenteral and Enteral Nutrition (A.S.P.E.N.). *JPEN-Parenter Enter.* 2009;33(3):277–316.
7. Staun M, Pironi L, Bozzetti F, et al. ESPEN guidelines on parenteral nutrition: home parenteral nutrition (HPN) in adult patients. *Clin Nutr.* 2009;28(4):467–479.
8. Gianotti L, Meier R, Lobo DN, et al. ESPEN guidelines on parenteral nutrition: pancreas. *Clin Nutr.* 2009;28(4):428–435.
9. Singer P, Berger MM, Van den Berghe G, et al. ESPEN guidelines on parenteral nutrition: intensive care. *Clin Nutr.* 2009;28(4):387–400.
10. Brown RO, Compher C, American Society for Parenteral and Enteral Nutrition Board of Directors. A.S.P.E.N. clinical guidelines: nutrition support in adult acute and chronic renal failure. *JPEN J Parenter Enteral Nutr.* 2010;34(4):366–377.
11. August DA, Huhmann MB, American Society for Parenteral and Enteral Nutrition (A.S.P.E.N.) Board of Directors. A.S.P.E.N. clinical guidelines: nutrition support therapy during adult anticancer treatment and in hematopoietic cell transplantation. the *JPEN J Parenter Enteral Nutr.* 2009;33(5):472–500.
12. Braga M, Ljungqvist O, Soeters P, et al. ESPEN guidelines on parenteral nutrition: surgery. *Clin Nutr* 2009;28(4):378–386.
13. Van Gossum A, Cabre E, Hébuterne X, et al. ESPEN Guidelines on Parenteral Nutrition: gastroenterology. *Clin Nutr.* 2009; 28(4):415–427.
14. Plauth M, Cabre E, Campillo B, et al. ESPEN guidelines on parenteral nutrition: hepatology. *Clin Nutr.* 2009;28(4):436–444.
15. Cano NJM, Aparicio M, Brunori G, et al. ESPEN guidelines on parenteral nutrition: adult renal failure. *Clin Nutr.* 2009;28(4):401–414.
16. Bozzetti F, Arends J, Lundholm K, et al. ESPEN guidelines on parenteral nutrition: non-surgical oncology. *Clin Nutr.* 2009;28(4):445–454.
17. Anker SD, Laviano A, Filippatos G, et al. ESPEN guidelines on parenteral nutrition: on cardiology and pneumology. *Clin Nutr.* 2009;28(4):455–460.
18. Sobotka L, Schneider SM, Berner YN, et al. ESPEN guidelines on parenteral nutrition: geriatrics. *Clin Nutr.* 2009;28(4):461–466.
19. Cangelosi MJ, Auerbach HR, Cohen JT. A clinical and economic evaluation of enteral nutrition. *Curr Med Res Opin.* 2011;27(2):413–422.
20. Good P, Cavenagh J, Mather M, Ravenscroft P. Medically assisted nutrition for palliative care in adult patients. *Cochrane Database Syst Rev,* 2008;(4):CD006274.
21. Murray SM, Pindoria S. Nutrition support for bone marrow transplant patients. *Cochrane Database Syst Rev.* 2009;(1):CD002920.
22. Fan B-G. Parenteral nutrition prolongs the survival of patients associated with malignant gastrointestinal obstruction. *JPEN J Parenter Enteral Nutr.* 2007;31(6):508–510.
23. Hasenberg T, Essenbreis M, Herold A, Post S, Shang E. Early supplementation of parenteral nutrition is capable of improving quality of life, chemotherapy-related toxicity and body composition in patients with advanced colorectal carcinoma undergoing palliative treatment: results from a prospective, randomized clinical trial. *Colorectal Dis.* 2010;12(10 online):e190–e199.
24. McClave SA, Martindale RG, Vanek VW, et al. Guidelines for the provision and assessment of nutrition support therapy in the adult critically ill patient: Society of Critical Care Medicine (SCCM) and American Society for Parenteral and Enteral Nutrition (A.S.P.E.N.). *JPEN J Parenter Enteral Nutr.* 2009;33(3):277–316.

25. Cano NJM, Fouque D, Roth H, et al. Intradialytic parenteral nutrition does not improve survival in malnourished hemodialysis patients: a 2-year multicenter, prospective, randomized study. *J Am Soc Nephrol.* 2007;18(9):2583–2591.
26. Young T, Busgeeth K. Home-based care for reducing morbidity and mortality in people infected with HIV/AIDS. *Cochrane Database Syst Rev.* 2010;(1):CD005417.
27. Steiner N. Methods of hydration in palliative care patients. *J Palliat Care.* 1998;14(2):6–13.
28. A.S.P.E.N. Ethics Position Paper Task Force, Barrocas A, Geppert C, et al. A.S.P.E.N. ethics position paper. *Nutr Clin Pract.* 2010;25(6):672–679.

PSYCHIATRIC SYMPTOMS

Chapter 32

How Does One Assess for Psychiatric Illness in Patients With Advanced Disease?

KIMBERLY G. KLIPSTEIN AND DEBORAH B. MARIN

INTRODUCTION AND SCOPE OF THE PROBLEM

Depression and anxiety, frequent illnesses in their own right, are even more common in patients with serious illness. The Epidemiologic Catchment Area Study found the lifetime prevalence of mood disorders to be 12.9% in medically ill patients compared to 8.9% in healthy aged-matched controls.[1] Additionally, it has been shown that patients with a greater number of comorbid medical illnesses[2] and those with a greater severity of medical illness[3] have even higher rates of depressive disorders. Rates also increase with the acuity of the medical illness, with depression in primary care settings ranging from 5% to 10% compared to 15% to 30% in hospital settings.[4]

Anxiety disorders show a similar association. The lifetime prevalence of any anxiety disorder is 11.9% among persons with comorbid medical illness compared to 6% in those without such comorbidity.[1] Associations with specific medical illnesses have also been found—stroke, Parkinson disease, multiple sclerosis,[5] cancer, diabetes, and myocardial infarction show a particularly high comorbidity with depressive disorders,[6] whereas arthritis, diabetes, chronic lung disease, and heart disease show a particularly high comorbidity with anxiety disorders.[7]

Although much debate exists as to how to properly diagnose depression and anxiety in the setting of serious illness, there is no doubt that psychiatric illness is underdiagnosed and undertreated in this patient population. Furthermore, it is clear that this lack of recognition and lack of treatment often leads to negative outcomes, including increased health care utilization,[8] poor quality of life, increased interference with medical treatment, poor medical compliance, and increased morbidity and mortality in a variety of disease states.[9]

RELEVANT DIAGNOSTIC PARADIGMS

In the absence of clear-cut biological markers, diagnosing psychiatric illness can be difficult. Psychiatric diagnosis is clinical and based solely on descriptive symptom clusters or criteria found in the *Diagnostic and Statistical Manual of Mental Disorders,* Fourth Edition (DSM-IV). Common psychiatric disorders seen in patients with serious illness include major depressive disorder (MDD), generalized anxiety disorder (GAD), and the adjustment disorders.[10] DSM-IV diagnostic criteria for MDD and GAD can be found in Tables 32-1 and 32-2, respectively. Two important principles to keep in mind when diagnosing psychiatric illness is that (1) the symptoms must cause significant distress or social and occupational dysfunction to qualify as a disorder and (2) all primary psychiatric illnesses are diagnoses of exclusion. This means that all other possible causes of the symptoms at hand must be ruled out before a patient can be diagnosed with a primary psychiatric diagnosis. For example, if there is evidence from the history, physical examination or laboratory findings that the symptoms are a direct physiological result of a general medical condition, a diagnosis of GAD or MDD is not given and instead patients are said to have either an anxiety disorder or a depressive disorder secondary to a general medical condition.[11] This is an important distinction because it is often the case that treating the underlying medical condition, as opposed to treating the psychiatric symptoms with psychiatric agents, leads to resolution of symptoms. A good example of this is a patient with hypothyroidism who experiences depressive symptoms. Antidepressants may not help the condition, but thyroid supplementation often resolves the depressive symptomatology completely.

Adjustment disorders, common in the medically ill, are considered subthreshold diagnoses whose essential feature is "the development of clinically significant emotional or behavioral symptoms in response to an identifiable stressor or stressors"[12] (Table 32-3). Anxiety and depressive symptoms in medically ill patients that do not meet the full criteria for GAD or MDD and that do not directly result from the physiological effects of a medical condition or a substance may fall into the category of adjustment disorder, with the medical illness acting as the stressor. These

TABLE 32-1. Diagnostic Criteria for Major Depressive Episode

A. Five (or more) of the following symptoms have been present for at least 2 weeks; at least one of the symptoms is either (1) depressed mood or (2) loss of interest or pleasure:
   1. Depressed mood most of the day, nearly every day, as indicated by either subjective report or observation by others
   2. Markedly diminished interest or pleasure in activities
   3. Significant weight loss or weight gain or decrease or increase in appetite nearly every day
   4. Insomnia or hypersomnia
   5. Psychomotor agitation or retardation as observed by others
   6. Fatigue or loss of energy
   7. Feelings of worthlessness or excessive or inappropriate guilt
   8. Difficulty concentrating or indecisiveness
   9. Recurrent thoughts of death, recurrent suicidal ideation without a specific plan, or a suicide attempt or a specific plan for committing suicide
B. The symptoms do not meet criteria for a Mixed Episode (i.e., an episode in which the patient has elements of both depression and mania).
C. The symptoms cause clinically significant distress or impairment in social, occupational, or other important areas of functioning.
D. The symptoms are not due to the direct physiological effects of a substance or a general medical condition
E. The symptoms are not better accounted for by bereavement (i.e., after the loss of a loved one); the symptoms persist for longer than 2 months or are characterized by marked functional impairment, morbid preoccupation with worthlessness, suicidal ideation, psychotic symptoms, or psychomotor retardation.

From American Psychiatric Association. *Diagnostic and Statistical Manual of Mental Disorders*. 4th ed. Text revision. Washington, DC: American Psychiatric Association; 2000:356.

TABLE 32-2. Diagnostic Criteria for Generalized Anxiety Disorder

A. At least 6 months of "excessive anxiety and worry," occurring more days than not, about a variety of events and situations in one's life.
B. The person has difficulty controlling the anxiety and worry.
C. The anxiety and worry are associated with three or more of the following symptoms:
   1. Feeling restless, keyed up, or on edge
   2. Easily fatigued
   3. Concentration problems
   4. Irritability
   5. Muscle tension
   6. Difficulty falling or staying asleep or restless sleep
D. The symptoms are not part of another mental disorder.
E. The symptoms cause "clinically significant distress" or impairment in social, occupational, or other important areas of functioning in daily life.
F. The condition is not due to the direct physiological effects of a substance or a general medical condition.

From American Psychiatric Association. *Diagnostic and Statistical Manual of Mental Disorders*. 4th ed. Text revision. Washington, DC: American Psychiatric Association; 2000:476.

TABLE 32-3. Diagnostic Criteria for Adjustment Disorder

A. The development of emotional or behavioral symptoms in response to an identifiable stressor(s) occurring within 3 months of the onset of the stressor(s).
B. These symptoms or behaviors are clinically significant as evidenced by either of the following:
   1. Marked distress that is in excess of what would be expected from exposure to the stressor
   2. Significant impairment in social or occupational functioning
C. The stress-related disturbance does not meet the criteria for another specific mental disorder.
D. The symptoms do not represent bereavement.
E. Once the stressor (or its consequences) has terminated, the symptoms do not persist for more than an additional 6 months.

Specify if:
Acute: If the disturbance lasts less than 6 months
Chronic: If the disturbance lasts for 6 months or longer

With Depressed Mood
With Anxiety
With Mixed Anxiety and Depressed Mood
With Disturbance of Conduct
With Mixed Disturbance of Emotions and Conduct
Unspecified

From American Psychiatric Association. *Diagnostic and Statistical Manual of Mental Disorders*. 4th ed. Text revision. Washington, DC: American Psychiatric Association; 2000:683.

DIAGNOSTIC CHALLENGES

Diagnosing psychiatric disorders in medically ill populations is challenging for several reasons. First, many of the symptoms of depression and anxiety overlap with those of advanced medical illness. For example, the neurovegetative criteria for MDD, including weight loss, changes in sleep, fatigue, and loss of energy, can all be direct manifestations of physical disease. Likewise, autonomic hyperactivity and vegetative symptoms often seen in anxiety disorders can occur as a direct result of a medical illness.[13] Therefore basing the diagnosis of depression or anxiety on these symptoms can lead to false positive diagnoses. An example of this is a patient with gastric cancer who demonstrates early satiety, poor appetite, fatigue, and low energy. A novice clinician might mistakenly attribute this to depression and start an antidepressant without further medical workup, when in reality the symptoms are more likely due to the cancer itself.

Complicating this matter further is the fact that depression and anxiety disorders themselves have associated somatic symptomatology, even in patients without medical illness. "Masked depression" is a historical term used to describe depression and anxiety symptoms that manifest primarily in the form of physical complaints as opposed to psychological distress. Many patients visit their primary care physicians with somatic symptoms, both physical and psychological in origin, making accurate diagnosis extremely difficult.[14]

Another challenge in assessing psychiatric illness in medically ill populations is that the boundary between sadness and a psychiatric disorder is

disorders tend to be self-limited and do not last longer than 6 months after the stressor has terminated. However, if the stressor persists beyond 6 months, as is often the case in serious illness, the disorders can become chronic.

often hard to distinguish. Nonpsychiatric physicians, patients, and families alike often view depression or anxiety in the setting of a serious medical illness as a "typical emotional response" as opposed to a disease state. In such circumstances, clinicians may miss the opportunity to treat significant psychiatric morbidity and alleviate suffering. Conversely, sadness, depressed mood, crying, nervousness, and even passive suicidal ideation can be normal psychological reactions to a serious medical illness and thus may not constitute a clinical psychiatric disorder requiring intervention. The symptom of passive suicidal ideation is a good example of this dilemma; in some circumstances, it is not clear whether suicidal ideation in an individual near the end of life is a symptom of depression or a rational wish to escape pain and suffering.[15] Jones and colleagues[16] found that the desire for hastened death occurred in up to 4% of hospitalized cancer patients and that in those patients with more advanced disease, this wish was not always accompanied by depression. This suggests that passive suicidal ideation in the severely medically ill may not be a reliable criterion on which to base a diagnosis of depression.

Anhedonia, the absence of interest and pleasure in activities and a characteristic symptom of depression, may not be a useful criterion for diagnosing depression in those with serious medical illness either. Advanced medical illness alone can lead to malaise, pain, and physical disability that would make participating in pleasurable activities unenjoyable. Therefore a lack of involvement in social or pleasurable activities that is out of proportion to physical disability is a better indicator of depression in these patients.[17]

DIAGNOSING DEPRESSION AND ANXIETY IN THE SERIOUSLY MEDICALLY ILL

When assessing for psychiatric illness in medical patient populations, it is essential to consider the differential diagnosis and to rule out other possible causes of the symptoms before arriving at a formal psychiatric diagnosis. Organic causes, including the direct effects of a medical illness or a side effect of a medication implicated in causing psychiatric symptoms, must first be ruled out. Vitamin deficiencies, electrolyte disturbances, illicit substance use, and neurological conditions such as seizures, dementia, and delirium should also be considered.

Many diagnostic schemes have been proposed to find more reliable criteria for diagnosing depression and anxiety in the seriously medically ill, although none have been routinely adopted in clinical practice. Approaches may be "exclusive" in nature, attempting to exclude symptoms that overlap with physical illness such as fatigue or weight loss.[18] This approach has been found useful in research studies because it has a high degree of specificity but appears to be less useful clinically. Substitutive approaches, in which neurovegetative symptoms are substituted

for cognitive symptoms such as irritability, tearfulness, or social withdrawal, are favored by some clinicians.[19] Clark and colleagues[20] showed that somatic symptoms were unhelpful in diagnosing depression in medically ill patients and suggested instead a focus on cognitive symptoms such as loss of interest, sense of failure, sense of punishment, and suicidal ideation. In a more recent study, demoralization as defined by feelings of hopelessness, helplessness, and despair was found to be a good predictor of MDD in medically ill patients.[21] Similarly, McKenzie and associates[22] found that pessimism may be a good indicator of depressive disorders in patients with advanced medical illness.

A more inclusive approach to psychiatric diagnosis, in which all symptoms in the DSM are included regardless of whether they overlap with symptoms of medical illness, appears to be the approach used most widely in routine clinical care. Many clinicians prefer this approach, believing that the risk for overdiagnosis of depression or anxiety in the medically ill is small and that the benefits of psychiatric treatment far outweigh the risks associated with failure to treat.[23] Finally, simple history taking to assess for a personal or family history of psychiatric illness can greatly assist in making a correct diagnosis in this patient population, given that psychiatric illnesses tend to be recurrent and often have genetic underpinnings. In cases in which diagnostic challenges remain, treatment trials of psychotropic medications may be indicated.

Many screening instruments have been proposed and used to help with psychiatric diagnoses in this patient population. The instruments that have been validated and used most often in the medically ill are the Center for Epidemiological Studies of Depression (CES-D) scale, which assesses only for depression, and the Hospital Anxiety and Depression Scale (HADS) and the Patient Health Questionnaire (PHQ-9), which evaluate for both depression and anxiety.[18] Although these instruments have been shown to improve detection of psychiatric illness in the medically ill, they have not necessarily led to better management of symptoms or improved patient outcomes over time.[24] Patients with significant medical illness, pain, and fatigue, as well as those facing death, may also find the screening instruments burdensome or unempathic. Furthermore, hidden costs of screening have been shown to negatively affect both patient outcomes and health care delivery systems.[25] Despite these drawbacks, however, the judicial use of screening instruments in this patient population has a role in assessment of complicated cases.

KEY MESSAGES TO PATIENTS AND FAMILIES

The palliative care clinician can help patients and families understand that there is a natural coping reaction associated with the diagnosis of serious illness and that many symptoms that they may be experiencing are in fact normal. On the other hand, it is important to explain to patients that debilitating symptoms of depression and anxiety may signify a more serious psychiatric illness that requires evaluation and treatment. Furthermore, treatment of these symptoms may improve their quality of life regardless of the course of their underlying medical illness. To be able to properly assess and treat psychiatric illness in this population, clinicians should strive to create an environment in which patients can feel comfortable talking openly and honestly about their feelings and symptoms, even if this includes thoughts of suicide.

CONCLUSION AND SUMMARY

Depression and anxiety are common psychiatric afflictions seen in high rates in medically ill populations with far-reaching consequences, including increased morbidity and mortality in medically ill patients. Unfortunately, both illnesses are underrecognized and undertreated in the advanced medically ill. Psychiatric illness in general is difficult to diagnose given a lack of biological markers and a reliance on the DSM-IV, which categorizes illnesses based on patterns of manifest symptoms, observed by the clinician or reported by the patient, that tend to cluster. In patients with chronic medical illness, psychiatric diagnosis is even more challenging because of the overlap of many neurovegetative symptoms with symptoms of physical disease. Some clinicians rely less on somatic symptoms and more on cognitive symptoms in making a diagnosis of depression or anxiety in this patient population, whereas others take a more inclusive approach, counting all possible symptoms as criteria for a depressive or anxiety disorder, even if they might be caused directly by the physical illness. This latter approach may cause more false positive psychiatric diagnoses but avoids possible undertreatment of depression and anxiety in the medically ill. Screening instruments may be useful aids in this patient population; however, negative patient attitudes toward these instruments, poor outcome data, and hidden costs may deter their use in routine clinical care.

SUMMARY RECOMMENDATIONS

- Given the high prevalence and undertreatment rates of depression and anxiety in patients with advanced illness, clinicians should screen all patients for these psychiatric disorders.
- Because symptoms of anxiety and depression may overlap with those of advanced disease, clinicians should carefully distinguish between psychiatric illness and those features related to the underlying disease.
- Psychiatric diagnoses are always diagnoses of exclusion; clinicians must first exclude organic causes of these symptoms.

- Depression and anxiety are never "normal" in advanced illness, and palliative care clinicians must strive to make sure that patients, families, and other clinicians understand that this is a medical illness that should be treated to improve symptoms and quality of life.
- Because these disorders may be difficult to treat in the setting of serious illness, clinicians may consider using screening instruments. However, inherent limitations in these instruments hinder their use.

REFERENCES

1. Wells KB, Golding JM, Burnam MA. Psychiatric disorder in a sample of the general population with and without chronic medical conditions. *Am J Psychiatry.* 1988;145:976–981.
2. Kessler RC, Zhao S, Blazer DG, et al. Prevalence, correlates and course of minor depression and major depression in the national comorbidity survey. *J Affect Disord.* 1997;45(1):19–30.
3. Casem EH. Depression and anxiety secondary to medical illness. *Psychiatr Clin North Am.* 1990;13:597–612.
4. Katon W, Sullivan M. Depression and chronic medical illness. *J Clin Psychiatry.* 1990;51(suppl 6):3–11.
5. Suh Y, Weikert M, Dlugonski D, et al. Physical activity, social support, and depression: possible independent and indirect associations in persons with multiple sclerosis. *Psychol Health Med.* 2012;17(2):196–206.
6. Sutor B, Rummans TA, Jowsey SG, et al. Major depression in medically ill patients. *Mayo Clin Proc.* 1998;73(4):329–337.
7. Wells KB, Golding JM, Burnam MA. Chronic medical conditions in a sample of the general population with anxiety, affective, substance use disorders. *Am J Psychiatry.* 1989; 146:1440–1446.
8. Simon GE, Ormel J, BonKorff M, et al. Health care costs associated with depressive and anxiety disorders in primary care. *Am J Psychiatry.* 1995;152:352–357.
9. Schulz R, Beach S, Ives D, et al. Association between depression and mortality in older adults: the Cardiovascular Health Study. *Arch Intern Med.* 2000;160:1761–1768.
10. Sartorius N, Ustun TB, Lecrubier Y, et al. Depression comorbid with anxiety: results from the WHO study on psychological disorders in primary health care. *Br J Psychiatry.* 1996;168 (suppl 30):38–43.
11. American Psychiatric Association. *Diagnostic and statistical manual of mental disorders.* 4th ed. Text revision. Washington, DC: American Psychiatric Association; 2000:683.
12. American Psychiatric Association. *Diagnostic and statistical manual of mental disorders.* 4th ed. Text revision. Washington, DC: American Psychiatric Association; 2000.
13. Noyes R, Carney C. Anxiety. In: Blumenfeld M, Strain JJ, eds. *Psychosomatic Medicine.* Philadelphia: Lippincott Williams and Wilkins; 2006:411–432.
14. Kroenke K. Patients presenting with somatic complaints: epidemiology, psychiatric comorbidity and management. *Int J Methods Psychiatr Res.* 2003;12(1):34–43.
15. Rodin G, Nolan R, Katz M. Depression. In: Levenson J, ed. *Textbook of Psychosomatic Medicine.* Richmond, VA: American Psychiatric Publishing; 2005:193–217.
16. Jones JM, Huggins MA, Tydall AC, et al. Symptomatic distress, hopelessness, and the desire for hastened death in hospitalized cancer patients. *J Psychosom Res.* 2003;55:411–418.
17. Rodin G, Nolan R, Katz M. Depression. In: Levenson J, ed. *Textbook of Psychosomatic Medicine.* Richmond, VA: American Psychiatric Publishing; 2005:193–217.
18. Cohen-Cole, Brown FW, McDaniel JS. Assessment of depression and grief reactions in the medically ill. In: Stoudemire A, Fogel BS, eds. *Psychiatric Care of the Medical Patient.* New York: Oxford University Press; 1993:53–69.
19. Cavanaugh S, Clark DC, Gibbons RD. Diagnosing depression in the hospitalized medically ill. *Psychosomatics.* 1983;24:809–815.

20. Clark DC, vonAmmon Cavanaugh S, Gibbons RD. The core symptoms of depression in the medically ill: a comparison of self-report measures, clinician judgment, and DSM-IV diagnosis. *J Nerv Men Dis*. 1983;171(12):705–713.

21. Clark DM, Smith GC, Dowe DL, et al. An empirically-derived taxonomy of common distress syndromes in the medical ill. *J Psychosom Res*. 2003;54:323–330.

22. McKenzie DP, Clarke DM, Forbes AB, et al. Pessimism, worthlessness, anhedonia, and thoughts of death identify DSM-IV major depression in hospitalized, medically ill patients. *Psychosomatics*. 2010;51:302–311.

23. Kathol RG, Mutgi A, Williams J, et al. Diagnosis of major depression in cancer patients according to four sets of criteria. *Am J Psychiatry*. 1990;147(8):1021–1024.

24. Schade CP, Jones Jr ER, Wittlin BJ. A ten-year review of the validity and clinical utility of depression screening. *Psychiatr Serv*. 1998;49:55–61.

25. Palmer SC, Coyne JC. Screening for depression in medical care: pitfalls, alternatives, and revised priorities. *J Psychosom Res*. 2003;54(4):279–287.

Chapter 33

What Treatments Are Effective for Depression in the Palliative Care Setting?

Scott A. Irwin and Susan Block

INTRODUCTION AND SCOPE OF THE PROBLEM

Depression is a profoundly distressing emotional experience for both patients and family members. Especially in the setting of serious illness, depression is amplified by physical symptoms, fear of dying, family distress, and grief. It has effects not just on the patient but also on the entire family, both in real time and during bereavement. Depression impairs the patient's ability to enjoy life, interferes with connection, is associated with feelings of emptiness and meaninglessness, and causes anguish to family and friends.[1] In addition, depression is associated with decreased adherence to treatment, prolonged hospital stays, and reduced quality of life.[2,3] It is a major risk factor for suicide and for requests to hasten death[4] and influences will-to-live in patients with cancer who are receiving palliative care.[5] It also has been increasingly recognized as a powerful factor in affecting survival in several cancers.[6-8] A meta-analysis examined both mortality and disease progression in patients with cancer, finding that patients with minor or major depression are at 39% higher risk for death and patients with depressive symptoms were at a 26% higher risk than patients without, even after adjusting for a variety of prognostic factors, suggesting that depression may be an independent risk factor for mortality in patients with cancer.[9] Thus appropriate treatment of patients with depression and advanced disease is a critical function of the palliative care clinician.

RELEVANT PATHOPHYSIOLOGY

Possible Mechanisms

Illness-related stresses induce chronic activation of the hypothalamic pituitary axis (HPA), which is thought to be a possible mediator that explains the effects of depression on cancer progression. In turn, activation of the HPA axis is thought to modulate immune function, which protects the "host" against tumor growth. HPA dysfunction associated with depression is also associated with activation of cytokines; immune regulatory substances, such as interleukin 1 and 2; and tumor necrosis factor alpha, which are thought to increase depression and other sickness-related symptoms (e.g., fatigue, sleep disorder). HPA dysfunction also can increase cellular inflammatory activity, growth-enhancing cytokines, and angiogenic factors that promote tumor growth. Other biological factors that may play a role in the effects of depression on cancer include hormonal and autonomic dysregulation.[10,11]

Prevalence, Types, and Theories About Depression in Advanced Illness

Psychological distress is a major cause of suffering among patients with advanced, life-threatening illness and is highly associated with decreased quality of life. More than 60% of patients with cancer report experiencing distress. Understanding the causes of this normative distress associated with illness and differentiating it from distress associated with psychiatric disorders requires an appreciation of the clinical characteristics and prevalence of psychiatric disorders. Failure to differentiate between these types of distress may result in clinicians ignoring a critically serious psychiatric disorder that can erode physical, psychological, social, and spiritual well-being.

Depression in Cancer Diagnoses. Prevalence rates of depression in patients with cancer range widely, depending on diagnostic criteria used and patient population studied. Symptoms of depression have been reported in up to 58% of patients with cancer. Rates of major depression range as high as 38% among these patients.[12-15] The wide variability in reported rates is explained by the lack of agreement on appropriate criteria for diagnosis of depression, differences in patient populations (in relation to both disease and staging), and variation in assessment methods used. Studies using structured psychiatric interviews suggest prevalence ranges of 5% to 26% for major depression, and recent reviews suggest that the median prevalence of major depression in patients with "advanced disease" is approximately 15%.[13,16,17] Research by Derogatis and colleagues[18] showed that 47% of patients with cancer (all types, all stages) fulfilled diagnostic criteria for a psychiatric disorder. Of that 47%, 68% had adjustment disorders with depressed or anxious mood, 13% had major depression, and 8% had organic mental disorders. Akechi and colleagues,[19] in a prospective study in a Japanese palliative care setting, found that, using the Structured Clinical Interview for *Diagnostic and Statistical Manual of Mental Disorders* (DSM), 16% of patients had adjustment disorder and 7% had major depression. At follow-up (median 58 days), changes were made in the diagnoses in 31% of the patients and 11% were found to have an adjustment disorder and 12% major depression. More recent data, using the Structured Clinical Interview for DSM-IV and including diverse patient populations showed that 39% of patients with advanced cancer either fulfilled criteria for a major psychiatric disorder and/or used mental health services for psychological distress after the cancer diagnosis. Twelve percent of the patients met criteria for a major psychiatric disorder: 7% major depression and 11% minor depression. Over one third of patients with a psychiatric diagnosis met criteria for two or more diagnoses.[20] Prevalence rates appear to increase as patients become sicker.[21,22] The highest rates of depression are seen in patients with cancers of the pancreas, oropharynx, and breast,[23] although no causative relationships have been established. As many as 59% of patients requesting assisted suicide are depressed.[4,24,25] Lloyd-Williams[25] carried out a prospective study to evaluate the incidence of suicidal ideation in a palliative care population, mostly with very late stage disease, and found that 3% had such thoughts often, 10% experienced them sometimes, 17% hardly ever experienced them, and 70% never had thoughts of self-harm. Younger patients were more likely to report suicidal thoughts. Several studies suggest that the prevalence of depression in cancer has declined over the past 20 years, perhaps related to improvements in medical care and outcomes[26] and destigmatization of the diagnosis of cancer.[27]

Depression in Noncancer Diagnoses. The experience of patients with advanced cancer, congestive heart failure, and chronic obstructive pulmonary disease (COPD) tend to be more similar than different.[28] Like patients with cancer, those with other medical illnesses also appear to have elevated rates of depression.[21,29] Depression prevalence ranges of up to 42% have been reported in palliative medicine settings.[16,30] Patients seeking to stop dialysis have rates of depression of between 5% and 25%[31]; those with end-stage heart disease are reported to have prevalence rates of 36% for major depression and 22% for minor depression.[32] Patients with congestive heart failure and COPD were found to have higher rates of depression than a population of patients with cancer with similar estimated survival estimates. Patients with a higher disease burden in all three diseases had more depression.[28] In a longitudinal study of patients with heart failure, worsening symptoms of depression were associated with hospitalizations for heart disease and death.[33] Fewer than half of patients with advanced heart disease received treatment for depression.[34]

Rates of Mental Health Service Use. A small number of studies have examined how clinicians assess and manage mental health issues in patients with advanced disease. Data suggest that palliative care clinicians and oncologists tend to underrecognize and underestimate the severity of patient depression.[35-37] An older study reported that only about 3% of patients with end-stage cancer were receiving antidepressant medications.[38] Although this may be improving, major depression is still untreated or undertreated in this population.[17] One more recent study of over 1000 patients receiving palliative care demonstrated that only 10% of patients received an antidepressant and of those, 76% were prescribed during the last 2 weeks of the patient's life.[39] Lawrie and colleagues[40] found that 73% of palliative care physicians routinely assess patients for depression and that 75% prescribed selective serotonin reuptake inhibitors (SSRIs), 25% prescribed tricyclic antidepressants, 6% prescribed psychostimulants, and 3% prescribed St. John's wort. When asked whether they would prescribe complementary or psychological therapies for depression, 35% reported that they would refer patients for aromatherapy and only 8% would refer for counseling. Fewer than half of patients with advanced heart disease receive treatment for depression.[34] Kadan-Lottick and colleagues[20] found that nearly half of patients who met criteria for psychiatric illness did not receive mental health services and that nonwhite patients were significantly less likely to receive mental health care than white patients.[20,41]

SUMMARY OF EVIDENCE REGARDING TREATMENT RECOMMENDATIONS

Contrary to much popular and professional opinion, depression is a treatable condition, even in patients who are terminally ill. However, effective treatment of depression in the context of distressing symptoms is difficult; thus the first step in treating depression is effectively controlling physical symptoms.[42] Some patients may be concerned that being labeled as "depressed" will lead their physicians to take their physical problems less seriously, to treat them less aggressively, or to stigmatize them; thus it is often essential for the physician to address these issues before the patient is able to accept treatment. A combination of antidepressant medication, supportive psychotherapy, and patient and family education are viewed as the gold standard of treatment.[43,44] Effective treatment of depression has been shown to improve symptoms of both patients and their caregivers.[45]

Psychotherapeutic Interventions

An accumulating body of evidence suggests that psychotherapeutic interventions are effective in reducing depressive symptoms in patients with advanced cancer; in particular, cognitive-behavioral therapy appears to offer significant benefit to this population.[46–48]

In a large randomized, controlled trial, Chochinov and colleagues[48] evaluated whether a dignity therapy intervention, focused on memories, hopes, wishes for loved ones, ways they wanted to be remembered, and lessons they wished to pass on, had an impact on distress and depression. In a population of patients with an estimated prognosis of less than 6 months, who were receiving palliative care and who had relatively low levels of baseline distress, dignity therapy did not reduce overall distress or depression, although patients found it to be a positive experience.[48] Another pilot randomized trial of an intervention designed to improve end-of-life preparation and life completion suggested that patients experience improvement in depressive symptoms, although the sample was quite small.[49]

Social Support Interventions

Group support interventions for patients with advanced cancer have shown conflicting results. Early studies of the effects of support groups on distress in women with breast cancer showed not only improvements in quality of life but also significantly improved survival.[50] Subsequent studies, including a large multicenter trial, showed that group psychosocial support improved mood but had no effect on survival.[51] A subsequent study demonstrated that group support appeared to improve survival only in patients with estrogen receptor–negative breast cancer, the subgroup of breast cancer with poorest prognoses.[52] A variety of other studies appear to suggest that longevity is prolonged for patients with melanoma, non–small cell lung cancer, leukemia, and gastrointestinal cancers when patients receive social support.[6]

Family Interventions

Several studies have examined relationships between patient and caregiver depressive symptoms.[53,54] Caregiver depressive symptoms, common in the setting of a loved one's advanced illness, are associated with patient unresponsiveness to depression treatments; in such circumstances, psychosocial support for caregivers, including appropriate medication, or family-oriented interventions may prove to be helpful.

Pharmacological Interventions

Because antidepressant therapy is usually relatively well-tolerated, expert consensus statements recommend having a low threshold for initiating treatment. Psychostimulants and SSRIs are the main pharmacological treatment modalities for depression at the end of life (Table 33-1). Evidence about the effectiveness of antidepressants in patients at the end of life is poor; although one study describes some effectiveness in as many as 80% of cancer patients,[55] lack of clear criteria for effectiveness and appropriate study design significantly compromise these data. Few randomized, controlled trials of antidepressants in the palliative care setting have been conducted. Because of these gaps in the evidence base, trials from primary care, general oncology, geriatrics, and human immunodeficiency virus (HIV) infection provide much of what we know about antidepressant effectiveness in palliative care.

Several randomized, controlled trials comparing antidepressants with placebo for depression in patients with cancer suggest a benefit of treatment,[56–58] but high dropout rates and narrow patient populations limit generalizability. A randomized, controlled study of paroxetine in an ambulatory oncology population demonstrated effectiveness for fatigue and depression.[59] A trial of an algorithm-based symptom screening tool for depression followed by oncologist-conducted clinical interviews and fluoxetine treatment for depressed patients demonstrated improvement in patient quality of life and depressive symptoms.[60] Open-label trials have demonstrated positive effects of paroxetine, sertraline, and mirtazapine,[61] and one case-control study suggests that duloxetine is effective for patients with cancer, with side effects similar to a control group without cancer.[62] Randomized, controlled trials (RCTs) in primary care have demonstrated the effectiveness of mirtazapine and paroxetine.[63] RCTs in geriatric settings demonstrate the effectiveness of combined modalities (community-based psychosocial interventions and antidepressant medication) for major and minor depression[64,65]; the results of these studies have been incorporated in recent treatment guidelines and algorithms for geriatric depression.[66–68] A meta-analysis of SSRIs for the treatment of HIV-associated depression suggested some therapeutic benefit and acceptable tolerability, but did not identify any agent(s) as particularly effective.[69] Other investigators demonstrated effectiveness of treatment with sertraline, paroxetine, and mirtazapine in open-label trials in patients with acquired immunodeficiency syndrome (AIDS) and HIV.[70]

The STAR*D trial, involving more than 4000 patients with chronic or recurrent depression from psychiatric and primary care settings, demonstrated a response rate of approximately 30% after 8 weeks of therapy

TABLE 33-1. Antidepressants for Patients With Advanced Illness

AGENTS	EVIDENCE QUALITY	ADVANTAGES	DISADVANTAGES	ONSET OF ACTION	DOSAGE	SIDE EFFECTS	SCHEDULE	COST
Psychostimulants	Anecdotal reports, retrospective case reviews, small controlled prospective trials[88,89]	Rapid onset of action; well-tolerated in elderly and debilitated patients; effective adjuvant analgesics[90,91]; counter opioid-induced sedation; improve appetite[92] and energy level; effectiveness 70%[93] to 82%[94]; useful in treating cognitive impairment in AIDS[95]	Cardiac decompensation can occur in elderly patients, those with heart disease; confusion in older or cognitively impaired patients[96]; tolerance may develop infrequently	<24 hr	Start low, titrate upward q1-2 days. *Methylphenidate starting dose:* 2.5-10 mg/day, usual dose 10-20 mg/day *Dextroamphetamine starting dose:* 5-10 mg/day, usual dose: 10-30 mg/day	Increased confusion; restlessness, nervousness, agitation, dizziness, nightmares, insomnia, palpitations, anorexia, arrhythmia, tremor, dry mouth, psychosis	Upon awakening and 4 hours later; some patients may need half dose in late afternoon	Low
SSRIs (general)	Double-blind, controlled studies show superiority over placebo in depression,[97–102] HIV-associated depression,[103] depression with heart disease,[104] and as effective as TCAs for depression[105–111]	Few drug interactions; easy to titrate; minimal cardiac side effects	Inhibit P450/2D6 causing some interactions with other drugs	4-8 wk	Start low, titrate upward q5-7 days	Nausea, GI distress, insomnia, activation, headache, sexual dysfunction, anorexia, dizziness, dry mouth, headache	Once a day	
Citalopram		Well-tolerated, effective for anxiety; few side effects; low risk for withdrawal[112]; fewer sexual side effects[113]	Risk of QT prolongation at higher doses[114]; 2011 FDA warning that doses >40 mg should not be used		10-20 mg/day *Usual therapeutic dose:* 20-40 mg/ day		Once a day	Low
Sertraline					*Starting dose:* 25-50 mg/day *Usual dose:* 50-100 mg/day		Once a day	Low
Escitalopram					*Starting dose:* 5-10 mg/day *Usual dose:* 10-15 mg/day		Once a day	High
Fluoxetine		Longer acting	Less well tolerated than sertraline[115]		*Starting dose:* 10 mg/day *Usual dose:* 20-40 mg/day		Once a day	Low
Paroxetine			Withdrawal effects a major issue; sedating		*Starting dose:* 10 mg/day *Usual dose:* 20-40 mg/day		Once a day	Low

Drug	Evidence/Notes	Additional notes	Onset	Dose	Adverse effects	Administration	Cost
SNRIs (general)	No trials in terminal illness	Comparable in effectiveness to SSRIs, TCAs	4-8 wk				
Venlafaxine	May be activating[116]	Withdrawal effects can be minimized with use of long-acting preparation		Starting dose: 37.5 mg/day; Usual dose: 75-225 mg/day	Asthenia, GI symptoms, dizziness, dry mouth, headache, insomnia, somnolence	Morning	Med-High
Duloxetine	May have some[117] benefits for patients with pain		4-8 wk	Starting dose: 30 mg/day; Usual dose: 60-120 mg/day		Once a day	High
Other agents							
Bupropion	Mechanism of action unknown	May be activating		Starting dose: 75 mg/day; Usual dose: 150-450 mg/day	Agitation, constipation, dizziness, insomnia, dry mouth, headache	Morning	Low
Mirtazapine	Helpful for patients with insomnia; associated with weight gain; antinausea effects noted; these effects can be noted within days[118]	Sedating		Starting dose: 7.5-15 mg/day; Usual dose: 30-45 mg/day	Somnolence, dizziness, weight gain	Bedtime	High
Tricyclic antidepressants	Multiple studies demonstrate efficacy in depressed medically ill patients[119]	May have benefits for patients with pain[120]; therapeutic response often seen at low dose; drug levels can be monitored[121]. Nortriptyline and desipramine are better tolerated than amitriptyline and imipramine[122]	4-8 wk		Adverse effects occur in as many as 34% of patients with cancer[123]; not well tolerated in terminally ill because of anticholinergic side effects (dry mouth, delirium, constipation, etc.)		
Desipramine				Starting dose: 25 mg/day; Usual dose: 75-150 mg/day		Bedtime	Low
Nortriptyline				Starting dose: 25 mg/day; Usual dose: 50-100 mg/day		Bedtime	Low

Cost Key is based on Consumer Reports Drug Comparison. Available at http://www.consumerreports.org/health/resources/pdf/best-buy-drugs/2pager_Antidepress.pdf. Accessed September 9, 2012.
Low, <$40/month; medium, $40-100/month; high, >$100/month.
AIDS, Acquired immunodeficiency syndrome; *FDA,* Food and Drug Administration; *GI,* gastrointestinal; *HIV,* human immunodeficieny virus; *SSRIs,* selective serotonin reuptake inhibitors; *TCAs,* tricyclic antidepressants.

with SSRIs. A substantial number of patients required at least 6 weeks to determine therapeutic efficacy. Nonresponding patients who were switched to a second antidepressant or received augmentation by the addition of a second agent had response rates in the 20% to 30% range. The 51% of patients in the trial who had anxious depression demonstrated lower responsiveness to antidepressant medications.[71-75]

The relatively low rates of response found here, even in patients who were, in general, much less medically ill than the average patient in palliative care, has important implications for our thinking about prescription of antidepressants in the palliative care setting. Certainly, depressed patients with short survival horizons are not good candidates for treatment with SSRIs. Second, we should recognize that SSRI trials should be extended for 8 to 12 weeks, before determining efficacy. For many patients in our palliative care population, this represents a large proportion (if not all) of their likely survival duration, rendering these drugs much less useful. The benefits found in the STAR*D trial from augmentation of SSRIs with other agents deserve consideration. Although not studied in that trial, psychostimulants may be effective agents for SSRI augmentation and providing rapid relief from depressive symptoms for patients with severe depression and short anticipated survival. Modafinil has also been shown to be effective in augmenting partial responses to SSRIs, particularly for patients with fatigue and sleepiness.[76,77]

Psychostimulants. Because of their rapid onset of action, psychostimulants (methylphenidate, dextroamphetamine) deserve special consideration in treating depression near the end of life. Therapeutic benefits can be achieved within 24 to 48 hours of starting medication. Several nonrandomized studies document the effectiveness of methylphenidate for depression in patients with cancer[78,79]; however, one RCT found no improvement in fatigue and quality of life from treatment with dextroamphetamine,[80] although this study did not look at depression. In patients with HIV infection, one RCT has shown stimulants to be effective in patients with a low energy level and apathy.[81] Another double-blind, randomized, controlled trial of psychostimulants for fatigue in patients with HIV showed statistically significant improvements in fatigue, quality of life, and psychological distress (including depression), with minimal side effects.[82] An open-label study of HIV-positive patients that evaluated modafinil as a treatment for fatigue showed evidence of effectiveness for both fatigue and depression.[83]

Choosing an Antidepressant. Several factors should be considered in choosing an antidepressant (Figure 33-1). First, has the patient had a good response to a particular antidepressant in the past? If not, have any of the patient's first-degree relatives responded well to a particular antidepressant? Beyond these two predictors of good response, half-life, side-effect profile, and cytochrome p450 enzyme interactions should be considered. Agents with a longer half-life (e.g., fluoxetine) might expose patients to

side effects that take longer to remit on discontinuation, whereas agents with a shorter half-life (e.g., paroxetine) can expose patients to withdrawal syndromes if suddenly discontinued. These same two agents have the most cytochrome p450 interactions, as well, but drug–drug interactions with the patient's current medications should always be checked before starting an antidepressant. Some agents tend to be more sedating (e.g., mirtazapine, paroxetine) and may help with sleep. Others tend to be more activating and may help with energy (e.g., fluoxetine, bupropion, duloxetine, venlafaxine) but may increase anxiety. The non-SSRIs and non–serotonin and norepinephrine reuptake inhibitors (SNRIs) tend not to have sexual side effects. Tricyclic antidepressants, SNRIs, and SSRIs (in that order) can help with neuropathic pain to some degree. As mentioned previously, prognosis should play a role in choosing between psychostimulants and other types of antidepressants.

Other Agents. Another group of medications that affect depression exists, including mirtazapine, bupropion, duloxetine, and venlafaxine. Like SSRIs in the general population, they are thought to be about as effective as tricyclic antidepressants, but most have less risk for adverse effects.

Bupropion and venlafaxine may have a positive impact on pain syndromes and can be energizing in patients with fatigue or psychomotor retardation.[84] Mirtazapine may help with pain syndromes, is an effective antidepressant, tends to be sedating at lower doses, and has been associated with increased appetite. It may be particularly helpful in patients who are depressed, have trouble sleeping, and also have a suppressed appetite. Duloxetine has also been found, in case-control studies, to have benefits for patients with cancer who have depression.[62]

The tricyclic antidepressants are not first-line agents for depression in the terminally ill; they are not as well tolerated as SSRIs because of autonomic and sedating effects. If used, dosages must be titrated to levels effective to target depression. Tricyclic antidepressants are effective for controlling neuropathic pain at much lower doses than for treating depression. Amitriptyline and doxepin are typically more sedating than desipramine and nortriptyline. These medications are associated with various side effects and should be adjusted when negative side effects occur. The therapeutic range is wide, and drug levels can be monitored for most tricyclic antidepressants.

Electroconvulsive Therapy. Electroconvulsive therapy is a highly effective treatment for depression and should be considered in patients with psychotic depression, those who cannot tolerate antidepressant medications, and those with treatment-resistant depression who have a prognosis of several months or more.[85,86]

Treatment-Resistant Depression

Refractory, treatment-resistant depression may occur in the palliative care setting. Comprehensive end-of-life care is best provided by an interdisciplinary team

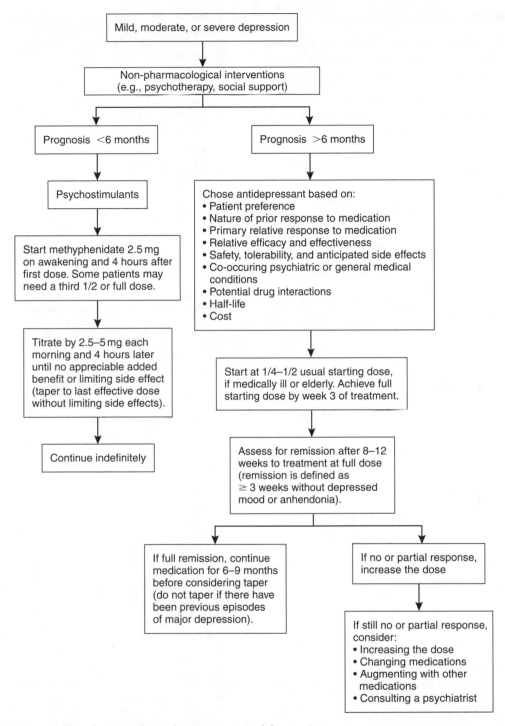

FIGURE 33-1. Decision tree for pharmacological management of depression.

that includes physicians, nurses, mental health clinicians, and spiritual counselors because these patients and their families have a broad array of needs and no single clinician is likely to be able to manage them all. In general, patients with suicidal ideation, treatment-resistant depression, diagnostic uncertainty, comorbid psychiatric disorder (e.g., anxiety, substance abuse, etc.), or physical symptoms greater than expected or refractory to maximal intervention should be referred to a psychiatrist.[87] Appropriate treatment planning for such patients requires not only an intensive interdisciplinary dialog, including a psychiatrist, but also involvement of the patient and patient's family in defining appropriate care. Very occasionally, in spite of state-of-the-art medication, psychotherapy, and palliative care, depression may be intractable; in such circumstances, clinicians are called on to respond to depression as part of a terminal illness syndrome that is causing profound suffering. In these rare circumstances, limitation of further aggressive intervention, as well as other palliative care approaches (e.g., palliative sedation), in the patient with extreme and irremediable suffering maybe considered in collaboration with mental health experts.

KEY MESSAGES TO PATIENTS AND FAMILIES

Depression is a treatable illness, even when a patient is seriously ill. Treating it may alleviate both physical and psychological suffering. Working with clinicians who are well versed in the therapies available to treat depression can ensure that appropriate treatments are chosen to improve symptoms and quality of life in patients with advanced illness and their caregivers.

CONCLUSION AND SUMMARY

Symptoms of depression are a common source of suffering in patients with advanced, life-threatening illness and their families. Careful assessment of depressed mood as a potential source of distress is warranted. Untreated, depression can have a negative impact on physical health and quality of life for patients and their families. A multimodal treatment that uses nonpharmacological treatments and, when necessary, the addition of medications can provide significant relief. Prognosis should be taken into account when choosing a medication.

SUMMARY RECOMMENDATIONS

- Recognize that symptoms of depression are a common source of suffering in patients with advanced, life-threatening illness.
- Screen and assess for depression on a regular basis.
- Do not assume depression is a normal part of a patient's end of life.
- Utilize a multimodal treatment strategy that uses nonpharmacological treatments and, when necessary, medications to provide relief.
- Take prognosis into account when choosing a medication.

REFERENCES

1. Block SD. Psychological issues in end-of-life care. *J Palliat Med.* 2006;9:751–772.
2. Pelletier G, Verhoef MJ, Khatri N, Hagen N. Quality of life in brain tumor patients: the relative contributions of depression, fatigue, emotional distress, and existential issues. *J Neurooncol.* 2002;57(1):41–49.
3. Breitbart W, Bruera E, Chochinov H, Lynch M. Neuropsychiatric syndromes and psychological symptoms in patients with advanced cancer. *J Pain Symptom Manage.* 1995;10(2):131–141.
4. Chochinov HM, Wilson KG, Enns M, et al. Desire for death in the terminally ill. *Am J Psychiatry.* 1995;152(8):1185–1191.
5. Chochinov HM, Tataryn D, Clinch JJ, Dudgeon D. Will to live in the terminally ill. *Lancet.* 1999;354(9181):816–819.
6. Spiegel D. Mind matters in cancer survival. *JAMA.* 2011;305(5):502–503.
7. Giese-Davis J, Collie K, Rancourt KM, Neri E, Kraemer HC, Spiegel D. Decrease in depression symptoms is associated with longer survival in patients with metastatic breast cancer: a secondary analysis. *J Clin Oncol.* 2011;29(4):413–420.
8. Temel JS, Greer JA, Muzikansky A, et al. Early palliative care for patients with metastatic non-small-cell lung cancer. *N Engl J Med.*19 2010;363(8):733–742.
9. Satin JR, Linden W, Phillips MJ. Depression as a predictor of disease progression and mortality in cancer patients: a meta-analysis. *Cancer.* 2009;115(22):5349–5361.
10. Reiche EM, Nunes SO, Morimoto HK. Stress, depression, the immune system, and cancer. *Lancet Oncol.* 2004;5(10):617–625.
11. Seruga B, Zhang H, Bernstein LJ, Tannock IF. Cytokines and their relationship to the symptoms and outcome of cancer. *Nat Rev Cancer.* 2008;8(11):887–899.
12. Massie MJ. Prevalence of depression in patients with cancer. *J Natl Cancer Inst Monogr.* 2004;(32):57–71.
13. Hotopf M, Chidgey J, Addington-Hall J, Ly KL. Depression in advanced disease: a systematic review. I. Prevalence and case finding. *Palliat Med.* 2002;16(2):81–97.
14. Pirl WF. Evidence report on the occurrence, assessment, and treatment of depression in cancer patients. *J Natl Cancer Inst Monogr.* 2004;(32):32–39.
15. Potash M, Breitbart W. Affective disorders in advanced cancer. *Hematol Oncol Clin North Am.* 2002;16(3):671–700.
16. Wilson KG, Chochinov H, de Faye BJ, Breitbart W. Diagnosis and management of depression in palliative care. In: Chochinov HM, Breitbart W, eds. *Handbook of Psychiatry in Palliative Medicine.* Oxford: Oxford University Press; 2000:25–50.
17. Wilson KG, Chochinov HM, Skirko MG, et al. Depression and anxiety disorders in palliative cancer care. *J Pain Symptom Manage.* 2007;33(2):118–129.
18. Derogatis LR, Morrow GR, Fetting J, et al. The prevalence of psychiatric disorders among cancer patients.*JAMA.* 1983;249(6):751–757.
19. Akechi T, Okuyama T, Sugawara Y, Nakano T, Shima Y, Uchitomi Y. Major depression, adjustment disorders, and post-traumatic stress disorder in terminally ill cancer patients: associated and predictive factors. *J Clin Oncol.* 2004;22(10):1957–1965.
20. Kadan-Lottick NS, Vanderwerker LC, Block SD, Zhang B, Prigerson HG. Psychiatric disorders and mental health service use in patients with advanced cancer: a report from the coping with cancer study. *Cancer.* 2005;104(12):2872–2881.
21. Evans DL, Staab JP, Petitto JM, et al. Depression in the medical setting: biopsychological interactions and treatment considerations. *J Clin Psychiatry.* 1999;60(suppl 4):40–55 discussion.
22. Ciaramella A, Poli P. Assessment of depression among cancer patients: the role of pain, cancer type and treatment. *Psychooncology.* 2001;10(2):156–165.
23. McDaniel JS, Musselman DL, Porter MR, Reed DA, Nemeroff CB. Depression in patients with cancer: diagnosis, biology, and treatment. *Arch Gen Psychiatry.* 1995;52(2):89–99.
24. Emanuel EJ, Fairclough DL, Emanuel LL. Attitudes and desires related to euthanasia and physician-assisted suicide among terminally ill patients and their caregivers. *JAMA.* 2000;284(19):2460–2468.
25. Lloyd-Williams M. How common are thoughts of self-harm in a UK palliative care population? *Support Care Cancer.* 2002;10(5):422–424.
26. van't Spijker A, Trijsburg RW, Duivenvoorden HJ. Psychological sequelae of cancer diagnosis: a meta-analytical review of 58 studies after 1980. *Psychosom Med.* 1997;59(3):280–293.
27. Spiegel D, Giese-Davis J. Depression and cancer: mechanisms and disease progression. *Biol Psychiatry.* 1 2003;54(3):269–282.
28. Steinhauser KE, Arnold RM, Olsen MK, et al. Comparing three life-limiting diseases: does diagnosis matter or is sick, sick? *J Pain Symptom Manage.* 2011;42(3):331–341.
29. Cassem EH. Depressive disorders in the medically ill: an overview. *Psychosomatics.* 1995;36(2):S2–S10.
30. Patrick DL, Ferketich SL, Frame PS, et al. National Institutes of Health State-of-the-Science Conference Statement: symptom management in cancer: pain, depression, and fatigue. *J Natl Cancer Inst Monogr.* 2004;(32):9–16.
31. Cohen LM, Dobscha SK, Hails KC, Pekow PS, Chochinov HM. Depression and suicidal ideation in patients who discontinue the life-support treatment of dialysis. *Psychosom Med.* 2002;64(6):889–896.
32. Gibbs JS, McCoy AS, Gibbs LM, Rogers AE, Addington-Hall JM. Living with and dying from heart failure: the role of palliative care. *Heart.* 2002;88(suppl 2):ii36–ii39.
33. Sherwood A, Blumenthal JA, Hinderliter AL, et al. Worsening depressive symptoms are associated with adverse clinical outcomes in patients with heart failure. *J Am Coll Cardiol.* 2011;57(4):418–423.
34. Koenig HG. Depression in hospitalized older patients with congestive heart failure. *Gen Hosp Psychiatry.* 1998;20(1):29–43.
35. Meyer HA, Sinnott C, Seed PT. Depressive symptoms in advanced cancer. I. Assessing depression: the Mood Evaluation Questionnaire. *Palliat Med.* 2003;17(7):596–603.

36. Meyer HA, Sinnott C, Seed PT. Depressive symptoms in advanced cancer. II. Depression over time; the role of the palliative care professional. *Palliat Med.* 2003;17(7):604–607.

37. Passik SD, Dugan W, McDonald MV, Rosenfeld B, Theobald DE, Edgerton S. Oncologists' recognition of depression in their patients with cancer. *J Clin Oncol.* 1998;16(4):1594–1600.

38. Goldberg RJ, Mor V. A survey of psychotropic use in terminal cancer patients. *Psychosomatics.* 1985;26(9):745–748 751.

39. Lloyd-Williams M, Friedman T, Rudd N. A survey of antidepressant prescribing in the terminally ill. *Palliat Med.* 1999;13(3):243–248.

40. Lawrie I, Lloyd-Williams M, Taylor F. How do palliative medicine physicians assess and manage depression. *Palliat Med.* 2004;18(3):234–238.

41. Vanderwerker LC, Laff RE, Kadan-Lottick NS, McColl S, Prigerson HG. Psychiatric disorders and mental health service use among caregivers of advanced cancer patients. *J Clin Oncol.* 2005;23(28):6899–6907.

42. Breitbart W. Cancer pain and suicide. In: Foley KM, Bonica JJ, Ventafridda V, eds. *Advances in Pain Research and Therapy.* New York: Raven; 1990:23–33.

43. Work Group on Major Depressive Disorder. *American Psychiatric Association Practice Guideline for the Treatment of Patients with Major Depressive Disorder.* 3rd ed. Arlington, VA: American Psychiatric Association Press; 2010:1–152.

44. Block SD. Assessing and managing depression in the terminally ill patient. ACP-ASIM End-of-Life Care Consensus Panel. American College of Physicians, American Society of Internal Medicine. *Ann Intern Med.* 2000;132(3):209–218.

45. Martire LM, Schulz R, Reynolds CF, Morse JQ, Butters MA, Hinrichsen GA. Impact of close family members on older adults' early response to depression treatment. *Psychol Aging.* 2008;23(2):447–452.

46. Akechi T, Okuyama T, Onishi J, Morita T, Furukawa TA. Psychotherapy for depression among incurable cancer patients. *Cochrane Database Syst Rev.* 2008;(2): CD005537.

47. Moorey S, Cort E, Kapari M, et al. A cluster randomized controlled trial of cognitive behaviour therapy for common mental disorders in patients with advanced cancer. *Psychol Med.* 2009;39(5):713–723.

48. Chochinov HM, Kristjanson LJ, Breitbart W, et al. Effect of dignity therapy on distress and end-of-life experience in terminally ill patients: a randomised controlled trial. *Lancet Oncol.* 2011;12(8):753–762.

49. Steinhauser KE, Alexander SC, Byock IR, George LK, Olsen MK, Tulsky JA. Do preparation and life completion discussions improve functioning and quality of life in seriously ill patients? Pilot randomized control trial. *J Palliat Med.* 2008;11(9):1234–1240.

50. Spiegel D, Bloom JR, Kraemer HC, Gottheil E. Effect of psychosocial treatment on survival of patients with metastatic breast cancer. *Lancet.* 1989;2(8668):888–891.

51. Goodwin PJ, Leszcz M, Ennis M, et al. The effect of group psychosocial support on survival in metastatic breast cancer. *N Engl J Med.* 2001;345(24):1719–1726.

52. Spiegel D, Butler LD, Giese-Davis J, et al. Effects of supportive-expressive group therapy on survival of patients with metastatic breast cancer: a randomized prospective trial. *Cancer.* 2007;110(5):1130–1138.

53. Bambauer KZ, Zhang B, Maciejewski PK, et al. Mutuality and specificity of mental disorders in advanced cancer patients and caregivers. *Soc Psychiatry Psychiatr Epidemiol.* 2006;41(10):819–824.

54. Siminoff LA, Wilson-Genderson M, Baker Jr. S. Depressive symptoms in lung cancer patients and their family caregivers and the influence of family environment. *Psychooncology.* 2010;19(12):1285–1293.

55. Chaturvedi SK, Maguire P, Hopwood P. Antidepressant medications in cancer patients. *Psychooncology.* 2007;3(1):57–60 1994.

56. Razavi D, Allilaire JF, Smith M, et al. The effect of fluoxetine on anxiety and depression symptoms in cancer patients. *Acta Psychiatr Scand.* 1996;94(3):205–210.

57. van Heeringen K, Zivkov M. Pharmacological treatment of depression in cancer patients: a placebo-controlled study of mianserin. *Br J Psychiatry.* 1996;169(4):440–443.

58. Theobald DE, Kirsh KL, Holtsclaw E, Donaghy K, Passik SD. An open label pilot study of citalopram for depression and boredom in ambulatory cancer patients. *Palliat Support Care.* 2003;1(1):71–77.

59. Morrow GR, Hickok JT, Roscoe JA, et al. Differential effects of paroxetine on fatigue and depression: a randomized, double-blind trial from the University of Rochester Cancer Center Community Clinical Oncology Program. *J Clin Oncol.* 2003;21(24):4635–4641.

60. Passik SD, Kirsh KL, Theobald D, et al. Use of a depression screening tool and a fluoxetine-based algorithm to improve the recognition and treatment of depression in cancer patients: a demonstration project. *J Pain Symptom Manage.* 2002;24(3):318–327.

61. Theobald DE, Kirsh KL, Holtsclaw E, Donaghy K, Passik SD. An open-label, crossover trial of mirtazapine (15 and 30 mg) in cancer patients with pain and other distressing symptoms. *J Pain Symptom Manage.* 2002;23(5):442–447.

62. Torta R, Leombruni P, Borio R, Castelli L. Duloxetine for the treatment of mood disorder in cancer patients: a 12-week case-control clinical trial. *Hum Psychopharmacol.* 2011;26(4–5):291–299.

63. Wade A, Crawford GM, Angus M, Wilson R, Hamilton L. A randomized, double-blind, 24-week study comparing the efficacy and tolerability of mirtazapine and paroxetine in depressed patients in primary care. *Int Clin Psychopharmacol.* 2003;18(3):133–141.

64. Ciechanowski P, Wagner E, Schmaling K, et al. Community-integrated home-based depression treatment in older adults: a randomized controlled trial. *JAMA.* 2004;291(13):1569–1577.

65. Bruce ML, Ten Have TR, Reynolds 3rd CF, et al. Reducing suicidal ideation and depressive symptoms in depressed older primary care patients: a randomized controlled trial. *JAMA.* 2004;291(9):1081–1091.

66. Alexopoulos GS, Katz IR, Reynolds 3rd CF, Carpenter D, Docherty JP, Ross RW. Pharmacotherapy of depression in older patients: a summary of the expert consensus guidelines. *J Psychiatr Pract.* 2001;7(6):361–376.

67. Mulsant BH, Alexopoulos GS, Reynolds 3rd CF, et al. Pharmacological treatment of depression in older primary care patients: the PROSPECT algorithm. *Int J Geriatr Psychiatry.* 2001;16(6):585–592.

68. Lapid MI, Rummans TA. Evaluation and management of geriatric depression in primary care. *Mayo Clin Proc.* 2003;78(11): 1423–1429.

69. Caballero J, Nahata MC. Use of selective serotonin-reuptake inhibitors in the treatment of depression in adults with HIV. *Ann Pharmacother.* 2005;39(1):141–145.

70. Ferrando SJ, Goldman JD, Charness WE. Selective serotonin reuptake inhibitor treatment of depression in symptomatic HIV infection and AIDS. Improvements in affective and somatic symptoms. *Gen Hosp Psychiatry.* 1997;19(2):89–97.

71. Trivedi MH, Rush AJ, Wisniewski SR, et al. Evaluation of outcomes with citalopram for depression using measurement-based care in STAR*D: implications for clinical practice. *Am J Psychiatry.* 2006;163(1):28–40.

72. Rush AJ, Trivedi MH, Wisniewski SR, et al. Bupropion-SR, sertraline, or venlafaxine-XR after failure of SSRIs for depression. *N Engl J Med.* 2006;354(12):1231–1242.

73. Trivedi MH, Fava M, Wisniewski SR, et al. Medication augmentation after the failure of SSRIs for depression. *N Engl J Med.* 2006;354(12):1243–1252.

74. Fava M, Rush AJ, Wisniewski SR, et al. A comparison of mirtazapine and nortriptyline following two consecutive failed medication treatments for depressed outpatients: a STAR*D report. *Am J Psychiatry.* 2006;163(7):1161–1172.

75. Fava M, Rush AJ, Alpert JE, et al. Difference in treatment outcome in outpatients with anxious versus nonanxious depression: a STAR*D report. *Am J Psychiatry.* 2008; 165(3):342–351.

76. Stoll AL, Pillay SS, Diamond L, Workum SB, Cole JO. Methylphenidate augmentation of serotonin selective reuptake inhibitors: a case series. *J Clin Psychiatry.* 1996;57(2):72–76.

77. Fava M, Thase ME, DeBattista C, Doghramji K, Arora S, Hughes RJ. Modafinil augmentation of selective serotonin reuptake inhibitor therapy in MDD partial responders with persistent fatigue and sleepiness. *Ann Clin Psychiatry.* 2007;19(3):153–159.

78. Olin J, Masand P. Psychostimulants for depression in hospitalized cancer patients. *Psychosomatics.* 1996;37(1):57–62.

79. Macleod AD. Methylphenidate in terminal depression. *J Pain Symptom Manage.* 1998;16(3):193–198.
80. Auret KA, Schug SA, Bremner AP, Bulsara M. A randomized, double-blind, placebo-controlled trial assessing the impact of dexamphetamine on fatigue in patients with advanced cancer. *J Pain Symptom Manage.* 2009;37(4):613–621.
81. Wagner GJ, Rabkin R. Effects of dextroamphetamine on depression and fatigue in men with HIV: a double-blind, placebo-controlled trial. *J Clin Psychiatry.* 2000;61(6):436–440.
82. Breitbart W, Rosenfeld B, Kaim M, Funesti-Esch J. A randomized, double-blind, placebo-controlled trial of psychostimulants for the treatment of fatigue in ambulatory patients with human immunodeficiency virus disease. *Arch Intern Med.* 2001;161(3):411–420.
83. Rabkin JG, McElhiney MC, Rabkin R, Ferrando SJ. Modafinil treatment for fatigue in HIV+ patients: a pilot study. *J Clin Psychiatry.* 2004;65(12):1688–1695.
84. Schatzberg AF, Cole JO, DeBattista C. *Manual of Clinical Psychopharmacology.* 7th ed. Washington, DC: American Psychiatric Publishing; 2010:35–136.
85. Bosworth HB, McQuoid DR, George LK, Steffens DC. Time-to-remission from geriatric depression: psychosocial and clinical factors. *Am J Geriatr Psychiatry.* 2002;10(5):551–559.
86. O'Connor MK, Knapp R, Husain M, et al. The influence of age on the response of major depression to electroconvulsive therapy: a C.O.R.E. report. *Am J Geriatr Psychiatry.* 2001;9(4):382–390.
87. Lebowitz BD, Pearson JL, Schneider LS, et al. Diagnosis and treatment of depression in late life. Consensus statement update. *JAMA.* 1997;278(14):1186–1190.
88. Masand PS, Tesar GE. Use of stimulants in the medically ill. *Psychiatr Clin North Am.* 1996;19(3):515–547.
89. Fernanez F, Adams F, Holmes VF, Levy JK, Neidhart M. Methylphenidate for depressive disorders in cancer patients: an alternative to standard antidepressants. *Psychosomatics.* 1987;28(9):455–462.
90. Bruce R, Fainsinger R, MacEachern T, Hanson J. The use of methylphenidate in patients with incident cancer pain receiving regular opiates: a preliminary report. *Pain.* 1992;50(1):75–77.
91. Forrest WH, Brown BW, Brown CR, et al. Dextroamphetamine with morphine for the treatment of postoperative pain. *N Engl J Med.* 1977;296(13):712–715.
92. Silverstone T. The clinical pharmacology of appetite-its relevance to psychiatry. *Psychol Med.* 1983;13(2):251–253.
93. Woods SW, Tesar GE, Murray GB, Cassem NH. Psychostimulant treatment of depressive disorders secondary to medical illness. *J Clin Psychiatry.* 1986;47(1):12–15.
94. Masand P, Pickett P, Murray GB. Psychostimulants for secondary depression in medical illness. *Psychosomatics.* 1991;32:203–208.
95. Fernandez F, Adams F, Levy JK, Holmes VF, Neidhart M, Mansell PW. Cognitive impairment due to AIDS-related complex and its response to psychostimulants. *Psychosomatics.* 1998;29:38–46.
96. Angrist B, d'Hollosy M, Sanfilipo M, et al. Central nervous system stimulants as symptomatic treatments for AIDS-related neuropsychiatric impairment. *J Clin Psychopharmacol.* 1992;12:268–272.
97. Kasper S, Fuger J, Moller HJ. Comparative efficacy of antidepressants. *Drugs.* 1992;43(suppl 2):11–22.
98. Geddes JR, Freemantle N, Mason J, Eccles MP, Boynton J. SSRIs versus other antidepressants for depressive disorder. *Cochrane Database Syst Rev.* 2000:CD001851.
99. Barbui C, Hotopf M, Freemantle N, et al. Selective serotonin reuptake inhibitors versus tricyclic and heterocyclic antidepressants: comparison of drug adherence. *Cochrane Database Syst Rev.* 2000;(2): CD002791.
100. Kennedy SH, Andersen HF, Lam RW. Efficacy of escitalopram in the treatment of major depressive disorder compared with conventional selective serotonin reuptake inhibitors and venlafaxine XR: a meta-analysis. *J Psychiatry Neurosci.* 2006;31:122–131.
101. Murdoch D, Keam SJ. Escitalopram: a review of its use in the management of major depressive disorder. *Drugs.* 2005;65:2379–2404.
102. Gartlehner G, Gaynes BN, Hansen RA. Comparative benefits and harms of second-generation antidepressants: background paper for the American College of Physicians. *Ann Intern Med.* 2008;149:734–750.
103. Elliot AJ, Uldall KK, Bergam K, Russo J, Claypoole K, Roy-Byrne PP. Randomized, placebo-controlled trial of paroxetine versus imipraminie in depressed HIV-positive outpatients. *Am J Psychiatry.* 1998;155:367–372.
104. Roose SP, Laghrissi-Thode F, Kennedy JS, et al. Comparison of paroxetine and nortriptyline in depressed patients with ischemic heart disease. *JAMA.* 1998;279:287–291.
105. Preskorn SH, Burke M. Somatic therapy for major depressive disorder: selection of an antidepressant. *J Clin Psychiatry.* 1992;53 (suppl): 5–18.
106. Mendels J. Clinical experie3nce with serotonin reuptake inhibiting antidepressants. *J Clin Psychiatry.* 1987;48 (suppl): 26–30 .
107. Cipriani A, Brambilla P, Furukawa T. Fluoxetine versus other types of pharmacotherapy for depression. *Cochrane Database Syst Rev.* 2005:CD004185.
108. Anderson IM. Selective serotonin reuptake inhibitors versus tricyclic antidepressants: a meta-analysis of efficacy and tolerability. *J Affect Disord.* 2000;58:19–36.
109. Montgomery SA. A meta-analysis of the efficacy and tolerability of paroxetine versus tricyclic antidepressants in the treatment of major depression. *Int Clin Psychopharmacol.* 2001;16(3):169–178.
110. Macgillivray S, Arroll B, Hatcher S. Efficacy and tolerability of selective serotonin reuptake inhibitors compared with tricyclic antidepressants in depression treated in primary care: systematic review and meta-analysis. *BMJ.* 2003;326(7397):1014.
111. Arroll B, Elley CR, Fishman T. Antidepressants versus placebo for depression in primary care. *Cochrane Database Syst Rev.* 2009;(30): CD00794.
112. Pato MT. Beyond depression: citalopram for obsessive-compulsive disorder. *Int Clin Psychopharmacol.* 1999;14(suppl 2):S19–S26.
113. Mendels J, Kiev A, Fabre LF. Double-blind comparison of citalopram and placebo in depressed outpatients with melancholia. *Depress Anxiety.* 1999;9(2):54–60.
114. Kelly CA, Dhaun N, Laing WJ, Strachan FE, Good AM, Bateman DN. Comparative toxicity of citalopram and the newer antidepressants after overdose. *J Toxicol Clin Toxicol.* 2004;42(1):67–71.
115. Rifkin A, Reardon G, Siris S, et al. Trimipramine in physical illness with depression. *J Clin Psychiatry.* 1985;46(2 Pt2):4–8.
116. Nemeroff CB, Entsuah R, Benattia I, Demitrack M, Sloan DM, Thase ME. Comprehensive analysis of remission (COMPARE) with venlafaxine versus SSRIs. *Biol Psychiatry.* 2008;63(4):424–434.
117. Thase ME, Pritchett YL, Ossanna MJ, Swindle RW, Xu J, Detke MJ. Efficacy of duloxetine and selective serotonin reuptake inhibitors: comparisons as assessed by remission rates in patients with major depressive disorder. *J Clin Psychopharmacol.* 2007;27(6):672–676.
118. Kim SW, Shin IS, Ki JM, et al. Effectiveness of mirtazapine for nausea and insomnia in cancer patients with depression. *Psychiatr Clin Neurosci.* 2008;62(1):75–83.
119. France RD. The future for antidepressants: treatment of pain. *Psychopathology.* 1987;20 (suppl): 99–113.
120. Preskorn SH, Jerkovich GS. Central nervous system toxicity of tricyclic antidepressants: phenomenology, course, risk, factors, and role of therapeutic drug monitoring. *J Clin Psychopharmacol.* 1990;10(2):88–95.
121. Preskorn SH. Recent pharmacologic advances in antidepressant therapy for the elderly. *Am J Med.* 1993;94(5A):2S–12S.
122. Lewis-Fernandez R, Kleinman A. Cultural psychiatry: theoretical, clinical, and research issues. *Psychiatr Clin North Am.* 1995;18:433–448.
123. Chaturvedi SK, Maguire P, Hopwood P. Antidepressant medications in cancer patients. *Psychooncology.* 1994;3:57–60.

Chapter 34

What Treatments Are Effective for Anxiety in Patients With Serious Illness?

SCOTT A. IRWIN, LORI P. MONTROSS, AND HARVEY M. CHOCHINOV

INTRODUCTION AND SCOPE OF THE PROBLEM

This chapter focuses on anxiety in patients with serious illness. First, anxiety is defined and its prevalence discussed. The major types of anxiety disorders are then reviewed, and the difficult task of diagnosing anxiety is addressed. Important differential diagnoses are summarized throughout. Finally, pharmacological and nonpharmacological treatments for anxiety in this population are reviewed.

Defining Anxiety

Anxiety is an expected, normal, transient response to stress.[1] Its evolutionary function was to warn of danger or the need to cope with a stressor.[1] Pathological anxiety is an excessive response to external stress or a response to an unidentified internal stress. It is often autonomous, with no recognizable trigger. Its intensity often exceeds a person's ability to cope. Pathological anxiety is often persistent, rather than transient, and leads to impaired coping behaviors such as avoidance or withdrawal.[2] The symptoms of pathological anxiety are physical (autonomic arousal with resulting tachycardia, tachypnea, diaphoresis, diarrhea, dizziness), emotional (edginess, terror, feelings of impending doom), behavioral (avoidance, compulsions, psychomotor agitation), and cognitive (worry, apprehension, fear, dread, uncertainty, obsession). In some instances, these symptoms lead to various forms of anxiety-related disorders.

Prevalence of Anxiety

Anxiety disorders are the most common psychiatric disorders in the general population, with up to 29% of the U.S. population suffering from an anxiety disorder at some point in their lifetime.[3,4] Often, no previous history of anxiety exists. Only a small percentage of people have any symptoms of anxiety before cancer diagnosis or treatment.[5] Symptoms of anxiety are thought to occur in more than 70% of medically ill patients, especially those with cancer or those approaching the end of life.[6–15]

Types of Anxiety Disorders

Several types of anxiety disorders exist. The most common anxiety disorders seen among patients with serious illness include adjustment disorder with anxious features, panic disorder, posttraumatic stress disorder, and generalized anxiety disorder.

Generalized anxiety disorder is a state of excessive anxiety or worry lasting at least 6 months and affecting day-to-day activities.[16–19] People suffering with generalized anxiety are often described as worriers by their friends and families.

A panic attack is the sudden onset of intense terror, apprehension, fearfulness, or a feeling of impending doom, usually occurring with symptoms such as shortness of breath, palpitations, chest discomfort, a sense of choking, and fear of "going crazy" or losing control, often in unexpected situations.[19] Panic attacks are discrete in nature and time-course, usually lasting 15 to 20 minutes. A panic disorder is diagnosed when multiple panic attacks occur or fear of another attack significantly reduces psychosocial functioning.[19]

Anxiety often co-occurs with adjustment disorders. An adjustment disorder is a psychological response to an identifiable stressor that results in the development of clinically significant emotional or behavioral symptoms, but does not qualify for a diagnosis of an anxiety disorder.[19] Many people with serious medical illness may have trouble psychologically adjusting to their diagnosis, prognosis, or treatment regimens.

Some patients may develop hyperarousal associated with their diagnosis or treatments and meet the criteria for the diagnosis of posttraumatic stress

TABLE 34-1. Questions to Ask Patients When Assessing Elements of Care Relating to Psychological Symptoms

ELEMENTS OF CARE	SAMPLE QUESTIONS TO ASK WHEN ASSESSING THE ELEMENT OF CARE
Anxiety symptoms	"Do you worry a lot?" "Are you often fearful?" "Do you feel anxious, nervous, or on edge?"
Developmental issues	"What is it like to be at this point in your life and facing a serious illness?"
Meaning, hope, and impact of illness	"How have you made sense of why this is happening to you?"
Coping style	"How have you coped with hard times in the past?"
Impact on sense of self	"How is your illness affecting your sense of self?"
Relationships	"Who are the most important people in your life?" "Who else will be affected by what is happening to you?"
Stressors	"What things are causing the most stress in your life right now?" "What are the things that are concerning you the most at this time?"
Spiritual resources	"What role does faith play in your life?"
Economic circumstances	"How much of a concern are financial matters for you right now and for the future?"
Physician–patient relationship	"How do you want me as your physician to help you?" "How can we best work together?" "I can only imagine what you must be going through."

Modified from Block SD. Psychological issues in end-of-life care. *J Palliat Med.* 2006;9:751-772; Emanuel LL, Ferris FD, von Gunten CF, Von Roenn J. *EPEC-O: Education in Palliative and End-of-Life Care for Oncology. Module 3c: Symptoms—Anxiety.* Chicago: The EPEC Project; 2005; and Chochinov HM. Dignity and the essence of medicine: the A, B, C, and D of dignity conserving care. *BMJ.* 2007;335:184-187.

disorder[20]; that is, they reexperience a traumatic event with symptoms of increased arousal, nightmares, intrusive memories, hypervigilance, and avoidance of reminders of the traumatic event.[19]

Anxiety disorders should be differentiated from other psychiatric disorders, such as depression or anxiety. Common symptoms in depression, such as loss of appetite, decreased libido, and insomnia may also be part of anxiety states.[21]

ASSESSMENT OF ANXIETY

Anxiety often goes undiagnosed or underdiagnosed. Recognizing anxiety can be particularly difficult because patients with serious illness often have a complex mix of physical, psychological, and psychiatric issues.[21] For these patients, anxiety frequently presents with somatic symptoms that overshadow psychological and cognitive manifestations.[22] A psychiatrist can be instrumental in helping clinicians who work with patients with serious illness understand these symptoms and can also help diagnose and treat an underlying anxiety disorder, if one exists.[19]

Assessing for Anxiety

Assessing for anxiety is critical because if left untreated, it leads to a poor prognosis. Anxiety can lead to significant impairments in physical and psychosocial functioning, as well as decreased quality of life.[23] Anxiety disorders are associated with increased alcohol use, marital problems, work-related problems, and suicide.[24-26]

In patients with advanced life-threatening illness and symptoms of anxiety, distress may be related to uncertainty regarding physical, psychological, social, spiritual, practical, end-of-life, and loss issues.[21,22] In this group, fear of uncontrolled symptoms or dependency is sometimes accompanied by a heightened interest in hastened death.[21]

Interdisciplinary team members can help facilitate these important discussions with patients, and a detailed history and appropriate physical examination and laboratory investigation is the gold standard of anxiety assessment. Input from patients, their family, and friends can be invaluable. Such inquiry takes time, so learning to ask *salient* questions that lead to an accurate assessment of the patients' circumstances and clinical picture are key. Clinicians can use the Hospital Anxiety and Depression Scale,[27] Profile of Mood States,[28] or Generalized Anxiety Disorder Screener (GAD-7)[29,30] to help screen for anxiety related issues.

Table 34-1 presents questions designed to guide conversations and aid clinicians in their assessment of anxiety, as well as other related clinical areas. Each question corresponds to an element of care; when these questions are asked in a comforting environment, they may lead to vital information about other domains.

Listen for Key Words. Although patients with serious illness often experience anxiety,[9,31] many patients may not directly express these symptoms to care providers or articulate their experiences in terms of readily identifiable diagnostic criteria. As a result, it behooves clinicians to listen for key words that can often signal underlying anxiety. For example, Anderson and colleagues[32] completed audio recordings of 415 visits between patients with advanced cancer and oncologists and found anxiety and fear were the most common types of emotion expressed within those visits. Patients most frequently used the words "concerned," "scared," "worried," and "nervous" to convey their experience of anxiety or fear. Being aware of these key words and noting if they occur during conversations with patients can aid clinicians in pinpointing the presence of anxiety.

It is also critical to note the interpersonal style of patients being treated for serious illness. Patients with anxiety may seem confused and unable to take in information. These patients may ask the same questions repeatedly or demonstrate difficulty making decisions, both of which may cause frustration for the treatment team. Patients with anxiety also may appear inconsistent or even suspicious.[33] Thus how the patient appears to the team or even what responses the patient evokes from the treatment team can be useful indicators of underlying patient distress. However, these also can be signs of other disorders, such as delirium, so care must be taken in coming to a diagnosis based on these observations.

Physiological Causes of Anxiety

Symptoms of anxiety may occur as a result of physiological abnormalities rather than from a primary anxiety disorder or psychological state, making discernment even more difficult.[34] It is worthwhile to have a high level of suspicion for physiological causes if the symptom onset is after age 35, personal or family history of anxiety is lacking, or the patient has a poor response to anxiolytic treatment. Common physiological causes of anxiety are listed in Table 34-2.

It is also important to be aware of disorders or physical symptoms that often coincide with anxiety. For example, head and neck cancers lead to changes in body appearance and image, thus contributing to anxiety. Head and neck cancers can also involve difficulty swallowing and ensuing weight loss, which further alters patients' self-image. For these patients, the frequent recurrence rate may also heighten anxiety as they vigilantly wonder if the "cancer is back."[35] As a result, patients with head and neck cancers should be carefully monitored for anxiety.

Dyspnea can also cause discomfort, fear, and anxiety.[36] The experience of air hunger has been shown to evoke anxiety and fear, even among healthy subjects who were fully aware that they were not in imminent danger.[37] The discomfort associated with shortness of breath is so pervasive that clinicians are well advised to evaluate its impact frequently among these patients.[36]

SUMMARY OF EVIDENCE REGARDING TREATMENT RECOMMENDATIONS

Treating Anxiety in Patients With Serious Illness

If treated, most patients with anxiety will improve; however, few achieve full or sustained remission. This is particularly the case in the context of unremitting or advancing life-limiting illness, thereby highlighting the importance of ongoing assessment and maintenance therapy.[38]

TABLE 34-2. Common Physiological Causes of Anxiety

Neurological
  Seizures
  Stroke
  Pain
Endocrine
  Hyperthyroidism
  Hyperparathyroidism
  Hyperadrenalism
Drug induced
  Caffeine
  Cocaine
  Amphetamine
  Theophylline
  Corticosteroids
  Thyroid hormone
  Antipsychotics (akathisia)
  Selective serotonin reuptake inhibitors (akathisia)
  Drug withdrawal
  Alcohol
  Sedative-hypnotics
  Opioids
  Nicotine
Toxic–metabolic abnormalities
  Acidosis
  Hyperthermia
  Electrolyte imbalances
Hypoxia (cerebral anoxia)
  Respiratory
    Chronic obstructive pulmonary disease
    Respiratory distress
    Pulmonary embolism
  Cardiovascular
    Arrhythmias
    Angina
    Congestive heart failure
    Anemia
    Myocardial infarction

Care Tenor. In treating patients with serious illness and with anxiety, the importance of care tenor cannot be overstated. Treating patients with compassion, respect, and dignity can serve as the foundation of effective care.[39] It also buffers self-worth and resilience, thereby mitigating feelings of anxiety that often emerge in the face of serious illness. Popa-Velea and associates[40] studied the specific effects of providing a compassionate, patient-centered treatment approach in patients with advanced colon cancer. The patient-centered treatment in this study involved frequent meetings with the doctor, the opportunity for patients to be involved in treatment decisions, ample information to be given about diagnosis and prognosis, and psychological support provided to the patient and family as needed. This type of engaged and personalized approach was found to not only improve quality of life but also lower anxiety. When a complete assessment has been performed using an appropriate tenor of care and anxiety has been found to be present, the physician and treatment team have several treatment options. The team may proceed with nonpharmacological or pharmacological interventions; often a combination thereof is most effective.[33,41]

Nonpharmacologic Interventions. For patients with serious illness, nonpharmacologic treatments can be particularly effective, especially for mild to moderate symptoms. They can enhance a sense of mastery and coping, while offering the advantage of avoiding the polypharmacy often seen in this population. Nonpharmacological options include individual or group psychotherapies, complementary therapies, and behavioral interventions.

Psychotherapies that are empirically based or evidenced-based treatments for anxiety include supportive psychotherapy, cognitive-behavioral therapy, and interpersonal therapy (see Table 34-3 for a more detailed description of each treatment).[33,42] These therapies have shown benefit when evaluated for anxiety in a broad context, although their effectiveness among patients with serious illness continues to be studied.

Several other therapies have been designed specifically for treatment of patients who are seriously ill or in palliative care. These therapeutic modalities include Managing Cancer and Living Meaningfully (CALM),[43] Dignity Therapy,[44,45] and Meaning-Centered Therapy.[46] The benefit of these treatments is the targeted applicability for seriously ill populations, but their specificity for managing anxiety has not yet been determined.

In addition to psychotherapy, numerous alternative therapies can be used when attempting to decrease anxiety among patients with serious illness. Viable complementary therapies include music therapy,[47] relaxation training,[42] acupuncture,[48] mindfulness meditation,[49] aromatherapy, massage, and art therapy.[50] Music therapy appears to show considerable promise for decreasing anxiety and improving quality of life in patients receiving hospice and palliative care.[47] Relaxation training is widely applied, particularly because it often can be provided at relatively low cost and has long-term effects if the techniques are practiced consistently over time.[42]

Several behavioral options exist for nonpharmacological intervention with seriously ill patients who are experiencing anxiety. Physical exercise can prove beneficial, even among the seriously ill. Exercise can decrease worry and anxiety while improving overall functioning. Exercise may also serve an important role in providing a sense of autonomy, control, or success. Patients who are bed-bound can engage in activities that provide exercise, even it if is only providing passive range of motion.[51]

Patients with serious illness who are experiencing anxiety may also benefit from a detailed assessment of their daily caffeine and alcohol intake. Learning about patients' consumption of these substances can help determine if lowering levels of each would diminish concomitant anxiety and may serve to educate the patient about the implications of such lifestyle behaviors. Similarly, a sleep hygiene protocol may be implemented to help regulate anxiety without pharmacological intervention. Finally, providing psychoeducation about the general course of serious illness and what to expect at

TABLE 34-3. Potential Nonpharmacological Interventions for Anxiety Among Patients With Serious Illness

INTERVENTION	BRIEF DESCRIPTION
Psychotherapies for Anxiety	
Supportive psychotherapy	Therapy focused on the provision of empathic, compassionate, and nonjudgmental listening
Cognitive-behavioral therapy (CBT)	Therapy based on modifying dysfunctional thoughts, feelings, and behaviors
Interpersonal therapy (IPT)	Therapy emphasizing the role of social dysfunction in creating or maintaining psychological distress; goal is improved relational adjustment
Psychotherapies for Palliative Care	
Managing Cancer and Living Meaningfully (CALM)	Structured therapy to relieve distress and promote psychological growth
Dignity Therapy	Therapy involving a life reflection interview and the subsequent creation of a tangible legacy document
Meaning-Centered Therapy	Therapy designed to enhance a sense of purpose in life through the exploration of meaning, values, suffering, humor, and other affective experiences
Complementary Therapies	
Music therapy	Recorded or performed music provided at the patient's bedside
Relaxation training	Describing and performing successive muscle relaxation or guided imagery with patients and families
Acupuncture	Traditional Chinese medicine practice of inserting thin needles into targeted points of the body
Mindfulness meditation	Meditation techniques used to raise contemplative awareness of the present moment while enhancing nonattachment and acceptance
Aromatherapy	Therapeutic use of plant-derived, aromatic essential oils to promote comfort and well-being
Massage	Touch stimulation throughout parts of the body
Art therapy	Encouragement of self-expression and creativity through painting, drawing, or craft activities
Other Interventions	
Exercise	Engagement in activity requiring physical effort
Decreased caffeine and alcohol consumption	Monitored caffeine and alcohol intake with modifications as necessary
Sleep hygiene protocol	The creation of a lifestyle regimen with habits conducive to sound sleep and rest
Psychoeducation	Providing information about the typical course of illness; the implications of diagnosis and prognosis

each stage may further decrease patients' levels of anxiety and worry.[41]

Pharmacological Interventions. Management of anxiety is usually most effective when psychotherapeutic and pharmacological approaches are combined. As with all things in palliative care, patients' overall functional status, life expectancy, and target symptoms need to be taken into account to discern the most prudent and likely successful management strategy. Although little high-level evidence exists on the role of antianxiety medications in seriously medically ill patients, the following discussion provides some clinical guidance on managing anxiety among these patients.

Standard anxiolytic pharmacotherapies often either carry significant risk for adverse events in those with advanced life-threatening illness or do not work quickly enough. Gabapentin, starting at 100 mg orally every hour as needed, to a maximum daily dose of 3600 mg, and trazodone, starting at 25 mg orally every hour as needed for anxiety or agitation or 25 to 100 mg orally at bedtime (for insomnia), are often effective alternatives and carry less risk for adverse events (Table 34-4). These medications can be given on a scheduled basis, as well.

In instances in which anxiety is acute and immediate relief is desired, benzodiazepines are often considered the first-line treatment in those who are medically well. However, as noted earlier, they need to be applied judiciously, in that excessive use can result in mental status changes—particularly in patients with preexisting cognitive impairment (e.g., confusion, reduced concentration, impaired memory). These changes are particularly concerning in the elderly, patients who are taking other central nervous system depressant medications, or patients with liver impairment. Like anticholinergics, benzodiazepines may worsen or induce delirium, especially in the elderly.

In most instances, benzodiazepines are selected based on the desired half-life. The longer the half-life, the more sustained the effect of the medication (e.g., clonazepam [$t_{1/2}$=30-40 hours] 0.5-2 mg orally daily or twice daily as needed). Medications with a half-life that extends beyond a day or two, such as clonazepam or diazepam, may accumulate, causing mounting side effects and toxicity.

Shorter-acting benzodiazepines, such as lorazepam ($t_{1/2}$=12 hours) 0.25 to 2 mg orally or sublingually every hour as needed can be dosed more frequently and not only are useful for anxiety but also can alleviate nausea and panic attacks. Benzodiazepines with a very short half-life (e.g., alprazolam $t_{1/2}$=11.2 hours, oxazepam $t_{1/2}$=2.8-8.6 hours, triazolam $t_{1/2}$=1.5-5.5 hours) are not suitable for treating anxiety because they remain effective for limited periods and are associated with a higher risk for rebound anxiety and withdrawal syndromes.

Patients with compromised hepatic function may do better with lorazepam, oxazepam, or temazepam, given these drugs are metabolized by conjugation and have no active metabolites.

TABLE 34-4. Anxiolytic Medications Used in Patients With Serious Illness

GENERIC NAME	APPROXIMATE DAILY DOSAGE RANGE (mg)*
Alternatives	
Trazodone	*PO:* 25 mg q1h, not to exceed 500 mg in 24 hr
Gabapentin	*PO:* 100 mg q1h, not to exceed 3600 mg in 24 hr
Benzodiazepines	
Very short acting	
Midazolam	*IV/subcutaneously:* 0.5-5 mg/hr infusion
Short Acting	
Lorazepam	*PO, SL, IV, IM:* 0.5-2 mg bid-tid
Intermediate acting	
Chlordiazepoxide	*PO, IM:* 10-50 mg tid-qid
Long acting	
Diazepam	*PO, IV, IM, PR:* 2-10 mg daily-bid
Clonazepam	*PO:* 0.25-3.0 mg daily-bid
Serotonin Specific Reuptake Inhibitors	
Paroxetine	*PO:* 10-60 mg daily
Citalopram	*PO:* 10-60 mg daily
Escitalopram	*PO:* 5-20 mg daily

Bid, Two times per day; *IM,* intramuscularly; *IV,* intravenously; *PO,* orally; *SL,* sublingually; *tid,* three times per day; *qid,* four times per day.
*Parenteral doses are generally twice as potent as oral doses. Intravenous bolus injections or infusions should be administered slowly.

The selective serotonin reuptake inhibitors (SSRIs) are now considered the drugs of choice in managing chronic anxiety in the medically well and those with a longer life-expectancy. The utility of antidepressants, including SSRIs, for treating anxiety is often limited in the seriously ill patient because they require weeks to achieve therapeutic effect. In these patients, clinicians must weigh the need to relieve symptoms in the short term against choosing a class of medications that requires several weeks to take effect. For severe anxiety, SSRIs, nonstandard approaches (as described earlier), and benzodiazepines can be used together, with the latter stopped once the former has reached therapeutic level.

Paroxetine (10-50 mg daily) is often chosen to address chronic anxiety; compared to some of the other SSRIs, it tends to be more sedating and calming. Other frequent choices of SSRIs in this population include citalopram (10-60 mg daily) and escitalopram (5-20 mg daily). Sedating antidepressants such as trazodone and mirtazapine may help patients with persistent anxiety and insomnia.

At times, symptoms of anxiety may be driven by other processes, such as delirium or shortness of breath. In these cases, the anxiety can be addressed by using treatments appropriate to these processes, such as reversing the cause of a delirium and treating distress with an antipsychotic or using opiates to treat shortness of breath.

KEY MESSAGES TO PATIENTS AND FAMILIES

Anxiety may be common in patients with advanced disease, and this is especially true for those with preexisting anxiety disorders. Patients and families should understand the importance of discussing this symptom with the clinical team because there are effective treatments for anxiety. These therapies include pharmacological and nonpharmacological treatments, and clinicians should explain that the therapies chosen depend on the sources of the anxiety, the patient's underlying medical condition(s), and the patient's life expectancy.

CONCLUSION AND SUMMARY

Symptoms of anxiety are a common source of suffering in patients with advanced life-threatening illness. Careful assessment of anxiety as a potential source of distress is warranted. Untreated, anxiety can negatively affect physical health and quality of life. A multimodal treatment that uses nonpharmacological treatments and when necessary includes the addition of pharmacological treatments can provide vital relief.

SUMMARY RECOMMENDATIONS

- Symptoms of anxiety can be common in medically ill patients, but frequently undiagnosed or underdiagnosed. Untreated anxiety can lead to a poor prognosis, considerable functional impairment, and decreased quality of life among patients. For all of these reasons, clinicians should ask about anxiety when treating all patients with serious illness.
- Anxiety can have numerous physiological causes, which need to be carefully assessed.
- Manage anxiety using a combination of psychotherapeutic and/or pharmacological treatments, all provided in a compassionate, patient-centered environment.
- Recommended nonpharmacological treatments for anxiety include individual or group psychotherapies, complementary therapies, and behavioral interventions.
- When used judiciously, psychopharmaceutical drugs play an important role in reducing anxiety that occurs in the context of terminal illness.

REFERENCES

1. Beck AT, Emery G. *Anxiety Disorders and Phobias: A Cognitive Perspective*. Cambridge, MA: Basic Books; 2005.
2. Alici Y, Levin TT. Anxiety disorders. In: Holland JC, Breitbart WC, Jacobsen PB, et al., eds. *Psychooncology*. New York: Oxford University Press; 2010:324.
3. Kessler RC, Chiu WT, Demler O, Merikangas KR, Walters EE. Prevalence, severity, and comorbidity of 12-month DSM-IV disorders in the National Comorbidity Survey Replication. *Arch Gen Psychiatry*. 2005;62:617–627.
4. Kessler RC, Berglund P, Demler O, Jin R, Merikangas KR, Walters EE. Lifetime prevalence and age-of-onset distributions of DSM-IV disorders in the National Comorbidity Survey Replication. *Arch Gen Psychiatry*. 2005;62:593–602.
5. Shalev AY, Schreiber S, Galai T, Melmed RN. Post-traumatic stress disorder following medical events. *Br J Clin Psychol*. 1993;32(Pt 2):247–253.
6. Portenoy RK, Thaler HT, Kornblith AB, et al. Symptom prevalence, characteristics and distress in a cancer population. *Qual Life Res*. 1994;3:183–189.
7. Portenoy RK, Thaler HT, Kornblith AB, et al. The Memorial Symptom Assessment Scale: an instrument for the evaluation of symptom prevalence, characteristics and distress. *Eur J Cancer*. 1994;30A:1326–1336.
8. Breitbart W, Bruera E, Chochinov H, Lynch M. Neuropsychiatric syndromes and psychological symptoms in patients with advanced cancer. *J Pain Symptom Manage*. 1995;10:131–141.
9. Wilson KG, Chochinov HM, Skirko MG. Depression and anxiety disorders in palliative cancer care. *J Pain Symptom Manage*. 2007;33:118–129.
10. Derogatis LR, Morrow GR, Fetting J, et al. The prevalence of psychiatric disorders among cancer patients. *JAMA*. 1983;249:751–757.
11. Roy-Byrne PP, Davidson KW, Kessler RC, et al. Anxiety disorders and comorbid medical illness. *Gen Hosp Psychiatry*. 2008;30:208–225.
12. Moorey S, Greer S, Watson M, et al. The factor structure and factor stability of the hospital anxiety and depression scale in patients with cancer. *Br J Psychiatry*. 1991;158:255–259.
13. Carroll BT, Kathol RG, Noyes Jr. R, Wald TG, Clamon GH. Screening for depression and anxiety in cancer patients using the Hospital Anxiety and Depression Scale. *Gen Hosp Psychiatry*. 1993;15:69–74.
14. Roth A, Nelson CJ, Rosenfeld B. Assessing anxiety in men with prostate cancer: further data on the reliability and validity of the Memorial Anxiety Scale for Prostate Cancer (MAX-PC). *Psychosomatics*. 2006;47:340–347.
15. Kissane DW, Grabsch B, Love A, Clarke DM, Bloch S, Smith GC. Psychiatric disorder in women with early stage and advanced breast cancer: a comparative analysis. *Aust N Z J Psychiatry*. 2004;38:320–326.
16. Smith MY, Redd W, DuHamel K, Vickberg SJ, Ricketts P. Validation of the PTSD Checklist-Civilian Version in survivors of bone marrow transplantation. *J Trauma Stress*. 1999;12:485–499.
17. Kangas M, Henry JL, Bryant RA. Posttraumatic stress disorder following cancer: a conceptual and empirical review. *Clin Psychol Rev*. 2002;22:499–524.
18. Andrykowski MA, Kangas M. Posttraumatic stress disorder associated with cancer diagnosis and treatment. In: Holland JC, Breitbart WC, Jacobsen PB, et al., eds. *Psychooncology*. New York: Oxford University Press; 2010:348.
19. American Psychiatric Association. *Diagnostic and Statistical Manual of Mental Disorders*. Text revision 4th ed Washington, DC: American Psychiatric Association; 2000.
20. Alter CL, Pelcovitz D, Axelrod A, et al. Identification of PTSD in cancer survivors. *Psychosomatics*. 1996;37:137–143.
21. Payne DK, Massie MJ. Anxiety in palliative care. In: Chochinov HM, Breitbart W, eds. *Handbook of Psychiatry in Palliative Medicine*. New York: Oxford University Press; 2000:435.
22. Atkinson Jr. JH, Grant I, Kennedy CJ, Richman DD, Spector SA, McCutchan JA. Prevalence of psychiatric disorders among men infected with human immunodeficiency virus: a controlled study. *Arch Gen Psychiatry*. 1988;45:859–864.
23. von Gunten CF, Sloan PA, Portenoy RK, Schonwetter RS. Physician board certification in hospice and palliative medicine. *J Palliat Med*. 2000;3:441–447.
24. Fawcett J. The detection and consequences of anxiety in clinical depression. *J Clin Psychiatry*. 1997;58(suppl 8):35–40.
25. Conway KP, Compton W, Stinson FS, Grant BF. Lifetime comorbidity of DSM-IV mood and anxiety disorders and specific drug use disorders: results from the National Epidemiologic Survey on Alcohol and Related Conditions. *J Clin Psychiatry*. 2006;67:247–257.

26. Bauer MS, Altshuler L, Evans DR, Beresford T, Williford WO, Hauger R. Prevalence and distinct correlates of anxiety, substance, and combined comorbidity in a multi-site public sector sample with bipolar disorder. *J Affect Disord.* 2005;85:301–315.

27. Ibbotson T, Maguire P, Selby P, Priestman T, Wallace L. Screening for anxiety and depression in cancer patients: the effects of disease and treatment. *Eur J Cancer.* 1994;30A:37–40.

28. Cella DF, Jacobsen PB, Orav EJ, Holland JC, Silberfarb PM, Rafla S. A brief POMS measure of distress for cancer patients. *J Chronic Dis.* 1987;40:939–942.

29. Spitzer RL, Kroenke K, Williams JB, Lowe B. A brief measure for assessing generalized anxiety disorder: the GAD-7. *Arch Intern Med.* 2006;166:1092–1097.

30. Lowe B, Decker O, Muller S, et al. Validation and standardization of the Generalized Anxiety Disorder Screener (GAD-7) in the general population. *Med Care.* 2008;46:266–274.

31. Fava GA, Porcelli P, Rafanelli C, Mangelli L, Grandi S. The spectrum of anxiety disorders in the medically ill. *J Clin Psychiatry.* 2010;71:910–914.

32. Anderson WG, Alexander SC, Rodriguez KL, et al. "What concerns me is…": expression of emotion by advanced cancer patients during outpatient visits. *Support Care Cancer.* 2008;16:803–811.

33. Block SD. Psychological issues in end-of-life care. *J Palliat Med.* 2006;9:751–772.

34. Bruera E, Miller L, McCallion J, Macmillan K, Krefting L, Hanson J. Cognitive failure in patients with terminal cancer: a prospective study. *J Pain Symptom Manage.* 1992;7:192–195.

35. Goldstein NE, Genden E, Morrison S. Palliative care for patients with head and neck cancer. *JAMA.* 2008;299:1818–1825.

36. Gilman SA, Banzett RB. Physiologic changes and clinical correlates of advanced dyspnea. *Curr Opin Support Palliat Care.* 2009;3:93–97.

37. Banzett RB, Pedersen SH, Schwartzstein RM, Lansing RW. The affective dimension of laboratory dyspnea: air hunger is more unpleasant than work/effort. *Am J Respir Crit Care Med.* 2008;177:1384–1390.

38. Gorman JM. Treatment of generalized anxiety disorder. *J Clin Psychiatry.* 2002;63(suppl 8):17–23.

39. Chochinov HM. Dignity and the essence of medicine: the A, B, C, and D of dignity conserving care. *BMJ.* 2007;335:184–187.

40. Popa-Velea O, Cernat B, Tambu A. Influence of personalized therapeutic approach on quality of life and psychiatric comorbidity in patients with advanced colonic cancer requiring palliative care. *J Med Life.* 2010;3:343–357.

41. Emanuel LL, Ferris FD, von Gunten CF, Von Roenn J. *EPEC-O: Education in Palliative and End-of-Life Care for Oncology. Module 3c: Symptoms—Anxiety.* Chicago: The EPEC Project, 2005.

42. Ayers CR, Sorrell JT, Thorp SR, Wetherell JL. Evidence-based psychological treatments for late-life anxiety. *Psychol Aging.* 2007;22:8–17.

43. Freeman EC, Lo C, Hales S, Rodin G. *Overcoming adversity: are positive changes possible after an advanced cancer diagnosis?* Canadian Virtual Hospice. Available at http://www.virtualhospice.ca/ Accessed September 14, 2012.

44. Chochinov HM. Dignity-conserving care: a new model for palliative care. *JAMA.* 2002;287:2253–2260.

45. Chochinov HM, Hack T, Hassard T, Kristjanson LJ, McClement S, Harlos M. Dignity therapy: a novel psychotherapeutic intervention for patients near the end of life. *J Clin Oncol.* 2005;23:5520–5525.

46. Breitbart W. Spirituality and meaning in supportive care: spirituality and meaning-centered group psychotherapy interventions in advanced cancer. *Support Care Cancer.* 2001;10:272–280.

47. Hilliard RE. Music therapy in hospice and palliative care: a review of the empirical data. *eCAM.* 2005;2:173–178.

48. Pilkington K, Kirkwood G, Rampes H, Cummings M, Richardson J. Acupuncture for anxiety and anxiety disorders: a systematic literature review. *Acupunct Med.* 2007;25:1–10.

49. Jain S, Shapiro S, Swanick S, et al. A randomized controlled trial of mindfulness meditation versus relaxation training: effects on distress, positive states of mind, rumination, and distraction. *Ann Behav Med.* 2007;33:11–21.

50. Barraclough J. ABC of palliative care: depression, anxiety, and confusion. *BMJ.* 1997;315:1365–1368.

51. MacDonald N. Physical activity as a supportive care intervention in palliative care patients. *J Support Oncol.* 2009;7:36–37.

DELIRIUM

Chapter 35

What Is Delirium?

MICHELLE T. WECKMANN AND R. SEAN MORRISON

INTRODUCTION AND SCOPE OF THE PROBLEM

Symptoms of delirium have been reported since the time of Hippocrates. The word *delirium* is derived from the Latin term meaning "off track." Delirium has many descriptors (acute confusion, altered mental status, confused, sundowning, intensive care unit [ICU] psychosis, organic psychosis, acute brain failure, toxic metabolic state, cerebral insufficiency, encephalopathy). All of these terms are used to describe an acute cognitive impairment associated with medical illness, which is more correctly labeled delirium. The American Psychiatry Association *Diagnostic and Statistical Manual of Mental Disorders,* Fourth Edition (DSM-IV) provides the most widely used and recognized definition (Table 35-1). Briefly, delirium is a transient, usually reversible cause of cerebral dysfunction that can manifest clinically with a wide range of neuropsychiatric abnormalities. The clinical hallmarks of delirium are decreased attention span and waxing and waning confusion.

Although delirium is a transient global disorder of cognition, affect and behavior are often involved. The increased morbidity and mortality rates make delirium a medical emergency. Therefore early diagnosis and resolution of symptoms are correlated with the best outcomes.[1] Unfortunately, delirium often is unrecognized or misdiagnosed.[2,3] It is commonly mistaken for dementia or depression, is attributed to hospitalization, or considered a part of old age (patients who are elderly are expected to become confused in the hospital).[4,5] The tendency of delirium to be mistaken for other psychiatric illnesses makes recognition and timely treatment difficult.

Prevalence

The prevalence of delirium depends on the population being studied. Delirium is present in 10% to 22% of elderly patients at the time of admission, with an additional 10% to 30% of cases developing after admission.[6-8] Certain subsets of patients have higher incidences of delirium, including the hospitalized elderly (15%-50%),[9,10] hospitalized cancer patients (25%-50%),[11-13] patients on a palliative care unit (28%-42%),[13,14] orthopedic patients (5%-61%),[6,15-19] patients in the ICU (80%), and patients near the end of life (up to 88%).[20-22] Additionally, delirium is extremely common among nursing home residents, with anywhere between 22% to 89% of nursing home residents with dementia developing delirium. No prospective studies have evaluated delirium prevalence in patients receiving home hospice care, although a study asking hospice nurses if their patient was confused during the previous week revealed that 50% of the patients were confused during that time.[23] This incidence is significantly higher than the 18% found by a chart review of 2716 patients in hospice care.[24] This review only looked for patients with the specific diagnosis of delirium in the chart, which may explain why the number is low, given that delirium is typically underrecognized, underdiagnosed, and rarely listed in the medical diagnoses for a patient.

Morbidity and Mortality

Delirium is associated with a host of negative outcomes, including a much greater mortality risk, longer hospital stays, and decreased ability to care for self, which increases both caregiver burden and nursing home placement.[25-27] Additionally, patients with delirium are not capable of accurately reporting physical symptoms, which can affect treatment decisions such as appropriate medical management of pain and lead to higher hospital charges.[28] In specific studies looking at elderly patients and patients during the postoperative period, delirium resulted in prolonged hospital stays, increased complications, increased cost, increased long-term disability, and worsening cognitive function.[29,30] In addition, patients who recover from delirium report recalling the experience with distress and are more likely to experience

TABLE 35-1. Diagnostic Criteria for Delirium

A. Disturbance of consciousness (i.e., reduced clarity of awareness of the environment) with reduced ability to focus, sustain, or shift attention.

B. A change in cognition or the development of a perceptual disturbance that is not better accounted for by a preexisting, established, or evolving dementia.

C. Disturbance that develops over a short period of time (usually hours to days) and tends to fluctuate during the course of the day.

D. There is evidence from the history, physical examination, or laboratory findings that the disturbance is caused by the direct physiological consequences of a general medical condition.

From American Psychiatric Association: *Diagnostic and Statistical Manual of Mental Disorders*. 4th ed. Text revision. Washington, DC, American Psychiatric Association, 2000; 143.

lasting psychological sequelae, including depression and posttraumatic stress disorder (PTSD).[31–34]

Perhaps the most striking complication of delirium is the increase in mortality. Patients who are admitted to the hospital with delirium have mortality rates 10% to 26% higher than similar patients without delirium at the time of admission.[35] Patients who develop delirium during hospitalization have a mortality rate of 22% to 76% and a high rate of death during the months following discharge.

Unfortunately, the impact of delirium often extends beyond the patient to affect the caregiver as well.[36] For example, nurses report that delirious patients are more challenging to care for and a study has shown a correlation between the level of caregiver distress and antipsychotic usage.[37,38] Family members also report distress related to a loved one experiencing delirium.[34,37,39,40] This distress can have long-lasting consequences for the caregiver, including decreased quality of life and increased risk for developing anxiety disorders.[41] Additionally, delirium is the most common reason palliative sedation is requested, emphasizing how distressing delirium can be to both the patient and observers.[42]

RELEVANT PATHOPHYSIOLOGY

Delirium results from a wide variety of both physiological and structural insults, but the overall mechanism of delirium is still not fully understood.[43] The main hypothesis involves reversible impairment of cerebral oxidative metabolism and multiple neurotransmitter abnormalities.[44] The two main neurotransmitters believed to be involved are high dopaminergic tone and low cholinergic tone.[45] Dopamine increase in mesolimbic and mesocortical tracts may cause agitation and delusions, whereas acetylcholine decrease in hippocampal and basal forebrain regions may lead to disorientation, hallucinations, and memory impairment.[46] Clinically this hypothesis is supported by the tendency for anticholinergic medications to cause acute confusional states, especially in patients with impaired cholinergic transmission, such as in Alzheimer disease, and in patients with postoperative delirium who have increased serum anticholinergic activity.[47,48] Additional support for this hypothesis is provided by the fact that symptomatic relief can be seen with the administration of neuroleptics, such as haloperidol, which are dopamine-blockers.[49] Other neurotransmitters (serotonin, γ-aminobutyric acid, cortisol, melatonin) are also believed to play a role in delirium, but their role is less clearly defined.[50,51] No specific neuronal pathways causing delirium have been identified; however, imaging studies of metabolic (e.g., hepatic encephalopathy) and structural (e.g., traumatic brain injury, stroke) factors support the hypothesis that certain anatomical pathways may play a more important role than others.[52,53] Additionally, disruptions in the blood–brain barrier can allow neurotoxic agents and inflammatory cytokines to enter the brain, which may cause delirium.[54–56]

Delirium Prevention

Several studies have shown that prevention of delirium is possible by both nonpharmacological and pharmacological interventions. A recent systematic literature review summarizes delirium prevention interventions for hospitalized patients.[57] The majority of the studies reviewed used a surgical population; patient ages were older than 40 years, and 10 studies were randomized controlled trials. Pharmacological and nonpharmacological methods were shown to be equally effective. The higher the incidence of delirium, the more likely the intervention was to be effective. This leads to the thought that delirium prevention should be undertaken in high-risk patient populations. Identified patient risk factors for delirium include dementia, cognitive impairment, medical illness, advanced age, sensory impairment, functional impairment, medications, preoperative psychoactive drug use, other psychiatric illnesses, institutional residence, abnormal kidney function, and alcohol abuse.[58,59] The rapidity of disease onset, disease severity, and treatment load should also be considered.[60] The strongest evidence exists for an association between delirium and cognitive impairment, psychotropic drug use, advanced age, and medical illness. Predictive models for the identification of delirium may be useful clinical tools to stratify the risk for delirium and have been validated for specific patient populations: elderly hospitalized patients,[61] after elective noncardiac surgery,[62] and after cardiac surgery.[63] However, it is important to note that delirium risk factors seem to vary across populations.

Assessment and Workup

Classification. Delirium is not a disease but rather a syndrome with many causes that result in a similar constellation of symptoms. Although delirium is a derangement primarily of cognition, affect and behavior are also involved, which gives rise to three described states of arousal (hyperactive, hypoactive, mixed). Hyperactive delirium is more commonly observed in patients in a state of alcohol withdrawal or intoxication with stimulants or hallucinogens. Hypoactive delirium is observed in patients in states of hepatic encephalopathy and hypercapnia and is more common in elderly patients. Mixed delirium is the most common and involves fluctuations between hypoactive and hyperactive states; these individuals commonly display daytime sedation with nocturnal agitation and behavioral problems. Some evidence suggests that the subtypes result in a different prognosis; dementia patients with hypoactive delirium have a worse prognosis.[64] Regardless of the behavioral manifestations of delirium, it can be useful to classify delirium as reversible or irreversible. This designation as reversible or irreversible should be determined in part by patient and family goals of care. Reversible delirium potentially can be treated by identifying and treating the underlying medical condition, whereas irreversible delirium is often a harbinger of death and is expected to continue until the person dies.

Screening. To diagnosis delirium, a clinician needs a low threshold for screening. Delirium is a bedside diagnosis; there are no laboratory values or scans that indicate that a patient is delirious. Therefore, to make a diagnosis of delirium, it is essential to obtain a thorough history and perform a comprehensive physical examination. Because of the patient's altered mental state, it is often necessary to obtain information from family, caregivers, or nurses. Hypoactive delirium is commonly mistaken for depression, which is complicated by the fact that patients with depressive symptoms are at higher risk for developing delirium.[65] Table 35-2 illustrates the differences among delirium, depression, and dementia. Although delirium is commonly misdiagnosed, it is more common to not even consider delirium as part of the differential. Once delirium is part of the differential diagnosis, having a low threshold for delirium screening can improve identification. Numerous easy-to-use delirium screening tools are available in the public domain. A comprehensive review is beyond the scope of this chapter, but recent reviews have been published.[66,67] The Confusion Assessment Method (CAM) is one of the most commonly used instruments for delirium screening, but its sensitivity tends to fluctuate based on the training and education level of the evaluator and the validity is poor for nonstandardized observations.[66] A recent study based on the principle that single-question depression screening has been shown to be an effective screen for depression,[68] demonstrated that the same approach may be useful for delirium screening.[69] A single question "Do you feel that [patient's name] has been more confused lately?" directed at the patient's caregiver or nurse had a specificity 71% and sensitivity of 80% in 21 general oncology inpatients. This may be a good way to quickly screen patients for delirium, with a more formal evaluation if the answer is yes.

History. When obtaining a history in a patient with delirium, timing is important and often provides the best clues as to cause. Specific attention should be paid to medication changes, substance intoxication or withdrawal, and evidence of infection. It is also important to determine the patient's baseline mental and cognitive status to rule out dementia and depression. A good mental status examination, including level of consciousness and attention, is essential. Easy bedside tests for attention include digit span, the number tapping test, recitation of the months of the year or days of the week backward, and alternating alphabet recitation and numbers (verbal trails B test). Common abnormal findings in the neurological examination include myoclonus, asterixis, unilateral weakness, hyperreflexia, Babinski reflexes, abnormal gait, and frontal release signs (grasp, snout, palmomental, suck, glabellar).[70]

TABLE 35-2. Differential Diagnosis for Dementia, Depression, and Delirium

CLINICAL FEATURE	DEMENTIA	DEPRESSION	DELIRIUM
Onset	Insidious (months to years)	Acute or insidious (weeks to months)	Acute (hours to days)
Duration	Months to years	Months to years	Hours to weeks
Course	Chronic and progressive	May be chronic	Fluctuating
Progression	Irreversible	Usually reversible	Usually reversible
Level of consciousness	Usually clear	Clear	Altered
Orientation	Disoriented	Oriented	Variable
Attention	Intact except in late stage	May be decreased	Impaired
Concentration	Intact except in late stage	May be decreased	Impaired
Speech	Coherent until late stage	Coherent (may be latent in severe)	May be incoherent or latent
Thought process	Limited	Organized	Disorganized
Perception	May have hallucinations (paranoia more common)	Mood congruent hallucinations in severe cases	Hallucinations are common (often visual)
Psychomotor activity	Variable	May be slowed in severe cases	Variable
Sleep pattern	Variable	Often increased but may have early morning awakenings	Variable, days and nights commonly confused

Delirium results from an underlying medical problem, and because a majority of delirium can be reversed once it is identified, it is essential to attempt to identify the cause (which is usually multifactorial). It is important to remember that not all patients and families find delirium distressing and they may not want the delirium reversed. Therefore discussion of prognosis and goals after the diagnosis of delirium has been made should occur before a complex workup for causes. Clinically, it is useful to divide causes into two groups—those that are immediately life threatening resulting from a readily identifiable cause (Table 35-3) and those that have a more complex and comprehensive differential diagnosis (Table 35-4). After a thorough history has been taken and a detailed physical examination performed, ordering a basic laboratory panel (Table 35-5) is recommended. If evaluation is suggestive of a specific pathology, additional workup to confirm or deny should be undertaken if consistent with patient and family goals.

SUMMARY OF EVIDENCE REGARDING TREATMENT RECOMMENDATIONS

All delirium treatment decisions should be made with patient and family goals of care in mind. Delirium has been shown to cause distress to everyone it touches and can have long-lasting mental health affects on bereaved family members.[34,40,71] Thus after the diagnosis of delirium is made it is essential to provide delirium education and support to the patient, caregivers, and members of the health care team.

Concurrent with providing education and support, it can be useful to initiate nonpharmacological measures (Table 35-6) while placing the delirium in the context of the medical illness and exploring goals for further medical care. Please see Chapter 36 for a more complete description of pharmacological measures; Chapter 37 provides a more comprehensive discussion of nonpharmacologic treatments for delirium. At this time it can be helpful to view the delirium as (potentially) reversible or irreversible, because each has different management strategies. Because delirium can be reversed more than 50% of the time, identify and treat potentially reversible causes. While doing this, it is important to palliate distressing symptoms (breathlessness, pain, agitation) while further workup is being undertaken.

TABLE 35-3. Immediately Life-Threatening Causes of Delirium: WHHHIMP

Wernicke encephalopathy
Hypoxia
Hyperglycemia
Hypertensive encephalopathy
Intracerebral hemorrhage
Meningitis and encephalitis
Poisoning

TABLE 35-4. More Comprehensive Differential of Delirium Causes: I WATCH DEATH

Infection	Urinary, encephalitis, meningitis, syphilis, HIV infection, sepsis, pneumonia
Withdrawal	Alcohol, benzodiazepines, barbiturates
Acute metabolic	Acidosis, alkalosis, electrolytes, glucose, liver or kidney failure
Trauma	Closed head injury, postoperative, burns, fractures
CNS pathology	Abscess, hemorrhage, hydrocephalus, subdural hematoma, infection, seizure, stroke, tumors, vasculitis
Hypoxia	Anemia, carbon monoxide poisoning, hypotension, heart failure
Deficiencies	Malnutrition (low albumin); vitamins B_1 (thiamine), B_3 (niacin), B_9 (folate), B_{12} (cyanocobalamin)
Endocrine	Overactivity or underactivity of thyroid, parathyroid, adrenal glands
Acute vascular	Severe hypertension, stroke, arrhythmia, shock
Toxins or drugs	Medications, illicit drugs, anesthetics, pesticides, solvents
Heavy metals	Lead, manganese, mercury

CNS, Central nervous system; *HIV*, human immunodeficiency virus.

TABLE 35-5. Basic Laboratory Evaluation of Delirium*

INITIAL INVESTIGATION	SPECIFIC TESTS IN SELECTED PATIENTS	RATIONALE FOR SPECIFIC TESTS
Complete blood count	Electrocardiogram	Existing cardiac disease
Blood urea and nitrogen levels	C-reactive protein and erythrocyte sedimentation rate	Suspected inflammatory disease
Electrolytes	Urinalysis, urine and blood cultures, chest radiography	Suspected infection
Blood sugar	Urine toxicology screen	Suspected drug use
Liver function	Vitamin B_{12}, folate	Malnutrition
Thyroid function	Electroencephalogram	Suspected seizures
Arterial blood gases	Computed tomography scan or magnetic resonance imaging scan of the brain	Suspected cerebral cause (stroke or brain metastasis)
	Lumbar puncture	Suspected meningitis

*The initial investigation (left column) should be considered for all patients. The "Specific Tests" column is ordered only when there is a particular rationale (right column).

The symptom of agitation should always be treated aggressively, especially if it is causing distress or endangering the patient or caregivers. Dopamine-blockers, such as first-generation antipsychotics, are typically the medication of choice in patients with hyperactive (agitated) delirium (Table 35-7). Schedule the dose based on the half-life and dose breakthroughs, depending on the time to achieve maximum concentration (typically 60 minutes when given orally and 30 minutes when given subcutaneously, intramuscularly, or intravenously). If antipsychotics are unsuccessful in treating severe agitation, benzodiazepines can be tried but should not be used as first-line treatment because of evidence that they can worsen delirium.[72,73] The one exception is irreversible terminal delirium, in which the goal is sedation; in these cases agents such as benzodiazepines, phenobarbital, and propofol are often used as first-line treatment to relieve the distress of delirium.[74] A full discussion of delirium at the end of life (also known as terminal delirium) can be found in Chapter 38. Hypoactive delirium also can be distressing, but little evidence exists to guide treatment. Trials have looked at using both antipsychotics and stimulants, but evidence supporting their efficacy for patients with hypoactive delirium is sparse.[75,76]

KEY MESSAGES TO PATIENTS AND FAMILIES

Patients and families should understand that delirium is a unique diagnosis often related to but separate from underlying medical conditions. Although dependent on the overall goals of care, the workup and treatment of delirium can ultimately improve the outcomes for the patient and family. The exception to this is patients with delirium at the end of life, and this may need to be explained to the patient's family. Clinicians should explain which causes may be reversible and which may not, so the patient or family can better understand the potential for reversing the condition.

CONCLUSION AND SUMMARY

Delirium is a common medical condition that causes significant distress to both patients and caregivers and often goes unrecognized and untreated. A high level of suspicion is needed to identify delirium, but when identified, it can be successfully treated in more than half of cases, even in patients with immediately life-threatening illnesses. Even if the delirium cannot be reversed, the symptoms often can be managed with both nonpharmacological and pharmacological measures.

TABLE 35-6. Nonpharmacological Interventions for Delirium Treatment

Frequent orientation (familiar objects/pictures, introductions, orientation board)
Cognitive exercises
Oral rehydration (beverage of choice available and within reach, frequent prompts to drink)
Attention to lighting (natural lighting, dim lighting at night)
Sensory aides (glasses, hearing aides)
Consistent caregivers (constant companions, sitters, family visits)
Sleep hygiene
Daily routine
Range of motion or physical activity
Limit immobilization (Foley catheters, intravenous lines, restraints)

SUMMARY RECOMMENDATIONS

- Given that delirium is associated with significant morbidity and mortality, high-risk patients should be routinely screened for delirium.
- All patients with delirium need a thorough medical evaluation with treatment of identified underlying causes and the initiation of nonpharmacological strategies.
- Treatment should be undertaken with patient and family goals clearly defined.
- Distressing symptoms (such as agitation) should be managed with antipsychotics. Haloperidol is the most commonly used antipsychotic drug.

TABLE 35-7. Pharmacological Treatment for Potentially Reversible Delirium

AGENT	DOSE*	ADVERSE EFFECTS [†]	COMMENTS [‡]
Haloperidol	*PO:* 0.5-2 mg bid and q1h prn *IV, subcutaneously:* 0.5-2 mg q30min prn	Extrapyramidal symptoms (especially in doses >4.5 mg/day)	Usual agent of choice based on studies and clinical guidelines
Chlorpromazine	*PO:* 25-50 mg bid and q1h prn *IV, subcutaneously:* 10-50 mg q30min prn	More anticholinergic, greater sedation	May be more effective for a highly agitated patient
Lorazepam	*PO:* 0.5-1 mg q2h prn *IV, subcutaneously:* 0.5-1 mg q30min prn	May worsen symptoms of delirium	Second-line agent Use for patients with agitation already on antipsychotics or when the cause of delirium is alcohol or benzodiazepine withdrawal

bid, Twice daily; *IV,* intravenously, *PO,* orally; *prn,* as needed.
*Can double prn dose if ineffective. Rethink diagnosis, doses, medication if ineffective after three prn doses.
[†]All antipsychotics have the potential for cardiac conduction effects. For a more detailed discussion of this and other risks associated with the use of antipsychotics, see chapter 36.
[‡]All antipsychotics may decrease nausea.

REFERENCES

1. Lundstrom M, Edlund A, Karlsson S, Brannstrom B, Bucht G, Gustafson Y. A multifactorial intervention program reduces the duration of delirium, length of hospitalization, and mortality in delirious patients. *J Am Geriatr Soc.* 2005;53(4):622–628.
2. Wada T, Wada M, Onishi H. Characteristics, interventions, and outcomes of misdiagnosed delirium in cancer patients. *Palliat Support Care.* 2010;8(2):125–131.
3. Breitbart W. Identifying patients at risk for, and treatment of major psychiatric complications of cancer. *Support Care Cancer.* 1995;3(1):45–60.
4. Inouye SK. The dilemma of delirium: clinical and research controversies regarding diagnosis and evaluation of delirium in hospitalized elderly medical patients. *Am J Med.* 1994;97(3):278–288.
5. Kishi Y, Kato M, Okuyama T, et al. Delirium: patient characteristics that predict a missed diagnosis at psychiatric consultation. *Gen Hosp Psychiatry.* 2007;29(5):442–445.
6. Bruce AJ, Ritchie CW, Blizard R, Lai R, Raven P. The incidence of delirium associated with orthopedic surgery: a meta-analytic review. *Int Psychogeriatr.* 2007;19(2):197–214.
7. Milisen K, Foreman MD, Godderis J, Abraham IL, Broos PL. Delirium in the hospitalized elderly: nursing assessment and management. *Nurs Clin North Am.* 1998;33(3):417–439.
8. Schuurmans M. The measurement of delirium: review of scales. *Res Theory Nurs Pract.* 2003;17(3):207–224.
9. Pompei P, Foreman M, Rudberg MA, Inouye SK, Braund V, Cassel CK. Delirium in hospitalized older persons: outcomes and predictors. *J Am Geriatr Soc.* 1994;42(8):809–815.
10. Inouye SK. Delirium in older persons. *N Engl J Med.* 2006; 354(11):1157–1165.
11. Fann JR, Alfano CM, Burington BE, Roth-Roemer S, Katon WJ, Syrjala KL. Clinical presentation of delirium in patients undergoing hematopoietic stem cell transplantation. *Cancer.* 2005; 103(4):810–820.
12. Breitbart W, Bruera E, Chochinov H, Lynch M. Neuropsychiatric syndromes and psychological symptoms in patients with advanced cancer. *J Pain Symptom Manage.* 1995;10(2):131–141.
13. Lawlor PG, Gagnon B, Mancini IL, et al. Occurrence, causes, and outcome of delirium in patients with advanced cancer: a prospective study. *Arch Intern Med.* 2000;160(6):786–794.
14. Leonard M, Agar M, Mason C, Lawlor P. Delirium issues in palliative care settings. *J Psychosom Res.* 2008;65(3):289–298.
15. Brauer C, Morrison RS, Silberzweig SB, Siu AL. The cause of delirium in patients with hip fracture. *Arch Intern Med.* 2000;160(12):1856–1860.
16. Kagansky N, Rimon E, Naor S, Dvornikov E, Cojocaru L, Levy S. Low incidence of delirium in very old patients after surgery for hip fractures. *Am J Geriatr Psychiatry.* 2004;12(3):306–314.
17. Kalisvaart K. Haloperidol prophylaxis for elderly hip-surgery patients at risk for delirium: a randomized placebo-controlled study. *J Am Geriatr Soc.* 2005;53:1658–1666.
18. Marcantonio ER, Juarez G, Goldman L, et al. The relationship of postoperative delirium with psychoactive medications. *JAMA.* 1994;272(19):1518–1522.
19. Morrison RS, Magaziner J, Gilbert M, et al. Relationship between pain and opioid analgesics on the development of delirium following hip fracture. *J Gerontol A Biol Sci Med Sci.* 2003;58(1):76–81.
20. Lawlor PG, Fainsinger RL, Bruera ED. Delirium at the end of life: critical issues in clinical practice and research. *JAMA.* 2000;284(19):2427–2429.
21. Gagnon B. Delirium in terminal cancer; a prospective study using daily screening, early diagnosis, and continuous monitoring. *J Pain Symptom Manage.* 2000;19(6):412–426.
22. Massie MJ, Holland J, Glass E. Delirium in terminally ill cancer patients. *Am J Psychiatry.* 1983;140(8):1048–1050.
23. Nowels D. Estimation of confusion prevalence in hospice patients. *J Palliat Med.* 2002;5(5):687–695.
24. Irwin SA, Rao S, Bower KA, et al. Psychiatric issues in palliative care: recognition of delirium in patients enrolled in hospice care. *Palliat Support Care.* 2008;6(2):159–164.
25. Witlox J, Eurelings LS, de Jonghe JF, Kalisvaart KJ, Eikelenboom P, van Gool WA. Delirium in elderly patients and the risk of postdischarge mortality, institutionalization, and dementia: a meta-analysis. *JAMA.* 2010;304(4):443–451.
26. Siddiqi N, House AO, Holmes JD. Occurrence and outcome of delirium in medical in-patients: a systematic literature review. *Age Ageing.* 2006;35(4):350–364.
27. Bickel H, Gradinger R, Kochs E, Forstl H. High risk of cognitive and functional decline after postoperative delirium: a three-year prospective study. *Dement Geriatr Cogn Disord.* 2008;26(1):26–31.
28. Leslie DL, Marcantonio ER, Zhang Y, Leo-Summers L, Inouye SK. One-year health care costs associated with delirium in the elderly population. *Arch Intern Med.* 2008;168(1):27–32.
29. Marcantonio ER, Kiely DK, Simon SE, et al. Outcomes of older people admitted to postacute facilities with delirium. *J Am Geriatr Soc.* 2005;53(6):963–969.
30. Fong TG, Jones RN, Shi P, et al. Delirium accelerates cognitive decline in Alzheimer disease. *Neurology.* 2009;72(18): 1570–1575.
31. Fleminger S. Remembering delirium. *Br J Psychiatry.* 2002; 180:4–5.
32. Griffiths RD, Jones C. Delirium, cognitive dysfunction and posttraumatic stress disorder. *Curr Opin Anaesthesiol.* 2007;20(2):124–129.
33. DiMartini A, Dew MA, Kormos R, McCurry K, Fontes P. Posttraumatic stress disorder caused by hallucinations and delusions experienced in delirium. *Psychosomatics.* 2007;48(5): 436–439.
34. Bruera E, Bush SH, Willey J, et al. Impact of delirium and recall on the level of distress in patients with advanced cancer and their family caregivers. *Cancer.* 2009;115(9):2004–2012.
35. McCusker J, Cole M, Abrahamowicz M, Primeau F, Belzile E. Delirium predicts 12-month mortality. *Arch Intern Med.* 2002;162(4):457–463.
36. O'Malley G, Leonard M, Mcagher D, O'Keeffe ST. The delirium experience: a review. *J Psychosom Res.* 2008;65(3):223–228.
37. Breitbart W, Gibson C, Tremblay A. The delirium experience: delirium recall and delirium-related distress in hospitalized patients with cancer, their spouses/caregivers, and their nurses. *Psychosomatics.* 2002;43(3):183–194.
38. Hui D, Bush SH, Gallo LE, Palmer JL, Yennurajalingam S, Bruera E. Neuroleptic dose in the management of delirium in patients with advanced cancer. *J Pain Symptom Manage.* 2010;39(2):186–196.
39. Morita T, Akechi T, Ikenaga M, et al. Terminal delirium: recommendations from bereaved families' experiences. *J Pain Symptom Manage.* 2007;34(6):579–589.
40. Morita T, Hirai K, Sakaguchi Y, Tsuneto S, Shima Y. Family-perceived distress from delirium-related symptoms of terminally ill cancer patients. *Psychosomatics.* 2004;45(2):107–113.
41. Buss MK, Vanderwerker LC, Inouye SK, Zhang B, Block SD, Prigerson HG. Associations between caregiver-perceived delirium in patients with cancer and generalized anxiety in their caregivers. *J Palliat Med.* 2007;10(5):1083–1092.
42. Mercadante S, Porzio G, Valle A, Fusco F, Aielli F, Costanzo V. Palliative sedation in patients with advanced cancer followed at home: a systematic review. *J Pain Symptom Manage.* 2011;41(4):754–760.
43. Mittal V, Muralee S, Williamson D, et al. Delirium in the elderly: a comprehensive review. *Am J Alzheimers Dis Other Demen.* 2011;26(2):97–109.
44. Maldonado JR. Pathoetiological model of delirium: a comprehensive understanding of the neurobiology of delirium and an evidence-based approach to prevention and treatment. *Crit Care Clin.* 2008;24(4):789–856 ix.
45. Trzepacz PT. Is there a final common neural pathway in delirium? Focus on acetylcholine and dopamine. *Semin Clin Neuropsychiatry.* 2000;5(2):132–148.
46. Murray AM, Levkoff SE, Wetle TT, et al. Acute delirium and functional decline in the hospitalized elderly patient. *J Gerontol.* 1993;48(5):M181–M186.
47. Hshieh TT, Fong TG, Marcantonio ER, Inouye SK. Cholinergic deficiency hypothesis in delirium: a synthesis of current evidence. *J Gerontol A Biol Sci Med Sci.* 2008;63(7):764–772.
48. Han L, McCusker J, Cole M, Abrahamowicz M, Primeau F, Elie M. Use of medications with anticholinergic effect predicts clinical severity of delirium symptoms in older medical inpatients. *Arch Intern Med.* 23 2001;161(8):1099–1105.

49. Campbell N, Boustani MA, Ayub A, et al. Pharmacological management of delirium in hospitalized adults: a systematic evidence review. *J Gen Intern Med.* 2009;24(7):848–853.

50. Yager JR, Magnotta VA, Mills JA, et al. Proton magnetic resonance spectroscopy in adult cancer patients with delirium. *Psychiatry Res.* 2011;191(2):128–132.

51. Shigeta H, Yasui A, Nimura Y, et al. Postoperative delirium and melatonin levels in elderly patients. *Am J Surg.* 2001;182(5):449–454.

52. Maclullich AM, Ferguson KJ, Miller T, de Rooij SE, Cunningham C. Unravelling the pathophysiology of delirium: a focus on the role of aberrant stress responses. *J Psychosom Res.* 2008;65(3):229–238.

53. Soiza RL, Sharma V, Ferguson K, Shenkin SD, Seymour DG, Maclullich AM. Neuroimaging studies of delirium: a systematic review. *J Psychosom Res.* 2008;65(3):239–248.

54. Rudolph JL, Ramlawi B, Kuchel GA, et al. Chemokines are associated with delirium after cardiac surgery. *J Gerontol A Biol Sci Med Sci.* 2008;63(2):184–189.

55. Fricchione GL, Nejad SH, Esses JA, et al. Postoperative delirium. *Am J Psychiatry.* 2008;165(7):803–812.

56. Ebersoldt M, Sharshar T, Annane D. Sepsis-associated delirium. *Intensive Care Med.* 2007;33(6):941–950.

57. Hempenius L, van Leeuwen BL, van Asselt DZ, et al. Structured analyses of interventions to prevent delirium. *Int J Geriatr Psychiatry.* 2011;26(5):441–450.

58. Elie M, Cole MG, Primeau FJ, Bellavance F. Delirium risk factors in elderly hospitalized patients. *J Gen Intern Med.* 1998;13(3):204–212.

59. Inouye SK. Predisposing and precipitating factors for delirium in hospitalized older patients. *Dement Geriatr Cogn Disord.* 1999;10(5):393–400.

60. Noimark D. Predicting the onset of delirium in the post-operative patient. *Age Ageing.* 2009;38(4):368–373.

61. Inouye SK, Charpentier PA. Precipitating factors for delirium in hospitalized elderly persons: predictive model and interrelationship with baseline vulnerability. *JAMA.* 1996;275(11):852–857.

62. Marcantonio ER, Goldman L, Mangione CM, et al. A clinical prediction rule for delirium after elective noncardiac surgery. *JAMA.* 1994;271(2):134–139.

63. Rudolph JL, Jones RN, Levkoff SE, et al. Derivation and validation of a preoperative prediction rule for delirium after cardiac surgery. *Circulation.* 2009;119(2):229–236.

64. Yang FM, Marcantonio ER, Inouye SK, et al. Phenomenological subtypes of delirium in older persons: patterns, prevalence, and prognosis. *Psychosomatics.* 2009;50(3):248–254.

65. Leonard M, Spiller J, Keen J, MacLullich A, Kamholtz B, Meagher D. Symptoms of depression and delirium assessed serially in palliative-care inpatients. *Psychosomatics.* 2009;50(5):506–514.

66. Wong CL, Holroyd-Leduc J, Simel DL, Straus SE. Does this patient have delirium? Value of bedside instruments. *JAMA.* 2010;304(7):779–786.

67. Adamis D, Sharma N, Whelan PJ, Macdonald AJ. Delirium scales: a review of current evidence. *Aging Ment Health.* 2010;14(5):543–555.

68. Chochinov HM, Wilson KG, Enns M, Lander S. "Are you depressed?" Screening for depression in the terminally ill. *Am J Psychiatry.* 1997;154(5):674–676.

69. Sands MB, Dantoc BP, Hartshorn A, Ryan CJ, Lujic S. Single Question in Delirium (SQiD): testing its efficacy against psychiatrist interview: the Confusion Assessment Method and the Memorial Delirium Assessment Scale. *Palliat Med.* 2010;24(6):561–565.

70. Amos JJ, Robinson RG, eds. *Psychosomatic Medicine: An Introduction to Consultation-Liason Psychiatry.* Cambridge: Cambridge University Press; 2010: 66.

71. Buss MK VL, Inouye SK, Zhang B, Block SD, Prigerson HD. Associations between caregiver-perceived delirium in cancer patients and generalized anxiety in their caregivers. *J Palliat Med.* 2007;10(5):1083–1092.

72. Breitbart W, Marotta R, Platt MM, et al. A double-blind trial of haloperidol, chlorpromazine, and lorazepam in the treatment of delirium in hospitalized AIDS patients. *Am J Psychiatry.* 1996;153(2):231–237.

73. Maldonado JR. Delirium in the acute care setting: characteristics, diagnosis and treatment. *Crit Care Clin.* 2008;24(4):657–722, vii.

74. Kehl KA. Treatment of terminal restlessness: a review of the evidence. *J Pain Palliat Care Pharmacother.* 2004; 18(1):5–30.

75. Platt MM, Breitbart W, Smith M, Marotta R, Weisman H, Jacobsen PB. Efficacy of neuroleptics for hypoactive delirium. *J Neuropsychiatry Clin Neurosci.* 1994;6(1):66–67.

76. Gagnon P, Allard P, Gagnon B, Merette C, Tardif F. Delirium prevention in terminal cancer: assessment of a multicomponent intervention. *Psychooncology.* 2012;21(2):187–194.

Chapter 36

What Pharmacological Treatments Are Effective for Delirium?

MICHELLE T. WECKMANN AND R. SEAN MORRISON

INTRODUCTION AND SCOPE OF THE PROBLEM

Delirium is an acute confusional state characterized by an alteration of consciousness with reduced ability to focus, sustain, or shift attention, resulting in cognitive failure. Delirium develops over a short time (usually hours to days) and tends to fluctuate during the course of the day. Delirium is typically caused by a medical condition, substance intoxication, or medication side effect. It is chiefly a cognitive disorder and often has associated emotional and behavioral components that can range from extreme lability and agitation to a loss of affect and extreme somnolence.

Delirium is the most common psychiatric disorder among patients with severe medical illness and particularly among older patients. It is not surprising that delirium is common in older patients because it is a multifactorial disorder. Factors that increase the risk for delirium can be classified into those that increase baseline vulnerability (predisposing factors) and those that precipitate the disorder (precipitating factors). Table 36-1 shows predisposing and precipitating factors related to the development of delirium.

Delirium can be difficult to recognize, and clinicians should maintain a high index of suspicion. In reality, delirium is frequently missed or misdiagnosed, particularly in younger patients.[1] Much of our knowledge of delirium comes from observational studies because systemic studies and clinical trials are difficult to perform in patients with cognitive impairment (i.e., delirium); therefore the management of delirium is primarily based on expert consensus and observational studies. No medications are approved by the Food and Drug Administration (FDA) for the treatment of delirium, and few randomized, controlled trials have been conducted.

RELEVANT PATHOPHYSIOLOGY

The pathophysiology of delirium is not yet fully understood. The neurotransmitters and receptors involved in wakefulness and consciousness are thought to be involved; these include acetylcholine, dopamine, norepinephrine, serotonin, histamine, orexin, and γ-aminobutyrie acid.[2] Additionally, acetylcholine depletion and dopamine excess are believed to play a critical role in the development of delirium[3,4] and a majority of the pharmacological trials have involved manipulation of those two neurotransmitters.

SUMMARY OF EVIDENCE REGARDING TREATMENT RECOMMENDATIONS

Prevention and therapy involve four basic principles: (1) avoid factors known to cause or aggravate delirium, (2) identify and treat underlying illness, (3) provide support and restorative care to prevent further physical and cognitive decline, and (4) control dangerous and disruptive behaviors. With the exception of identify and treat the underlying illness, these principles always should be applied to patients with delirium. In general, patients and families want the underlying medical illness identified and treated, but occasionally (e.g., when the patient is actively dying) the goals of care may be focused solely on comfort and thus identification of underlying causes of delirium will be more burdensome than beneficial and should not be undertaken. A more complete discussion of terminal delirium can be found in Chapter 38.

Prevention Strategies

Interventions to reduce the risk for developing delirium by managing modifiable risk factors are effective.[5] Delirium interventions are typically multicomponent and use standardized protocols to screen and control for risk factors. Sample elements of these interventions include orientation protocols, environmental modifications, nonpharmacological sleep aides, early mobilization, visual and hearing aides (if needed), oral volume repletion, staff education about delirium, and medication review.[6–9]

Prophylactic use of cholinesterase inhibitors has been proposed to prevent delirium, but clinical trials have not supported their use in either the prevention or treatment of delirium.[10–12] Studies have examined the use of antipsychotic agents (haloperidol, risperidone, olanzapine) and anticonvulsants (specifically

TABLE 36-1. Precipitating and Predisposing Factors for Delirium

Precipitating Factors

Medications (polypharmacy, anticholinergics, opioids, benzodiazepines)

Infection

Metabolic disturbances

Dehydration

Immobility (restraints, intravenous lines, catheters)

Malnutrition

Untreated pain and inadequate analgesia

Being in an intensive care unit

Increased number of room changes

Predisposing Factors

Cognitive impairment (dementia, Parkinson disease, stroke)

Advanced age

Need for surgery

Psychiatric symptoms

Medical comorbidity

Poor renal or liver function

Sensory impairment (hearing and vision loss)

Advanced cancer

Being near death

Data from References 53–58.

gabapentin) for the prevention of delirium. Although many of these agents look promising, the evidence is not yet sufficiently strong to support their routine use as a preventive measure for patients at high risk for developing delirium.[13–16]

Initial Delirium Treatment

Initial treatment of delirium should begin with providing support and education to the patient and family and initiation of nonpharmacological interventions (discussed in detail in Chapter 37). The presence and meaning of the delirium should be discussed in the context of the underlying medical comorbidities, overall prognosis, and patient and family goals. If desired, initial workup should be undertaken to find reversible medical causes of the delirium. Delirium can be reversed 50% to 80% of the time in patients with terminal illnesses[17,18] and studies of delirium incidence have shown that a certain percentage resolves spontaneously without intervention beyond standard medical care. If reversible causes are found, it is common to treat those and not initiate additional medications unless the associated behaviors of delirium are problematic. The most frequent reason to initiate a pharmacological agent is agitation, followed by disturbing hallucinations.[19,20]

Management of Agitation in Delirium

Managing disruptive behavior (commonly termed hyperactive delirium) is often the most challenging aspect of delirium therapy. Hyperactive delirium is more common in younger patients. In older patients, delirium tends to be hypoactive or mixed (patients fluctuate between being agitated and being somnolent).[21,22] Hyperactive behaviors can put both the patient and caregivers at risk for injury. These behaviors can be difficult to control, but, if at all possible, physical restraints should be avoided because they have been shown to worsen and prolong delirium.[23] Mild agitation can be controlled with nonpharmacological measures, and frequent reassurances, touch, and verbal orientation from familiar persons have been shown beneficial. If the patient is a danger to self or others, or the symptoms of delirium are very distressing for the patient or family, a cautious trial of an antipsychotic agent might be indicated.

Antipsychotic Agents for Delirium

Unfortunately, limited data are available to guide antipsychotic use or dosing. Numerous studies have been performed, but most are of poor quality because of the methods used and small sample size. Based on available evidence, most guidelines and specialists recommend that haloperidol be used for the management of delirium-associated agitation or distress (with the exception of delirium in Parkinson disease, in which an atypical antipsychotic, such as quetiapine should be used).[24] Typical starting doses of haloperidol are 2 mg (orally, intramuscularly, intravenously, subcutaneously) for mild agitation, 5 mg for moderate agitation, and 7.5 to 10 mg for severe agitation. In the elderly, doses should be reduced to approximately one third (i.e., 0.5-1 mg in mild agitation). Doses should be repeated every 30 minutes until the patient is calm yet arousable to normal voice. When serious agitation persists, the previous dosage can be doubled 30 minutes later; this approach of successful doubling can be repeated. The goal is to treat the agitation as any breakthrough symptom would be treated, to get the agitation under control as quickly as possible, because some evidence indicates that partial treatment may prolong the delirium.[25] When symptom control is achieved, the amount of drug used in 24 hours should be calculated and that dose given either once per day or divided twice daily. If the agitation is difficult to control with haloperidol alone, the addition of lorazepam (1-2 mg every 2-4 hours) can be beneficial because lorazepam may reduce the extrapyramidal side effects of haloperidol.[26,27]

Patients should have at least two normal assessments (no evidence of delirium) before an attempt is made to discontinue antipsychotics. Ideally, the antipsychotic dose should be slowly decreased over 5 to 7 days, monitoring closely for signs of delirium recurrence. If the delirium recurs, the antipsychotic should be increased to the last effective dose and remain at that dose until the patient again experiences a delirium-free period. It is important to remember that resolution of delirium can lag behind resolution of the medical condition, particularly in patients with underlying dementia. This time lag is often unappreciated by clinicians, and it is not uncommon for a physician to declare a patient better despite evidence of a residual delirium. Discharging a patient with partially resolved delirium increases the burden on caregivers and increases the risk for placement in an institution outside of the home.[28,29]

Small studies examining the newer atypical antipsychotic agents (quetiapine, risperidone, ziprasidone, aripiprazole, olanzapine) appear to show efficacy similar to that of haloperidol, with possibly fewer side effects.[24,30–36] Currently, insufficient evidence exists to recommend use of atypical antipsychotics over more traditional agents. Caution must be exercised when using antipsychotics with a higher anticholinergic effect (e.g., chlorpromazine, olanzapine) because data indicate that these agents can precipitate delirium.[37,38] Table 36-2 summarizes typical and atypical antipsychotic doses and side effects.

Hypoactive delirium has the potential to cause just as much distress to patients and families as agitated delirium and may have a worse overall prognosis, but less evidence is available to guide pharmacological treatment. Psychostimulants have been used with some success to increase alertness and improve mental function in patients with hypoactive delirium; however, insufficient data exist to recommend their routine use.[39,40] Haloperidol (in similar doses) appears to be the most effective option and should be tried first.[41,42]

Potential Risks of Antipsychotic Agents

Antipsychotics have numerous side effects related to their receptor profiles. All can cause a rare condition called neuromalignant syndrome, characterized by fever, rigidity, and catatonia. Additionally, alternation to the cardiac conduction system is a serious side effect seen with all antipsychotics. It has long been known that antipsychotics, including haloperidol, can cause a dose-dependent increase in QTc prolongation that can increase the risk for sudden death.[43] A meta-analysis showed an increased risk for sudden death of elderly patients with dementia who were treated with antipsychotics.[44] It was shown that use of atypical antipsychotics for more than 8 to 12 weeks resulted in a small increased risk for death (odds ratio, 1.6-1.7), which was revealed only when trials were pooled. The risk seen was equal to 1 death in the group treated with atypical antipsychotics for every 100 patients who received that treatment for 10 to 12 weeks, leading to a risk ratio of 1.5, which was believed to be true across all atypical antipsychotics and is likely also true for typical antipsychotics.[45] This finding prompted the FDA to add a black box warning to all antipsychotics detailing the risk for increased cardiovascular adverse events and death in elderly patients with dementia. However, in a study of 326 elderly patients with delirium, antipsychotic use was not associated with increased mortality.[46] Currently, electrocardiographic monitoring is recommended before initiation of a long-term, high-dose antipsychotic, but it

is not yet the standard of care. Literature supports electrocardiographic monitoring before haloperidol administration, with consideration to not initiating treatment if the QTc interval is greater than 450 msec and discontinuation of treatment if the QTc increases 25% over baseline after treatment is initiated. The choice to obtain an electrocardiogram to guide treatment should be viewed in the context of the patient's overall condition, prognosis, expected mortality, distress level, and goals of care. Usually the benefits of treating delirium outweigh the risks.

Other known complications of using antipsychotics include extrapyramidal symptoms and sedation; however, most occur when high doses of antipsychotics are used for prolonged periods. Extrapyramidal symptoms have been seen when haloperidol is used for treatment of delirium in doses greater than 4.5 mg per day, but it is typically described as mild and resolves when treatment is discontinued.

Use of Benzodiazepines

It is not uncommon for an antipsychotic alone to be insufficient to control delirium-related agitation. In the case of agitated delirium refractory to antipsychotic therapy, it is recommended practice to add a sedating agent. Benzodiazepines are frequently used for this purpose, and lorazepam is most frequently used.[47] Lorazepam can be given by the oral, subcutaneous, parenteral, and intramuscular routes. Common starting doses are 0.5 to 2 mg orally every hour as needed. Much like haloperidol, the dose or lorazepam can be doubled every 30 minutes until effective. When an effective dose is achieved it can be repeated every 3 to 4 hours as needed. Of note, benzodiazepines used alone without an antipsychotic agent have been shown to increase the severity of delirium and precipitate delirium in the elderly.[48–50]

Sedation for Refractory Delirium

Delirium is an independent prognostic sign of a shortened life expectancy and a common reason for patients and families to request palliative sedation.[51] When the symptoms of distressing, agitated delirium cannot be controlled with a combination of antipsychotics and benzodiazepines, it is reasonable to consider a deeper means of sedation. Before initiating sedation it is important to have a conversation with the family to elicit goals and explain the irreversible and terminal nature of the delirium. The goal of sedation is symptom control; therefore it should be achieved with the minimally effective doses necessary. It is possible to induce and maintain sedation without shortening life, and this point should be made clear to families when discussing the use of sedation.[52] Common medications for deeper sedation include phenobarbital and propofol. Additional details can be found in Chapter 38.

TABLE 36-2. Suggested Antipsychotic Doses for Older Patients With Delirium*

AGENT	ADVANTAGES	DISADVANTAGES	ONSET OF ACTION	STARTING DOSE	USUAL DAILY DOSE	SIDE EFFECTS
Haloperidol	*Routes:* PO, IM, IV, subcutaneous, liquid Can decrease nausea Less sedation	May cause restlessness or EPS in doses >4.5 mg PO q24h (few to no EPS with subcutaneous or IV administration)	*PO:* 30-60 min *IV, subcutaneously:* 5-15 min	0.5-1 mg q1h prn	1-5 mg over 24 hr	Increased risk for death in older patients with dementia
Chlorpromazine	*Routes:* PO, rectal, IM, IV, subcutaneous, liquid Can decrease nausea and treat hiccups	Can cause sedation, confusion, falls, dry mouth, hypotension May precipitate delirium	*PO:* 30-60 min *IV, subcutaneously:* 15-30 min	*PO:* 25-50 mg q1h prn *Subcutaneously:* 5-10 mg q30min	*PO:* 50 mg tid *Subcutaneously:* 5-50 mg/hr	Hypotension, constipation, and dry mouth more common NMS and prolonged QTc rare Irritating for the skin when given subcutaneously (flushing site daily with 1 mg of dexamethasone can decrease irritation)
Risperidone	*Routes:* PO, IM, liquid, oral dissolving tablet	EPS	30-60 min	0.5-1 mg q1h prn	1 mg bid	Increased risk for death in older patients with dementia
Olanzapine	*Routes:* PO, IM, oral dissolving tablet May decrease nausea, pain, and oral secretions May increase appetite	Can cause sedation, confusion, and hypotension	30-60 min	2.5-5 mg q1h prn	5 mg bid	Increased risk for sudden cardiac death, dizziness, and insomnia Metabolic dysfunction, hyperglycemia
Quetiapine	*Route:* PO May decrease oral secretions May be best option in patients with Parkinson disease Least amount of EPS	Can cause sedation, confusion, and hypotension	30-60 min	12.5-25 mg q1h prn	50 mg bid	Increased risk for death in older patients with dementia
Aripiprazole	*Routes:* PO, IM, liquid, oral dissolving tablet May improve cognition and attention	Minimally sedating	30-60 min	5 mg q1h prn	10 mg daily	Negligible QTc prolongation Increased risk for death in older patients

EPS, extrapyramidal symptoms; *IM,* intramuscularly; *IV,* intravenously; *NMS,* neuromalignant syndrome; *prn,* as needed; *tid,* three times a day.
* Effective doses are often higher in younger patients. Note that all antipsychotic medications have a risk for QTc prolongation and NMS. See text for precautions in the use of these medications. *bid,* Twice daily;

KEY MESSAGES TO PATIENTS AND FAMILIES

Confusion is a medical emergency and should not be ignored, because it can be successfully treated even in the last weeks of life. The most common cause of confusion is delirium, which is cognitive failure associated with medical illness. Delirium can complicate care and is often distressing to both the patient and the family. Agitation is a common symptom of delirium and can usually be managed with an antipsychotic medication, such as haloperidol. Antipsychotic medications do have side effects, but the side effects from untreated delirium are often worse. If the antipsychotic alone is unsuccessful at controlling the agitation, a second sedating agent, lorazepam, can be added. Sometimes clinicians are unable to control the symptoms of delirium with usual treatments; in these cases, use of stronger medications should be discussed that have the side effect of sedation such that the patient will be unable to eat or talk.

CONCLUSION AND SUMMARY

Delirium is an acute confusional state characterized by alteration of consciousness with reduced ability to focus, sustain, or shift attention. It is distressing to the patient and family and has significant short-term and long-term complications. Treatment should be determined in the context of the medical condition, prognosis, and goals of care. When delirium cannot be reversed by nonpharmacological treatment or treatment of the underlying medical cause, or dangerous agitation is present, antipsychotics should be used, with haloperidol being the preferred agent. Atypical antipsychotics are increasingly regarded to be of equal efficacy, but the lack of a parenteral route and cost limits their use in advanced disease. Antipsychotic medications have numerous potentially life-limiting side effects, so caution is warranted in their use.

SUMMARY RECOMMENDATIONS

- Delirium treatment is effective, even at the end of life.
- Initial delirium treatment should involve non-pharmacological management strategies, clarification of patient and family goals, and reversal of the underlying cause if possible.
- Delirium that does not resolve with conservative measures or has dangerous (or distressing) symptoms, such as agitation, should be aggressively treated using antipsychotics, with haloperidol being the agent of choice.
- Delirium that is difficult to treat may require a combination of both an antipsychotic and a benzodiazepine for symptom control.
- Some of the medications used to treat delirium have serious side effects (including death), so clinicians must be clear that the benefits of these medications outweigh their risks when employing their use in patients with advanced illness.

REFERENCES

1. Wada T, Wada M, Onishi H. Characteristics, interventions, and outcomes of misdiagnosed delirium in cancer patients. *Palliat Support Care.* 2010;8(2):125–131.
2. Caraceni A, Simonetti F. Palliating delirium in patients with cancer. *Lancet Oncol.* 2009;10(2):164–172.
3. Trzepacz PT. Anticholinergic model for delirium. *Semin Clin Neuropsychiatry.* 1996;1(4):294–303.
4. Trzepacz PT. Is there a final common neural pathway in delirium? Focus on acetylcholine and dopamine. *Semin Clin Neuropsychiatry.* 2000;5(2):132–148.
5. Hempenius L, van Leeuwen BL, van Asselt DZ, et al. Structured analyses of interventions to prevent delirium. *Int J Geriatr Psychiatry.* 2011;26(5):441–450.
6. Inouye SK, Bogardus Jr ST, Charpentier PA, et al. A multicomponent intervention to prevent delirium in hospitalized older patients. *N Engl J Med.* 1999;340(9):669–676.
7. Caplan GA, Harper EL. Recruitment of volunteers to improve vitality in the elderly: the REVIVE study. *Intern Med J.* 2007;37(2):95–100.
8. Wong CP, Chiu PK, Chu LW. Zopiclone withdrawal: an unusual cause of delirium in the elderly. *Age Ageing.* 2005;34(5):526–527.
9. Tabet N, Hudson S, Sweeney V, et al. An educational intervention can prevent delirium on acute medical wards. *Age Ageing.* 2005;34(2):152–156.
10. Sampson EL, Raven PR, Ndhlovu PN, et al. A randomized, double-blind, placebo-controlled trial of donepezil hydrochloride (Aricept) for reducing the incidence of postoperative delirium after elective total hip replacement. *Int J Geriatr Psychiatry.* 2007;22(4):343–349.
11. Gamberini M, Bolliger D, Lurati Buse GA, et al. Rivastigmine for the prevention of postoperative delirium in elderly patients undergoing elective cardiac surgery: a randomized controlled trial. *Crit Care Med.* 2009;37(5):1762–1768.
12. Liptzin B, Laki A, Garb JL, Fingeroth R, Krushell R. Donepezil in the prevention and treatment of post-surgical delirium. *Am J Geriatr Psychiatry.* 2005;13(12):1100–1106.
13. Kalisvaart K. Haloperidol prophylaxis for elderly hip-surgery patients at risk for delirium: a randomized placebo-controlled study. *J Am Geriatr Soc.* 2005;53:1658–1666.
14. Leung JM, Sands LP, Rico M, et al. Pilot clinical trial of gabapentin to decrease postoperative delirium in older patients. *Neurology.* 2006;67(7):1251–1253.
15. Prakanrattana U, Prapaitrakool S. Efficacy of risperidone for prevention of postoperative delirium in cardiac surgery. *Anaesth Intensive Care.* 2007;35(5):714–719.
16. Larsen KA, Kelly SE, Stern TA, et al. Administration of olanzapine to prevent postoperative delirium in elderly joint-replacement patients: a randomized, controlled trial. *Psychosomatics.* 2010;51(5):409–418.
17. Lawlor PG, Gagnon B, Mancini IL, et al. Occurrence, causes, and outcome of delirium in patients with advanced cancer: a prospective study. *Arch Intern Med.* 2000;160(6):786–794.
18. Ljubisavljevic V, Kelly B. Risk factors for development of delirium among oncology patients. *Gen Hosp Psychiatry.* 2003; 25(5):345–352.
19. Someya T, Endo T, Hara T, Yagi G, Suzuki J. A survey on the drug therapy for delirium. *Psychiatry Clin Neurosci.* 2001;55(4):397–401.
20. Hui D, Bush SH, Gallo LE, Palmer JL, Yennurajalingam S, Bruera E. Neuroleptic dose in the management of delirium in patients with advanced cancer. *J Pain Symptom Manage.* 2010;39(2):186–196.
21. Peterson J. Delirium and its motoric subtypes: a study of 614 critically ill patients. *J Am Geriatr Soc.* 2006;54(3):479–484.
22. Yang FM, Marcantonio ER, Inouye SK, et al. Phenomenological subtypes of delirium in older persons: patterns, prevalence, and prognosis. *Psychosomatics.* 2009;50(3):248–254.
23. Inouye SK, Charpentier PA. Precipitating factors for delirium in hospitalized elderly persons: predictive model and interrelationship with baseline vulnerability. *JAMA.* 1996;275(11): 852–857.
24. Lonergan E, Britton AM, Luxenberg J, Wyller T. Antipsychotics for delirium. *Cochrane Database Syst Rev.* 2007;(2): CD005594.
25. Amos JJ, Robinson RG, eds. *Psychosomatic Medicine: An Introduction to Consultation-Liason Psychiatry.* Cambridge: Cambride University Press; 2010: 68–69.

26. Menza MA, Murray GB, Holmes VF, Rafuls WA. Decreased extrapyramidal symptoms with intravenous haloperidol. *J Clin Psychiatry*. 1987;48(7):278–280.

27. Adams F, Fernandez F, Andersson BS. Emergency pharmacotherapy of delirium in the critically ill cancer patient. *Psychosomatics*. 1986;27(1 suppl):33–38.

28. Witlox J, Eurelings LS, de Jonghe JF, Kalisvaart KJ, Eikelenboom P, van Gool WA. Delirium in elderly patients and the risk of postdischarge mortality, institutionalization, and dementia: a meta-analysis. *JAMA*. 2010;304(4):443–451.

29. Kat MG, Vreeswijk R, de Jonghe JF, et al. Long-term cognitive outcome of delirium in elderly hip surgery patients: a prospective matched controlled study over two and a half years. *Dement Geriatr Cogn Disord*. 2008;26(1):1–8.

30. Parellada E, Baeza I, de Pablo J, Martinez G. Risperidone in the treatment of patients with delirium. *J Clin Psychiatry*. 2004;65(3):348–353.

31. Skrobik YK, Bergeron N, Dumont M, Gottfried SB. Olanzapine vs haloperidol: treating delirium in a critical care setting. *Intensive Care Med*. 2004;30(3):444–449.

32. Devlin JW, Roberts RJ, Fong JJ, et al. Efficacy and safety of quetiapine in critically ill patients with delirium: a prospective, multicenter, randomized, double-blind, placebo-controlled pilot study. *Crit Care Med*. 2010;38(2):419–427.

33. Horikawa N, Yamazaki T, Miyamoto K, et al. Treatment for delirium with risperidone: results of a prospective open trial with 10 patients. *Gen Hosp Psychiatry*. 2003;25(4):289–292.

34. Alao AO, Soderberg M, Pohl EL, Koss M. Aripiprazole in the treatment of delirium. *Int J Psychiatry Med*.2005;35(4):429–433.

35. Sipahimalani A, Masand PS. Olanzapine in the treatment of delirium. *Psychosomatics*. 1998;39(5):422–430.

36. Han CS, Kim YK. A double-blind trial of risperidone and haloperidol for the treatment of delirium. *Psychosomatics*. 2004;45(4):297–301.

37. Lim CJ, Trevino C, Tampi RR. Can olanzapine cause delirium in the elderly? *Ann Pharmacother*. 2006;40(1):135–138.

38. Gaudreau JD, Gagnon P, Harel F, Roy MA, Tremblay A. Psychoactive medications and risk of delirium in hospitalized cancer patients. *J Clin Oncol*. 2005;23(27):6712–6718.

39. Stiefel F, Bruera E. Psychostimulants for hypoactive-hypoalert delirium? *J Palliat Care*. 1991;7(3):25–26.

40. Elie D, Gagnon P, Gagnon B, Giguere A. Using psychostimulants in end-of-life patients with hypoactive delirium and cognitive disorders: a literature review. *Can J Psychiatry*. 2010;55(6):386–393.

41. Platt MM, Breitbart W, Smith M, Marotta R, Weisman H, Jacobsen PB. Efficacy of neuroleptics for hypoactive delirium. *J Neuropsychiatry Clin Neurosci*. 1994;6(1):66–67.

42. Breitbart W, Marotta R, Platt MM, et al. A double-blind trial of haloperidol, chlorpromazine, and lorazepam in the treatment of delirium in hospitalized AIDS patients. *Am J Psychiatry*. 1996;153(2):231–237.

43. Zareba W, Lin DA. Antipsychotic drugs and QT interval prolongation. *Psychiatr Q*. 2003;74(3):291–306.

44. Schneider LS, Dagerman KS, Insel P. Risk of death with atypical antipsychotic drug treatment for dementia: meta-analysis of randomized placebo-controlled trials. *JAMA*. 2005;294(15):1934–1943.

45. Mittal V, Muralee S, Williamson D, et al. Delirium in the elderly: a comprehensive review. *Am J Alzheimers Dis Other Demen*. 2011;26(2):97–109.

46. Elie M, Boss K, Cole MG, McCusker J, Belzile E, Ciampi A. A retrospective, exploratory, secondary analysis of the association between antipsychotic use and mortality in elderly patients with delirium. *Int Psychogeriatr*. 2009;21(3):588–592.

47. Cook I. *Guideline Watch: Practice Guideline for the Treatment of Patients With Delirium*. Arlington, VA: American Psychiatric Association; 2004: 24–25.

48. Gandreu J. Psychoactive medications and risk of delirium in hospitalized cancer patients. *J Clin Oncol*. 2005;23(27):6712–6718.

49. Clegg A, Young JB. Which medications to avoid in people at risk of delirium: a systematic review. *Age Ageing*. 2011;40(1):23–29.

50. Pisani MA, Murphy TE, Araujo KL, Slattum P, Van Ness PH, Inouye SK. Benzodiazepine and opioid use and the duration of intensive care unit delirium in an older population. *Crit Care Med*. 2009;37(1):177–183.

51. Sykes N, Thorns A. Sedative use in the last week of life and the implications for end-of-life decision making. *Arch J Intern Med*. 2003;163(3):341–344.

52. Morita T, Chinone Y, Ikenaga M, et al. Efficacy and safety of palliative sedation therapy: a multicenter, prospective, observational study conducted on specialized palliative care units in Japan. *J Pain Symptom Manage*. 2005;30(4):320–328.

53. McCusker J, Cole M, Abrahamowicz M, Han L, Podoba JE, Ramman-Haddad L. Environmental risk factors for delirium in hospitalized older people. *J Am Geriatr Soc*. 2001;49(10):1327–1334.

54. Morrison RS, Magaziner J, Gilbert M, et al. Relationship between pain and opioid analgesics on the development of delirium following hip fracture. *J Gerontol A Biol Sci Med Sci*. 2003;58(1):76–81.

55. Pisani MA, Murphy TE, Van Ness PH, Araujo KL, Inouye SK. Characteristics associated with delirium in older patients in a medical intensive care unit. *Arch Intern Med*. 2007;167(15):1629–1634.

56. Robinson TN, Raeburn CD, Tran ZV, Angles EM, Brenner LA, Moss M. Postoperative delirium in the elderly: risk factors and outcomes. *Ann Surg*. 2009;249(1):173–178.

57. Rudolph JL, Jones RN, Rasmussen LS, Silverstein JH, Inouye SK, Marcantonio ER. Independent vascular and cognitive risk factors for postoperative delirium. *Am J Med*. 2007;120(9):807–813.

58. Inouye SK, Schlesinger MJ, Lydon TJ. Delirium: a symptom of how hospital care is failing older persons and a window to improve quality of hospital care. *Am J Med*. 1999;106(5):565–573.

Chapter 37

What Nonpharmacological Treatments Are Effective for Delirium?

Michelle T. Weckmann and R. Sean Morrison

INTRODUCTION AND SCOPE OF THE PROBLEM

Delirium is a highly prevalent and deleterious disorder in medically ill patients that affects large numbers of individuals each year. Delirium is chiefly a disturbance of cognition with associated changes in the ability to shift, focus, or maintain attention and fluctuating levels of consciousness. Other features commonly associated with delirium include behavioral changes such as restlessness, agitation, lethargy, reversed sleep–wake cycle, and affect changes such as irritability, emotional lability, anger, and euphoria. Given the range of symptoms in delirium it is not surprising that it generates a high degree of distress for patients, families, and clinicians.[1-4] Delirium is associated with a host of negative outcomes, including persistent functional and cognitive decline, longer hospital stays, higher rates of nursing home placement, increased health care costs, and higher mortality rates.[5-7]

Multiple studies examining the risk factors for delirium have had varied results, suggesting that different populations have different risks for developing delirium. The exceptions are advanced age and previously impaired cognition, which appear to place all patients at risk.[8] Table 37-1 details the delirium risk factors for various populations. In general, the risk factors for delirium fall into two categories: predisposing and precipitating. Predisposing factors are innate to the person and often hard to modify (these include age, presence of a cognitive deficit, medical disease severity, sensory deficits, gender). Precipitating factors are insults to the person that make it more likely delirium will develop (e.g., use of restraints, polypharmacy, infections, hip fractures). A combination of predisposing and precipitating factors determine a person's risk for developing delirium. The more predisposing factors a person has, the fewer precipitating factors that are needed to initiate an episode of delirium and vice versa. For example, an older patient with dementia and visual impairment may develop delirium with just a single insult (such as developing a urinary tract infection), whereas a younger patient without cognitive impairment may need a much bigger insult (e.g., developing the combination of urinary sepsis with hypotension and acute renal failure) before delirium develops.

RELEVANT PATHOPHYSIOLOGY

The pathophysiology of delirium is unknown, and many different hypotheses have been proposed, including involvement of the thalamus,[9] cholinergic deficiency,[10] dopamine excess,[11] impairment of cerebral oxidative metabolism,[12] and cellular damage resulting from neurotoxic and inflammatory agents.[13-15] The pathophysiology of delirium is likely multifactorial, much like its causes. Although some patients may develop delirium secondary to a single medical reason (e.g., the older patient with dementia who develops delirium after developing a urinary tract infection), they are in the minority. The majority of patients have multiple potential causes for their delirium. In a study of 571 older patients with hip fracture, the cause of delirium was attributed to one or more comorbid conditions 61% of the time.[16] Studies of inpatients with cancer show an average of two or three causes.[17,18] More detailed discussion of the causes of delirium can be found in Chapter 35.

Delirium is typically classified as hypoactive, hyperactive, or mixed, and these classifications have importance for detection, treatment, and outcome. Delirium often remains undetected. This is of particular importance in older patients and patients admitted to an inpatient palliative care unit, where hypoactive delirium is more common.[19-22] This lack of detection is important because hypoactive delirium has an increased mortality over hyperactive delirium.[20,21] Compared to hyperactive delirium, hypoactive delirium has the potential to cause as much, if not more, distress because it typically impairs a person's ability to communicate, and patients and family consistently rate being able to communicate and being mentally aware as critical elements at the end of life.[3,23] Detection of delirium can be improved by both staff education and instituting formal delirium screening,[24-26] potentially leading to earlier treatment and improved outcomes. The Confusion Assessment Methods (CAM)[27] is a validated and well-received

TABLE 37-1. Risk Factors for Developing Delirium*

RISK FACTOR TYPE	PATIENTS WITH CANCER	PATIENTS AT THE END OF LIFE	GENERAL MEDICAL INPATIENTS	POSTSURGICAL PATIENTS
Predisposing				
Advanced age	+[43,44]		+[8,45,46]	+[8,47,48]
Gender	+[44]		+[46]	+[49]
Previously impaired cognition	+[43,50]		+[8,45,46]	+[8,16,48,49,51]
Severity of illness		+[52]	+[8,46]	+[48]
Previous delirium	+[53]		+[46]	+[45,54]
Depression		+[55]	+[46]	+[48,51]
Sensory deficits (visual or hearing impairment)			+[8,46]	+[16,48]
Functional impairment			+[8,46]	+[8,47,48,56]
Alcohol abuse			+[46]	+[8,47,51]
Precipitating				
Hypoxia	+[2,17,18,57]	+[52,58]	+[46]	
Metabolic abnormalities	+[17,18,50,57]	+[52,58]	+[8,46]	+[8,47]
Low albumin (malnutrition)	+[43]	+[52]	+[46]	
Bone metastasis	+[43]			
Hematological cancer	+[17,43]			
Brain involvement (metastasis, stroke)	+[1,2,17,57]	+[52,58]	+[46]	
Polypharmacy			+[46]	+[16]
Opioids	+[1,2,18,44,50,53]	+[52,58]		+[49,56]
Corticosteroids	+[2,18,53,57]	+[52]		
Benzodiazepines	+[17,18,53]	+[52]		
Infection	+[1,2,17,57]	+[52,58]	+[8]	+[16]
Dehydration	+[1,2,17,18]	+[52,58]	+[46]	+[56]
Immobility/use of restraints			+[46]	+[56]

*A + indicates that a relationship exists between the factor and the development of delirium in the specific population noted. References are provided for the reader who wants to access the actual studies demonstrating this relationship.

diagnostic tool and one of the most commonly used for formal delirium screening. However, to improve validity, a cognitive test should be completed along with it.[28] Common cognitive tests include the Folstein Mini Mental Status Examination (MMSE),[29] Blessed Memory Orientation and Concentration test (BOMC),[30] and the Mini-Cog.[31]

SUMMARY OF EVIDENCE REGARDING TREATMENT RECOMMENDATIONS

Nonpharmacological Prevention Strategies

An estimated 30% to 40% of delirium cases are preventable. Multiple interventions to prevent delirium have been developed.[32] The majority of interventions are designed to target modifiable risk factors for delirium. Interventions range from single interventions (e.g., use of exercise or psychotherapy) to multicomponent interventions targeting multiple risk factors.[33,34] Patients at high risk for development of delirium have been targeted with the use of geriatric consultation, multidisciplinary teams, specific units with specialized delirium training, and nurse-driven multicomponent interventions (e.g., Hospital Elder Life Program and the Stop Delirium! project).[35–38] The studies using nonpharmacological methods to prevent delirium have overall been positive, and the consensus is that they are at least somewhat effective at reducing the incidence of delirium, particularly if the incidence of delirium is greater than 30% in the targeted population. Additionally, multicomponent interventions may be more effective than single-component interventions.[34]

Treatment of Delirium

Before delirium can be treated it needs to be diagnosed. Diagnosis involves maintaining a high index of suspicion and routinely screening for delirium. When delirium has been identified, several steps should occur concurrently, including (1) family and patient education and support, (2) clarification of goals of care and workup for potentially reversible causes, (3) institution of nonpharmacological treatment measures, and (4) management of any dangerous or distressing symptoms such as agitation. Education and support of families has been shown to decrease delirium-related distress and should be repeated frequently through the course of the delirium.[39,40] Delirium can be reversed, even in patients who are in the last week of life,[17] and evaluation for and treatment of potential causes should always be undertaken. The intensity of the evaluation should be based on the overall prognosis and goals of care. Even when delirium is felt to be terminal and irreversible, a basic noninvasive evaluation (e.g., reviewing medications or assessing for physical causes of delirium such as constipation) can be beneficial. More detail on performing a workup for the causes of delirium can be found in Chapter 35. Regardless of the cause of delirium or the suspected

TABLE 37-2. Common Nonpharmacological Interventions for Delirium

TYPE OF INTERVENTIONS	EXAMPLES
Reorientation	Reminders to date and time Calendars Orientation boards
Behavioral	Clear, simple instructions Frequent eye contact Proper introduction by all staff
Sensory	Apply working glasses and hearing aids
Avoid physical restraints	Limit or remove Foley catheters, intravenous lines, oxygen Use oral rehydration
Environmental	Limit room and staff changes Display familiar objects and pictures Allow uninterrupted sleep
Minimize medications	Sleep protocol (warm milk or herbal tea, relaxation tapes or music, back massage)[60] Use consulting pharmacists for medication review
Staff education	Workshops, lectures, poster presentations, training in screening tools

Data from References 38, 41, 59.

prognosis, nonpharmacological methods for treatment have been shown to be beneficial, with no risk for side effects for the patient or family.

The nonpharmacological methods designed to treat delirium are essentially the same ones recommended to prevent delirium, and most of them target the causes and modifiable risk factors associated with delirium. They include frequent reorientation, providing a calm environment that avoids both sensory deprivation and overstimulation, using clear verbal instructions, providing emotional support and avoiding confrontation (do not confront delusional beliefs, focus on emotions not content, use distraction), promoting a normal sleep–wake cycle, correcting sensory deficits (glasses and hearing aids available and working), minimizing the use of physical restraints (including discontinuing or avoiding intravenous and urinary catheters), minimizing room and staff changes, and requesting that family members bring in familiar items and sit with the patient (Table 37-2).[32,41,42]

KEY MESSAGES TO PATIENTS AND FAMILIES

Delirium is a disturbance of thinking that is common in patients with medical illnesses. It often has distressing behavioral symptoms ranging from agitation to sedation. Strategies designed to decrease the risk factors for delirium by managing the environment and providing education are able to both make it less likely that delirium will occur and improve the symptoms of delirium if it develops. These nonpharmacological strategies pose no risk to the patient and do not involve the use of medications.

CONCLUSION AND SUMMARY

Delirium is common and distressing but often not diagnosed. Clinicians should have a high index of suspicion, particularly in older patients and in patients with a life-limiting illness. Delirium can be prevented in high-risk populations with nonpharmacological multicomponent interventions. All patients with delirium should have an initial evaluation for causes. Treatment for suspected causes should be based on prognosis and goals of care. All patients can benefit from the institution of nonpharmacological management that can improve outcome without side effects. Common nonpharmacological strategies include reorientation, correction of sensory impairments, avoidance of physical restraints, and behavioral and environmental interventions.

SUMMARY RECOMMENDATIONS

- Nonpharmacological interventions should be used to prevent delirium in high-risk populations.
- Nonpharmacological interventions should be initiated in all patients with delirium.
- Underlying causes of delirium should be identified if possible and treated as is congruent with patient and family goals of care.
- Distressing or dangerous symptoms, such as agitation, should be treated aggressively with pharmacological management.

REFERENCES

1. Bruera E, Bush SH, Willey J, et al. Impact of delirium and recall on the level of distress in patients with advanced cancer and their family caregivers. *Cancer.* 2009;115(9):2004–2012.
2. Breitbart W, Gibson C, Tremblay A. The delirium experience: delirium recall and delirium-related distress in hospitalized patients with cancer, their spouses/caregivers, and their nurses. *Psychosomatics.* 2002;43(3):183–194.
3. Morita T, Hirai K, Sakaguchi Y, Tsuneto S, Shima Y. Family-perceived distress from delirium-related symptoms of terminally ill cancer patients. *Psychosomatics.* 2004;45(2):107–113.
4. O'Malley G, Leonard M, Meagher D, O'Keeffe ST. The delirium experience: a review. *J Psychosom Res.* 2008;65(3):223–228.
5. Siddiqi N, House AO, Holmes JD. Occurrence and outcome of delirium in medical in-patients: a systematic literature review. *Age Ageing.* 2006;35(4):350–364.
6. Cole MG, Ciampi A, Belzile E, Zhong L. Persistent delirium in older hospital patients: a systematic review of frequency and prognosis. *Age Ageing.* 2009;38(1):19–26.
7. Mittal V, Muralee S, Williamson D, et al. Delirium in the elderly: a comprehensive review. *Am J Alzheimers Dis Other Demen.* 2011;26(2):97–109.
8. Caraceni A, Simonetti F. Palliating delirium in patients with cancer. *Lancet Oncol.* 2009;10(2):164–172.
9. Gaudreau JD, Gagnon P. Psychotogenic drugs and delirium pathogenesis: the central role of the thalamus. *Med Hypotheses.* 2005;64(3):471–475.
10. Hshieh TT, Fong TG, Marcantonio ER, Inouye SK. Cholinergic deficiency hypothesis in delirium: a synthesis of current evidence. *J Gerontol A Biol Sci Med Sci.* 2008;63(7):764–772.
11. Trzepacz PT. Update on the neuropathogenesis of delirium. *Dement Geriatr Cogn Disord.* 1999;10(5):330–334.
12. Maldonado JR. Pathoetiological model of delirium: a comprehensive understanding of the neurobiology of delirium and an

evidence-based approach to prevention and treatment. *Crit Care Clin.* 2008;24(4):789–856 ix.

13. Rudolph JL, Ramlawi B, Kuchel GA, et al. Chemokines are associated with delirium after cardiac surgery. *J Gerontol A Biol Sci Med Sci.* 2008;63(2):184–189.

14. Fricchione GL, Nejad SH, Esses JA, et al. Postoperative delirium. *Am J Psychiatry.* 2008;165(7):803–812.

15. Ebersoldt M, Sharshar T, Annane D. Sepsis-associated delirium. *Intensive Care Med.* 2007;33(6):941–950.

16. Brauer C, Morrison RS, Silberzweig SB, Siu AL. The cause of delirium in patients with hip fracture. *Arch Intern Med.* 2000;160(12):1856–1860.

17. Lawlor PG, Gagnon B, Mancini IL, et al. Occurrence, causes, and outcome of delirium in patients with advanced cancer: a prospective study. *Arch Intern Med.* 2000;160(6):786–794.

18. Sagawa R, Akechi T, Okuyama T, Uchida M, Furukawa TA. Etiologies of delirium and their relationship to reversibility and motor subtype in cancer patients. *Jpn J Clin Oncol.* 2009;39(3):175–182.

19. Inouye SK, Foreman MD, Mion LC, Katz KH, Cooney Jr LM. Nurses' recognition of delirium and its symptoms: comparison of nurse and researcher ratings. *Arch Intern Med.* 2001;161(20):2467–2473.

20. Yang FM, Marcantonio ER, Inouye SK, et al. Phenomenological subtypes of delirium in older persons: patterns, prevalence, and prognosis. *Psychosomatics.* 2009;50(3):248–254.

21. Robinson TN, Raeburn CD, Tran ZV, Brenner LA, Moss M. Motor subtypes of postoperative delirium in older adults. *Arch Surg.* 2011;146(3):295–300.

22. Spiller JA. Hypoactive delirium: assessing the extent of the problem for inpatient specialist palliative care. *Palliat Med.* 2006;1(20):17–23.

23. Steinhauser KE, Christakis NA, Clipp EC, McNeilly M, McIntyre L, Tulsky JA. Factors considered important at the end of life by patients, family, physicians, and other care providers. *JAMA.* 2000;284(19):2476–2482.

24. Wong CL, Holroyd-Leduc J, Simel DL, Straus SE. Does this patient have delirium? Value of bedside instruments. *JAMA.* 2010;304(7):779–786.

25. Vidan MT, Sanchez E, Alonso M, Montero B, Ortiz J, Serra JA. An intervention integrated into daily clinical practice reduces the incidence of delirium during hospitalization in elderly patients. *J Am Geriatr Soc.* 2009;57(11):2029–2036.

26. Ramaswamy R, Dix EF, Drew JE, Diamond JJ, Inouye SK, Roehl BJ. Beyond grand rounds: a comprehensive and sequential intervention to improve identification of delirium. *Gerontologist.* 2011;51(1):122–131.

27. Inouye S. Clarifying confusion: the confusion assessment method: a new method for detection of delirium. *Ann Intern Med.* 1990;113(12):941–948.

28. Adamis D, Sharma N, Whelan PJ, Macdonald AJ. Delirium scales: a review of current evidence. *Aging Ment Health.* 2010;14(5):543–555.

29. Folstein MF, Folstein SE, McHugh PR. "Mini-mental state": a practical method for grading the cognitive state of patients for the clinician. *J Psychiatr Res.* 1975;12(3):189–198.

30. Katzman R, Brown T, Fuld P, Peck A, Schechter R, Schimmel H. Validation of a short Orientation-Memory-Concentration Test of cognitive impairment. *Am J Psychiatry.* 1983;140(6):734–739.

31. Borson S, Scanlan JM, Chen P, Ganguli M. The Mini-Cog as a screen for dementia: validation in a population-based sample. *J Am Geriatr Soc.* 2003;51(10):1451–1454.

32. Fong TG, Tulebaev SR, Inouye SK. Delirium in elderly adults: diagnosis, prevention and treatment. *Nat Rev Neurol.* 2009;5(4):210–220.

33. Tatematsu N, Hayashi A, Narita K, Tamaki A, Tsuboyama T. The effects of exercise therapy on delirium in cancer patients: a retrospective study. *Support Care Cancer.* April 30, 2010.

34. Hempenius L, van Leeuwen BL, van Asselt DZ, et al. Structured analyses of interventions to prevent delirium. *Int J Geriatr Psychiatry.* 2011;26(5):441–450.

35. Inouye SK. Prevention of delirium in hospitalized older patients: risk factors and targeted intervention strategies. *Ann Med.* 2000;32(4):257–263.

36. Siddiqi N, Young J, House AO, et al. Stop Delirium! A complex intervention to prevent delirium in care homes: a mixed-methods feasibility study. *Age Ageing.* 2011;40(1):90–98.

37. Featherstone I, Hopton A, Siddiqi N. An intervention to reduce delirium in care homes. *Nurs Older People.* 2010;22(4):16–21.

38. Tabet N, Howard R. Non-pharmacological interventions in the prevention of delirium. *Age Ageing.* 2009;38(4):374–379.

39. Gagnon P, Charbonneau C, Allard P, Soulard C, Dumont S, Fillion L. Delirium in advanced cancer: a psychoeducational intervention for family caregivers. *J Palliat Care.* 2002;18(4):253–261.

40. Morita T, Akechi T, Ikenaga M, et al. Terminal delirium: recommendations from bereaved families' experiences. *J Pain Symptom Manage.* 2007;34(6):579–589.

41. Cook I. *Guideline Watch: Practice Guideline for the Treatment of Patients With Delirium.* Arlington, VA: American Psychiatric Association; 2004.

42. Hogan DBG, Bruto V, Burne D, et al. National guidelines for seniors' mental health: the assessment and treatment of delirium. *Can J Geriatr.* 2006;9(suppl 2):42–52.

43. Ljubisavljevic V, Kelly B. Risk factors for development of delirium among oncology patients. *Gen Hosp Psychiatry.* 2003;25(5):345–352.

44. Shiiba M, Takei M, Nakatsuru M, et al. Clinical observations of postoperative delirium after surgery for oral carcinoma. *Int J Oral Maxillofac Surg.* 2009;38(6):661–665.

45. Fick DM, Agostini JV, Inouye SK. Delirium superimposed on dementia: a systematic review. *J Am Geriatr Soc.* 2002;50(10):1723–1732.

46. Inouye SK. Delirium in older persons. *New Engl J Med.* 2006;354(11):1157–1165.

47. Marcantonio ER, Goldman L, Mangione CM, et al. A clinical prediction rule for delirium after elective noncardiac surgery. *JAMA.* 1994;271(2):134–139.

48. Dasgupta M, Dumbrell AC. Preoperative risk assessment for delirium after noncardiac surgery: a systematic review. *J Am Geriatr Soc.* 2006;54(10):1578–1589.

49. Morrison RS, Magaziner J, Gilbert M, et al. Relationship between pain and opioid analgesics on the development of delirium following hip fracture. *J Gerontol A Biol Sci Med Sci.* 2003;58(1):76–81.

50. Fann JR, Hubbard RA, Alfano CM, Roth-Roemer S, Katon WJ, Syrjala KL. Pre- and post-transplantation risk factors for delirium onset and severity in patients undergoing hematopoietic stem-cell transplantation. *J Clin Oncol.* 2011;29(7):895–901.

51. Minden S. Predictors and outcomes of delirium. *Gen Hosp Psychiatry.* 2005;27(3):209–214.

52. Michaud L, Burnand B, Stiefel F. Taking care of the terminally ill cancer patient: delirium as a symptom of terminal disease. *Ann Oncol.* 2004;15(suppl 4):iv199–iv203.

53. Gandreu J. Psychoactive medications and risk of delirium in hospitalized cancer patients. *J Clin Oncol.* 2005;23(27):6712–6718.

54. Sharma P. Recovery room delirium predicts postoperative delirium after hip-fracture repair. *Anesth Analg.* 2005;101(4):1215–1220.

55. Leonard M, Spiller J, Keen J, MacLullich A, Kamholtz B, Meagher D. Symptoms of depression and delirium assessed serially in palliative-care inpatients. *Psychosomatics.* 2009;50(5):506–514.

56. Robinson S, Vollmer C. Undermedication for pain and precipitation of delirium. *Medsurg Nurs.* 2010;19(2):79–83 quiz 84.

57. Olofsson SM, Weitzner MA, Valentine AD, Baile WF, Meyers CA. A retrospective study of the psychiatric management and outcome of delirium in the cancer patient. *Support Care Cancer.* 1996;4(5):351–357.

58. Morita T. Underlying pathologies and their associations with clinical features in terminal delirium of cancer patients. *J Pain Symptom Manage.* 2001;22(6):997–1006.

59. Fossa SD, Cvancarova M, Chen L, et al. Adverse prognostic factors for testicular cancer-specific survival: a population-based study of 27,948 patients. *J Clin Oncol.* 2011;29(8):963–970.

60. McDowell JA, Mion LC, Lydon TJ, Inouye SK. A nonpharmacologic sleep protocol for hospitalized older patients. *J Am Geriatr Soc.* 1998;46(6):700–705.

Chapter 38

What Are the Differences When Treating a Patient at the End of Life With Delirium (Terminal Delirium)?

MICHELLE T. WECKMANN AND R. SEAN MORRISON

INTRODUCTION AND SCOPE OF THE PROBLEM

Delirium is an acute alteration in attention and cognition with associated behavioral and emotional manifestations. Delirium can strike at any point in a disease cycle but is most common when a person is near the end of life. Up to 88% of patients suffer symptoms consistent with delirium in the days or weeks leading up to their death.[1] Behavioral manifestations of delirium often include restlessness and agitation and when unmanaged have been cited as the most common reason a family requests palliative sedation.[2]

Unfortunately, a lack of consensus exists on the definition of terminal delirium. The literature uses terms such as confusion at the end of life, terminal anguish, terminal delirium, and terminal restlessness to refer to a similar cluster of symptoms. Some attribute the altered cognition and sensorium a person experiences while dying to a normal part of the dying process whereas others pathologize it and label it delirium. Some say that terminal delirium can be identified only in retrospect after a patient has died; others say it can be diagnosed prospectively. For this chapter, the term terminal delirium will describe an irreversible delirium that occurs when a patient has an expected prognosis of days to weeks.

RELEVANT PATHOPHYSIOLOGY

The causes of delirium at the end of life are similar to the causes at other times in a disease process and include medications, withdrawal, dehydration, metabolic disturbances, organ failure, and sepsis. It is important to remember that the medications commonly given for symptom control at the end of life (i.e., scopolamine, metoclopramide, opioids) can also cause delirium.[3] Additionally, other common causes of delirium, such as metabolic derangements, electrolyte abnormalities, and alterations in renal function, are regular findings during the dying process.

Treatment of the underlying medical causes of delirium has been shown efficacious in improving or resolving delirium, even in the last weeks of life.[1,4,5] If congruent with patient and family goals, treatment of potential causes of delirium should always be attempted because delirium has been shown to have a long-lasting, deleterious impact on bereaved caregivers. The negative effects of delirium on families and caregivers include dissatisfaction with the dying process, increased incidence of anxiety disorders, and complicated bereavement.[6–9]

SUMMARY OF EVIDENCE REGARDING TREATMENT RECOMMENDATIONS

Initial treatment of delirium at the end of life is the same as treatment at any other time and should be undertaken with the goals of care elucidated as clearly as possible. It can be challenging to find an intermediate between an unduly fatalistic view and inappropriately aggressive medical investigation and treatment. Treatment should start with family and caregiver support and education while nonpharmacological methods are initiated.[10] In all cases, aggressive management of other symptoms (e.g., pain and dyspnea) is advised because control of distressing symptoms alone can help improve agitation. The overall poor prognosis and anticipate life expectancy should be clearly conveyed to the family because that knowledge is essential to create reasonable goals. Once goals are established, a directed workup can be undertaken for potentially correctable causes (factors such as opioids and dehydration). Opioid rotation has been shown to be beneficial in dying patients who have evidence of opioid-induced toxicity (myoclonus, escalating pain, allodynia).[11,12] When rotating opioids, methadone and fentanyl are the preferred opioids in patients with delirium at the end of life because they have been shown to reduce both pain and delirium.[13,14]

Dehydration is another common cause of terminal delirium. It is believed that dehydration results in the build-up of toxic metabolites of medications such as opioids and that this may lead to delirium.[13] In select patients with dehydration, oral rehydration can decrease delirium. Therefore in some situations it may be beneficial to do a time-limited trial of parental hydration (either intravenous or subcutaneous) because some of the symptoms of delirium can be relieved with fluids, even in patients close to death.[1,15] It is important to consider overall fluid status before initiating parenteral fluids, to avoid worsening other symptoms such as dyspnea or edema.[11,15]

When a patient has distressing symptoms related to terminal delirium it is critical that the goals of care drive the treatments selected. If the goal is to maximize alertness and the ability to interact with others, the initial treatment should start with institution of nonpharmacological management strategies, attention to potentially reversible causes, and the initiation of an antipsychotic agent. Haloperidol and chlorpromazine have the most evidence and therefore are recommended in most guidelines.[16,17] If control of agitation cannot be achieved with an antipsychotic alone, the addition of a benzodiazepine can be beneficial. Lorazepam and midazolam are the most commonly recommended. If the goal is to control agitation and provide rest or sedation (or if a combination of antipsychotics and benzodiazepines is ineffective), treatment should proceed with the use of a sedating agent such as midazolam, phenobarbital, or propofol. All of these agents are efficacious for the treatment of agitation associated with terminal delirium.[18,19] These sedating agents should be titrated to the point that symptom control is achieved and no further unless there has been a documented discussion and agreement with the family that the intent is palliative sedation. Table 38-1 lists the most common agents used to treat terminal delirium.

Agitation is a common reason families request help in caring for a patient with delirium. Agitation related to delirium should be treated as a psychiatric emergency and managed aggressively. The recommended treatment for agitation associated with terminal delirium is the same as treatment of agitation for any delirium. Further discussion of pharmacological treatment of delirium can be found in Chapter 36. The difference is that higher doses of antipsychotics are often needed. In addition, first-line medications are not as successful as for patients who are not at the very end of life, thus necessitating the addition of other sedating agents such as benzodiazepines.[20]

The majority of research has focused on patients with hyperactive delirium because agitation is often perceived as more distressing than somnolence. The prevalence of hypoactive delirium in the final days to weeks of life is unknown, in part because it can mimic the comatose state many patients go through as they die. Very limited evidence exists to guide treatment of hypoactive delirium at the end of life. Psychostimulants have been used with some success to increase alertness and improve mental function in patients with hypoactive delirium; however, insufficient data are available to recommend their routine use.[21,22] Still, if the hypoactive delirium is distressing and has not improved with a trial of haloperidol, it may be worth trying a stimulant. Case reports have shown improvement with doses of methylphenidate 10 to 60 mg per day.[23,24] Although risks are noted in using a stimulant in medically ill patients (hallucinations, agitation, hypertension, tachycardia), they are believed to be small. Caution should be used when prescribing

TABLE 38-1. Pharmacological Management of Terminal Delirium*

DRUG CATEGORY	INDICATIONS	EXAMPLES	BENEFITS
Antipsychotics	First-line treatment	Haloperidol—*PO, IM, IV, SL, subcutaneously:* 0.5-5 mg q30min prn	Wide therapeutic window Available in oral, rectal, parenteral forms Assists with nausea
		Chlorpromazine—*PO, IV, SL, PR, subcutaneously:* 12.5-25 mg q30min prn	Wide therapeutic window Available in oral, rectal, parenteral forms Assists with nausea and hiccups More sedating than haloperidol IV form can cause hypotension, especially if given too rapidly
Benzodiazepines (should be combined with an antipsychotic agent)	Additional treatment of delirium Use in aggressive or agitated patients unresponsive to antipsychotics alone	Lorazepam—*PO, IV, SL, subcutaneously:* 0.5-5 mg q60min prn	Can treat myoclonus and seizures
Sedatives	Goal is sedation Use if continued aggression or agitation with antipsychotic and benzodiazepine treatment	Midazolam—*IV, subcutaneously:* 0.5-5 mg bolus then 0.5-10 mg/hr continuous	Short half-life Can treat myoclonus and seizures
		Propofol—*IV:* 2.5-5 mcg/kg/min (titrate q10min)	Short half-life and rapid onset of action Causes muscle relaxation and bronchodilation
		Phenobarbital—*IV, subcutaneously:* 200 mg loading dose, then 0.5 mg/kg/hr continuous	Can treat seizures

Data from References 25–27.
IM, Intramuscularly; *IV,* intravenously; *PO,* orally; *PR,* per rectum; *SL,* sublingually.
*Titrate dose to effect in all regimens. See Chapter 36 for a discussion of the precautions to consider when prescribing antipsychotic medications to patients.

methylphenidate for a patient with underlying cardiac disease, and the lowest effective dose should always be used in this population.

KEY MESSAGES TO PATIENTS AND FAMILIES

Confusion (delirium) is a common finding during a patient's final days or weeks of life. Terminal delirium can be very upsetting and can cause a patient to be agitated and restless and experience upsetting hallucinations. It may also make a patient very sedated and unable to communicate. Even when a patient is close to death, delirium can be treated in more than 50% of cases, and if the delirium is not reversed, medications can improve the symptoms. These medications include antipsychotics such as haloperidol and sedating agents such as lorazepam. Occasionally the symptoms of delirium are severe and are not well controlled with these medications. In these cases, clinicians should discuss using a more sedating medication to reduce both patient and family distress.

CONCLUSION AND SUMMARY

Terminal delirium is a nearly uniform experience at the end of life, occurring in the majority of patients (up to 88%) during the final days or weeks of life. The symptoms of delirium often cause incredible distress to both the patient and caregivers and can prevent a family and patient from experiencing a "peaceful" death, thus leading to potential long-term complications for caregivers. The symptoms of delirium in a dying patient should be managed aggressively, especially if the patient is agitated. The goals of care should guide symptom management and include treatment of potentially reversible causes, nonpharmacological strategies, and pharmacological management. In terminal delirium, higher doses of antipsychotics are often needed and are often unsuccessful alone. It is not uncommon to need to include a benzodiazepine to assist with agitation control.

SUMMARY RECOMMENDATIONS

- A majority of terminal delirium can be improved by treating underlying medical causes.
- Haloperidol is the recommended medication for symptom control but often needs to be augmented with a benzodiazepine (e.g., lorazepam) to control distressing agitation.
- It is not uncommon for patients with terminal delirium to require sedation for symptom control.

REFERENCES

1. Lawlor PG, Gagnon B, Mancini IL, et al. Occurrence, causes, and outcome of delirium in patients with advanced cancer: a prospective study. *Arch Intern Med.* 2000;160(6):786–794.

2. Mercadante S, Porzio G, Valle A, Fusco F, Aielli F, Costanzo V. Palliative sedation in patients with advanced cancer followed at home: a systematic review. *J Pain Symptom Manage.* 2011;41(4):754–760.

3. White C, McCann MA, Jackson N. First do no harm... Terminal restlessness or drug-induced delirium. *J Palliat Med.* 2007;10(2):345–351.

4. Leonard M, Raju B, Conroy M, et al. Reversibility of delirium in terminally ill patients and predictors of mortality. *Palliat Med.* 2008;22(7):848–854.

5. Gagnon B. Delirium in terminal cancer: a prospective study using daily screening, early diagnosis, and continuous monitoring. *J Pain Symptom Manage.* 2000;19(6):412–426.

6. Buss MK VL, Inouye SK, Zhang B, Block SD, Prigerson HD. Associations between caregiver-perceived delirium in cancer patients and generalized anxiety in their caregivers. *J Palliat Med.* 2007;10(5):1083–1092.

7. Morita T, Akechi T, Ikenaga M, et al. Terminal delirium: recommendations from bereaved families' experiences. *J Pain Symptom Manage.* 2007;34(6):579–589.

8. Breitbart W, Gibson C, Tremblay A. The delirium experience: delirium recall and delirium-related distress in hospitalized patients with cancer, their spouses/caregivers, and their nurses. *Psychosomatics.* 2002;43(3):183–194.

9. Bruera E, Bush SH, Willey J, et al. Impact of delirium and recall on the level of distress in patients with advanced cancer and their family caregivers. *Cancer.* 2009;115(9):2004–2012.

10. Gagnon P, Charbonneau C, Allard P, Soulard C, Dumont S, Fillion L. Delirium in advanced cancer: a psychoeducational intervention for family caregivers. *J Palliat Care.* 2002;18(4):253–261.

11. Centeno C, Sanz A, Bruera E. Delirium in advanced cancer patients. *Palliat Med.* 2004;3(18):184–194.

12. McNicol E, Horowicz-Mehler N, Fisk RA, et al. Management of opioid side effects in cancer-related and chronic noncancer pain: a systematic review. *J Pain.* 2003;4(5):231–256.

13. Moyer DD. Terminal delirium in geriatric patients with cancer at end of life. *Am J Hosp Palliat Care.* 2011;28(1):44–51.

14. Fine PG. Clinical approaches to special issues related to opioid therapy. *Semin Oncol Nurs.* 2009;25(2 suppl 1):S20–S28.

15. Morita T, Hyodo I, Yoshimi T, et al. Association between hydration volume and symptoms in terminally ill cancer patients with abdominal malignancies. *Ann Oncol.* 2005;16(4):640–647.

16. Jackson KC, Lipman AG. Drug therapy for delirium in terminally ill patients. *Cochrane Database Syst Rev.* 2004;(2):CD004770.

17. Breitbart W, Marotta R, Platt MM, et al. A double-blind trial of haloperidol, chlorpromazine, and lorazepam in the treatment of delirium in hospitalized AIDS patients. *Am J Psychiatry.* 1996;153(2):231–237.

18. Casarett DJ, Inouye SK. Diagnosis and management of delirium near the end of life. *Ann Intern Med.* 2001;135(1):32–40.

19. Kehl KA. Treatment of terminal restlessness: a review of the evidence. *J Pain Palliat Care Pharmacother.* 2004;18(1):5–30.

20. Fang CK, Chen HW, Liu SI, Lin CJ, Tsai LY, Lai YL. Prevalence, detection and treatment of delirium in terminal cancer inpatients: a prospective survey. *Jpn J Clin Oncol.* 2008;38(1):56–63.

21. Stiefel F, Bruera E. Psychostimulants for hypoactive-hypoalert delirium? *J Palliat Care.* 1991;7(3):25–26.

22. Elie D, Gagnon P, Gagnon B, Giguere A. Using psychostimulants in end-of-life patients with hypoactive delirium and cognitive disorders: a literature review. *Can J Psychiatry.* 2010;55(6):386–393.

23. Gagnon B, Low G, Schreier G. Methylphenidate hydrochloride improves cognitive function in patients with advanced cancer and hypoactive delirium: a prospective clinical study. *J Psychiatry Neurosci.* 2005;30(2):100–107.

24. Morita T, Otani H, Tsunoda J, Inoue S, Chihara S. Successful palliation of hypoactive delirium due to multi-organ failure by oral methylphenidate. *Support Care Cancer.* 2000;8(2):134–137.

25. de Graeff A, Dean M. Palliative sedation therapy in the last weeks of life: a literature review and recommendations for standards. *J Palliat Med.* 2007;10(1):67–85.

26. Lynch M. Palliative sedation. *Clin J Oncol Nurs.* 2003;7(6):653–657 667.

27. Burke AL, Diamond PL, Hulbert J, Yeatman J, Farr EA. Terminal restlessness: its management and the role of midazolam. *Med J Aust.* 1991;155(7):485–487.

SYMPTOMS AT THE END OF LIFE

Chapter 39

How Do Symptoms Change for Patients in the Last Days and Hours of Life?

Lorie N. Smith and Vicki A. Jackson

INTRODUCTION AND SCOPE OF THE PROBLEM

Many patients faced with a life-threatening illness wonder what the last days and hours of their life will entail. They may express concerns that their symptoms will be difficult to control or that they will suffer at the very end of life. Equally concerning to patients is the fear that their loved ones will be burdened by their care or that observing their death will be traumatic. Patients in a study by Singer and colleagues[1] identified five domains of good end-of-life care: (1) receiving adequate pain and symptom management, (2) avoiding inappropriate prolongation of dying, (3) achieving a sense of control, (4) relieving burden on others, and (5) strengthening relationships with loved ones. Patients should be reassured that management of their symptoms will be of utmost priority and that they will be treated with dignity and respect, both during and after the dying process.

Most health care providers are not trained in palliative care and perhaps have not cared for a patient in the last hours of life. The last days and hours of life represent a unique period in a person's life that deserves special attention. The dying process is not simply a continuation of what has come before, but rather a vulnerable period with new physical and emotional challenges for both patients and their loved ones. Care plans need to recognize and adapt to these changes. Unaddressed suffering in the last days or hours of life is often remembered by relatives and can be a significant source of distress even months after their loved one has died.

RELEVANT PATHOPHYSIOLOGY

Given the nature of this chapter, what follows in this section is a general discussion related to identifying when patients enter the last phase of life. Outlining the key signs that a patient is actively dying may be helpful to families so they will know what to expect. However, the discussion of the pathophysiology of particular symptoms is covered in the next section.

When educating family members on approaching death, it is helpful to describe what has been termed the "transitional phase" of the dying process.[2] This phase usually occurs in the last weeks to days of life. Signs that indicate the beginning of this phase include the following:
- Increasing somnolence
- Weakness
- Decreased interest in surroundings
- Loss of appetite
- Confusion
- Falls
- Incontinence

Although a patient may have exhibited any one of these signs at different points in an illness, when observed simultaneously it likely signals that the patient is entering the last days of life. It is important to educate family and friends about these changes for several reasons. If unprepared, relatives might mistakenly think the patient has control over these changes and experience anger or frustration toward the patient. Throughout the patient's illness, family members have often been a source of encouragement, a cheering coach of sorts, during difficult temporary setbacks. With the understanding that these changes represent the natural progression of the dying process rather than a temporary change, they can refocus their efforts as caregivers. A more practical reason for identifying for families when a patient has entered the transitional phase is that families often have limited ability to be with their loved one full time because of their own work or personal responsibilities. Knowing that the patient has entered this transitional phase allows them to plan appropriately.

SUMMARY OF EVIDENCE REGARDING TREATMENT RECOMMENDATIONS

Caring for the Patient

To best address all sources of suffering at the end of life and prepare the patient and patient's family members for what to expect during this time, it is important for health care providers to understand how symptoms change at the end of life. Symptom management in a patient's last days can often be challenging. The Study to Understand Prognoses and Preferences for Outcomes and Risks of Treatments (SUPPORT) demonstrated that family members often felt that patients' symptoms were not adequately controlled. Indeed, family members of patients who were conscious reported that 40% had undertreated severe pain and, of those with cancer with superimposed multisystem organ failure, 70% had severe dyspnea and 25% had moderate anxiety or dysphoria.[3]

Pain. Up to 75% of dying patients will experience pain requiring opioid analgesics when they enter the terminal phase.[4] Cancer pain has been extensively studied, and moderate to severe pain is experienced by at least 70% of patients with advanced cancer.[5] Similarly, pain at the end of life was recorded in more than 93% of patients dying from human immunodeficiency virus (HIV) infection or acquired immunodeficiency syndrome (AIDS), although pain prevalence has declined with the introduction of antiretroviral therapies.[6] Other studies have suggested that as many as 75% of patients with heart failure experience pain, often related to comorbid conditions such as osteoarthritis or diabetes.[7]

Pain in terminally ill patients has many causes. The general causes of pain in patients with life-threatening illnesses are addressed elsewhere in this book. Although many patients may have experienced pain previously, more than half will experience a new pain as they enter the terminal phase, requiring careful observation on the part of the health care provider. For patients who had preexisting pain conditions, it is important to continue treatment even when the patient is no longer able to verbally report pain. New pain may be related to disease progression or a new problem related to the dying process. Examples include the following:

- Change in pain medication or route of administration leading to uncontrolled pain
- New pathological fracture resulting from movement of the patient
- Development of oral thrush
- Development of urinary retention or constipation
- Development of pressure ulcers

The assessment of pain can be challenging in the last days or hours of life. Often patients are no longer able to verbally report pain. Nonverbal signs of pain such as grimacing, moaning, and withdrawing from stimuli are often good indicators of pain and should be monitored closely. In addition, eliciting the observations of those closest to the patient (nurses, aides, family members) can be useful when assessing for pain. Careful physical examination of patients at the end of life also will help identify potential new sources of pain. For instance, the recognition of urinary retention on suprapubic examination when the clinician palpates a full bladder can be easily alleviated with the placement of a urinary catheter. A distended abdomen may signify constipation, which can be treated with suppositories. A careful skin examination and communication with nurses can reveal the existence of pressure ulcers, the pain of which may be relieved with local anesthetic gels. Frequently, new pain will require both opioids and nonopioid adjuvant medications for pain control. The practice of providing analgesics immediately before the patient is turned, moved, or cleaned can help reduce incident pain and should be standard practice in the dying patient.

One study showed that 60% of patients were able to swallow until their death.[8] For patients unable to swallow, it is necessary to use alternative methods of medication administration to ensure continued treatment of pain. A patient unable to take pills can receive opioid pain medication by the buccal, sublingual, rectal, or transdermal routes. In some instances, however, a patient may require subcutaneous or intravenous infusion. Patient-controlled analgesia is generally inappropriate as the terminal phase advances because the dying patient will likely not be able to use it properly or reliably. Additionally, family members can be tempted to administer bolus doses to the patient themselves, which can result in the patient receiving inappropriately high opioid doses and can be a burdensome task to families sitting vigil at the bedside.

Oral solutions of morphine or oxycodone can be given by buccal or sublingual routes with a dropper. Concentrated oral solutions of morphine or oxycodone are available for patients who can tolerate larger doses of opioids. Patients requiring multiple doses per day may benefit from transition to a long-acting opioid. Although not approved by the Food and Drug Administration (FDA), rectal administration of sustained-release morphine has been demonstrated to have equivalent absorption to oral morphine. Patients can receive sustained-release morphine 15 to 30 mg rectally every 12 hours. Alternatively, if higher doses are required, or if the family would prefer alternative modes of administration, a fentanyl patch can be placed. Liquid or rectal opioid should be provided for the first 12 hours after placement of the patch, to allow absorption into the bloodstream for adequate pain control.

Some adjuvant medications also can be given rectally or subcutaneously. If a patient had previously benefited from oral acetaminophen or nonsteroidal antiinflammatory drug therapy, both acetaminophen and indomethacin are available in suppository form. Similarly, patients receiving corticosteroids for bone or nerve pain can be given subcutaneous or intravenous dexamethasone. Oral tricyclic antidepressants, often used for neuropathic pain, can be replaced with rectal doxepin.

Nearly half of all dying patients will need an increase in their opioid dose during their last days.[8] If the required opioid dose is too large to be given by the sublingual, rectal, or transdermal routes, the medication can be given by subcutaneous infusion (or intravenous infusion, if access is already available). Both types of infusion can be used in the home environment with the aid of hospice or other home nurses. When infusing opioid medications, the starting dose for a patient with well-controlled pain should be the intravenous equivalent of the oral dose; if the pain is not well-controlled, administer a dose that is 25% to 100% higher depending on the level of distress.

Opioid doses occasionally need to be reduced. Health care providers should consider lowering opioid doses when a patient has become significantly more somnolent when previously alert and is known to be drinking less and becoming oliguric. These findings suggest that morphine metabolites are accumulating and a reduced opioid dose might be appropriate. An alternative to dose reduction is to decrease the frequency with which opioids are administered (e.g., changing from every 4 hours to every 6 hours, particularly in older patients).

Dyspnea. Dyspnea, or the subjective sensation of breathlessness, is a common distressing symptom for patients with serious illness. In a study of patients with end-stage heart failure in hospice care, 75% had dyspnea on exertion and 53% at rest. Studies in patients with cancer demonstrate prevalence rates ranging from 20% to 60%.[9] By the time patients have reached the terminal phase, all treatable causes of dyspnea have likely been addressed. At this stage, the most common causes of dyspnea include the following:
- Extensive lung metastases
- Secondary pneumonia
- Pulmonary edema
- Anxiety or panic
- Stridor from extratracheal pressure from nodes
- Large pleural effusions
- Large pericardial effusions with tamponade
- Anemia
- Metabolic acidosis from organ failure

Some of the more invasive treatments (e.g., draining an effusion) that might have served a palliative role at an earlier stage are no longer appropriate when death is imminent. Similarly, antibiotics usually are not beneficial at this stage. The symptomatic management of dyspnea in the terminal phase may include nonpharmacological and pharmacological methods and is the same as that for patients at earlier stages of the disease. Simple repositioning may be effective. Patients with chronic obstructive pulmonary disease may be more comfortable sitting up, whereas patients with unilateral lung disease may prefer lying on one side more than the other. Oxygen or cool air from a fan can reduce the sensation of breathlessness regardless of whether clinical hypoxia is present.[10] Sometimes oxygen provided by a facemask exacerbates dyspnea by contributing to a feeling of claustrophobia, thereby increasing anxiety. Dyspnea experienced in the home setting can be exacerbated by warm, dry rooms. Families should be advised to open windows, reposition patients to benefit from a stream of air, use fans, and humidify the ambient air with a humidifier or by placing a bowl of water in the room.[11]

Pharmacological management of dyspnea relies on the use of opioids, usually morphine, titrated to effect. As in the management of pain (see earlier discussion), morphine can be given orally or if the patient is unable to take oral medications, as a suppository or by subcutaneous administration. In addition to opioids, anxiolytics should be used to treat the panic that frequently accompanies the sensation of breathlessness. Lorazepam (0.5-2 mg q4-6 hours prn) can be given sublingually for anxiety related to dyspnea. For refractory anxiety, a low dose of diazepam (2-10 mg at bedtime or divided BID/TID) can be administered orally or rectally as needed or midazolam (5-10mg q4-6 hours prn) can be administered subcutaneously. Chlorpromazine (25 mg orally or rectally or 12.5 mg intravenously) also can be useful as needed.[12]

As patients approach the last hours or days of life, changes in breathing patterns may occur that family members interpret as dyspnea and suffering. Rapid shallow breathing, periods of apnea, and a Cheyne-Stokes respiratory pattern are common observations at the end of life[13] (see later discussion of the final hours). Relatives of patients should be educated that this is a natural part of the dying process and that the patient does not experience these breathing patterns as dyspnea. If, despite reassurance, the family perceives the patient to be distressed, offering low-dose opioids or benzodiazepines as needed may be appropriate.

Anorexia and Decreased Oral Intake. Families often struggle with a patient's lack of interest in eating and drinking. Preparing food for an ill family member can have significant cultural, familial, or personal significance. When a patient is no longer interested in eating, the family may experience this as a rejection of their love or support. Additionally, families may worry that by not providing nutrition or hydration they are contributing to their loved one's suffering and ultimately to the patient's death. Health care providers can help educate families about the natural loss of appetite and the diminished benefit of nutrition at this stage in a patient's illness because of the inability to metabolize food. A study by McCann and colleagues[14] demonstrated that comfort could be achieved with sips of fluid, moistening the lips, and excellent oral care, obviating the need for intravenous hydration in the dying patient. Furthermore, health care professionals can remind families of the other meaningful ways to demonstrate their love and support.

Delirium and Restlessness. Terminal delirium is a common finding among dying patients and occurs with a frequency of 85% to 90% during the final 24 to 48 hours of life in patients with terminal cancer.[15,16] Delirium typically presents as a fluctuating level of consciousness that can vary from hour to hour. In addition, patients may experience restlessness, insomnia, agitation, nightmares, combative behavior, or sensory distortions. They may report seeing or speaking to loved ones who have died or other visual or auditory hallucinations. Delirium can be distressing to the patient, family, and staff and is the main contributing factor to a family's inability to continue caring for a patient in the home.[17]

Potential causes of delirium include untreated pain, urinary retention, constipation or fecal impaction, dyspnea, anxiety, medication side effects, electrolyte disturbances, and organ dysfunction. In other patients, unresolved psychological, spiritual, or social problems may be contributing to the distress. An interdisciplinary approach, including visits from chaplaincy, social workers, and psychologists, may be useful in easing a patient's restlessness. If the underlying cause cannot be identified or reversed, and the symptoms are distressing to the patient, they should be managed both nonpharmacologically and pharmacologically.

Nonpharmacological interventions are important to remember when caring for the delirious patient at end of life. Maintaining a balance between sensory deprivation and sensory overload is a key component to a successful intervention. Nursing staff, family members, and clinicians all play an important role in maintaining this environment. Ensuring a consistent environment (e.g., avoiding room or bed changes, maintaining patient routines, and, when possible, promoting continuity of staff) help reduce the risk for delirium. Equally important to keeping a consistent environment is paying close attention to the characteristics of the environment. Avoiding ambiguous lighting helps prevent illusions and hallucinations enhanced by shadowing, and therefore a well-lit room is preferable. The ambient noise level should be limited to below 45 dB (think of a quiet library) during the day and below 20 dB (akin to rustling leaves in the distance) at night.[18] Eyeglasses and hearing aids should be available to prevent complete sensory deprivation, and personal items such as comforters and pillows can be brought in by family members to help promote a familiar environment. Additionally, noxious stimuli should be removed (e.g., catheters) and medical testing avoided. If the patient becomes agitated by visitors, reducing the number of visitors and the number of visits is appropriate. Clinicians should communicate with the patient in a simple and reassuring manner and use simple questions to elicit symptoms or signs of distress.

Pharmacological interventions may be necessary to treat distressing agitation or restlessness. Haloperidol or other antipsychotics (e.g., olanzapine) are the drugs of choice in the treatment of terminal delirium. Haloperidol helps treat the agitation associated with delirium and allows the patient to rest once a response is achieved. If using haloperidol, typical dosing is 0.5 to 1 mg intravenously or 1 to 2 mg orally every 6 hours, with a similar dose scheduled every 2 hours as needed until either the agitation resolves or 20 mg has been given within a 24-hour period. For refractory patients who can take oral or sublingual medications, olanzapine, 2.5 to 5 mg orally twice per day and every 4 hours as needed, can be helpful. See Chapter 36 for a discussion of the precautions to consider when prescribing antipsychotic medications to patients with delirium.

Terminal Secretions. When a patient is no longer able to swallow or expectorate saliva, the secretions will collect at the back of the throat. This pooling leads to a noisy gurgling, often referred to as the "death rattle," and can occur in 31% to 92% of dying patients.[19] Patients are usually unconscious at this point, so are not troubled by the noise, and there is no reason to think the secretions are causing discomfort to these patients. However, as one might imagine, the noise can be quite alarming to family members at the patient's bedside. They may worry that their loved one is being suffocated by the secretions. Education of the family may help, as might repositioning the patient in a lateral recumbent position, but often it is useful to reduce the secretions with medications.

Most patients benefit from one of the anticholinergic or drying agents, such as hyoscyamine, a transdermal scopolamine patch, intravenous or nebulized glycopyrrolate, or atropine drops administered sublingually (Table 39-1). Although standard palliative care practices are generally effective at symptom relief, 22% to 50% of cases of terminal secretions are refractory. Bennett[20] proposed two subtypes of the symptom: type 1, related to declined conscious levels, which responds to antimuscarinic medications, and type 2, caused by increased bronchial secretion, resulting in poor symptom control. A prospective study performed on hospice inpatients further supported the theory that refractory symptoms were significantly associated with pulmonary pathology.[21] In these cases, educating those at the bedside of the patient is of utmost importance.

Spiritual Suffering. Terminally ill patients are often confronted with severe existential symptoms and spiritual distress that can challenge health care providers. The spiritual aspects of dying are particularly challenging in that there is a lack of consensus on the

TABLE 39-1. Medications Available to Treat Uncontrolled Secretions at the End of Life (the "Death Rattle")

DRUG	TRADE NAME	DOSING	ONSET
Hyoscyamine	Levsin	*PO, SL:* 0.125 mg tid to qid	30 min
Scopolamine	Transdermal Scopolamine	*Patch (1.5 mg):* 1-3 patches q72h	~12 hr (24 hr to steady state)
Glycopyrrolate	Robinul	*PO, IV, subcutaneously:* 0.2-0.6 mg tid	*PO:* 30 min
			IV, subcutaneously: 1 min
Glycopyrrolate		*Nebulizer:* 04.-0.8 mg tid	
Atropine	Atropine	*Subcutaneously:* 0.1-0.4 mg q4-6h as needed	1 min
Atropine (drops)	Multiple	*SL:* 1 gtt (1% ophthalmic solution) q4-6h as needed	30 min

IV, Intravenously; *PO,* orally; *qid,* four times daily; *tid,* three times daily.

definition of spirituality, who should be addressing spiritual issues at end of life, and the appropriate interventions to implement. Despite this lack of clarity, the importance of spirituality in the care of the seriously ill is increasingly acknowledged by clinicians, and the Institute of Medicine lists spiritual well-being as one of six domains of quality supportive care of the dying.

Little empirical evidence is available on how dying patients define spirituality. However, Chao and colleagues studied six Buddhist and Christian terminally ill patients in Taiwan, asking them what the essence of spirituality meant to them. Ten themes in four broad categories emerged: communion with self (self-identity, wholeness, inner peace), communion with others (love, reconciliation), communion with nature (inspiration, creativity), and communion with a higher being (faithfulness, hope, gratitude).[22]

Conventional symptom distress may therefore cross over into the realm of spiritual or existential distress when a patient experiences loss of control, feeling burdensome to others, a sense of isolation or hopelessness, or an intense fear of dying. Spiritual suffering may manifest as symptoms in any area of a person's experience—physical (e.g., intractable pain), psychological (e.g., anxiety, depression, hopelessness), religious (e.g., crisis of faith), or social (e.g., breakdown of human relationships). Spiritual pain toward the end of life also may take the form of losing one's will to live or expressing a heightened desire for death.

Perhaps the best intervention for spiritual distress is merely the acknowledgment of its existence. Puchalski and Romer[23] recommend the mnemonic FICA as a way of approaching spiritual inquiry. FICA stands for **F**aith or beliefs, **I**mportance and influence, **C**ommunity, and **A**ddress. Some specific questions in each category include: What is your faith or belief? What role do your beliefs play in influencing your health? Are you part of a spiritual community? How should these issues be addressed by the health care provider? The goal of this inquiry is to demonstrate an acceptance of ongoing dialog regarding spiritual concerns. Kearney and Mount[24] describe a more formal approach to spiritual distress through "surface-work" and "depth-work" as psychotherapeutic responses to spiritual pain. Surface-work refers to interventions aimed at alleviating distress at the conscious level of the individual's experience. Depth-work helps the patient reconnect with simple and ordinary aspects of life that, in the past, brought that person a sense of satisfaction. Examples of depth-work interventions include art and music therapy, image work, dream work, and meditation. Furthermore, Chochinov and colleagues[25] developed a therapeutic intervention termed Dignity Therapy, which targets depression and suffering and enhances a sense of meaning and purpose in patients at end of life. Briefly, Dignity Therapy allows patients to address grief-related issues, offer comfort to loved ones they will leave behind, or provide instructions to friends and families by offering patients an opportunity to recall aspects of their lives that were most meaningful, identify personal history they most want remembered, and say the things that need to be said. Most of this work should be started before the last days and hours of life, but can be continued throughout the last days if the patient is able to participate.

Special Considerations

Hemorrhage. Major bleeding at the end of life is an emergent situation that can cause distress to all involved—patient, family, and health care providers. Major bleeding may be caused by disorders of the blood vessels, qualitative or quantitative platelet abnormalities, or coagulation disorders. Acute terminal hemorrhage occurs in up to 10% of patients with cancer, and in patients with advanced hematological malignancies, major bleeding has been reported in up to 30% of patients. In patients with solid tumors, bleeding depends on the type and location of the tumor, but patients with a mediastinal or head and neck tumor, a fistulating pelvic tumor, or a fungating tumor surface have a higher risk for bleed. To minimize distress, it is helpful to plan for bleeding events in advance through good explanation and communication with the patient, family, and caregivers.

In noncatastrophic bleeds, adrenaline-soaked tamponades, tranexamic acid, and desmopressin might reduce bleeding. When more catastrophic bleeding is anticipated, it is prudent to have dark-colored towels (and perhaps sheets and blankets) available to minimize the visual effect of blood-stained bed sheets. One might also consider placement of a peripherally inserted central catheter line, when there is not already established intravenous access, in those patients with a high risk for bleed to provide intravenous sedation. For such situations, a fast-acting sedative drug such as midazolam (5-20 mg intravenously, depending on whether the patient was already on that medication) should be given for immediate sedation. Alternatively, rectal diazepam solution 10 to 20 mg or rectal lorazepam 2 mg can be given in the home by relatives previously instructed on proper administration. A major bleeding event often results in death within minutes.

Airway Obstruction. Patients known to have tumors involving the trachea might develop acute stridor at end of life because of either hemorrhage into the tumor or progression of tumor growth causing further compression of the trachea. This situation requires rapid sedation with either intravenous midazolam 5 to 20 mg or rectal diazepam solution 10 to 20 mg, both of which are effective within minutes.

Opioid-Induced Neurotoxicity. Opioid-induced neurotoxicity is a multifactorial syndrome that causes a spectrum of symptoms ranging from mild confusion or drowsiness to myoclonus, hallucinations, hyperalgesia, and seizures. It can occur with any opioids, but is more likely to occur when using opioids with active metabolites such as meperidine, codeine, morphine, (and to a lesser degree) hydromorphone. These metabolites, excreted by the kidney, may build up with dehydration or decreasing renal function. Myoclonus, the uncontrollable twitching and jerking of muscles or muscle groups, is one early manifestation of neurotoxicity that may be seen at the end of life. Although patients may be unaware of the symptom, it may be noticed by the patient's family members and cause them concern.

Patients who are experiencing neurotoxicity are at risk for developing other extreme symptoms that can cause intense suffering at the end of life. Many clinicians believe there is no upper limit of opioid dosing for patients in the final hours and days of life. In fact, opioid dosing is often limited by neurotoxicity. Paradoxical hyperalgesia, which is the increased experience of pain in the setting of patients receiving rapidly increasing doses of opioids, is a diagnosis that cannot be missed in the dying patient.

Addressing neurotoxicity in the last days or hours of life is imperative. If the patient is not disturbed by the myoclonus and satisfied with current therapy, explaining the cause and progression of symptoms may be sufficient. Benzodiazepines are the treatment of choice for myoclonus and usually manage this more minor sign of neurotoxicity. However, if more concerning symptoms are present, such as hyperalgesia, the toxicity must be managed more aggressively.

Neurotoxicity is best managed by opioid rotation, decreasing the opioid dose, use of adjuvant analgesics, or judicious use of intravenous hydration. Adjuvant analgesics (e.g., anticonvulsants, antidepressants, corticosteroids) or nondrug therapies (e.g., acupuncture, heat, cold) may allow for opioid dose reduction, with preservation of analgesia. Rotation to a different opioid may help, keeping in mind the advantages and disadvantages of changing opioid therapies in the terminal phase of the dying process. Rotating to a lower dose of a structurally dissimilar opioid will often reduce myoclonus and other neurotoxic effects within 24 hours, while maintaining comparable pain control. Traditionally, methadone and fentanyl have been considered to have less association with myoclonus because they have fewer active metabolites (which are implicated in the neuroexcitatory effects of other opioids). Unfortunately, a recent systematic review examining the management of opioid-induced central nervous system side effects reported poor-quality evidence for any specific treatment recommendations.[26] At times, neurotoxicity can be so severe and refractory that palliative sedation must be considered.

Reviewing and Discontinuing Medications

As patients enter the terminal phase of life, clinicians should reassess the medications they are receiving. Polypharmacy is not uncommon in the palliative care setting, because patients are often receiving not only medications for symptom control such as analgesics, laxatives, antiemetics, and anxiolytics, but also medications for chronic medical problems such as cardiac medications, oral hypoglycemics, or thyroid hormones. A careful review can lead to the elimination of unnecessary medications and the potential

for associated pill burden or adverse effects. It can be difficult for health care providers to recognize which medications are no longer necessary and to explain to the patient and family the reason medications are being discontinued.

When considering the discontinuation of a medication, it is important to remember that in the final days of life, natural physiological changes make previously necessary medications unnecessary. At the end of life, the workload on the heart is usually decreased and most cardiac medications can be discontinued. Similarly, advanced cancer or other disease processes lower blood pressure, and antihypertensives can be stopped. As food intake decreases in the last days of life, hypoglycemic agents become unnecessary. Health care providers should review all medications in this way, remembering how physiology changes during the dying process and discontinuing medications that are no longer benefitting the patient. Two potential exceptions to this would be the withdrawal of long-term antiarrhythmics or corticosteroids, because sudden withdrawal may be more harmful and uncomfortable to the patient.

Perhaps more challenging than the recognition of medications that are no longer necessary is the explanation to patients and families of the rationale behind these decisions. Family members may interpret the withdrawal of certain long-term medications as an attempt to expedite death or save money. It is important to recognize this concern and carefully educate both patients and relatives on the decisions being made.

The medications that are most commonly used in the last days of life address symptoms and include analgesics, anticonvulsants, and anxiolytics. The goal is to administer these medications to address patient distress without causing unnecessary discomfort. As patients transition from the early stages of the dying process to the final stages, there is often a further decline in mental status. Patients may become obtunded and therefore unable to swallow medications. The inability to take oral medications necessitates finding alternative routes for medication administration to ensure comfort. It often becomes necessary to administer medications through the sublingual, rectal, subcutaneous, or parenteral route. Realizing that the route of administration of a medication will likely need to change in the final days underscores the importance of administering only essential medications and eliminating those that are unnecessary. The route chosen depends on whether care is being provided in the home or in a hospital-like setting, who is administering the medication, and which alternative routes are available for a particular medication (Tables 39-2 and 39-3).

The Final Hours

Clinicians have termed the constellation of symptoms at the very end of life the "syndrome of imminent death" and refer to a patient experiencing these

TABLE 39-2. Medications Available in Sublingual Form*

DRUG	AVAILABLE STRENGTHS
Morphine	10 mg/5 mL, 20 mg/5 mL, 20 mg/mL
Hydromorphone	1 mg/mL
Oxycodone	5 mg/5 mL, 20 mg/mL
Methadone	5 mg/5 mL, 10 mg/5 mL, 10 mg/mL
Hyoscyamine (Levsin SL)	0.125 mg
Lorazepam (Ativan)	2 mg/mL
Olanzapine (Zyprexa, Zydis)	5 mg, 10 mg, 15 mg, 20 mg

*This list offers options for medications that can be used to treat symptoms in patients who may have difficulty swallowing at the end of life.

TABLE 39-3. Medications Available in Suppository Form*

DRUG	AVAILABLE STRENGTHS
Opium and Belladonna	15 mg
B & O Supprettes nos., 15A, 16A	30 mg, 60 mg
Oxymorphone	5 mg
Morphine	5 mg, 10 mg, 20 mg, 30 mg
Hydromorphone	3 mg
Thiethylperazine	10 mg
Trimethobenzamide	100 mg, 200 mg (FDA approval withdrawn for lack of efficacy)
Chlorpromazine	25 mg, 100 mg

B & O, Belladonna and opium; FDA, Food and Drug Administration.
*This list offers options for rectal administration of medications that can be used to treat symptoms in patients who cannot swallow.

symptoms as "actively dying." In the final stages of the dying process, patients exhibit certain signs indicating they have hours left to live. One indication is the change in temperature and appearance of the skin. The skin gets colder, starting from the periphery and moving inward. The skin may also feel clammy. Family members who have been at the bedside over time may notice this change as they touch their loved one's hands. The color of the skin of the extremities and around the mouth becomes slightly cyanotic or mottled. There is also a noticeable change in the breathing pattern. Respirations become more shallow, slower, and irregular, often with long apneic periods and in a Cheyne-Stokes pattern. Caregivers may observe a decrease in urinary output as the kidneys stop functioning. Although monitoring vital signs in a dying patient is unnecessary (because it will not contribute to the care plan), the pulse does get weaker and the blood pressure gradually falls. Eventually all signs of cardiac, respiratory, and brainstem function cease.

Health care providers should gently educate family members at the bedside about these changes to avoid misinterpretations of their observations and to allow the family to prepare for the impending death. Clinicians may step out of the room to allow families to be alone with their loved one during this time, making sure the family knows how to reach them if they have any concerns.

Family Support

Although the main focus of end-of-life care should of course be the patient, providing family support is critical to good end-of-life care. Relatives of patients will likely have their own questions about the symptoms experienced by patients at the end of life. Many family members have watched their loved one decline over time and wonder how they will recognize when death is approaching and worry about what they will witness. They also look for guidance on their role and how to focus their care. This can be a frightening time for families. Many have not seen a dying person, and they worry about their abilities to care for their loved one and remain emotionally stable at such a challenging time. After conducting interviews, Hampe[27] identified eight needs of spouses of dying patients in the hospital setting: (1) to be with the dying person; (2) to be helpful; (3) to be assured of the comfort of the dying person; (4) to be informed of the person's condition; (5) to be informed of impending death; (6) to express emotions; (7) to be comforted and supported by family members; and (8) to be accepted, supported, and comforted by health care professionals.

Some families may actually pose their questions and concerns to health care professionals, but more often than not, families will remain silent. It is therefore important for providers to anticipate their concerns and address them even when not asked directly. Several studies examining bereaved family members' experience of end-of-life care demonstrate that poor communication between health care provider and family leads to increased distress among the bereaved.[28,29] Whenever possible, family members should be prepared for the sequence of events and reassured about what their loved one will experience.

Interacting with a patient who is less attentive or exhibiting changes in mental status can contribute to family members questioning their abilities to support a patient at end of life. They may ask the health care provider, "Can he hear me?" or "What should I say?" It is believed that hearing and touch are senses that remain until a person is very near death. Even when the exact content is not understood, the sound of a familiar voice can be soothing to a patient. Loving words and touch provided by a family member may comfort the patient, encouraging a continuing relationship.[30] Assuring family members that the patient may still be able to hear them can empower them psychologically in the face of the patient's death.[3] In the book *Dying Well*,[31] Dr. Ira Byock describes "Five Things" that both the dying patient and the family member can benefit from hearing: (1) I forgive you, (2) forgive me, (3) thank you, (4) I love you, and (5) good-bye. Different family members will have varying levels of comfort in sharing these sentiments, but most will be able to express at least one.

To best support family members during this time, it is important to recognize the role they have likely filled throughout their loved one's illness. Many relatives have been informal caregivers at home as well as the eyes and ears for clinicians, reporting symptoms and keeping records of laboratory values, vital signs, and medications. As their loved one approaches the end of life, it will be necessary to address their changing role. Although they can still be helpful in reporting observed symptoms or signs of distress, the other tasks can be relinquished. Rather, they should be encouraged to focus on their relationship with the patient, an equally important role, and participate in shared stories and discussions about life meaning and help with legacy development.

KEY MESSAGES TO PATIENTS AND FAMILIES

The end of a patient's life can be frightening and unfamiliar for both the patient and the family. One of the key jobs of the palliative care clinician is to educate both patients and families about the signs and symptoms that indicate the patient is coming to the end of life and ensure that both comfort and dignity can be maintained throughout the entire process of dying. Given the prevalence of these concerns, it is often helpful to preemptively deliver some of this information because families are often too overwhelmed to be able to ask questions such as these. Delivering this information must be done in a compassionate manner and only after checking to determine how much information the family wants to know. Ensuring nonabandonment from all members of the clinical team is also important at this time because families are often particularly vulnerable given the impending loss of a loved one.

CONCLUSION AND SUMMARY

As patients enter the last days and hours of life, a new set of questions, concerns, and symptoms may arise. Providers need to be prepared for this and provide support and reassurance to both patients and their family members. Educating patients and their loved ones about the natural dying process alleviates unnecessary distress and often allows them to optimize quality time together. Anticipating potential complications at the end of life enables providers to quickly recognize and manage the associated symptoms, thereby minimizing suffering.

SUMMARY RECOMMENDATIONS

- The last days and hours of life can present new physical and emotional challenges for both the patient and loved ones. It is important for providers to be aware of these changes and have the skills needed to properly address them.
- Preparing and educating patients' families is necessary for good end-of-life care. Families will often need guidance as to how best to support their dying loved one and how to recognize when death is approaching.

- Symptom management in a patient's last days can be challenging. Frequently, patients develop new or worsening pain, dyspnea, secretions, and delirium. Recognizing these symptoms and knowing the available nonpharmacological and pharmacological therapies can reduce suffering at the end of life.
- Hemorrhage, airway obstruction, and neurotoxicity are end-of-life emergencies that, when possible, should be anticipated and then quickly addressed.
- Health care providers should reassess the medications being administered to patients in the last days of life, to eliminate unnecessary pill burden and adverse effects.

REFERENCES

1. Prendergast TJ, Luce JM. Increasing incidence of withholding and withdrawal of life support from the critically ill. *Am J Crit Care Med.* 1997;155(1):15–20.
2. Doyle-Brown M. The transitional phase: the closing journey for patients and family caregivers. *Am J Hosp Palliat Care.* 2000;17(5):354–357.
3. Lynn J, Teno JM, Phillips RS, et al. Perceptions by family members of the dying experience of older and seriously ill patients. *Ann Intern Med.* 1997;126(2):97–106.
4. Lichter I, Hunt E. The last 48 hours of life. *J Palliat Care.* 1990;6(4):7–15.
5. Van den Beuken-van Everdingen MH, de Rijke JM, Kessels AG, Schouten HC, van Kleef M, Patijen J. High prevalence of pain in patients with cancer in a large population-based study in the Netherlands. *Pain.* 2007;132(3):312.
6. Kimball LR, McCormick WC. The pharmacologic management of pain and discomfort in persons with AIDS near the end of life: use of opioid analgesia in the hospice setting. *J Pain Symptom Manage.* 1996;11:88–94.
7. Nordgren L, Sorensen S. Symptoms experienced in the last six months of life in patients with end-stage heart failure. *Eur J Cardiovasc Nurs.* 2003;2(3):213–217.
8. Twycross RG, Lack S. *Symptom Control in Far-Advanced Cancer: Pain Relief.* London: Pitman; 1983; 305.
9. End of Life Online curriculum Project. *Prevalence of dyspnea. End of life curriculum project: a joint project of the US Veterans Administration and SUMMIT, Stanford University Medical School.* Available at http://endoflife.stanford.edu/ Accessed September 9, 2012.
10. Spiller J, Alexander D. Domiciliary care: a comparison of the views of terminally ill patients and their family caregivers. *Palliat Med.* 1993;7(2):109–115.
11. Schwartzstein RM, Lahive K, Pope A, et al. Cold facial stimulation reduces breathlessness in normal subjects. *Am Rev Respir Dis.* 1987;136(1):58–61.
12. McIver B, Walsh D, Nelson K. The use of chlorpromazine for symptom control in dying cancer patients. *J Pain Symptom Manage.* 1994;9(5):341–345.
13. Emanuel LL, von Gunten CF, Ferris FF, eds. Module 12: last hours of living. In: *EPEC (Education on Palliative and End-of-Life Care) Participant's Handbook. EPEC Project.* Princeton Township, NJ: Robert Wood Johnson Foundation; 1999; M12-10.
14. McCann R, Hall W, Groth-Juncker A. Comfort care for terminally ill patients: the appropriate use of nutrition and hydration. *JAMA.* 1994;272(16):1263–1266.
15. Macleod AD. The management of terminal delirium. *Indian J Palliat Care.* 2006;12(1):22–28.
16. Bruera E, Bush SH, Willey J, et al. Impact of delirium and recall on the level of distress in patients with advanced cancer and their family caregivers. *Cancer.* 2009;115(9):2004–2012.
17. Cobb JL, Glantz MJ, Nicholas PK, et al. Delirium in patients with cancer at the end of life. *Cancer Pract.* 2000;8(4):172–177.

18. Moyer D. Terminal delirium in geriatric patients with cancer at end of life. *Am J Hosp Palliat Med.* 2011;28:44–51.

19. Hugel H, Ellershaw J, Gambles M. Respiratory tract secretions in the dying patient: a comparison between glycopyrronium and hyoscine hydrobromide. *J Palliat Care Med.* 2006;9:279–284.

20. Bennett MI. Death rattle: an audit of hyoscine (scopolamine) use and review of management. *J Pain Symptom Manage.* 1996;12(4):229–233.

21. Morita T, Tsunoda J, Inoue S, et al. Risk factors for death rattle in terminally ill cancer patients: a prospective exploratory study. *Palliat Med.* 2000;14(1):19–23.

22. Chao CC, Chen C, Yen M. The essence of spirituality of terminally ill patients. *J Nurs Res.* 2002;10(4):237–244.

23. Puchalski CM, Romer AL. Taking a spiritual history allows clinicians to understand patients more fully. *J Palliat Med.* 2000;3(1):129–137.

24. Kearney M, Mount B. Spiritual care of the dying patient. In: Cochinov MH, Breitbar W, eds. *Handbook of Psychiatry in Palliative Medicine.* New York: Oxford University Press; 2000:357–373.

25. Chochinov HM. Dignity conserving care: a new model for palliative care. *JAMA.* 2002;287:2253–2260.

26. Stone P, Minton O. European Palliative Care Research Collaborative pain guidelines: central side-effects management—what is the evidence to support best practice in the management of sedation, cognitive impairment and myoclonus? *Palliat Med.* 2010;25(5):431–441.

27. Hampe SO. Needs of the grieving spouse in a hospital setting. *Nurs Res.* 1975;2(2):113–120.

28. Shinjo T, Morita T, Hirai K, et al. Care for imminently dying cancer patients: family members' experiences and recommendations. *J Clin Oncol.* 2010;28(1):142–148.

29. Hanson L, Danis M, Garrett J. What is wrong with end-of-life care? Opinions of bereaved family members. *JAGS.* 1997;45(11):1339–1344.

30. Heyland DK, Dodek P, Rocker G, et al. What matters most in end-of-life care: perceptions of seriously ill patients and their family members. *CMAJ.* 2006;174:627–633.

31. Byock I. *Dying Well-Peace and Possibilities at the End of Life.* New York: The Berkley Publishing Group; 1997; 139–140.

COMMUNICATION

Chapter 40

What Is Known About Prognostication in Advanced Illness?

ROBERT GRAMLING, THOMAS CARROLL, AND RONALD M. EPSTEIN

And it [the effect of prognostication on outcomes] is one of the main reasons prognosis in medicine has both metaphysical significance and ethical implications; the effectiveness of prediction gives physicians greater clinical power and greater ethical obligations.

—*N. A. Christakis in Daedalus.[1]*

[T]he most fundamental medical choice patients with [serious illness] face—the decision between life-extending therapy and comfort care—may be highly influenced by their understanding of their prognoses.[2]

—*Study to Understand Prognoses and Preferences for Outcomes and Risks of Treatments (SUPPORT) Study Investigators*

INTRODUCTION AND SCOPE OF THE PROBLEM

Prognostication—the process of addressing "what to expect" for an individual's disease course—is essential for meaningful decision-making[3,4] and end-of-life planning[3,5] in advanced illness.[6–8] Despite the compelling reasons for communicating about prognosis, health professionals are often uncomfortable with prognostic uncertainty. That discomfort, and a culture of "ritualized optimism"[1] in medicine, are among myriad factors creating a health care environment in which prognostic conversations with seriously ill patients too infrequently occur.[1,7,9,10] For the many patients with advanced illness who wish to participate in decision making about their treatment options, the established practice of avoiding timely, balanced, and sensitive prognosis conversations presents a major challenge to patient-centered care.[11,12]

Promoting patient-centered communication in medical care is endorsed by the Institute of Medicine and the National Priorities Partnership as a major goal for twenty-first century health care.[11,12] "Patient-centered care" is a specific concept; it is something more than just "being nice" or doing what the patient asks. Patient-centered care considers the patient's unique experience of illness on equal ground with the physician's perspective; it directs clinicians to see the world both through the patient's eyes and through a clinical lens. Patient-centered care ultimately promotes meaningful involvement in care and decisions that reflect each patient's unique clinical context, personal values, and preferences.[13–15] Good communication is the cornerstone of patient-centered care, and promoting prognostic conversations that facilitate patient-centered communication with seriously ill patients is a timely issue facing society.

Mounting evidence that palliative care leads to substantial benefits in both quality and quantity of life[16,17] is accelerating an already steady growth of palliative care services in the United States.[18–20] Given its central focus on supporting patient-centered communication and decision-making,[21–23] palliative care will likely serve to catalyze the reemergence of prognostication in the practice of medicine.[2] Therefore palliative care requires ongoing and vigorous attention to the procedure of prognostication as clinicians establish, challenge, and reestablish best practices for this emerging discipline.

Improving communication in serious illness is difficult,[24] but it can be done.[25–29] Facilitating meaningful conversations in the emotionally charged, value-laden, and highly personal context of serious illness requires understanding and supporting communication behaviors for all participants (i.e., patients, family members, clinicians).[27] Therefore models of communication that address the dynamic "ecology" that conversation participants and contexts create are needed.

Note: Portions of this chapter have been published in Holloway RG, Gramling R, Kelly AG. Estimating and communicating prognoses in neurological disease. *Neurology.* 2012; in press.

ECOLOGICAL MODEL OF PROGNOSIS CONVERSATIONS

This chapter proposes an Ecological Model of Prognostic Conversations (EMPC) to address the specific content of prognosis conversations as well as the mutual influences among clinicians, patients, and their family members that contribute to effective information-seeking, comprehension, and deliberation. The communicational behaviors (shown in Figure 40-1 and described later) are dynamic factors crafted by all participants in the conversation. Each individual element has variable importance to promoting patient-centered conversations, depending on patient and caregiver interests, preferences, and readiness; the nature of suffering in need of immediate attention; and the salience to clinical management decisions.

EMPC identifies four main communication tasks for promoting patient-centered conversations about prognosis: *engaging* at desired levels of participation in decision-making and discussion of prognosis; mutually *informing* each other's understanding and opinions about the patient's prognosis; *responding* to emotions; and balanced *framing* of prognostic uncertainty. Evidence demonstrates that these behaviors result in psychological well-being, improved quality of life, better symptom management, better adherence to treatment, greater patient satisfaction, and lower levels of caregiver bereavement.[27]

Conversations about prognosis always involve uncertainty, and the degree of uncertainty can be substantial. Managing that prognostic uncertainty often assumes paramount importance to patients, their families, and their doctors as they balance complex issues of treatment burdens and benefits, comfort, function, location of care, bereavement, estate planning, relationship and spiritual reconciliation, and, ultimately, how to spend the remaining life. Disease trajectories are often challenging in predicting for individual patients, and the outcome of that uncertainty can be terrifying (i.e., suffering, death); thus the communicational skills for managing prognostic uncertainty in serious illness require attention to cognitive, emotional, and existential aspects of uncertainty near the end of life.

Currently there is a lack of adequate empirical understanding of best practices that effectively manage prognostic uncertainty, balance issues of hope and "realism" in serious illness,[30,31] and lead to patient-centered care. However, the existing empirical data demonstrate important barriers to the communication tasks proposed by the EMPC. Therefore this chapter is organized in two sections, Summary of Evidence and Suggestions for Practice, each of which is then further subdivided into the four conceptual domains: *Engaging, Informing, Responding,* and *Framing.*

SUMMARY OF EVIDENCE

Engaging

Prognosis conversations happen too infrequently, despite patient and family interest in having them. Seriously ill patients and their families do not object to prognostic discussions[32]; in fact, most want to have these conversations.[5,6,33–40] Most patients and clinicians favor full disclosure of prognosis, yet many clinicians fear that patients will be harmed by such discussions. Reassuringly, although patients often experience anxiety immediately after such discussions, evidence suggests that the anxiety is short-lived and that they are not harmed by discussing a poor prognosis with their doctor.[41] In fact, many are hurt more by perceived dishonesty about prognosis.[42–44]

Therefore communicating with patients and families about "what to expect" regarding the disease course, symptom and function trajectory, and remaining survival time is expected of clinicians who care for patients with serious illness.[3,6,45,46] Nonetheless, clinicians frequently avoid discussing poor or uncertain prognoses altogether.[7,9,47,48]

Although clinician knowledge and access to prognosis estimates are real barriers to engaging in such conversations, the SUPPORT study experience suggests that this does not fully explain reasons for avoidance. In the SUPPORT trial, physicians were provided with prognosis estimates nearly daily for more than 4500 seriously ill hospitalized patients. After 2 weeks of hospitalization, patients in the intervention group reported discussing prognosis with their physicians as infrequently as those in the control group (41% versus 39%). Even fewer (approximately 15%) participating physicians recalled any discussion of prognosis. Among those patients reporting no prognosis conversation, nearly half (42% among those in the intervention group, 44% in the control group) reported wanting to discuss prognosis.[47] These data suggest that avoidance of prognosis conversations is a multifaceted aspect of modern medical culture and not merely lack of

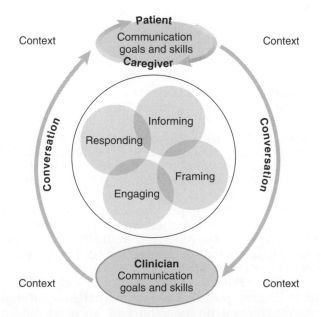

FIGURE 40-1. Ecological model of prognosis conversations.

access to prognosis estimates or patient or family desire for such discussions.

Palliative care is likely to address some of these gaps in communication about prognosis among the seriously ill.[3,8,23,49] Although few direct-observation data exist to describe palliative care communication practices, the authors recently observed and audio-recorded 75 palliative care inpatient consultations. Ninety-three percent contained direct conversations about prognosis.

Informing

When conversations do occur, participants enter the conversation with an understanding about prognosis that is often optimistic. Christakis[50,51] describes prognostication as a procedure involving forecasting and foretelling, both of which are vulnerable to optimistic biases. Forecasting is the clinician's or patient's estimate of the patient's prognosis. Forecasting estimates by both clinicians[51,52] and patients[53] tend to be optimistically biased. Among seriously ill hospitalized patients, Weeks and colleagues[2,47] observed that physicians overestimated patient survival, that patients were even more optimistic than physicians, and that patients' optimistic forecasting biases predict more aggressive, cure-oriented treatment.[2,47]

Responding

Conversations about prognosis are laden with emotion, yet clinicians typically fail to recognize or respond to patient cues for empathic responses. Fear, sadness, worry, joy, and hope are among the many human emotional experiences that prognosis conversations can elicit. These may manifest directly and in easily recognizable ways (e.g., "I'm afraid of dying."). However, patients often express important emotions indirectly (e.g., humor, sarcasm, nervousness, withdrawal).[27] To be patient-centered, clinicians need to attend to these indirect cues and thus uncover psychological and existential suffering. By recognizing emotions, clinicians can enhance their understanding of the person and acknowledge the role of emotions in their decision making.

Cues to explore or acknowledge emotion often go unnoticed for patients with advanced illness.[27,54] For example, Pollak and colleagues[54] audiorecorded 398 office visit conversations between 51 oncologists and 270 patients with advanced cancers. They identified 292 "empathic opportunities" of expressed negative emotions, of which two thirds were direct cues (e.g., "I'm scared about…"[54]) and one third were indirect cues (e.g., "Oh no. What do we do now?"[54]). Physicians responded to fewer than one third of the empathic opportunities with attempts to name, understand, respect, support, or explore the emotion, regardless of whether the cue was indirect or direct.

Framing

Participants craft conversations that place an additional optimistic frame on their already optimistic

understanding. Foretelling refers to the prognosis that the clinician communicates to the patient; often clinicians indicate to the patient a more optimistic estimate than the clinician actually believes.[7,52] Optimistic framing can include the manner of presenting (1) probabilistic information (e.g., "likely," "soon," relative risk, absolute risk); (2) what is to be gained or lost relating to the decision for which prognosis is being discussed (e.g., gain: "Choosing hospice allows us to focus all of our energy on enhancing the quality of your life, however long that is."); or merely (3) the frequency of optimistic versus pessimistic statements made during the conversation.[55–58] One of the few studies of the impact that framing has on treatment decisions among the seriously ill was done by Robinson and colleagues,[58] who observed conversations between 51 oncologists and 141 outpatients with advanced cancer. Patients were eligible if the oncologist "would not be surprised" if they died within 1 year. This work produced two main findings: (1) oncologists made nearly three times as many optimistic remarks as pessimistic ones, and (2) the absence of pessimistic remarks made by the oncologist was associated with patients reporting optimistically biased expectations for cure at 1 week follow-up.[58] This combination of forecasting and foretelling biases often sets the patient up for doubly optimistic information in prognostic discussions.[43,50,52]

SUGGESTIONS FOR PRACTICE

Due to its brevity, this chapter can provide only some general suggestions based on the empirical observations described in the previous section. Clinicians at all stages of practice should continually seek opportunities for communication training, mentoring, and skill maintenance.

Engaging

For clinicians who wish to engage in prognosis conversations with patients but are concerned that prognosis information is not desired by seriously ill patients and their families, the literature should be reassuring here. Most patients with advanced illness want at least some prognostic information from their physicians.[6,35–38,43] Of importance to clinicians preparing for these conversations, most of these patients want at least some control as to the timing, amount of information, manner of presentation, and who should be present during discussions.[6,36–38,43,59] Therefore clinicians should ask patients and families if they would like to discuss prognosis and then, if desired, inquire about patient preferences for timing, who should be there, the roles they would like to take with regard to important decisions, and the level of detail and format of the information.

Question Prompt Lists (QPLs) can help patients and families participate. To be patient-centered, clinicians need an ongoing and accurate understanding of the patient's perspective, values, and needs—some of which are quite dynamic and can even evolve during a single conversation. Patients may need help clarifying their questions, concerns, and hopes regarding prognosis before conversations with their physicians. A tool such as a QPL[60,61] can help patients and families contemplate what they wish to know, identify whether they are ready, express how they would like to discuss prognosis and be involved in decisions, determine when they would like information, and state how much information they want to receive and in what form they would like that information. An example section of a QPL that focuses on prognosis communication is shown in Box 40-1.

Many patients will not have had a meaningful conversation about prognosis. A QPL can help patients and families clarify what they wish to know about prognosis. However, a QPL is neither necessary nor sufficient for achieving a complete understanding of information preferences and perspectives; this remains an essential part of the human interaction in the conversation. The time spent in this endeavor will depend on the demands of the clinical situation—the degree to which patients demonstrate interest and capacity and the degree of distress that may be caused by attempting to define preferences. Many, if not most, conversations begin with one understanding of information preferences and evolve, sometimes quickly, toward a substantially different set of information preferences and needs. Clinicians will need flexibility and should remain mindful of both cognitive and emotional cues for changing information needs during the conversation. Others have recently characterized this patient-centered skill as a delicate balance of "sharing *versus* caring"—meaning that attending to emotional and existential well-being may at times preclude, delay, or abort the sharing of information when caring for persons in often terrifying

decision-making contexts, such as advanced or serious illness.[62]

In some instances, prognostic uncertainty represents an unnecessary barrier to decision making in prognosis conversations. The clinician should be aware of three such situations. The first is to identify the dimensions regarding "what to expect" that are most important to the patient. For example, sometimes survival prognoses are highly uncertain, yet trajectories of functional decline are more predictable. In such cases, clarity about expected function can be very important for patient decision

---

BOX 40-1. Question Prompt List for Prognosis Conversations (Oncology Visit Example)

Introduction

Most people who see their oncologist have questions and concerns, particularly when there are changes. It's very common to forget important questions during an office visit, only to wish you had remembered to ask them later.

We put this list of questions together after discussion with patients, their families, and their caregivers, as well as doctors and other health care professionals. This list can help your doctor answer any questions you have now or may have in the future.

What can I expect?
• What can I expect to be able to do in the future?
• Will this cancer shorten my life?
• Is it possible to give me a timeframe?
• What is the best-case scenario? The worst-case scenario?
• Notes:

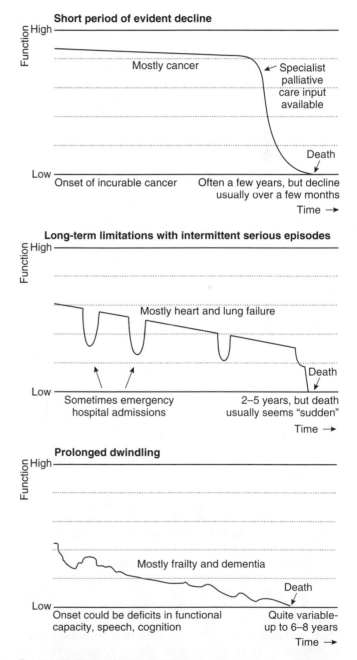

FIGURE 40-2. Common function trajectories in palliative care. (*Modified from Lynn J, Adamson DM. Living Well at the End of Life: Adapting Health Care to Serious Chronic Illness in Old Age. Washington, DC: Rand Health; 2003:8.*)

making. Figure 40-2 presents examples of functional trajectories that can be shared directly (as pictures) or explained in the context of conversations in which patients desire such information.

In the second situation, the clinician should understand what a "good" outcome would be for an individual patient. For example, in many clinical contexts (e.g., severe head injury, stroke, massive myocardial infarction), clinicians are very uncertain whether a person might live or be able to perform any basic functions (e.g., talking, eating, dressing), but quite certain that returning to independent living is extremely unlikely. For some decisions facing patients, surrogates, and families, the chance that the patient will return to full and independent function (which is nearly certain) might be of greater importance than estimates of survival time or lesser functioning (which is quite uncertain).

Third, clinicians should consider timeframes and levels of precision that are relevant to patients and families. For example, clinicians often find it challenging to estimate whether a patient with advanced illness is likely to live for 1, 2, or 3 months. Often, this struggle leads to more prognostic testing or avoidance of prognosis conversations with patients or other members of a multidisciplinary clinical team who are trying to weigh treatment recommendations. However, the patient and family may still be considering prognosis in terms of "cure" or years of survival. In such situations, it may be sufficient to adjust the patients' and families' general sense that the likely horizon is far closer than they imagined. This information is often enough to inform treatment decisions; prioritize spiritual, existential, and relationship healing efforts; prepare family and caregivers; and initiate end-of-life planning. Sensitively asking patients (and those family members or caregivers patients wish to be part of the conversation) to share their intuitions and understanding of their prognosis, as well as the degree of clarity they would find helpful often can avoid these mismatches.

Responding

Physicians who desire to improve their skills for responding to empathic opportunities can do so.[25,28,63,64] Particularly for busy clinicians in practice, brief communication training programs that directly observe conversations with standardized patients, followed by immediate feedback, coaching, and practice may be helpful.[26,65]

For clinicians to continually recognize and respond to empathic opportunities in practice, this requires ongoing nurturing. Clinicians will have many individual strategies for maintaining the reservoir of attention, compassionate energy, and self-awareness that is required to maintain effective empathic communication in practice. For those seeking further resources, recent evidence finds that mindfulness-based training opportunities are particularly effective for helping clinicians avoid burnout and improve empathy in practice.[66]

Framing

"Foretelling" within a conversation is a collective venture that is vulnerable to imbalance, depending on the understanding, motivations, and personalities of the conversation participants. As the expert participant in the conversation, clinicians need to maintain ongoing attention to the evolving frame of the prognosis "picture" that arises during the conversation. If the frame becomes imbalanced, clinicians will need to consider carefully whether the degree of imbalance is appropriate to the patient's personal and decisional context. This can be challenging and requires a high degree of self-awareness on the part of the clinician. Although it is convenient (and true) to state that "dishonesty" is ethically unjustified, three points should be considered when framing imbalance and honesty. First is that intentional dishonesty is nearly always hurtful to the patient and family, even if such dishonesty provides immediate comfort. For example, a well-meaning clinician may allow a conversation to be heavily flavored with optimism and feel good about instilling hope or even joy, yet then not bear witness the utter devastation and indignity that patients and families can feel when they realize that their hopes were, in fact, drastically misinformed. Second, "dishonesty" reflects misrepresentation rather than retrospective inaccuracy. For nearly all illness trajectories, some subsets of people live substantially longer and some live substantially shorter than the common course; often patients ask clinicians to evaluate their chances of being in the favorable (or unfavorable) group. When clinicians communicate their thoughtful appraisal that an individual is likely to do better or worse than the norm, such actions are honest, regardless of whether this proves untrue in time. Third, "bluntness" is also hurtful; clinicians who wish to bring balance to overly optimistic (or overly pessimistic) prognosis conversations need not do so in insensitive or dismissive ways. Gramling and Epstein[30] and Back and colleagues[31] describe one effective strategy for balancing optimism and realism in prognostic conversations.

NEXT STEPS FOR RESEARCH

Communicating about prognosis requires probabilistic thinking on the part of all participants. Such conversations are not objective procedures of shuttling data from "transmitters" to "receivers"; it is subjective, emotional, and relational. Little is known about which clinician communication behaviors constitute "best practices" for the rapidly emerging field of palliative care. Establishing such standards will require, at a minimum, a stronger empirical understanding of how characteristics of prognosis conversations shape participants' perceptions and processes of deliberation; match treatment decisions to preferences and values; ameliorate suffering; and enhance quality of life.

SUMMARY RECOMMENDATIONS

- Palliative care clinicians should develop and maintain skills in estimating and discussing prognosis in order to engage patients and families in high quality conversations.
- Using a concrete model of communication will help ensure that communication about prognosis meets the highest standards of patient-centered care.
- More research is needed to establish a stronger empirical understanding about the prognosis communication behaviors that ultimately support patient-centered care.

REFERENCES

1. Christakis NA. Prognostication and bioethics. *Daedalus.* 1999;128(4):197–214.
2. Weeks JC, Cook EF, O'Day SJ, et al. Relationship between cancer patients' predictions of prognosis and their treatment preferences. *JAMA.* 1998;279(21):1709–1714.
3. Glare PA, Sinclair CT. Palliative medicine review: prognostication. *J Palliat Med.* 2008;11(1):84–103.
4. Norton SA, Bowers BJ. Working toward consensus: providers' strategies to shift patients from curative to palliative treatment choices. *Res Nurs Health.* 2001;24(4):258–269.
5. Steinhauser KE, Christakis NA, Clipp EC, McNeilly M, McIntyre L, Tulsky JA. Factors considered important at the end of life by patients, family, physicians, and other care providers. *JAMA.* 2000;284(19):2476–2482.
6. Parker SM, Clayton JM, Hancock K, et al. A systematic review of prognostic/end-of-life communication with adults in the advanced stages of a life-limiting illness: patient/caregiver preferences for the content, style, and timing of information. *J Pain Symptom Manage.* 2007;34(1):81–93.
7. Christakis NA, Iwashyna TJ. Attitude and self-reported practice regarding prognostication in a national sample of internists. *Arch Intern Med.* 1998;158(21):2389–2395.
8. Goodlin SJ, Hauptman PJ, Arnold R, et al. Consensus statement: palliative and supportive care in advanced heart failure. *J Cardiac Failure.* 2004;10(3):200–209.
9. White DB, Engelberg RA, Wenrich MD, Lo B, Curtis JR. Prognostication during physician-family discussions about limiting life support in intensive care units. *Crit Care Med.* 2007;35(2):442–448.
10. White DB, Engelberg RA, Wenrich MD, Lo B, Curtis JR. The language of prognostication in intensive care units. *Med Decis Making.* 2008;30:76–83.
11. National Priorities Partnership. *National Priorities and Goals: Aligning Our Efforts to Transform America's Healthcare.* Washington, DC: National Quality Forum; 2008.
12. Institute of Medicine Committee on Quality of Health Care in America. *Crossing the Quality Chasm: A New Health System for the 21st Century.* Washington, DC: National Academies Press; 2001; 360.
13. McWhinney IR. Why we need a new clinical method. *Scand J Prim Health Care.* 1993;11(1):3–7.
14. Epstein RM, Campbell TL, Cohen-Cole SA, McWhinney IR, Smilkstein G. Perspectives on patient-doctor communication. *J Fam Pract.* 1993;37(4):377–388.
15. Epstein RM, Franks P, Fiscella K, et al. Measuring patient-centered communication in patient-physician consultations: theoretical and practical issues. *Soc Sci Med.* 2005;61(7):1516–1528.
16. Temel JS, Greer JA, Muzikansky A, et al. Early palliative care for patients with metastatic non-small-cell lung cancer. *N Engl J Med.* 2010;363(8):733–742.
17. Bakitas M, Lyons KD, Hegel MT, et al. Effects of a palliative care intervention on clinical outcomes in patients with advanced cancer: the Project ENABLE II randomized controlled trial. *JAMA.* 2009;302(7):741–749.
18. National Palliative Care Research Center. *Growth of Hospital Based Palliative Care Programs Since 1998.* www.npcrc.org. Accessed September 10, 2012.
19. Morrison RS, Maroney-Galin C, Kralovec PD, Meier DE. The growth of palliative care programs in United States hospitals. *J Palliat Med.* 2005;8(6):1127–1134.
20. Center to Advance Palliative Care. *New analysis shows hospitals continue to implement palliative care programs at rapid pace: new medical subspecialty fills gap for aging population.* Available at www.capc.org; 2008. Accessed September 10, 2012.
21. Homsi J, Walsh D, Nelson KA, et al. The impact of a palliative medicine consultation service in medical oncology. *Support Care Cancer.* 2002;10(4):337–342.
22. Manfredi PL, Morrison RS, Morris J, Goldhirsch SL, Carter JM, Meier DE. Palliative care consultations: how do they impact the care of hospitalized patients? *J Pain Symptom Manage.* 2000;20(3):166–173.
23. Weissman DE. Consultation in palliative medicine. *Arch Intern Med.* 1997;157(7):733–737.
24. Covinsky KE, Fuller JD, Yaffe K, et al. Communication and decision-making in seriously ill patients: findings of the SUPPORT project. The Study to Understand Prognoses and Preferences for Outcomes and Risks of Treatments. *J Am Geriatr Soc.* 2000;48(5 suppl):S187–S193.
25. Back AL, Arnold RM, Baile WF, et al. Efficacy of communication skills training for giving bad news and discussing transitions to palliative care. *Arch Intern Med.* 2007;167(5):453–460.
26. Back AL, Arnold RM, Tulsky JA, Baile WF, Fryer-Edwards KA. Teaching communication skills to medical oncology fellows. *J Clin Oncol.* 2003;21(12):2433–2436.
27. Epstein RM, Street RL. *Patient-Centered Communication in Cancer Care.* Bethesda, MD: National Institutes of Health; 2007; 203.
28. Lewin SA, Skea ZC, Entwistle V, Zwarenstein M, Dick J. Interventions for providers to promote a patient-centred approach in clinical consultations. *Cochrane Database Syst Rev.* 2001;(4) CD003267.
29. Rao JK, Anderson LA, Inui TS, Frankel RM. Communication interventions make a difference in conversations between physicians and patients: a systematic review of the evidence. *Med Care.* 2007;45(4):340–349.
30. Gramling R, Epstein R. Optimism amid serious illness: clinical panacea or ethical conundrum? *Arch Intern Med.* 2011; 171(10):935–936.
31. Back AL, Arnold RM, Quill TE. Hope for the best, and prepare for the worst. *Ann Intern Med.* 2003;138(5):439–443.
32. Shah S, Blanchard M, Tookman A, Jones L, Blizard R, King M. Estimating needs in life threatening illness: a feasibility study to assess the views of patients and doctors. *Palliat Med.* 2006;20(3):205–210.
33. Horne G, Payne S. Removing the boundaries: palliative care for patients with heart failure. *Palliat Med.* 2004;18(4):291–296.
34. Apatira L, Boyd EA, Malvar G, et al. Hope, truth, and preparing for death: perspectives of surrogate decision makers. *Ann Intern Med.* 2008;149(12):861–868.
35. Butow PN, Dowsett S, Hagerty R, Tattersall MH. Communicating prognosis to patients with metastatic disease: what do they really want to know? *Support Care Cancer.* 2002; 10(2):161–168.
36. Hagerty RG, Butow PN, Ellis PA, et al. Cancer patient preferences for communication of prognosis in the metastatic setting. *J Clin Oncol.* 2004;22(9):1721–1730.
37. Hagerty RG, Butow PN, Ellis PM, Dimitry S, Tattersall MH. Communicating prognosis in cancer care: a systematic review of the literature. *Ann Oncol.* 2005;16(7):1005–1053.
38. Hagerty RG, Butow PN, Ellis PM, et al. Communicating with realism and hope: incurable cancer patients' views on the disclosure of prognosis. *J Clin Oncol.* 2005;23(6):1278–1288.
39. Hancock K, Clayton JM, Parker SM, et al. Truth-telling in discussing prognosis in advanced life-limiting illnesses: a systematic review. *Palliat Med.* 2007;21(6):507–517.
40. Hancock K, Clayton JM, Parker SM, et al. Discrepant perceptions about end-of-life communication: a systematic review. *J Pain Symptom Manage.* 2007;34(2):190–200.
41. Weiner JS, Roth J. Avoiding iatrogenic harm to patient and family while discussing goals of care near the end of life. *J Palliat Med.* 2006;9(2):451–463.

42. Clayton JM, Butow PN, Tattersall MH. The needs of terminally ill cancer patients versus those of caregivers for information regarding prognosis and end-of-life issues. *Cancer.* 2005;103(9):1957–1964.

43. Fallowfield LJ, Jenkins VA, Beveridge HA. Truth may hurt but deceit hurts more: communication in palliative care. *Palliat Med.* 2002;16(4):297–303.

44. Norton SA, Tilden VP, Tolle SW, Nelson CA, Eggman ST. Life support withdrawal: communication and conflict. *Am J Crit Care.* 2003;12(6):548–555.

45. Bruera E, Neumann CM, Mazzocato C, Stiefel F, Sala R. Attitudes and beliefs of palliative care physicians regarding communication with terminally ill cancer patients. *Palliat Med.* 2000;14(4):287–298.

46. Lamont EB, Christakis NA. Complexities in prognostication in advanced cancer: "to help them live their lives the way they want to." *JAMA.* 2003;290(1):98–104.

47. The SUPPORT Principal Investigators. A controlled trial to improve care for seriously ill hospitalized patients. The Study to Understand Prognoses and Preferences for Outcomes and Risks of Treatments (SUPPORT). *JAMA.* 1995;274(20):1591–1598.

48. White DB, Engelberg RA, Wenrich MD, Lo B, Curtis JR. Prognostication during physician-family discussions about limiting life support in intensive care units. *Crit Care Med.* 2007;35(2):442–448.

49. Clayton JM, Hancock KM, Butow PN, et al. Clinical practice guidelines for communicating prognosis and end-of-life issues with adults in the advanced stages of a life-limiting illness, and their caregivers. *Med J Aust.* 2007;186(12 suppl):S77–S108.

50. Christakis NA. *Death Foretold: Prophecy and Prognosis in Medical Care.* Chicago: University of Chicago Press; 1999; 374.

51. Christakis NA, Lamont EB. Extent and determinants of error in doctors' prognoses in terminally ill patients: prospective cohort study. *BMJ.* 2000;320(7233):469–472.

52. Lamont EB, Christakis NA. Prognostic disclosure to patients with cancer near the end of life. *Ann Intern Med.* 2001;134(12):1096–1105.

53. Allen LA, Yager JE, Funk MJ, et al. Discordance between patient-predicted and model-predicted life expectancy among ambulatory patients with heart failure. *JAMA.* 2008;299(21):2533–2542.

54. Pollak KI, Arnold RM, Jeffreys AS, et al. Oncologist communication about emotion during visits with patients with advanced cancer. *J Clin Oncol.* 2007;25(36):5748–5752.

55. Rothman AJ, Kiviniemi MT. Treating people with information: an analysis and review of approaches to communicating health risk information. *J Natl Cancer Inst Monogr.* 1999;25:44–51.

56. Rothman AJ, Salovey P. Shaping perceptions to motivate healthy behavior: the role of message framing. *Psychol Bull.* 1997;121(1):3–19.

57. Sulls J, Wallston KA. *Social Psychological Foundations of Health and Illness.* Malden, MA: Blackwell; 2003:608.

58. Robinson TM, Alexander SC, Hays M, et al. Patient-oncologist communication in advanced cancer: predictors of patient perception of prognosis. *Support Care Cancer.* 2008;16(9):1049–1057.

59. Clayton JM, Butow PN, Arnold RM, Tattersall MH. Discussing life expectancy with terminally ill cancer patients and their carers: a qualitative study. *Support Care Cancer.* 2005;13(9): 733–742.

60. Butow PN, Dunn SM, Tattersall MH, Jones QJ. Patient participation in the cancer consultation: evaluation of a question prompt sheet. *Ann Oncol.* 1994;5(3):199–204.

61. Dimoska A, Tattersall MH, Butow PN, Shepherd H, Kinnersley P. Can a "prompt list" empower cancer patients to ask relevant questions? *Cancer.* 2008;113(2):225–237.

62. Smith A, Juraskova I, Butow P, et al. Sharing vs. caring: the relative impact of sharing decisions versus managing emotions on patient outcomes. *Patient Educ Couns.* 2011;82(2):233–239.

63. Platt FW, Keller VF. Empathic communication: a teachable and learnable skill. *J Gen Intern Med.* 1994;9(4):222–226.

64. Gysels M, Richardson A, Higginson IJ. Communication training for health professionals who care for patients with cancer: a systematic review of effectiveness. *Support Care Cancer.* 2004;12(10):692–700.

65. Gysels M, Richardson A, Higginson IJ. Communication training for health professionals who care for patients with cancer: a systematic review of training methods. *Support Care Cancer.* 2005;13(6):356–366.

66. Krasner MS, Epstein RM, Beckman H, et al. Association of an educational program in mindful communication with burnout, empathy, and attitudes among primary care physicians. *JAMA.* 2009;302(12):1284–1293.

67. Lynn J, Adamson DM. *Living Well at the End of Life: Adapting Health Care to Serious Chronic Illness in Old Age.* Washington, DC: Rand Health; 2003:8.

Chapter 41

What Is a Useful Strategy for Estimating Survival in Palliative Care Settings for Persons With Advanced Cancer?

THOMAS CARROLL, RONALD M. EPSTEIN, AND ROBERT GRAMLING

ANTICIPATING
ANCHORING
TAILORING
DEBIASING
CLINICAL SCENARIO
    Step 1: Anticipating
    Step 2: Anchoring
    Step 3: Tailoring
    Step 4: Debiasing

The goal of this chapter is to provide a framework for clinicians to efficiently and accurately estimate survival prognoses in preparation for patient-centered conversations. This chapter describes a four-step clinical process of "anticipating," "anchoring," "tailoring," and "debiasing."

ANTICIPATING

Clarifying preferences for timing and desired types of prognostic information is a relational process that occurs during a conversation or series of conversations. Nonetheless, clinicians will need to prepare some basic information about prognosis for an initial conversation. In preparation, clinicians will need to make judgments about the types of survival information that appear to fit the urgency and types of decisions facing the patient and family. Clinicians will need to confirm or adapt these initial assumptions upon meeting the patient/family and evaluating the clinical situation more closely.

In general, estimating survival in terms of "usual," "best case," and "worst case" can be useful for prognostic discussions. Therefore the following Anchoring and Tailoring sections are organized to provide basic survival prognosis for the usual course of disease (i.e., median survival, 25%-75% range of survival), best case (i.e., 25% surviving the longest period), and worst case (i.e., 25% surviving the shortest period).

Clinicians will note that the usual course of survival can be quite broad. For some clinical situations, further prognostic tests (including passage of time) can add some precision to prognosis estimates. Pursuit of further testing will generally delay conversations and often add burden to patients. Therefore clinicians must anticipate how much precision is warranted to engage patients in conversation about prognosis. In some situations simple tests or short periods of clinical observation can help refine extremely imprecise and often meaningless estimates (e.g., "it could be days, it could be years"). On the other hand, available data can generally inform prognosis estimates with less extreme degrees of imprecision and be useful for initial conversations. For example, some patients and families may find merely knowing that usual survival is on the order of "weeks to a few months" quite useful to orienting decision making. Some patients and families will seek more efforts to refine such estimates with further testing, whereas others will not.

ANCHORING

Predicting the natural history for a patient's clinical course first requires an "anchored"[1] understanding of the illness trajectory at the population level. Population-level descriptions about the usual illness course arise by aggregating the observations from single or multiple epidemiological studies. One critical judgment for clinicians to make about population-based prognosis estimates is whether the patient's clinical condition is similar enough to that of the reference population (i.e., the theoretical group of people represented by the individual studies) to provide useful comparison. Most reference populations have been defined by the disease and stage of disease. However, many advanced illnesses have similar survival trajectories as functional status declines,[2] and function-based survival data are becoming increasingly more available to palliative care clinicians.

This chapter presents "anchors" for several cancers using both disease-specific and function-specific reference populations (Tables 41-1 and 41-2). These function-based data use the Palliative Performance Scale (PPS) for determining functional status (Table 41-3). The anchored survival estimates are organized to fit the anticipated information needs described previously—usual course (median, 25%-75% range), best case (25% surviving the longest period), and worst case (25% surviving the shortest period).

TAILORING

Often, population data alone are useful for decision making, but patients and clinicians ultimately struggle to predict "what to expect" for the individual patient.

Note: Portions of this chapter have been published in Holloway RG, Gramling R, Kelly AG. Estimating and communicating prognoses in neurological disease. *Neurology.* 2012; in press.

TABLE 41-1. Benchmark Anchors for Advanced Cancers Commonly Encountered in Palliative Care

CANCER SITE	TYPE	INDICATORS OF ADVANCED STAGE	TREATMENT STATUS*	SURVIVAL TIME (MO)[†]														
				≤1	2	4	6	8	10	12	14	16	18	20	22	24	>24	>36
Lung	NSCLC[4,5]	Distant mets	B/C			4												
	SCLC[4]	Distant mets	C					8										
Head/neck[6,7]	Laryngeal	Advanced	A															36
Gastro-intestinal	Colon AdenoCA[8]	Distant mets	C							12								
	Pancreatic[9]	Inoperable	A						10									
	Pancreatic[9]	Inoperable	B				5											
	Esophageal[10]	Inoperable	A						10									
	Hepatocellular[11]	Inoperable	B				6											
	Gastric[12]	Distant mets	B			5												
	Ampullary[13]	Node positive	A											20				
Renal[14]	RCC	Stage IV, measurable lesions	A							12								
Breast[15]	Invasive breast cancer	Distant mets	B															36
Prostate[16]	Hormone resistant	Any metastasis	A								15							
Intracranial[17]	GBM, age <50 yr	New diagnosis	A					8										
	GBM, age >80 yr		A		3													
Cutaneous[18]	Melanoma[19]	Distant mets, abnormal LDH	C				6											
		Distant mets, normal LDH	C												22			
Hemato-logical	AML[20]	Second relapse	A		3													
	AML[21]	First relapse	A					8										
Unknown primary[22]	Adenocarcinoma	Liver mets or alb <3.5	A, B				6											
	Adenocarcinoma	No liver mets and alb >3.5	A, B					8										

The treatment bars represent the usual survival range (i.e., that representative of 25%-75% of patients with the condition as described). The area to the right of the bars is the best case scenario (i.e., a survival expectation above the 75th percentile). The area to the left of the bars is the worst case scenario (i.e., a survival expectation less than the 25th percentile). The bold numbers superimposed on each of the bars represent the median survival time (rounded, in months) for the condition as described.
AdenoCA, Adenocarcinoma; *alb*, albumin; *AML*, acute myelogenous leukemia; *GBM*, glioblastoma multiforme; *mets*, metastasis; *NSCLC*, non–small cell lung cancer; *RCC*, renal cell carcinoma; *SCLC*, small cell lung cancer.
*Treatments status: A, Active disease-moderating treatment; B, no or minimal active disease-moderating treatment; C, undefined.
[†]Rounded to the nearest 2-mo interval; most values were manually extrapolated from published Kaplan-Meier Survival curves and are approximate.

TABLE 41-2. Function-Based Anchors of Survival Time in a Population Receiving Palliative Care Services

REFERENCE POPULATION[24]	SAMPLE SIZE	PPS CATEGORY (%)	SURVIVAL TIME (WK)*														
			<1	1	2	3	4	5	6	7	8	9	10	11	12	>12	≥16	≥24
People enrolled in Canadian hospice for home, acute, or respite palliative care	150	70											10					
	487	60							6									
	1055	50						5										
	1647	40			2													
	1420	30		1														
	737	20	<1															

The treatment bars represent the usual survival range (i.e., that representative of 25%-75% of patients with the condition as described). The area to the right of the bars is the best case scenario (i.e., a survival expectation above the 75th percentile). The area to the left of the bars is the worst case scenario (i.e., a survival expectation less than the 25th percentile). The bold numbers superimposed on each of the bars represent the median survival time (rounded, in months) for the condition as described.
PPS, Palliative Performance Scale.
*Extrapolated from Kaplan-Meier survival curves. Similar pattern of median and worst case survival times observed in a meta-analysis of other palliative care cohorts; best case were similar or a little longer.[23]

TABLE 41-3. Palliative Performance Scale

PPS LEVEL (%)	AMBULATION	ACTIVITY AND EVIDENCE OF DISEASE	SELF-CARE	INTAKE	CONSCIOUS LEVEL
100	Full	Normal activity and work No evidence of disease	Full	Normal	Full
90	Full	Normal activity and work Some evidence of disease	Full	Normal	Full
80	Full	Normal activity with effort Some evidence of disease	Full	Normal or reduced	Full
70	Reduced	Unable to perform normal job/work Significant disease	Full	Normal or reduced	Full
60	Reduced	Unable to do hobby/house work Significant disease	Occasional assistance necessary	Normal or reduced	Full or confusion
50	Mainly sit/lie	Unable to do any work Extensive disease	Considerable assistance required	Normal or reduced	Full or confusion
40	Mainly in bed	Unable to do most activity Extensive disease	Mainly assistance	Normal or reduced	Full or drowsy +/– confusion
30	Totally bed bound	Unable to do any activity Extensive disease	Total care	Normal or reduced	Full or drowsy +/– confusion
20	Totally bed bound	Unable to do any activity Extensive disease	Total care	Minimal to sips	Full or drowsy +/– confusion
10	Totally bed bound	Unable to do any activity Extensive disease	Total care	Mouth care only	Drowsy or coma +/– confusion
0	Dead	—	—	—	—

From Ho F, Lau F, Downing MG, Lesperance M. A reliability and validity study of the Palliative Performance Scale. *BMC Palliat Care.* 2008;7:10.

Some of this tailoring process can occur before the initial conversation, but the bulk will occur as the clinician gets to know the patient and the clinical situation. Tailoring usually stretches epidemiological data (i.e., finite amount of reference populations that can never truly represent a patient's unique context) and mathematical assumptions (i.e., applying probabilities to an individual). Nonetheless, this can be accomplished with a reasonable level of clinical utility. Tailoring procedures involve modeling of data from empirically observed populations and/or heuristically integrating clinical experience and judgment.

Modeling calculates the probability of survival for an imaginary individual that is defined by the factors available in the observed data (i.e., age, gender, stage, etc.). Disease-specific calculators (e.g., Seattle Heart Failure) are most common; however, some setting-specific models (e.g., Acute Physiology and Chronic Health Evaluation [APACHE] for the intensive care unit) are also available. The PPS is a palliative care setting–specific model[3] for calculating a tailored survival estimate based on functional status, age, gender, disease category, and clinical setting. The nomogram calculator for tailoring survival estimate using the PPS is shown in Table 41-1.

Clinical judgment is always present to varying degrees in prognosis estimation. Such judgments can be quite accurate depending on the proximity from death and the skill of the clinician. However, clinical judgment is also subject to substantial optimistic biases as described in Chapter 40. Thus debiasing is an important final step in prognosis estimation, particularly when such judgments are heavily based on clinical heuristics.

DEBIASING

Understanding the factors that promote sound prognostic judgment remain poorly understood; however, there are some strategies for addressing the observed tendency to systematically overestimate survival. (The process of debiasing also will help avoid systematically underestimating survival, as well.) First, use anchors and tailoring calculators based in representative populations. Second, ask questions that can help free clinicians to contemplate their prognostic judgments without the undue burden of "needing to be certain" before considering that death is approaching. For example, asking, "Would I be surprised if this person died in the next few days?" or "Would I be surprised if this person lived for 3 months?" can help to ground expectations. These "would I be surprised if…" estimates do require clinical experience to inform the judgment and might not work as well for clinicians who are newer to caring for people with advanced illnesses. Third, institute systematic practice with both survival and functional predictions and model these efforts for trainees. One approach might involve privately committing to a prognostic estimate (i.e., recording it in a personal notebook) and systematically comparing the estimate to the observed clinical course, starting first with shorter time horizons and moving toward longer predictions as accuracy improves.

CLINICAL SCENARIO

The following clinical scenario will walk the reader through a hypothetical case of a patient with cancer and demonstrate how to use the techniques outlined in this chapter.

Your palliative care team is asked by the oncology team to help address goals of care for a hospitalized patient with advanced pancreatic cancer. You review the hospital chart, speak with her nurse, and call the oncology attending to clarify the clinical situation. You learn that the patient, J. L., is a 48-year-old woman who was diagnosed with advanced pancreatic cancer approximately 3 months ago. Her oncologist is not recommending any further disease-moderating therapies, and chemotherapy was recently stopped because the burdens outweighed the expected benefits. Her functional status has been declining rapidly over the past 2 months; from the description you estimate her PPS to be 40%. She was admitted 3 days ago for pain and failure to thrive at home. The nursing chart documents 4 to 6 on a pain rating scale of 0 to 10 consistently since admission. Her advanced directives are not documented. Her husband, sister, and grown children have been present during the hospitalization and are expected to be present today. The hospitalist attending is unsure if J.L.'s primary oncologist has already discussed prognosis, but the hospital team has not. J.L. has had full decision-making capacity during this hospitalization.

Step 1: Anticipating

You foresee the possibility that your initial conversation will at least touch on treatment choices (i.e., advance directives) and care planning, for which prognosis information is of potential importance. You also appreciate that her current symptoms of pain will require attention and may take precedence over any prognosis conversation today. You decide that being able to accurately estimate survival in general timeframes (e.g., "days to a few weeks," "weeks to a few months," "many months to more than a year," or "many years") is reasonable preparation for your initial meeting with J. L. You are ready to modify these assumptions as you get to know her and her clinical situation better.

Step 2: Anchoring

You reference two types of populations to anchor your survival estimate. The first is a population of people with advanced pancreatic cancer who are not undergoing active disease-moderating treatment (Table 41-1), observing a median survival of 5 months, 25% living longer than 8 months (best case), and 25% dying within 4 months (worst case). The second is palliative care population with similar levels of function (Table 41-2; PPS 40%), observing a median survival of 2 months, 25% living longer than 4 months (best case), and 25% dying within 1 month (worst case). You note the degree of discrepancy and recognize that you are leaning more toward the palliative care population estimate, given what you have been told and read about her level of functional decline and clinical condition. You wait to confirm with your clinical assessment.

Step 3: Tailoring

You are able to quickly access sufficient clinical data for further tailoring your function-based anchor. You refer to the PPS nomogram (Figure 41-1) and sum the points attributed to each of the tailoring variables (0 [gender] + 0 [age] + 14 [main disease type] + 3 [care setting] + 31 [PPS score of 40%] = 48). You note that the total score of 48 predicts a median survival of 3 weeks, with 25% surviving fewer than 7 days and 25% surviving longer than 2 months.

Step 4: Debiasing

You recognize that you have chosen an anchor and tailoring model that predicts shorter survival times than the disease-specific anchor data. You are ready to challenge this decision as you evaluate the patient. In preparation for your evaluation, you prompt the oncology attending and floor nurse with your tailored estimates. From what they have experienced with J. L., both would be surprised if J.L. died within the next few days but quite surprised if she survived longer than 2 months. You estimate her survival is likely to be less than 2 months, and communicating in terms of the usual course (25% to 75%) being in timeframe of weeks. You are ready to challenge this estimate and communication approach on evaluating J. L.

SUMMARY RECOMMENDATIONS

- Use the four-step process outlined in this chapter to estimate survival for patients with advanced cancer. The four steps are:
  - *Anticipating* involves clarifying the types of descriptors (e.g., usual trajectory, likelihood of 6-month survival, best case and worst case probabilities) and levels of precision (e.g., within days, within weeks, within months, etc.) required for engaging patients and families in an initial conversation. This is based on the urgency and types of decisions facing the patient and family. Clinicians will need to confirm and/or adapt these initial assumptions when meeting the patient and family.
  - *Anchoring* the estimate by defining the "ballpark" range of survival for patients with similar stages of advanced illness. This is done by identifying an appropriate reference population for whom survival time has been observed and reported.
  - *Tailoring* involves estimating where the individual patient's survival is likely to fall within the range of population anchor. This is done using modeling (i.e., extrapolation) of the reference population data (i.e., calculators) and clinical judgment.
  - *Debiasing* is used to avoid systematic errors in judgment, typically overestimation of survival. When estimates are based on representative anchors and tailoring models that reflect the patient's clinical context, less debiasing effort is required.

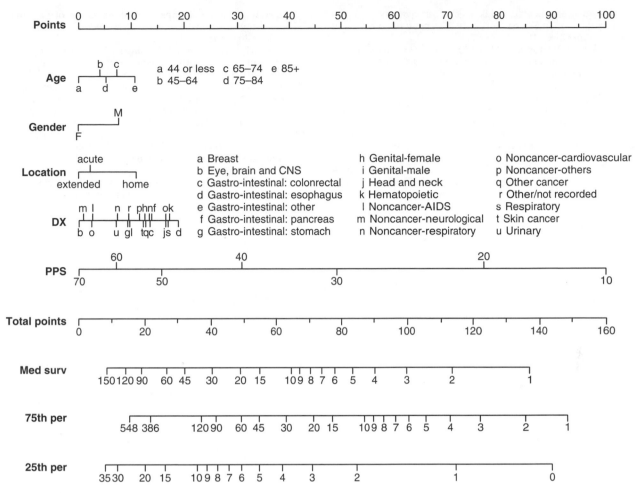

FIGURE 41-1. Nomogram for tailoring survival estimates using the Palliative Performance Scale. To use the survival nomogram, first use the patient's clinical criteria (i.e., age, gender, current location, diagnosis, and PPS) to determine the total number of points assigned to the patient. This is done by drawing a straight line from the nomogram for each of the characteristics to the uppermost line labeled *Points*. Add points up for all of these factors, and then draw a line on the *Total points* scale from this total score downward. Where this line crosses the *Med Surv* line demonstrates that patient's median survival in days. Where this line crosses the *75th per* line is the number of days the patient can be expected to survive if the patient is in the upper 75th percentile of survival. Likewise, where the line crosses the *25th per* line is the number of days the patient can be expected to survive if the patient is in the lower 25th percentile of survival. *(From Lau F, Downing M, Lesperance M, Karlson N, Kuziemsky C, Yang J. Using the Palliative Performance Scale to provide meaningful survival estimates.* J Pain Symptom Manage. *2009;38[1]:134–144.)*

REFERENCES

1. Downing GM. "Who Knows?" 10 Steps to Better Prognostication. In: Emanuel L, Librach L, eds. *Palliative Care: Core Skills and Clinical Competencies*. New York: Saunders; 2011:68–78.
2. Lunney JR, Lynn J, Foley DJ, et al. Patterns of functional decline at the end of life. *JAMA*. 2003;289(18):2387–2392.
3. Anderson F, Downing GM, Hill J, et al. Palliative performance scale (PPS): a new tool. *J Palliat Care*. 1996;12(1):5–11.
4. Edge SB, Byrd DR, Compton CC, et al. *American Joint Committee on Cancer (AJCC) Cancer Staging Manual*. 7 ed. New York: Springer; 2010:261.
5. Non-small Cell Lung Cancer Collaborative Group. Chemotherapy in non-small cell lung cancer: a meta-analysis using updated data on individual patients from 52 randomised clinical trials. *BMJ*. 1995;311(7010):899–909.
6. Woodard TD, Oplatek A, Petruzzelli GJ. Life after total laryngectomy: a measure of long-term survival, function, and quality of life. *Arch Otolaryngol Head Neck Surg*. 2007;133(6):526–532.
7. Duffy SA, Ronis DL, McLean S, et al. Pretreatment health behaviors predict survival among patients with head and neck squamous cell carcinoma. *J Clin Oncol*. 2009;27(12):1969–1975.
8. Edge SB, Byrd DR, Compton CC, et al. *American Joint Committee on Cancer (AJCC) Cancer Staging Manual*. 7 ed. New York: Springer; 2010:154.
9. Krzyzanowska MK, Weeks JC, Earle CC. Treatment of locally advanced pancreatic cancer in the real world: population-based practices and effectiveness. *J Clin Oncol*. 2003;21(18):3409–3414.
10. Chau I, Norman AR, Cunningham D, et al. The impact of primary tumour origins in patients with advanced oesophageal, oesophago-gastric junction and gastric adenocarcinoma: individual patient data from 1775 patients in four randomised controlled trials. *Ann Oncol*. 2009;20(5):885–891.
11. Dollinger MM, Lautenschlaeger C, Lesske J, et al. Thymostimulin versus placebo for palliative treatment of locally advanced or metastasised hepatocellular carcinoma: a phase III clinical trial. *BMC Cancer*. 2010;10:457.
12. Glimelius B, Ekstrom K, Hoffman K, et al. Randomized comparison between chemotherapy plus best supportive care with best supportive care in advanced gastric cancer. *Ann Oncol*. 1997;8(2):163–168.
13. Brown KM, Tompkins AJ, Yong S, et al. Pancreaticoduodenectomy is curative in the majority of patients with node-negative ampullary cancer. *Arch Surg*. 2005;140(6):529–532 discussion 532–523.

14. Motzer RJ, Mazumdar M, Bacik J, et al. Survival and prognostic stratification of 670 patients with advanced renal cell carcinoma. *J Clin Oncol.* 1999;17(8):2530–2540.

15. Johnstone PA, Norton MS, Riffenburgh RH. Survival of patients with untreated breast cancer. *J Surg Oncol.* 2000;73(4):273–277.

16. Halabi S, Small EJ, Kantoff PW, et al. Prognostic model for predicting survival in men with hormone-refractory metastatic prostate cancer. *J Clin Oncol.* 2003;21(7):1232–1237.

17. Ohgaki H, Dessen P, Jourde B, et al. Genetic pathways to glioblastoma: a population-based study. *Cancer Res.* 2004;64(19):6892–6899.

18. Edge SB, Byrd DR, Compton CC, et al. *American Joint Committee on Cancer (AJCC) Cancer Staging Manual.* 7th ed. New York: Springer; 2010.

19. Edge SB, Byrd DR, Compton CC, et al. *American Joint Committee on Cancer (AJCC) Cancer Staging Manual.* 7 ed. New York: Springer; 2010:334.

20. Giles F, O'Brien S, Cortes J, et al. Outcome of patients with acute myelogenous leukemia after second salvage therapy. *Cancer.* 2005;104(3):547–554.

21. Breems DA, Van Putten WL, Huijgens PC, et al. Prognostic index for adult patients with acute myeloid leukemia in first relapse. *J Clin Oncol.* 2005;23(9):1969–1978.

22. Seve P, Ray-Coquard I, Trillet-Lenoir V, et al. Low serum albumin levels and liver metastasis are powerful prognostic markers for survival in patients with carcinomas of unknown primary site. *Cancer.* 2006;107(11):2698–2705.

23. Downing M, Lau F, Lesperance M, et al. Meta-analysis of survival prediction with Palliative Performance Scale. *J Palliat Care.* 2007;23(4):245–252; discussion 252–244.

24. Lau F, Downing M, Lesperance M, et al. Using the Palliative Performance Scale to provide meaningful survival estimates. *J Pain Symptom Manage.* 2009;38(1):134–144.

Chapter 42

What Is a Useful Strategy for Estimating Survival for Persons With Advanced Non–Cancer-Related Illness in Palliative Care Settings?

THOMAS CARROLL, RONALD M. EPSTEIN, AND ROBERT GRAMLING

ANCHORING ESTIMATES IN NON–CANCER-RELATED ILLNESSES
CLINICAL SCENARIO
  Step 1: Anticipating
  Step 2: Anchoring
  Step 3: Tailoring
  Step 4: Debiasing

This chapter, based on the content outlined in Chapter 41, describes an approach for estimating survival prognoses in non-cancer related illness. The concepts of anticipating, anchoring, tailoring, and debiasing, as described in the last chapter, are similarly valid in noncancer populations and have been summarized in Table 42-1. There are unique challenges in defining these concepts in noncancer populations, however, as discussed in this chapter.

ANCHORING ESTIMATES IN NON–CANCER-RELATED ILLNESSES

The accuracy of anchoring depends on two important elements: population data that are representative of advanced stages of illness and clinically useful

Note: Portions of this chapter have been published in Holloway RG, Gramling R, Kelly AG. Estimating and communicating prognoses in neurological disease. *Neurology.* 2012; in press.

indicators that the illness is, in fact, advanced. In cancer, one often relies on staging, response to prior courses of treatment, and performance status. This process produces identifiable groups (e.g., those who failed first-line chemotherapy) at standardized time points. Such systematic classification is useful. It allows for efficient identification and standardized definitions of populations for natural history studies on which to base prognosis estimates. It also provides timely tools for clinicians to estimate the individual patient's stage of illness and for referencing to population data.

These signposts of advancing illness are often more subtle and less systematically identified in non–cancer-related settings. Therefore natural history data defining clinically useful definitions of "advanced" are often hard to find in non–cancer-related illnesses. Similarly, recognizing when an individual patient's illness has reached an advanced stage is challenging and often that realization occurs at very late stages of illness (i.e., when patients are actively dying).

Two resources are provided to address these challenges to anchoring. First are disease-specific and population-based anchors for illnesses commonly encountered in palliative care settings (Table 42-2). The clinical indicators of "advanced" that characterize the reference population and organize the survival estimates are similar to those in Chapter 41 (median

---

TABLE 42-1. Process for Estimating Prognosis in Advanced Illness

STEP	PURPOSE
Anticipating	To clarify the types of descriptors (e.g., usual trajectory, likelihood of 6-month survival, best case/worst case probabilities) and precision (e.g., within days, within weeks, within months, etc.) that are required for engaging patients/families in an initial conversation. This is based on the urgency and types of decisions facing the patient/family. Clinicians will need to confirm and/or adapt these initial assumptions when meeting the patient/family.
Anchoring	To define the "ballpark" range of survival for patients with similar stages of advanced illness. This is done by identifying an appropriate reference population for whom survival time has been observed and reported.
Tailoring	To estimate where the individual patient's survival is likely to fall within the range of population anchor. This is done using modeling (i.e., extrapolation) of the reference population data (i.e., calculators) and clinical judgment.
Debiasing	To acknowledge and overcome the pervasive tendency to overestimate survival. When estimates are based on representative anchors and tailoring models that take into account clinical course (i.e., functional decline), less debiasing effort is required.

TABLE 42-2. Survival Estimate Anchors for Advanced Non–Cancer-Related Illnesses Commonly Encountered in Palliative Care

DISEASE	PRIMARY INDICATORS OF ADVANCED STATUS	TREATMENT STATUS[*]	SURVIVAL TIME IN MONTHS[†]
			≤2 — 3 — 6 — 9 — 12 — 15 — 18 — 21 — 24 — 27 — 30 — 33 — 36 — >36
Heart failure[‡]	NYHA class IV, AHA/ACC stage D[1]	A (VAD)	**14** (bar ~3–24)
	NYHA class IV, AHA/ACC stage D[1]	A (no VAD)	**5** (bar ≤2–9)
	NYHA class IV, AHA/ACC stage C/D[2]	A	Median and 75% not reached after 12 mo
	NYHA class IV, AHA/ACC sage C/D[2]	B[§]	**5** (bar ≤2–12); 75% not reached after 12 mo
COPD[3]	Chronic hypercapnia	A	**24** (bar ~6–30)
Dementia[4]	Nursing home	C	**16** (bar ~3–30)
	with eating problem	C	**8** (bar ≤2–24)
End-stage renal disease[5]	>75 yr, GFR <15 mL/min	A (dialysis)	**>36** (bar ~24–>36)
	>75 yr, GFR <15 mL/min	B (no dialysis)	**18** (bar ~9–33)
Cirrhosis[6]	Child C[‖]	A	**5** (bar ≤2–12)
AIDS[7]	CD4 <25 after 3 yr of cART	A	Median and 75% not reached after 24 mo

The treatment bars represent the usual survival range (i.e., that representative of 25%-75% of patients with the condition as described). The area to the right of the bars is the best case scenario (i.e., a survival expectation above the 75th percentile). The area to the left of the bars is the worst case scenario (i.e., a survival expectation less than the 25th percentile). The bold numbers superimposed on each of the bars represent the median survival time (rounded, in months) for the condition as described.

AHA/ACC, American Heart Association/American College of Cardiology; AIDS, acquired immunodeficiency virus; cART, combination antiretroviral therapy; COPD, chronic obstructive pulmonary disease; GFR, glomerular filtration rate; INR, international normalized ratio; NYHA, New York Heart Association; VAD, ventricular assist device.

[*]Reference population: A, Active disease moderating treatment; B, no/minimal active disease moderating treatment; C, undefined.
[†]Rounded to the nearest 3-mo interval.
[‡]NYHA class IV = dyspnea at rest; stage C = structural heart disease with current or recent heart failure symptoms; stage D = refractory, end-stage heart failure. In the stage D sample, <⅔ were on intravenous inotropes at baseline.[8]
[§]Receiving diuretics; not receiving angiotensin-converting enzyme inhibitor or vasodilators.
[‖]Child-Pugh score is used to estimate prognosis in liver failure.[9] Points are assigned based on total bilirubin, serum albumin, INR, ascites, and hepatic encephalopathy.

survival, 25%-75% "usual" range; 25% "best case"; 25% "worst case"). The second resource provides estimates that are function-specific and arise from observations of palliative care clinical populations (see Table 41-2). These function-based anchors are stratified using the Palliative Performance Scale (PPS) (see Table 41-3).

CLINICAL SCENARIO

The following clinical scenario will walk the reader through a hypothetical case of a patient and demonstrate how to use the techniques outlined in this chapter.

You are preparing to see H. M. in an outpatient palliative care consultation at the request of his family physician. You review the referral letter and learn that he is a 72-year-old retired manager with New York Heart Association class IV, stage D heart failure, who is ineligible for a ventricular assist device or cardiac transplant (determined at last hospitalization 1 month ago). He had been living alone, but his function has declined substantially over the past 6 months. He is now living with his adult daughter, spends most of the day in a chair, is oxygen dependent, and requires help with many daily activities. They are familiar with hospice care because his wife died of cancer 5 years ago, and had asked their family doctor if "hospice is even an option at this point." He is here to see you with his daughter.

Step 1: Anticipating

You note the type of decision that H. M. and his daughter are considering (i.e., hospice) and know that the survival eligibility criteria often request clinicians to report expectations in terms of months. You believe that being able to discuss survival in terms of "months" will also help you engage H. M. and his daughter in an initial conversation. You also remind yourself that patterns of functional decline in late-stage heart failure (see Figure 40-2) involve accelerating frequency of acute exacerbations, any of which might bring about death.

Step 2: Anchoring

You consider two types of populations to anchor your survival estimate. The first is in a disease-specific population (see Table 42-2, stage D/no ventricular assist device), observing a median survival of 5 months, 25% living longer than 1 year (best case), and 25% dying within 2 months (worst case). The second is in a palliative care population with similar levels of function (see Table 42-2). You review two such reference populations and observe the trajectories to be quite similar. From the available description in the referral letter, you estimate his PPS score (see Table 41-3) to be 50%. These predict a median survival of approximately 1.5 months, with 25% living longer than 2 to 3 months (best case) and 25% dying within 1 month (worst case).

Step 3: Tailoring

You are able to quickly access sufficient clinical data for further tailoring your function-based anchor. You refer to the PPS nomogram (see Figure 41-1) and sum the points attributed to each of the tailoring variables (8 [gender] + 7 [age] + 3 [main disease type] + 10 [care setting] + 15 [PPS 50%] = 43). You note that the total score of 43 predicts a median survival of approximately 1 month, with 25% surviving more than 2.5 months (best case) and 25% surviving 1 week or less.

Step 4: Debiasing

You recognize that you have chosen to tailor a function-based anchor estimate that predicts shorter survival times than the disease-specific anchor data. You are ready to challenge this decision as you evaluate the patient. Under either choice of anchor (disease-based or function-based) it is reasonable to attest that he is not likely to survive longer than 6 months (i.e., for hospice eligibility).

SUMMARY RECOMMENDATIONS

- Use the four-step process outlined in this chapter to estimate survival for patients with non-cancer-related advanced illness.
- Use palliative care reference populations that are based on functional decline in advanced non-cancer-related illnesses, as these hold particular promise for anchoring and tailoring estimates.

REFERENCES

1. Rose EA, Gelijns AC, Moskowitz AJ, et al. Long-term use of a left ventricular assist device for end-stage heart failure. *N Engl J Med.* 2001;345(20):1435–1443.
2. The CONSENSUS Trial Study Group. Effects of enalapril on mortality in severe congestive heart failure: results of the Cooperative North Scandinavian Enalapril Survival Study (CONSENSUS). *N Engl J Med.* 1987;316(23):1429–1435.
3. Costello R, Deegan P, Fitzpatrick M, et al. Reversible hypercapnia in chronic obstructive pulmonary disease: a distinct pattern of respiratory failure with a favorable prognosis. *Am J Med.* 1997;102(3):239–244.
4. Mitchell SL, Teno JM, Kiely DK, et al. The clinical course of advanced dementia. *N Engl J Med.* 2009;361(16):1529–1538.
5. Murtagh FE, Marsh JE, Donohoe P, et al. Dialysis or not? A comparative survival study of patients over 75 years with chronic kidney disease stage 5. *Nephrol Dial Transplant.* 2007;22(7):1955–1962.
6. Albers I, Hartmann H, Bircher J, et al. Superiority of the Child-Pugh classification to quantitative liver function tests for assessing prognosis of liver cirrhosis. *Scand J Gastroenterol.* 1989;24(3): 269–276.
7. May M, Sterne JA, Sabin C, et al. Prognosis of HIV-1-infected patients up to 5 years after initiation of HAART: collaborative analysis of prospective studies. *AIDS.* 2007;21(9):1185–1197.
8. Hunt SA, Abraham WT, Chin MH, et al. 2009 focused update incorporated into the ACC/AHA 2005 guidelines for the diagnosis and management of heart failure in adults: a report of the American College of Cardiology Foundation/American Heart Association Task Force on Practice Guidelines, developed in collaboration with the International Society for Heart and Lung Transplantation. *Circulation.* 2009;119(14): e391–e479.
9. Child C, Turcotte J. *Surgery and Portal Hypertension.* Philadelphia: Saunders; 1964;50–58.

SETTING GOALS AND COMMUNICATING SERIOUS NEWS

Chapter 43

What Are the Key Elements to Having a Conversation About Setting Goals and Communicating Serious News?

LYNN B. O'NEILL AND ANTHONY L. BACK

INTRODUCTION AND SCOPE OF THE PROBLEM

The two most common communication tasks faced by palliative care clinicians are communicating serious news and discussing transitions in goals of care. Although these tasks are often taught in medical and nursing schools, the way they present for palliative care clinicians is generally more complex (Table 43-1). A palliative care consultation often involves both communicating serious news and discussing goals of care; however, the literature separates these into two distinct communication tasks. This chapter provides a discussion of the communication science surrounding these tasks; a summary of the key elements for each of these tasks, including the evidence for the recommendations when available; and suggested language for palliative medicine clinicians.

TABLE 43-1. Common Conversations in Palliative Care

Shifting focus from cure to managing the disease

Shifting focus from quantity of life to quality of life

Shifting focus from managing the disease to preparing for death

Discussing prognosis when time is short

Shifting goals when the patient's initial goals are not achievable

Discussing patient's desire to return home but patient cannot

Discussing patient's desire to live to see a particular event, but unlikely given life expectancy

---

RELEVANT COMMUNICATION SCIENCE

The science surrounding the tasks of communicating serious news and discussing transitions in goals of care represents two different perspectives—that of the patient and that of the clinician.

From the patient's perspective, hearing serious news provokes various emotions, including shock, fright, acceptance, and sadness.[1] A patient's future emotional adjustment to the illness is affected by two factors: (1) the manner in which the patient is told the serious news[2] and (2) the manner in which the clinician responds to the emotion provoked by the serious news.[1]

Patients' preferences vary in their desire for how serious news is discussed.[1,3–12] Commonly, studies have found that most but not all patients prefer to have a close relative or friend present,[1,4,5,9,11,12] but they differ on whether patients desire the presence of other health professionals such as a chaplain or social worker.[5,9,12] This heterogeneity of patient preferences regarding how to best communicate serious news suggests that each individual patient should be asked about preferences as part of the preparatory work for a serious news conversation.

The manner in which the clinician responds to the patient's emotion, the second factor affecting a patient's future emotional adjustment, depends on the clinician's ability to recognize emotions expressed during the conversation. From the clinician's perspective, the emotionally charged nature of communicating serious news and discussing transitions in goals of care makes these communication tasks especially challenging. Existing studies indicate that physicians commonly overlook emotional cues and make few empathic responses when talking to patients.[13] Because emotion can be expressed at any point in the conversation, the skillful clinician will be ready to respond to this emotion in an empathic manner whenever it arises. Empathic responses to emotion align the clinician with the patient and seem to help patients and family members process what is happening so they can hear more of what the clinician says.

The few existing communication guidelines organize the best available medical evidence into a stepwise approach to these tasks of communicating serious news and discussing transitions in goals of care while also taking into account factors affecting a patient's future emotional adjustment.[14-16]

SUMMARY OF EVIDENCE REGARDING COMMUNICATION RECOMMENDATIONS

This chapter consolidates the existing data to present a stepwise guide of elements to consider before, during, and after an encounter. Although medical encounters in which either serious news is delivered or in which a transition in the goals of care are discussed are rarely linear,[17] stepwise guidelines offer several advantages for the learner, the medical educator, and the clinician. First, these stepwise approaches serve as useful cognitive frameworks for learners who may be asked to observe one of these encounters. In reflecting on such an observed encounter, the learner who has been primed with a short didactic describing a stepwise approach will be able to scaffold observations into clear steps. For the medical educator, stepwise guidelines translate to skills that can be taught, observed, and evaluated (see Chapter 44). Finally, for the advanced palliative care practitioner, stepwise guidelines serve as the foundation on which to build a wider breadth of advanced communication skills. These may be particularly important for the experienced practitioner to draw on when faced with complex or challenging communication interactions.

This discussion will illustrate these skills using a palliative care family meeting. These recommendations are also relevant to a clinician preparing for a one-on-one conversation with a patient. In addition, it should be noted that this chapter covers both communicating serious news and discussing transitions in goals of care. These represent two distinct communication tasks that may or may not be covered in a single conversation depending on the situation and the patient's cognitive and emotional capacity to continue after hearing the serious news. This chapter will present these two tasks in sequence.

Before the Meeting

Two major tasks must be undertaken before sitting down for the family meeting—planning the meeting and the premeeting.

Planning the Meeting. Every attempt should be made to plan the meeting in advance. For this to happen, the clinician must first recognize that a serious piece of information must be conveyed to the patient. In so doing, the clinician identifies this piece of information as important and sufficiently serious that it should be discussed at a time set aside specifically for that purpose.

Planning the meeting in advance offers three main advantages. First, it ensures adequate time and privacy, key components of all clinician–patient communication.[18] Second, planning the meeting in advance will allow the clinician to consider questions such as who should be involved in the meeting and where it will occur. Regarding the former, this may involve asking who the patient would like to have present at the meeting. Having a significant other present to hear the serious news has been associated with lower levels of patient anxiety.[19] Alternatively, in the case of a patient who does not have capacity and will be unable to participate in the meeting, the clinician should determine if there is a health care proxy, health care power of attorney or other "family" member ("family" as defined by the patient) who should be present for the conversation. In addition, the palliative medicine consultant must consider which other clinicians should be present for the meeting, including members of the primary team, other subspecialty consultants, and other members of the interdisciplinary team, such as the primary care nurse, social worker, and chaplain.

The Premeeting. The second major task to be completed before the family meeting is the premeeting with the clinicians who will attend the conference. The two primary goals of the premeeting are negotiating roles and discussing the prognostic information and treatment options to be presented. In negotiating roles, the clinicians involved should decide who will lead the meeting, who will serve as content experts, and what role others in the room will play. The process of negotiating roles for the meeting should take into account the patient's prior relationship with the individual clinicians, the nature and content of the serious news to be delivered, and the preference of the primary physician. The palliative medicine consultant often serves at the request of the primary physician, and therefore the primary physician wishing to lead the family meeting should be allowed to do so. A useful approach in these situations can be for the palliative medicine clinician to assist the primary clinician by opening the meeting. For example, a palliative medicine clinician might say in the premeeting that, "I absolutely agree that, because you are the patient's oncologist, you should be the one to share with the patient that no further chemotherapeutic options exist. I often find it helpful before sharing the serious news to make sure that everyone in the room has been introduced and also to allow patients to share their understanding of where things currently stand. Would it be okay if I start off the meeting with those two things and then turn it over to you to share the information about no further chemotherapy? I'll be there for other issues that might come up." In this way, the palliative medicine clinician is respecting the primary physician's prior relationship with the patient while also ensuring that the meeting will go as smoothly as possible by making a recommendation on how to help facilitate the beginning of the meeting.

After roles have been negotiated, the clinicians should discuss the prognostic information and treatment options to be presented. If differing opinions exist, these should be discussed before entering the meeting room and a consensus reached. Communication skills are required to negotiate and mediate the conflict that can inevitably occur between clinicians with differing opinions.[20] As the palliative medicine consultant, approaching apparent conflict with a respectful curiosity can be useful. "Respectful curiosity" assumes respect for the others' opinions and the expertise on which those opinions are based and sincere interest (or curiosity) in hearing how others have arrived at those conclusions. In the same spirit of collegiality, the palliative medicine consultant can then offer an opinion on the issue at hand. Through this type of open communication, all clinicians should be able to agree on the information to be delivered during the meeting or at least a mechanism to explain that differences of opinion may exist about a particular topic.

During the Meeting

The content of the meeting itself can be divided into three major portions—introductions and patient's perception, delivering the serious news, and discussing transitions in goals of care.

Introductions and Eliciting Patient Perception of Illness. As the meeting begins, the clinician leading the meeting should confirm with the patient that this is still a good time for this conversation. When this has been established, all in the room should be asked to introduce themselves. Taking down these names as they are spoken will allow the clinician to refer to both family members and other health care professionals by name as the meeting progresses and will promote more thorough documentation of the meeting afterward.

After introduction of those in the room, the clinician leading the meeting can briefly introduce the purpose of the family meeting before assessing patient perception of the illness and the clinical course to this point.[14] As the patient responds, the skilled palliative medicine clinician will observe and listen to the patient on two levels—cognitive and emotional (Table 43-2). The cognitive level refers to the actual information that the patient relates and the language used to express it. The clinician will learn about the patient's depth of understanding and

level of health literacy and any misconceptions the patient may have. On the cognitive level the clinician may detect clues in the patient's speech that suggest denial, such as wishful thinking, omission of essential but unfavorable details of the illness, or unrealistic expectations.[21] On the emotional level the clinician will note the emotional state of the patient and others in the room and displays of emotion (verbal or nonverbal) in relation to particular issues or areas of concern that warrant further discussion. Emotional data may also begin to give the clinician an idea of what the patient and family values as important. By dividing observations into cognitive and emotional data, the clinician will be better able to use these data to help inform strategy in leading the meeting as it progresses.

Once the patient has defined his or her perception of the illness, the clinician may want to clarify or correct any factual differences or misconceptions that become apparent as the patient is speaking. Before doing this, however, the clinician may ask other family members in the room what their understanding is, if they have anything to add, or if they understood anything differently. Often, other family members will correct the misconception through stating their own understanding. When summarizing the collective understanding of the patient and family, the clinician can highlight the correct information, thus deemphasizing the misperceptions.

Delivering the Serious News. Before providing new information, particularly of the serious variety, the clinician should determine the patient's preference for amount of information (and with whom it should be shared). Information needs and preferences may change throughout the disease trajectory,[22] so the clinician should check with the patient before providing new information. In addition, family caregivers and patients may have varied information preferences and needs especially in relation to prognosis.[23] Therefore the clinician should check with all in the room before sharing key information. For example, if a patient's wife asks about prognosis, it would be worthwhile to first ask the patient if this is information that would be helpful to him. If the patient declines to hear about prognosis, the clinician may ask the patient if it would be appropriate to discuss this with his wife at a later time.

When all in the room are prepared to hear the serious news, the clinician should provide the information in small portions, allowing space between these pieces of information for the patient to mentally process and verbally respond with either emotion or questions. Information should be provided using lay language, being careful to avoid the use of jargon or euphemisms. One study demonstrated that a substantial proportion of the general public do not understand medical terms such as "metastasis" and "spots in the liver."[24] Therefore the clinician can use cognitive-level observations in hearing the patient's perception to guide the language used to impart serious news, taking care to use the patient's chosen words when describing new information about the illness.

TABLE 43-2. Guide to Organizing Observations During a Family Meeting

Cognitive level
  Depth of understanding of the illness
  Health literacy and the language used to describe the illness
  Misconceptions about the diagnosis or treatments
  Clues that suggest denial
    Wishful thinking
    Omission of unfavorable details of illness
    Unrealistic expectations
Emotional level
  Emotional state of patient and family
  Displays of emotion in relation to particular issues
  May begin to have clues as to what the patient and the family value as important

When communicating serious news, a potential pitfall is for clinicians to be so focused on what they are saying and how they say it that they miss the emotional-level data a patient is providing in the form of nonverbal reaction to the information. An observational study indicated that when nurses responded to a patient's emotional cues more often, the patient's informational recall improved.[25] Although it is important to track the emotional response of the patient and family members throughout the encounter, it is perhaps most crucial to attend to this when the serious news is being imparted. To appropriately respond to emotion, the clinician must first recognize the patient's emotion and then name the emotion.[26] The instinct to fix or quiet the patient's emotion is often a reflection of the clinician's own worries. Pausing long enough to note this internal concern will allow the clinician to reflect on those worries and resist the urge to "fix" the patient's emotion.[20] Finally, the clinician should acknowledge the emotion explicitly by demonstrating empathy. Empathy can by conveyed either nonverbally through touch, nodding, silence, or eye contact or verbally through an empathic statement.[20] The value of clinician empathy is that it aligns the clinician with the patient and allows the patient to express more about the thoughts or feeling of the moment. The NURSE acronym is a useful summary of verbal ways that clinicians can respond empathically[18] (Table 43-3).

After imparting the serious news and responding to emotion, the clinician has two options for how to proceed. Guidelines specific to the communication task of discussing serious news suggest that the next action is to summarize the conversation and plan for the next steps.[14] However, a second option would be to move on to a discussion of the patient's goals of care in light of the serious news that was just imparted. Patients' preferences vary in regard to the timing of conversations on transitions in goals of care and who should initiate this discussion.[27] Therefore, the clinician can best determine how to proceed by employing a patient-centered approach in which the clinician asks whether the patient wants to discuss further care options now or later.[28] If the patient opts for further discussion later, the clinician can bring the meeting to a close by summarizing the discussion and strategizing the next steps, including the timing of a follow-up meeting.[14]

Discussing Transitions in Goals of Care. If the patient indicates a willingness to discuss goals of care now, the clinician can shift focus to this second main communication task. Discussing transitions in goals of care consists of four key elements: (1) eliciting concerns, (2) eliciting values and goals, (3) balancing realism and hope, and (4) making a recommendation.

The first key element of a discussion of goals of care is eliciting concerns. Having just heard serious news, the patient is likely to have a high degree of uncertainty about the future and anxiety and worries about the worst case scenarios.[29] These concerns can be elicited by asking open-ended questions. Allowing the patient to disclose concerns is useful in that even simply talking about the concerns can help defuse them.[30] It is important for the clinician to recognize that it is the eliciting of the concerns and allowing them to be articulated that is helpful, even if these concerns cannot be "fixed." Using some or all of the following open-ended questions will invite the patient to disclose concerns.[20,31]

- "What concerns you most right now?" or "As you think about the future, what concerns you most?"
- "What has been most difficult about this illness for you?" or "What is the hardest part?"
- "What's your biggest fear?" or "What would be your worst case scenario?"

Asking questions such as these can be anxiety-provoking for the patient. Empathic communication reduces a patient's level of anxiety.[32,33] Therefore, use of empathic statements (see Table 43-3) is just as important in this stage of the meeting as it was during the discussion of the serious news.

The second key element of a discussion of goals of care is eliciting the patient's values and goals. Sometimes in allowing the patient to discuss concerns, the clinician will begin to get a picture of what the patient values. However, additional open-ended questions with this particular aim in mind may be necessary.[20]

- "As you think about the future, what is most important to you?" or "What are your biggest goals?
- "What is going on in your life outside the hospital right now?" or "What about your life is most valuable right now?"
- "What are you hoping for?"

The third key element in a discussion of transitions in goals of care is maintaining hope while being honest and realistic. From the clinician's perspective, asking what the patient is hoping for holds an inherent

---

TABLE 43-3. NURSE: An Acronym for Verbal Expressions of Empathy

Example of a patient's emotional statement:
"What do you mean no more chemo? Chemo's all I've got."

EMPATHIC CLINICIAN RESPONSES		SAMPLE LANGUAGE
N	*NAME* the emotion	"You seem angry."
U	*UNDERSTAND* the emotion	"I can only imagine how upsetting this must be."
R	*RESPECT* (praise) the patient	"I'm so impressed with the determination and strength you've exhibited during your chemotherapy up to this point."
S	*SUPPORT* the patient	"I will continue to be here for you."
E	*EXPLORE* the emotion	"Tell me more about what the chemo means to you."

Modified from Smith RC, Hoppe RB. The patient's story: integrating the patient- and physician-centered approaches to interviewing. *Ann Intern Med.* 1991;115(6):470–477.

risk that the patient is hoping for something that is not achievable. Patients identify both communicating hope and providing honest information as important when discussing issues such as prognosis.[34] One way to nurture hope while discussing end-of-life issues is to emphasize what can be done, including symptom control, emotional support, preservation of dignity, and practical support.[23] In this way, the clinician is expanding the spectrum of things for which the patient might be hopeful. If the patient does express hope, for instance, for a cure when this is not achievable, the clinician can again employ empathic statements to align with the patient and hear more about what a cure means to the patient. A wish statement is a skill that the clinician can use in response to the patient's hope for a cure: "I wish things were different."[35] This statement acknowledges the patient's hope and aligns the clinician with the patient while implicitly reiterating that a cure is not likely.

After the clinician has explored the patient's goals and values in the context of day-to-day life, the final element in a discussion of transitions in goals of care is making a recommendation. Making a recommendation can be subdivided into three important steps—invitation, proposal, and seeking feedback.[20] The invitation involves asking the patient's permission before making the recommendation. The proposal is a suggested plan based on what the patient has identified as hopes, goals, and values. The plan will likely be multipronged and will include each goal and the steps that the physician will take to attempt to achieve each goal. Note that the focus is on what can be done. The statement "nothing can be done for you" should be avoided because it is associated with high emotional distress and considerable dissatisfaction when used in discussing a transition in goals of care.[36] Finally, after presenting a proposed plan, the clinician should seek feedback from the patient on the plan and be willing to rethink and modify the plan to better meet the patient's goals.[20]

After the Meeting

When the meeting has concluded, the clinicians involved should take time for debriefing of the meeting. This debriefing should include a discussion of the process, content of the meeting, and clinicians' reflections on their own emotions related to the meeting.

Just as the content of this family meeting has been emotional for the patient and family, it will also have incited emotions in each clinician who was present.[37] On conclusion of the meeting, the palliative medicine clinician can serve as a role model by reflecting on emotions experienced during the meeting and feelings now that the meeting is over.[38] Unexamined emotions can over time result in physician distress, disengagement, burnout, and poor judgment.[37] The discussion of the process and content of the meeting is especially important for any learners who were present. This is further discussed in Chapter 44.

KEY MESSAGES TO PATIENTS AND FAMILIES

The key messages to patients and families when discussing serious news and transitions in goals of care are explicit. The clinician has outlined new information for the patient and family and has partnered with them to craft a plan going forward that is based on the patient's values and goals. Success in this case is defined as an improvement in patient understanding. The feedback that the clinician receives after making a recommendation in the form of the patient's thoughts about this plan will provide the clinician with data about the patient's current level of understanding. Absorbing serious news takes time, and a complete understanding and acceptance should not be the measure of success after a single family meeting. This meeting represents one in a series of conversations that will take place over time among the patient, the family, and the team of clinicians caring for the patient.

CONCLUSION AND SUMMARY

Communicating serious news and discussing transitions in goals of care are common communication tasks in palliative care. The complexity of these tasks requires the palliative medicine clinician to bring to bear skills of honest, empathic communication with patients, negotiation with colleagues, and introspective awareness of one's own emotions. By having a mental model of the process for leading these conversations (Table 43-4), the clinician can be best prepared to handle the intricacies of individual patient and family responses to the serious news and the prospect of a transition in the goals of care. In this way, patients and families will be provided with the information they need to make plans going forward and the support they require to cope with the prospect of a future that is different from what they had envisioned.

SUMMARY RECOMMENDATIONS

- Clinicians should ensure that conversations in which serious news is communicated or transitions in goals of care are discussed include the patient, any other family members the patient would like included, and other clinicians whose presence will be important given the content of the meeting.
- All clinicians who will be present in the meeting should gather for a premeeting to negotiate roles and clarify the information to be presented to the patient and family.
- Clinicians should closely observe the reactions of the patient and family members to the information, gathering both cognitive and emotional data that may help inform the conversation as it moves into a discussion of values and goals of care.
- Clinicians should make a recommendation about the plan going forward based on the patient's stated values and goals.

TABLE 43-4. Considerations in Communicating Serious News and Discussing Transitions in Goals of Care

I. Before the meeting
    A. Plan the meeting
        1. Who will be involved in the meeting?
            a. Who would the patient like to have present?
            b. If the patient does not have capacity, is there a health care proxy or health care power of attorney who should be present?
            c. Who is included in this patient's definition of "family" and who of that group is able to be present for the conversation?
            d. What other clinicians should be present for the meeting (members of the primary team [if palliative care is not primary team], subspecialty consultants, primary care nurse, social worker, chaplain)?
        2. Where will the meeting occur?
            a. Is there adequate space and adequate seating?
            b. Is it private and quiet?
    B. Premeeting
        1. Negotiate roles for the meeting
            a. Who will lead the meeting?
            b. Who will serve as content experts?
            c. How will other team members, such as social workers, nurses, or chaplains, be involved?
            d. What role will learners play in this encounter?
        2. Discussing the prognostic information and treatment options to be presented
            a. What information should be obtained during the course of the meeting? What information from the patient and/or family do the clinicians need to help guide treatment recommendations?
            b. What is the information to be delivered? Do all of the clinicians agree on the information to be delivered?
II. During the meeting
    A. Introductions and patient's perception
        1. Introductions
            a. Write down names and relationships to the patient for easy reference later in the meeting
            b. Describe purpose of the meeting
        2. Patient's perception
            a. Organize observations into cognitive and emotional data
            b. Ask for others' understanding of the illness first before clarifying misconceptions
    B. Delivering the serious news
        1. Inquire about patient's preference for amount of information
        2. Impart the serious news
            a. Deliver information in small portions and use clear, lay language
            b. Avoid jargon and euphemisms
         3. Respond to emotion
            a. Recognize the emotion
            b. Name it silently to yourself
            c. Avoid the urge to "fix" the emotion
            d. Respond empathically (see Table 43-3, for the NURSE acronym)
        4. Checkpoint: Ask whether patient would like to discuss goals of care in light of this serious news.
            a. If not, summarize and strategize (including planning a time for the next meeting)
    C. Discussing transitions in goals of care
        1. Elicit concerns
            a. *What concerns you most right now?* or *As you think about the future, what concerns you most?*
            b. *What has been most difficult about this illness for you?* or *What is the hardest part?*
            c. *What's your biggest fear?* or *What would be your worst case scenario?*
        2. Elicit values and goals
            a. *As you think about the future, what is most important to you?* or *What are your biggest goals?*
            b. *Tell me what is going on in your life outside the hospital right now.* or *Tell me what about your life is most valuable right now.*
            c. *What are you hoping for?*
        3. Balance realism and hope
            a. Emphasize what can be done
            b. Consider using a "wish" statement *"I wish things were different."*
        4. Make a recommendation
            a. Invitation: Offer to make a recommendation
            b. Proposal: Present goals and a plan for each goal based on the patient's values
            c. Seek feedback from the patient and modify the plan based on this feedback
III. After the meeting
    A. Discuss the process and content of the meeting
    B. Reflect on clinicians' emotions and debrief as a group

REFERENCES

1. Butow PN, Kazemi JN, Beeney LJ, et al. When the diagnosis is cancer: patient communication experiences and preferences. *Cancer.* 1996;77(12):2630–2637.
2. Omne-Ponten M, Holmberg L, Sjoden P-O. Psychosocial adjustment among women with breast cancer stages I and II: Six-year follow-up of consecutive patients. *J Clin Oncol.* 1994;12(9):1778–1782.
3. Tobias JS, Souhami RL. Fully informed consent can be needlessly cruel. *BMJ.* 1993;307(6913):1199–1201.
4. Peteet JR, Abrams HE, Murray Ross D, et al. Presenting a diagnosis of cancer: patients' views. *J Fam Pract.* 1991;32(6):577–581.
5. Fallowfield L. Giving sad and bad news. *Lancet.* 1993; 341(8843):476–478.
6. Maguire P, Faulkner A. Communicate with cancer patients. I. Handling bad news and difficult questions. *BMJ.* 1988; 297(6653):907–909.
7. Maguire P, Faulkner A. Communicate with cancer patients. II. Handling uncertainty, collusion and denial. *BMJ.* 1988; 297(6654):972–974.

8. Brewin TB. Three ways of giving bad news. *Lancet.* 1991; 37(8751):1207–1209.

9. Roberts CS, Cox CE, Reintgen MD, et al. Influence of doctor communication on newly diagnosed breast patients' psychologic adjustment and decision-making. *Cancer.* 1994; 74(suppl):336–341.

10. Lind SE, Good MD, Seidel S, et al. Telling the diagnosis of cancer. *J Clin Oncol.* 1989;7(5):583–589.

11. Holland JC. Now we tell—but how well? *J Clin Oncol.* 1989;7(5): 557–559.

12. Sardell AN, Trierweiler SJ. Disclosing the cancer diagnosis. *Cancer.* 1993;72(11):3355–3365.

13. Butow PN, Brown RF, Cogar S, et al. Oncologists' reaction to cancer patients' verbal cues. *Psychooncology.* 2002;11(1):47–58.

14. Baile WF, Buckman R, Lenzi R, et al. SPIKES: a six-step protocol for delivering bad news—application to the patient with cancer. *Oncologist.* 2000;5(4):302–311.

15. Girgis A, Sanson-Fisher RW. Breaking bad news: consensus guidelines for medical practitioners. *J Clin Oncol.* 1995;13(9): 2449–2456.

16. Buckman R, Kason Y. *How to Break Bad News: A Guide for Health Care Professionals.* Baltimore, MD: Johns Hopkins University Press; 1992.

17. Eggly S, Penner L, Albrecht TL, et al. Discussing bad news in the outpatient oncology clinic: rethinking current communication guidelines. *J Clin Oncol.* 2006;24(4):716–719.

18. Smith RC, Hoppe RB. The patient's story: integrating the patient- and physician-centered approaches to interviewing. *Ann Intern Med.* 1991;115(6):470–477.

19. Schofield PE, Butow PN, Thompson JF, et al. Psychological responses of patients receiving a diagnosis of cancer. *Ann Oncol.* 2003;14(1):48–56.

20. Back A, Arnold R, Tulsky J. *Mastering Communication with Seriously Ill Patients: Balancing Honesty with Empathy and Hope.* New York: Cambridge University Press; 2009.

21. Lubinsky MS. Bearing bad news: dealing with the mimics of denial. *Genet Couns.* 1999;3:5–12.

22. Jenkins V, Fallowfield L, Saul J. Information needs of patients with cancer: results from a large study in UK cancer centres. *Br J Cancer.* 2001;84(1):48–51.

23. Clayton JM, Butow PN, Arnold RM, et al. Fostering coping and nurturing hope when discussing the future with terminally ill cancer patients and their caregivers. *Cancer.* 2005;103(9): 1965–1975.

24. Chapman K, Abraham C, Jenkins V, et al. Lay understanding of terms used in cancer consultations. *Psychooncology.* 2003;12(6): 557–566.

25. Jansen J, van Weert JC, de Groot J, et al. Emotional and informational patient cues: the impact of nurses' responses on recall. *Patient Educ Couns.* 2010;79(2):218–224.

26. Ptacek JT, Eberhardt TL. Breaking bad news: a review of the literature. *JAMA.* 1996;276(6):496–502.

27. Hagerty RG, Butow PN, Ellis PA, et al. Cancer patient preferences for communication of prognosis in the metastatic setting. *J Clin Oncol.* 2004;22(9):1721–1730.

28. Schofield P, Carey M, Love A, et al. 'Would you like to talk about your future treatment options?' discussing the transition from curative cancer treatment to palliative care. *Palliat Med.* 2006;20(4):397–406.

29. Evans WG, Tulsky JA, Back AL, et al. Communication at times of transitions: how to help patients cope with loss and redefine hope. *Cancer J.* 2006;12(5):417–424.

30. Heaven CM, Maguire P. Disclosure of concerns by hospice patients and their identification by nurses. *Palliat Med.* 1997;11(4):283–290.

31. Lo B, Quill T, Tulsky J. Discussing palliative care with patients. ACP-ASIM end-of-life care consensus panel. American College of Physicians – American Society of Internal Medicine. *Ann Inter Med.* 1999;130(9):744–749.

32. Roter DL, Hall JA, Kern DE, et al. Improving physicians' interviewing skills and reducing patients' emotional distress: a randomized clinical trial. *Arch Intern Med.* 1995;155:1877–1884.

33. Fogarty LA, Curbow BA, Wingard JR, et al. Can 40 seconds of compassion reduce patient anxiety? *J Clin Oncol.* 1999; 17(1):371–379.

34. Butow PN, Dowsett S, Hagerty R, et al. Communicating prognosis to patients with metastatic disease: what do they really want to know? *Support Care Cancer.* 2002;10(2):161–168.

35. Quill TE, Arnold RM, Platt F. "I wish things were different": expressing wishes in response to loss, futility, and unrealistic hopes. *Ann Intern Med.* 2001;135(7):551–555.

36. Morita T, Akechi T, Ikenaga M, et al. Communication about the ending of anticancer treatment and transition to palliative care. *Ann Oncol.* 2004;15(10):1551–1557.

37. Meier DE, Back AL, Morrison RS. The inner life of physicians and care of the seriously ill. *JAMA.* 2001;286(23):3007–3014.

38. Smith RC, Dwamena FC, Fortin AH 6th. Teaching personal awareness. *J Gen Intern Med.* 2005;20(2):201–207.

Chapter 44

What Do Palliative Care Clinicians Need to Know About Teaching Communication?

LYNN B. O'NEILL AND ANTHONY L. BACK

INTRODUCTION AND SCOPE OF THE PROBLEM

Being a clinician who is a skilled communicator does not guarantee that the clinician can teach others to be similarly skilled. Palliative medicine clinicians must frequently take on the dual role of expert communicator and teacher of communication, being asked to both facilitate a difficult conversation with a patient and family and attend to the educational needs of one or more learners. If the clinician communicates expertly but does not engage and debrief the learner, the learner can easily develop the misperception that the palliative medicine clinician is just innately a good communicator. This misperception leads learners to believe that this "magic" of communication is something that one either possesses or does not and that if one falls into the latter category, there is little hope to be able to effectively communicate in these particularly difficult situations. In fact, studies have shown that educational interventions can be designed to effectively improve the communication skills of learners.[1-5] This chapter reviews the method of deliberate practice and how it relates to communication skills acquisition, delineates how teachers can structure their encounters with learners to help foster deliberate practice, and elucidates how teachers can use deliberate practice to improve their teaching of communication skills.

This chapter is geared toward palliative care clinicians who teach advanced communication skills. The learners may be fellows in palliative medicine, geriatrics, oncology, and other subspecialties; nurse practitioner students specializing in palliative care; and

perhaps advanced senior residents. Although some of the theories presented here may have some application for teachers of medical students, in this chapter, when the term *learners* is used, it is assumed that the learner has basic interviewing and history-taking skills. The chapter draws on research in how professionals acquire expertise to establish recommendations and a cognitive map for teaching communication. For learners wanting to improve their own communication skills, a summary of tips can be found in Table 44-1.

SCIENCE OF EXPERTISE ACQUISITION

Taking on the perspective of a teacher requires knowledge of how professionals acquire expertise. The current literature on expertise acquisition demonstrates that although one needs experience to become an expert, experience alone does not lead to the acquisition of expertise.[6] This science of expertise acquisition provides a useful framework for guiding how teachers should act. This chapter uses the theory of deliberate practice as the framework for teaching communication skills.

Deliberate Practice Theory of Skill Acquisition

Ericsson and colleagues[7] proposed a framework called "deliberate practice" to explain individual variation in skill attainment and development without

TABLE 44-1. A Learner's Guide to Deliberate Practice

Practice deliberately
    Goals of deliberate practice:
        Improve existing skills
        Extend reach and range of your skills
    But what makes practice deliberate practice?
        Out of your comfort zone
        In a simulated setting
Set aside time to review a particular encounter
        What worked?
        Where did I go wrong?
        How can I improve?
Find a mentor who can:
        Provide supervision for your deliberate practice
        Offer constructive feedback
        Help you identify your learning edge*

*A learning edge is the aspect of performance that will need to be improved to get an individual to the next skill level.

relying solely on innate factors. They developed this framework through study of superior performance in various skill-based fields, including chess, typing, and music. They posit that experts in multiple domains share two major things—the quality of the practice and the amount of practice.

First, the quality of the practice that these expert chess players and musicians engage in is deliberate. The goals of deliberate practice are to both improve one's existing skills and to extend the reach and range of one's skills.[7] The key elements of deliberate practice are threefold. First, the learner must aim to improve some aspect of performance of a well-defined task.[7] Second, the learner must have a coach or teacher available to provide immediate feedback on the performance and to help guide the learner to set new, higher goals.[6] Third, the learner must have ample opportunities to improve performance gradually by performing the same or similar tasks repeatedly.[7] This process of deliberate practice also encourages learners to think deliberately.[8] Deliberate thought involves the ability to reflect on one's actions and assess where they went wrong and determine how to avoid future errors. This reflection on action allows learners to continually work on eliminating weaknesses.[9]

In addition to the importance of the quality of practice, the quantity of practice is also paramount. The amount of practice required to become an expert in a given field has been studied and found to be similar across multiple domains. All performers in sports, science, and the arts need a minimum of 10 years of intense involvement before they reach an international level.[7] Indeed, most take much longer.

Although these elements of deliberate practice are true across multiple unrelated domains, medicine is different in several ways. First, individuals do not begin their medical or nursing studies until at least their early 20s. Therefore, they have a knowledge and skills base, acquired through years of life and non-medical education, which they will then look to apply to new tasks they are asked to perform. Learners must acquire new skills and adapt previously acquired skills to better meet the needs of these new medically related tasks. Some aspects of these preexisting skills and knowledge structures may not be easily modified, making it more difficult for some individuals to attain a high level of performance.[6] Contrast this with expert pianists who begin the study of piano at a very young age with limited preexisting knowledge or skills that can be applied to their task, and who, by the age of 20, have amassed approximately 10,000 hours of practice.[10] The difference here is that all young pianists start as complete novices and, therefore their eventual level of expertise is based in large part on the quality and amount of practice.

Applying Deliberate Practice to Medicine

Although deliberate practice cannot completely modify the level of expertise acquisition in medicine,

teachers can structure curricula so as to encourage deliberate practice among their learners. First, teachers can identify superior, reproducible behavior for representative tasks in the associated domain.[6] For learners, identifying this optimal performance will provide them with a clear picture of expertise and the potential range of attainable skill level. For teachers, predefining what constitutes various levels of excellence will aid in providing valid skills-based feedback. Second, teachers can structure training that is individualized and tailored to the learner's preexisting skill level.[6] Finally, teachers can emphasize that skill acquisition does not end with graduation from residency or fellowship but requires life-long learning and practice. Deliberate practice must extend beyond the formal medical education structure in order for clinicians to continue to acquire and perfect skills and to avoid arrested development of previously acquired skills.[6]

Until so-called ordinary individuals recognize that sustained effort is necessary to reach expert performance, they will continue to misattribute their inability to attain expert achievement rapidly to a lack of natural talent and will, thus, fail to reach their highest attainable level.[6]

SUMMARY OF EVIDENCE REGARDING RECOMMENDATIONS FOR TEACHING ADVANCED COMMUNICATION SKILLS

Although theories of expertise acquisition have received little empirical testing in the setting of medical communication skills, this chapter uses the theory of deliberate practice to scaffold recommendations for teaching communication skills. For this discussion, these teaching skills are illustrated using an example of a palliative care family meeting in which the teacher is a palliative care attending physician and the learner is a palliative care fellow. The goal of this particular family meeting is to communicate serious news.

Defining Optimal Performance

Before asking learners to perform a new task or to extend their reach and attempt to perform a familiar task in a different way than what might be comfortable for them, it is helpful to provide a cognitive road map of the task. For the common palliative medicine communication tasks of giving bad news and discussing transitions to palliative care, cognitive road maps have been developed[11] based on empirical studies of patient preferences.[12-18] This evidence base of patient preferences provides guidance for some of the key skills on which teachers and learners can focus their skill acquisition efforts. Chapter 43 of this book provides a review of the empirical evidence and a cognitive road map for the tasks of communicating serious news and discussing transitions in goals of care.

Knowing the steps of a cognitive road map and being able to perform them does not constitute optimal performance, however. True expertise comes with the ability to analyze and self-correct one's skills in real time when faced with a situation that does not lend itself to straightforward use of the cognitive road map.[8] This type of expertise in communication is difficult to replicate and measure. Therefore the old paradigm of "watching the expert in action"[19] does have utility when teaching advanced communication skills. The success of this teaching strategy, however, will be determined by the quality of the setup and the debriefing.

In our scenario of a palliative care family meeting, the clinician might be faced with a situation in which the fellow will primarily be an observer. The teacher can set the fellow up for a successful learning encounter by framing the conversation and then asking what the fellow finds difficult. "In today's family meeting, we will primarily be discussing the results of the CT scan with the patient and her family. What about these types of meetings is hardest for you? Where do you find that you get stuck?" The fellow shares that he does not know how to respond when the patient or a family member becomes visibly upset or starts crying in response to the news. The next step is to inquire about the fellow's knowledge of specific tools that might be used to respond to emotion. "Have you learned any specific skills or tools aimed at responding to emotion either in your fellowship didactics or during your work with other members of the palliative care team?" The fellow has just attended a lecture that introduced the NURSE acronym[20] (see Chapter 43, Table 43-3) as a tool for responding to emotion, but the fellow has yet to see it used in practice or use it himself. The teacher can then give the fellow a specific task for observation related to his "stuck point" and his new tool. "Watch how I respond to emotion. You might make note of specific phrases I use that are examples of naming, understanding, respecting, supporting, or exploring statements. It may even be helpful to jot down some notes as you are observing so that we can talk about the exact language I use during our debriefing afterward." Here, the teacher has given the fellow a specific observational task, reviewed the NURSE mnemonic, and given permission to take notes, something that is not normally done during a patient encounter but that can be of great help to those learning through observation.

In the debriefing after the encounter, the teacher's questions can focus on the skill that he was specifically hoping to observe. "What emotion did you notice in the patient and when?" The fellow observed that the patient seemed like she was in a state of shock when she heard the news that the cancer had spread. "And how did I respond?" The fellow was able to identify a naming statement that the teacher used: "You seem shocked." "And what did the patient do in response?" The fellow recognized that the patient concurred with this emotion and then went on to say more about how she was receiving this serious news.

"Right. So by responding to the patient's emotion with a naming statement, I aligned myself with the patient and provided implicit permission for her to speak more about her feelings. Do you have a take-home point from this family meeting?" After the fellow offers his take-home point, the teacher can take it a step further and ask the fellow for a commitment. "Do you have a new skill or tool that you would like to commit to trying sometime over the next week?" In this way, a pure observation can be transformed into a learner-centered experience that enables the learner to see the cognitive road map in practice performed by a skilled clinician, to work collaboratively with that skilled clinician to further define optimal performance, and to develop an action plan for the near future.

Individualized Learning

The second assumption of deliberate practice is that training is individualized and tailored to the learner's preexisting skill level.[6] For a scenario in which the fellow will be an active and vocal participant in the family meeting, the teacher's job is to set the fellow up for a successful encounter using three primary skills—fellow engagement, goal setting, and reflective feedback.[19] Through their work with attending physicians in oncology, Back and colleagues[19] developed a cognitive road map for a teaching encounter based on expertise acquisition theory that defined specific teaching tasks that occur before, during, and after an encounter (Table 44-2). In the deliberate practice model, the teacher is more guide than expert.[8] An expert would tell learners what they should be doing, whereas a guide will coach learners to achieve that next level of desired performance.[19] This requires that the teacher recognize that the learner is moving along a developmental path in relation to these specific communication skills and that the goal of any single teaching encounter is to move the learner one step closer to achieving a high level of performance.[19]

Before the Encounter

Just as it is important to have a premeeting for purposes of negotiating the goals of the meeting from the varying viewpoints of all of those who will be in attendance, it is also important that this premeeting include a focus on the learner who will be involved in the meeting. The key tasks of the teacher–learner interaction before the encounter are to engage the learner, identify realistic learning goals for the encounter, and discuss how the learner will measure success.[19]

Take the case of the fellow who actively observed the earlier family meeting. The fellow will now be the primary facilitator of a family meeting with the same patient, during which the team plans to discuss goals of care and to introduce the possibility of hospice care for the patient. The task of engaging the learner

TABLE 44-2. Considerations for Teaching Advanced Communication Skills

1. Define optimal performance by allowing the learner to observe the teacher.
   a. Set up the encounter.
      - What's difficult about this type of encounter?
      - Inquire about specific skills in the learner's toolbox that might be used if this difficulty is encountered.
      - Briefly review the skill identified by the learner (or provide a brief didactic about a specific tool if the learner does not already know of one that might be utilized).
      - Give the learner a specific observational task and give permission to take notes while observing.
   b. Debrief the encounter.
      - What did the learner observe in regard to the specific observational task?
      - What did skills did the teacher use?
      - How did the patient respond?
      - Ask the learner for the take-home point.
      - Have the learner develop an action plan for the future by making a commitment to practice the skill within the coming days or weeks.
2. Promote individualized learning by allowing the learner to practice a specific skill during a communication encounter.
   a. Before the encounter.
      - Engage the learner.
      - Identify realistic learning goals for the encounter.
      - Discuss how the learner will measure success.
   b. During the encounter.
      - Collect observations.
      - Identify a learning edge.
      - Ensure a positive outcome for both the learner and the patient and family.
   c. After the encounter.
      - Begin with an emotional check-in, which encourages reflection.
      - Provide goal-directed feedback using the learner's goals.
      - Leave the learner with a sense of accomplishment by eliciting the take-home point.

aims to involve the fellow in the process of individualized learning from the very beginning of the teaching encounter. "In thinking about the goals of this meeting related to discussing goals of care and hospice, I am wondering what about this type of conversation is most difficult for you." A focused, open-ended question such as this will allow the fellow to identify problem areas in these types of encounters. This sets the stage for the goal setting that immediately follows.

The goal setting for a specific teaching encounter such as this one will be grounded in the fellow's broader learning goals for the rotation. As the attending, you will have gathered data about this fellow's learning goals during your previous interactions. For example, from the earlier active observation exercise, the teacher knows that one of the fellow's goals was to be better able to respond to patient emotion. To help the fellow be as specific as possible in developing learning goals for this encounter, the teacher can refer back to this previous experience with the fellow. "During the last family meeting with the patient, you identified responding to emotion as an area of focus. Given that experience earlier this week, is there something specific you would

like to focus on today?" The fellow identifies practicing responding to emotion and would like to have an opportunity to do this after saying the word "hospice"; the fellow has seen several patients and families have strong responses to this word in the past.

To determine how the fellow will measure accomplishing this goal, the teacher will want to continue to ask questions that require the fellow to be more specific about how he will respond to emotion.[21] "Is there a specific skill that you would like to try to use when responding to the patient's emotion?" The fellow indicates practice using NURSE statements. "Are there one or two particular types of NURSE statements that you feel that you have employed less frequently in the past that you would like to try today?" The fellow relates normally making a lot of support statements but has not used naming or understanding statements as often. "Okay. So I'll plan to watch how you respond to emotion and specifically your use of naming and understanding statements."

During the Encounter

During the encounter, the teacher has three main tasks: collect observations, identify a learning edge, and ensure a positive outcome for both the learner and the patient and family.[19]

First, the teacher should carefully observe the learner, especially in relation to the learner's predetermined goals. Writing down the fellow's words and the patient's response will allow the teacher to provide more robust feedback after the encounter.[19]

In observing, the teacher is also trying to identifying the fellow's "learning edge"—the aspect of the fellow's performance that will need to be improved to achieve the next skill level.[22] A related and important question for the teacher to consider during the encounter is, "Where is the fellow in professional development?"[19] Identifying the fellow's stage of professional development and learning edge will allow the teacher to more successfully frame the fellow's learning point from this encounter during the debriefing after the encounter.

Finally, the unique role of the attending physician in this context is that of both teacher and clinician. The attending has two main goals that may not always be in alignment—teaching and patient care.[23,24] The attending physician should track the fellow's behavior and the patient's behavior closely during the encounter.[19] The decision to intervene is one that should not be taken lightly and is an advanced teaching skill that is beyond the scope of this chapter.[25]

After the Encounter

After the encounter, the goals of the teacher during the debriefing time with the learner are threefold: (1) providing goal-directed feedback using the learner's goals, (2) leaving the learner with a sense of what has been accomplished, and (3) encouraging reflection.[19]

The goal of encouraging reflection is something that can be accomplished throughout the debriefing. If the meeting has been particularly emotionally charged, it may be appropriate to begin the debriefing with an emotional check-in.[26] This could be in the form of a general observation such as, "That seemed really emotional," or a specific empathic statement aimed at attending to the fellow's emotion such as, "You seem really drained." Beginning the debriefing with this type of check-in both allows the teacher to model the empathic response the fellow is encouraged to use with patients and allows the fellow time and space to process emotions related to the encounter.[26] If emotionally overwhelmed from the meeting, the fellow may find it challenging to focus on feedback and learning.

After attending to the fellow's emotions, the teacher can ask about discussing more specifically the fellow's involvement in the meeting. The first step in providing feedback is asking the learner for a self-assessment, focusing on the aspects that the fellow did well before moving to problem areas.[26] "What things do you think you did well during the meeting?" Learners will often make general comments such as thinking it went well overall or may make one or two positive comments before quickly moving on to areas in which they think they could have done better. As the guide, the teacher should gently redirect the learner back to what was done well. If the teacher wants to highlight specific behaviors or tools that the fellow does not mention, those can be shared with the fellow. "You've identified several things that you did very well. I agree with everything you have said. May I point out one other thing you did well?" If the fellow agrees, you may proceed. "Your goal was to use naming and understanding statements, right? Well, I heard you use an understanding statement in the beginning of the encounter. You said [reading from your notes], 'I can only imagine how difficult the past couple of days must have been since our last meeting.' The effect on the patient was that she then told us more about her emotional state over the past couple of days. I think this really added to the overall effectiveness of today's meeting by aligning yourself with the patient early through an empathic statement." Note that this feedback is specific, related to the learner's goals, and addresses the way in which this choice to use an understanding statement early in the discussion may have affected the interaction as a whole.

When the things that the fellow did well have been delineated, the feedback can then move to what the fellow thinks could have gone better. The fellow thinks the discussion about hospice did not go as smoothly as desired. "What did you notice about the patient's nonverbal cues after you used the word hospice?" The fellow correctly identifies that the patient seemed to "shut down." "I'm wondering if you had a hypothesis at that moment about why the patient was shutting down." The fellow reports assuming that the patient held common misperceptions about hospice being only for the very end of life. "Can you think of a tool that you could have used to check out that assumption?" Given the learner's goals, hopefully his response to this question will be some sort of response to the patient's emotion of shutting down. If the fellow gives an answer that does not involve responding to the patient's emotion, it may be worthwhile to ask the fellow to think about what effect the proposed tactic would have had on the patient. If the fellow is not able to give an answer that relates to responding to emotion, the guide may choose to refer the fellow back to the goals. "What were you hoping to practice again during this encounter?" When the fellow recalls wanting to practice naming and understanding statements, you might say, "Yeah. I'm wondering if one of those might have been helpful here. How would you have used a naming statement when it looked like the patient was shutting down?" In this way, the teacher is serving as a guide by helping the fellow brainstorm words for how the situation might have been handled differently.

To achieve the second teaching goal of the debriefing—leaving the learner with a sense of accomplishment, the teacher can elicit the learner's take-home point. "Do you have a take-home point from today's meeting?" The important thing to remember here is that whatever the learner identifies as the take-home point is nonnegotiable. As the teacher, you hope that the fellow's take-home point will be that responding to patient's emotion is a method to check out assumptions about why the patient might be displaying a particular emotion. However, the fellow's take-home point may be something entirely different. The potential pitfall here is to correct the fellow's take-home point. Instead, use the information gleaned from what the fellow identifies as the take-home point as data for where the fellow is in professional development and to help guide future teaching encounters with this fellow.

Promoting Lifelong Learning

Although the acquisition of new skills and the need to continually practice these skills does not end with completion of formal medical education, the presence of a teacher often does. On completion of training, newly minted palliative medicine clinicians will begin their career without the physical presence of the teachers who previously provided guidance. In the model of deliberate practice, learners will, after enough deliberate thought and practice, become their own inner coach. As teachers, the goal is to provide the learners with the communication skills and an understanding of the importance of self-reflection on their own practice. With this knowledge, the hope is that the fellow will continue to set personal learning goals in order to continue to acquire the next level of expertise with each successive communication encounter.

Applying the Theory of Deliberate Practice to Teaching

In the same way that educators are encouraging learners to practice and think deliberately to improve their skills in communication, the educators themselves can engage in deliberate practice of their teaching skills. The deliberate thought and practice of teaching can be conceptualized in three stages of reflection: (1) planning and anticipatory reflection, (2) teaching and reflection in action, and (3) reflection on action.[9] The first stage of planning and anticipatory reflection occurs before the teaching opportunity and includes preparing adequately, limiting content, creating a positive atmosphere, and considering how to tailor instruction to the unique skill level of the learner.[27] The second stage of teaching and reflection in action involves the process of thinking or problem solving while directly engaged in teaching. This stage requires monitoring one's own actions as the teacher, as well as the learner's reactions, and being flexible enough to make adjustments in the teaching strategy during the encounter.[27] The third stage of reflection on action occurs after the teaching encounter and involves a deliberate process of evaluation of one's own actions as the teacher. Although it is common to engage in a process of evaluation and reflection after a self-perceived teaching failure,[9] it is equally as important to engage in this process after a successful teaching encounter as well.[27] Failures provide a powerful emotional motivator for major changes in one's teaching strategy,[9] and reflection on successes allows for continuous incremental quality improvement of one's teaching.[27] In the process of reflection on action, the teacher can examine what went well, what behaviors or techniques were employed to contribute to success, and what modifications can be made to effect an even better result the next time. When thinking about strategies that were not as effective, the teacher may consider what factors led to the lack of effectiveness. It may be that the strategy itself was not flawed, but rather that the implementation of the strategy needs to be slightly modified for it to be more successful.[9]

KEY MESSAGES TO LEARNERS

To become an expert in anything, including communication, a tremendous amount of practice is required. Success has several keys when trying to improve pre-existing skills. These include practicing deliberately, thinking deliberately, and finding a mentor. These elements are summarized in Table 44-1.

CONCLUSION AND SUMMARY

Palliative medicine clinicians are commonly called on to be both an expert communicator and a teacher of communication. The duality of these roles requires the palliative medicine clinician to attend to the needs of the learners, the patient, and the family as part of any communication encounter. By having a mental model of the process by which to engage, observe, and debrief the learner every time, the teacher can aim to provide an individualized learning experience for each learner that promotes deliberate practice. Through elicitation of the learner's goals

and close observation, the teacher will be able to help the learner identify what the learner does well, where difficulties lie, and what needs to be worked on to move to the next level of expertise as a communicator. By promoting this type of deliberate practice by learners over time, the teacher will instill a culture of lifelong learning and continued deliberate practice so learners will develop the ability to reflect on their own communication skills, continuously rising to the next level of expertise even after their formal medical education is complete.

SUMMARY RECOMMENDATIONS

- Teachers should have an interaction with the learner before a communication encounter in which they engage the learner, identify realistic learning goals for the encounter, and discuss how the learner will measure success.
- During the encounter, teachers should closely observe the learner to identify the learner's learning edge while also ensuring a positive outcome for both the learner, the patient, and the family.
- During the debriefing with the learner after the encounter, teachers should provide goal-directed feedback using the learner's goals, leave the learner with a sense of accomplishment, and encourage reflection.
- When beginning to debrief the encounter, it can often be helpful to start with an emotional check-in—an empathic statement that attends to the emotion of the learner.
- The learner's take-home point is nonnegotiable and can be used by the teacher as data to help guide future teaching encounters with this learner.

REFERENCES

1. Back AL, Arnold RM, Baile WF, et al. Efficacy of communication skills training for giving bad news and discussing transitions to palliative care. *Arch Intern Med.* 2007;167(5):453–460.
2. Fallowfield L, Jenkins V, Farewell V, et al. Efficacy of a Cancer Research UK communication skills training model for oncologists: a randomised controlled trial. *Lancet.* 2002; 359(9307):650–656.
3. Roter DL, Larson S, Shinitzky H, et al. Use of an innovative video feedback technique to enhance communication skills training. *Med Educ.* 2004;38(2):145–157.
4. Roter DL, Hall JA, Kern DE, et al. Improving physicians' interviewing skills and reducing patients' emotional distress: a randomized clinical trial. *Arch Intern Med.* 1995;155(17):1877–1884.
5. Levinson W, Roter D. The effects of two continuing medical education programs on communication skills of practicing primary care physicians. *J Gen Intern Med.* 1993;8(6):318–324.
6. Ericsson KA. Deliberate practice acquisition of maintenance of expert performance in medicine and related domains. *Acad Med.* 2004;79(suppl 10):S70–S81.
7. Ericsson KA, Krampe RT, Tesch-Romer C. The role of deliberate practice in the acquisition of expert performance. *Psychol Rev.* 1993;100:363–406.
8. Ericsson KA, Prietula MJ, Cokely ET. The making of an expert. *Harv Business Rev.* July-August 2007:115–121.

9. Pinksy LE, Irby DM. "If at first you don't succeed": using failure to improve teaching. *Acad Med.* 1997;72(11):973–976.

10. Krampe RT, Ericsson KA. Maintaining excellence: deliberate practice and elite performance in young and older pianists. *J Exp Psychol Gen.* 1996;125(4):331–359.

11. Back AL, Arnold R, Baile W, et al. Approaching difficult communication tasks in oncology. *CA Cancer J Clin.* 2005;55(3):164–177.

12. Morita T, Akechi T, Ikenaga M, et al. Communication about the ending of anticancer treatment and transition to palliative care. *Ann Oncol.* 2004;15(10):1551–1557.

13. Hagerty RG, Butow PN, Ellis PM, et al. Communicating with realism and hope: incurable cancer patients' views on the disclosure of prognosis. *J Clin Oncol.* 2005;23(6):1278–1288.

14. Girgis A, Sanson-Fisher RW. Breaking bad news. I. current best advice for clinicians. *Behav Med.* 1998;24(2):53–59.

15. Girgis A, Sanson-Fisher RW. Breaking bad news: consensus guidelines for medical practitioners. *J Clin Oncol.* 1995;13(2):2449–2456.

16. Thorne SE, Bultz BD, Baile WF. Is there a cost to poor communication in cancer care? A critical review of the literature. *Psychooncology.* 2005;14(10):875–884.

17. Walsh RA, Girgis A, Sanson-Fisher RW. Breaking bad news. II. What evidence is available to guide clinicians? *Behav Med.* 1998;24(2):61–72.

18. Griffith III CH, Wilson JF, Langer S, et al. House staff nonverbal communication skills and standardized patient satisfaction. *J Gen Intern Med.* 2003;18:170–174.

19. Back AL, Arnold RM, Baile WF, et al. Faculty development to change the paradigm of communication skills teaching in oncology. *J Clin Oncol.* 2009;27:1137–1141.

20. Smith RC, Hoppe RB. The patient's story: integrating the patient- and physician-centered approaches to interviewing. *Ann Intern Med.* 1991;115(6):470–477.

21. Fryer-Edwards K, Arnold RM, Baile W, et al. *Tough Talk: Helping Doctors Approach Difficult Conversations.* http://depts.washington.edu/toolbox; Accessed September 24, 2012.

22. Fryer-Edwards K, Arnold R, Baile W, et al. Reflective teaching practices: an approach to teaching communication skills in a small-group setting. *Acad Med.* 2006;81(7):638–644.

23. Coldicott Y, Pope C, Roberts C. The ethics of intimate examinations: teaching tomorrow's doctors. *BMJ.* 2003;326:97–101.

24. Reiser SJ. The ethics of learning and teaching medicine. *Acad Med.* 1994;69(11):872–876.

25. Back AL, Arnold RM, Tulsky JA, et al. "Could I add something?": teaching communication by intervening in real time during a clinical encounter. *Acad Med.* 2010;85(6):1048–1051.

26. Thomas JD, Arnold RM. Giving feedback. *J Palliat Med.* 2011;14(2):233–239.

27. Pinksy LE, Monson D, Irby DM. How excellent teachers are made: reflecting on success to improve teaching. *Adv Health Sci Educ.* 1998;3(3):207–215.

ADVANCE CARE PLANNING

Chapter 45

What Are Advance Care Plans and How Are They Different From Advance Directives?

GORDON WOOD AND ROBERT M. ARNOLD

INTRODUCTION AND SCOPE OF THE PROBLEM
ADVANCE DIRECTIVES
ADVANCE CARE PLANS
KEY MESSAGES TO PATIENTS AND FAMILIES
CONCLUSION AND SUMMARY

INTRODUCTION AND SCOPE OF THE PROBLEM

When asked what is important at the end of life, people say that they want to be comfortable and in control. They want to relieve burden on their families, strengthen relationships, and communicate well with their physicians. Finally, most want to avoid unhelpful life support and do not want to inappropriately prolong the dying process.[1,2] Unfortunately, for too many a mismatch exists between the care they want and the care they receive. For example, despite wanting to die at home with family, the most common location of death is the hospital.[3]

One solution to this problem is to encourage earlier discussions with patients about how they want to approach treatments in the setting of serious illness, a process called advance care planning. Encouraging patients to verbalize their goals early in the course of their illness ensures greater clarity about what is important to the patient. In addition, these conversations allow the surrogates to know the patient's wishes, thus decreasing their guilt and ambivalence when the patient is actually dying. This process should, therefore, increase understanding of the patient's values, raise the probability the patient's values guide decision-making, and decrease surrogate emotional burden.

The push for advance care planning has been ongoing for more than 25 years. Early on, the focus was on the creation of a document describing the patient's preferences, called an advance directive. Over time, many advocated for a more comprehensive approach to advance care planning that stresses ongoing conversations among the clinician, the patient, and the surrogate and results in a goal and value-based advance care plan. This chapter focuses on differentiating between advance directives and advance care plans. Subsequent chapters describe essential elements to

effective advance care planning (Chapter 46) and the evidence supporting the assertion that advance care planning changes outcomes (Chapter 47).

ADVANCE DIRECTIVES

Many trace the origin of the advance directive to 1969, when Louis Kutner, an Illinois attorney, proposed a "living will" as a document by which people could put their wishes for future medical care in writing, thereby allowing these wishes to be followed even if the person could not communicate.[4] Over time, different types of documents were prepared and the general term *advance directive* came to cover any type of written document stating a patient's wishes for how to address future medical decisions (Table 45-1 lists some of the many forms of advance directives available, and Table 45-2 provides information to access state-specific advance directives). Two general forms of directives exist (although some directives contain both forms). Substantive directives, or living wills, allow patients to state their values and treatment preferences should they become incapacitated. Process directives, or health care proxies, allow patients to say whom they would want to make decisions for them should they become incapacitated.

Advance directives slowly gained popularity, and many hoped that they would be the solution to the troubling situation of unwanted treatments at the end of life. Heavily publicized cases of conflict regarding withdrawal of life support, such as those of Karen Ann Quinlan, Nancy Cruzan, and Terry Schiavo, have fueled the push for advance directive completion.[5,6] In 1990, Congress approved the Patient Self Determination Act requiring hospitals and other health care institutions to ask whether patients had an advance directive on admission. The facility was also required to educate health care staff about advance directives and educate patients about their decision-making rights, including the right to make an advance directive and refuse any medical treatment. By 2005, 29% of Americans had completed a living will, up from 12% in 1990. In patients 78 to 92 years of age, 57% had completed a living will, up from 19% in 1990.[7]

TABLE 45-1. Key Advance Care Planning Documents

DOCUMENT	DESCRIPTION
Substantive Directives *Also known as...* • Living will • Five Wishes • Personal wishes statement	Allows a patient to specify wishes for future care May also include a section to designate a proxy decision-maker
Process Directives *Also known as...* • Health care power of attorney • Health care proxy • Durable power of attorney for health care	Designates a surrogate decision-maker Does not specify wishes for care
Physician Orders for Life Sustaining Treatment	Document containing physician orders regarding cardiopulmonary resuscitation and medical interventions, including antibiotics and artificial nutrition and hydration Travels with a patient across care sites and is legally valid as an order in transit
Code status	Order or document in a particular institution specifying whether to perform cardiopulmonary resuscitation in the event of clinical decompensation

TABLE 45-2. Advance Care Planning Resources

RESOURCE	DESCRIPTION	WEB ADDRESS*
Massachusetts Medical Society: End of Life Care	Instructional website for patients that discusses advance care planning with a focus on designation of a health care proxy. Includes a Massachusetts Health Care Proxy Form.	www.healthcareproxy.org
Better Ending	Guides for patients in Massachusetts regarding how to do advance care planning. Includes videos and guides in multiple languages.	www.betterending.org
Aging with Dignity	Five Wishes distribution site. Samples are available for review, and hard copies can be purchased. Next Steps, a companion guide for how to discuss Five Wishes, is also available.	www.agingwithdignity.org
Americans for Better Care of the Dying	National nonprofit organization that advocates for better end-of-life care through policy change and reform of current systems. Website also offers excerpts from the book *Handbook for Mortals* that may be helpful to patients.	www.abcd-caring.org
The POLST Paradigm	Website centered on the Physician Orders for Life Sustaining Treatment form and how to use it and access it in each state.	www.polst.org
American Bar Association: Consumer's Toolkit for Health Care Advance Planning	Toolkit for patients regarding all aspects of advance care planning. Includes excellent list of resources, including books that patients might find helpful.	www.abanet.org/aging (select under resources)
Caring Connections	Guide for patients from the National Hospice and Palliative Care Organization (NHPCO) that includes a link to download state-specific advance directives.	www.caringinfo.org
Respecting Choices	Offers national online and onsite courses for medical professionals in advance care planning. From the group at Gunderson Lutheran Medical Foundation in LaCrosse, Wisconsin.	www.respectingchoices.org

*Websites accessed October 1, 2012.

Unfortunately, little benefit has been seen from advance directives alone, with most studies focused on substantive directives.[3,8] The Study to Understand Prognoses and Preferences for Outcomes and Risks of Treatment (SUPPORT) trial, released in 1995, revealed that advance directives appeared to have no impact on communication or decisions about end-of-life care.[3,9] A follow-up meta-analysis confirmed these findings.[10]

Advance directives alone are ineffective for several reasons. First, people find it difficult to predict the type of care they would want to receive in a future hypothetical state of health. In one study, 45% reported being uncertain about what they would want, even in the scenario of being in a very compromised state of health and being told that the outcome of life support would be poor.[11] Second, concern exists that patients will change their minds, undercutting the directive power of the advance directive. In fact, studies show that up to half of elderly patients with serious illnesses may have end-of-life preferences that vary over time.[12] This is a barrier also recognized by surrogates and physicians.[13,14] Preferences may change because health states that seem unacceptable when the patient is doing well may become palatable when they are actually experienced. For example, a patient with amyotrophic lateral sclerosis (ALS) may say that he would not want to live with certain degrees of disability but, as he slowly gets worse, each state becomes acceptable and the next level of disability is then thought to be the point at which the patient would not want to live.[15] Alternatively, preferences may change over time because patients slowly come to peace with their diagnosis and become more accepting of comfort-focused care.[16] This is especially true in patients with cancer, who tend to favor more aggressive care shortly after the diagnosis but tend to focus more on quality of life as the disease progresses.[17]

Third, the content of substantive directives leads to practical problems. If the language is too specific, it is often difficult to extrapolate to the inherently more complex current medical condition.[8,18,19] For example, if a patient with cancer states that she does not want intubation but then has an aspiration event while taking contrast for a computed tomography scan, should she be intubated given that she is likely to make a full recovery? On the other hand, broad value statements in isolation are often too vague to guide specific medical care.[8,19] Because of these issues, both providers and surrogates have difficulty interpreting how an advance directive should be applied to certain scenarios of clinical care.[8,20] In fact, surrogates incorrectly predict a patient's wishes in a third of cases and having an advance directive does not improve their accuracy.[8,21] In addition, even with an advance directive, surrogates must interpret what the patient meant. Without talking with the patient about the patient's overarching goals, this interpretation may be based on factors that include their own values, beliefs, and preferences for end-of-life care.[22]

In addition to these conceptual issues with advance directives, implementation issues have limited their efficacy. Patients may have wishes for their care, but they often do not discuss them with their doctors[23] or create an advance directive.[24,25] If an advance directive is created, it is often not documented appropriately in the medical record[26,27] or transferred between different sites of care.[28] Finally, legal shortcomings of advance directives limit their implementation, including readability issues and witness and notary requirements.[29]

ADVANCE CARE PLANS

In response to the numerous conceptual and implementation issues that have limited the efficacy of advance directives alone, more recent attention has focused on more comprehensive advance care plans. Advance care planning is a broader construct that focuses on conversations about eliciting goals rather than the creation of a document. The conversations among clinicians, patients, and families should attend to relationships, as well as the emotions of decision-making.[30] The focus is on getting the patient and the surrogate together; ensuring a shared understanding of the diagnosis, prognosis, treatment options, and the relevant goals and values; and then establishing a plan to make sure the treatment plan matches the goals.[30] The specific details of care are addressed when appropriate and include both biomedical interventions and the preferred site of end-of-life care.[31] Preparations

are made to ensure the plans can be enacted and that expected complications are appropriately addressed, such as making sure that medications are available to treat dyspnea if intubation is to be avoided.[32] Any special instructions about how to involve family and how to address spiritual or religious issues should also be discussed over the course of the patient's illness.[32]

The modern conception of advance care planning specifically addresses the uncertainty inherent in planning for the future and focuses on preparing the patient and surrogate for "in-the-moment" decision-making.[33] Knowing that the patient is likely to be incapacitated during the dying process, advance care planning tries to ensure the surrogate is intimately involved in the conversations. The clinician explicitly discusses how decisions will be made when they arise, including open discussion about the leeway the patient wants to allow the surrogate in decision-making. Finally, rather than being viewed as a static document, advance care planning is viewed as a flexible process that occurs over the course of the illness. This allows changing preferences and values to be integrated into the ongoing conversation.[33]

Although the focus of an advance care plan is the conversation, the results of the discussions do still need to be documented. They should be described in detail in the physician's notes. A written advance directive should also be prepared. The difference, however, is that this document is only one piece of an effective advance care plan. The most important function that the written advance directive serves is designation of the surrogate with whom these careful discussions have taken place. This can be done on a health care power of attorney or health care proxy form. To a certain degree, the content of the discussion can also be transferred to substantive advance directives, most of which also contain a proxy designation section. One particularly popular version of an advance directive that tries to combine eliciting patient goals and documenting substantive and process decisions is called Five Wishes. It is considered a legal document in 40 states and serves as a workbook that goes through what the patient wishes regarding who will make decisions for the patient, what treatment the patient wants or does not want, how comfortable the patient wants to be, how the patient wants to be treated by others, and what the patient wants loved ones to know. Another document in which particular wishes near the end of life may be documented is the Physician Orders for Life Sustaining Treatment (POLST).[34] This document operationalizes a patient's wishes as physician orders regarding cardiopulmonary resuscitation and medical interventions such as antibiotics and artificial nutrition and hydration. POLST forms have been shown to influence treatment decisions by emergency medical technicians[35] and are used commonly in nursing homes[35] and in patients in hospice care.[36] Many hospitals and other institutions will translate a POLST into a code status order that appears in the patient's medical record to direct how the staff should respond in the setting of the need for resuscitation.

This current construct of advance care planning is in keeping with what patients say they want. When asked what they saw as the purpose of advance care planning, 48 patients on hemodialysis thought it was to prepare for death and dying, including exercising some degree of control and relieving burdens. They prioritized discussions with family over filling out forms.[37] A survey of 64 caregivers of deceased patients suggests that surrogates want similar things from advance care planning. They wanted the process to facilitate communication between the patient and the caregivers, recognizing that preferences may fluctuate and considering decisions other than treatment decisions, such as preferred site of end-of-life care.[31]

KEY MESSAGES TO PATIENTS AND FAMILIES

Patients and families should understand that participating in the preparation of comprehensive advance care plans with their physician can help patients receive the care desired and help relieve the burden on their loved ones. Although the completion of an advance directive may seem irrelevant to the patient who has talked to family about these issues, a more comprehensive process guided by a skilled clinician can prepare everyone for the challenging decisions that are likely to lie ahead.

CONCLUSION AND SUMMARY

Many patients now die while unresponsive after decisions made by surrogates and physicians. End-of-life care often does not match patient preferences. Advance directives alone have been unsuccessful at changing this reality because of conceptual and implementation issues. A more comprehensive advance care planning process is now advocated and supported by positive patient outcomes (see Chapter 47). The next chapter reviews, in more detail, how to perform this type of advance care planning, including specifics on how to hold the conversation to create an advance care plan that gives the patient and the surrogate what they need in the difficult moments that come at the end of life.

SUMMARY RECOMMENDATIONS

- Do not focus advance care planning discussions solely on the creation of an advance directive, because it alone is unlikely to change patient outcomes.
- Advance care planning should focus on getting the surrogate and patient to a shared understanding of the disease, prognosis, goals, and values.
- Advance care plans should be devised to make sure care is directed at achieving these goals, including practical preparations and discussions of uncertainty and acceptable leeway in decision making.
- Advance directives should be only one part of a comprehensive advance care plan.

REFERENCES

1. Strachan PH, Ross H, Rocker GM, et al., Canadian Researchers at the End of Life Network (CARENET), Mind the gap: opportunities for improving end-of-life care for patients with advanced heart failure. *Can J Cardiol.* 2009;25(11):635–640.
2. Singer PA, Martin DK, Kelner M. Quality end-of-life care: patients' perspectives. *JAMA.* 1999;281(12):163–168.
3. Teno J, Lynn J, Wenger N, et al. Advance directives for seriously ill hospitalized patients: effectiveness with the patient self-determination act and the SUPPORT intervention. SUPPORT Investigators. Study to Understand Prognoses and Preferences for Outcomes and Risks of Treatment. *J Am Geriatr Soc.* 1997;45(4):500–507.
4. Kutner L. Due process of euthanasia: the living will, a proposal. *Indiana Law J.* 1969;44:539–554.
5. Racine E, Karczewska M, Seidler M, et al. How the public responded to the Schiavo controversy: evidence from letters to editors. *J Med Ethics.* 2010;36(9):571–573.
6. Annas GJ. "Culture of life" politics at the bedside: the case of Terri Schiavo. *N Engl J Med.* 2005;352(16):1710–1715.
7. *More Americans discussing—and planning—end-of-life treatment.* The Pew Research Center. http://people-press.org/files/legacy-pdf/266.pdf; 2006 Updated. Accessed October 1, 2012.
8. Ditto PH, Danks JH, Smucker WD, et al. Advance directives as acts of communication: a randomized controlled trial. *Arch Intern Med.* 2001;161(3):421–430.
9. The SUPPORT principal investigators. A controlled trial to improve care for seriously ill hospitalized patients. The Study to Understand Prognoses and Preferences for Outcomes and Risks of Treatments (SUPPORT). *JAMA.* 1995;274(3):1591–1598.
10. Hanson LC, Tulsky JA, Danis M. Can clinical interventions change care at the end of life? *Ann Intern Med.* 1997;126(5):381–388.
11. Sudore RL, Schillinger D, Knight SF, et al. Uncertainty about advance care planning treatment preferences among diverse older adults. *J Health Commun.* 2010;15(suppl 2):159–171.
12. Fried TR, O'Leary J, Van Ness P, et al. Inconsistency over time in the preferences of older persons with advanced illness for life-sustaining treatment. *J Am Geriatr Soc.* 2001;55(7):1007–1014.
13. Knauft E, Nielsen EL, Engelberg RA, et al. Barriers and facilitators to end-of-life care communication for patients with COPD. *Chest.* 2005;127:2188–2196.
14. Fried TR, O'Leary JR. Using the experiences of bereaved caregivers to inform patient- and caregiver-centered advance care planning. *J Gen Intern Med.* 2008;23(10):1602–1607.
15. Silverstein MD, Stocking CB, Antel JP, et al. Amyotrophic lateral sclerosis and life-sustaining therapy: patients' desires for information, participation in decision making, and life-sustaining therapy. *Mayo Clin Proc.* 1991;66(9):906–913.
16. Wittink MN, Morales KH, Meoni LA, et al. Stability of preferences for end-of-life treatment after 3 years of follow-up: the Johns Hopkins Precursors Study. *Arch Intern Med.* 2008;168(19):2125–2130.
17. Voogt E, van der Heide A, Rietjens JA, et al. Attitudes of patients with incurable cancer toward medical treatments in the last phase of life. *J Clin Oncol.* 2005;23(9):2012–2019.
18. Brett AS. Limitations of listing specific medical interventions in advance directives. *JAMA.* 1991;266(6):825–828.
19. Coppola KM, Ditto PH, Danks JH, et al. Accuracy of primary care and hospital-based physicians' predictions of elderly outpatients' treatment preferences with and without advance directives. *Arch Intern Med.* 2001;161(3):431–440.
20. Thompson T, Barbour R, Schwartz L. Adherence to advance directives in critical decision making: vignette study. *BMJ.* 2003;327(7422):1011.
21. Shalowitz DL, Barrett-Mayer E, Wendler D. The accuracy of surrogate decision makers: a systematic review. *Arch Intern Med.* 2006;166(5):493–497.
22. Vig EK, Taylor JS, Starks H, et al. Beyond substituted judgment: how surrogates navigate end-of-life decision-making. *J Am Geriatr Soc.* 2006;54(11):1688–1693.
23. Fried TR, Redding CA, Robbins ML, et al. Stages of change for the component behaviors of advance care planning. *J Am Geriatr Soc.* 2010;58(12):2329–2336.

24. Go RS, Hammes BA, Lee JA, et al. Advance directives among health care professional at a community-based cancer center. *Mayo Clin Proc.* 2007;82(12):1487–1490.

25. Camhi SL, Mercado AF, Morrison RS, et al. Deciding in the dark: advance directives and continuation of treatment in chronic critical illness. *Crit Care Med.* 2009;37(3):919–925.

26. Yung VY, Walling AM, Min L, et al. Documentation of advance care planning for community-dwelling elders. *J Palliat Med.* 2010;13:861–867.

27. Ternel JS, Greer JA, Admane S, et al. Code status documentation in the outpatient electronic medical records of patients with metastatic cancer. *J Gen Intern Med.* 2009;25(2): 150–153.

28. Daaleman TP, Williams CS, Preisser JS, et al. Advance care planning in nursing homes and assisted living communities. *J Am Med Dir Assoc.* 2009;10(4):243–251.

29. Castillo LS, Williams BA, Hooper SM, et al. Lost in translation: the unintended consequences of advance directive law on clinical care. *Ann Intern Med.* 2011;154(2):121–128.

30. Tulsky JA. Beyond advance directives: importance of communication skills at the end of life. *JAMA.* 2005;294(3): 359–365.

31. Fried TR, O'Leary JR. Using the experiences of bereaved caregivers to inform patient- and caregiver-centered advance care planning. *J Gen Intern Med.* 2008;23(10):1602–1607.

32. Lynn J, Goldstein NE. Advance care planning for fatal chronic illness: avoiding commonplace errors and unwanted suffering. *Ann Intern Med.* 2003;138(10):812–818.

33. Sudore RL, Fried TR. Redefining the "planning" in advance care planning: preparing for end-of-life decision-making. *Ann Intern Med.* 2010;153(4):256–261.

34. Bomba PA, Vermilyea D. Integrating POLST into palliative care guidelines: a paradigm shift in advance care planning in oncology. *J Natl Compr Canc Netw.* 2006;4(8):819–829.

35. Schmidt TA, Hickman SE, Tolle SW, et al. The physician orders for life-sustaining treatment program: Oregon emergency medical technicians' practical experiences and attitudes. *J Am Geriatr Soc.* 2004;52(9):1430–1434.

36. Hickman SE, Nelson CA, Moss AH, et al. Use of the physician orders for life-sustaining treatment (POLST) paradigm program in the hospice setting. *J Palliat Med.* 2009;12(2):133–141.

37. Singer PA, Martin DK, Lavery JV, et al. Reconceptualizing advance care planning from the patient's perspective. *Arch Intern Med.* 1998;158(8):879–884.

Chapter 46

What Elements Are Essential to Effective Advance Care Planning?

GORDON WOOD AND ROBERT M. ARNOLD

INTRODUCTION AND SCOPE OF THE PROBLEM

One of the best examples of community-wide advance care planning is currently in LaCrosse, Wisconsin, where 90% of the population has an advance directive, 99.4% of those are in the medical record at patient death, and 99.5% of people receive care in keeping with their wishes at the end of life.[1] These impressive numbers were achieved through a comprehensive program known as Respecting Choices,[2] implemented by the local health system. Although this is not the only way to approach advance care planning, its five essential elements are common to most successful advance care planning interventions. These five elements include (1) trained facilitators, (2) patient-centered discussions, (3) involvement of surrogates in the discussions, (4) correctly filed documentation, and (5) systematic education of doctors. This chapter focuses on operationalizing these principles for the individual palliative care practitioner (steps 2-4). Particular attention is paid to how to have a patient-centered conversation that involves the surrogate and is correctly documented, because these are within the control of individual practitioners. The system-level aspects regarding training of facilitators and systematic physician education about advance care planning will be addressed more fully in the following chapter in a discussion about barriers to system-wide improvements and their possible solutions. The stepwise approach to the conversation presented in the following section should be familiar to clinicians because it is the same approach used for many palliative care discussions.[3] Table 46-1 summarizes these steps and includes sample phrasings a clinician might use to achieve each step.

STEP 1: PREPARE FOR THE CONVERSATION: THE PREMEETING

The steps taken before any discussion are often the key to its success. Some call this the premeeting. The premeeting for an advance care planning discussion includes many of the standard tasks before any meeting: making sure the diagnosis, prognosis, and treatment options are clear and agreed upon by all of the clinicians; getting the relevant people in the room (including the surrogate); setting up a suitable physical setting that is quiet, private, and uninterrupted and has seating and tissues; clarifying the goal for the meeting; and having a plan for how to run the discussion, including who will lead if there are multiple clinicians.[4] However, certain aspects of the premeeting deserve particular attention.

When to Discuss Advance Care Planning

The first aspect to consider is when to bring up advance care planning. The Respecting Choices program considers three different types of discussions for three different times in a patient's life.[5] The first is when the patient is healthy and the goals are to name a surrogate and define wishes if the patient develops severe neurological injury and is unlikely to recover. The second is when the patient has a life-threatening illness and is starting to progress. The third conversation is for people likely in the last 12 months of life. Because the focus of this text is on the palliative care clinician, this chapter will focus on the latter two types of discussion. In these populations, the topic of advance care planning should be brought up with all patients and is often done as part of the normal routine of care. Many clinicians choose to discuss advance care planning at a visit when the patient is doing well so there is time to talk and recognize the discussion can stretch out over multiple visits.[6]

Some triggers should prompt more urgent discussions of advance care planning in patients with life-threatening illness. Worsening clinical status, declining functional status, frequent hospitalizations, or imminent expected complications should trigger an advance care planning discussion. For example, some clinicians may use hospitalizations as a trigger

TABLE 46-1. The Advance Care Planning Conversation

STEPS AND GOALS	SAMPLE PHRASINGS
Step 1: Prepare for the conversation Who will be present? What are the facts about the illness and what are the cultural or spiritual norms that may be relevant? When is it appropriate to discuss advance care planning? Where can the discussion be held? Why is the discussion occurring (are there specific goals)? How will the discussion be run if multiple clinicians are present?	N/A
Steps 2 and 3: Determine what the patient knows and wants to know	
Introduce the topic	*"One thing I like to do with all of my patients is to discuss advance care planning. Do you know what that means?"* *"Because it was such a difficult hospitalization, I think it might be helpful to take some time to discuss what we should do if you get sick again."*
Assess readiness to discuss and address barriers as needed	*"Is this something you would feel comfortable discussing today?"* *"Most patients, at some point, are unable to make their own decisions. Giving your spouse some direction about what to do if that happens can make it much easier on him."* *"Are there specific reasons that you find this difficult to discuss?"*
Choose and involve a decision-maker	*"If you were unable to make your own decisions, who should I turn to if something needs to be decided?"* *"Let's set up a visit when he can be here to specifically talk about advance care planning. Here are some materials for you to read and think about before that visit."*
Assess what they know	*"So I know where to begin, tell me what you know about what's going on with you medically."*
Step 4: Deliver any new information	
Correct any misunderstandings	*"You told me that you wanted to hear it straight so I'll do that. Although the chemotherapy may prolong your life, I'm afraid that we cannot cure your cancer."*
Discuss prognosis	*"We are really bad at giving exact estimates, and the best I can give you is a range. Unfortunately, I think we're talking about somewhere between weeks and months, not years."*
Step 5: Notice and respond to emotions	
Convey empathy	*"This is really hard."*
Allow the patient and surrogate to process the emotions enough to engage in further planning	*"Anyone in your situation would be upset by news like this."* *"You've done all the right things."* *"No matter what happens, I'll walk this road with you."* *"Tell me more about what worries you."* *"Do you think you're ready to discuss what we do now?"*
Step 6: Determine goals of care and treatment priorities	
Establish overall goals and values that can subsequently guide formation of an advance care plan	*"Given what I've told you about the prognosis, what is most important for you in the time that you have?"*
Discuss valued life activities	*"What gives your life meaning?"*
Discuss acceptable health states	*"When you think about what lies ahead, what do you hope for? Is there anything you want to avoid?"*
Discuss specific scenarios as appropriate	*"If your breathing were to get worse again, we should talk about whether you would want to go back on the breathing machine, because there are other options."*
Discuss "hopeless" scenario	*"It may sound silly that I would even ask this, but ... many patients say that if they got into a situation in which they were unable to communicate and were dying without any hope of improving, that they would not want their death prolonged with machines, whereas other people feel differently. Is this something you have thought about?"*
Step 7: Agree on a plan	
Offer value-centered recommendations	*"Given that your goal is to die at home, I would not recommend putting you on machines if you got sicker. Rather, I would recommend treating what we can with medicines in your home."*
Make specific plans for expected complications	*"If your breathing gets short again, we will have morphine in the sealed box in your refrigerator."*
Discuss decision-making uncertainty and leeway	*"Although we plan the best we can, things can get tricky when they actually happen. Sometimes families need to decide to go against these plans so it works out best for everyone. If we had to do that, would it be OK with you? Are there any things we've discussed that you would consider nonnegotiable?"*
Discuss how decisions will need to be readdressed over time	*"Your wishes may change over time, and that is normal. We will readdress this periodically, and you should always feel comfortable bringing it up with me again."*
Explain how to use any documents	*"Keep the living will somewhere convenient at home so you can take it with you if you ever need to go to the hospital."*

for initiating an advance care planning discussion. Many consider these to be teachable moments, and patients generally seem open to the discussion in this setting.[7,8] Also, certain vulnerable populations should trigger the clinician to talk about surrogate decision-makers. These populations are at high risk for not having the decision-maker they want if they do not engage in advance care planning, such as same-sex couples, common-law couples, and single people. Without formal declaration of a surrogate, the decision-maker will be chosen by a state's surrogacy laws, which generally base the designation on blood relations. Fortunately, public awareness campaigns and physician efforts seem to be conveying this message and many people in these groups have participated in advance care planning.[9]

Although some physicians worry about bringing up advance care planning too soon, patients generally want to have these discussions earlier than physicians realize.[10] In fact, disease severity appears to have no correlation to a patient's desire to engage in end-of-life discussions.[11] Rather, it may be more related to personal preferences and level of comfort.[6]

Cultural and Religious and Spiritual Norms

Before starting a meeting about advance care planning, it also can be helpful to consider whether any cultural, spiritual, or religious norms have an impact on the discussion. Although the clinician should never assume that all members of a group have the same beliefs, knowledge of some of the norms can aid in the discussion. For example, a recent study suggests that elderly Latinos appear to prefer less aggressive end-of-life care but rarely complete an advance directive or participate in advance care planning[12] and thus receive more aggressive care[13] perhaps because of this lack of planning. Literacy and language-appropriate documents may increase advance care planning in this population.[14] Indo-Caribbean Hindus have similar positive attitudes toward advance care planning and negative attitudes toward life-sustaining measures, but also rarely complete advance directives.[15] African-Americans are also less likely to engage in advance care planning but, in contrast to Latinos and Hindus, seem to desire the aggressive use of life-sustaining treatments they tend to receive at the end of life.[13,16] Unfortunately, the majority of clinicians are unaware of common end-of-life preferences in African-American patients.[17] Spiritual beliefs in the African-American community that may affect advance care planning include God is responsible for health and the doctor is God's tool; only God determines when someone dies; and divine interventions and miracles do occur.[18] In fact, positive religious coping (drawing strength from one's faith) in general is associated with more intensive medical treatment near death and a desire for all measures to prolong life.[19,20] However, a small body of literature suggests that information and education, such as watching videos of patients with dementia, may result in a preference for less aggressive end-of-life care.[21,22]

Although a knowledge of these groups' general preferences can be helpful, knowing what the individual patient wants or is even willing to discuss cannot be predicted. The only way to know is to ask in a nonjudgmental, patient-centered manner.[23] Possible phrasings that may be considered if these issues seem relevant include the following:
- How do your religious or spiritual beliefs influence your goals for your medical care near the end of your life?
- Are there any cultural, spiritual, or religious factors that I should know about as we talk about the care you would want if you got sicker?

STEPS 2 AND 3: DETERMINE WHAT THE PATIENT KNOWS AND WANTS TO KNOW

When the premeeting considerations have been discussed, it is time to begin the advance care planning discussion. Please refer to Table 46-1 for sample phrasings for each step. The majority of the first part of the conversation involves introducing the topic and seeing what the patient understands about advance care planning, assessing readiness to discuss, getting the surrogate present, then seeing what everyone knows about the illness. The general principle for this entire segment of the conversation is to ask before you tell, because it gives an idea of where to begin.

Introducing the Topic

The topic of advance care planning is usually brought up in one of two ways. The first is to normalize it as something you discuss with all of your patients. The second is to bring it up in the context of the patient's particular illness. For example, if the patient has just been in the intensive care unit for respiratory failure, the clinician may reference that stay and bring up the need for a discussion of what to do should that happen again. Although the task of introducing the topic may seem trivial, the mere act of a clinician broaching the discussion and explaining its importance has been associated with a higher rate of advance directive completion.[24,25]

Assess Readiness to Discuss

Once the topic has been broached, the next task is to determine if the patient is ready to discuss advance care planning. If the patient is not ready or experiences strong emotion in regard to the conversation, this can be addressed at the outset. Many advocate a "stages of change" model similar to other health behaviors.[26] Recent data suggest that patients may be at different stages of change for different parts of the advance care planning process (e.g., talking to the doctor, talking to the family, completing an advance directive, etc.) so asking about each step may be helpful.[27] Advance care planning behavior change seems to start with contemplation, then progresses to the patient having a discussion, most often with family first. The patient then progresses to documentation or discussion with the physician. Talking with friends and family seems to be the key step and may predict the patient's future discussion with clinicians and completion of advance directives.[14] If a patient is not ready to discuss, the clinician may consider educating, motivating, and addressing barriers, depending on the situation.[28] See Table 46-1 for examples of how this may be done.

Choose and Involve the Surrogate Decision-Maker

When patients are ready to engage in a discussion about advanced care planning, the first task is to ask if they would choose a surrogate decision-maker. The surrogate would be involved in representing their wishes should they become incapacitated. Many people choose their spouse, and some data suggest that the spouse may be most accurate at predicting patient wishes. Proxies with less family conflict also tend to be more accurate.[29] It is important to note that many people, especially in certain cultures, prefer to have more than one person involved in decision making, so this should be asked about directly.[12,30] When the surrogate or surrogates are chosen, the clinician should ask the patient if it is acceptable to include them in the discussion. Most patients prefer to have family present at the discussions and, as discussed earlier, may even favor discussing these issues with family over physicians.[31] Involving the surrogate helps ensure that all have the same understanding of the patient's wishes should the patient become sicker and unable to communicate. When starting the discussion with the surrogate decision-maker, it can be helpful to describe how decision making would occur if needed in the future, including an explicit description of the principle of substituted judgment, in which the family's job is to convey what the patient would want instead of what they would want.

Assess What They Know

When everyone is assembled and the purpose of the discussion is described, the next step is to assess what everyone knows about advance care planning and what they know and want to know about the illness, including prognosis. According to palliative care patients and their caregivers, this creates the optimal context for a discussion about the end of life.[32]

STEP 4: DELIVER ANY NEW INFORMATION

If, when the clinician asks what the patient and surrogate know about the illness, major knowledge gaps exist, they must be addressed before any discussion of advance care planning can occur. Accurate information, including prognosis, helps patients and surrogates make decisions that are consistent with their values. For example, if a patient understands that prognosis is short, the patient is more likely to favor a comfort approach to care.[33,34]

STEP 5: NOTICE AND RESPOND TO EMOTIONS

If new information is conveyed, especially regarding a poor prognosis, emotional responses are likely. A growing body of literature supports the importance of monitoring for emotions and responding empathically.[34,35] It is a difficult but attainable skill that builds relationships and allows the patient and surrogate to process the emotions enough to fully engage in the subsequent steps of advance care planning. See Chapter 43 for more information about recognizing and responding to emotions in conversations about goals of care.

STEP 6: DETERMINE GOALS OF CARE AND TREATMENT PRIORITIES

Determining the goals of care and treatment priorities is the key step in current recommendations for how to approach advance care planning.[28,35,36] Instead of focusing on creating a document describing what the patient does not want, the focus is on a discussion among the patient, surrogate, and clinician about what is important to the patient and what the patient *does* want. Then a plan can be created to maximize the chance of achieving these goals.

Goals of care can be established by asking what gives the patient's life meaning and what is truly important to the patient in the time remaining, given the conversation just held about prognosis. It appears to be more helpful to patients to discuss what sort of health state would be acceptable and what activities are really valued, rather than asking about specific medical interventions.[37] Sometimes, however, specific situations need to be discussed, especially as the patient gets closer to the end of life. This can be done in the context of prior experiences the patient has had with illness. For example, an episode on a ventilator often triggers discussion of what would happen if respiratory failure developed again. In considering specific interventions, such as cardiopulmonary resuscitation (CPR), recent studies suggest that having a patient watch a video can be helpful in conveying the realities of the various care options.[22,38,39] In some states, it can be particularly important to discuss artificial nutrition and hydration because of laws requiring "clear and convincing evidence" that a patient would not want artificial nutrition and hydration to allow it to be withheld or withdrawn.

Another specific situation that is often addressed in this discussion is the hopeless scenario described in many advance directives. Although it is difficult to determine exactly when someone is in a terminal condition with no reasonable hope of recovery,[28] most patients agree that some states are worse than death.[10] Having discussed this scenario is often helpful when meeting with families at the end of a patient's life, because it decreases their guilt and allows them to feel they have done "everything." If the physician can tell the family that the patient has entered that hopeless state, many families seem to find comfort in the belief that they are only following the patient's wishes when they consent to withdrawal of life-sustaining therapies.

STEP 7: AGREE ON A PLAN

Once the goals and priorities are established, the final step is for the clinician to help develop a treatment plan to meet those goals. Although recent ethical precepts stress the importance of autonomy, patients and their families often have a poor understanding of the complex medical situations that arise at the end of life. It can be helpful for physicians to offer recommendations based not on paternalistic impressions of what they think is right but on their understanding of how best to approach care to achieve the patient's goals and values.[40] See Table 46-1 for an example of how such a value-centered recommendation can be phrased so the reasoning is transparent to patients and families. In doing this, it is important to realize that some patients may not want physicians to make the final decisions, but they almost always want to hear the physician's opinion and may then subsequently want further discussion.[41]

When approaching these discussions, it is helpful to start with what can be done to achieve the patient's goals and then discuss what should not be done because it will not help promote these goals. Many junior clinicians start by talking about what should not be done, for example, CPR, but feel uncomfortable offering recommendations. This tends to result in decisions with which the clinician disagrees and poor patient understanding.[42] If the clinician, instead, is able to recommend, for example, avoiding CPR in the patient who wishes to die at home, it is more likely that care can be structured to help patients meet their goals.

Specific plans should be made to account for expected complications so the overall advance care plan can be successful.[36] This includes making sure that symptom medications are available and that both site of care and support of the medical team are discussed. Site of care while dying can be a particularly important discussion. Despite a patient's desire to die at home, it may be logistically difficult for the family.[43] Having discussed this initially will allow an honest conversation about the burden and may allow the patient to alleviate the family's guilt.

Finally, the amount of leeway the patient wants to grant the surrogate in making decisions in keeping with the predetermined goals should be discussed. One way to approach this is to explore which wishes are nonnegotiable and which the patient might be willing to let the surrogate and doctor change if they both believed it was in the best interest of the patient or family.[28]

Making the plan also includes some form of documentation. The discussion should be recorded in the medical record. A health care power of attorney form may also be needed, especially if the surrogate is someone other than the default decision-maker by the state's surrogacy laws. A substantive advance directive may also be useful, especially if specific treatment wishes have been expressed. Care at the end of life is often not with the same clinician who has the advance care planning discussion; therefore having a document can be helpful, if only to clearly name the surrogate or for the "hopeless" statement referenced earlier, which can be of use during an end-of-life family meeting. Near the end of life, a Physician Orders for Life-Sustaining Treatment (POLST) form can operationalize specific wishes regarding CPR and other medical interventions as doctor's orders that are transportable between settings. When a document is created, it is important to specifically address how to use it. It should be readily available and not in a safe deposit box, and the patient and family should bring it to all hospitalizations.

Finally, it is important to discuss the need to readdress over time. It can be helpful to normalize that preferences may change regarding treatment[44] and even regarding who the patient wants to help with decision-making.[45]

KEY MESSAGES TO PATIENTS AND FAMILIES

Patients and families should expect to engage in advance care planning discussions with their physicians or other members of the clinical team. They should carefully choose a surrogate decision-maker who knows them well and whom they feel could represent their wishes were they unable to communicate. This surrogate should come to the advance care planning visit and actively participate. Spending some time thinking about what is important to them and what gives their lives meaning can help facilitate the discussion. When patients and surrogates have decided what is important and what they want to avoid, it may be helpful for the clinicians to make recommendations about what is most likely to achieve these goals. When a plan is established, they should record it in some sort of document that is readily available, which they bring to any hospitalization or any significantly involved new provider. They should also expect to readdress the plan over time.

CONCLUSION AND SUMMARY

An advance care planning discussion follows a pattern similar to that in many other conversations in palliative care. It begins with a careful premeeting during which preparations for the discussion are made. The clinician then starts the meeting by determining what the patient knows about advance care planning and assists in choosing a surrogate, who is included in the discussion. Both the patient and surrogate are asked what they know about the illness, including prognosis. Any misunderstandings or gaps are addressed, and emotions are attended to throughout. The clinician then explores the patient's goals and values and structures an advance care plan that helps meet those goals. Specific situations are discussed as needed, and the clinician offers recommendations based on the patient values. The final plan includes attention to practical details to ensure it will work. It also includes discussion of future decision making, with attention to uncertainty and leeway in decision-making and the need to readdress over time.

SUMMARY RECOMMENDATIONS

- Advance care planning should be discussed with all patients with life-threatening illness, but more urgently in those at risk for having an unwanted decision-maker, such as those not in a traditional marriage
- The clinician should be aware of cultural, religious, and spiritual norms but not assume that a particular patient follows those norms.
- The topic of advance care planning should be introduced by normalizing or by referencing the patient's illness.
- Advance care planning should be thought of as a health behavior with stages of change.
- The surrogate decision-maker should be involved in discussions on advance care planning.
- The clinician should discuss prognosis with those who want to know.
- The clinician should notice and respond to emotions.
- The discussion should elicit goals and values.
- The clinician should offer recommendations and form an advance care plan based on patient goals and values.
- Practicalities such as medication availability should be considered as part of the advance care plan.
- Specifically discuss uncertainty and leeway in decision-making.
- The discussion should be documented and readdressed periodically.

REFERENCES

1. Hammes BJ, Rooney BL, Gundrum JD. A comparative, retrospective, observational study of the prevalence, availability, and specificity of advance care plans in a county that implemented an advance care planning microsystem. *J Am Geriatr Soc.* 2010;58(7):1249–1255.
2. Detering KM, Hancock AD, Reade MC, et al. The impact of advance care planning on end of life care in elderly patients: randomized controlled trial. *BMJ.* 2010;340:c1345.
3. Von Gunten CF, Ferris FD, Emanuel LL. Ensuring competency in end-of-life care: communication and relational skills. *JAMA.* 2000;284(23):3051–3057.
4. Baile WF, Buckman R, Lenzi R, et al. SPIKES: a six step protocol for delivering bad news—application to the patient with cancer. *Oncologist.* 2000;5(4):302–311.
5. Stages of Planning. *Respecting Choices.* 2011. Updated http://www.respectingchoices.org/faqs/stages_of_planning; Accessed October 1, 2012.
6. Kahana B, Dan A, Kahana E, et al. The personal and social context of planning for end-of-life care. *J Am Geriatr Soc.* 2004;52(7):1163–1167.
7. Dow LA, Matsuyama RK, Ramakrishnan V, et al. Paradoxes in advance care planning: the complex relationship of oncology patients, their physicians, and advance medical directives. *J Clin Oncol.* 2009;28(2):299–304.
8. Reilly BM, Magnussen CR, Ross J, et al. Can we talk? Inpatient discussions about advance directives in a community hospital—attending physicians' attitudes, their inpatients' wishes, and reported experience. *Arch Intern Med.* 1994;154(20):2299–2308.
9. Clark MA, Boehmer U, Rogers ML, et al. Planning for future care needs: experiences of unmarried heterosexual and sexual minority women. *Women Health.* 2010;50(7):599–617.
10. Johnston SC, Pfeifer MP, McNutt R. The discussion about advance directives: patient and physician opinions regarding when and how it should be conducted. End of Life Study Group. *Arch Intern Med.* 1995;155(10):1025–1030.
11. Pfeifer MP, Mitchell CK, Chamberlain L. The value of disease severity in predicting patient readiness to address end-of-life issues. *Arch Intern Med.* 2003;163(5):609–612.
12. Kelley AS, Wenger NS, Sarkisian CA. Opiniones: end-of-life care preferences and planning of older Latinos. *J Am Geriatr Soc.* 2010;58(6):1109–1116.
13. Kelley AS, Ettner SL, Morrison RS, et al. Determinants of medical expenditures in the last 6 months of life. *Ann Intern Med.* 2011;154(4):235–242.
14. Sudore RL, Schickedanz AD, Landefeld CS, et al. Engagement in multiple steps of the advance care planning process: a descriptive study of diverse older adults. *J Am Geriatr Soc.* 2008;56(6):1006–1013.
15. Rao AS, Dephande OM, Jamoona C, et al. Elderly Indo-Caribbean Hindus and end-of-life care: a community-based exploratory study. *J Am Geriatr Soc.* 2008;56(6):1129–1133.
16. Smith AK, McCarthy EP, Paulk E, et al. Racial and ethnic differences in advance care planning among patients with cancer: impact of terminal illness acknowledgment, religiousness, and treatment preferences. *J Clin Oncol.* 2008;26(25):4131–4137.
17. Wallace MP, Weiner JS, et al. Physician cultural sensitivity in African American advance care planning: a pilot study. *J Palliat Med.* 2007;10(3):721–727.
18. Johnson KS, Elbert-Avila KI, Tulsky JA. The influence of spiritual beliefs and practices on the treatment preferences of African-Americans: a review of the literature. *J Am Geriatr Soc.* 2005;53(4):711–719.
19. Phelps AC, Maciejewski PK, Nilsson M, et al. Religious coping and use of intensive life-prolonging care near death in patients with advance cancer. *JAMA.* 2009;301(11):1140–1147.
20. Balboni TA, Vanderwerker LC, Block SD, et al. Religiousness and spiritual support among advanced cancer patients and associations with end-of-life treatment preferences and quality of life. *J Clin Oncol.* 2007;25(5):555–560.
21. Allen RS, Allen JY, Hilgeman MM, et al. End-of-life decision-making, decisional conflict, and enhanced information: race effects. *J Am Geriatr Soc.* 2008;56(10):1904–1909.
22. Volandes AE, Lehmann LS, Cook ES, et al. Using video images of dementia in advance care planning. *Arch Intern Med.* 2007;167(8):828–833.
23. Yardley SJ, Walshe CE, Parr A. Improving training in spiritual care: a qualitative study exploring patient perceptions of professional educational requirements. *Palliat Med.* 2009;23(7):601–607.
24. Alano GJ, Pekmezaris R, Tai JY, et al. Factors influencing older adults to complete advance directives. *Palliat Support Care.* 2010;8(3):267–275.
25. Gordon NP, Shade SB. Advance directives are more likely among seniors asked about end-of-life care preferences. *Arch Intern Med.* 1999;159(7):701–704.
26. Fried TR, Bullock K, Iannone L, et al. Understanding advance care planning as a process of health behavior change. *J Am Geriatr Soc.* 2009;57(9):1547–1555.
27. Fried TR, Redding CA, Robbins ML, et al. Stages of change for the component behaviors of advance care planning. *J Am Geriatr Soc.* 2010;58(12):2329–2336.

28. Sudore RL, Fried TR. Redefining the "planning" in advance care planning: preparing for end-of-life decision-making. *Ann Intern Med.* 2010;153(4):256–261.

29. Parks SM, Winter L, Santana AJ, et al. Family factors in end-of-lie decision-making: family conflict and proxy relationship. *J Palliat Med.* 2011;14(2):179–184.

30. Dizon DS, Gass JS, Bandera C, et al. Does one person provide it all? Primary support and advanced care planning for women with cancer. *J Clin Oncol.* 2007;25(11):1412–1416.

31. Hines SC, Glover JJ, Holley JL, et al. Dialysis patients' preferences for family-based advance care planning. *Ann Intern Med.* 1999;130(10):825–828.

32. Clayton JM, Butow PN, Tattersall MH. When and how to initiate discussion about prognosis and end-of-life issues with terminally ill patients. *J Pain Symptom Manage.* 2005;30(2):132–144.

33. Murphy DJ, Burrows D, Santilli S, et al. The influence of probability of survival on patients' preferences regarding cardiopulmonary resuscitation. *N Engl J Med.* 1994;330(8):545–549.

34. Weeks JC, Cook EF, O'Day SJ, et al. Relationship between cancer patients' predictions of prognosis and their treatment preferences. *JAMA.* 1998;279(2):1709–1714.

35. Tulsky JA. Beyond advance directives: importance of communication skills at the end of life. *JAMA.* 2005;294(3):359–365.

36. Lynn J, Goldstein NE. Advance care planning for fatal chronic illness: avoiding commonplace errors and unwanted suffering. *Ann Intern Med.* 2003;138(10):812–818.

37. Rodriguez KL, Young AJ. Patients' and healthcare providers' understanding of life-sustaining treatment: are perceptions of goals shared or divergent. *Soc Sci Med.* 2006;62(1):125–133.

38. El-Jawahri A, Podgurski LM, Eichler AF, et al. Use of video to facilitate end-of-life discussion with patients with cancer: a randomized controlled trial. *J Clin Oncol.* 2010;28(2):305–310.

39. Volandes AE, Paasche-Orlow MK, Barry MJ, et al. Video decision support tool for advance care planning in dementia: a randomized controlled trial. *BMJ.* 2009;338:b1964.

40. Quill TE, Brody H. Physician recommendations and patient autonomy: finding a balance between physician power and patient choice. *Ann Intern Med.* 1996;125(9):763–769.

41. Johnson SK, Bautista CA, Hong SY, et al. An empirical study of surrogates' preferred level of control over value-laden life support decisions in intensive care units. *Am J Respir Crit Care Med.* 2011;183(7):915–921.

42. Deep KS, Griffith CH, Wilson JF. Communication and decision making about life-sustaining treatment: examining the experiences of resident physicians and seriously ill hospitalized patients. *J Gen Intern Med.* 2008;23(11):1877–1882.

43. Nakamura S, Kuzuya M, Funaki Y, et al. Factors influencing death at home in terminally ill cancer patients. *Geriatr Gerontol Int.* 2010;10(2):154–160.

44. Voogt E, van der Heide A, Rietjens JA, et al. Attitudes of patients with incurable cancer toward medical treatments in the last phase of life. *J Clin Oncol.* 2005;23(9):2012–2019.

45. Dizon DS, Schutzer ME, Politi MC, et al. Advance care planning decisions of women with cancer: provider recognition and stability of choices. *J Psychosoc Oncol.* 2009;27(4):38–395.

What Is the Evidence That Advance Care Plans Change Patient Outcomes?

GORDON WOOD AND ROBERT M. ARNOLD

INTRODUCTION AND SCOPE OF THE PROBLEM

As outlined in Chapter 45, much of the original research about advance care planning focused on the advance directive. Early studies focused on increasing the advance directive completion rate, and those were successful.[1] From 1996 to 2004, the nursing home advance directive completion rates rose from 53% to 70%.[2] Other studies focused on improving surrogate and physician understanding of patient wishes. They used techniques such as structured interviews, scenario-based advance directives, motivational counseling, and provider cues to discuss advance care planning. Although these studies showed improved surrogate–patient and provider–patient concordance regarding patient wishes,[3-6] improving patient outcomes was more difficult.[7] Advance directives alone do not seem to have an impact on care because of both conceptual (difficulty predicting future wishes, changing wishes, ability to adapt to previously undesired health states) and practical (discussions not held or not documented, documents not transferred between sites or not followed) issues.

Recently, however, a body of literature has emerged showing positive outcomes of advance care planning.[8] Two possible reasons exist for these positive outcomes. First, the more recent articles have considered a broader range of outcomes of advance care planning, looking at how this process influences surrogate decision making and caregiver burden.[9]

A second reason is that recent studies have moved away from looking at the effects of written advanced directives and have begun examining the results of intensive interventions based on more comprehensive advance care plans. These interventions involve training health care providers how to discuss advance care planning, institutionalizing patient-centered discussions of goals and values with both patients and surrogates, and operationalizing how these values translate into clinical decisions. They also involve system change to make sure these plans can be implemented.

This chapter reviews this literature and concludes with a discussion of the barriers that still exist to implementing these intensive interventions on a population level and how these barriers might be overcome. Table 47-1 summarizes some of the key studies showing positive patient outcomes with advance care planning.

BROADER OBJECTIVES FOR ADVANCE CARE PLANNING

Part of the problem with the early studies of advance directives is that they focused on the health care provider point of view and thus looked primarily at the impact of advance care planning on intensity of therapy at the end of life. More recent studies have begun to look at advance care planning from the patient and family point of view and examine a broader range of outcomes.

First, studies have looked at how advance care planning influences surrogates' experience of end-of-life communication. For example, in one randomized controlled trial, the group who had undergone three 60- to 90-minute advance care planning sessions reported less conflict and overall better quality of communication than the control group, who participated in discussions about different topics.[10]

Second, studies have looked at caregiver burden. Anecdotally, many providers see the major benefit of advance care planning in how it informs family meetings with surrogates when a patient is at the end of life. Often, being able to refer to a conversation or a document about end-of-life wishes allows families to make the difficult decisions to change to comfort-focused care because they believe it is in keeping with the patient's wishes. Many families state that they could not have made such a decision without knowledge of these wishes.[11] A recent systematic review found that making treatment decisions is associated with a high degree of caregiver burden.[12] In the majority of the included studies, knowing the patient's wishes lessened this burden. Interestingly, conflict between what the surrogate believes is best for the patient and the patient's wishes is associated with higher emotional burden.[12]

Third, studies have looked at "dying in place." Dying in the patient's site of choice is considered a quality measure of end-of-life care because most patients prefer dying at home, avoiding last minute transfers to the hospital.[13] Advance care planning can help achieve this for patients. For example, a study of 539 patients found that having a living will decreased

TABLE 47-1. Selected Studies Showing Positive Patient Outcomes From Advance Care Planning

SOURCE	DESIGN	SETTING	PARTICIPANTS	INTERVENTION	RESULTS
Degenholtz,[14] 2004	Secondary data analysis of a national longitudinal study	Community and nursing home	539 proxies for patients who died at an age >70	N/A	Having a living will decreased the probability of dying in the hospital from 0.65 to 0.52 for patients living in the community and from 0.35 to 0.13 for patients living in a nursing home.
Ratner,[15] 2001	Case series	Urban home health agency	84 adult patients receiving home care other than hospice	Structured social work visits to discuss end-of-life issues and communication of results to nurses and physicians	99% participated in ACP. Of the 64% who had a preference for site of terminal care, 82% wanted it to be at home. 75% of deaths occurred at home or in a hospice residence.
Lyon,[10] 2009	Randomized, controlled trial	2 hospital-based outpatient clinics	38 adolescents with HIV and their caregivers	Three 60- to 90-minute ACP sessions by trained interviewer using Lyon Advance Care Planning Survey, Respecting Choices and Five Wishes	Intervention group had higher congruence of wishes, decreased conflict and enhanced perceived quality of communication.
Hammes,[16] 2010	Retrospective chart review	All health care organizations in LaCrosse, Wisconsin	540 adults who died in 1995-1996 and 400 adults who died in 2007-2008	Systematic ACP approach using Respecting Choices since 1993 with continuous quality improvement	At the latter date, 90% had an advance directive, 99.4% of those were in the chart, and care was concordant in 99.5%.
Detering,[17] 2010	Randomized, controlled trial	University hospital in Melbourne, Australia	309 inpatients age ≥80 or more	Facilitated ACP session by a nurse or allied health worker using Respecting Choices model	Of the 56 who died, those in the intervention group were more likely to have wishes known and followed (25/29 vs. 8/27).
Molloy,[18] 2000	Randomized, controlled trial	6 nursing homes in Ontario, Canada	1292 nursing home residents	Staff, patient, family education and facilitated ACP discussions by trained nurses	Intervention nursing homes had lower average total cost per patient ($3490 vs. $5239 CAN) and fewer hospitalizations per resident (0.27 vs. 0.48).
Morrison,[19] 2005	Controlled clinical trial	New York City nursing home	139 newly admitted patients	Ongoing ACP discussions by trained social workers, review of goals of care at team meetings, flagging of advance directives on patients' charts, feedback to health care providers regarding congruence of care with wishes	Intervention residents more likely to have preferences documented in the chart compared to usual care (e.g., 40% vs. 20% for CPR) and less likely to receive discordant care (5% vs. 18%).
Hanson,[20] 1999	Cross sectional interviews	Decedents in 12 North Carolina counties identified by death certificates	461 informants and 240 treating physicians	N/A	78.2% of informants recalled discussing treatment options with physicians. 72% of these were a month or more before death. Having a living will was an independent predictor of less aggressive end-of-life care.
Wright,[21] 2008	Prospective longitudinal cohort study	7 different outpatient cancer clinics	638 adult patients with advanced cancer and a caregiver	N/A	37% had end-of-life discussions. These were not associated with worse depression, anxiety, or PTSD but were associated with less aggressive care and earlier hospice referral. Aggressive care was associated with worse caregiver bereavement outcomes.
Hickman[23] 2009	Cross-sectional interview and chart review	All hospice programs in Wisconsin, Oregon, and West Virginia	71 hospice staff member and 373 chart reviews.	N/A	Majority (97%) found the POLST useful in preventing unwanted resuscitations (97%). Treatment preferences respected in 98%.
Silveira,[37] 2010	Retrospective review of longitudinal survey	Nationally representative cohort	3746 patients 60 or older who died between 2000 and 2006	N/A	Of those who needed decision-making, 68% had an advance directive. Wishes on the advance directive either for aggressive or limited care were strongly associated with care received.

ACP, Advance care planning; *CPR,* cardiopulmonary resuscitation; *POLST,* Physician Orders for Life Sustaining Treatment; *PTSD,* posttraumatic stress disorder.

the chance of dying in the hospital for nursing home resident and community-dwelling patients.[14] Similarly, 84 patients who received a social work visit to complete advance care planning had a higher likelihood of dying at home, in keeping with their preferences.[15]

SPECIFIC ADVANCE CARE PLANNING INTERVENTIONS WITH POSITIVE OUTCOMES

In addition to the studies discussed earlier showing positive outcomes from the patient and family point of view, a growing number of intensive advance care planning interventions show positive clinical outcomes across a variety of clinical sites.

The classic example of this is the LaCrosse, Wisconsin experience, where a community-wide intervention called Respecting Choices produced remarkable outcomes. This methodology stresses a patient-centered discussion with the surrogate present and system-wide physician education. With this approach, almost 100% of the population had an advance directive in the medical record and received care in keeping with preferences. The majority of the advance care plans for these patients specifically addressed their wishes regarding cardiopulmonary resuscitation (CPR) and hospitalization.[16] This same methodology was applied in Melbourne, Australia in a randomized, controlled fashion for 309 patients admitted to the hospital. Of patients who died, 86% of those in the intervention arm had wishes that were known and followed, compared to 30% in the usual care arm. Intervention families had less stress, anxiety, and depression and higher satisfaction.[17]

A similar comprehensive Canadian nursing home-based program called "Let Me Decide" had comparable results. In a randomized, controlled trial of 1292 patients, patients in the intervention arm had fewer hospitalizations and less resource use, despite a similar number of deaths and similar satisfaction.[18] Similar results have been found in nursing homes in New York using a slightly different but still comprehensive social worker intervention.[19]

Comprehensive advance care planning also improves outcomes in community-based primary care practices. A survey of 165 surrogates for deceased patients found that 78% remembered discussing treatment options with the physician, mostly a month before the death, suggesting the kind of ongoing, patient-centered discussions advocated in the Respecting Choice program. Many of the discussions were documented in a living will, and having a living will was associated with less aggressive treatment before death. Physicians found that advance care planning and good relationships were the key factors in good decision making at the end of life.[20]

Advance care planning also has been found to improve care among patients very close to death. In a prospective cohort study of 332 terminally ill patients with cancer who died a median of 4 months after the start of study, patient recollection of having end-of-life discussions with their physician was associated with less aggressive end-of-life care, earlier hospice referral, better perceived quality of life near death, and better bereavement outcomes for their surrogates.[21] The Physician Orders for Life Sustaining Treatment (POLST) can be particularly helpful at translating the results of advance care planning discussions for those near the end of life into physician orders.[22] In one hospice setting, none of the patients with a POLST received unwanted intubation, care in an intensive care unit, or feeding tubes.[23]

BARRIERS TO POPULATION-LEVEL IMPROVEMENTS

Given the impressive results in specific populations noted earlier, it may seem surprising how infrequently population-level interventions have been implemented. Unfortunately, there are numerous provider, system, patient, and media barriers (summarized along with possible solutions in Table 47-2) that must

---

TABLE 47-2. Barriers to Advance Care Planning Changing Patient Outcomes

BARRIER	POTENTIAL SOLUTION
Provider	
Lack of training	Communication skills training sessions
Fear of doing harm by discussing dying	Education about data demonstrating lack of harm
System	
Lack of time, lack of reimbursement for time spent	Change in reimbursement structure to support dedicated advance care planning visits
Lack of systematic reminder and lack of transfer of wishes across settings	Electronic medical record modifications to support reminders and clearly display results of advance care planning discussions
Patient	
Not wanting to discuss; not perceiving importance; worry about burdening family; perceived lack of physician time; uncertain which physician to talk to; lacking a primary care physician; perceived unwillingness of physician to talk about the topic; and a lack of knowledge about the interventions and advance care planning as a whole	Education of clinicians regarding how to uncover and address these barriers Media campaigns Systems changes to ensure each patient sees a primary care physician
Media	
Charged and inaccurate descriptions of advance care planning	Coordinated, accurate media campaign

be overcome before the lessons from these studies can be applied to society in general.

Providers cite a lack of training in how to hold these conversations as one of their major barriers.[24,25] Fortunately, it is becoming increasingly clear that these skills are teachable[26] and that the teaching can influence behaviors. For example, residents who receive feedback about how they perform advance care planning discussions were more likely to engage in these discussions in the future.[27] Another barrier cited by providers as a reason not to talk about advance care planning is their concern that bringing up this difficult subject will cause patients emotional distress or result in their losing hope. Data suggest that these concerns are unfounded. Patients who engage in end-of-life discussions do not have worse physical or psychological outcomes.[21] In one study of patients who had undergone stem cell transplant, the advance care planning group had a lower mortality rate.[28] Advance care planning also does not seem to extinguish hope or cause psychological distress.[21] In a study of patients with end-stage renal disease, advance care planning actually enhanced rather than diminished patients' sense of hope.[29]

System barriers also may impede the dissemination of advance care planning. Physicians note the lack of time and reimbursement for these time-intensive conversations.[24,30] Busy clinicians also may forget to initiate the conversations.[24] Clinician reminders plus patient mailings have been shown to increase advance directive completion rates.[31] In addition, the lack of a unified electronic medical record can make communication of advance care plans difficult.

Patients also cite barriers, some of which mirror physician concerns. Some patients simply do not want to discuss the topic, preferring a wait-and-see approach. Others perceive advance care planning as irrelevant, state they are too busy, or worry about the effect of the conversation on their family. In addition, patients may want their physician to initiate the discussion but may not have a primary care physician or know with which of their many doctors they should have this discussion. Alternatively, they may simply not know about advance care planning, what end-of-life options exist, and what type of care they would want.[32–34]

Finally, the media can present barriers by inappropriately characterizing the process of advance care planning using inaccurate or charged language.[35] On the other hand, positive exposure to media campaigns has been associated with increased rates of advance directive completion.[36]

To overcome these barriers and see population-level changes similar to those seen with the studies discussed earlier, system-wide change is needed. Clinicians need to be trained in how to have these discussions. Decision aids and videos should be widely available and accessible, as should better, standardized, culturally sensitive, literacy-appropriate advance directives. Health care systems should implement automated reminders and could consider more active tracking of advance care planning as a quality measure. The electronic medical record must also be improved so that the results of these discussions are readily available across sites. The media can play a positive role in stimulating this process. Finally, a reimbursement structure is needed that allows time for discussion of advanced care planning by trained physician or nonphysician personnel.

KEY MESSAGES TO PATIENTS AND FAMILIES

Patients and families should understand that advance care planning, when performed properly within an appropriate system, can help them receive the care they want at the end of their lives. It can also decrease burden on their family, improve communication between their family and their clinicians, and make it more likely they will die in their site of choice.

CONCLUSION AND SUMMARY

Although the early data that focused on advance directives generally failed to show any impact on patient outcomes, recent data have been more positive. Advance care planning has been associated with decreased caregiver burden, improved family perceptions of communication, and dying in the preferred place. In specific settings in which a comprehensive system-wide intervention is enacted, including trained facilitators who carry out patient-centered discussions focused on values, advance care planning has also been shown to ensure that care received is concordant with patient preferences. Although numerous barriers exist to translating these smaller experiences into population-wide changes in end-of-life care, these barriers are not insurmountable. As a positive sign that a more comprehensive view of advance care planning is taking hold, a 2010 study reversed the findings of multiple previous studies and found that advance directives were associated with care received at the end of life.[37] Hopefully, system change can continue, these results can be replicated, and patients throughout the country can take comfort in knowing that they will not receive care at the end of life that does not match their preferences.

SUMMARY RECOMMENDATIONS

- Clinicians should engage in advance care planning with their patients because it can decrease caregiver burden, increase the chance of dying in the preferred place, and improve surrogate perception of communication at the end of life.
- Personal or system-wide training in advance care planning should be initiated because a coordinated system enacted by trained facilitators has been associated with care in keeping with preferences, reduced costs, and improved bereavement outcomes.
- Clinicians should be aware of common provider, patient, system, and media barriers to engaging in advance care planning.

REFERENCES

1. Patel RV, Sinuff T, Cook DJ. Influencing advance directive completion rates in non-terminally ill patients: a systematic review. *J Crit Care.* 2004;19(1):1–9.
2. Resnick HE, Schuur JD, Heineman J, et al. Advance directives in nursing home residents aged > or = 65 years: United Sates 2004. *Am J Hosp Palliat Care.* 2009;25(6):476–482.
3. Kirchoff KT, Hammes BJ, Kehl KA, et al. Effect of a disease-specific planning intervention on surrogate understanding of patient goals for future medical treatment. *J Am Geriatr Soc.* 2010;58(7):1233–1240.
4. Coppola KM, Ditto PH, Danks JH, et al. Accuracy of primary care and hospital-based physicians' predictions of elderly outpatients' treatment preferences with and without advance directives. *Arch Intern Med.* 2001;161(3):431–440.
5. Schwarz CE, Wheeler HB, Hammes B, et al. Early intervention in planning end-of-life care with ambulatory geriatric patients: results of a pilot trial. *Arch Intern Med.* 2002;162(14): 1611–1618.
6. Pearlman RA, Sarks H, Cain KC, et al. Improvements in advance care planning in the veterans affairs system: results of a multifaceted intervention. *Arch Intern Med.* 2005;165(6):667–674.
7. Hanson LC, Tulsky JA, Danis M. Can clinical interventions change care at the end of life? *Ann Intern Med.* 1997;126(5): 381–388.
8. Lorenz KA, Lynn J, Dy SM, et al. Evidence for improving palliative care at the end of life: a systematic review. *Ann Intern Med.* 2008;148(2):147–159.
9. Kolarik RS, Arnold RM, Fischer GS, et al. Objectives for advance care planning. *J Palliat Med.* 2002;5(5):697–704.
10. Lyon ME, Garvey PA, McCarter R, et al. Who will speak for me? Improving end-of-life decision-making for adolescents with HIV and their families. *Pediatrics.* 2009;123(2):e199–e206.
11. Fried TR, O'Leary JR. Using the experiences of bereaved caregivers to inform patient- and caregiver-centered advance care planning. *J Gen Intern Med.* 2008;23(10):1602–1607.
12. Wendler D, Rid A. Systematic review: the effect of surrogates of making treatment decisions for others. *Ann Intern Med.* 2011;154(5):336–346.
13. Tang ST. When death is imminent: where terminally ill patients with cancer prefer to die and why. *Cancer Nurs.* 2003;26(3):245–251.
14. Degenholtz HB, Rhee Y, Arnold RM. Brief communication: the relationship between having a living will and dying in place. *Ann Intern Med.* 2004;141(2):113–117.
15. Ratner E, Norlander L, McSteen K. Death at home following a targeted advance-care planning process at home: the kitchen table discussion. *J Am Geriatr Soc.* 2001;49(6):778–781.
16. Hammes BJ, Rooney BL, Gundrum JD. A comparative, retrospective, observational study of the prevalence, availability, and specificity of advance care plans in a county that implemented an advance care planning microsystem. *J Am Geriatr Soc.* 2010;58(7):1249–1255.
17. Detering KM, Hancock AD, Reade MC, et al. The impact of advance care planning on end of life care in elderly patients: randomized controlled trial. *BMJ.* 2010;340:c1345.
18. Molloy DW, Guyatt GH, Russon R, et al. Systematic implementation of an advance directive program in nursing homes: a randomized controlled trial. *JAMA.* 2000;283(11):1437–1444.
19. Morrison RS, Chichin E, Carter J, et al. The effect of a social work intervention to enhance advance care planning documentation in the nursing home. *J Am Geriatr Soc.* 2005;53(2):290–294.
20. Hanson LC, Earp JA, Garrett J, et al. Community physicians who provide terminal care. *Arch Intern Med.* 1999;159(10):1133–1138.
21. Wright AA, Zhang B, Ray A, et al. Associations between end-of-life discussions, patient mental health, medical care near death, and caregiver bereavement adjustment. *JAMA.* 2008;300(14):1665–1673.
22. Schmidt TA, Hickman SE, Tolle SW, et al. The physician orders for life-sustaining treatment program: Oregon emergency medical technicians' practical experiences and attitudes. *J Am Geriatr Soc.* 2004;52(9):1430–1434.
23. Hickman SE, Nelson CA, Moss AH, et al. Use of the physician orders for life-sustaining treatment (POLST) paradigm program in the hospice setting. *J Palliat Med.* 2009;12(2):133–141.
24. Tung EE, North F. Advance care planning in the primary care setting: a comparison of attending staff and resident barriers. *Am J Hosp Palliat Care.* 2010;26(6):456–463.
25. Selman L, Harding R, Beynon T, et al. Improving end-of-life care for patients with chronic heart failure: "let's hope it'll get better, when I know in my heart of hearts it won't". *Heart.* 2007;93(8):963–967 9.
26. Alexander SC, Keitz SA, Sloane R, et al. A controlled trial of a short course to improve residents' communication with patients at the end of life. *Acad Med.* 2006;81(11):1008–1012.
27. Smith AK, Ries AP, Zhang G, et al. Resident approaches to advance care planning on the day of hospital admission. *Arch Intern Med.* 2006;166(15):1597–1602.
28. Ganti AK, Lee SJ, Vose JM, et al. Outcomes after hematopoietic stem-cell transplantation for hematologic malignancies in patients with or without advance care planning. *J Clin Oncol.* 2007;25(35):5643–5648.
29. Davison SN, Simpson C. Hope and advance care planning in patients with end-stage renal disease: qualitative interview study. *BMJ.* 2006 Oct 28;333(7574):886.
30. Emanuel L. Structured advance planning. Is it finally time for physician action and reimbursement. *JAMA.* 1995;275(6):598.
31. Heiman H, Bates DW, Fairchild D, et al. Improving completion of advance directives in the primary care setting: a randomized controlled trial. *Am J Med.* 2004;117(5):318–324.
32. Knauft E, Nielsen EL, Engelberg RA, et al. Barriers and facilitators to end-of-life care communication for patients with COPD. *Chest.* 2005;127(6):2188–2196.
33. Schickedanz AD, Schillinger D, Landefeld CS, et al. A clinical framework for improving the advance care planning process: start with the patients' self-identified barriers. *J Am Geriatr Soc.* 2009;57(1):31–39.
34. Morrison RS, Meier DE. High rates of advance care planning in New York City's elderly population. *Arch Intern Med.* 2004;164(22):2421–2426.
35. Racine E, Amaram R, Seidler M, et al. Media coverage of the persistent vegetative state and end-of-life decision-making. *Neurology.* 2008;71(13):1027–1032.
36. Alano GJ, Pekmezaris R, Tai JY, et al. Factors influencing older adults to complete advance directives. *Palliat Support Care.* 2010;8(3):267–275.
37. Silveira MJ, KIM SYH, Langa KM. Advance directives and outcomes of surrogate decision making before death. *N Engl J Med.* 2010;362(13):1211–1218.

DISEASE-SPECIFIC TOPICS

CANCER

Chapter 48

What Is the Role for Palliative Care in Patients With Advanced Cancer?

KAVITHA J. RAMCHANDRAN AND JAMIE H. VON ROENN

INTRODUCTION AND SCOPE OF THE PROBLEM
SCREENING FOR PALLIATIVE CARE
SUMMARY OF EVIDENCE REGARDING TREATMENT
  RECOMMENDATIONS
KEY MESSAGES TO PATIENTS AND FAMILIES
CONCLUSION AND SUMMARY

Palliative care is given throughout a patient's experience with cancer. It should begin at diagnosis and continue through treatment, follow-up care, and the end of life.

The National Cancer Institute Fact Sheet
on Palliative Care

INTRODUCTION AND SCOPE OF THE PROBLEM

The World Health Organization (WHO) defines palliative care as "an approach that improves the quality of life of patients and their families facing the problems associated with life-threatening illness, through the prevention and relief of suffering by means of early identification and impeccable assessment and treatment of pain and other problems, physical, psychosocial and spiritual ... [palliative care] is applicable early in the course of illness, in conjunction with other therapies that are intended to prolong life ...."[1]

Palliative care is based on an interdisciplinary team approach (nursing, social work, physician, chaplaincy) with the goal of caring for the patient unit (patient, family, and caregivers) throughout the course of advanced illness from diagnosis to death or cure. As the burden of cancer increases, in terms of both numbers (WHO estimates 15 million cancer cases by 2020) and suffering, it is clear that palliative care will be a much needed component of cancer care for all patients.[2]

Unfortunately, although rapid growth has occurred in the number of hospitals with palliative care services, access in the United States is still limited. A report by the Center to Advance Palliative Care (CAPC) found that among hospitals in the United States with 50 or more beds, approximately 60% had a palliative care service. In larger hospitals (>300 beds) the prevalence improves to 80%.[3] The current state of integration of palliative care into U.S. cancer centers is also variable. A recent study published in the *Journal of the American Medical Association* evaluated the integration of palliative care into U.S. cancer centers. The authors found that palliative care was more likely to be present in National Cancer Institute (NCI)-designated cancer centers and the majority of palliative care services were inpatient based. Only 59% of NCI-designated cancer centers and 22% of non–NCI-designated cancer centers had an outpatient palliative care clinic or team. Critical endeavors such as research programs, palliative care fellowships, and mandatory palliative care training for oncologists are even more limited.[4] Despite the variability in palliative care services, it is clear that palliative care should be a component of cancer care for all patients. This chapter provides guidance on how best to integrate oncological therapy with palliative care.

SCREENING FOR PALLIATIVE CARE

Palliative care is appropriate for patients in four key areas. Optimal care for these patients would be concurrent palliative care with oncological care from the time of initial cancer diagnosis.

1. Advanced disease with a prognosis less than 1 year
2. Significant symptom burden from disease or from treatment
3. Significant social or psychological distress
4. Eastern Cooperative Oncology Group (ECOG) performance status of 3 or above (see Chapter 50)

For patients who may not meet initial screening criteria, frequent palliative care screens for symptom burden, change in performance status, and change in disease trajectory or goals of care is appropriate. For example, the National Comprehensive Cancer Network (NCCN) Distress Thermometer is an effective, well-validated tool to evaluate for untreated distress—physical, social, or psychological.[5-9] The Distress Thermometer is a rapid use tool for patients to rate distress from 0 to 10 and then designate particular areas of concern (Figure 48-1). A recent study by Mitchel and colleagues found that these types of tools have a much higher negative predictive value (93.4%) than positive predictive value (34.2%) and may be better at excluding possible causes of depression but poor at confirming a diagnosis.[6] However, these test characteristics are likely appropriate for

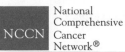

NCCN Guidelines™ Version 2.2012
Distress Management

National
Comprehensive
Cancer
Network®

SCREENING TOOLS FOR MEASURING DISTRESS

Instructions: First please circle the number (0-10) that best describes how much distress you have been experiencing in the past week including today.

Extreme distress — 10

9

8

7

6

5

4

3

2

1

No distress — 0

Second, please indicate if any of the following has been a problem for you in the past week including today. Be sure to check YES or NO for each.

YES NO Practical Problems
☐ ☐ Child care
☐ ☐ Housing
☐ ☐ Insurance/financial
☐ ☐ Transportation
☐ ☐ Work/school
☐ ☐ Treatment decisions

Family Problems
☐ ☐ Dealing with children
☐ ☐ Dealing with partner
☐ ☐ Ability to have children
☐ ☐ Family health issues

Emotional Problems
☐ ☐ Depression
☐ ☐ Fears
☐ ☐ Nervousness
☐ ☐ Sadness
☐ ☐ Worry
☐ ☐ Loss of interest in usual activities

☐ ☐ **Spiritual/religious concerns**

Other Problems: _____

YES NO Physical Problems
☐ ☐ Appearance
☐ ☐ Bathing/dressing
☐ ☐ Breathing
☐ ☐ Changes in urination
☐ ☐ Constipation
☐ ☐ Diarrhea
☐ ☐ Eating
☐ ☐ Fatigue
☐ ☐ Feeling swollen
☐ ☐ Fevers
☐ ☐ Getting around
☐ ☐ Indigestion
☐ ☐ Memory/concentration
☐ ☐ Mouth sores
☐ ☐ Nausea
☐ ☐ Nose dry/congested
☐ ☐ Pain
☐ ☐ Sexual
☐ ☐ Skin dry/itchy
☐ ☐ Sleep
☐ ☐ Tingling in hands/feet

FIGURE 48-1. National Comprehensive Cancer Network Guidelines for Distress Management. *(Reproduced with permission from the NCCN Clinical Practice Guidelines in Oncology [NCCN Guideline] for Distress Management V.2.2012. © 2012. © 2010 National Comprehensive Cancer Network, Inc. All rights reserved. The NCCN Guidelines™ and illustrations herein may not be reproduced in any form, for any purpose, without the express written permission of the NCCN. To view the most recent and complete version of the NCCN Guidelines, go online to NCCN.org. NATIONAL COMPREHENSIVE CANCER NETWORK®, NCCN®, NCCN GUIDELINES™, and all other NCCN Content are trademarks owned by the National Comprehensive Cancer Network, Inc.).*

an initial screen. Patients who screen positive would merit further evaluation by a palliative care consultation team to assess for symptoms of physical and psychological distress.

Certain physical symptoms may also merit palliative care referral. A recent retrospective Canadian study of more than 18,000 patients in the last 6 months of life found that symptoms such as pain, nausea, anxiety, and depression were relatively stable. Alternatively, symptoms such as dyspnea, drowsiness, decreased well-being, anorexia, and fatigue increased over the last month of life.[10] The hypothesis for this is that the former symptoms are often assessed and treated effectively by the primary oncologist. This is due to adequate training of oncologists in treating chemotherapy toxicities (e.g., nausea) and availability of effective prescription medications for these symptoms (e.g., morphine for pain). However, the latter symptoms, which include fatigue, decreased overall well-being, and anorexia, often require a multidisciplinary approach to care, and available prescription

medications are less effective. These symptoms would best be served by a team approach and palliative care. Finally, when symptoms are poorly controlled or refractory to front-line medications (e.g., refractory nausea and vomiting, bowel obstruction), a palliative care team can be beneficial.

Certain symptoms and clinical findings portend a poor prognosis. The National Hospice Organization looked at five symptoms and performance status and found that a KPS of less than 50 and the presence of anorexia, weight loss, dysphagia, dry mouth, and dyspnea predicted for a median survival of 6 weeks.[11] Other symptoms or signs of advanced disease include hypercalcemia, malignant effusions, spinal cord compression, brain metastases, and laboratory abnormalities, such as elevated bilirubin or decreased albumin levels.[12] These physical signs and symptoms of advanced disease not only require intensive monitoring and titration of medications but also require appropriate communication about their implication on a patient's prognosis. A palliative care team can be effective in helping both the patient and primary provider address these issues.

A change in performance status that is not considered to be reversible with anticancer therapy is another indicator for palliative care involvement. Both the Karnofsky Performance Status (KPS) scale and the ECOG Performance Status scale have been validated in patients with cancer to correlate with survival (described in Chapter 50). A KPS of 40 or an ECOG score of greater than 3 are associated with survival of 3 months or less.[11,13–17]

Finally, a change in treatment trajectory determined by the clinician or the patient may warrant palliative care involvement. Examples include toxicity from treatment (e.g., grade IV graft-versus-host disease in a patient who has received a bone marrow transplant), refractory disease (i.e., disease that is no longer treatment-sensitive), new significant comorbid illness (e.g., myocardial infarction, stroke), or a reluctance on the part of the patient to continue with anticancer therapy because of the burdens of treatment.

SUMMARY OF EVIDENCE REGARDING TREATMENT RECOMMENDATIONS

The impact of palliative care integration with cancer care has been studied in various settings. However, the now landmark trial published by Temel and colleagues[18] sets the benchmark with regard to the impact of a concurrent model of care integrating palliative care into standard oncological care. The study included 151 patients with stage IV lung cancer randomized to usual oncology care versus usual oncology care plus concurrent palliative care. Patients in the usual care arm were allowed to receive palliative care by a standard referral-based approach. The study found that patients in the concurrent care arm had a sustained improvement in symptoms, mood, end-of-life care, and survival (8.9 versus 11.6 months, $p = .02$). Other studies have shown a similar impact of an integrated care approach on quality of life, mood, symptom intensity, and improved quality of end-of-life care (Table 48-1).[19–24]

TABLE 48-1. Studies Evaluating the Impact of Palliative Care Integration Into Oncologic Care

STUDY	INTERVENTION	STUDY DESIGN	OUTCOMES
Follwell,[22] 2009	Oncology Palliative Care Clinic for Advanced Cancer, with regular symptom assessment by ESAS	Phase II prospective study 150 patients with metastatic cancer	Significant improvements in pain, fatigue, nausea, depression, anxiety, drowsiness, appetite, insomnia, and constipation ($p = .005$) and family satisfaction ($p = .0001$)
Bakitas,[28] 2009	Case management, educational approach with monthly shared medical appointments	RCT 322 patients with cancer (GI, GU, breast)	Higher QoL ($p = .02$), lower symptom intensity ($p = .06$), and depressed mood ($p = .02$), no change in hospital, ICU utilization, ED admissions
Temel,[18] 2010	Early concurrent palliative care for advanced lung cancer	RCT: Usual care vs. early palliative care 151 patients with advanced lung cancer (stage IIIB, IV)	Improve QoL ($p = .03$), mood ($p = .01$), less aggressive end-of life-care ($p = .05$), and longer survival ($p = .02$)
Casarett,[29] 2008	Telephone interview of caregivers of veterans who had received palliative care vs. those who had not during their last month of life	Retrospective study 524 caregivers	PC patients had higher scores in almost all domains—symptoms, care at the time of death, spiritual support, access to benefits and services
Strasser,[23] 2004	MD palliative care vs. pain and symptom management clinic for patients with advanced cancer	Case control Patients with advanced cancer 138 referred to MD palliative care clinic 77 referred to pain and symptom management clinic	MD palliative care group had improvements in pain, nausea, depression, anxiety, sleep, dyspnea, and well-being, but not in fatigue, anorexia, or drowsiness
Rabow,[30] 2004	Outpatient palliative care for patients with advanced disease (cancer and non–cancer-related diagnoses) compared to usual care	Case control Patients with advanced cancer, COPD, and CHF 50 intervention 40 control (usual care)	PC patients had less dyspnea ($p = .01$) and anxiety ($p = .05$) and improved sleep quality ($p = .05$) and spiritual well-being ($p = .007$), but no change in pain ($p = .41$), depression ($p = .28$), quality of life ($p = .43$), or satisfaction with care ($p = .26$).
Meyers[31] 2004	"Simultaneous Care" (SC): A home-based care program focused on symptoms and care-giving needs, compared to usual care (UC)	Case control Advanced cancer on phase I or II investigational therapies 44 patients in SC 20 patients in UC	The SC group improved compared to the UC group but did not reach a significant difference A statistically significant difference (increase) in referral to hospice was seen in the SC group ($p = .034$)

CHF, Congestive heart failure; *COPD,* chronic obstructive pulmonary disease; *ED,* emergency department; *ESAS,* Edmonton System Assessment System; *GI,* gastrointestinal; *GU,* genitourinary; *ICU,* intensive care unit; *MD,* multidisciplinary; *PC,* palliative care; *QoL,* quality of life; *RCT,* randomized, controlled trial; *SC,* simultaneous care; *UC,* usual care.

Policy and guidelines also support an integrated palliative care–oncology model. The American Society of Clinical Oncology's (ASCO's) vision of personalized medicine includes the specific biology of a disease and incorporation of evidence-based medicine. More importantly, however, it incorporates patient's preferences and goals to help direct discussion regarding anticancer and palliative care options. With this in mind, personalized medicine can be best achieved in collaboration with palliative medicine.[25] The NCCN, which publishes a widely recognized national set of guidelines, integrates palliative care into anticancer therapy.[12] A recent American Society of Clinical Oncology–European Society for Medical Oncology consensus statement on quality cancer care, included "pain management, supportive and palliative care" as one of their key goals.[26] Finally, the recently developed Quality Oncology Practice Initiatives, supported by ASCO, incorporates a wide array of palliative care measures as quality indicators, including impeccable symptom control, attention to emotional well-being, and quality of end-of-life care.[27]

It should be recognized that oncologists can provide some components of palliative care (e.g., antiemetics for nausea, opioids for pain control). However, key components to palliative care that span the psychological, social, and spiritual areas are best addressed with a palliative care multidisciplinary team approach. These include refractory physical symptoms; symptoms that are best handled with a team approach (e.g., depression); communication around the meaning and impact of advanced illness in a physical, social, and spiritual context; and transitions in care (e.g., anticancer therapy to hospice care).

KEY MESSAGES TO PATIENTS AND FAMILIES

Palliative care is an integral component of cancer care and should be a part of all active cancer therapies. The extent of integration is variable and depends on disease trajectory, symptom burden, and social factors. Frequent assessment of palliative care needs is imperative because palliative care has been shown to improve outcomes in terms of survival and clinical outcomes such as symptom burden and psychosocial support.

The following are sample questions for oncology providers to consider discussing with their patients. An emphasis on collaboration between the two teams, with the goals and values of the patient being central, should be emphasized.

1. Would you like to learn more about how palliative care might help you and your family?
2. Do you have unanswered questions about your prognosis and its implications? A palliative care team, in conjunction with ours, is a good resource for discussing your concerns further.
3. Do you have uncontrolled symptoms (physical, psychological, or social)? A palliative care team approach may be effective to help manage these symptoms.

CONCLUSION AND SUMMARY

The intersection of palliative care and anticancer care should be frequent and encompassing. Ideally, collaboration occurs at the time of diagnosis and continues throughout therapy, with adjustments for individual and disease-related factors. This integration is supported by both clinical evidence and policy. The next steps include appropriate growth both in quantity and quality of palliative care services to support this vision.

SUMMARY RECOMMENDATIONS

- Palliative care should be an integrated component of anticancer therapy for all patients and their families.
- The scope of palliative care services available to patients varies geographically because of a scarcity of resources and trained providers.
- Palliative care should be introduced at the time of cancer diagnosis.
- The evidence base for palliative care demonstrates that it improves control of physical and psychological symptoms, quality of care for both patient and family, and survival.

REFERENCES

1. World Health Organization. *National Cancer Control Programmes: Policies and Managerial Guidelines.* 2nd ed. Geneva: World Health Organization; 2002.
2. Boyle P, Levin B. *World Cancer Report 2008.* Geneva: World Health Organization; 2009.
3. Grant M, Elk R, Ferrell B, et al. Current status of palliative care: clinical implementation, education, and research. *CA Cancer J Clin.* 2009;59(5):327–335.
4. Hui D, Elsayem A, De la Cruz, et al. Availability and integration of palliative care at US cancer centers. *JAMA.* 2010;303(11):1054–1061.
5. Zwahlen D, Hagenbuch N, Carley MI, et al. Screening cancer patients' families with the distress thermometer (DT): a validation study. *Psychooncology.* 2008;17(10):959–966.
6. Mitchell AJ. Pooled results from 38 analyses of the accuracy of Distress Thermometer and other ultra-short methods of detecting cancer-related mood disorders. *J Clin Oncol.* 2007;25(29):4670–4681.
7. Ransom S, Jacobsen PB, Booth-Jones M. Validation of the Distress Thermometer with bone marrow transplant patients. *Psychooncology.* 2006;15(7):604–612.
8. Jacobsen PB, Ransom S. Implementation of NCCN distress management guidelines by member institutions. *J Natl Compr Canc Netw.* 2007;5(1):99–103.
9. Hegel MT, Collins ED, Kearing S, et al. Sensitivity and specificity of the Distress Thermometer for depression in newly diagnosed breast cancer patients. *Psychooncology.* 2008;17(6):556–560.
10. Seow H, Barbera L, Sutradhar R, et al. Trajectory of performance status and symptom scores for patients with cancer during the last six months of life. *J Clin Oncol.* 2011;29(9):1151–1158.
11. Reuben DB, Mor V, Hiris J. Clinical symptoms and length of survival in patients with terminal cancer. *Arch Intern Med.* 1988;148(7):1586–1591.
12. Levy MH, Back A, Benedetti C, et al. NCCN clinical practice guidelines in oncology: palliative care. *J Natl Compr Canc Netw.* 2009;7(4):436–473.
13. Evans C, McCarthy M. Prognostic uncertainty in terminal care: can the Karnofsky index help? *Lancet.* 1985;1(8439):1204–1206.

14. Maltoni M, Nanni O, Derni S, et al. Clinical prediction of survival is more accurate than the Karnofsky Performance Status in estimating life span of terminally ill cancer patients. *Eur J Cancer.* 1994;30A(6):764–766.
15. Maltoni M, Pirovano M, Scarpi E, et al. Prediction of survival of patients terminally ill with cancer: results of an Italian prospective multicentric study. *Cancer.* 1995;75(10):2613–2622.
16. Morita T, Tsunoda J, Inoue S, et al. Validity of the palliative performance scale from a survival perspective. *J Pain Symptom Manage.* 1999;18(1):2–3.
17. Llobera J, Esteva M, Rifá J, et al. Terminal cancer: duration and prediction of survival time. *Eur J Cancer.* 2000;36(16):2036–2043.
18. Temel JS, Greer JA, Muzikansky A, et al. Early palliative care for patients with metastatic non-small-cell lung cancer. *N Engl J Med.* 2010;363(8):733–742.
19. Bakitas M, Lyons KD, Hegel MT, et al. Effects of a palliative care intervention on clinical outcomes in patients with advanced cancer: the Project ENABLE II randomized controlled trial. *JAMA.* 2009;302(7):741–749.
20. Jordhoy MS, Fayers P, Saltnes T, et al. A palliative-care intervention and death at home: a cluster randomised trial. *Lancet.* 2000;356(9233):888–893.
21. Jordhoy MS, Fayers P, Loge JH, et al. Quality of life in palliative cancer care: results from a cluster randomized trial. *J Clin Oncol.* 2001;19(18):3884–3894.
22. Follwell M, Buman D, Le LW, et al. Phase II study of an outpatient palliative care intervention in patients with metastatic cancer. *J Clin Oncol.* 2009;27(2):206–213.
23. Strasser F, Sweeney C, Willey J, et al. Impact of a half-day multidisciplinary symptom control and palliative care outpatient clinic in a comprehensive cancer center on recommendations, symptom intensity, and patient satisfaction: a retrospective descriptive study. *J Pain Symptom Manage.* 2004;27(6):481–491.
24. Casarett DJ, Hirschman KB, Coffey JF, et al. Does a palliative care clinic have a role in improving end-of-life care? Results of a pilot program. *J Palliat Med.* 2002;5(3):387–396.
25. Peppercorn JM, Smith TJ, Helft PR, et al. American Society of Clinical Oncology statement: toward individualized care for patients with advanced cancer. *J Clin Oncol.* 2011;29(6):755–760.
26. American Society of Clinical Oncology–European Society for Medical Oncology. Consensus statement on quality cancer care. *Ann Oncol* 2006;17(7):1063–1064.
27. McNiff KK, Neuss MN, Jacobson JO, et al. Measuring supportive care in medical oncology practice: lessons learned from the quality oncology practice initiative. *J Clin Oncol.* 2008;26(23):3832–3837.
28. Bakitas M, Lyons KD, Hegel MT, et al. The project ENABLE II randomized controlled trial to improve palliative care for rural patients with advanced cancer: baseline findings, methodological challenges, and solutions. *Palliat Support Care.* 2009;7(1):75–86.
29. Casarett D, Pickard A, Bailey FA, et al. Do palliative consultations improve patient outcomes? *J Am Geriatr Soc.* 2008;56(4):593–599.
30. Rabow MW, Dibble SL, Pantilat SZ, et al. The comprehensive care team: a controlled trial of outpatient palliative medicine consultation. *Arch Intern Med.* 2004;164(1):83–91.
31. Meyers FJ, Linder J, Beckett L, et al. Simultaneous care: a model approach to the perceived conflict between investigational therapy and palliative care. *J Pain Symptom Manage.* 2004;28(6):548–556.

Chapter 49

What Is the Clinical Course of Advanced Cancer?

KAVITHA J. RAMCHANDRAN AND JAMIE H. VON ROENN

INTRODUCTION AND SCOPE OF THE PROBLEM

Approximately 12 million patients are living with cancer in the United States.[1] Fortunately, deaths from cancer have been on the decline, with survival rates increasing.[2] Advances have been made in survival in breast, colon, prostate, and lung cancer. Figures 49-1 and 49-2 depict a decrease in age-adjusted cancer death rates across all major cancer sites in both men and women, with the exception of lung cancer in women. This also can be depicted as number of deaths avoided based on an overall decrease in mortality rate (Figure 49-3). Because patients with cancer are living longer, they are more likely to die with

advanced disease. This chapter discusses the clinical trajectory of cancer, as well as symptoms associated with advanced disease.

The care of patients with cancer throughout the course of their illness should include an integrated approach with palliative care. Studies have shown that an integrated model of care improves outcomes for patients across multiple domains (physical, psychological, social), improves quality of care, and may have an impact on survival.[3-6] The role of palliative care in advanced cancer is covered in further detail in Chapter 48.

RELEVANT PATHOPHYSIOLOGY

Illness Trajectory of Advanced Cancer

The clinical course of advanced cancer differs from the course of other chronic illnesses such as heart failure, end-stage renal disease, chronic pulmonary disease, or dementia. Many chronic illnesses exhibit a sine wave pattern—periods of wellness alternating with periods of illness, with small progressive stepwise declines over time. In contrast, patients with advanced cancer generally have a period of relatively stable health followed by a rapid decline (Figure 49-4). The trajectory of illness for patients with cancer varies based on primary site of disease, responsiveness

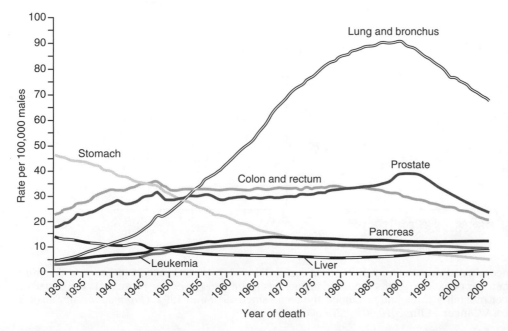

FIGURE 49-1. Annual age-adjusted cancer death rates among males for selected cancers, United States, 1930 to 2006. Rates are age-adjusted to the 2000 U.S. standard population. Because of changes in International Classification of Diseases (ICD) coding, numerator information has changed over time. Rates for cancers of the lung and bronchus, colon, and rectum, and liver are affected by these changes. (*Based on data from U.S. Mortality Data, 1960 to 2006 and U.S. Mortality Vol. 1930 to 1959, 2011. Bethesda, MD: National Center for Health Statistics, Centers for Disease Control and Prevention.*)

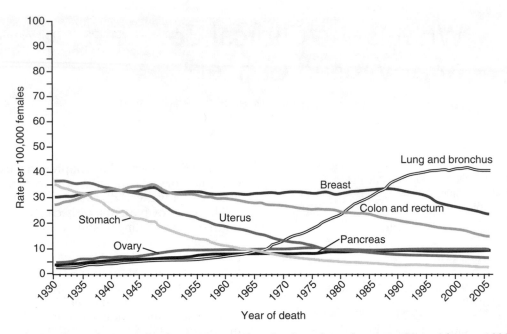

FIGURE 49-2. Annual age-adjusted cancer death rates among females for selected cancers, United States, 1930 to 2006. Rates are age-adjusted to the 2000 U.S. standard population. Because of changes in International Classification of Diseases (ICD) coding, numerator information has changed over time. Rates for cancers of the lung and bronchus, colon and rectum, and liver are affected by these changes. *(Based on data from U.S. Mortality Data 1960 to 2006 and U.S. Mortality Vol. 1930 to 1959, 2011. Bethesda, MD: National Center for Health Statistics, Centers for Disease Control and Prevention.)*

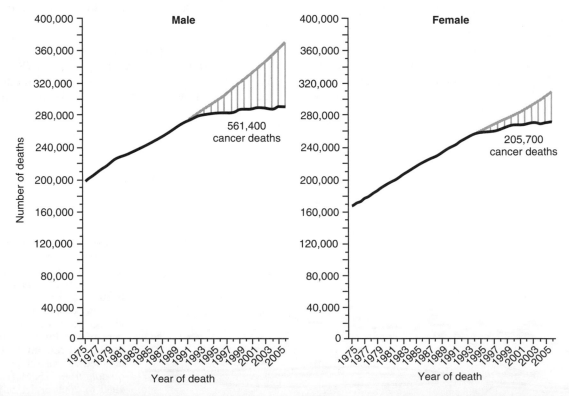

FIGURE 49-3. Total number of cancer deaths avoided from 1991 to 2006 in males and from 1992 to 2006 in females. The *main black line* represents the actual number of cancer deaths recorded in each year; the *gray upper line* represents the expected number of cancer deaths if cancer mortality rates had remained the same since 1990 and 1991. *(From Jemal A, Siegel R, Xu J, et al. Cancer statistics, 2010. CA Cancer J Clin. 2010;60(5):277-300.)*

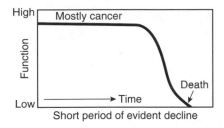

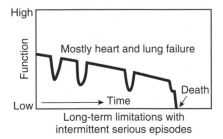

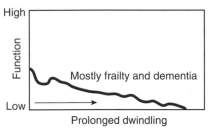

Figure 49-4. Comparison of chronic illness trajectory curves. *(From Lynn J, Adamson DM.* Living Well at the End of Life: Adapting Health Care to Serious Chronic Illness in Old Age. *Washington, DC: Rand Health, 2003;8)*

to therapy, disease-free interval, and patient performance status. Having a clear understanding of these subtleties helps identify transition points for families and health care practitioners.

Advanced disease in patients with cancer will have a different trajectory based on responsiveness to treatment, disease-free interval, and performance status. We will divide these into the following four categories (Table 49-1):

1. Responsive to therapy, long progression-free/ overall survival (PFS/OS), treatment sensitive with prolonged periods of wellness (good functional status, quality of life).

TABLE 49-1. Trajectories of Illness in Advanced Cancer			
RESPONSIVE LONG PFS/OS	**RESPONSIVE SHORT PFS/OS**	**NOT RESPONSIVE LONG PFS/OS**	**NOT RESPONSIVE SHORT PFS/OS**
Breast	Small cell lung	Indolent lymphoma	Non–small cell lung
Prostate	Aggressive lymphoma		Pancreas
Anal			Gastric
Uterine			Bladder
Good-risk leukemia			Colon
Myeloma			Esophageal
Ovary			Kidney
			Poor-risk leukemia
			Liver

PFS/OS, Progression-free/overall survival.

*NOTE: These are based on advanced (or metastatic) cancer presentations.

2. Responsive to therapy, short progression-free/ overall survival (PFS/OS), treatment sensitive, but response is short-lived, and patients experience a short period of wellness followed by rapid decline.
3. Not responsive to therapy, short progression-free/overall survival (PFS/OS), treatment resistant, with short survival, rapid decline.
4. Not responsive to therapy, long progression free/overall survival (PFS/OS), treatment resistant; however, disease biology is indolent and patients can still have a prolonged period of wellness.
5. Performance status precludes treatment.

Table 49-1 provides common examples.

Although discussing all of the various malignancies and their trajectories is beyond the scope of this chapter, it is important to collaborate with the oncology team to understand in which subgroup a particular disease falls. This will allow for better prognostication and thus improved guidance of clinical decisions based on patient goals.

Performance Status

The clinical course of all patients with advanced cancer is influenced by performance status. Patients with a performance status of Eastern Cooperative Oncology Group (ECOG) greater than 2, more that 50% of time in bed or in a chair, may not be candidates for and may not benefit from anticancer therapy. Multiple studies have demonstrated that patients with a performance status greater than 2 have increased toxicity from treatment and thus do not derive clinical benefit from anticancer therapy.[7-14] As performance status continues to deteriorate, survival is affected. Patients with an ECOG Performance Status score of 3 and/or a Karnofsky Performance Status score of 30 to 40 have a median survival of 8 to 50 days. Patients with an ECOG score of 4 and/or Karnofsky score of 10 to 20 have a median survival of 7 to 16 days.[15-20] Please refer to Chapter 50 for more details on how performance status influences treatment decisions.

Physical Symptoms

In some cases, physical symptoms can be treated with anticancer therapy. For example, in advanced lung cancer, symptoms such as dyspnea, anorexia, and cough are improved with chemotherapy and/or targeted treatment.[21-24] In the Initiating Dialysis Early and Late (IDEAL) trial, gefitinib, an epidermal growth factor receptor (EGFR) inhibitor, resulted in a rapid improvement in symptoms such as dyspnea and fatigue within 3 weeks of starting therapy.[25] Although the responses with chemotherapy are less rapid, similar improvements in symptom burden can occur. Anticancer treatment effects are also seen in breast cancer, in which some symptoms, including pain and fatigue, are ameliorated by effective anticancer therapy.[26-29]

Certain symptoms, however, are an indicator of end-stage disease and will likely not be reversed with anticancer treatment. Symptoms such as dysphagia, xerostomia, cognitive dysfunction, and anorexia have been shown in some studies to correlate with decreased survival. Table 49-2 depicts the prevalence of these symptoms, based on a study of 1000 patients with cancer.[30] A study by Maltoni and colleagues found that the presence of significant dyspnea or dysphagia predicted a median survival of 30 days or less.[17] A recent retrospective Canadian study of more than 18,000 patients with cancer patients in the last 6 months of life found that symptoms such as pain, nausea, anxiety, and depression were relatively stable. Alternatively, symptoms such as dyspnea, drowsiness, decreased well-being, anorexia, and fatigue increased over the last month of life.[31]

Another observation in patients with advanced disease is symptom clusters. The term *symptom clusters* refers to several symptoms that are related to each other but may or may not share a common cause.[32] Common symptom clusters are described in Table 49-3.[33] Some debate exists in the literature as to whether symptom clusters truly exist; however, studies point to clusters by disease type, treatment, and patient demographics (e.g., clusters in patients from the United States versus clusters in patients from China).[2] For example, different symptom clusters likely occur for patients with breast cancer versus lung cancer. Symptom clusters may also be classified based on underlying common physiology or treatment (e.g., small bowel obstruction, taxane-based treatment).[34,35] Further research on symptom

TABLE 49-3. Common Symptom Clusters Seen in Cancer Patients

Anxiety/Agitation/Delirium

Cough/Breathlessness/Fatigue

Depression/Anxiety

Fatigue/Anorexia-Cachexia

Fatigue/Drowsiness/Nausea/Decreased Appetite/Dyspnea

Fatigue/Pain/Anxiety/Depression

Fatigue/Somnolence

Nausea/Anorexia/Dehydration

Nausea/Appetite Loss/Constipation

Pain/Depression/Fatigue

Pain/Dyspnea/Numbness

From Esper P. Symptom clusters in individuals living with advanced cancer. *Semin Oncol Nurs.* 2010;26(3):168-174, Table 3.

clusters has the potential to inform both symptom assessment and treatment decisions.

Knowing when anticancer treatment can ameliorate symptoms and understanding the prognostic significance of symptoms such as dyspnea and dysphagia allow clinicians to provide appropriate information and counseling to patients and families regarding overall goals of therapy.

Psychological, Social, and Spiritual Factors

Advanced cancer also presents psychological, social, and spiritual challenges. Patients with advanced disease who have physical symptoms (e.g., pain) have greater psychological distress.[36,37] Existential and social concerns also contribute to suffering in advanced cancer. A study of 381 patients with cancer found that whereas physical problems accounted for approximately half (49.5%) of patient reports of suffering, psychological, existential, and social concerns accounted for 14.0%, 17.7%, and 18.8%, respectively.[38] Of note, often patients with depression or anxiety have smaller social networks and less participation in spiritual or religious communities.[39] An integrated palliative care approach can ensure adequate assessment and treatment of psychological, social, and spiritual distress.

Hematological Malignancies

A special note needs to be made in regard to the hematological malignancies, such as leukemia, aggressive lymphoma, and multiple myeloma. Patients often present with advanced variants of these diseases, and, in spite of this, treatment may achieve the goal of cure or prolonged survival. These patients are referred to palliative care later than their counterparts with solid organ disease and often die in the hospital.[40–42] Patients have a significant symptom burden, with an increase in symptoms such as delirium and drowsiness.[43] They are also prone to additional complications such as infection and bleeding.

TABLE 49-2. Prevalence of Symptoms in Advanced Cancer

SYMPTOM	%
Pain	84
Fatigue	69
Weakness	66
Anorexia	66
Xerostomia	57
Constipation	52
Early satiety	51
Dyspnea	50
Weight loss	50
Sleep problems	49
Depression	41
Cough	38
Nausea	36
Edema	28
Taste change	28
Hoarseness	24
Anxiety	24
Vomiting	23
Confusion	21

Modified from Walsh D, Donnelly S, Rybicki L. The symptoms of advanced cancer: relationship to age, gender, and performance status in 1,000 patients. *Support Care Cancer.* 2000;8(3):175-179, Table 3.

Quality Palliative Care

In 2005 the American Society of Clinical Oncology (ASCO) commissioned the Quality Oncology Practice Initiative (QOPI) to develop key quality indicators for cancer care.[44] QOPI covers a wide array of quality measures, including documentation of diagnosis, assessment of symptoms, implementation of guideline-based care, appropriate follow-up, and resource usage. The goals are guidance and transparency around quality care for all patients with cancer.

QOPI has key quality measures for palliative care for patients with cancer. These were studied and documented by McNiff and colleagues in 2008,[45] including assessment of symptoms such as pain and nausea.[45] Constipation, dyspnea, and emotional well-being have been included in the most recent set of core measures.[46] Finally, appropriate use of hospice and active-cancer therapy is also being evaluated. For example, chemotherapy within 2 weeks of death would be inappropriate, as would lack of hospice referral for a patient who has no further anticancer treatment options.[47] Many of the key measures can be effectively met with an integrated palliative care approach.

Although QOPI is currently a voluntary effort on the part of both community and academic practitioners, it will likely soon set the standard by which institutions are judged and compared. It is a means to better understand the quality of care provided for patients with cancer on local, regional, and national levels.

SUMMARY OF EVIDENCE REGARDING TREATMENT RECOMMENDATIONS

Advanced cancer is complex, in terms of both understanding unique illness trajectories and dealing with a symptom burden that encompasses the physical, social, emotional, and spiritual domains. Treatment must address this complexity. An approach that integrates palliative care into the treatment plan for patients with advanced disease will reduce the overall symptom burden, improve quality of life, and possibly improve survival.[19-23] Integrated care is best provided by a multidisciplinary team, including but not limited to, a nurse, social worker, chaplain, and physician. Chapter 48 discusses in more depth the integration of palliative care into anticancer care.

KEY MESSAGES TO PATIENTS AND FAMILIES

Patients with advanced cancer may survive only days or as long as years. The prediction of survival is difficult but may be estimated based on the prior responsiveness of the cancer to treatment, available therapies, and individual patient characteristics (e.g., age, other illnesses, ability to do daily tasks). Physical symptoms are almost always present and should be treated aggressively regardless of the prognosis. Palliative care, ideally involving an interdisciplinary team with integrated oncology care provides optimal cancer care.

Often it is difficult for patients and families to navigate the terrain of cancer treatment and to ask the right questions to begin planning for the future. Sample questions for patients to pose to their oncology team include the following:

1. Is my cancer treatable?
2. What is the goal of treatment—cure or palliation?
3. Will treatment improve the symptoms of my disease?
4. What is the appropriate time to stop treatment and to focus on goals such as quality of life or comfort?
5. How will my psychological, spiritual, and social concerns be addressed both during and after treatment?

CONCLUSION AND SUMMARY

With approximately 12 million patients living with cancer in the United States, and with survival continuing to increase, the number of patients living with advanced cancer as a chronic disease will also continue to rise. Although the trajectory of illness for these patients may initially be variable, most of them will experience a significant burden of symptoms—physical, social, psychological, and spiritual. A concurrent care model with palliative care always and anticancer therapy when appropriate offers patients the best care.

SUMMARY RECOMMENDATIONS

- Advanced cancer can take many trajectories; understanding the trajectory of illness is key to understanding the goal of anticancer treatment.
- Performance status can help guide treatment decisions, as well as provide important information about prognosis.
- Treatment of symptoms (physical, social, psychological, and spiritual) is important when treating advanced disease.
- An integrated palliative care and oncology approach is best practice to provide quality care that is in line with patient-centric goals and values.

REFERENCES

1. Howlader N, Noone AM, Krapcho M, et al., eds. *SEER Cancer Statistics Review, 1975-2008*. Bethesda, MD: National Cancer Institute; 2011. http://seer.cancer.gov/csr/1975_2008/, based on November 2010 SEER data submission, posted to the SEER website.
2. Jemal A, Siegal R, Ward E, et al. Cancer statistics, 2009. *CA Cancer J Clin*. 2009;59(4):225–249.
3. Bakitas M, Lyons KD, Hegel MT, et al. The project ENABLE II randomized controlled trial to improve palliative care for rural patients with advanced cancer: baseline findings, methodological challenges, and solutions. *Palliat Support Care*. 2009;7(1):75–86.

4. Temel JS, Greer JA, Muzikansky A, et al. Early palliative care for patients with metastatic non-small-cell lung cancer. *N Engl J Med.* 2010;363(8):733–742.

5. Follwell M, Burman D, Le LW, et al. Phase II study of an outpatient palliative care intervention in patients with metastatic cancer. *J Clin Oncol.* 2009;27(2):206–213.

6. Muir JC, Daly F, Davis MS, et al. Integrating palliative care into the outpatient, private practice oncology setting. *J Pain Symptom Manage.* 2010;40(1):126–135.

7. Albain KS, Crowley JJ, LeBlanc M, et al. Survival determinants in extensive-stage non-small-cell lung cancer: the Southwest Oncology Group experience. *J Clin Oncol.* 1991;9(9):1618–1626.

8. Sengeløv L, Kamby C, Geertsen P, et al. Predictive factors of response to cisplatin-based chemotherapy and the relation of response to survival in patients with metastatic urothelial cancer. *Cancer Chemother Pharmacol.* 2000;46(5):357–364.

9. Oshita F, Kurata T, Kasai T, et al. Prospective evaluation of the feasibility of cisplatin-based chemotherapy for elderly lung cancer patients with normal organ functions. *Jpn J Cancer Res.* 1995;86(12):1198–1202.

10. Firat S, Byhardt RW, Gore E. Comorbidity and Karnofksy performance score are independent prognostic factors in stage III non-small-cell lung cancer: an institutional analysis of patients treated on four RTOG studies. Radiation Therapy Oncology Group. *Int J Radiat Oncol Biol Phys.* 2002;54(2):357–364.

11. Gupta D, Lammersfeld CA, Vashi PG, et al. Prognostic significance of Subjective Global Assessment (SGA) in advanced colorectal cancer. *Eur J Clin Nutr.* 2005;59(1):35–40.

12. Wang WS, Fan FS, Hsieh RK, et al. Factors predictive of response and survival in patients with metastatic colorectal cancer in Taiwan. *Jpn J Clin Oncol.* 1997;27(3):174–179.

13. Carey MS, Bacon M, Tu D, et al. The prognostic effects of performance status and quality of life scores on progression-free survival and overall survival in advanced ovarian cancer. *Gynecol Oncol.* 2008;108(1):100–105.

14. Ihde DC. Chemotherapy of lung cancer. *N Engl J Med.* 1992;327(20):1434–1441.

15. Evans C, McCarthy M. Prognostic uncertainty in terminal care: can the Karnofsky index help? *Lancet.* 1985;1(8439):1204–1206.

16. Maltoni M, Nanni O, Derni S, et al. Clinical prediction of survival is more accurate than the Karnofsky performance status in estimating life span of terminally ill cancer patients. *Eur J Cancer.* 1994;30A(6):764–766.

17. Maltoni M, Pirovano M, Scarpi E, et al. Prediction of survival of patients terminally ill with cancer: results of an Italian prospective multicentric study. *Cancer.* 1995;75(10):2613–2622.

18. Reuben DB, Mor V, Hiris J. Clinical symptoms and length of survival in patients with terminal cancer. *Arch Intern Med.* 1988;148(7):1586–1591.

19. Pirovano M, Maltoni M, Nanni O, et al. A new palliative prognostic score: a first step for the staging of terminally ill cancer patients. Italian Multicenter and Study Group on Palliative Care. *J Pain Symptom Manage.* 1999;17(4):231–239.

20. Llobera J, Esteva M, Rifà J, et al. Terminal cancer: duration and prediction of survival time. *Eur J Cancer.* 2000;36(16):2036–2043.

21. The Elderly Lung Cancer Vinorelbine Italian Study Group. Effects of vinorelbine on quality of life and survival of elderly patients with advanced non-small-cell lung cancer. *J Natl Cancer Inst.* 1999;91(1):66–72.

22. NSCLC Meta-Analyses Collaborative Group. Chemotherapy in addition to supportive care improves survival in advanced non-small-cell lung cancer: a systematic review and meta-analysis of individual patient data from 16 randomized controlled trials. *J Clin Oncol.* 2008;26(28):4617–4625.

23. Anderson H, Hopwood P, Stephens RJ, et al. Gemcitabine plus best supportive care (BSC) vs BSC in inoperable non-small cell lung cancer: a randomized trial with quality of life as the primary outcome. UK NSCLC Gemcitabine Group. Non-Small Cell Lung Cancer. *Br J Cancer.* 2000;83(4):447–453.

24. Ranson M, Davidson N, Nicolson M, et al. Randomized trial of paclitaxel plus supportive care versus supportive care for patients with advanced non-small-cell lung cancer. *J Natl Cancer Inst.* 2000;92(13):1074–1080.

25. Kris MG, Natale RB, Herbst RS, et al. Efficacy of gefitinib, an inhibitor of the epidermal growth factor receptor tyrosine kinase, in symptomatic patients with non-small cell lung cancer: a randomized trial. *JAMA.* 2003;290(16):2149–2158.

26. Wu Y, Amonkar MM, Sherill BH, et al. Impact of lapatinib plus trastuzumab versus single-agent lapatinib on quality of life of patients with trastuzumab-refractory HER2 + metastatic breast cancer. *Ann Oncol.* 2011;22(12):2582–2590.

27. Perez EA, Vogel CL, Irwin DH, et al. Multicenter phase II trial of weekly paclitaxel in women with metastatic breast cancer. *J Clin Oncol.* 2001;19(22):4216–4223.

28. Degner LF, Sloan JA. Symptom distress in newly diagnosed ambulatory cancer patients and as a predictor of survival in lung cancer. *J Pain Symptom Manage.* 1995;10(6):423–431.

29. Blum JL. The role of capecitabine, an oral, enzymatically activated fluoropyrimidine, in the treatment of metastatic breast cancer. *Oncologist.* 2001;6(1):56–64.

30. Walsh D, Donnelly S, Rybicki L. The symptoms of advanced cancer: relationship to age, gender, and performance status in 1,000 patients. *Support Care Cancer.* 2000;8(3):175–179.

31. Seow H, Barbera L, Sutradhar R, et al. Trajectory of performance status and symptom scores for patients with cancer during the last six months of life. *J Clin Oncol.* 2011;29(9):1151–1158.

32. Dodd MJ, Miaskowski C, Paul SM. Symptom clusters and their effect on the functional status of patients with cancer. *Oncol Nurs Forum.* 2001;28(3):465–470.

33. Esper P. Symptom clusters in individuals living with advanced cancer. *Semin Oncol Nurs.* 2010;26(3):168–174.

34. Honea N, Brant J, Beck SL. Treatment-related symptom clusters. *Semin Oncol Nurs.* 2007;23(2):142–151.

35. Gift AG. Symptom clusters related to specific cancers. *Semin Oncol Nurs.* 2007;23(2):136–141.

36. Kaasa S, Malt U, Hagen S, et al. Psychological distress in cancer patients with advanced disease. *Radiother Oncol.* 1993;27(3):193–197.

37. Mystakidou K, Tsilika E, Parpa E, et al. Psychological distress of patients with advanced cancer: influence and contribution of pain severity and pain interference. *Cancer Nurs.* 2006;29(5):400–405.

38. Wilson KG, Chochinov HM, McPherson CJ, et al. Suffering with advanced cancer. *J Clin Oncol.* 2007;25(13):1691–1697.

39. Wilson KG, Chochinov HM, Skirko MG, et al. Depression and anxiety disorders in palliative cancer care. *J Pain Symptom Manage.* 2007;33(2):118–129.

40. Maddocks I, Bentley L, Sheedy J. Quality of life issues in patients dying from haematological diseases. *Ann Acad Med Singapore.* 1994;23(2):244–248.

41. Fadul N, Elsayem A, Palmer JL, et al. Predictors of access to palliative care services among patients who died at a comprehensive cancer center. *J Palliat Med.* 2007;10(5):1146–1152.

42. Cheng WW, Willey J, Palmer JL, et al. Interval between palliative care referral and death among patients treated at a comprehensive cancer center. *J Palliat Med.* 2005;8(5):1025–1032.

43. Fadul NA, El Osta B, Dalal S, et al. Comparison of symptom burden among patients referred to palliative care with hematologic malignancies versus those with solid tumors. *J Palliat Med.* 2008;11(3):422–427.

44. Neuss MN, Desch CE, McNiff KK, et al. A process for measuring the quality of cancer care: the Quality Oncology Practice Initiative. *J Clin Oncol.* 2005;23(25):6233–6239.

45. McNiff KK, Neuss MN, Jacobson JO, et al. Measuring supportive care in medical oncology practice: lessons learned from the quality oncology practice initiative. *J Clin Oncol.* 2008;26(23):3832–3837.

46. Fan G, Hadi S, Chow E. Symptom clusters in patients with advanced-stage cancer referred for palliative radiation therapy in an outpatient setting. *Support Cancer Ther.* 2007;4(3):157–162.

47. Blayney DW, et al. Implementation of the Quality Oncology Practice Initiative at a university comprehensive cancer center. *J Clin Oncol.* 2009;27(23):3802–3807.

Chapter 50

What Is the Relationship Between Patient Performance Status and Ability to Offer Chemotherapeutic Treatments?

KAVITHA J. RAMCHANDRAN AND JAMIE H. VON ROENN

INTRODUCTION
RELEVANT SYSTEMS
SUMMARY OF EVIDENCE
KEY MESSAGES TO PATIENTS AND FAMILIES
CONCLUSION AND SUMMARY

INTRODUCTION

Performance status is the method physicians use to describe a patients' overall physical well-being, based on their ability to do everyday tasks such as bathing, walking, and performing other normal activities. In the treatment of patients with cancer it is a key component of determining whether patients will benefit from therapy.[1,2]

RELEVANT SYSTEMS

The two scales used most frequently to define performance status are the Eastern Cooperative Oncology Group (ECOG) scale, also known as the Zubrod scale, and the Karnofsky Performance Scale (KPS). The KPS ranges from 0 to 100%, with a performance status of 100% being normal with no symptoms of disease and a performance status of 0% being equal to death. The ECOG scale scores patient status from 0 to 5, with 0 referring to an asymptomatic patient with no signs of disease and 5 being equal to death. Table 50-1 details the elements of each of the scoring systems and correlates the two scales. The correlation has been validated in several studies.[3,4]

SUMMARY OF EVIDENCE

Performance status has been shown to correlate with survival. For example, a KPS of 50 or higher has been shown to correlate with patient survival of 50 to 90 days. A KPS of 30 to 40 correlates with median survival of 8 to 50 days, and a KPS of 10 to 20 correlates with survival of 7 to 16 days.[5–9] These data are extracted primarily from studies of patients with

TABLE 50-1. Comparison of Eastern Cooperative Oncology Group Scale (ECOG) and Karnofsky Performance Scale (KPS)

ECOG	ECOG = KPS	KPS
0: Asymptomatic (fully active, able to perform all predisease activities without restriction)	ECOG 0 = KPS 100; 90-100	100%: Normal, no complaints, no signs of disease 90%: Capable of normal activity, few symptoms or signs of disease
1: Symptomatic but completely ambulatory (restricted in physically strenuous activity but ambulatory and able to perform work of a light or sedentary nature, for example, light housework, office work)	ECOG 1 = KPS 80-90; 70-80	80%: Normal activity with some difficulty, some symptoms or signs 70%: Caring for self, not capable of normal activity or work
2: Symptomatic, <50% in bed during the day (ambulatory and capable of all self-care but unable to perform any work activities. Up and about more than 50% of waking hours)	ECOG 2 = KPS 60-70; 50-60	60%: Requiring some help, can take care of most personal requirements 50%: Requires help often, requires frequent medical care
3: Symptomatic, >50% in bed, but not bedbound (capable of only limited self-care, confined to bed or chair 50% or more of waking hours)	ECOG 3 = KPS 40-50; 30-40	40%: Disabled, requires special care and help 30%: Severely disabled, hospital admission indicated but no risk for death
4: Bedbound (completely disabled, cannot perform any self-care, totally confined to bed or chair)	ECOG 4 = KPS 20-30; 10-20	20%: Very ill, urgently requiring admission, requires supportive measures or treatment 10%: Moribund, rapidly progressive fatal disease processes
5: Dead	ECOG 5 = KPS 0	0%: Dead

Modified from Karnofsky DA, Burchenal JH. The clinical evaluation of chemotherapeutic agents in cancer. In: MacLeod CM (ed). *Evaluation of Chemotherapeutic Agents.* New York: Columbia University Press; 1949:196; Oken MM, Creech RH, Tomey DC. Toxicity and response criteria of the Eastern Cooperative Oncology Group. *Am J Clin Oncol.* 1982;5(6):649–655; Karnofsky DA, Ellison RR, Golbey RB. Selection of patients for evaluation of chemotherapeutic procedures in advanced cancer. *Cancer Chemother Rep.* 1962;16:73–77; Buccheri G, Ferrigno D, Tamburini M. Karnofsky and ECOG performance status scoring in lung cancer: a prospective, longitudinal study of 536 patients from a single institution. *Eur J Cancer.* 1996;32A(7):1135–1141.

advanced malignant disease who are no longer candidates for anticancer therapy and may not apply to patients with early-stage disease or those who are still receiving anticancer therapy.

Treatment of patients relative to their performance status is based on studies that demonstrate the correlations between performance status and response to treatment, survival, and quality of life.[10–13] For example, in patients with non–small cell lung cancer, cytotoxic therapy is not effective and may increase toxicity in patients with a ECOG performance status of 2 or greater.[10,14,15] This also holds true for patients with other solid tumors.[16–18] Similarly, in patients with leukemia and lymphoma, a poor performance status precludes aggressive therapies such as stem cell transplantation.[19–23] Further evidence of the importance of performance status is available from data collected in the geriatric patient population. Older adults with a good performance status have treatment outcomes similar to those of their younger counterparts.[23–25] Certain rare diseases are considered exquisitely chemosensitive (e.g., small cell lung cancer, Burkitt's lymphoma), and in these patients poor performance status may be reversed with appropriate cytotoxic therapy.[26–29] Of note, most of the data that correlate performance status to response to treatment are based on standard cytotoxic chemotherapeutics. The field of treatment has changed dramatically and now includes immune modulators, biological therapy ("targeted therapy") and hormone therapy. The data on performance status and these treatments are far from clear and continue to evolve. For example, patients with non–small cell lung cancer and a mutation in the epidermal growth factor receptor (EGFR) may benefit from treatment with erlotinib or gefitinib (an EGFR mutation inhibitor) regardless of performance status. A Japanese study showed that patients with a poor performance status still benefit from treatment targeted to this specific mutation. Poor performances status was defined as either a ECOG score of 3 or 4 in all comers; a score of 2 to 4 in patients older than 70; or in patients older than 80 with any performance status but with symptoms.[30] However, in contrast, a study conducted in North America was less definitive and showed only a non-statistical trend toward a benefit in survival for a similar patient population. These patients had an ECOG performance status of 2 or 3 (see Table 50-1) and were considered "unfit for chemotherapy." Additionally, the survival benefit was quite limited (3 months in both groups).[31] In patients with renal cell carcinoma, interleukin-2 may be an effective therapy for those with a good performance status but has a substantial risk for treatment-related mortality in patients with a poor performance status.[32–36] Interestingly, an alternative class of drugs for renal cell carcinoma, mammalian target of rapamycin (mTor) inhibitors, seem to be more effective in patients with poor risk factors, one of which is poor performance status.[37,38]

Hormone-based therapies may be quite effective in patients with hormone-sensitive prostate or breast cancer. Hormonal therapy may be considered even in patients with poor performance status (e.g., ECOG greater than 2, or KPS score less than 40).[39–41] The main issues to consider in an unfit, poor performance status group is cardiovascular and bone-related side effects (i.e., osteopenia, osteoporosis) of hormone manipulation.[42–44] Additionally, the less dangerous, but debilitating effects of arthralgias and joint pain may affect quality of life in this patient population.

The benefit and burden of therapies need to be weighed carefully in light of the goals and values of the patient. This is the juncture at which collaboration between palliative care and oncology becomes critical.

KEY MESSAGES TO PATIENTS AND FAMILIES

Performance status is a key indicator of response to therapy, survival, and overall quality of life. It is measured by a patient's ability to do basic activities such as bathing, eating, dressing, and walking (Karnofsky) or simply by determining what percent of time a patient is spending confined to a bed or a chair (ECOG). Palliative care and oncology providers routinely assess performance status to determine the safety and efficacy of potential treatments. As treatment options in oncology evolve and more targeted and less toxic treatments become available, it may become safer to offer treatment to patients with an ECOG performance status greater than 2.

CONCLUSION AND SUMMARY

Assessing performance status is an important first step in the evaluation of all patients before a recommendation for antineoplastic treatment. The evidence is well established that standard cytotoxic treatments are not effective and may be harmful in patients with a poor performance status. At this juncture, other options such as palliative care or alternative treatments should be considered. Newer treatment options, in particular targeted agents and hormone therapy are changing the field of cancer treatment and may allow for patients with a poor performance status to adequately tolerate and benefit from treatment.

SUMMARY RECOMMENDATIONS

- Performance status is the method clinicians use to describe patients' overall physical well-being, based on ability to do everyday tasks such as bathing, walking, and performing other normal activities. The two primary scales clinicians should use are the ECOG (Zubrod) and Karnofsky scales.
- Performance status correlates with survival and is a key metric used to determine whether anticancer therapy will be safe and effective. Explaining this can be helpful for patients and families.
- The paradigm of treatment is changing to include less toxic drugs. Clinicians can now consider using these agents when treating patients with a performance score higher 2.

REFERENCES

1. Oken MM, Creech RH, Tomey DC, et al. Toxicity and response criteria of the Eastern Cooperative Oncology Group. *Am J Clin Oncol.* 1982;5(6):649–655.
2. Karnofsky DA, Ellison RR, Golbey RB. Selection of patients for evaluation of chemotherapeutic procedures in advanced cancer. *Cancer Chemother Rep.* 1962;16:73–77.
3. Buccheri G, Ferrigno D, Tamburini M. Karnofsky and ECOG performance status scoring in lung cancer: a prospective, longitudinal study of 536 patients from a single institution. *Eur J Cancer.* 1996;32A(7):1135–1141.
4. Roila F, Lupattelli M, Sassi M, et al. Intra and interobserver variability in cancer patients' performance status assessed according to Karnofsky and ECOG scales. *Ann Oncol.* 1991;2(6):437–439.
5. Evans C, McCarthy M. Prognostic uncertainty in terminal care: can the Karnofsky index help? *Lancet.* 1985;1(8439):1204–1206.
6. Maltoni M, et al. Clinical prediction of survival is more accurate than the Karnofsky performance status in estimating life span of terminally ill cancer patients. *Eur J Cancer.* 1994;30A(6):764–766.
7. Maltoni M, Pirovano M, Scarpi E, et al. Prediction of survival of patients terminally ill with cancer: results of an Italian prospective multicentric study. *Cancer.* 1995;75(10):2613–2622.
8. Morita T, Tsunoda J, Inoue S, et al. Validity of the palliative performance scale from a survival perspective. *J Pain Symptom Manage.* 1999;18(1):2–3.
9. Llobera J, Esteva M, Rifà J, et al. Terminal cancer: duration and prediction of survival time. *Eur J Cancer.* 2000;36(16):2036–2043.
10. Albain KS, Crowley JJ, LeBlanc M, et al. Survival determinants in extensive-stage non-small-cell lung cancer: the Southwest Oncology Group experience. *J Clin Oncol.* 1991;9(9):1618–1626.
11. Sengeløv L, Kamby C, Geersten P, et al. Predictive factors of response to cisplatin-based chemotherapy and the relation of response to survival in patients with metastatic urothelial cancer. *Cancer Chemother Pharmacol.* 2000;46(5):357–364.
12. Firat S, Bousamra M, Gore E, et al. Comorbidity and KPS are independent prognostic factors in stage I non-small-cell lung cancer. *Int J Radiat Oncol Biol Phys.* 2002;52(4):1047–1057.
13. Cella D, Eton D, Hensing TA, et al. Relationship between symptom change, objective tumor measurements, and performance status during chemotherapy for advanced lung cancer. *Clin Lung Cancer.* 2008;9(1):51–58.
14. Ihde DC. Chemotherapy of lung cancer. *N Engl J Med.* 1992;327(20):1434–1441.
15. Oshita F, Kurata T, Kasai T, et al. Prospective evaluation of the feasibility of cisplatin-based chemotherapy for elderly lung cancer patients with normal organ functions. *Jpn J Cancer Res.* 1995;86(12):1198–1202.
16. Gupta D, Lammersfeld CA, Vashi PG, et al. Prognostic significance of Subjective Global Assessment (SGA) in advanced colorectal cancer. *Eur J Clin Nutr.* 2005;59(1):35–40.
17. Wang WS, Fan FS, Hsieh RK, et al. Factors predictive of response and survival in patients with metastatic colorectal cancer in Taiwan. *Jpn J Clin Oncol.* 1997;27(3):174–179.
18. Carey MS, Bacon M, Tu D, et al. The prognostic effects of performance status and quality of life scores on progression-free survival and overall survival in advanced ovarian cancer. *Gynecol Oncol.* 2008;108(1):100–105.
19. Klepin HD, Balducci L. Acute myelogenous leukemia in older adults. *Oncologist.* 2009;14(3):222–232.
20. Appelbaum FR, Gundacker H, Head DR, et al. Age and acute myeloid leukemia. *Blood.* 2006;107(9):3481–3485.
21. Kantarjian H, O'Brien S, Cortes J, et al. Results of intensive chemotherapy in 998 patients age 65 years or older with acute myeloid leukemia or high-risk myelodysplastic syndrome: predictive prognostic models for outcome. *Cancer.* 2006;106(5):1090–1098.
22. Malfuson JV, Etienne A, Tulure P, et al. Risk factors and decision criteria for intensive chemotherapy in older patients with acute myeloid leukemia. *Haematologica.* 2008;93(12):1806–1813.
23. Garg P, Rana F, Gupta R, et al. Predictors of toxicity and toxicity profile of adjuvant chemotherapy in elderly breast cancer patients. *Breast J.* 2009;15(4):404–408.
24. Sargent DJ, Goldberg RM, Jacobson SD, et al. A pooled analysis of adjuvant chemotherapy for resected colon cancer in elderly patients. *N Engl J Med.* 2001;345(15):1091–1097.
25. Folprecht G, Cunningham D, Ross P, et al. Efficacy of 5-fluorouracil-based chemotherapy in elderly patients with metastatic colorectal cancer: a pooled analysis of clinical trials. *Ann Oncol.* 2004;15(9):1330–1338.
26. Jennens RR, Rosenthal MA, Mitchell P, et al. Outcome of patients admitted to the intensive care unit with newly diagnosed small cell lung cancer. *Lung Cancer.* 2002;38(3):291–296.
27. Soares M, Darmon M, Salluh JI, et al. Prognosis of lung cancer patients with life-threatening complications. *Chest.* 2007;131(3):840–846.
28. Thomas DA, Faderl S, O'Brien S, et al. Chemoimmunotherapy with hyper-CVAD plus rituximab for the treatment of adult Burkitt and Burkitt-type lymphoma or acute lymphoblastic leukemia. *Cancer.* 2006;106(7):1569–1580.
29. Mead GM, Sydes MR, Walweski J, et al. An international evaluation of CODOX-M and CODOX-M alternating with IVAC in adult Burkitt's lymphoma: results of United Kingdom Lymphoma Group LY06 study. *Ann Oncol.* 2002;13(8):1264–1274.
30. Inoue A, Kobayashi K, Usui K, et al. First-line gefitinib for patients with advanced non-small-cell lung cancer harboring epidermal growth factor receptor mutations without indication for chemotherapy. *J Clin Oncol.* 2009;27(9):1394–1400.
31. Goss G, Ferry D, Wierbicki R, Laura SA, et al. Randomized phase II study of gefitinib compared with placebo in chemotherapy-naive patients with advanced non-small-cell lung cancer and poor performance status. *J Clin Oncol.* 2009;27(13):2253–2260.
32. Fyfe G, Fisher RI, Rosenberg SA, et al. Results of treatment of 255 patients with metastatic renal cell carcinoma who received high-dose recombinant interleukin-2 therapy. *J Clin Oncol.* 1995;13(3):688–696.
33. Fisher RI, Rosenberg SA, Fyfe G. Long-term survival update for high-dose recombinant interleukin-2 in patients with renal cell carcinoma. *Cancer J Sci Am.* 2000;6(suppl 1):S55–S57.
34. Rosenberg SA, Yang JC, White DE, et al. Durability of complete responses in patients with metastatic cancer treated with high-dose interleukin-2: identification of the antigens mediating response. *Ann Surg.* 1998;228(3):307–319.
35. Figlin RA, Pierce WC, Kaboo R, et al. Treatment of metastatic renal cell carcinoma with nephrectomy, interleukin-2 and cytokine-primed or CD8(+) selected tumor infiltrating lymphocytes from primary tumor. *J Urol.* 1997;158(3 Pt 1):740–745.
36. Joffe JK, Banks RE, Forbes MA, et al. A phase II study of interferon-alpha, interleukin-2 and 5-fluorouracil in advanced renal carcinoma: clinical data and laboratory evidence of protease activation. *Br J Urol.* 1996;77(5):638–649.
37. Motzer RJ, Escudier B, Oudard S, et al. Efficacy of everolimus in advanced renal cell carcinoma: a double-blind, randomised, placebo-controlled phase III trial. *Lancet.* 2008;372(9637):449–456.
38. Hudes G, Carducci M, Tomczak P, et al. Temsirolimus, interferon alfa, or both for advanced renal-cell carcinoma. *N Engl J Med.* 2007;356(22):2271–2281.
39. Freyer G, Ligneau B, Trillet-Lenoir VV. Palliative hormone therapy, low-dose chemotherapy, and bisphosphonate in breast cancer patients with bone marrow involvement and pancytopenia: report of a pilot experience. *Eur J Intern Med.* 2000;11(6):329–333.
40. Venturino A, Comandini D, Granetto C, et al. Formestane is feasible and effective in elderly breast cancer patients with comorbidity and disability. *Breast Cancer Res Treat.* 2000;62(3):217–222.
41. Basso U, Tonti S, Bassi C, et al. Management of frail and not-frail elderly cancer patients in a hospital-based geriatric oncology program. *Crit Rev Oncol Hematol.* 2008;66(2):163–170.
42. Crivellari D, Sun Z, Coates AS, et al. Letrozole compared with tamoxifen for elderly patients with endocrine-responsive early breast cancer: the BIG 1–98 trial. *J Clin Oncol.* 2008;26(12):1972–1979.
43. Coleman RE, Banks LM, Girgis SI, et al. Skeletal effects of exemestane on bone-mineral density, bone biomarkers, and fracture incidence in postmenopausal women with early breast cancer participating in the Intergroup Exemestane Study (IES): a randomised controlled study. *Lancet Oncol.* 2007;8(2):119–127.
44. Coombes RC, Kilburn LS, Snowdon CF, et al. Survival and safety of exemestane versus tamoxifen after 2–3 years' tamoxifen treatment (Intergroup Exemestane Study): a randomised controlled trial. *Lancet.* 2007;369(9561):559–570.

DEMENTIA

What Is the Clinical Course of Advanced Dementia?

Eric Widera and Kenneth E. Covinsky

INTRODUCTION AND SCOPE OF THE PROBLEM

Dementia is a clinical syndrome associated with significant changes in cognition, behavior, and functional status. It is characterized by the development of multiple cognitive and behavioral impairments involving at least two of the following domains: (1) memory, (2) executive function (reasoning, planning, judgment), (3) visuospatial ability, (4) language, (5) and personality or behavior.[1] Importantly, the decline in cognitive abilities must be severe enough to interfere with social or occupational functioning, and cannot be accounted for by other psychiatric conditions such as depression.

It is currently estimated that 24 million people worldwide have dementia.[2] The incidence increases with age, rising from 5% in those aged 71 to 79 years to more than 30% in those aged 90 and older.[3] Alzheimer disease represents the majority of these cases, accounting for over 50%. Others include vascular dementia, Lewy body dementia, dementia related to Parkinson disease, and frontotemporal dementia. These different types of dementia are associated with distinct symptom patterns, but often overlap exists (Table 51-1).

For the vast majority of dementias, the clinical course is relentlessly progressive, irreversible, and ultimately fatal. Initially, the decline in cognition may

TABLE 51-1. Dementia Syndromes and Key Features

TYPE OF DEMENTIA	CHARACTERISTICS
Alzheimer disease	Most common type of dementia
	Memory impairment, with difficulty remembering names and recent events often seen early in the disease
	Impaired behavior changes and difficulty speaking, swallowing, and walking seen later in disease
	Deposition of β-amyloid (plaques) and tau (tangles) in brain
Vascular dementia	Second most common type of dementia
	Criteria for dementia occurring in the setting of historical, physical, or neuroimaging evidence of cerebrovascular disease
	May present as an abrupt deterioration in cognitive function or in a fluctuating, stepwise manner.
Mixed dementia	Disease progression and pattern similar to that of Alzheimer disease and vascular dementia
Lewy body dementia	Progressive cognitive decline accompanied by well-formed visual hallucinations, parkinsonism, and fluctuating levels of alertness
	Notable sensitivity to neuroleptic medications
	Insoluble α-synuclein aggregations in brain are a key pathological feature
Parkinson disease	Distinguished by dementia occurring in the setting of well-established Parkinson disease rather than before or soon after parkinsonian symptoms developed
Frontotemporal dementia	A heterogeneous disorder characterized by focal atrophy of the frontal and temporal lobes
	Prominent features include personality and behavior change, with inappropriate social conduct, early loss of insight, and blunted emotional responses
	Often seen in individuals younger than those with Alzheimer's disease.
Normal pressure hydrocephalus	Pathologically enlarged ventricular size with normal opening pressures on lumbar puncture
	Associated with a classic triad of dementia, gait disturbance, and urinary incontinence
	Potentially reversible by the placement of a ventriculoperitoneal shunt

manifest itself as behavioral and mood changes, as well as the inability to perform instrumental activities of daily living, such as managing medications, using the telephone, shopping, and handling finances.[4] In the end stage of the disease, the different dementia syndromes can appear very similar, with individuals losing the ability to communicate, recognize loved ones, and ambulate. These individuals have a very poor prognosis and are likely to experience a high burden of illness such as dysphagia, aspiration pneumonia, and weight loss, as well as having increased risk for multiple burdensome interventions.

RELEVANT PATHOPHYSIOLOGY

The accumulation of extracellular amyloid plaques, formation of intracellular neurofibrillary tangles, and loss of neurons are characteristic findings seen at autopsy in individuals with advanced Alzheimer disease. Amyloid plaques are likely the result of abnormal metabolism of amyloid-β 40 and amyloid-β 42, leading to plaque accumulation. These plaques accumulate in areas of the brain responsible for learning and memory, most notably the hippocampus and entorhinal cortex. Neurofibrillary tangles consist mainly of hyperphosphorylated tau protein, a microtubule assembly protein. The mechanism for neuronal death and its relationship to neuritic plaques and neurofibrillary tangles continues to be an area of great controversy, because these pathological findings can be observed at autopsy in older adults who had no clinical evidence of dementia during their lifetime. More research is needed to distinguish whether plaques and tangles are the mediators or the by-products of the pathogenesis of Alzheimer disease.[5]

Classifying the Severity of Dementia

Decline in cognitive and functional ability in Alzheimer dementia can be viewed as passing through stages, although significant variation occurs among individuals and types of dementia. In mild dementia, individuals often have impairments with recent memories and difficulties with complex tasks, such as managing financial affairs.[4] As the disease progresses, individuals lose cognitive and physical function. They begin to have problems with disorientation, often getting lost in familiar places, and have increasing difficulty recognizing family and friends. Moderate dementia is commonly associated with significant deficits with complex tasks and an increased need for assistance with basic activities of daily living. In the most advanced stages, individuals with dementia become completely dependent on others, often requiring around-the-clock care. Loss of the ability to ambulate independently, to communicate with others, and to eat without assistance is characteristic of the end stage of the disease. The predominant functional trajectory for these individuals is a persistently severe disability, in which they are completely dependent in basic activities of daily living throughout the last year of life.[6]

Staging the severity of dementia may be aided by using standardize cognitive assessment tools, such as the Mini-Mental State Examination (MMSE),[7] and global severity scales. Two of the most commonly used global severity scales are the Functional Assessment Staging (FAST) scale and the Clinical Dementia Rating (CDR) scale.[8] The FAST scale measures functional status in dementia and consists of 7 major stages split into 16 different substages (Table 51-2). The CDR rates impairments in memory, orientation, judgment and problem solving, community affairs, home and hobbies, and personal care based on a semistructured interview with the patient and an informant. The CDR ranges from 0 to 3, with higher scores indicating a greater severity of impairment. Although no singular definition of advanced dementia exists, individuals generally must score 10 or less on the MMSE, meet criteria for stage 6 or 7 on the FAST, or score a 3 on the CDR (Table 51-3).

TABLE 51-2. Summary of Functional Assessment Staging (FAST)

Stage 1	No subjective or objective impairments in cognition
Stage 2	Mainly subject complains of forgetting names and misplacing objects
Stage 3	Objective evidence of memory impairment, impairment beginning to affect work performance
Stage 4	Moderate cognitive decline, with impairments in instrumental activities of daily living
Stage 5	Difficulty with naming current aspects of life and some disorientation
Stage 6 (a-e)	Difficulty dressing, bathing, toileting without assistance; later divisions include urinary (6d) and fecal (6e) incontinence
Stage 7 (a-f)	Speech declines from <6 intelligible words per day (7a) to ≤1 (7b); progressive loss of ability to ambulate (7c), sit up (7d), smile (7e), and hold head up (7f)

From The National Hospice Organization. Medical guidelines for determining prognosis in selected non-cancer diseases. *Hosp J.* 1996;11(2):47-63.

TABLE 51-3. Staging the Severity of Dementia

SEVERITY OR STAGE	REFERENCE	EXAMPLES OF DEFICITS
Mild	MMSE >18 FAST stage 4 CDR = 1	Difficulty with instrumental activities of daily living (IADLs) such as finances, shopping, medication management. May need prompting for personal care
Moderate	MMSE = 10 – 18 FAST stages 5 and 6 CDR = 2	Same as for mild, plus difficulties with simpler food preparation, household cleanup, and yard work; may require some assistance with some self-care
Severe	MMSE <10 FAST stages 6 and 7 CDR = 3	Requires near total assistance with ADLs such as bathing, dressing, toileting, transferring

SUMMARY OF EVIDENCE REGARDING TREATMENT RECOMMENDATIONS

Prognosis

Individuals with dementia are at increased risk for death. The median survival after the diagnosis of Alzheimer disease ranges from 4 to 6 years after diagnosis.[9] The prognosis is worse for those with more advanced cognitive and functional impairment.[9] For those with advanced disease who reside in a nursing home, the 6-month mortality rate is 25%, with a median survival in one study of only 478 days.[10] Despite evidence for a poor prognosis, health care providers have overly optimistic prognoses for individuals with advanced dementia. In one study of nursing home admissions, only 1% of residents were perceived to have life expectancy of less than 6 months. However, 71% died within that same period.[11]

Estimating when individuals with advanced Alzheimer disease will die is difficult because of the prolonged period of severe functional and cognitive impairment that occurs before death. Currently, hospice eligibility criteria for dementia are based largely on whether patients meet or exceed stage 7c on the FAST scale and whether they have at least one complication from their dementia. Unfortunately, these criteria do not accurately predict 6-month survival. The criteria also fail to account for the observation that dementia often does not progress in a sequential pattern as documented in the FAST. Other validated models have been developed to predict survival in advanced dementia, although their accuracy remains poor in predicting the risk for death within 6 months.[12] One notable model that can be used in nursing home residents with advanced dementia is the Advanced Dementia Prognostic Tool (ADEPT).[13] The ADEPT can help identify nursing home residents with advanced dementia at high risk for death within 6 months, although these criteria are only marginally better than current hospice eligibility guidelines.

Complications of advanced dementia are common, with eating problems, pneumonias, and other febrile episodes occurring frequently near the end of life. The development of these complications should serve as a marker of very poor short-term survival. In a recent prospective study of advanced dementia residing in a nursing home, the 6-month mortality rates after the development of pneumonia, a febrile episode, or eating problems was 47%, 45%, and 39%, respectively.[10] Similar findings are seen in individuals with advanced dementia who are admitted to the hospital with either pneumonia or a hip fracture, with 6-month mortality rates exceeding 50%.[14] These findings underscore the fact that patients with advanced dementia may survive for long periods with severe functional and cognitive decline and at the same time are at risk for sudden, life-threatening events such as respiratory and urinary tract infections.

Place of Death and Hospice Use

Almost all individuals with advanced dementia require nursing home level care at some point in their illness. For most of these individuals, the nursing homes also will be the site of their death, representing a significant shift from hospitals or homes as the site of death. In 2001, 67% of dementia-related deaths occurred in nursing homes, ranging from 40% in Texas to 89% in Rhode Island.[15] Higher rates of hospital deaths were seen in states with a greater number of hospital beds and fewer nursing home beds.[15]

Hospice use among individuals with advanced dementia is increasing over time, although access varies substantially across the United States. For instance, Miller and colleagues[17] found that hospice use tripled over the span of 7 years for nursing home decedents with advanced dementia, increasing from 15% in 1999 to 43% in 2006.[16] Mean stays in hospice in advanced dementia residents also rose from 46 days in 1999 to 118 days in 2006.[16] Even though these data are encouraging, this only tells part of the story. The hospice length of stay distribution was found to be bimodal in this study, with 25% of dementia residents having stays of 1 week or less and 20% having stays of over 6 months. This distribution is likely the result of the restrictive prognosis-based Medicare eligibility guidelines and the difficulty clinicians have in assessing prognosis in advanced dementia.[17]

Symptoms

Distressing signs and symptoms are common for individuals with advanced dementia and increase as death approaches. In one study of nursing home residents with advanced dementia, the proportions of residents who had distressing symptoms during the 18-month follow-up period was remarkably high, with 46% having dyspnea, 39% having pain 5 or more days per month, 39% having stage II or higher pressure ulcers, and 54% having agitation.[10] Furthermore, dyspnea, pain, pressure ulcers, and aspiration all increased in likelihood as the end of life approached.

The undertreatment of physical symptoms in patients with dementia is common.[18] For example, individuals with advanced dementia recovering from hip fracture surgery have been shown to receive only a third of the amount of opioid analgesia compared with cognitively intact adults.[19] Only a quarter of these individuals received any standing analgesia, despite the fact that pain is to be expected after hip surgery.[19] Furthermore, in a study of residents living in long-term care, documentation of pain and analgesic use decreased as cognitive impairment increased.[20] Community-dwelling individuals with dementia are also at highest risk for undertreatment of pain, with a 20% decreased probability of receiving analgesics for daily pain relative to patients with normal cognition.[21]

Burden of Medical Interventions

Individuals with advanced dementia frequently experience uncomfortable and aggressive interventions at the end of life. Mitchell and colleagues[11] found that 25% of residents with advanced dementia died with a feeding tube compared with 5% of residents with terminal cancer. This is despite a lack of evidence showing that feeding tubes improve survival or decrease complications for individuals with advanced dementia.[22] Most (68%) feeding-tube insertions are performed during an acute hospitalization, with the most common reasons for admission being pneumonia, dehydration, and dysphagia.[23] Median survival after insertion is short, at only 56 days.[23] Complications of feeding tube placement are high, with one in five tube-fed residents experiencing a tube-related complication necessitating a hospital transfer in the year following insertion.

Hospitalization is often considered when individuals with advanced dementia develop infections such as pneumonia.[24] Hospitalization for an infection should be thought of as a significant event in the course of advanced dementia because it heralds increased short-term morbidity and mortality. For instance, even if nursing home residents survive hospitalization for pneumonia, almost half (43%) develop another episode within 12 months.[25] Some literature suggests that among nursing home residents the hospital may not be the optimal setting for the treatment of pneumonia. Mortality rates appear similar whether treatment is provided in a nursing home or hospital, with some evidence suggesting greater functional decline in hospitalized residents.[26-28]

KEY MESSAGES TO PATIENTS AND FAMILIES

Discussions with patients and families about the clinical course of dementia should occur early in the course of the illness, preferably at the time of diagnosis. They should be made aware that dementia is a continuously progressive and ultimately fatal illness. In the advanced stages of the disease, patients may survive for long periods with severe functional and cognitive decline and at the same time are at risk for sudden, life-threatening events such as pneumonias. Without proper advance care planning, individuals with advanced dementia are likely to experience a high burden of illness and multiple burdensome interventions.

CONCLUSION AND SUMMARY

As the population continues to age, the prevalence of patients with dementia will increase. Research on the causes and treatments of dementia needs to continue so basic understanding and treatment of the disease improve, as does research on prognosis and treatment of symptoms and complications of the disease. Further education of patients and families about the progressive nature of the disease and its expected complications (e.g., difficulties with feeding near the end of life)

may improve outcomes while limiting procedures that are of little help. Likewise, the role of caregivers in the disease and the burden they experience when caring for an ill loved one with dementia needs to be further elucidated.

SUMMARY RECOMMENDATIONS

- Advanced dementia is a terminal illness and should be considered so when discussing treatment options and preferences with patients and family members.
- Although mortality rates are high in advanced dementia, no tools exist that accurately predict 6-month survival. Clinicians can, however, use scales to stage where patients are in the course of the disease, and this can assist in advance care planning.
- Symptoms such as pain and dyspnea should be recognized as common and treatable complications of advanced dementia.

REFERENCES

1. McKhann GM, Knopman DS, Chertkow H, et al. The diagnosis of dementia due to Alzheimer's disease: recommendations from the National Institute on Aging-Alzheimer's Association workgroups on diagnostic guidelines for Alzheimer's disease. *Alzheimers Dement.* 2011;7(3):263–269.
2. Ballard C, Gauthier S, Corbett A, Brayne C, Aarsland D, Jones E. Alzheimer's disease. *Lancet.* 2011;377(9770):1019–1031.
3. Plassman BL, Langa KM, Fisher GG, et al. Prevalence of dementia in the United States: the aging, demographics, and memory study. *Neuroepidemiology.* 2007;29(1–2):125–132.
4. Widera E, Steenpass V, Marson D, Sudore R. Finances in the older patient with cognitive impairment: "He didn't want me to take over". *JAMA.* 2011;305(7):698–706.
5. Querfurth HW, LaFerla FM. Alzheimer's disease. *N Engl J Med.* 2010;362(4):329–344.
6. Gill TM, Gahbauer EA, Han L, Allore HG. Trajectories of disability in the last year of life. *N Engl J Med.* 2010;362(13):1173–1180.
7. Folstein MF, Folstein SE, McHugh PR. Mini-Mental State: a practical method for grading the cognitive state of patients for the clinician. *J Psychiatr Res.* 1975;12(3):189–198.
8. Morris JC. The Clinical Dementia Rating (CDR): current version and scoring rules. *Neurology.* 1993;43(11):2412–2414.
9. Larson EB, Shadlen MF, Wang L, et al. Survival after initial diagnosis of Alzheimer disease. *Ann Intern Med.* 2004;140(7):501–509.
10. Mitchell SL, Teno JM, Kiely DK, et al. The clinical course of advanced dementia. *N Engl J Med.* 2009;361(16):1529–1538.
11. Mitchell SL, Kiely DK, Hamel MB. Dying with advanced dementia in the nursing home. *Arch Intern Med.* 2004;164(3):321–326.
12. Yaffe K. Treatment of Alzheimer disease and prognosis of dementia: time to translate research to results. *JAMA.* 2010;304(17):1952–1953.
13. Mitchell SL, Miller SC, Teno JM, Kiely DK, Davis RB, Shaffer ML. Prediction of 6-month survival of nursing home residents with advanced dementia using ADEPT vs hospice eligibility guidelines. *JAMA.* 2010;304(17):1929–1935.
14. Morrison RS, Siu AL. Survival in end-stage dementia following acute illness. *JAMA.* 2000;284(1):47–52.
15. Mitchell SL, Teno JM, Miller SC, Mor V. A national study of the location of death for older persons with dementia. *J Am Geriatr Soc.* 2005;53(2):299–305.
16. Miller SC, Lima JC, Mitchell SL. Hospice care for persons with dementia: The growth of access in US nursing homes. *Am J Alzheimers Dis Other Demen.* 2010;25(8):666–673.

17. Brickner L, Scannell K, Marquet S, Ackerson L. Barriers to hospice care and referrals: survey of physicians' knowledge, attitudes, and perceptions in a health maintenance organization. *J Palliat Med.* 2004;7(3):411–418.

18. Bernabei R, Gambassi G, Lapane K, et al. Management of pain in elderly patients with cancer: systematic assessment of geriatric drug use via epidemiology. SAGE Study Group. *JAMA.* 1998;279(23):1877–1882.

19. Morrison RS, Siu AL. A comparison of pain and its treatment in advanced dementia and cognitively intact patients with hip fracture. *J Pain Symptom Manage.* 2000;19(4):240–248.

20. Reynolds KS, Hanson LC, DeVellis RF, Henderson M, Steinhauser KE. Disparities in pain management between cognitively intact and cognitively impaired nursing home residents. *J Pain Symptom Manage.* 2008;35(4):388–396.

21. Landi F, Onder G, Cesari M, et al. Pain management in frail, community-living elderly patients. *Arch Intern Med.* 2001;161(22):2721–2724.

22. Sampson EL, Candy B, Jones L. Enteral tube feeding for older people with advanced dementia. *Cochrane Database Syst Rev.* 2009;(2):CD007209.

23. Kuo S, Rhodes RL, Mitchell SL, Mor V, Teno JM. Natural history of feeding-tube use in nursing home residents with advanced dementia. *J Am Med Dir Assoc.* 2009;10(4):264–270.

24. Volicer L, Hurley AC, Blasi ZV. Characteristics of dementia end-of-life care across care settings. *Am J Hosp Palliat Care.* 2003;20(3):191–200.

25. Muder RR, Brennen C, Swenson DL, Wagener M. Pneumonia in a long-term care facility: a prospective study of outcome. *Arch Intern Med.* 1996;156(20):2365–2370.

26. Fried TR, Gillick MR, Lipsitz LA. Whether to transfer? Factors associated with hospitalization and outcome of elderly long-term care patients with pneumonia. *J Gen Intern Med.* 1995;10(5):246–250.

27. Mylotte JM, Naughton B, Saludades C, Maszarovics Z. Validation and application of the pneumonia prognosis index to nursing home residents with pneumonia. *J Am Geriatr Soc.* 1998;46(12):1538–1544.

28. Fried TR, Gillick MR, Lipsitz LA. Short-term functional outcomes of long-term care residents with pneumonia treated with and without hospital transfer. *J Am Geriatr Soc.* 1997;45(3): 302–306.

Chapter 52

What Are Appropriate Palliative Interventions for Patients With Advanced Dementia?

ERIC WIDERA AND KENNETH E. COVINSKY

INTRODUCTION AND SCOPE OF THE PROBLEM

A growing body of literature shows that individuals with dementia receive suboptimal palliative care. Symptoms such as pain, dyspnea, and agitation are common, occurring in 40% to 50% of patients with advanced dementia. These symptoms become more common as dementia progresses and death nears.[1] Burdensome interventions, such as hospitalizations and parenteral therapy, are commonly seen in the last months of life. Those individuals with dementia who reside in a nursing home are further at risk for the undertreatment of symptoms and interventions that offer little evidence of benefit, including tube feeding and restraints.[2]

RELEVANT PALLIATIVE CARE ISSUES

Advanced dementia is the end stage of a progressive terminal illness in which individuals have significant impairments in both cognitive and functional status. Palliative care for individuals with advanced dementia should involve key interventions including advance care planning; hospice enrollment; caregiver support; management of symptoms, including pain and dementia-related behaviors; and avoidance of potentially inappropriate interventions. Improving the delivery of these palliative interventions can significantly improve the care given to individuals with dementia and their family members. In a study by Engel and colleagues,[3] greater satisfaction with care among decedents of nursing home residents with advanced dementia was associated with increased time spent discussing advance directives with the health care proxies, greater resident comfort, and less use of feeding tubes.

SUMMARY OF EVIDENCE REGARDING PALLIATIVE CARE INTERVENTIONS

Advance Care Planning

One of the most important aspects when caring for patients with dementia is to plan for continued disease progression. Advance care planning should occur as early as possible in the course of the illness, hopefully while patients maintain decision-making capacity for stating their values and preferences to guide decisions when they unable to speak for themselves. Specific aspects of care, such as artificial nutrition and hydration, intubation, cardiopulmonary resuscitation, and other common medical interventions at the end of life, should be explored with patients and their family members and documented in advance health care directives. However, taking a step back from the specifics and documenting overall values and goals, including whether the patient views comfort and quality of life as an overriding priority, may be more helpful for surrogate decision-makers when asked to weigh the risks and benefits of the many interventions frequently performed on patients with advanced dementia. This approach also highlights the importance of documenting a trusted designee to make decisions when an individual loses either medical or financial capacity through the use of a durable power of attorney for both health care and for financial matters.[4]

Verbally communicating aspects about the future course of dementia and asking what patients would want in the given scenario is the traditional method used for advance care planning. However, this type of advance planning may be difficult, because many patients may not understand what living with severe dementia is actually like. Using video-augmented advance care planning may help individuals who retain decision-making capacity make more informed decisions by allowing them to better envision future health states.[5] In one study, the use of videos helped focus decision making on patient-focused issues such as quality of life and effects on the family, rather than a conventional treatment-centric approach with an intent to preserve life as long as possible.[6] Individuals using the video decision support tool of advanced dementia are also more likely to choose a comfort-oriented approach compared with patients solely listening to a verbal narrative of the disease.[7]

Patient preferences are often not documented early in the disease, despite the anticipated loss of capacity that occurs with dementia. A common reason for this is that family members often do not realize the importance of discussing advance care plans with their loved one until it is too late to have the discussion.[8] When talking with family members of individuals with advanced dementia, it is important to frame these decisions in the context of having a terminal illness, because family members of nursing home residents with dementia who perceive that the patient's prognosis is poor have reduced likelihood of receiving burdensome interventions in the last 3 months of life.[1]

Hospice Enrollment

Hospice services should be considered for individuals with end-stage dementia. Hospice enrollment for individuals with end-stage dementia is associated with improved patient and caregiver outcomes compared to usual care.[9] Hospice enrollees are more likely than non–hospice enrollees to have better pain management and fewer hospitalizations during the last 30 days of life than those not receiving hospice services.[10] They are more likely to receive scheduled opioids for pain and symptomatic treatment for dyspnea, as well as have fewer unmet needs during the last 7 days of life.[11] Individuals with dementia are significantly more likely to die in their location of choice and less likely to die in the hospital if enrolled in hospice.[12] Furthermore, caregivers of individuals enrolled in hospice because of dementia also have greater satisfaction with end-of-life care.[12]

The current National Hospice and Palliative Care Organization (NHPCO) guidelines for hospice eligibility are of limited accuracy in predicting death within 6 months.[13] Nevertheless, it is important to note that effective use of hospice inevitably means that many patients who are referred will survive beyond 6 months and that appropriateness for hospice is not based on actual survival, but rather a reasonable expectation that survival will be less than 6 months. It would therefore be appropriate to refer to hospice individuals with advanced dementia who develop pneumonia, febrile episodes, or eating problems, because these are markers of a poor 6-month prognosis.

Caregiver Support

Informal caregivers provide the majority of care for patients with Alzheimer disease living in the community. As Alzheimer disease progresses and individuals become increasingly less functional, rates of informal care usage and caregiving hours increase substantially. Ultimately, patients require continuous supervision and care.[14] Many caregivers suffer adverse outcomes as a result of the extensive demands placed on them during the course of the disease. Caregivers are at greater risk for depression and anxiety, and some evidence suggests that they have an increased risk for mortality. In one study, nearly 43% of family caregivers who were providing care for patients with dementia had clinically significant levels of depression during the last few months of the patient's life.[15] Caregivers are at risk for adverse health outcomes not only while providing care at home but also after their loved one is moved to an institutional care environment. This is particularly true of spouses who place their relative in a long-term care facility, because they continue to have high rates of depression and anxiety.[15] For these family members, caregiving does not end with transfer to an institutional setting; many continue to visit their loved ones daily in institutional environments and continue to provide physical care during these visits.

Multicomponent interventions combining education, counseling, and support are effective in supporting caregivers and may improve outcomes, including well-being. Callahan and colleagues[16] tested a collaborative care approach led by advanced practice nurses who worked with caregivers and were integrated within primary care. This intervention led to significant improvements in the quality of care and in behavioral and psychological symptoms of dementia among primary care patients and their caregivers.[16] Another example of a caregiver support intervention is Resources for Enhancing Alzheimer's Caregiver Health (REACH II), which combines an individualized multicomponent home-based and telephone-based intervention designed to enhance caregivers' coping skills and management of dementia-related behaviors.[17] The REACH II intervention significantly improved caregiver quality of life in terms of burden, depression, self-care and healthy behaviors, social support, and management of patient problem behaviors. It also resulted in one extra hour per day that caregivers were not required to provide direct patient care. If multicomponent interventions are not available, clinicians can support caregivers by providing many of the components of these interventions, including advice about behavior management, or referral to respite care or adult day health programs.

Pain Management

The assessment and effective management of pain in advanced dementia presents clinicians with significant challenges. An often-cited fear of using opioids in individuals with dementia is that they may exacerbate comorbid illnesses or precipitate adverse effects such as delirium. However, good evidence indicates that undertreatment of pain is a greater risk factor for the development of delirium than the use of opioids.[18] A perception exists that individuals with dementia feel and experience less pain, because they commonly report less pain to their health care providers and caregivers. Inadequate assessment of pain as a result of poor patient recall and communication of painful symptoms is the most likely cause of the underreporting of symptoms, because numerous studies have shown that pain sensitivity and perceptual processing of pain remain largely intact with advanced dementia.[19]

The assessment of pain in dementia should include a combination of patient reports, caregiver reports, and direct observation of the patient. Even people with moderate to severe dementia may be able to communicate the presence and severity of pain currently experienced. Patients with advanced dementia may have difficulty with verbal rating scales; verbal descriptor scales, visual analog scales, pain thermometers, and the Wong-Baker Faces Pain Scales can be used as alternatives. Direct observations by the health care provider or caregivers are valuable in the assessment of pain in advanced dementia. Observational signs of distress may include changes in facial expressions, vocalizations, body movements, interpersonal interactions, activity patterns, and mental status. Agitation, irritability, and physical aggression may also occur, especially if exacerbation of pain occurs during caregiver tasks. Several observational scales have been developed to assess for pain. The best validated tools include the Pain Assessment in Advanced Dementia (PAINAD), the Pain Assessment Checklist for Seniors with Limited Ability to Communicate (PACSLAC), and the Doloplus-2 scale.[20]

The choice of an analgesic medication should be made based on the severity of pain, the previous responses to analgesic medications, the interaction of the analgesic with comorbid conditions, and the care setting and support services. Acetaminophen should be considered the first-line therapy for mild pain when caring for those with dementia. It should also be considered with new behavior changes even if the presence of pain is uncertain, because evidence suggests that acetaminophen may lead to improved activity levels and social engagement in nursing home residents with moderate to severe dementia.[21] The use of NSAIDs, including cyclooxygenase-2– selective inhibitors, should generally be avoided in this population because of the high risk for side effects, including renal failure, gastrointestinal irritation, and worsening heart failure.

Opioids remain an effective therapy for treating pain in dementia, although greater consideration should be given to drug selection and dosing frequency when prescribing these agents for patients with dementia. Impairments in renal or hepatic function are common with age, as are changes in the volume of distribution as a result of decreased muscle mass and increased body fat. These changes increase sensitivity to adverse effects from opioids in individuals with dementia. Opioids that should be avoided for these reasons include propoxyphene and meperidine; their metabolites often lead to adverse effects such as delirium. Individuals with severe cognitive impairment are also likely to be unable to request pain medications because of cognitive impairment, significantly decreasing the effectiveness of short-acting medications given only as needed for pain. Around-the-clock dosing and long-acting formulations are better alternatives, especially when managing chronic pain. As with all individuals treated with an opioid, constipation should be aggressively managed with a stimulant laxative, such as senna.

Interventions for Behavioral and Psychological Symptoms

The majority of individuals with Alzheimer disease will develop behavioral symptoms during their illness, including wandering, agitation, repetitive vocalization, or resistance to care.[22] Although these symptoms often occur earlier in the disease, many patients continue to have challenging behaviors in the later stages of dementia. Behavioral issues cause significant strain on caregivers and are associated with caregivers' decisions for nursing home admission.

The initial treatment of behavioral symptoms should focus on identifying a primary cause and creating a treatment plan to mitigate this cause. Other nonpharmacological interventions may include music therapy, massage, and physical activity.[23] Pharmacotherapy should be considered only when nonpharmacologic approaches have failed or the behaviors are severe enough to become a safety issue. Antipsychotics should generally be avoided in dementia because they are associated with significant increase in stroke and death.[24,25] Antipsychotic medications also help little in the way of improving behaviors except for some modest efficacy for the treatment of aggression and psychosis over a short 6- to 12-week course.[26] Limited evidence exists of any longer-term benefit. Little difference in effectiveness has been noted between first-generation antipsychotics (e.g., haloperidol) and second-generation agents. Valproic acid and divalproex are also frequently prescribed to treat dementia-related behaviors. However, these drugs are ineffective to treat agitation and have an unacceptable rate of adverse effects, including somnolence, thrombocytopenia, infection.[27]

Avoidance of Potentially Inappropriate Interventions

Cognitive Interventions. Acetylcholinesterase inhibitors, such as donepezil, galantamine, and rivastigmine, and the N-methyl-D-aspartate (NMDA) antagonist memantine are the classes of pharmacological agents currently available to modify the clinical manifestations of Alzheimer disease. Several studies suggest statistically significant improvements in cognitive, functional, and behavioral outcomes with the use of cholinesterase inhibitors and memantine in patients with moderate to severe dementia.[28] The clinical significance of this is less clear, especially in patients with more advanced disease. Furthermore, few of the trials on these agents include subjects with functional impairment substantial enough to meet hospice eligibility requirements. Despite the lack of evidence for their use in end-stage dementia, both cholinesterase inhibitors and memantine are commonly prescribed in this population. In one study of hospice enrollees with a primary hospice diagnosis of Alzheimer dementia, dementia, or cerebral degeneration, 21.3% were prescribed at least one of these medications.[29]

Adverse events are common with both cholinesterase inhibitors and memantine. Nearly a third of trial participants experience some type of adverse side effect, with nausea, vomiting, and diarrhea being the most common.[28] Use of acetylcholinesterase inhibitors is also associated with increased risks for syncope, bradycardia, permanent pacemaker insertion, and hip fracture in community-dwelling older adults.[30] Given the lack of proven benefit and the high rates of side effects, these agents should be used sparingly, if at all, in individuals with advanced disease who are near the end of life.

Nutritional Interventions. Feeding and eating difficulties become increasingly common as dementia progresses, often leading to progressive weight loss. It is important to rule out comorbid depression, medication side effects, dental issues, and functional difficulties as possible reversible causes of weight loss. For instance, apraxia may result in difficulty using utensils, making it difficult to impossible for individuals to feed themselves without significant caregiver assistance. Poor food intake may also be due to nonmodifiable factors, including the loss of appetite and satiety resulting from changes in limbic or hypothalamic function, or the development of impairments with the act of swallowing.[31]

When eating and swallowing difficulties arise, family members are often faced with the decision to administer food and fluids by nasogastric tube or percutaneous endoscopic gastrostomy (PEG) tube. Use of these feeding tubes has not been shown to improve survival for individuals with dementia.[32] No evidence has demonstrated that tube feeding prevents aspiration pneumonia, deceases the risk for pressure ulcers, improves patient comfort, or prolongs life.[31] In addition to possible postoperative complications, other significant harms that may arise from use of feeding tubes include decreased pleasure from tasting foods, likelihood of less caregiver contact during the mealtime, and possible need to use restraints to prevent feeding tube displacement.

Despite the lack of evidence for their effectiveness, PEG tubes are commonly placed in individuals with dementia, with more than one third of severely cognitively impaired residents in the United States having feeding tubes.[33,34] Placement of PEG tubes often occurs after transfer to an acute care facility for eating problems or pneumonia. It is therefore important to discuss and document preferences for and alternatives to artificial nutrition and hydration before any hospitalization, preferably on admission to the nursing home. Alternatives to PEG placement include careful hand feeding and proper oral care. In contrast to the paucity of data on PEG tubes, oral care has been shown to decrease incidence of pneumonia, number of febrile days, and death from pneumonia in nursing home residents.[35]

Antibiotics. Pneumonia is the most commonly identified cause of death among individuals with advanced Alzheimer disease. It has been debated whether antibiotic therapy for pneumonia is beneficial in individuals with advanced Alzheimer disease. In one recent prospective study of 323 nursing home residents with advanced dementia, antibiotic therapy for episodes of pneumonia did improve survival after pneumonia compared with no antibiotic treatment. However, treatment with antibiotics for pneumonia was associated with lower scores on the Symptom Management at End-of-Life in Dementia scale, indicating more discomfort compared to untreated residents.[36] If antibiotics are not given, comfort can adequately maintained with aggressive use of antipyretics, analgesics, and oxygen if hypoxic.

KEY MESSAGES TO PATIENTS AND FAMILIES

Educating patients and families about the progressive and terminal nature of dementia is a key palliative care intervention that may alter the treatments the patient receives and improve the coping of caregivers both during the illness and after the patient dies. Patients and families should be encouraged to have conversations about goals of treatments and desirable outcomes for their health early in the course of the disease, and it is important to document preferences through the use of comprehensive advance directives. Likewise, patients should designate an individual to act as their power of attorney for financial matters, because they are likely to be unable to manage them as the disease progresses.

CONCLUSION AND SUMMARY

Despite the fact that Alzheimer dementia is an incurable disease, patients and families should be made aware that many ways exist to preserve autonomy, relieve suffering, and maintain dignity as the disease progresses. Early use of hospice can improve the management of pain and other symptoms and should be considered for anyone who develops common complications of advanced dementia, such as pneumonia, recurrent fever, or eating problems. Health care providers should reassure caregivers that their well-being is an important aspect to the care of the patient and they too will be supported as the patient's disease progresses.

SUMMARY RECOMMENDATIONS

- Advance directives, including durable power of attorney forms for both health care and financial matters, should be documented soon after the diagnosis of dementia.
- Hospice referral should be considered for individuals with advanced dementia who develop pneumonia, febrile episodes, or difficulty eating, because these are markers of poor prognosis and limited life-expectancy.
- Multicomponent caregiver support interventions combining education, counseling, and support should be standard of care for community-dwelling individuals with dementia.
- Cholinesterase inhibitors and memantine offer little proven benefit in individuals with end-stage dementia and should be used sparingly.
- Permanent tube feeding is not recommended for individuals with advanced dementia who develop nutritional or feeding problems.

REFERENCES

1. Mitchell SL, Teno JM, Kiely DK, et al. The clinical course of advanced dementia. *N Engl J Med.* 2009;361(16):1529–1538.
2. Mitchell SL, Kiely DK, Hamel MB. Dying with advanced dementia in the nursing home. *Arch Intern Med.* 2004;164(3):321–326.
3. Engel SE, Kiely DK, Mitchell SL. Satisfaction with end-of-life care for nursing home residents with advanced dementia. *J Am Geriatr Soc.* 2006;54(10):1567–1572.
4. Widera E, Steenpass V, Marson D, Sudore R. Finances in the older patient with cognitive impairment: "He didn't want me to take over". *JAMA.* 2011;305(7):698–706.
5. Volandes AE, Lehmann LS, Cook EF, Shaykevich S, Abbo ED, Gillick MR. Using video images of dementia in advance care planning. *Arch Intern Med.* 2007;167(8):828–833.
6. Deep KS, Hunter A, Murphy K, Volandes A. "It helps me see with my heart": how video informs patients' rationale for decisions about future care in advanced dementia. *Patient Educ Couns.* 2010;81(2):229–234.
7. Volandes AE, Paasche-Orlow MK, Barry MJ, et al. Video decision support tool for advance care planning in dementia: randomised controlled trial. *BMJ.* 2009;338:b2159.
8. Hirschman KB, Kapo JM, Karlawish JH. Identifying the factors that facilitate or hinder advance planning by persons with dementia. *Alzheimer Dis Assoc Disord.* 2008;22(3):293–298.
9. Mitchell SL, Kiely DK, Miller SC, Connor SR, Spence C, Teno JM. Hospice care for patients with dementia. *J Pain Symptom Manage.* 2007;34(1):7–16.
10. Miller SC, Gozalo P, Mor V. Hospice enrollment and hospitalization of dying nursing home patients. *Am J Med.* 2001;111(1):38–44.
11. Kiely DK, Givens JL, Shaffer ML, Teno JM, Mitchell SL. Hospice use and outcomes in nursing home residents with advanced dementia. *J Am Geriatr Soc.* 2010;58(12):2284–2291.
12. Shega JW, Hougham GW, Stocking CB, Cox-Hayley D, Sachs GA. Patients dying with dementia: experience at the end of life and impact of hospice care. *J Pain Symptom Manage.* 2008;35(5):499–507.
13. Mitchell SL, Miller SC, Teno JM, Kiely DK, Davis RB, Shaffer ML. Prediction of 6-month survival of nursing home residents with advanced dementia using ADEPT vs hospice eligibility guidelines. *JAMA.* 2010;304(17):1929–1935.
14. Zhu CW, Scarmeas N, Torgan R, et al. Clinical characteristics and longitudinal changes of informal cost of Alzheimer's disease in the community. *J Am Geriatr Soc.* 2006;54(10):1596–1602.
15. Schulz R, Belle SH, Czaja SJ, McGinnis KA, Stevens A, Zhang S. Long-term care placement of dementia patients and caregiver health and well-being. *JAMA.* 2004;292(8):961–967.
16. Callahan CM, Boustani MA, Unverzagt FW, et al. Effectiveness of collaborative care for older adults with Alzheimer disease in primary care: a randomized controlled trial. *JAMA.* 2006;295(18):2148–2157.
17. Belle SH, Burgio L, Burns R, et al. Enhancing the quality of life of dementia caregivers from different ethnic or racial groups: a randomized, controlled trial. *Ann Intern Med.* 2006;145(10):727–738.
18. Morrison RS, Magaziner J, Gilbert M, et al. Relationship between pain and opioid analgesics on the development of delirium following hip fracture. *J Gerontol A Biol Sci Med Sci.* 2003;58(1):76–81.
19. Widera E, Smith A. Pain management in moderate and advanced dementia. *Geriatr Aging.* 2009;7(12):353–356.
20. Pargeon KL, Hailey BJ. Barriers to effective cancer pain management: a review of the literature. *J Pain Symptom Manage.* 1999;18(5):358–368.
21. Chibnall JT, Tait RC, Harman B, Luebbert RA. Effect of acetaminophen on behavior, well-being, and psychotropic medication use in nursing home residents with moderate-to-severe dementia. *J Am Geriatr Soc.* 2005;53(11):1921–1929.
22. Ballard CG, Gauthier S, Cummings JL, et al. Management of agitation and aggression associated with Alzheimer disease. *Nat Rev Neurol.* 2009;5(5):245–255.
23. Hulme C, Wright J, Crocker T, Oluboyede Y, House A. Non-pharmacological approaches for dementia that informal carers might try or access: a systematic review. *Int J Geriatr Psychiatry.* 2010;25(7):756–763.
24. Schneider LS, Dagerman KS, Insel P. Risk of death with atypical antipsychotic drug treatment for dementia: meta-analysis of randomized placebo-controlled trials. *JAMA.* 2005;294(15):1934–1943.
25. Sacchetti E, Turrina C, Valsecchi P. Cerebrovascular accidents in elderly people treated with antipsychotic drugs: a systematic review. *Drug Saf.* 2010;33(4):273–288.
26. Ballard C, Waite J. The effectiveness of atypical antipsychotics for the treatment of aggression and psychosis in Alzheimer's disease. *Cochrane Database Syst Rev.* 2006;(1): CD003476.
27. Lonergan E, Luxenberg J. Valproate preparations for agitation in dementia. *Cochrane Database Syst Rev.* 2009;(3): CD003945.
28. Birks J. Cholinesterase inhibitors for Alzheimer's disease. *Cochrane Database Syst Rev.* 2006;(1): CD005593.
29. Weschules DJ, Maxwell TL, Shega JW. Acetylcholinesterase inhibitor and N-methyl-D-aspartic acid receptor antagonist use among hospice enrollees with a primary diagnosis of dementia. *J Palliat Med.* 2008;11(5):738–745.
30. Gill SS, Anderson GM, Fischer HD, et al. Syncope and its consequences in patients with dementia receiving cholinesterase inhibitors: a population-based cohort study. *Arch Intern Med.* 2009;169(9):867–873.
31. Finucane TE, Christmas C, Travis K. Tube feeding in patients with advanced dementia: a review of the evidence. *JAMA.* 1999;282(14):1365–1370.
32. Sampson EL, Candy B, Jones L. Enteral tube feeding for older people with advanced dementia. *Cochrane Database Syst Rev.* 2009;(2):CD007209.
33. Mitchell SL, Kiely DK, Gillick MR. Nursing home characteristics associated with tube feeding in advanced cognitive impairment. *J Am Geriatr Soc.* 2003;51(1):75–79.
34. Ahronheim JC, Mulvihill M, Sieger C, Park P, Fries BE. State practice variations in the use of tube feeding for nursing home residents with severe cognitive impairment. *J Am Geriatr Soc.* 2001;49(2):148–152.
35. Yoneyama T, Yoshida M, Ohrui T, et al. Oral care reduces pneumonia in older patients in nursing homes. *J Am Geriatr Soc.* 2002;50(3):430–433.
36. Givens JL, Jones RN, Shaffer ML, Kiely DK, Mitchell SL. Survival and comfort after treatment of pneumonia in advanced dementia. *Arch Intern Med.* 2010;170(13):1102–1107.

ADVANCED LIVER DISEASE

Chapter 53

What Is the Clinical Course of Advanced Liver Disease and What Symptoms Are Associated With It?

ALUKO A. HOPE AND R. SEAN MORRISON

INTRODUCTION AND SCOPE OF THE PROBLEM

Chronic liver diseases (CLDs) are a set of diseases characterized by decreased hepatic function as a result of chronic inflammation or insult to the liver. At their most advanced stage, CLDs often lead to the development of cirrhosis, defined as the irreversible distortion of the liver architecture by fibrosis, scar, and abnormal nodules. With cirrhosis comes the risk for progressive liver dysfunction and complications of portal hypertension. Recent estimates suggest that approximately 5.5 million persons suffer from CLD worldwide and as many as 40,000 persons will die of its natural course or complications.[1] In the United States alone, CLD results in 4000 to 5000 deaths per year and 11,000 to 17,000 hospitalizations.[1] CLD is the twelfth leading cause of death in the United States.[2] Although liver transplantation can significantly improve the survival and quality of life for patients with advanced CLD, many patients are not eligible because of medical or social comorbidities and an additional 10% to 15% of eligible patients die waiting for a transplant because of the severe shortage of viable organs.[3] Patients with advanced CLD face a variety of symptoms that affect their survival and quality of life. Even those who receive a successful transplantation often experience complications associated with physical and emotional suffering and, in some cases, premature mortality.

Palliative care providers may be called in various settings to help manage symptoms or to help with communication, decision making, or care coordination for patients with CLD. Decision making and communication are complicated in this patient population due to the difficulty in predicting outcomes,[4] the patients' and families frequent misunderstandings of the life-limiting nature of the illness,[5] and the high risk of severe cognitive dysfunction that may impair decision-making capacity.[6,7] In contrast to diseases such as cancer, in which standard disease-modifying options often lose effectiveness even near the end of life, symptoms in patients with CLD can benefit from disease-specific treatments. This chapter discusses the common causes and symptoms of CLD. Chapter 54 discusses the special considerations needed for treating persons with CLD.

RELEVANT PATHOPHYSIOLOGY

Disorders Leading to Chronic Liver Disease

CLD and cirrhosis are the common final pathways in several different disorders. The majority of cases of CLD result from complications of alcohol and viral hepatitis, which together account for more than 75% of all cases.[8] Additional causes of CLD are in Table 53-1.

Alcohol. Chronic excessive alcohol use results in several diseases, including alcoholic hepatitis, fatty liver, and alcoholic cirrhosis.[9,10] Additionally, alcohol can exacerbate hepatic damage in the setting of other CLDs, including viral hepatitis, fatty liver disease secondary to obesity, and metabolic liver disease. Chronic alcohol use can result in the centrilobular, pericellular, or periportal fibrosis that disrupts the normal architecture of the liver. Ongoing fibrosis results in micronodular cirrhosis—a process that typically takes years to decades of ongoing alcohol-induced injury. Signs and symptoms of alcoholic liver disease are consistent with CLD and can be both nonspecific (e.g., right upper quadrant pain, nausea and vomiting, diarrhea, anorexia, generalized fatigue) or more liver specific (e.g., ascites, peripheral edema, anasarca, gastrointestinal hemorrhage). Occasionally, patients can present with late-stage jaundice or encephalopathy. The primary treatment of alcohol-related liver disease is cessation of alcohol use combined with enhanced nutrition. Transplantation is an option for those with end-stage disease, although most transplant programs

TABLE 53-1. Epidemiology of Chronic Liver Disease in the United States[8]

CAUSE	PERCENT NEWLY DIAGNOSED CASES OF CHRONIC LIVER DISEASE
Alcohol (alcohol liver disease [ALD])	8
Viral	
Hepatitis B	3
Hepatitis C alone	42
Hepatitis C with ALD	22
Biliary cirrhosis	
Primary biliary cirrhosis	1.5
Primary sclerosing cholangitis	1
Autoimmune cholangiopathy	<1
Miscellaneous causes	
Autoimmune hepatitis	1.5
Cardiac cirrhosis	<1
Cryptogenic cirrhosis	1
Metabolic liver diseases	<1
α_1-Antitrypsin deficiency	<1
Cystic fibrosis	1
Hemochromatosis	<1
Wilson's disease	9
Nonalcoholic steatohepatitis	
Undetermined	9

Data from Bell BP, Manos MM, Zaman A, et al. The epidemiology of newly diagnosed chronic liver disease in gastroenterology practices in the United States: results from population-based surveillance. *Am J Gastroenterol.* 2008;103:2727-2736.

require abstinence from alcohol for a period of 6 months before being considered for transplant. Five-year survival of patients who continue to consume alcohol in the setting of cirrhosis is less than 50%.[9,10]

Chronic Viral Hepatitis. Hepatitis B (HBV) and C (HCV) are now the leading cause of CLD both in the United States and in the world, although the prevalence ratios are markedly different. Worldwide, the ratio of hepatitis B/C carriers is 2:1, whereas in the United States, that ratio is reversed (1:2).[1] Recent estimates suggest that in the United States more than 1.25 million people are carriers of HBV and more than 2.5 million carriers of HCV (300-400 million and 170 million, respectively, worldwide).[1] Approximately 20% of CLD patients with HBV will eventually progress to cirrhosis.[1] Progression in the setting of chronic HCV is slightly higher, with 30% of patients with CLD eventually developing cirrhosis.[1] Approximately 15% of those with cirrhosis from viral hepatitis will develop hepatocellular carcinoma (HCC).[1] Liver damage from both HBV and HCV is similar. Damage is likely immune mediated, with the development of portal-based fibrosis and progression to a mixed micronodular and macronodular cirrhosis. Clinical signs and symptoms are those of CLD as described above. Antiviral treatment for HBV is quite effective and indeed can reverse decompensated liver disease. Currently available treatments include lamivudine, adefovir, telbivudine, entecavir, and tenofovir. Interferon-α also can be effective but should be avoided in the presence of cirrhosis. Treatment regimens for HCV are more problematic. Although highly effective when tolerated, dose-limiting cytopenias and severe side effects can result in discontinuation of both pegylated interferon and ribavirin therapies. Orthotopic liver transplantation is an accepted and effective treatment for viral CLD.

Hepatocellular Carcinoma. CLD is a major risk factor for hepatocellular carcinoma (HCC). HCC is the ninth leading cause of cancer deaths in the United States, the second leading cause of cancer deaths worldwide in men, and the sixth leading cause of death in women. Annual global incidence hovers around 1 million cases. In the United States, it has been shown to be the fastest growing cause of cancer-related death in men.[11] Infection with HBV or HCV is the major risk factor for HCC. Of all patients diagnosed with HCC, 80% have an underlying infection with HBV or HCV.[11] Progression from infection with HBC or HCV to cirrhosis takes approximately 20 to 40 years, and thereafter the annual risk for HCC is 2% to 3% for HBV and 1% to 7% for HCV.[12] In the setting of alcohol-induced HCC, the risk is approximately 1% per year.[12] Hepatocellular cancer can develop in the absence of cirrhosis in patients with HBV infection at a rate of 0.26% to 0.6% per year.[12]

Typically, patients with HCC are asymptomatic during the early stages of the disease; approximately 80% of diagnoses are made at advanced stages when prognosis is poor.[13] Median survival of untreated patients with newly diagnosed hepatocellular cancer is weeks to months.[12] Factors associated with worse outcome include male sex, advanced age, etiological agent (HCV worse than HBV), presence of more than one risk factor, size, number and doubling time of nodules, vascular invasion, and distant metastasis.[12] Surgical resection is the mainstay of treatment for most patients when technically possible. Keys to surgical eligibility include appropriate liver reserve following resection and the absence of portal hypertension. With these criteria, 60% to 70% 5-year survival rates have been reported. Seventy percent of patients will develop tumor recurrence by 5 years.[12] For the small group who qualify (i.e., patients with one solitary lesion <5 cm or three lesions each <3 cm), liver transplantation offers long-term survival benefits.[12] Whereas early experience with orthotopic liver transplantation for HCC was relatively dismal because of poor selection criteria (recurrence rates >80%), a landmark study confirmed that excellent outcomes can be achieved with orthotopic liver transplantation, with 5-year survival of 70% with recurrence rates as low as 15% for HCC if certain criteria are met (single lesion <5 cm, three lesions <3 cm in diameter, no extrahepatic metastasis, or no vascular invasion).[14]

Orthotopic Liver Transplantation

Orthotopic liver transplantation (OLT), first performed in 1963 has become a standard treatment for end-stage liver disease and select cases of HCC (see earlier discussion). Survival rates of 7 to 10 years for OLT range from 60% to 80% depending on the underlying disease.[1] Complications of transplantation relate to technical aspects of the transplantation, rejection (acute and chronic), consequences of long-term immunosuppression, and recurrence of the primary disease leading to transplantation. The disorders most commonly associated with recurrence include HBV and HCV infection and HCC, as noted earlier. The recent practice of administering hepatitis B immune globulin at the time of OLT and at regular intervals thereafter, in combination with other antivirals, has dramatically reduced the incidence of HBV recurrence to less than 10%.[1] Conversely, HCV viremia almost always occurs after OLT, although the progression of liver disease is highly variable, with some having indolent disease and others progressing to cirrhosis and recurrent liver failure. Treatment is unfortunately limited by toxicity.

SUMMARY OF EVIDENCE REGARDING TREATMENT RECOMMENDATIONS

Symptoms and Treatment in End-Stage Liver Disease

Pain. Data from the Study to Understand Prognoses and Preferences for Outcomes and Risk of Treatments (SUPPORT) suggest that severe pain is quite common and protracted in patients with CLD who are seriously ill.[15] Aggressive symptom control may improve quality of life in these patients.[16] The basic principles of pain assessment and management apply equally for patients with CLD. The standard World Health Organization ladder approach to pain management will need modification in patients with advanced CLD and cirrhosis because of the altered pharmacokinetics and pharmacodynamics that can occur in patients with decreased hepatic function.[17] For mild pain in patients with hepatic dysfunction, acetaminophen is preferred over the selective or nonselective antiinflammatory drugs (NSAIDS). NSAIDS, by suppressing the afferent vasodilatory effect of the renal prostaglandin, can lead to acute renal insufficiency in patients with cirrhosis.[17-19] In addition, the antiplatelet effect of the NSAIDS can precipitate a gastrointestinal hemorrhage. The preponderance of data does not suggest an increased risk for hepatic injury with short-term use of acetaminophen in the therapeutic range (≤ 4 g/day).[20] The multiple case reports describing worsening liver disease in patients with CLD after acetaminophen use are all in the context of acetaminophen overdose, either as a suicide gesture or through patients ingesting medications they did not know contain acetaminophen.[18] Although no prospective studies have assessed the long-term safety of acetaminophen in patients with cirrhosis or hepatic dysfunction, many experts recommend a reduced dose of 2 to 3 g/day for long-term acetaminophen use in nonalcoholic patients with hepatic dysfunction.[20] Extra caution may be warranted for both short-term and long-term use of acetaminophen in patients with a history of alcohol abuse and nonadherence to medications.[21,22]

For patients with moderate to severe pain, opioid analgesics can be safely used in the setting of hepatic dysfunction. The risks and benefits of starting opioids

should be discussed openly with the patient and all involved health care practitioners, particularly the providers in the liver transplant pr ogram, as applicable. Opioids are known to precipitate or contribute to hepatic encephalopathy (through the drug effect or through the opioid-induced constipation); therefore patients with CLD on who are on opioids and their families should have an action plan for the possibility of cognitive changes.

Codeine, dextropropoxyphene, meperidine, and tramadol should be avoided in patients with CLD because of decreased efficacy and increased risk for adverse events.[17] Oxymorphone is contraindicated in patients with moderate to severe hepatic dysfunction and is therefore best avoided in patients with CLD. It may be prudent to avoid morphine in patients with severe hepatic dysfunction or any element of impaired renal function. When starting opioids in patients with CLD, a generally followed approach is the "start low and go slow" method: decrease the typical starting dose by 25% to 50% and increase the frequency for short-acting opioids from every 4 hours to every 6 hours. Fentanyl, hydromorphone, and oxycodone are the preferred opioids in patients with CLD. The use of methadone in patients with CLD should be considered only if expert guidance is available given the wide interindividual variability in pharmacokinetics and the potential for significant drug interactions in seriously ill patients. The type of pain, its severity, and the risk for adverse drug events (including polypharmacy) are all considered when deciding on adjuvant analgesics (e.g., anticonvulsants and antidepressants) in patients with severe pain and CLD.

A high prevalence of prior or active substance abuse is found in patients with CLD. Although an approach to pain treatment in patients with a history of substance abuse is beyond the scope of this review, routine screening for a history of current or prior substance abuse, family history of substance abuse, and psychiatric disorders such as depression or anxiety may help palliative care providers in devising an individualized, comprehensive approach to pain treatment in patients with CLD. In patients on methadone maintenance, pharamacokinetic studies suggest that the doses in CLD can be safely maintained until very late into their illness trajectory.[23,24]

Pruritus. Pruritus is a complication of CLD that has been associated with poorer quality of life.[25] Although known to occur in CLD of any origin,[26] it is more common in patients with cholestatic liver diseases.[27] The pathogenesis of pruritus in CLD remains elusive, but it is thought to be mediated by some pruritogenic substance or substances that accumulate as a result of impaired biliary secretion.[27] These pruritogens may act at the nerve endings at the level of the skin or act centrally to mediate itching.

Therapeutic efforts to treat pruritus should first ensure that the underlying disease is adequately addressed. Pruritus from extrahepatic biliary obstruction is often effectively treated by endoscopic biliary stenting, percutaneous biliary drainage, or surgical biliodigestive anastomoses. Pruritus secondary to intrahepatic cholestasis is more challenging to treat and often requires careful empiric trials.

Nonabsorbable resins such as cholestyramine and cholestipol have been used extensively in patients with cholestasis-associated pruritus.[27] These agents binds anions and ampiphathic substances, including the bile salts and the putative pruritogens, thereby preventing reuptake in the terminal ileum and facilitating fecal excretion. Up to 80% of patients respond partially or completely to these agents.[27] The starting dose of cholestyramine is 4 g once or twice per day, which can be increased steadily to up to 16 g daily. Pruritogens are thought to accumulate in the gallbladder overnight; therefore the drug is usually given 30 minutes to 1 hour before and after breakfast.[27,28] These drugs decrease the absorption of multiple drugs and the fat-soluble vitamins and are thus taken 4 hours before any other medications. Adverse effects include abdominal discomfort, bloating, and diarrhea.[27,29]

Rifampicin is a semisynthetic antibiotic that has been shown to be an effective short-term treatment of pruritus[27,29] at doses of 300 to 600 mg per day. Long-term use is precluded by hepatotoxicity, severe idiosyncratic reactions such as hemolytic anemia, renal failure, and thrombocytopenic purpura.[27,29] Because it is an enzyme inducer, its use may have important implications in the efficacy of concomitantly administered drugs. In particular, patients on methadone maintenance will experience withdrawal symptoms when treated with rifampicin. Patients should be warned that the drug will change the color of their urine and tears to orange-red.[27,29]

Opioid antagonists have been shown in multiple studies to be an efficacious treatment for pruritus in CLD. Patients with CLD pruritus have high plasma levels of opioids and opioid receptor levels in the brain are decreased in cholestasis.[30] Both intravenous (naloxone 0.4 mg bolus followed by a continuous infusion) and oral (nalmefone at 60-120 mg/day and naltrexone at 25-50 mg/day) agents have been shown to be efficacious in CLD-associated pruritus.[31] The temporary opioid withdrawal reaction commonly seen in treating these patients can be treated by coadministration of clonidine during the first week of the treatment[32] or starting with a subtherapeutic dose of the opioid antagonist and slowly increasing to a therapeutic range. In using an oral opioid antagonist, it may even be necessary to start with a subtherapeutic intravenous infusion of naloxone, slowly increase the naloxone to therapeutic range, and then switch to small doses of an orally bioavailable opioid antagonist.[33] With long-term administration of these agents for pruritus, a breakthrough phenomenon has been observed in which the perception of pruritus is increased in the early weeks of treatment, likely mediated by the upregulation of the opiate receptors in the brain leading to an increased sensitivity to endogenous opioids.[27] This breakthrough phenomenon is treated by either an upward titration of the opioid antagonist[34] or with treatment interruption for 2 days every week.[35]

Opioid-receptor selectivity may be important in mediating the pruritus of CLD. Recent case reports suggest that butorphanol, a commercially available kappa-opioid agonist and mu-opioid antagonist, may have efficacy in intractable pruritus in patients with CLD.[28,36]

Ascites. Ascites is the most common complication of CLD and the most common reason for hospital admission.[37] Both the presence of ascites and the frequency of hospitalizations have been found to be important predictors of poor quality of life in patients with CLD.[25]

All patients with CLD and ascites should be maintained on a low-sodium diet, thereby delaying accumulation of fluid. Initial oral diuretic therapy usually consists of the aldosterone antagonist spironolactone alone or in combination with a loop diuretic. The combination of spironolactone and furosemide in a 5:2 ratio is associated with a lower risk for hyperkalemia and less time for fluid mobilization compared to spironolactone use alone.[38,39] Typically, spironolactone and furosemide are started at 100 mg and 40 mg daily, respectively, and are increased simultaneously to effect every 3 to 5 days. Furosemide may need to be held in patients with severe hypokalemia, and the dose of spironolactone may need to be decreased in patients with renal failure. For patients with tense ascites associated with significant abdominal distress, studies have suggested that a strategy of large volume paracentesis followed by maintenance diuretic therapy is faster at fluid removal (minutes) than oral diuretic therapy (days to weeks).[40,41] Intravenous diuretic therapy is associated with an increased risk for encephalopathy, renal failure, and electrolyte changes.[38] Patients whose clinical condition precludes oral diuretic treatment should be treated as if their ascites is refractory to treatment.

Refractory ascites, which occurs in 5% to 10% of patients with ascites, has two subtypes. Diuretic-resistant ascites is defined as a lack of response to sodium restriction and the maximum dose of diuretics; diuretic-intractable ascites is defined by the development of diuretic-induced complications that preclude the use of an effective diuretic dosage.[42] The medical management of refractory ascites is repeat large volume paracentesis combined with maintenance diuretic therapy. Large volume paracentesis is typically performed every 2 to 4 weeks; the procedure can be performed safely as an outpatient. Controversy continues regarding the need for volume expansion (e.g., with intravenous albumin) when removing ascites with large volume paracentesis because of the potential risk for circulatory dysfunction after fluid removal.[43] Given the cost of albumin, a reasonable approach is to forego volume expansion if less than 5 liters is removed.[37]

Transjugular intrahepatic portosystemic shunt (TIPS), by angiographically creating a low-resistance channel between the hepatic vein and the intrahepatic portion of the portal vein, effectively decompresses portal pressures and has been shown to be an effective treatment option for patients with CLD and refractory ascites.[44] The studies comparing TIPS with medical management in patients with advanced CLD suggest that TIPS is efficacious in controlling ascites but results in an increased risk (either in incidence or in frequency) for hepatic encephalopathy. Patients randomized to TIPS require fewer large volume paracentesis procedures and lower diuretic doses but at the cost of increased hospitalizations and the risk for increased confusion.[45] Patients with severe decompensated liver disease are likely at increased risk for worsening liver failure after TIPS, and therefore most of the studies of TIPS versus medical management have excluded these patients. TIPS may be considered even in those with a limited life expectancy if hepatic function is well preserved.

Near the end of life, medical management of ascites may become difficult. Case reports have described the use of indwelling catheters for drainage of ascites in patients with CLD.[46,47] The placement of these catheters can be complicated by infection, occlusion or accidental removal or leakage. Given the potential risks and the lack of controlled studies, these catheters should be considered near the end of life only in carefully selected patients.

Hepatic Encephalopathy. Hepatic encephalopathy is a spectrum of potentially reversible neuropsychiatric abnormalities in patients with significant liver dysfunction and a complication of CLD that significantly impairs quality of life.[48] Common precipitating factors for episodic hepatic encephalopathy include gastrointestinal hemorrhage, uremia, drugs, dietary changes, infections, constipation, and fluid and electrolyte changes. Persistent hepatic encephalopathy describes the cognitive and noncognitive deficits (e.g., sleep disturbances, extrapyramidal alterations) that have an impact on social and occupational functioning. Minimal hepatic encephalopathy describes patients with CLD without overt mental status changes who are found to have significant impairment (usually >2 standard deviations from the normative population) in a battery of psychometric tests thought to be specific for hepatic encephalopathy.[6] Minimal hepatic encephalopathy is highly prevalent in patients with CLD,[49] is associated with decreased ability to perform complex tasks and increased risk for overt hepatic encephalopathy,[49,50] and may portend a poorer prognosis.[51]

Even near the end of life, treatment of an episode of hepatic encephalopathy should focus first on identifying and treating the potential precipitating causes. In particular, new infections and drugs are common causes of worsened hepatic encephalopathy even with limited life expectancy. Empiric treatment for potential precipitants of hepatic encephalopathy is common practice when the burdens of invasive diagnostic testing outweigh potential benefits.

The nonabsorbable disaccharide lactulose remains the standard of care despite the poor quality of the multiple studies that tested its efficacy.[52] When oral medication is precluded by mental status, lactulose can be given rectally. Lactulose sometimes can be poorly tolerated because of abdominal discomfort and flatulence. Lactitol, dispensed as a crystalline powder is a better tolerated disaccharide that is as efficacious as lactulose.[53]

Second-line agents for hepatic encephalopathy include the nonabsorbable antibiotics. Oral neomycin, used alone (1-2 g/day) or combined with sorbitol, is one alternative, best used when the known increased risks for ototoxicity and nephrotoxicity are no longer of concern.[54] Rifaximin (at dosages of 1200 to 2400 mg/day) is an oral antibiotic with minimal side effects shown in multiple studies to be safe and efficacious in treating hepatic encephalopathy.[55,56] Oral metronidazole (250 mg two or three times daily) has been shown to be effective but is limited by metallic taste and significant peripheral neuropathy.[52]

Agitation and delirium in patients with CLD are not infrequent complications in late-stage disease. Principles of treatment are similar to those described in Chapters 35 to 38. Benzodiazepines should be avoided given the increased sensitivity of the γ-aminobutyric acid (GABA)-ergic neurotransmitter system in these patients[57] and the recent studies suggesting an increased risk for delirium after benzodiazepine use.[58]

Variceal Hemorrhage. For patients and families, acute variceal hemorrhage is likely the most frightening complication of CLD, therefore constituting a crisis for which palliative care providers need to prepare the patient, family, and caregivers.[59] Discussions about treatment preferences should address the appropriateness of continuing β-blockade to decrease the risk for variceal hemorrhage in selected patients. As part of crisis planning, palliative care providers should discuss openly with the patient and other providers the role of blood transfusions, emergency endoscopy, or TIPS in the event of an acute hemorrhage.[60]

Approaches to the management of variceal hemorrhage can be extrapolated from the literature on terminal hemorrhage in patients with cancer.[61] Nasal packing and dark towels might be helpful in reducing the alarming associations of blood-covered sheets. Patients with variceal hemorrhage can be treated with the somatostatin analog octreotride, either subcutaneously or by continuous infusion. The medication works by decreasing the splanchnic blood flow. Patients in an inpatient setting also may benefit from intravenous desmopressin or vasopressin, posterior pituitary hormones known to mediate splanchnic vasoconstriction. Regardless of setting, patients should be quickly sedated with short-acting benzodiazepines or other sedatives. If the patient is at home, families will need to be instructed on how to administer the medications subcutaneously.

Other Symptoms and Complications

Muscle cramps are common in patients with CLD and associated with poor quality of life.[25] No consensus guidelines are available on how to approach treatment in this population, so empiric treatment is indicated. A meta-analysis of all of the studies testing the efficacy of quinine (dose of 200-500 mg/day) in muscle cramps for older adults without cirrhosis found that the drug decreased the number of cramps but not the severity or the duration.[62] One small study found quinidine (400 mg/day) to be effective at decreasing the number of cramps in patients with cirrhosis.[63] Based on some evidence of low serum concentration of magnesium in patients with CLD, particularly in alcoholics, magnesium sulfate is often used to treat cramps in this population.

Depression is highly prevalent in this patient population: prevalence rates were 30% to 40% in one study that found depressed patients more likely to die waiting for a transplant.[64] For more on the treatment of depression, see Chapters 32 and 33. Fatigue is also common, particularly in patients with primary biliary cirrhosis and HCV infection.[56,65]

KEY MESSAGES TO PATIENTS AND FAMILIES

CLD encompasses a diverse group of diseases that share a common set of symptoms, pattern of liver damage, and outcomes. Whereas OLT has dramatically increased survival in this disease, many patients will experience significant symptoms before transplantation that can significantly impair quality of life and add to family distress. Palliative care consultation should be sought at the time of diagnosis to provide an extra layer of support to patients and families living with CLD and to improve symptom management. Additional roles of palliative care in this spectrum of diseases beyond symptom management are described in the subsequent chapter.

CONCLUSION AND SUMMARY

CLD presents with a unique symptom burden that is associated with many symptoms and complications. The high prevalence of encephalopathy and ineffective drug metabolism have a significant impact on symptom management and decision making in this disease. OLT, for those who are eligible and for whom a donor organ is available, provides a potentially curative approach to the many diseases that lead to CLD and HCC. Nevertheless, the number of patients who are not OLT eligible, the lack of available donors, and the high symptom burden and care needs of this patient population result in a critical need for palliative care. Additional research is critically needed to address symptoms other than pain, particularly delirium and encephalopathy. Chapter 54 describes the special role that palliative care can play in this disease.

SUMMARY RECOMMENDATIONS

- Acetaminophen is safe in nonalcoholic patients with chronic liver disease at doses of 2 to 3 g per day.
- Opioids can be safely used—start low and go slow. Preferred opioids include fentanyl, hydromorphone, and oxycodone. Avoid codeine, dextropropoxyphene, meperidine, and tramadol, and oxymorphone. Methadone should be used with extreme caution by expert clinicians only.

- The clinician should address the underlying cause of pruritus, if possible, by reducing biliary obstruction through stenting, percutaneous drainage, or surgical biliodigestive anastomoses.
- Nonabsorbable resins are effective in cholestatic-induced pruritus.
- Other alternatives for pruritus include rifampicin and opioid antagonists.
- All patients with ascites should be maintained on a low-sodium diet.
- The combination of spironolactone and furosemide (ratio of 5:2) has been shown to be the most effective diuretic regimen.
- Refractory ascites can be managed with low volume paracentesis or transjugular intrahepatic postosystemic shunts.
- The clinician should identify and address underlying causes of encephalopathy (infections, medications).
- Lactulose remains the standard of care for treatment of encephalopathy and can be administered orally or rectally.
- It is critical to address with patients and families and discuss the roles of transfusion, emergency endoscopy, and transjugular intrahepatic postosystemic shunts in regard to variceal hemorrhage.
- Pharmacological management for variceal hemorrhage includes subcutaneous octreotide; intravenous desmopressin, and vasopressin if in an inpatient setting.
- Patients with variceal hemorrhage should be rapidly sedated with short-acting benzodiazepines to address fear and anxiety.
- Effective treatments for muscle cramps are few, but include quinine and perhaps magnesium sulfate.

REFERENCES

1. Larson AM, Curtis JR. Integrating palliative care for liver transplant candidates: "too well for transplant, too sick for life". *JAMA*. 2006;295:2168–2176.
2. Murphy SL, Xu J, Kochanek KD. Deaths: preliminary data for 2010. *Nat Vital Stat Rep*. 2012;60:7.
3. The U.S. Organ Procurement and Transplantation Network, Scientific Registry of Transplant Recipients. *OPTN/SRTR 2010 Annual Data Report*. Rockville, MD, 2011.
4. Fox E, Landrum-McNiff K, Zhong Z, Dawson NV, Wu AW, Lynn J. Evaluation of prognostic criteria for determining hospice eligibility in patients with advanced lung, heart, or liver disease. SUPPORT Investigators: Study to Understand Prognoses and Preferences for Outcomes and Risks of Treatments. *JAMA*. 1999;282:1638–1645.
5. Guy V. Liver failure, life support, family support, and palliation: an inside story. *J Crit Care*. 2006;21:250–252.
6. Bajaj JS. Minimal hepatic encephalopathy matters in daily life. *World J Gastroenterol*. 2008;14:3609–3615.
7. Schomerus H, Hamster W. Quality of life in cirrhotics with minimal hepatic encephalopathy. *Metab Brain Dis*. 2001;16:37–41.
8. Bell BP, Manos MM, Zaman A, et al. The epidemiology of newly diagnosed chronic liver disease in gastroenterology practices in the United States: results from population-based surveillance. *Am J Gastroenterol*. 2008;103:2727–2736;quiz 37.

9. Basra G, Basra S, Parupudi S. Symptoms and signs of acute alcoholic hepatitis. *World J Hepatol.* 2011;3:118–120.

10. Basra S, Anand BS. Definition, epidemiology and magnitude of alcoholic hepatitis. *World J Hepatol.* 2011;3:108–113.

11. El-Serag HB, Rudolph KL. Hepatocellular carcinoma: epidemiology and molecular carcinogenesis. *Gastroenterology.* 2007;132:2557–2576.

12. Parikh S, Hyman D. Hepatocellular cancer: a guide for the internist. *Am J Med.* 2007;120:194–202.

13. Cahill BA, Braccia D. Current treatment for hepatocellular carcinoma. *Clin J Oncol Nurs.* 2004;8:393–399.

14. Mazzaferro V, Regalia E, Doci R, et al. Liver transplantation for the treatment of small hepatocellular carcinomas in patients with cirrhosis. *N Engl J Med.* 1996;334:693–699.

15. Roth K, Lynn J, Zhong Z, Borum M, Dawson NV. Dying with end stage liver disease with cirrhosis: insights from SUPPORT. Study to Understand Prognoses and Preferences for Outcomes and Risks of Treatment. *J Am Geriatr Soc.* 2000;48:S122–S130.

16. Devulder J, Richarz U, Nataraja SH. Impact of long-term use of opioids on quality of life in patients with chronic, non-malignant pain. *Curr Med Res Opin.* 2005;21:1555–1568.

17. Rhee C, Broadbent AM. Palliation and liver failure: palliative medications dosage guidelines. *J Palliat Med.* 2007;10:677–685.

18. Giovanni G, Giovanni P. Do non-steroidal anti-inflammatory drugs and COX-2 selective inhibitors have different renal effects? *J Nephrol.* 2002;15:480–488.

19. Murray MD, Brater DC. Renal toxicity of the nonsteroidal anti-inflammatory drugs. *Annu Rev Pharmacol Toxicol.* 1993;33:435–465.

20. Benson GD, Koff RS, Tolman KG. The therapeutic use of acetaminophen in patients with liver disease. *Am J Ther.* 2005;12:133–141.

21. Dart RC, Kuffner EK, Rumack BH. Treatment of pain or fever with paracetamol (acetaminophen) in the alcoholic patient: a systematic review. *Am J Ther.* 2000;7:123–134.

22. Kuffner EK, Green JL, Bogdan GM, et al. The effect of acetaminophen (four grams a day. *BMC Med.* 2007;5:13.

23. Novick DM, Kreek MJ, Fanizza AM, Yancovitz SR, Gelb AM, Stenger RJ. Methadone disposition in patients with chronic liver disease. *Clin Pharmacol Ther.* 1981;30:353–362.

24. Tegeder I, Lotsch J, Geisslinger G. Pharmacokinetics of opioids in liver disease. *Clin Pharmacokinet.* 1999;37:17–40.

25. Marchesini G, Bianchi G, Amodio P, et al. Factors associated with poor health-related quality of life of patients with cirrhosis. *Gastroenterology.* 2001;120:170–178.

26. Lebovics E, Seif F, Kim D, et al. Pruritus in chronic hepatitis C: association with high serum bile acids, advanced pathology, and bile duct abnormalities. *Dig Dis Sci.* 1997;42:1094–1099.

27. Kremer AE, Beuers U, Oude-Elferink RP, Pusl T. Pathogenesis and treatment of pruritus in cholestasis. *Drugs.* 2008;68:2163–2182.

28. Bergasa NV. Medical palliation of the jaundiced patient with pruritus. *Gastroenterol Clin North Am.* 2006;35:113–123.

29. Mela M, Mancuso A, Burroughs AK. Review article: pruritus in cholestatic and other liver diseases. *Aliment Pharmacol Ther.* 2003;17:857–870.

30. Marzioni M, Svegliati Baroni G, Alpini G, Benedetti A. Endogenous opioid peptides and chronic liver disease: from bedside to bench. *J Hepatol.* 2007;46:583–586.

31. Tandon P, Rowe BH, Vandermeer B, Bain VG. The efficacy and safety of bile acid binding agents, opioid antagonists, or rifampin in the treatment of cholestasis-associated pruritus. *Am J Gastroenterol.* 2007;102:1528–1536.

32. Thornton JR, Losowsky MS. Opioid peptides and primary biliary cirrhosis. *BMJ.* 1988;297:1501–1504.

33. Jones EA, Neuberger J, Bergasa NV. Opiate antagonist therapy for the pruritus of cholestasis: the avoidance of opioid withdrawal-like reactions. *QJM.* 2002;95:547–552.

34. Bergasa NV, Schmitt JM, Talbot TL, et al. Open-label trial of oral nalmefene therapy for the pruritus of cholestasis. *Hepatology.* 1998;27:679–684.

35. Carson KL, Tran TT, Cotton P, Sharara AI, Hunt CM. Pilot study of the use of naltrexone to treat the severe pruritus of cholestatic liver disease. *Am J Gastroenterol.* 1996;91:1022–1023.

36. Dawn AG, Yosipovitch G. Butorphanol for treatment of intractable pruritus. *J Am Acad Dermatol.* 2006;54:527–531.

37. Runyon BA. Treatment of patients with cirrhosis and ascites. *Semin Liver Dis.* 1997;17:249–260.

38. Runyon BA. Management of adult patients with ascites due to cirrhosis: an update. *Hepatology.* 2009;49:2087–2107.

39. Santos J, Planas R, Pardo A, et al. Spironolactone alone or in combination with furosemide in the treatment of moderate ascites in nonazotemic cirrhosis: a randomized comparative study of efficacy and safety. *J Hepatol.* 2003;39:187–192.

40. Gines P, Arroyo V, Quintero E, et al. Comparison of paracentesis and diuretics in the treatment of cirrhotics with tense ascites: results of a randomized study. *Gastroenterology.* 1987;93:234–241.

41. Salerno F, Badalamenti S, Incerti P, et al. Repeated paracentesis and i.v. albumin infusion to treat 'tense' ascites in cirrhotic patients: a safe alternative therapy. *J Hepatol.* 1987;5:102–108.

42. Cardenas A, Gines P. Management of refractory ascites. *Clin Gastroenterol Hepatol.* 2005;3:1187–1191.

43. Cardenas A, Gines P, Runyon BA. Is albumin infusion necessary after large volume paracentesis? *Liver Int.* 2009;29:636–640 discussion 40–41.

44. Colombato L. The role of transjugular intrahepatic portosystemic shunt (TIPS) in the management of portal hypertension. *J Clin Gastroenterol.* 2007;41(suppl 3):S344–S351.

45. Campbell MS, Brensinger CM, Sanyal AJ, et al. Quality of life in refractory ascites: transjugular intrahepatic portal-systemic shunting versus medical therapy. *Hepatology.* 2005;42:635–640.

46. Reisfield GM, Wilson GR. Management of intractable, cirrhotic ascites with an indwelling drainage catheter. *J Palliat Med.* 2003;6:787–791.

47. Rosenblum DI, Geisinger MA, Newman JS, et al. Use of subcutaneous venous access ports to treat refractory ascites. *J Vasc Interv Radiol.* 2001;12:1343–1346.

48. Ferenci P, Lockwood A, Mullen K, Tarter R, Weissenborn K, Blei AT. Hepatic encephalopathy: definition, nomenclature, diagnosis, and quantification—final report of the working party at the 11th World Congresses of Gastroenterology, Vienna, 1998. *Hepatology.* 2002;35:716–721.

49. Das A, Dhiman RK, Saraswat VA, Verma M, Naik SR. Prevalence and natural history of subclinical hepatic encephalopathy in cirrhosis. *J Gastroenterol Hepatol.* 2001;16:531–535.

50. Romero-Gomez M, Boza F, Garcia-Valdecasas MS, Garcia E, Aguilar-Reina J. Subclinical hepatic encephalopathy predicts the development of overt hepatic encephalopathy. *Am J Gastroenterol.* 2001;96:2718–2723.

51. Romero-Gomez M, Grande L, Camacho I. Prognostic value of altered oral glutamine challenge in patients with minimal hepatic encephalopathy. *Hepatology.* 2004;39:939–943.

52. Sundaram V, Shaikh OS. Hepatic encephalopathy: pathophysiology and emerging therapies. *Med Clin North Am.* 2009;93:819–836, vii.

53. Morgan MY, Alonso M, Stanger LC. Lactitol and lactulose for the treatment of subclinical hepatic encephalopathy in cirrhotic patients: a randomised, cross-over study. *J Hepatol.* 1989;8:208–217.

54. Atterbury CE, Maddrey WC, Conn HO. Neomycin-sorbitol and lactulose in the treatment of acute portal-systemic encephalopathy: a controlled, double-blind clinical trial. *Am J Dig Dis.* 1978;23:398–406.

55. Lumby J. Liver transplantation: the death/life paradox. *Int J Nurs Pract.* 1997;3:231–238.

56. van der Plas SM, Hansen BE, de Boer JB, et al. Generic and disease-specific health related quality of life in non-cirrhotic, cirrhotic and transplanted liver patients: a cross-sectional study. *BMC Gastroenterol.* 2003;3:33.

57. Laccetti M, Manes G, Uomo G, Lioniello M, Rabitti PG, Balzano A. Flumazenil in the treatment of acute hepatic encephalopathy in cirrhotic patients: a double blind randomized placebo controlled study. *Dig Liver Dis.* 2000;32:335–338.

58. Pandharipande P, Shintani A, Peterson J, et al. Lorazepam is an independent risk factor for transitioning to delirium in intensive care unit patients. *Anesthesiology.* 2006;104:21–26.

59. Nauck F, Alt-Epping B. Crises in palliative care: a comprehensive approach. *Lancet Oncol.* 2008;9:1086–1091.

60. Monti M, Castellani L, Berlusconi A, Cunietti E. Use of red blood cell transfusions in terminally ill cancer patients admitted to a palliative care unit. *J Pain Symptom Manage.* 1996;12:18–22.

61. Harris DG, Noble SI. Management of terminal hemorrhage in patients with advanced cancer: a systematic literature review. *J Pain Symptom Manage.* 2009;38(6):913–927.

62. Man-Son-Hing M, Wells G. Meta-analysis of efficacy of quinine for treatment of nocturnal leg cramps in elderly people. *BMJ.* 1995;310:13–17.

63. Lee FY, Lee SD, Tsai YT, et al. A randomized controlled trial of quinidine in the treatment of cirrhotic patients with muscle cramps. *J Hepatol.* 1991;12:236–240.

64. Singh N, Gayowski T, Wagener MM, Marino IR. Depression in patients with cirrhosis. *Impact on outcome. Dig Dis Sci.* 1997;42:1421–1427.

65. Kim SH, Oh EG, Lee WH. Symptom experience, psychological distress, and quality of life in Korean patients with liver cirrhosis: a cross-sectional survey. *Int J Nurs Stud.* 2006;43:1047–1056. 134.

Chapter 54

What Special Considerations Are Needed for Treating Patients With Chronic Liver Disease?

ALUKO A. HOPE AND R. SEAN MORRISON

INTRODUCTION AND SCOPE OF THE PROBLEM

Recent estimates suggest that approximately 5.5 million persons suffer from chronic liver disease (CLD) worldwide and as many as 40,000 persons will die of its natural course or complications.[1] In the United States alone, CLD results in 4000 to 5000 deaths per year and 11,000 to 17,000 hospitalizations.[1] Palliative care providers may be called in various settings to help with communication, decision making, or care coordination for patients with CLD. Decision making and communication are complicated in this patient population because of the difficulty in predicting outcomes,[1] frequent patient and family misunderstanding of the life-limiting nature of the illness,[2] and high risk for severe cognitive dysfunction that may impair decision-making capacity.[3,4] This chapter aims to improve the knowledge of palliative care providers around these particularly complex issues in patients with CLD so they can better integrate specialty palliative care with disease-specific and life-prolonging therapies for these patients. Specifically, the chapter addresses prognostication, special considerations around communication, and an integrated palliative care delivery model for persons with CLD.

RELEVANT PATHOPHYSIOLOGY

Predicting survival in patients with advanced CLD and cirrhosis is difficult because of the unpredictable disease trajectory that often involves episodic and acute exacerbations, frequent hospitalizations, and stabilizations.[5] The natural history of CLD and cirrhosis are characterized by an asymptomatic or compensated phase followed by a progressive phase marked by the development of the many complications of progressive liver dysfunction and portal hypertension.[6] The median survival of patients with compensated cirrhosis is more than 12 years, and most of these patients die either by transitioning to a decompensated state or from causes unrelated to their liver disease. Patients with compensated cirrhosis develop complications at a rate of 5% to 7% per year.[6,7]

Decompensated cirrhosis may be characterized by the development of jaundice, variceal hemorrhage, ascites, or hepatic encephalopathy, each with management challenges and implications for prognosis.[8] With the development of esophageal varices, median survival decreases to 7 years and these patients die from a variceal bleed or development of other complications of liver disease.[6] The disease-specific treatments available for patients with these events have decreased mortality over the years, but the hospital mortality per episode is still above 10%.[6]

Approximately 50% to 60% of patients with compensated cirrhosis will develop ascites over 10 years.[8] Ascites increases the risk for infection (e.g., spontaneous bacterial infection) and renal failure. When ascites becomes refractory to medical management, survival decreases from about 50% at 5 years to 15% without liver transplantation.[9,10] The development of hepatorenal syndrome (HRS) is an ominous sign in patients with cirrhosis. Type 2 HRS, characterized by moderate renal failure (serum creatinine 1.5-2.5 mg/dL), with a subacute, progressive course, is associated with a median survival of 6 months. Type 1 HRS, characterized by rapidly progressive renal failure (doubling of serum creatinine to a level >2.5 in <2 weeks), usually portends impending death in days to weeks, with a median survival of 1 to 2 weeks.[11,12]

Prognostication in Chronic Liver Disease

Multiple prognostic models and scoring systems have been developed to predict short-term and long-term outcomes in patients with CLD and cirrhosis. The two in most common use are the Child-Turcotte-Pugh Classification (CTP) and the Model for End Stage Liver Disease (MELD) score.

The Child-Turcotte-Pugh Classification. The Child-Turcotte score[13] was originally proposed more than 30 years ago and then subsequently modified 10 years later (Table 54-1). Patients are grouped into three classes based on the sum of the scores for each of five variables.[14] Patients can be classified into CTP Class A

TABLE 54-1. The Child-Turcotte-Pugh Score and Classification*

CRITERION	1 POINT	2 POINTS	3 POINTS
Bilirubin (mg/dL)[†]	<2	2-3	>3
Albumin	>3.5	2.8-3.5	<2.8
Prothrombin time and INR[‡]	<1.7	1.7-2.3	>2.3
Hepatic encephalopathy[§]	None	Stage 1-2	Stage 3-4
Ascites	None	Mild-moderate	Severe

INR, International normalized ratio.
*The classification is based on the sum of the scores for each of the five criteria: Class A (5-6 points), Class B (7-9 points), Class C (10-15 points).
[†]Normal total bilirubin <1.0 mg/dL.
[‡]The original cutoff values of 4 and 6 seconds for prothrombin time prolongation correspond to the INR of 1.7 and 2, respectively.
[§]Stage 1: shortened attention, euphoria, anxiety, impaired addition and subtraction; stage 2: increasing lethargy with disorientation of time, personality changes or inappropriate behavior; stage 3: somnolence to semistupor; stage 4: coma.

TABLE 54-2. Model for End Stage Liver Disease (MELD) Score

SCORE	3-MONTH MORTALITY (%)
40 or more	71
30-39	53
20-29	20
10-19	6
9 or less	2

From Wiesner R, Edwards E, Freeman R, et al. Model for end-stage liver disease (MELD) and allocation of donor livers. *Gastroenterology.* 2003;124(1):91-96.
MELD = 3.78[ln serum bilirubin* (mg/dL)] + 11.2[ln INR] + 9.57[ln serum creatinine[†] (mg/dL)] + 6.43.
*Any value <1 is given a value of 1 (e.g., if bilirubin is 0.8, a value of 1.0 is used) to prevent the occurrence of scores below 0 (i.e., the natural logarithm of 1 is 0, and any value <1 would yield a negative result)
[†]If the patient has been dialyzed twice within the last 7 days, then the value for serum creatinine used should be 4.0.

(5-6 points), which is associated with a 1- and 2-year median survival of 95% and 90%, respectively; CTP Class B (7-9 points), with a 1- and 2-year median survival of 80% and 70%, respectively; and CTP Class C (10-15 points) with a 1- and 2-year median survival of 45% and 38%, respectively.[10] Multiple studies have confirmed that the CTP class and score are independently associated with an increased mortality across multiple disease presentations and settings.[15,16]

The Model for End Stage Liver Disease. The MELD score was originally designed to predict 3-month mortality of patients with cirrhosis undergoing transjugular portosystemic intrahepatic shunt (TIPS).[17] Multivariable analysis found four independent variables that had an impact on survival. Subsequently, a modified model with three of the original variables (bilirubin, creatinine, and international normalized ration) was shown to accurately predict 3-month mortality in patients with cirrhosis listed for liver transplant.[18] Since its initial development, the MELD score has been validated as a robust marker of early and long-term survival in patients with CLD across a wide spectrum of disease causes and settings (Table 54-2).[6,11,19,20]

The strength of the MELD score as a prognostic model lies in its rigorous statistical foundation and its use of objective, readily available parameters. However, the MELD score does overestimate liver disease severity in patients with intrinsic renal disease, patients with hyperbilirubinemia secondary to Gilbert syndrome, and patients on anticoagulation therapy.[21] Studies also have suggested that a subset of patients with a low MELD score and refractory ascites and hyponatremia,[22–26] or complications such as hepatopulmonary syndrome,[27,28] mild portopulmonary hypertension, or ascites with large-volume pleural effusion are at high risk for death in the absence of a liver transplantation.[29]

Finally, when patients with cirrhosis are admitted to the intensive care unit (ICU) because of multiorgan failure, the prognosis is especially poor. Mortality in patients with cirrhosis admitted to the ICU with two or three organ systems failing ranges from 75% to 95%, respectively,[30] much higher than rates seen, for example, in severe sepsis without liver disease.[31]

SUMMARY OF EVIDENCE REGARDING TREATMENT RECOMMENDATIONS

Advance Care Planning and Decision Making in Chronic Liver Disease

Patients with CLD often develop or indeed present with compromised cognitive status as a result of hepatic encephalopathy, and therefore advance care planning is of critical importance. Chapters 45 and 46 present a detailed discussion on goals of care discussions and advance care planning. Given that the presence of even mild hepatic encephalopathy can impair decision-making capacity, it is of utmost importance that health care proxies or surrogates be identified at the earliest possible stage in the illness trajectory and that goals of care are clearly addressed with both patients and proxies.

The uncertainty of the clinical course in CLD makes addressing goals of care both increasingly important and also relatively difficult compared to other diseases. As described by Larson and Curtis,[32] patients and families ride a roller coaster of emotions; patients and families must expect and plan for multiple potential outcomes simultaneously—successful transplant, transplant ineligibility, catastrophic decline and death before transplant, lack of organ availability, or death from transplant complications. Helping patients maintain and preserve hope in the setting of these competing realities is an important role for palliative care teams. Hope has been described not as the wish for a certain outcome but as a process by which we expect something good in the future and make plans toward that goal.[33] One approach to preserving hope in the setting of prolonged uncertainty is the model of "hope for the best, prepare for the worst."[34] Using this model, clinicians can discuss the possibility of less desirable outcomes with patients who seem to be clinging to unrealistic hopes. This approach allows patients to engage in practical planning while not taking away hope for a good outcome (e.g., transplantation) and at the same time, permits patients to face undesirable outcomes and begin to engage in finding new hopes aside from cure.[35] Indeed, this approach permits multiple possibilities to be held at the same time, allowing discussion of difficult possibilities that otherwise could not be considered and aligning patients and physicians.

A Model of Palliative Care for Chronic Liver Disease

Patients with CLD who have a clinical indication to be evaluated for liver transplantation (presence of ascites, variceal hemorrhage, acute kidney injury, hepatic encephalopathy, hepatocellular cancer) should also have palliative care integrated into their traditional disease management. Although patients with ESLD often meet the prognostic guidelines for hospice and would benefit from hospice's approach to symptom management and quality of life, patients listed for liver transplantation are precluded from hospice in the United States under the current Medicare regulations because they are pursuing curative treatment with the potential for long-term survival.[32] Patients who are deemed not eligible for liver transplantation should be offered hospice.

Patients who are eligible for transplantation should have palliative care integrated into their routine medical care. Specifically, palliative care teams, by providing an added layer of support to the transplant team can assist with symptom management, help negotiate goals of care in the setting of progressive illness, and, if liver transplantation is not available or the patient is deemed ineligible for transplantation, provide timely end-of-life care. Timely integration of palliative care may help validate the time paradox for patients on the transplant list in which they are preparing both for their dying (without a transplant) and for their new life (after the transplant).[36] This integrated approach may also facilitate the continuation of disease-specific treatments that have an impact on quality of life even after the patient is deemed ineligible for transplant. The multidisciplinary nature of the transplant evaluation process makes it ripe for integration of formal palliative care consults for patients and families who might benefit.

KEY MESSAGES TO PATIENTS AND FAMILIES

CLD is a complex illness that requires patients and families to simultaneously live with two competing realities—the hope for liver transplantation and prolonged longevity versus the threat of dying from their underlying liver disease. Palliative care clinicians can help establish realistic understanding of prognosis, guide patients to establish goals of care, and help match treatments to those goals through honest and empathic communication. The "hope for the best, plan for the worst" approach is particularly relevant to CLD and allows patients and families to engage in practical outcomes without taking away hope for cure or prolonged longevity.

CONCLUSION AND SUMMARY

Research on palliative care in CLD is in its infancy—much more information is needed on the expectations, needs, and requirements of the patients living with CLD. A system of care that allows for better integration of the transplant evaluation with palliative care may ultimately provide us with the tools to make life and death as symptom-free and fulfilling as possible for patients with CLD.

SUMMARY RECOMMENDATIONS

- Advance care planning is critical in chronic liver disease given the very high prevalence of cognitive impairment resulting from encephalopathy.
- Because of the complexity of chronic liver disease and its uncertain prognosis, palliative care can help ensure that conversations about patients' understanding of their illness and the overall goals and values related to their health care are reassessed over time.
- The strategy of hoping for the best and planning for the worst is a particularly valuable communication strategy in the setting of chronic liver disease.

REFERENCES

1. Fox E, Landrum-McNiff K, Zhong Z, Dawson NV, Wu AW, Lynn J. Evaluation of prognostic criteria for determining hospice eligibility in patients with advanced lung, heart, or liver disease. SUPPORT Investigators: Study to Understand Prognoses and Preferences for Outcomes and Risks of Treatments. *JAMA*. 1999;282:1638–1645.
2. Guy V. Liver failure, life support, family support, and palliation: an inside story. *J Crit Care*. 2006;21:250–252.
3. Bajaj JS. Minimal hepatic encephalopathy matters in daily life. *World J Gastroenterol*. 2008;14:3609–3615.
4. Schomerus H, Hamster W. Quality of life in cirrhotics with minimal hepatic encephalopathy. *Metab Brain Dis*. 2001;16:37–41.
5. Roth K, Lynn J, Zhong Z, Borum M, Dawson NV. Dying with end stage liver disease with cirrhosis: insights from SUPPORT. Study to Understand Prognoses and Preferences for Outcomes and Risks of Treatment. *J Am Geriatr Soc* 2000;48:S122–S130.
6. D'Amico G, Garcia-Tsao G, Pagliaro L. Natural history and prognostic indicators of survival in cirrhosis: a systematic review of 118 studies. *J Hepatol*. 2006;44:217–231.
7. Garcia-Tsao G, Lim JK. Management and treatment of patients with cirrhosis and portal hypertension: recommendations from the Department of Veterans Affairs Hepatitis C Resource Center Program and the National Hepatitis C Program. *Am J Gastroenterol*. 2009;104:1802–1829.
8. Gines P, Quintero E, Arroyo V, et al. Compensated cirrhosis: natural history and prognostic factors. *Hepatology*. 1987;7:122–128.
9. Planas R, Montoliu S, Balleste B, et al. Natural history of patients hospitalized for management of cirrhotic ascites. *Clin Gastroenterol Hepatol*. 2006;4:1385–1394.
10. Runyon BA. Treatment of patients with cirrhosis and ascites. *Semin Liver Dis*. 1997;17:249–260.

11. Alessandria C, Ozdogan O, Guevara M, et al. MELD score and clinical type predict prognosis in hepatorenal syndrome: relevance to liver transplantation. *Hepatology*. 2005;41:1282–1289.

12. Arroyo V, Terra C, Gines P. Advances in the pathogenesis and treatment of type-1 and type-2 hepatorenal syndrome. *J Hepatol*. 2007;46:935–946.

13. Child CG. Surgery and portal hypertension. In: Child CG, ed. *The Liver and Portal hypertension*. Philadelphia: W. B. Saunders; 1964:50–72.

14. Pugh RN, Murray-Lyon IM, Dawson JL, Pietroni MC, Williams R. Transection of the oesophagus for bleeding oesophageal varices. *Br J Surg*. 1973;60:646–649.

15. Fernandez-Esparrach G, Sanchez-Fueyo A, Gines P, et al. A prognostic model for predicting survival in cirrhosis with ascites. *J Hepatol*. 2001;34:46–52.

16. Planas R, Balleste B, Alvarez MA, et al. Natural history of decompensated hepatitis C virus-related cirrhosis: a study of 200 patients. *J Hepatol*. 2004;40:823–830.

17. Malinchoc M, Kamath PS, Gordon FD, Peine CJ, Rank J, ter Borg PC. A model to predict poor survival in patients undergoing transjugular intrahepatic portosystemic shunts. *Hepatology*. 2000;31:864–871.

18. Kamath PS, Wiesner RH, Malinchoc M, et al. A model to predict survival in patients with end-stage liver disease. *Hepatology*. 2001;33:464–470.

19. Antaki F, Lukowski A. The model for end-stage liver disease (MELD) predicts survival of liver cirrhosis patients after discharge to hospice. *J Clin Gastroenterol*. 2007;41:412–415.

20. Chalasani N, Kahi C, Francois F, et al. Model for end-stage liver disease (MELD) for predicting mortality in patients with acute variceal bleeding. *Hepatology*. 2002;35:1282–1284.

21. Kamath PS, Kim WR. The model for end-stage liver disease (MELD). *Hepatology*. 2007;45:797–805.

22. Biggins SW, Rodriguez HJ, Bacchetti P, Bass NM, Roberts JP, Terrault NA. Serum sodium predicts mortality in patients listed for liver transplantation. *Hepatology*. 2005;41:32–39.

23. Kim WR, Biggins SW, Kremers WK, et al. Hyponatremia and mortality among patients on the liver-transplant waiting list. *N Engl J Med*. 2008;359:1018–1026.

24. Londono MC, Cardenas A, Guevara M, et al. MELD score and serum sodium in the prediction of survival of patients with cirrhosis awaiting liver transplantation. *Gut*. 2007;56:1283–1290.

25. Ruf AE, Kremers WK, Chavez LL, Descalzi VI, Podesta LG, Villamil FG. Addition of serum sodium into the MELD score predicts waiting list mortality better than MELD alone. *Liver Transpl*. 2005;11:336–343.

26. Sanyal AJ, Bosch J, Blei A, Arroyo V. Portal hypertension and its complications. *Gastroenterology*. 2008;134:1715–1728.

27. Schenk P, Schoniger-Hekele M, Fuhrmann V, Madl C, Silberhumer G, Muller C. Prognostic significance of the hepatopulmonary syndrome in patients with cirrhosis. *Gastroenterology*. 2003;125:1042–1052.

28. Swanson KL, Wiesner RH, Krowka MJ. Natural history of hepatopulmonary syndrome: impact of liver transplantation. *Hepatology*. 2005;41:1122–1129.

29. Durand F, Valla D. Assessment of prognosis of cirrhosis. *Semin Liver Dis*. 2008;28:110–122.

30. Wehler M, Kokoska J, Reulbach U, Hahn EG, Strauss R. Short-term prognosis in critically ill patients with cirrhosis assessed by prognostic scoring systems. *Hepatology*. 2001;34:255–261.

31. Dhainaut JF, Laterre PF, Janes JM, et al. Drotrecogin alfa (activated) in the treatment of severe sepsis patients with multiple-organ dysfunction: data from the PROWESS trial. *Intensive Care Med*. 2003;29:894–903.

32. Larson AM, Curtis JR. Integrating palliative care for liver transplant candidates: "too well for transplant, too sick for life". *JAMA*. 2006;295:2168–2176.

33. Von Roenn JH, von Gunten CF. Setting goals to maintain hope. *J Clin Oncol*. 2003;21:570–574.

34. Back AL, Arnold RM, Quill TE. Hope for the best, and prepare for the worst. *Ann Intern Med*. 2003;138:439–443.

35. Evans WG, Tulsky JA, Back AL, Arnold RM. Communication at times of transitions: how to help patients cope with loss and re-define hope. *Cancer J*. 2006;12:417–424.

36. Lumby J. Liver transplantation: the death/life paradox. *Int J Nurs Pract*. 1997;3:231–238.

BRAIN FUNCTION

Chapter 55

What Is the Role of Palliative Care in Stroke?

Mara Lugassy

INTRODUCTION AND SCOPE OF THE PROBLEM

Every year in the United States, approximately 795,000 people experience a stroke,[1] meaning someone has a stroke approximately every 40 seconds. Around 80% of strokes are ischemic, with the remainder being hemorrhagic. Stroke is the third leading cause of death in the United Sates, behind heart disease and cancer.[2] In 2007, stroke accounted for 1 in 18 deaths in the United States.[1] Over the past several decades, significant advances have been made in the prevention, acute treatment, and rehabilitation of stroke. Despite this, stroke remains a significant cause of morbidity and mortality and is the leading cause of significant disability in adults.[2] Among those who survive an acute stroke, the majority will be left with some degree of physical, cognitive, or psychological disability, with 15% to 30% remaining permanently disabled and 20% requiring institutional care at 3 months after the event.[1]

Because palliative care focuses on improving quality of life throughout the trajectory of serious illness, the role of palliative medicine in stroke has the potential to be significant—benefitting patients, families, and caregivers at multiple stages of illness and in multiple care settings.

Because of the varied outcomes and degree of disability in patients who have had a stroke, the role of palliative care may vary depending on whether the patient is in the acute poststroke period or has progressed to a more chronic, disabled state.

SUMMARY OF EVIDENCE REGARDING TREATMENT RECOMMENDATIONS

Palliative Care in the Acute Stroke Period

One aspect of stroke that makes it unique from the palliative care perspective is the rapidity of onset; a person can go from fully functional and seemingly healthy to completely disabled or even comatose in a matter of seconds. Other conditions commonly seen by palliative care practitioners, such as cancer, dementia, or advanced cardiopulmonary disease, typically have a more gradual progression. In these conditions, patients and their families may have had some time to reflect on their disease and at least have an opportunity to develop some form of advance care plan. With acute stroke, on the other hand, many patients and families may be in shock by the rapid turn of events and may have given little prior thought to goals in the setting of serious illness.

Little evidence exists in the literature about the intersection between palliative care and stroke, in terms of both patient and family preferences for goals of care (this is especially true for patients with stroke who suddenly come to the end of their lives) and available interventions. However, some data have been published regarding what patients and families consider the most salient issues to be addressed. A qualitative study involving semistructured interviews of stroke patients and their families revealed several principles important to this population, including the assurance of a peaceful and dignified death; maintenance of communication among the family, caregivers, and health care team (in terms of both style and content); and continuing to include families and caregivers in discussions and decisions even after the goals of care may have shifted.[3] In another retrospective study of bereaved relatives of patients who had a stroke, predictors of satisfaction with care in the last 3 months of life included the ability to discuss worries or fears about the condition, treatments, or tests and the feeling that medical staff knew enough about the patient's condition. In the final 3 days of life, predictors of satisfaction with care included the feeling that enough help was available to meet the patient's needs, that the family had sufficient involvement in decision making, and that the person had died in the right place.[4] It follows that palliative care is well suited to assist in addressing these issues, particularly in the acute setting, in which establishing goals of care is central to developing the treatment plan.

Prognostic information is important for families and caregivers involved in discussions of goals of care, and it ultimately helps to shape decisions. Predictors of early mortality after an acute hemorrhagic or ischemic stroke include coma lasting more than 3 days, with patients having abnormal brainstem responses, absent response to verbal stimulation, and absent withdrawal to painful stimuli. Other predictors of poor prognosis include serum creatinine greater than 1.5 mg per dL and age greater than 70 years.[5]

Even in situations in which the palliative care practitioner is not providing the specific prognostic information, the palliative care team may serve a significant role in assisting the family in reflecting on the prognostic information. This includes the important work of helping them to frame the prognosis in the context of the patient's and family's overall values, prior wishes, and goals of care.

In the acute poststroke setting, the potential withdrawal or withholding of artificial nutrition and hydration is often a central discussion point in the severely impaired patient. Palliative care clinicians are often integrally involved in these conversations.[6] This topic in particular may be a source of conflict for families. One retrospective study of 104 patient deaths on an acute stroke unit demonstrated conflict in this area with nearly half of all interactions between family and staff.[7] The palliative care team may serve as a bridge among families, caregivers, and health care providers. Palliative care practitioners may also be an important source of education for families regarding concerns about quality of life and symptoms in patients for whom artificial nutrition may be withheld or withdrawn.

Another key issue in which the palliative care team may be involved is the withdrawal of ventilator support in patients with devastating strokes. This may include helping the family make the decision about removal of life-sustaining treatments and managing postextubation symptoms, including dyspnea, stridor, and retained oral or respiratory secretions.[8] Survival times after extubation of patients with neurological stroke sequelae vary; one study of ventilator withdrawal in patients in a neurological intensive care unit demonstrated survival times ranging from 10 minutes to 11 days after extubation, with the majority (59%) experiencing agonal or labored breathing during this time.[9] In the same study, families who decided to withdraw ventilator support were surveyed 1 year later and noted quality of life, overall prognosis, and level of suffering to be important factors in their decision-making process. When asked, 75% of respondents felt that the decision to withdraw ventilator support should be made jointly by physicians and families.

Evidence shows that dyspnea in particular may be a significant issue in end-of-life care for patients with stroke. In a retrospective study of 42 patients dying from stoke who were referred to a hospital-based palliative care consult service, 81% exhibited dyspnea or dyspnea behaviors, including noisy bronchial secretions, tachypnea, and use of accessory muscles of respiration.[10] This symptom may have multiple causes, including aspiration pneumonia, cardiac failure, pulmonary embolus, or renal failure with associated pulmonary edema.[10] Respiratory failure may also be directly related to brain injury, with either brainstem injury or overall impaired level of consciousness resulting in loss of pharyngeal tone, cough, gag, and swallowing reflexes.[11] Dyspnea in patients who have had a stroke may respond to the same modalities of treatment as in other conditions and should be tailored to the underlying cause, with treatments including bronchodilators, antibiotics, and opioids.

Terminal secretions may occur early and prominently in patients who have had a stroke; the prevalence of dysphagia and the resultant accumulation of salivary secretions in the upper airway or oropharynx is high. This symptom responds to the same types of treatments for retained secretions seen in other conditions, including using anticholinergic medications, appropriate positioning, and limiting excessive fluid intake.

In addition to dyspnea and associated respiratory distress, patients who have had a stroke may experience specific changes in breathing patterns related to their underlying brain injury, such as Cheyne-Stokes respirations, central hyperventilation, and agonal breathing. These breathing patterns may be particularly prevalent in cases of bilateral cerebral dysfunction or brainstem compression. Although these altered respiratory patterns may be of great concern to family members and other caregivers, they do not necessarily indicate distress on the part of the patient but are instead a part of the natural progression of the brain injury. In addition to providing symptom management for dyspnea and respiratory distress, the palliative care practitioner can serve as an importance resource in terms of explaining these breathing patterns and educating families about their underlying meaning.

Although less common than many of the symptoms noted earlier, fever is often seen in the acute poststroke period. It may occur in more than half of patients[12] and is associated with significantly higher morbidity and mortality. Although fever may be secondary to infection in some cases, in many cases the cause is unclear and may be related to a central cause.[11] Fever may be controlled with acetaminophen, ibuprofen, aspirin, or external cooling methods.

Palliative Care in the Long-Term Management of Stroke

A significant number of patients who have had a stroke and survive the initial acute stroke are left with a range of disability. Even when the main focus becomes rehabilitation and maximizing function, the patient who has had a stroke is often left with a host of symptoms and issues that need to be addressed. The palliative care clinician can play a major role in managing these symptoms, and given that many patients may not be able to communicate well, practitioners should maintain a low threshold for their recognition.

Common manifestations of stroke result from the specific oxygen-deprived territory of the brain, as well as complications secondary to the initial disabilities. Common primary deficits related to the area of infarction include hemiparesis, sensory loss, aphasia, dysarthria, dysphagia, visual loss, neglect syndromes, and cognitive impairment. These deficits may in turn contribute to a multitude of symptoms that can be addressed in the palliative care setting. In a retrospective study of patients who had a stroke evaluated by a palliative care consult service in an inpatient setting, symptoms addressed included dyspnea (81%), pain or pain behaviors (69%), dry mouth (62%), constipation (38%), and anxiety or sadness (26%).[10] In another prospective study examining symptoms and complications in patients 1 year after a stroke, common symptoms noted included contractures (60%), pain (55%), shoulder pain (52%), depression (50%), and pressure sores (22%).[13]

Pain is an important issue in management of both early and later stages of stroke, and palliative care practitioners may have a role in both assessment and management. Approximately 42% to 72% of stroke patients report pain.[14] This may result from a variety of causes, including stroke-related headaches, central poststroke pain, shoulder-hand syndrome, and type II complex regional pain.[10] Patients may also have pain from previous underlying medical conditions such as arthritis.

Among stroke survivors, shoulder pain associated with hemiplegia is particularly common; some reports document a prevalence as high as 80%.[15] This may result from a variety of causes, including glenohumeral subluxation, flaccidity, spasticity, and prior shoulder pathology. Management of these conditions often requires require careful attention to positioning, range-of-motion exercise, and appropriate use of analgesics.

A particular type of pain often noted in the poststroke period is shoulder-hand syndrome, which may occur in 20% to 30% of patients despite optimal rehabilitation programs.[16] It is characterized by pain and edema in the shoulder, wrist, and hand and may be followed by trophic skin changes, muscle atrophy, and contracture. Emphasis should be placed on range-of-motion activities to provide normal motion of the humerus and scapula. A short course of oral steroids[16,17] or tricyclic antidepressants may be helpful.

Also unique to patients who have had a stroke is central poststroke pain, which is believed to be secondary to the brain lesion itself, although the exact pathophysiology is yet unknown. Previously termed thalamic pain, it is now widely believed that lesions anywhere along the sensory tract can cause this syndrome. Poststroke pain typically has a delayed onset, occurring weeks to months after the acute stroke. It is often associated with dysesthetic-type sensations such as burning, squeezing, aching, or cold.[18] Some evidence suggests that adrenergic antidepressants such as amitriptyline can be effective in central poststroke pain,[19] although the effects can be limited and side effects can be prohibitive.[8] More recently, a randomized controlled study

demonstrated the efficacy of lamotrigine in central poststroke pain,[20] and medications such as gabapentin and pregabalin also may be potentially useful.[18]

Of particular importance in management of pain in patients who have had a stroke is the assessment of pain in patients with impaired communication, whether from aphasia, dysarthria, or overall altered level of consciousness. Evidence indicates that pain may be underrecognized and undertreated in nonverbal patients who have had a stroke. In a retrospective review of 207 patients with stroke admitted to a rehabilitation hospital, comparing the as-needed usage of pain medications in patients with and without aphasia, it was found that although the amount of medication *prescribed* to the different groups was the same, the patients with aphasia ultimately *received* significantly less pain medication than those without aphasia during their hospital course.[21] Although to date no studies have specifically examined the use of as-needed versus routine scheduled pain medications in patients with stroke, it seems logical that consideration should be given to the use of scheduled pain medications, particularly in the setting of aphasia or other communication deficits.

Limited evidence exists on assessment of pain in nonverbal patients with stroke, with much of the assessment strategies currently in use extrapolated from patients with dementia. However, evidence does indicate that patients with poststroke aphasia may be able to use a visual analog scale to communicate different levels of stimulus intensity.[22] This may provide a novel way for these patients to effectively communicate differing levels of pain.

Depression is also common in patients with stroke and may be related to a variety of causes, including psychosocial stress from loss of function and changes in the neurotransmitter systems. A meta-analysis of 51 studies examining poststroke depression demonstrated that approximately 33% of all stroke survivors experience depression, although this may well be a conservative estimate given the potential for underreporting or underrecognition in patients with cognitive or communication deficits.[23] For all of these reasons, depression may be easy to miss in patients who have had a stroke and can be severely disabling and result in worsened outcomes in terms of functional recovery, morbidity, and mortality. Thus palliative care clinicians should maintain a low threshold for recognition and treatment of depression in patients with stroke.[2] Because of the interdisciplinary nature of palliative care, the team may be well suited to manage depression in this population through the use of counseling, psychotherapy, and pharmacotherapy. Although various antidepressants can be effective in treating poststroke depression, consideration should be given to the side effect profile of medications given the patient's underlying condition. For example, the anticholinergic aspects of some antidepressants (e.g., tricyclics) can exacerbate symptoms already common in patients with stroke, such as sedation, constipation, and urinary retention. For these reasons, selective serotonin reuptake inhibitors may be a better first-line agent in many of these patients.

Dysphagia occurs in 37% to 78% of patients with stroke and is a risk factor for stroke-associated pneumonia and poor outcomes. Aspiration resulting from dysphagia can be suspected when patients cough or choke while eating; have a wet, gurgly voice; or have recurrent pneumonias. It is important to remember, however, that approximately half of all aspirations are "silent," with no associated symptoms.[2] Dysphagia can sometimes be managed in the acute setting by dietary modifications, although with more severe dysphagia, placement of a nasogastric tube may be considered. Dysphagia can sometime resolve quickly; if persistent, however, discussions about more permanent feeding options, such as a percutaneous endoscopic gastrostomy tube, may need to be initiated. Given the complexity of these conversations in patients with serious stroke, the palliative care team may play an important role in facilitating these discussions.

Spasticity is common in patients who have had a stroke, occurring in up to 60% of cases.[2] Spasticity involves overactivity of muscles in which the muscles overrespond to stretch reflexes. This typically may result in forcing the arms to involuntarily flex and pronate and the legs to extend and adduct.[16] Spasticity may be a source of great distress to patients, resulting in painful spasms, uncontrollable clonus, and abnormal posturing. These conditions may ultimately lead to contractures that can interfere with hygiene and other aspects of care. Nonpharmacological treatments of spasticity include positioning, stretch exercises, and splinting. Systemic medications such as baclofen and benzodiazepines can have sedating effects and thus must be considered in the context of the overall condition and goals of care of the patient. Local therapy with botulinum toxin injections is an alternative that has been shown to be safe and well tolerated and may prevent contractures, improve range of motion, and make aspects of care such as grooming and positioning easier.[24]

Pressure ulcers are a common complication of stroke. A study of 122 severely disabled stroke survivors in the year after stroke showed a prevalence of pressure ulcers of 22%.[13] Because the immobility commonly experienced by severely disabled patients with stroke can lead to skin breakdown and pressure ulcers, meticulous attention needs to be paid to prevention and management of skin breakdown. This includes practices such as preventing friction, reducing pressure, and eliminating maceration of skin over bony prominences. Skin breakdown may also be worsened by incontinence. In cases of advanced ulceration in which no hope remains of curing the skin breakdown, emphasis can be placed on preventing further exacerbation of the wound and maintaining optimal comfort levels.

Constipation is extremely common after stroke and can be related to a variety of causes, including decreased oral intake and motor impairment. Medications may also play a role in constipation for patients after a stroke. For example, opioids given for pain, anticholinergics for bladder dysfunction, tricyclic antidepressants, and antiemetics that decrease gut motility may all lead to constipation.[25] Constipation of this nature can be a significant source of distress for patients and can contribute to overflow fecal incontinence, ultimately worsening skin breakdown. Advanced age, large and disabling strokes, and impaired consciousness are all predictors of fecal incontinence.[25] This cycle frequently can be prevented by adequate fluid intake, adequate fiber (if taking substances by mouth), and an appropriate laxative regimen.[16] Bowel movements should be closely monitored, especially in patients with impaired communication skills.

Urinary incontinence is also common in the poststroke period, with prevalence rates between 38% and 60% in the early poststroke period. Urinary incontinence is often an important factor in determining whether stroke survivors are cared for in a home or in an institutional setting.[2] Although urinary incontinence and retention often result from lack of control of the detrusor reflex, the simple inability of a patient to communicate the need to void, either from aphasia or other disability, can result in incontinence as well. In such cases, it is important to keep the surrounding skin clean and dry to prevent further maceration and breakdown. In some cases, catheterization (preferably intermittently) may be indicated.[16]

KEY MESSAGES TO PATIENTS AND THEIR FAMILIES

Stroke is a common condition that can result in a range of disability and symptoms. Palliative care can play an important role in improving quality of life in stroke, both immediately after the stroke and on a longer-term basis. These services include helping the patient and family make decisions, better understanding the patient's prognosis, and ameliorating difficult to control symptoms.

CONCLUSION AND SUMMARY

Research into the intersection between stroke and palliative care remains in the early stages. However, given the underlying principles of the field, it is clear that palliative care clinicians can play a significant role in the care of patients who have had a stroke. Interventions that the team can provide range from facilitating end-of-life decisions in cases of devastating brain damage to managing chronic symptoms and improving quality of life in stroke survivors. Patients with stroke may exhibit a wide range of symptoms and complications, and the palliative care clinician should remain vigilant in monitoring for these symptoms and have a low threshold for treatment.

SUMMARY RECOMMENDATIONS

- Palliative care may play a significant role throughout the trajectory of the acute and chronic phases of a patient's poststroke period.
- Facilitating communication about goals of care discussions in relationship to withdrawal of mechanical ventilation and artificial nutrition and hydration is a key role for the palliative care team.
- Dyspnea and terminal secretions occur frequently and early in severe stroke and should be addressed aggressively with anticholinergic medications, positioning, and limiting excess fluids.
- A high frequency of pain is present in the poststroke period, and it is especially important to monitor for pain in patients with aphasia and other communication impairments.
- Urinary and fecal incontinence are common, and one of the goals of treatment is to prevent skin breakdown.

REFERENCES

1. Roger VL, Go AS, Lloyd-Jones DM, et al. Heart disease and stroke stastics: 2011update—a report from the American Heart Association. *Circulation.* 2011;123(4):e240.
2. Good D, Bettermann K, Reichwein R. Stroke rehabilitation. *Continuum.* 2011;17(3):545–567.
3. Payne S, Burton C, Addington-Hall J, Jones A. End of life issues in acute stroke care: a qualitative study of the experiences and preferences of patients and families. *Palliat Med.* 2010;24(2):146–153.
4. Young AJ, Rogers A, Dent L, Addington-Hall JM. Experiences of hospital care reported by bereaved relatives of patients after a stroke: a retrospective survey using the VOICES questionnaire. *J Adv Nurs.* 2009;65:2161–2174.
5. Kurent J. Palliative care of patients with specific neurological diseases. *Continuum.* 2005;11(6):33–77.
6. Wee B, Adams A, Eva G. Palliative and end of life care for people with stroke. *Curr Opin Support Palliat Care.* 2010;4:229–232.
7. Blacquiere DP, Gubitz GJ, Dupere D, McLeod D, Phillips S. Evaluating an organized palliative care approach in patients with severe stroke. *Can J Neurol Sci.* 2009;36(6):731–734.
8. Simmons B, Parks S. Intracerebral hemorrhage for the palliative care provider: what you need to know. *J Palliat Med.* 2008;11(10):1336–1339.
9. Mayer AM, Kossoff SB. Withdrawal of life support in the neurological intensive care unit. *Neurology.* 1999;52:1602–1609.
10. Mazzocato C. The last days of dying stroke patients referred to a palliative care consult team in an acute hospital. *Eur J Neurol.* 2010;17(1):73–77.
11. Zazulia AR. Critical care management of acute ischemic stroke. *Continuum.* 2009;15(3):68–82.
12. Hajat C, Hajat S, Sharma P. Effects of poststroke pyrexia on stroke outcome: a meta-analysis of studies in patients. *Stroke.* 2000;31(2):410–414.
13. Sackley C, Brittle N, Patel S, et al. The prevalence of joint contracture, pressure sores, painful shoulder, other pain, falls, and depression in the year after a severely disabling stroke. *Stroke.* 2008;39(12):3329–3334.
14. Kong KH, Woon VC, Yang SY. Prevalence of chronic pain and its impact on health related quality of life in stroke survivors. *Arch Phys Med Rehabil.* 2004;85(1):35–40.
15. Dromerick A, Edwards D, Dumar A. Hemiplegic shoulder pain syndrome: frequency and characteristics during inpatient stroke rehabilitation. *Arch Phys Med Rehabil.* 2008;89(8):1589–1593.
16. Volpe BT. Palliative treatment for stroke. *Neurol Clin.* 2001;19(4):903–920.
17. Braus DF, Krauss JK, STrobel J. The shoulder–hand syndrome after stroke: a prospective clinical trial. *Ann Neurol.* 1994;36(5):728–733.
18. Kim JS. Post stroke pain. *Expert Rev Neurother.* 2009;9(5):711–721.
19. Leijon G, Boivie J. Central post-stroke pain: a controlled trial of amitriptyline and carbamazepine. *Pain.* 1989;36(1):27–36.
20. Vestergaard K, Andersen G, Gottrup H, Kristensen BT, Jensen TS. Lamotrigine for central poststroke pain: a randomized controlled trial. *Neurology.* 2001;56(2):184–190.
21. Kehayia E, Korner-Bitensky N, Singer F, et al. Differences in pain medication use in stroke patients with aphasia and without aphasia. *Stroke.* 1997;28(10):1867–1870.
22. Korner-Bitensky N, Kehayia E, Tremblay N, et al. Eliciting information on differential sensation of heat in those with and without post stroke aphasia using a visual analogue scale. *Stroke.* 2006;37(2):471–475.
23. Hackett ML, Yapa C, Parag V, Anderson CS. Frequency of depression after stroke: a systematic review of observational studies. *Stroke.* 2005;36(6):1330–1340.
24. Simpson DM, Gracies JM, Graham HK, et al. Assessment: botulinum neurotoxin for the treatment of spasticity (an evidence-based review)—report of the Therapeutics and Technology Assessment Subcommittee of the American Academy of Neurology. *Neurology.* 2008;70(19):1691–1698.
25. Kumar S, Selim MH, Caplan LR. Medical complications after stroke. *Lancet Neurol.* 2010;9(1):105–118.

| Chapter 56 | What Special Considerations Are Needed for Individuals With Amyotrophic Lateral Sclerosis, Multiple Sclerosis, or Parkinson Disease? |

ELIZABETH LINDENBERGER AND DIANE E. MEIER

INTRODUCTION AND SCOPE OF THE PROBLEM

Neurodegenerative diseases affect adults of all ages and are associated with complex physical and neuropsychiatric symptoms, progressive functional impairments, and high levels of personal and caregiver suffering. Although amyotrophic lateral sclerosis (ALS), multiple sclerosis (MS), and Parkinson disease (PD) are distinct disease entities varying in prevalence and disease trajectories, they share numerous characteristics and care needs. All are associated with multiple domains of loss and profound disruptions of patient roles and relationships. The loss of the ability to eat and communicate, for example, significantly affects quality of life and yet is often not addressed by standard medical care. Critical concerns identified by patients and caregivers include staying connected, enduring financial hardship, managing physical challenges and caregiver burden, and finding help for advanced disease.[1,2]

Palliative care aims to relieve suffering and improve quality of life for patients with serious illnesses and their families. Palliative care services are underused in MS and PD compared to ALS,[3] due in large part to differences in disease trajectories. Whereas ALS is a relentlessly progressive and rapidly fatal condition, MS and PD are chronic conditions that generally progress slowly over a period of many years (Table 56-1). Other barriers to palliative care include uncertain prognosis and lack of recognition by health providers, patients, and families about the meaning and benefits of palliative care.[3] Core palliative care tasks include communication with patients and families, management of symptoms, psychosocial support, and coordination of medical and social services.[4] These tasks may take place over a short time for a rapidly progressive disease such as ALS or over many years for MS or PD (Table 56-2).

Patients with neurodegenerative diseases require a comprehensive multispecialty approach and care coordination. Patients commonly have difficulties accessing coordinated care. Interdisciplinary team care is most widely accepted as the evidence-based standard of care for ALS and is associated with quality of life and survival benefits.[5,6] More than 70 multidisciplinary ALS clinics operate in the United States certified by voluntary disease organizations, including the ALS Association (ALSA) and Muscular Dystrophy Association (MDA). Although interdisciplinary clinics for MS and PD care are also becoming more common and increasingly recognized as optimal care models, many patients lack access to this type of coordinated care team. Furthermore, these disease-specific clinics rarely formally incorporate palliative care specialists. In a survey of ALS certified centers and clinics, for example, 41% reported that their center provided no grief or bereavement support.[7] Interdisciplinary palliative care teams play an important role in supporting patients and families throughout the disease course.

Epidemiology and Disease Trajectory

Neurodegenerative diseases vary greatly in their prevalence, risk factors, typical onset age, and disease trajectories (see Table 56-1). Even within a particular disease, there may be considerable variation in presentation and course. Recognizing disease patterns and expected future trajectories is essential to helping patients plan for the future.

ALS is an uncommon disease with a relative short survival compared to MS and PD. Median survival is 3 to 5 years, but 5% to 10% of patients survive more

TABLE 56-1. Epidemiology of Amyotrophic Lateral Sclerosis, Multiple Sclerosis, and Parkinson Disease

CHARACTERISTICS	ALS	MS	PD
Prevalence in the United States	0.03 million	0.3 million	1.5 million
Incidence of death per 100,000	1.8	1.8	24
Median survival	3-5 years (longer if patients receive tracheostomy and invasive mechanical ventilation)	30 + years (high variability)	16 years (high variability)
Mean age of onset	60	30	60
Risk factors for disease	Older age, family history (10% familial, 90% sporadic), cigarette smoking, pesticide and heavy metal exposure, factory work, military history	Female sex, northern European descent, family history, personal history of autoimmune disease	Older age, male sex, and certain occupational exposures such as pesticides and heavy metals
Risk factors for decreased survival	Older age, rapid early disease course, bulbar or respiratory onset	Primary progressive form	Older age, male sex, severe motor symptoms, psychotic symptoms, and dementia

Data from Liao S, Arnold RM. Attitudinal differences in neurodegenerative disorders. *J Palliat Med.* 2007;10(2):430-432; and Elman LB, Houghton DJ, Wu GF, Hurtig HI, Markowitz CE, McCluskey L. Palliative care in amyotrophic lateral sclerosis, Parkinson's disease, and multiple sclerosis. *J Palliat Med.* 2007;10(2):433-457.
ALS, Amyotrophic lateral sclerosis; *MS,* multiple sclerosis; *PD,* Parkinson disease.

TABLE 56-2. Coordination of Care for Stages of Neurodegererative Disease*

PALLIATIVE CARE SERVICES	EARLY STAGE	MIDDLE STAGE	LATE STAGE
Advance care planning	1. Assess decision-making capacity for advance care planning 2. Identify health care proxy and encourage completion of advance directive 3. Discuss diagnosis, prognosis, likely course of illness, including disease-modifying therapies and future disease-specific decisions that may arise 4. Elicit patient-centered goals, hopes, expectations	Review steps 1-4 as in Early Stage Additionally: 5. Review patient's understanding of prognosis 6. Review efficacy and burden ratio of disease-modifying or life-prolonging treatments 7. Prepare patient and family for a shift in goals	Review steps 1-7 Additionally: 8. Help patient and family explicitly plan for a peaceful death 9. Encourage completion of important tasks and increased attention to relationships and financial affairs
Programmatic support	1. Assess personal care and equipment needs 2. Advise patients regarding options for visiting nurse, home care, case management services, and disease-specific support organizations 3. Offer care from certified multidisciplinary centers when available	Review steps 1-3 as in Early Stage Additionally: 4. Advise patients regarding options for palliative care and hospice services	Review steps 1-4 Additionally: 5. Consider nursing home placement with hospice if patient's home caregivers are overwhelmed
Financial planning	1. Advise patient to seek help in planning for financial, long-term care, and insurance needs; refer to lawyer experienced in health issues 2. Assess eligibility for SSDI, SSI, Medicare, Medicaid, and VA services 3. Encourage completion of durable power of attorney	Review steps 1-3 as in Early Stage Additionally: 4. For rapidly progressive disease (e.g., ALS), consider hospice referral	Review steps 1-3 Additionally: 5. Recommend hospice and review its advantages
Caregiver support	1. Listen to concerns 2. Ask about health and well-being of caregivers 3. Ask about practical support needs (e.g., transportation, prescription drug coverage, respite care, and personal care) 4. Encourage support or counseling of family caregivers; inform patient and family about practical resources, including disease-specific support groups	Review steps 1-4 as in Early Stage Additionally: 5. Raise the possibility of hospice and discuss its benefits 6. Identify respite resources and recommend help from family and friends	Review Steps 1-6 Additionally: 7. Encourage out-of-town family to visit 8. After death, send bereavement card and call after 1-2 wk; screen for complicated bereavement; offer bereavement support through hospice

Modified from Morrison RS, Meier DE. Clinical practice: palliative care. *N Engl J Med.* 2004;350(25):2582-2590.
ALS, Amyotrophic lateral sclerosis; *MS,* multiple sclerosis; *PD,* Parkinson disease; *SSDI,* Social Security Disability Insurance; *SSI,* Supplemental Security Income.
*Early stage refers to the stage of disease at time of diagnosis, middle stage to progressive disease and increasing functional decline, and late stage to the stage when death is imminent.

than 10 years.[8] Bulbar-onset ALS, presenting with dysarthria or dysphagia without significant spinal involvement, has a particularly poor prognosis, with a median survival time of 2 years. The vast majority of patients die from respiratory failure. For the small minority of patients undergoing tracheostomy with long-term mechanical ventilation, life expectancy may be 15 years or longer. Riluzole, the only drug approved as a disease-modifying therapy for ALS, increases life expectancy by approximately 2 to 3 months

Unlike ALS, the typical MS course spans decades, and although the disease typically causes progressive disability over years, many patients will eventually die of other causes. Compared to the general population, however, MS patients have a threefold increased risk for death and a 10-year shorter life expectancy.[9] One population-based study demonstrated a median survival time of 38 years from symptoms onset and mean age at death of 65. Cause of death was related to MS in 58% of patients, and the most common cause of death was respiratory disease.[10]

The majority of MS cases are the relapsing-remitting type (80%-90%), characterized by periods of progression punctuated by periods of plateau. This phase typically lasts two decades and is followed by a secondary progressive phase that lacks periods of significant remission. Approximately 15% of patients present with primary-progressive MS, which progresses relentlessly without prolonged plateaus. A small subgroup of MS patients has a benign form that never relapses. Disease-modifying therapies, including interferon-β1a, interferon-β1b, glatiramer acetate, and natalizumab, decrease the rates of relapse and disease progression in relapsing-remitting MS. Acute attacks, or relapses, are typically treated with corticosteroids. As with other serious progressive illnesses, effective palliative care for MS includes helping patients weigh the potential benefits and burdens of disease-modifying therapies on an ongoing basis throughout the disease course.

In contrast to ALS and MS, PD is a common neurodegenerative disease. PD predominantly affects older people and is characterized by gradually worsening motor and nonmotor symptoms over a period of years. PD commonly causes swallowing impairment in advanced disease, and aspiration pneumonia accounts for up to 70% of PD deaths.[11]

RELEVANT PATHOPHYSIOLOGY

ALS is the most common motor neuron disease and is characterized by upper and lower motor neuron loss. ALS nerve degeneration causes progressive limb, axial, and neck paralysis; dysarthria; dysphagia; and respiratory failure. The cause of ALS is unknown. Upper motor neuron symptoms, including spasticity and hyperreflexia, result from degeneration of motor neurons running from the motor strip of the frontal cortex to the spinal cord. Common upper motor neuron symptoms include stiffness and spasticity with gait instability and poor balance, Lower motor neuron symptoms, including weakness, atrophy, and fasciculations, result from degeneration of neurons connecting the brainstem and spinal cord with muscle fibers. Bulbar symptoms such as dysarthria and dysphagia may be caused by both upper and lower motor neuron dysfunction.

MS is an inflammatory demyelinating disease of the central nervous system. Although the cause of MS is unknown, it is most widely believed to be autoimmune in origin. The disease causes axonal injury, loss of myelin and oligodendrocytes, diffuse brain inflammation, and cerebral atrophy. MS may present with any variety of neurological signs or symptoms, but the most common are sensory symptoms, visual loss, and muscle weakness. Typically, sensory symptoms are described as numbness, tingling, electrical, cold, or itching. Lesions of the descending motor tracts of the spinal cord may lead to spasticity, hyperreflexia, and weakness of the legs.

PD is a complex motor system disorder associated with a wide array of nonmotor symptoms. The cardinal features of PD are tremor, rigidity, and bradykinesia. Postural instability is also a common feature of PD that generally occurs later in the disease. Like ALS and MS, the cause of PD is unknown. Dopamine depletion causes disruption of the basal ganglia circuits, resulting in bradykinesia and other parkinsonian symptoms. Although Lewy bodies are a key pathological feature of PD and found throughout the brain and other organs, they are relatively nonspecific findings.

SUMMARY OF EVIDENCE REGARDING TREATMENT RECOMMENDATIONS

Motor Symptoms

Amyotrophic Lateral Sclerosis and Multiple Sclerosis: Weakness and Spasticity. Patients with ALS develop progressive weakness that spreads gradually throughout all muscle groups but usually spares sphincter control and eye movement. Most patients with ALS present with asymmetrical limb weakness in the upper or lower extremities. In MS, limb weakness is typically more common and severe in the lower than in the upper extremities. Spasticity is a common and disabling symptom among patients with MS and generally worsens with advanced disease. Increased tone in the legs may lead to difficulty walking and pain. Spasticity can also be a problem for patients with ALS with prominent upper motor neuron symptoms. Treatment aims at improving mobility and function and reducing the risk for falls and fall-related injury.

Parkinson Disease: Tremor, Rigidity, Bradykinesia. In contrast to the weakness and spasticity of ALS and MS, the primary motor symptoms of PD include bradykinesia, tremor, and rigidity. Motor symptoms are generally asymmetrical and progress gradually over time. Bradykinesia, a generalized slowness of movement, presents as slowed walking with short steps and progresses to festination and gait freezing. PD tremors are resting, often characterized as "pill-rolling." Although bradykinesia is usually the most disabling symptom, tremor can be highly disabling if it affects the dominant hand.

Symptomatic treatment for PD is generally begun when patients develop gait impairment or when symptoms interfere with activities of daily living or social function. Patients may vary greatly in their preferences and goals regarding pharmacological therapy. Levodopa is the most effective therapy for PD and is the mainstay of treatment. Although particularly effective in treating bradykinesia, levodopa may also decrease symptoms of tremor and rigidity. A subset of patients with parkinsonism do not respond to high-dose levodopa, and a diagnosis of atypical parkinsonism, for example, progressive subranuclear palsy or multiple system atrophy, should be considered in these cases.

Levodopa is administered in combination with a decarboxylase inhibitor to prevent peripheral conversion of levodopa to dopamine, which results in nausea. The combination of carbidopa, a decarboxylase inhibitor, and levodopa is marketed in the United States as immediate-release Sinemet. Adverse central nervous system effects of levodopa are particularly common among older patients and include confusion, hallucinations, delusions, agitation, and psychosis. Other drugs used to treat symptomatic PD include dopamine agonists, monoamine oxidase inhibitors, catecholamine O-methyltransferase (COMT) inhibitors, anticholinergic agents, and amantadine. Dopamine agonists are often used as initial monotherapy in younger patients with PD because they are associated with a decreased risk for dyskinesia and motor fluctuations compared to levodopa. However, dopamine agonist therapy is associated with more hallucinations, somnolence, dizziness, edema, and nausea compared to levodopa therapy.[12]

Parkinson Disease Motor Complications: Dykinesias and Motor Fluctuations. More than 50% of patients with PD who have received levodopa for longer than 5 years experience motor complications, and these symptoms are most common in young-onset PD.[13] Motor complications are categorized in two subgroups: dyskinesias and motor fluctuations. Patients with motor fluctuations experience alternating "on" periods when response to medication is good and "off periods" when there is little response. Interestingly, many of the nonmotor symptoms of PD, including neuropychiatric symptoms and pain, also may fluctuate between "on" and "off" states, and treatment strategies are generally the same as for PD motor symptoms (Table 56-3).

Early in PD, patients typically have a long, that is, greater than 4-hour, response to levodopa. As the disease advances, this "on" period becomes progressively shorter. First-line pharmacological strategies to decrease wearing "off" periods include increasing the dose or the dosing frequency of levodopa (e.g., decrease the dosing interval by 30-60 minutes). Other strategies include adding a COMT inhibitor such as entacapone or adding an oral dopamine agonist such as pramipexole or ropinirole. Sustained-release carbidopa/levodopa has not been shown to decrease "off" time.[14]

Levodopa-induced dyskinesias are also common in advanced PD and may include not only choreiform movements (most common) but also dystonia or myoclonus. Dystonia, which can be painful, may involve any part of the body, including the head, neck, limbs, or respiratory muscles. Dystonia also may be a feature of untreated PD; therefore a careful clinical history will help distinguish between "on" phenomenon dystonia (too much levodopa) or "off" dystonia (too little levodopa). Although dyskinesias are treatable by decreasing or eliminating levodopa, finding an effective balance between decreasing parkinsonian symptoms and minimizing dyskinesias may be difficult. As PD advances, the therapeutic window for levodopa dosing decreases and patients may fluctuate between "off" periods with parkinsonian symptoms and "on" periods with dyskinesias. Most PD patients prefer the "on" periods with dyskinesia to the alternative rigid, bradykinetic state.[13] Deep brain stimulation of the subthalamic nucleus and globus pallidus interna are effective in treating motor fluctuations and may improve quality of life. Nevertheless, many patients with advanced PD are too frail to undergo this procedure.

Pain

Pain is among the most common symptoms reported by patients with neurodegenerative diseases. When assessing pain, it is essential to address not only physical causes but also psychological, spiritual, or emotional factors that may be affecting the patient. Many pain syndromes are multifactorial in cause and require a multidisciplinary approach to treatment (Table 56-4).

In ALS the major causes of pain are immobility, spasticity, and leg cramps. ALS does not directly cause sensory symptoms or sensory pain syndromes. Patients unable to change position may experience pain along pressure points. Pain in MS may be due to an acute paroxysmal attack or may be subacute or chronic. Pain is reported among more than 50% of patients with advanced MS.[15] Similar to ALS, patients with advanced MS experience immobility and spasticity-related pain. Unlike ALS, however, these patients experience a variety of complex sensory pain syndromes throughout the disease course. Like in ALS and MS, pain in PD is common and results from multiple causes. Pain was reported by 85% of patients in one community-based survey and reported as severe in 42% of patients with end-stage PD in a caregiver survey study.[16,17] Pain resulting from rigidity, dystonia, and dyskinesia is common, and treatment focuses on motor symptom control (see Table 56-4)

Dyspnea

Dyspnea is common in ALS because of progressive respiratory muscle weakness (see later discussion of respiratory failure and ALS). Although it is generally a less common problem in PD, these patients

TABLE 56-3. Neuropsychiatric and Cognitive Symptoms

PROBLEM	DISEASE	CHARACTERISTICS	NONPHARMACOLOGICAL TREATMENTS	PHARMACOLOGICAL TREATMENTS
Cognitive impairment	ALS	Frontotemporal cognitive dysfunction (in 30%) or dementia (15%), apathy, impaired executive function, impaired language, and inappropriate behaviors	Caregiver education and support	No proven treatments for cognitive symptoms; SSRIs may be helpful for inappropriate behaviors
	MS	Mild symptoms common, dementia uncommon, attention, information processing speed, visual spatial abilities, short-term memory, and verbal fluency	Cognitive rehabilitation programs and environmental adaptations may help	Cholinesterase inhibitors (e.g., donepezil, galantamine) may provide small benefit; discontinue medications that may exacerbate symptoms (e.g., benzodiazepines, anticholinergics)
	PD	Dementia common in advanced disease (30%); mild symptoms in early disease; executive dysfunction and visuospatial impairments are common	Caregiver education and support	Cholinesterase inhibitors may provide small benefit; discontinue medications that may exacerbate symptoms (e.g., benzodiazepines, anticholinergics)
Depression	ALS	Transient depressive symptoms are common	Psychotherapy, support groups	SSRIs and TCAs
	MS	Common, often cluster with symptoms of fatigue, anxiety, and cognitive impairment; may occur as side effect of interferon immunomodulatory therapies	Cognitive behavioral therapy, support groups, psychotherapy, mindfulness training	SSRIs and TCAs; consider trial off of immunomodulatory therapies
	PD	Common; masked facies and stooped posture may mimic depression in a nondepressed patient	Psychotherapy, support groups	SSRIs and TCAs
Anxiety	ALS	May be associated with dyspnea or nighttime immobility and insomnia	BPAP if dyspnea contributing; psychotherapy; support groups; home support	SSRIs and benzodiazepines
	MS	Common, especially among patients with pain and fatigue	Psychotherapy; support groups	SSRIs and benzodiazepines
	PD	May manifest as agitation, irritability, restlessness, dysphoria. May occur as fluctuating symptom, complication of levodopa therapy	Psychotherapy for patients without dementia	SSRIs; caution with benzodiazepines because they may lead to confusion, falls. Treat as for motor fluctuations of PD (adjust dopaminergic medications)
Pseudobulbar effect	ALS	Common (20%–50% of patients); characterized by uncontrolled laughing or crying	Educate patient and family regarding the symptom, that it is not a mood disorder	SSRIs and TCAs as first-line therapy; alternative is fixed combination of dextromethorphan hydrobromde 20mg with quinidine sulfate 10mg orally twice daily
	MS	10% of patients	As for ALS	As for ALS
	PD	<10% of patients	As for ALS and MS	As for ALS and MS
Psychotic and behavioral	ALS	May occur in patients with frontotemporal dementia	Caregiver education and support, respite	Antidepressants may improve symptoms in frontotemporal dementia; antipsychotic medications if needed for severe symptoms
	MS	Uncommon, but epidemiological evidence of increased prevalence of psychotic disorders in MS	Caregiver education and support, respite	Antipsychotic medications if needed for severe symptoms
	PD	Visual hallucinations and paranoid delusions are most common; may be exacerbated by dopaminergic medications	Caregiver education and support, respite	Evaluate for delirium and potential medical cause if acute change; decrease levodopa and consider discontinuing dopamine agonists; if antipsychotic medications needed, quetiapine and clozapine are preferred (lower risk for motor side effects)

TABLE 56-4. Common Physical Symptoms

PROBLEM	DISEASE	CAUSES AND CHARACTERISTICS	NONPHARMACOLOGICAL TREATMENTS	PHARMACOLOGICAL TREATMENTS
Motor, gait instability, falls	ALS	Weakness	Assistive devices, adaptive equipment, ankle-foot orthotics	None
		Spasticity	Stretching, splinting, ROM, massage	Baclofen, tizanidine, gabapentin, dantrolene, benzodiazepines (monitor for sedation) Intrathecal baclofen pump or botulinum injection into affected muscle for severe cases
	MS	Weakness and spasticity	As for ALS	Corticosteroids for acute attacks; treat spasticity if present (as for ALS)
	PD	Bradykinesia, rigidity, tremor, shuffling gait, freezing, festination	Assistive devices and rehabilitation therapies	Dopaminergic agents
		Falls resulting from orthostasis	Increase salt and fluid intake; educate about effects of eating, bathing, warm weather, and rising quickly from lying down	Discontinue antihypertensive medications if possible; consider trial of fludrocortisone or midodrine
		Dyskinesias and motor fluctuations	Avoid taking levodopa with high-protein meals	Adjust PD dopaminergic medications (see section on PD motor complications); consider deep brain stimulation
Pain	ALS	Immobility, including joint pain (e.g., shoulder, neck) because of impaired mobility	Frequent repositioning, ROM exercises; massage; supportive mattresses and wheelchair cushions; neck support and collar when needed	Acetaminophen and NSAIDS for mild pain; opioid analgesics for moderate to severe pain
		Leg cramps	Calf muscle stretching; tonic water contains variable levels of quinine and may be helpful	Consider quinine sulfate for severe cases (FDA warning against routine use because of adverse effects)
	MS	Neuropathic pain syndromes (e.g., lower extremity dysesthesias, burning pain of legs and feet), Lhermitte's phenomenon, and trigeminal neuralgia; painful tonic spasms	Stress reduction, TENS, avoidance of heat exposure if heat-exacerbated symptoms	Anticonvulsants (e.g., gabapentin, pregabalin, carbamazepine; TCAs; duloxetine)
		Immobility-related pain in advanced disease	As for ALS	Same as for ALS
	PD	Rigidity, dystonias, dyskinesias	Physical therapy	Adjust levodopa or dopamine agonists TCAs, anticonvulsants
		Neuropathic pain syndromes (e.g., numbness or paresthesias of arms/legs)	As for MS	
		Immobility-related pain in advanced disease	As for ALS and MS	As for ALS and MS
Dyspnea	ALS	Progressive respiratory muscle weakness	Noninvasive ventilation (BPAP)	Opioids; benzodiazepines when coexisting anxiety or for advanced disease; avoid supplemental oxygen as may worsen hypercapnia symptoms such as headaches and confusion
		Terminal phase respiratory failure	Room fans, supplemental oxygen, repositioning	Opioids; benzodiazepines if needed
	MS	Terminal phase pneumonias	As for ALS	As for ALS
	PD	Restrictive syndromes (e.g., neck and trunk dystonias)	Physical therapy, exercise, stretching, massage	Botulinum toxin injections; adjust dopaminergic agents; opioids if needed
		Nonmotor fluctuating symptom ("on" or "off"), complication of levodopa therapy		Treat as for motor fluctuations of PD (adjust dopaminergic medications)
		Terminal phase pneumonias	As for ALS and MS	As for ALS and MS
Sialorrhea	ALS	Results from poor handling of saliva	Mechanical suction devices if desirable to patient Cough assist devices for clearing secretions when cough is weak	Anticholinergic medications; consider an anticholinergic TCA such as amitriptyline if there is a second indication as well (e.g., treatment of depression or pseudobulbar affect); salivary gland botulinum injections or radiation therapy for severe cases
	MS	As for ALS	As for ALS	As for ALS
	PD	As for ALS and MS	As for ALS and MS	As for ALS and MS; caution with anticholinergic medications because they may cause confusion, falls

Symptom	Disease	Description	Nonpharmacologic management	Pharmacologic management
Fatigue, low energy, and sleep disorders	ALS	Increased effort needed to function because of immobility and respiratory muscles weakness	Energy conservation techniques; BPAP for hypoventilation	Consider modafinil
		Fatigue may be side effect of riluzole Sleep disturbance because of dyspnea, difficulty turning in bed, or pain	Treat underlying causes	Trial off riluzole Treat underlying causes
	MS	Primary fatigue is common and may be disabling; associated with high lesion load in the brain	Exercise, energy conservation techniques, complementary therapies such as mindfulness and yoga	Amantadine, SSRIs, modafinil, amphetamines; possible role for high-dose aspirin (1300 mg daily); treat depression if present
	PD	Fatigue commonly associated with depression	Counseling, support groups for depression	SSRIs for depression; consider methylphenidate for fatigue
		Rapid eye movement (REM) behavior disorder (RBD)	Educate patient and sleep partners; reduce nighttime safety risks	Low dose benzodiazepines at night; (dopaminergic medications make it worse); melatonin
		Restless leg syndrome (RLS)	Stretching of posterior leg muscles before sleep	Nighttime carbidopa/levodopa, benzodiazepines, gabapentin, or opioids
Constipation and bowel incontinence	ALS	Constipation resulting from immobility	Increase fiber and fluid intake	Laxatives and suppositories titrated to achieve a daily bowel movement
	MS	Constipation Bowel incontinence	High-fiber diet with increased fluids; exercise Avoid high-fiber foods, caffeine, artificial sweeteners; biofeedback	Laxatives and suppositories titrated to achieve a daily bowel movement Regulate a timed bowel schedule with laxatives and suppositories
	PD	Constipation resulting from decreased motility and immobility	High-fiber diet with increased fluids; exercise	Laxatives and suppositories
Nausea	ALS	Potential side effect of riluzole or opioids		Trial off riluzole; haloperidol for opioid-induced nausea
	MS	Potential side effect of activating medications (e.g., modafinil, amphetamines)		Discontinue medications that may cause nausea
	PD	Delayed gastric emptying Potential side effect of levodopa and dopamine agonists	Frequent, small meals; low-fat, low-fiber diet Take with meal or snack	Domperidone (not available in United States); erythromycin; possible role for botulinum injection into pyloric sphincter Start low doses; increase carbidopa dose with levodopa
Urinary symptoms	ALS	Some patients have urgency	Frequent, timed voiding; pelvic floor training; limit caffeine and alcohol intake	Oxybutinin, tolterodine, and other antimuscarinics
	MS	Urgency common	Frequent, timed voiding; pelvic floor training; limit caffeine and alcohol intake	Oxybutinin, tolterodine, and other antimuscarinics
		Urinary retention in severe disease, may cause overflow incontinence	Monitor postvoid residual volume; intermittent catheterization or suprapubic catheter for severe chronic retention	
	PD	Urgency (especially nocturia), frequency, and incontinence	Timed voiding; decrease nighttime fluid intake	Oxybutynin, tolterodine, and other antimuscarinics (caution: potential for side effect of impaired gastric emptying or confusion)

ALS, Amyotrophic lateral sclerosis; *BPAP,* bilevel positive airway pressure; *FDA,* Food and Drug Administration; *MS,* multiple sclerosis; *NSAIDs,* nonsteroidal anti-inflammatory drugs; *PD,* Parkinson disease; *ROM,* range of motion; *SSRI,* selective serotonin reuptake inhibitors; *TCA,* tricyclic antidepressant; *TENS,* transcutaneous electrical nerve stimulation.

also may experience troublesome dyspnea throughout the course of disease. PD-related dyspnea may be due to rigidity and bradykinesia of respiratory muscles or the dropped head, truncal flexion, or neck and trunk dystonias that impair chest expansion and lung volumes.[11] Dyspnea in PD may occur as a complication of long-term levodopa therapy, fluctuating as an "on" or "off" phenomenon (see Table 56-4). Respiratory failure in PD is rare and generally results from upper airway obstruction from vocal cord palsy, laryngospasm, or dystonia of oropharyngeal and cervical muscles.

Dyspnea is less common in the last month of life for PD compared to ALS.[16,17] However, in the active dying phase, patients with PD may develop dyspnea as a result of aspiration pneumonia. Although not generally a significant problem for patients with MS, dyspnea may be experienced with all neurodegenerative diseases during acute respiratory tract infections, including aspiration pneumonias, and during the active dying process. Low-dose opioid medications are safe and highly effective in treating dyspnea. For opioid-naïve patients, a typical starting dose of morphine 5 mg, or its equivalent, orally every 4 hours as needed is usually effective.

Respiratory Failure and Amyotrophic Lateral Sclerosis

In ALS, progressive weakness of respiratory muscles causes dyspnea and eventually death from respiratory failure. Advance care planning must begin early after diagnosis and include discussions of preferences regarding tracheostomy with invasive mechanical ventilation. The majority of patients with ALS choose to forego this procedure and die from respiratory failure.

Although many patients worry about "suffocating" or "choking to death," the vast majority of ALS caregivers surveyed report that their loved ones experience a peaceful death.[18]

In the United States, approximately 2% to 10% of patients with ALS undergo tracheostomy and unfortunately many receive this intervention emergently, without prior advance care planning discussions. Although invasive mechanical ventilation prolongs life indefinitely through automated mechanical breathing, disease progression continues. Home care costs and caregiver burden are high. For patients who choose this option, it is important to ask under what circumstances death would be preferable to life with severe impairment. Some patients with ALS choosing invasive mechanical ventilation state, for example, that if they progress to a "locked in" state, that is, unable to communicate even by eye movement, they would want their ventilator support withdrawn.[19]

Evidence-based guidelines recommend regular respiratory monitoring for patients with ALS.[20] Forced vital capacity (FVC) and maximal inspiratory pressure (MIP, or negative inspiratory force) are commonly used and predictive of ALS survival time. Monitoring respiratory function is important in guiding medical interventions and advance care planning discussions. Results may guide decisions about respiratory interventions such as noninvasive mechanical ventilation and tracheostomy, feeding tube placement, and hospice referrals (Figure 56-1)

Early respiratory symptoms include orthopnea, dyspnea on exertion, and nighttime hypoventilation resulting in hypoxia and hypercapnea. Nighttime hypoventilation may cause frequent awakenings, morning headaches, daytime fatigue, cognitive impairment, and uncontrolled hypertension. Noninvasive

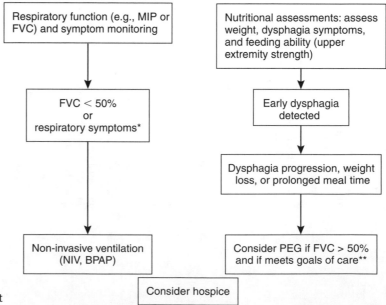

Figure 56-1. Respiratory and nutritional management in amyotrophic lateral sclerosis. (*BPAP*, Bilevel positive airway pressure; *FVC*, forced vital capacity; *MIP*, maximal inspiratory force; *NIV*, noninvasive ventilation; *PEG*, Percutaneous endoscopic gastrostomy.)

* dyspnea, orthopnea, or symptomatic hypercapnea
**if FVC < 50% and patient desires gastrostomy tube, may consider strategies to decrease procedure-related risk, e.g. respiratory support during PEG or radiologically inserted PEG

mechanical ventilation is the most effective intervention for ALS-associated hypoventilation and alleviates symptoms of dyspnea, insomnia, anxiety, and hypoxia-related cognitive dysfunction. Noninvasive mechanical ventilation is associated with improved survival and quality of life and does not significantly increase caregiver burden or stress.[21,22] Greatest survival benefit is seen among patients who use bilevel positive airway pressure (BPAP) for more than 4 hours per day. Because of the potential for worsening hypoventilation, supplemental oxygen is generally contraindicated in ALS except if paired with BPAP or if needed during the active dying phase.

Challenges related to BPAP include bulbar and facial weakness resulting in poor mask fitting, excessive drooling, and weak arms that impair patients' abilities to self-adjust the mask. Cognitive impairment may also make using BPAP a challenge in patients. Compliance with BPAP is highest when initiated early in the course of respiratory failure. Patients may be advised to start with 1 or 2 hours of BPAP on going to sleep at night or during a nap and titrate up to 4 or more hours at night.

Respiratory and bulbar muscle weakness may also lead to a weak cough and difficulty managing secretions. Cough augmentation strategies include manually assisted cough and mechanical insufflation-exsufflation (MIE). Weak evidence demonstrates MIE may improve clearance of upper airway secretions among patients with ALS with reduced cough flow.[20] MIE may be particularly clinically useful during acute respiratory tract infections or aspiration events.

Dysphagia and Weight Loss

Dysphagia is common in ALS, particularly among patients with bulbar-prominent disease. Choking is a frightening symptom for patients and caregivers and may lead to malnutrition and weight loss. Weight loss may also be caused by muscle wasting and arm weakness leading to difficulties with self-feeding. Dysphagia and arm weakness may cause meals to be prolonged and exhausting for patients and their caregivers. Percutaneous endoscopic gastrostomy (PEG) may for some patients decrease the stress of prolonged meals and allay fears of choking. Many patients may continue to eat small amounts of food by mouth but supplement with enteral feedings by PEG.

Class II and Class III studies have demonstrated benefit of PEG for weight stabilization in ALS.[20] Although studies examining the impact of PEG on ALS survival have had mixed results, Class II studies using appropriate controls have demonstrated survival benefit.[20] Because PEG placement becomes risky once patients have significant respiratory impairment, some patients may have a short window of safe PEG timing after dysphagia develops but respiratory function remains good. Evidence-based guidelines recommend minimizing risk by offering PEG placement when FVC remains above 50%[20] (see Figure 56-1). For patients with FVC less than 50% who desire feeding

tube placement, radiologically inserted gastrostomy or PEG with noninvasive ventilation assistance may reduce procedure-related risk. In advanced disease with significant respiratory failure, PEG is unlikely to benefit patients and may expose them to unnecessary burdens and risk.

Among patients with ALS counseled about the option of PEG, 80% decline. Thirteen percent of patients with ALS receive a PEG, with significant variation across clinical sites, suggesting great variation in how the topic is presented by physicians.[23] Given the great variation in disease forms and course, many patients with ALS will not develop dysphagia and will continue to eat a normal diet at the time of death.

Although generally less severe than in ALS, dysphagia is a common symptom in PD and MS. PD-related dysphagia may be caused by impairments in all swallowing phases, that is, oral, pharyngeal, and esophageal. In one randomized clinical trial of patients with PD, honey-thickened liquids were the most rapidly effective intervention, followed by nectar-thickened liquids and chin-down posture.[24] Dysphagia that significantly impairs nutritional intake in MS is rare. In these unusual circumstances, PEG placement may be considered if consistent with a patient's goals and values. Severe dysphagia is common among patients with end-stage PD with dementia, and in this setting no evidence exists for survival or quality of life benefits of PEG placement.

Speech Impairment

Speech impairment is a common, disabling, and socially isolating symptom. In ALS, speech impairment is due to bulbar damage and respiratory weakness. Speech rehabilitation and voice amplifiers can be helpful early in the disease course. When impairment becomes severe, high-technology augmentive and alternative communication becomes necessary. Numerous options are available for computer control, including dynamic touch screens that respond to head or eye-tracking and produce synthetic voice. In PD, speech impairment is common and characterized by a monopitch, soft, hoarse voice with a variable rate.[25] Helpful interventions include speech rehabilitation, voice amplifiers and alphabet supplementation. In MS, dysarthria from bulbar and cerebellar damage occurs in approximately 50% of patients and is typically most severe in advanced disease. Speech rehabilitation is often beneficial. In contrast to ALS, total speech loss is uncommon in MS and PD.

Other Physical Symptoms

Sialorrhea (excessive drooling) is a common and often embarrassing problem among patients with ALS, MS, and PD. This symptom may be even more burdensome for patients with arm weakness that prevents them from wiping their mouths. Sialorrhea is due to poor handling of saliva rather than increased production. In ALS, PD, and MS, this may be caused by weakened or bradykinetic orofacial muscles and dysphagia. Treatment strategies are outlined in Table 56-4.

Fatigue and low energy are common in neurodegenerative disease, and the causes are often multifactorial. Fatigue affects more the 50% of patients with MS, is associated with high lesion load in the brain, and is often reported as the most disabling symptom. Fatigue has been identified as part of a symptom cluster that includes depression, pain, perceived cognitive impairments, and quality of life.[26] Treatment strategies are outlined in Table 56-4.

Sleep disturbances are especially common in ALS and PD and may cause daytime fatigue (see Table 56-4). Nighttime hypoventilation, impaired bed mobility, and pain may lead to poor-quality sleep. Finally, fatigue and low energy may affect patients with respiratory and motor impairments from any cause as a result of increased work necessary to carry out activities of daily living. Management of fatigue may target underlying causes when possible. Energy conservation techniques, for example, pacing and prioritizing activities, may be helpful for fatigue and low energy of any cause.

Constipation is a common distressing symptom among patients with neurodegenerative disease. Immobility is a major contributor to constipation for patients with advanced ALS, MS, and PD. In PD, decreased colonic transit time is common and may occur early in the disease course. Patients with PD may also experience difficulty with the act of defecating because of difficulties with muscle coordination. In MS, constipation may be directly disease-related as a result of neurogenic bowel. Constipation is a side effect of medications such as opioid analgesics and anticholinergic agents. Approximately 30% to 50% of patients with MS experience bowel incontinence.[27] Treatment strategies are outlined in Table 56-4.

In PD, gastroparesis is a common cause of nausea and bloating. For patients with any neurodegenerative disease experiencing nausea, attention should first be given to potential medication side effects. In ALS, nausea or poor appetite may be a side effect of riluzole. In MS, activating medications such as modafinil may cause nausea. Opioids, which may be used for pain or dyspnea, may cause nausea, particularly early in opioid therapy. In PD, dopaminergic medication is the most common cause of nausea. Starting with low doses of levodopa, titrating up slowly, and adding carbidopa if needed, all help decrease nausea.

Urinary symptoms may affect patients with all neurodegenerative diseases and are particularly common and severe in MS. Among patients who have had MS for more than 10 years, nearly 100% have bladder dysfunction.[27] Bladder symptoms may worsen during relapses. The most common urinary symptom is urgency caused by hyperreflexic bladder. In more advanced disease, sacral spinal cord damage may lead to urinary retention. Urinary frequency and incontinence may occur as a result of hyperreflexic bladder or as an overflow phenomenon from urinary retention. Bladder function should be monitored regularly in patients with MS, with particular attention to residual urinary volumes. Similar to patients with MS, those with PD commonly experience urgency, frequency, and incontinence because of a hyperreflexic bladder. More than 50% of patients with PD experience urinary symptoms, which have a significant detrimental impact on quality of life.[28] Treatment strategies are described in Table 56-4.

Cognitive Impairment

Cognitive impairment is among the most burdensome and disabling symptoms of neurodegenerative disease (see Table 56-3). Cognitive impairment meeting criteria for dementia is most common in PD and least common in MS. MS-related cognitive impairments are common, with 50% of patients having cognitive symptoms during their disease course.[27] Although symptoms are often mild, they may present early in disease. Because patients with MS are generally younger and may live for decades, unemployment resulting from cognitive disabilities is a major concern. Cognitive impairment may also result in social isolation and difficult role changes.[27]

Approximately 15% of patients with ALS develop frontotemporal dementia (FTD). Dementia may be difficult to diagnose in patients with severe ALS if communication and physical function are highly impaired. Dementia is common in PD, particularly among older patients and those with longer disease duration.[13] Although dementia is uncommon in the first 5 years of PD diagnosis, mild cognitive impairment and hallucinations are common. If a patients presents with dementia early in the disease course, Lewy body dementia is a likely alternative diagnosis.

Neuropsychiatric Symptoms

Depression and anxiety are common among patients with neurodegenerative diseases. Complex causes include the stressors of chronic disabling illnesses, direct effects of frontal or subcortical white matter disease, and medication side effects, for example, fluctuations with levodopa in PD or depression as an immunomodulatory therapy side effect in MS. Table 56-3 describes treatment strategies.

Pseudobulbar affect is a neurological disorder characterized by uncontrollable episodes of laughing and crying. This symptom is sometimes misunderstood as a mood disorder and may cause embarrassment and social isolation. Although the exact cause is not known, the condition is thought to be due to degeneration of the corticobulbar tracts.

Occurrence of psychotic and behavioral symptoms is greatest among patients with PD. Of patients with PD, 20% experience hallucinations, with the highest risk in older patients and those with dementia. They may present at any stage of PD and frequently occur as side effects of antiparkinsonian or other psychoactive medications. Typically they are visual and often nonthreatening hallucinations of people or pets.[13] Hallucinations may be a presenting feature of delirium from a medical cause; therefore acute reversible medical conditions such as infection or fecal impaction should be considered when assessing new-onset hallucinations. Patients with PD who have dementia may experience agitation and paranoid delusions. Behavioral symptoms are rare in ALS except in the context of FTD. In MS, epidemiological studies demonstrate a 2 to 3 times higher prevalence of psychotic symptoms compared to the general population.[29] Although not well-characterized, numerous case reports describe symptoms such as hallucinations, paranoid delusions, irritability, and agitation among patients with MS.

Functional Impairment

Functional disability is a major concern for patients with neurodegenerative diseases. Lower extremity weakness (ALS and MS), ataxia (MS), and motor symptoms of PD may all impair ambulation. Falls are common and often multifactorial, because of gait instability, orthostatic hypotension in PD, or medications such as anticholinergic drugs or benzodiazepines. Assistive devices such as canes and walkers are essential for maximizing ambulation and safety. Other devices, such as ankle foot orthotics for foot drop, also may improve walking ability. Interventions to reduce falls and fall-related injury include physical therapy, home safety evaluations, and reduction of medications that may increase fall risk.

Patients with advanced neurodegenerative diseases may lose transfer ability and become confined to a wheelchair or bed. Transfer devices are critical in helping nonambulatory patients mobilize safely. Complications of immobility include pressure ulcers, pain, constipation, thromboembolic disease, social isolation, and depression. Strategies to decrease risk include therapeutic wheelchair cushions and mattresses, range-of-motion exercises, and attention to constipation, pain, and psychological symptoms.

Neurodegenerative diseases may impair any activities of daily living. In ALS and MS, upper extremity weakness may impair self-feeding, toileting, bathing turning in bed, and writing. In PD, bradykinesia, tremor, and rigidity may lead to similar impairments in all of these domains. Occupational therapists may assess patient needs and offer equipment to maximize independence and function. Examples include specialized utensils to improve grip for self-feeding, raised toilet seats, grab bars, and shower chairs and transfer devices for bathing.

Psychosocial Adjustment and Coping

Patients with neurodegenerative diseases may suffer emotionally, socially, spiritually, and financially. Progressive physical disability may lead to a relentless process of loss (of physical function, social contacts, relationship roles, employment). Many seriously disabled patients rely on a spouse for personal care, and the relationship shift from partner to patient may cause significant distress. Disease-related sexual dysfunction may also negatively affect spousal and other intimate relationships. Patients who are younger at diagnosis, for example, in MS, may also experience difficulties with normal developmental experiences such as career and family building. Inquiring routinely about patients' overall well-being is extremely important. Psychological counseling and disease-specific support groups can be helpful. Offering support regarding community resources, home care, and financial planning throughout the disease trajectory is essential (see Table 56-2).

Caregiver Burden

Caregiver burden results from the multiple physical, psychological, social, and financial stressors associated with caregiving. Burden is particularly high in neurodegenerative diseases, given the progressive disability that may occur over years. In a survey study of PD caregivers, 40% reported that their health had suffered from caregiving and 65% reported that their social life suffered.[30] Compared to ALS caregivers, PD caregivers report a higher level of isolation from loved ones. This is likely explained by the fact that PD patients are generally older at the time of death, have outlived many of their peers, have often suffered a long chronic course involving dementia, and are more likely to die in nursing homes because no one is able to care for them in their own homes.[17]

Caregivers report excessive time spent on personal care needs of their loved ones and low satisfaction with insurance coverage of needed home and community-based services.[1,31] Although home care and respite services are essential to reducing caregiver burden, health insurance coverage of home aide and attendant services is often limited. Table 56-2 summarizes resources available for caregiver support.

Financial Burdens and Resources

Patients with neurodegenerative diseases commonly experience financial hardship, due not only to loss of employment but also to high costs of personal care, medical care, and equipment. Table 56-2 outlines an approach to financial counseling throughout the disease trajectory.

For younger patients who are facing loss of employment due to disability, it is important to assess eligibility for Social Security Disability Insurance (SSDI), a cash benefit for people under age 65 who have paid a qualifying amount into the social security system throughout their working years. Typically patients may begin receiving Medicare coverage after a 24-month waiting period after SSDI initiation. This waiting period is waived, however, for ALS. Supplemental Security Income (SSI) disability, in contrast to SSDI, is a monthly benefit for people who are over age 65, blind, or disabled and have limited income. People receiving SSI are often eligible for Medicaid as well.

In addition to the Medicare waiting period waiver, patients with ALS may be eligible for other benefits or expedited processing. Patients with ALS meet Social Security disability criteria based on diagnosis alone, that is, "presumptive disability." Patients with other disabling diseases, including MS and PD, must demonstrate that they have disease-related disability to receive disability benefits from Social Security. Finally, because ALS is considered a "presumption of service connection" diagnosis by the Department of Veterans Affairs (VA), veterans with ALS are eligible for many VA benefits, including disability payments, adaptive equipment, eligibility for VA long-term care, palliative care, and home care services, among others.

Advance Care Planning: Special Issues

Advance care planning is an ongoing process that should begin at diagnosis and continue throughout the disease process (see Table 56-2). Given the high prevalence of cognitive impairment among patients with neurodegenerative disease, it is important to assess decision-making capacity for advance care planning discussions. Decision-making capacity may be determined by any physician and is decision-specific. For example, a patient with PD and mild dementia may have capacity to name a health care proxy but may lack capacity to make a more complex decision such as undergoing cardiopulmonary resuscitation in the event of catastrophic illness.

Advance care planning discussions should focus on eliciting patients' goals and values. It is important for physicians to have open discussions with patients regarding the likely course of their disease and likely decisions that will arise. In the case of ALS, for example, the natural disease course for nearly all patients is death from respiratory failure. Therefore open discussions regarding tracheostomy and long-term invasive mechanical ventilation should be addressed early with patients and families, well in advance of crisis. Conversations should address quality of life concerns, hopes and fears, and potential financial and caregiver burdens. It is important to recognize that advance care planning is a long-term process, and it is normal for patients' perspectives and decisions to change over time.

Hospice

The Medicare Hospice Benefit provides interdisciplinary comfort-oriented care for patients with a life expectancy of 6 months or less. Hospice services are highly beneficial for patients in the end stages of neurodegenerative disease. Compared to those without hospice, those patients receiving hospice are more likely to die in their preferred location, receive morphine during the dying process, and have a better understanding of their illness.[1] Patients who are receiving hospice care must relinquish Medicare-reimbursed services focused on prolongation of life or cure. Patients with ALS receiving invasive mechanical ventilation, for example, are generally not eligible for hospice care for ALS. Furthermore, hospice agencies are frequently unable to pay for expensive equipment such as power wheelchairs or computerized communication devices. Such equipment should ideally be offered to patients before hospice enrollment.

Medicare hospice eligibility criteria for ALS include critically impaired breathing, rapid progression and critical nutritional impairment, or rapid progression and life-threatening complications. These criteria are likely overly restrictive, because they exclude many patients who will die within 6 months.[32] Determining prognosis may be particularly challenging for chronic diseases of long duration such as PD or MS. Compared to patients with ALS, those with PD have shorter hospice enrollments, possibly because of lack of recognition of end-stage disease and difficulties of prognostication.[17] No specific Medicare criteria exist for determining hospice readiness for PD or MS. Improved prognostic tools for all advanced neurodegenerative diseases are needed promote increased and earlier access to hospice services.

KEY MESSAGES TO PATIENTS AND FAMILIES

Palliative care offers critical support for patients with ALS, PD, and MS to relieve suffering, maximize patient control and choice, and promote quality of life throughout the disease course. Optimal care is interdisciplinary and coordinated, meeting and anticipating patient and family needs throughout the care continuum. Numerous resources, including programmatic and support group information, are available through disease-specific organizations such as the ALSA, Muscular Dystrophy Association ALS Division, Parkinson's Disease Foundation and National Muscular Sclerosis Society. Hospice services are beneficial to patients and families at the end stages of disease.

CONCLUSION AND SUMMARY

Although unique diseases with diverse pathophysiology and disease trajectories, ALS, MS, and PD share numerous characteristics and care needs. All are associated with complex physical and neuropsychiatric symptoms, progressive functional impairments, and high levels of prolonged personal suffering and caregiver burden. Palliative care is underused for neurodegenerative diseases, particularly for long-term chronic diseases such as MS and PD. Coordinated, interdisciplinary care that incorporates palliative care throughout the disease trajectory is essential for relieving suffering and improving quality of life.

SUMMARY RECOMMENDATIONS

- Although disease trajectories vary greatly, palliative care should be an integral component of interdisciplinary coordinated care for patients at all stages of neurodegenerative disease.
- Burdensome symptoms are common, and ongoing assessments should include attention to complex motor, cognitive, and neuropsychiatric symptoms.
- Home equipment and assistive devices are essential in promoting quality of life in the face of progressive functional losses.
- Advance care planning should be addressed early and often, with special attention to disease-specific challenges.
- Financial and caregiver burdens are numerous. Identifying supportive community, insurance, and legal and financial planning services is essential.

REFERENCES

1. Ganzini L, Johnston WS, Silveira MJ. The final month of life in patients with ALS. *Neurology.* 2002;59(3):428–431.
2. Hudson PL, Toye C, Kristjanson LJ. Would people with Parkinson's disease benefit from palliative care? *Palliat Med.* 2006;20(2):87–94.
3. Liao S, Arnold RM. Attitudinal differences in neurodegenerative disorders. *J Palliat Med.* 2007;10(2):430–432.
4. Morrison RS, Meier DE. Clinical practice: palliative care. *N Engl J Med.* 2004;350(25):2582–2590.
5. Van den Berg JP, Kalmijn S, Lindeman E, et al. Multidisciplinary ALS care improves quality of life in patients with ALS. *Neurology.* 2005;65(8):1264–1267.
6. Traynor BJ, Alexander M, Corr B, Frost E, Hardiman O. Effect of a multidisciplinary amyotrophic lateral sclerosis (ALS) clinic on ALS survival: a population based study, 1996–2000. *J Neurol Neurosurg Psychiatry.* 2003;74(9):1258–1261.
7. Hebert RS, Lacomis D, Easter C, Frick V, Shear MK. Grief support for informal caregivers of patients with ALS: a national survey. *Neurology.* 2005;64(1):137–138.
8. Chio A, Logroscino G, Hardiman O, et al. Prognostic factors in ALS: a critical review. *Amyotroph Lateral Scler.* 2009;10(5–6):310–323.
9. Tremlett H, Zhao Y, Rieckmann P, Hutchinson M. New perspectives in the natural history of multiple sclerosis. *Neurology.* 2010;74(24):2004–2015.
10. Hirst C, Swingler R, Compston DA, Ben-Shlomo Y, Robertson NP. Survival and cause of death in multiple sclerosis: a prospective population-based study. *J Neurol Neurosurg Psychiatry.* 2008;79(9):1016–1021.
11. Mehanna R, Jankovic J. Respiratory problems in neurologic movement disorders. *Parkinsonism Relat Disord.* 2010;16(10):628–638.
12. Stowe RL, Ives NJ, Clarke C, et al. Dopamine agonist therapy in early Parkinson's disease. *Cochrane Database Syst Rev.* 2008;(2): CD006564.
13. Olanow CW, Watts RL, Koller WC. An algorithm (decision tree) for the management of Parkinson's disease (2001): treatment guidelines. *Neurology.* 2001;56(11 suppl 5):S1–S88.
14. Pahwa R, Factor SA, Lyons KE, et al. Practice parameter: treatment of Parkinson disease with motor fluctuations and dyskinesia (an evidence-based review): report of the Quality Standards Subcommittee of the American Academy of Neurology. *Neurology.* 2006;66(7):983–995.
15. Higginson IJ, Hart S, Silber E, Burman R, Edmonds P. Symptom prevalence and severity in people severely affected by multiple sclerosis. *J Palliat Care.* 2006;22(3):158–165.
16. Lee MA, Prentice WM, Hildreth AJ, Walker RW. Measuring symptom load in idiopathic Parkinson's disease. *Parkinsonism Relat Disord.* 2007;13(5):284–289.
17. Goy ER, Carter J, Ganzini L. Neurologic disease at the end of life: caregiver descriptions of Parkinson disease and amyotrophic lateral sclerosis. *J Palliat Med.* 2008;11(4):548–554.
18. Neudert C, Oliver D, Wasner M, Borasio GD. The course of the terminal phase in patients with amyotrophic lateral sclerosis. *J Neurol.* 2001;248(7):612–616.
19. Mitsumoto H, Rabkin JG. Palliative care for patients with amyotrophic lateral sclerosis: "prepare for the worst and hope for the best". *JAMA.* 2007;298(2):207–216.
20. Miller RG, Jackson CE, Kasarskis EJ, et al. Practice parameter update: the care of the patient with amyotrophic lateral sclerosis: drug, nutritional, and respiratory therapies (an evidence-based review): report of the Quality Standards Subcommittee of the American Academy of Neurology. *Neurology.* 2009;73(15):1218–1226.
21. Bourke SC, Tomlinson M, Williams TL, Bullock RE, Shaw PJ, Gibson GJ. Effects of non-invasive ventilation on survival and quality of life in patients with amyotrophic lateral sclerosis: a randomised controlled trial. *Lancet Neurol.* 2006;5(2):140–147.
22. Mustfa N, Walsh E, Bryant V, et al. The effect of noninvasive ventilation on ALS patients and their caregivers. *Neurology.* 2006;66(8):1211–1217.
23. Ganzini L. Artificial nutrition and hydration at the end of life: ethics and evidence. *Palliat Support Care.* 2006;4(2):135–143.
24. Logemann JA, Gensler G, Robbins J, et al. A randomized study of three interventions for aspiration of thin liquids in patients with dementia or Parkinson's disease. *J Speech Lang Hear Res.* 2008;51(1):173–183.
25. Cohen SM, Elackattu A, Noordzij JP, Walsh MJ, Langmore SE. Palliative treatment of dysphonia and dysarthria. *Otolaryngol Clin North Am.* 2009;42(1):107–121, x.
26. Motl RW, Suh Y, Weikert M. Symptom cluster and quality of life in multiple sclerosis. *J Pain Symptom Manage.* 2010;39(6):1025–1032.
27. Ben-Zacharia AB. Therapeutics for multiple sclerosis symptoms. *Mt Sinai J Med.* 2011;78(2):176–191.
28. Martinez-Martin P, Rodriguez-Blazquez C, Kurtis MM, Chaudhuri KR. The impact of non-motor symptoms on health-related quality of life of patients with Parkinson's disease. *Mov Disord.* 2011;26(3):399–406.
29. Patten SB, Svenson LW, Metz LM. Psychotic disorders in MS: population-based evidence of an association. *Neurology.* 2005;65(7):1123–1125.
30. Schrag A, Hovris A, Morley D, Quinn N, Jahanshahi M. Caregiver-burden in parkinson's disease is closely associated with psychiatric symptoms, falls, and disability. *Parkinsonism Relat Disord.* 2006;12(1):35–41.
31. Buchanan R, Radin D, Chakravorty BJ, Tyry T. Perceptions of informal care givers: health and support services provided to people with multiple sclerosis. *Disabil Rehabil.* 2010;32(6):500–510.
32. McCluskey L, Houseman G. Medicare hospice referral criteria for patients with amyotrophic lateral sclerosis: a need for improvement. *J Palliat Med.* 2004;7(1):47–53.

Chapter 57

What Is the Clinical Course of Advanced Heart Failure and How Do Implanted Cardiac Devices Alter This Course?

NATHAN E. GOLDSTEIN AND DEBORAH D. ASCHEIM

INTRODUCTION AND SCOPE OF THE PROBLEM

Heart failure is a chronic and progressive illness frequently associated with multiple comorbidities, and it is a leading cause of death in the United States. Reaching epidemic numbers, nearly 6 million people have heart failure, with the incidence approaching 1 in 100 adults over the age of 65.[1] Data from 2005 indicate that heart failure is implicated in some manner in 1 in 8 deaths in the United States.[2] The majority of these individuals (approximately 70%) have systolic heart failure, which is associated with impaired contractility or ejection of the ventricles. The remaining have diastolic heart failure, which is associated with impaired relaxation or filling of the heart.[3] Despite medical and surgical advances, 5-year adjusted survival for patients with heart failure remains approximately 50%.[4,5] The estimated costs of heart failure in the United States in 2009 were in excess of $37 billion.[2] Heart failure adversely affects quality of life because of its relatively high burden of symptoms,[6] and as patients live longer with the disease, the population living with end-stage heart failure and symptoms refractory to medical therapy continues to grow.

Many clinicians may be familiar with the New York Heart Association Classification as a tool for staging the severity of a patient's heart failure.[7,8] This scheme consists of classes I to IV as follows[9]:

Class I: Asymptomatic—patients have no limitation of physical activity, and ordinary physical activity does not cause shortness of breath or other symptoms.

Class II: Mild heart failure—patients have slight limitations in function; they will be comfortable at rest, but ordinary physical activity creates symptoms.

Class III: Moderate heart failure—these patients have marked limitations of their activity; although they are comfortable at rest, less than ordinary activity will cause symptoms.

Class IV: Severe—patients cannot undertake any physical activity without discomfort and have symptoms of heart failure at rest.

Although this scale is widely known and useful, the relatively new American Heart Association/American College of Cardiology system of Heart Failure Stage is being used with increasing frequency[10]:

Stage A: Patients who are at risk but do not have symptoms; may include patients with hypertension, coronary artery disease, and diabetes. The goal of this stage is to identify these individuals early to modify risk factors to prevent them from developing heart failure.

Stage B: Patients who are asymptomatic but have developed some element of heart failure. These may be patients with a previous myocardial infarction or left ventricular systolic dysfunction, for example.

Stage C: Patients with symptomatic heart failure. They have known structural heart disease and may have reduced exercise tolerance as a result of shortness of breath and fatigue.

Stage D: Patients with refractory end-stage heart failure. These individuals have marked symptoms at rest and minimal exertion despite maximal medical therapy.

RELEVANT PATHOPHYSIOLOGY

A comprehensive review of the relevant pathophysiology of heart failure or coronary artery disease is beyond the scope of this text. This chapter focuses on the key pathophysiological elements relative to the practice of palliative medicine—mechanisms behind the symptoms seen most commonly in patients with advanced heart failure, the reasons that the trajectory of heart failure is so difficult to predict, and the influence of new advanced medical technologies on this trajectory.

The relationship between the progression of heart failure and symptoms is a complex one, but it is important for palliative care clinicians to understand so they can proactively plan for future symptoms a patient might have and educate patients and their families. As a patient's heart disease progresses to its end stages, the symptom burden will increase. Volume overload may be the prominent symptom and can result in abdominal bloating or discomfort, constipation, and altered mobility resulting from lower extremity edema.[11] Dyspnea is one of the more common symptoms and may be seen in more than 85% of patients.[12] It may be due to volume overload related to pulmonary congestion, as well as hypoperfusion.[13] Data have shown that up to half of patients with heart failure will have pain, and this may include uncontrolled pain in specific regions (e.g., abdomen, chest, joints, legs) as well as a generalized pain syndrome.[13,14] Although still not completely understood, the cause of this generalized pain syndrome may be inflammatory mediators and dysregulation of hormonal modulators and cytokines.[13] Abdominal pain is more commonly related to hepatic congestion and consequent swelling of the liver capsule, and it may also be related to hypoperfusion of the abdominal viscera. Indeed it is important for the palliative care clinician to remember that heart failure is a systemic disease that affects multiple bodily systems and not just a disease of a single organ. This is particularly apparent given that as many as 90% of patients may exhibit signs of fatigue, cachexia, and anorexia—all of which are related to the systemic effects of heart failure.[13] Insomnia and disrupted sleep are also common symptoms in patients with advanced heart failure, and many patients suffer from daytime somnolence and fatigue related to undiagnosed sleep apnea.[13] Finally, psychological symptoms are significant, particularly anxiety and depression. Feelings of social isolation may also be increased in patients with heart failure, most likely related to their fatigue and reduced exercise tolerance making it difficult for them to leave their home and socialize with others.

The second key element important for the palliative care clinician to understand is the complex, unpredictable nature of heart failure. Unlike patients with cancer, who will maintain their functional state for a prolonged period of time and then have rapid decline in function that is often an indicator that death is imminent, the trajectory of heart failure exacerbations is not as predictable (Figure 57-1).[15,16] Over their final years and months of life patients with heart failure may have multiple acute periods of decline, but it may be difficult (if not impossible) to determine which of these exacerbations may be their last. This infuses a significant degree of uncertainty into the care of patients with advanced heart failure. Indeed, although multiple prognostic models have been developed to predict mortality in a

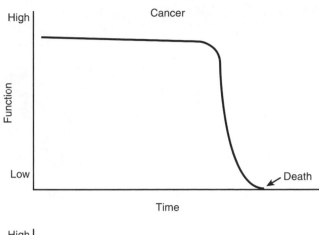

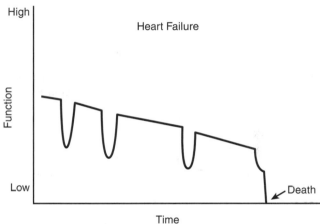

FIGURE 57-1. The top graph is the cancer trajectory, in which patients have a period of preserved function over time, until the patient approaches the end of life and has a rapid decline in function until death. The lower trajectory exemplifies the heart failure trajectory, in which patients have periods of disease exacerbation with functional status decreasing abruptly but then improving somewhat. *(From Goldstein NE, Lynn J. Trajectory of end-stage heart failure: the influence of technology and implications for policy change.* Perspect Biol Med. *2006;49[1]:10-18.)*

group of patients with heart failure, these models do not always work well at the bedside when applied to a particular patient. This uncertainty can make discussions about advance care planning particularly complicated.[11] Put another way, when can one be sure that a patient—no matter how ill the patient appears at a particular moment in time—is in what may be the "final exacerbation?" This not only makes planning itself difficult but also carries an emotional toll for patients and their caregivers. Each exacerbation may be a patient's terminal hospitalization, leaving the patient and caregiver in a sort of emotional limbo, hoping for the best, but terrified that the patient may die.

The Role of Implantable Devices

The trajectory of the course of heart failure is made even more complicated by current implantable cardiac devices (Figure 57-2). One such device is the implantable cardiac defibrillator (ICD). These devices

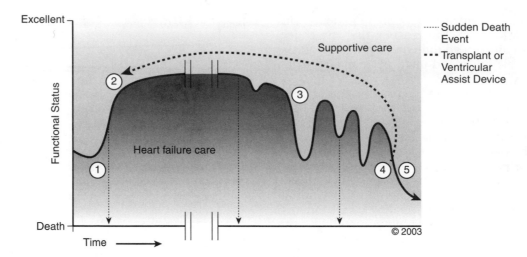

FIGURE 57-2. Implantable cardiac devices make the trajectory of advanced heart failure more complicated to predict. As the diagram shows, the initial symptoms are present at the time the patient develops heart failure (1). However the disease will plateau over a prolonged period (2), followed by periods of disease exacerbation (3). Some patient may receive a transplant or ventricular assist device (4), and these patients often return to the "plateau" phase for a prolonged time. However, for many patients with heart failure, the end of life (5) comes eventually as a result of the disease or its complications. Please visit our website at "http://www.expertconsult.com" to view this image in color. *(Used with permission, © Sarah Goodlin, MD, Patient-centered Education and Research.)*

continually monitor the heart rhythm and can terminate potentially lethal arrhythmias (i.e., ventricular fibrillation and unstable ventricular tachycardia) in patients with advanced heart disease. Multiple studies have shown that ICDs reduce sudden cardiac death.[17-20] At late stages of advanced disease, however, an ICD may no longer prolong a life of acceptable quality and can instead contribute to suffering and distress. In this circumstance the device may actually prolong the patient's inevitable death. Patients report that receiving shocks from an ICD is comparable to being "kicked or punched" in the chest.[21-23] ICDs shock without warning, and these shocks have been associated with the development of adjustment disorders, depression, posttraumatic stress disorder, and panic disorder.[24-26] Family caregivers who observe patients being shocked report feelings of fear, worry, and helplessness and have been shown to have increased rates of depression and anxiety.[27-30]

For these reasons, it is appropriate to have a conversation with patients and their families about deactivation of the shocking function of ICDs as patients approach the end of life. A discussion about ICD deactivation is inherently about prognosis, with physicians acknowledging that patients could die from their underlying disease(s). Previous work has shown that discussions about prognosis in patients with heart disease rarely occur.[31] When an ICD is implanted, it is appropriate at that particular time given the patient's clinical status and goals. An ICD that is indicated at one point may become inappropriate later, and a new benefit versus burden calculation becomes necessary. Discussing ICD deactivation is of such importance that several cardiology societies have begun to address the issue. Recent guidelines of the American Heart Association, the European Society of Cardiology, and the Heart Rhythm Society all state

that deactivation of ICDs should be addressed for all patients near the end of life.[32-34]

Another device that may change the complex trajectory for heart failure patients is the ventricular assist device (VAD). A VAD, or mechanical circulatory support device, is surgically implanted in the patient's chest and abdomen and augments the pumping function of the heart. Originally approved as a temporary therapy to "bridge" patients as they waited for cardiac transplantation, VADs are now implanted in patients with advanced heart failure whose eligibility for transplant is unclear (bridge to candidacy) or who are ineligible for transplantation (destination therapy).[35,36]

In terms of palliative care issues related to the VAD, patients may have symptoms of discomfort related to the device, such as neck, shoulder, and back pain resulting from the need to carry batteries and the controller for the VAD; collectively these elements weigh approximately 7 pounds.[37] Although patients who receive VADs have improved cardiac output and quality of life, good data on prevalence of pain after implantation are lacking. In terms of psychological symptoms, maintenance of the VAD and the crucial requirement for a continuous power supply may create anxiety and a sense of vulnerability to mishap. The physical presence of the external driveline and peripheral equipment constantly reminds patients they are dependent on a life-saving device. This may result in anxiety or depression.

SUMMARY OF EVIDENCE REGARDING TREATMENT RECOMMENDATIONS

The evidence base for the benefits of palliative care for patients with cancer is well established, but the evidence base demonstrating the ways palliative care can influence outcomes and quality of care in patients with heart failure is still lacking.[38–43] In general the best symptom control for patients with heart failure are those disease-directed therapies that treat the exacerbation itself (e.g., intravenous furosemide, inotropic therapy, or vasodilators during an acute exacerbation). Studies have demonstrated the role of comprehensive case management in the care of patients with advanced heart failure, and these studies show that this type of intensive case management results in reduction in hospitalizations and emergency department use.[44–46] One can extrapolate these findings to palliative care, but it should be noted that although similar, palliative care is not the same as comprehensive outpatient case management for these patients. One small randomized, controlled trial of palliative care for 107 patients with chronic illness, 50% of whom had heart failure, demonstrated no difference in symptoms or satisfaction with care.[47] Despite the current lack of evidence demonstrating the benefits of palliative care for patients with heart failure, numerous professional societies have called for the continued and earlier integration of palliative care for patients with advanced heart disease.[11,32,34]

To be clear, this is not to say there is no benefit of palliative care for patients with advanced heart disease. Instead, it simply means that in terms of examining the evidence base for palliative care for heart failure as compared to the benefits of palliative care for patients with other forms of chronic illness, definitive evidence is lacking. Numerous excellent reviews have been written on the benefits of palliative care for patients with heart failure, however, and these often rely on extrapolating evidence from other fields and illnesses to those patients with heart failure.[11,13,43]

One of the particularly challenging aspects of heart failure relates to the complex and unpredictable trajectory. Palliative care specialists are experts when it comes to improving conversations with patients and families, and so their expertise in communicating about goals of care may be of particular benefit to these individuals. Indeed patients with advanced heart failure and their families often have difficulty understanding the complex trajectory and may benefit from the palliative care approach to "hope for the best and plan for the worst." In this context, the role of palliative care can be to continue to work with the primary medical and heart failure teams to ensure that patients' symptoms are controlled at baseline and during exacerbations, while at the same time having conversations to determine the overall goals of care for these patients. Thus, when the patient is finally at the point of the illness when the current exacerbation cannot be reversed, the conversation about what the patient wants in terms of overall goals and wishes has already occurred. Although the treatments desired will still need to be reviewed with the patient and the family, at least the conversations have begun and can be reviewed as opposed to having to start them from scratch at a time an emergent medical decision may need to be made.

The Evidence for Palliative Care for Patients With Implanted Devices

In terms of the management of ICDs for patients nearing the end of life, previous data have demonstrated that conversations about deactivating the shocking function of ICDs rarely occurs and patients receive shocks from their devices at the end of life.[48,49] In addition, patients do not know that deactivating the shocking function may eventually be necessary[50] and they are often confused about the role of the device in their overall health care.[51] Likewise, physicians agree that these conversations are important but admit that they rarely have them or have concerns about them.[52–54] Numerous calls have been made to move conversations about ICD deactivation upstream, so that the conversations occur at the time of device implant and not at the time when the patient is actively dying or receiving repeated shocks from the device.[34] It also has been suggested that the conversation around informed consent when a device is implanted not cover just the risks of the procedure itself but also the future tradeoffs related to the device as the patient nears the end of life.[34,55] Regardless, it is clear that conversations about the management of implantable defibrillators are complicated and therefore should not be one-time events. Instead they need to be part of a larger discussion about patients' goals and values for their health care, and these conversations should be revisited as patients' disease trajectories change over time.

In terms of VADs, although anecdotal evidence exists that some centers are integrating palliative care into the clinical team caring for these patients and their families,[56] no formal studies have evaluated the impact of palliative care services on outcomes such as symptoms, usage, and documentation of patient preferences for care. It has been proposed that palliative care should be introduced into the routine care of these individuals, and indeed palliative care helps meet many of the Joint Commission requirements necessary for certification of VAD centers.[37,56]

KEY MESSAGES TO PATIENTS AND FAMILIES

Clinicians should help patients and families understand that heart failure is a chronic, relapsing illness with a complex and unpredictable trajectory. This means that although the focus is on life-sustaining treatments, a time will come when patients have an exacerbation from which they will not recover. The role of palliative care in these cases is to "hope for the best and plan for the worst," that is, to ensure symptom control and provide emotional and psychosocial support for the patient and family while at the same time continuing to have conversations about advance care planning over time. In terms of the use of advanced technologies and implanted devices, clinicians need to help patients and families understand the risks and benefits not only at the time of implantation but also later in the course of the patient's life. Although the benefits of these treatments often far outweigh the burdens, a better understanding of the nuances of these treatments and how the balance may change in the future helps to ensure better informed decision making and may make future decisions easier for the patient and family.

CONCLUSION AND SUMMARY

Heart failure is a complex illness with an unpredictable trajectory. New technologies have made it even more difficult to predict life expectancy for patients with implanted cardiac devices. The evidence is clear that these devices save lives and (in the case of VADs) improve quality of life, but they are not without burdens. Thus the role of palliative care is to support patients with advanced heart failure by ensuring symptom control and providing support while at the same time making sure that conversations about goals of care and patients' understanding of their heart disease occur over time.

SUMMARY RECOMMENDATIONS

- Heart failure is a chronic illness, with an unpredictable trajectory. This trajectory is punctuated by periods of disease exacerbation that are marked by increased symptoms, poor functional status, and decreased quality of life.
- Implantable cardiac devices may change the course of this disease trajectory. Although these devices are life-saving, they may be associated with significant burdens that patients and families may not fully understand at the time of implantation.
- The role of the palliative care clinician is to ensure that physical and psychological symptoms are always controlled while providing additional psychosocial support for families and their caregivers, regardless of where the patient is on the illness trajectory.
- Because of the complexity of the heart failure trajectory and its unpredictable nature, palliative care can help ensure that conversations about patients' understanding of their illness as well as the overall goals and values related to their health care are reassessed over time.

REFERENCES

1. Rosamond W, Flegal K, Friday G, et al. Heart disease and stroke statistics: 2007 update—a report from the American Heart Association Statistics Committee and Stroke Statistics Subcommittee. *Circulation.* 2007;115(5):e69–e171.
2. Lloyd-Jones D, Adams R, Carnethon M, et al. Heart disease and stroke statistics: 2009 update—a report from the American Heart Association Statistics Committee and Stroke Statistics Subcommittee. *Circulation.* 2009;119(3):480–486.
3. Lilly L. *Pathophysiology of Heart Disease: A Collaborative Project of Medical Students and Faculty.* 3rd ed. Baltimore, MD: Lippincott Williams & Wilkins; 2002; 216–243.
4. Levy D, Kenchaiah S, Larson MG, et al. Long-term trends in the incidence of and survival with heart failure. *N Engl J Med.* 2002;347(18):1397–1402.
5. Roger VL, Weston SA, Redfield MM, et al. Trends in heart failure incidence and survival in a community-based population. *JAMA.* 2004;292(3):344–350.
6. Bekelman DB, Rumsfeld JS, Havranek EP, et al. Symptom burden, depression, and spiritual well-being: a comparison of heart failure and advanced cancer patients. *J Gen Intern Med.* 2009;24(5):592–598.
7. The Criteria Committee of the New York Heart Association. *Nomenclature and Criteria for Diagnosis of Diseases of the Heart and Great Vessels.* 9th ed. Boston: Little, Brown & Co; 1994; 253–256.
8. Carbajal E, Deedwania P. Congestive heart failure. In: Crawford M, ed. *Current Diagnosis & Treatment: Cardiology.* New York: McGraw-Hill; 2009; 217–250.
9. Heart Failure Society of America. *NYHA Classification: the stages of heart failure.* http://www.abouthf.org/questions_stages.htm; Accessed February 15, 2012.
10. Hunt S, Baker D, Chin M, et al. ACC/AHA guidelines for the evaluation and management of chronic heart failure in the adult: executive summary. *Circulation.* 2001;104(24):2996–3007.
11. Adler ED, Goldfinger JZ, Kalman J, Park ME, Meier DE. Palliative care in the treatment of advanced heart failure. *Circulation.* 2009;120(25):2597–2606.
12. Nordgren L, Sorensen S. Symptoms experienced in the last six months of life in patients with end-stage heart failure. *Eur J Cardiovasc Nurs.* 2003;2(3):213–217.
13. Goodlin SJ. Palliative care in congestive heart failure. *J Am Coll Cardiol.* 2009;54(5):386–396.
14. Desbiens N, Wu A. Pain and suffering in seriously ill hospitalized patients. *J Am Geriatr Soc.* 2000;48(5):S183–S186.
15. Goldstein NE, Lynn J. Trajectory of end-stage heart failure: the influence of technology and implications for policy change. *Perspect Biol Med.* 2006;49(1):10–18.
16. Lunney JR, Lynn J, Hogan C. Profiles of older Medicare decedents. *J Am Geriatr Soc.* 2002;50(6):1108–1112.
17. Buxton AE, Lee KL, Fisher JD, Josephson ME, Prytowsky EN, Hafley G. A randomized study of the prevention of sudden death in patients with coronary artery disease. *N Engl J Med.* 1993;341(25):1882–1890.
18. Moss AJ, Hall WJ, Cannom DS, et al. Improved survival with an implanted defibrillator in patients with coronary disease at high risk for ventricular arrhythmia. *N Engl J Med.* 1996;335(26):1933–1940.
19. Moss AJ, Zareba W, Hall WJ, et al. Prophylactic implantation of a defibrillator in patients with myocardial infarction and reduced ejection fraction. *N Engl J Med.* 2002;346(12):877–883.
20. Bardy GH, Lee KL, Mark DB, et al. Amiodarone or an implantable cardioverter-defibrillator for congestive heart failure. *N Engl J Med.* 2005;352(3):225–237.
21. Glikson M, Friedman PA. The implantable cardioverter defibrillator. *Lancet.* 2001;357:1107–1117.
22. Eckert M, Jones T. How does an implantable cardioverter defibrillator (ICD) affect the lives of patients and their families? *Int J Nurs Pract.* 2002;8:152–157.
23. Sears SF, Conti J. Quality of life and psychological functioning of ICD patients. *Heart.* 2002;87:488–493.
24. Morris PL, Badger J, Chmielewski C, Berger E, Goldberg RJ. Psychiatric morbidity following implantation of the automatic implantable cardioverter defibrillator. *Psychosomatics.* 1991;32(1):58–64.
25. Ladwig KH, Baumert J, Marten-Mittag B, Kolb C, Zrenner B, Schmitt C. Posttraumatic stress symptoms and predicted mortality in patients with implantable cardioverter-defibrillators: results from the prospective living with an implanted cardioverter-defibrillator study. *Arch Gen Psychiatry.* 2008;65(11):1324–1330.
26. Kapa S, Rotondi-Trevisan D, Mariano Z, et al. Psychopathology in patients with ICDs over time: results of a prospective study. *Pacing Clin Electrophysiol.* 2010;33(2):198–208.
27. Pedersen SS, Van Den Berg M, Erdman RA, Van Son J, Jordaens L, Theuns DA. Increased anxiety in partners of patients with a cardioverter-defibrillator: the role of indication for ICD therapy, shocks, and personality. *Pacing Clin Electrophysiol.* 2009;32(2):184–192.

28. Dougherty CM. Psychological reactions and family adjustment in shock versus no shock groups after implantation of internal cardioverter defibrillator. *Heart Lung.* 1995;24(4):281–291.

29. Dougherty CM, Pyper GP, Benoliel JQ. Domains of concern of intimate partners of sudden cardiac arrest survivors after ICD implantation. *J Cardiovasc Nurs.* 2004;19(1):21–31.

30. Dunbar SB, Warner CD, Purcell JA. Internal cardioverter defibrillator device discharge: experiences of patients and family members. *Heart Lung.* 1993;22(6):494–501.

31. Fried T, Bradley E, Towle V, Allore H. Understanding the treatment preferences of seriously ill patients. *N Engl J Med.* 2002;346(14):1061–1066.

32. Hunt SA, Abraham WT, Chin MH, et al. 2009 Focused update incorporated into the ACC/AHA 2005 guidelines for the diagnosis and management of heart failure in adults a report of the American College of Cardiology Foundation/American Heart Association Task Force on Practice Guidelines Developed in Collaboration With the International Society for Heart and Lung Transplantation. *J Am Coll Cardiol.* 2009;53(15):e1–e90.

33. Jaarsma T, Beattie JM, Ryder M, et al. Palliative care in heart failure: a position statement from the palliative care workshop of the Heart Failure Association of the European Society of Cardiology. *Eur J Heart Fail.* 2009;11(5):433–443.

34. Lampert R, Hayes DL, Annas GJ, et al. HRS expert consensus statement on the management of cardiovascular implantable electronic devices (CIEDs) in patients nearing end of life or requesting withdrawal of therapy. *Heart Rhythm.* 2010;7(7):1008–1026.

35. Sayer G, Naka Y, Jorde UP. Ventricular assist device therapy. *Cardiovasc Ther.* 2009;27(2):140–150.

36. Rose EA, Gelijns AC, Moskowitz AJ, et al. Long-term mechanical left ventricular assistance for end-stage heart failure. Randomized Evaluation of Mechanical Assistance for the Treatment of Congestive Heart Failure (REMATCH) Study Group. *N Engl J Med* 2001;345(20):1435–1443.

37. Goldstein NE, May CW, Meier DE. Comprehensive care for mechanical circulatory support: a new frontier for synergy with palliative care. *Circ Heart Fail.* 2011;4(4):519–527.

38. Jordhoy MS, Fayers P, Loge JH, Ahlner-Elmqvist M, Kaasa S. Quality of life in palliative cancer care: results from a cluster randomized trial. *J Clin Oncol.* 2001;19(18):3884–3894.

39. El-Jawahri A, Podgurski LM, Eichler AF, et al. Use of video to facilitate end-of-life discussions with patients with cancer: a randomized controlled trial. *J Clin Oncol.* 2010;28(2):305–310.

40. Temel JS, Greer JA, Muzikansky A, et al. Early palliative care for patients with metastatic non-small-cell lung cancer. *N Engl J Med.* 2010;363(8):733–742.

41. Back AL, Li YF, Sales AE. Impact of palliative care case management on resource use by patients dying of cancer at a Veterans Affairs medical center. *J Palliat Med.* 2005;8(1):26–35.

42. Elsayem A, Swint K, Fisch MJ, et al. Palliative care inpatient service in a comprehensive cancer center: clinical and financial outcomes. *J Clin Oncol.* 2004;22(10):2008–2014.

43. Goodlin SJ, Hauptman PJ, Arnold R, et al. Consensus statement: palliative and supportive care in advanced heart failure. *J Card Fail.* 2004;10(3):200–209.

44. Bird S, Noronha M, Sinnott H. An integrated care facilitation model improves quality of life and reduces use of hospital resources by patients with chronic obstructive pulmonary disease and chronic heart failure. *Aust J Prim Health.* 2010;16(4):326–333.

45. Whellan DJ, Hasselblad V, Peterson E, O'Connor CM, Schulman KA. Metaanalysis and review of heart failure disease management randomized controlled clinical trials. *Am Heart J.* 2005;149(4):722–729.

46. Riegel B, Carlson B, Kopp Z, LePetri B, Glaser D, Unger A. Effect of a standardized nurse case-management telephone intervention on resource use in patients with chronic heart failure. *Arch Intern Med.* 2002;162(6):705–712.

47. Pantilat SZ, O'Riordan DL, Dibble SL, Landefeld CS. Hospital-based palliative medicine consultation: a randomized controlled trial. *Arch Intern Med.* 2010;170(22):2038–2040.

48. Goldstein NE, Carlson M, Livote E, Kutner JS. Management of implantable defibrillators in hospice: a nationwide survey. *Ann Intern Med.* 2010;152(2):296–299.

49. Goldstein NE, Lampert R, Bradley EH, Lynn J, Krumholz HM. Management of implantable cardioverter defibrillators in end-of-life care. *Ann Intern Med.* 2004;141:835–838.

50. Kirkpatrick JN, Gottlieb M, Sehgal P, Patel R, Verdino RJ. Deactivation of implantable cardioverter defibrillators in terminal illness and end of life care. *Am J Cardiol.* 2012;109(1):91–94.

51. Goldstein NE, Mehta D, Siddiqui S, et al. "That's like an act of suicide" patients' attitudes toward deactivation of implantable defibrillators. *J Gen Intern Med.* 2008;23(suppl 1):7–12.

52. Goldstein NE, Bradley E, Zeidman J, Mehta D, Morrison RS. Barriers to conversations about deactivation of implantable defibrillators in seriously ill patients: results of a nation wide survey comparing cardiology specialists to primary care physicians. *J Am Coll Cardiol.* 2009;54(3):371–373.

53. Goldstein NE, Mehta D, Teitelbaum E, Bradley EH, Morrison RS. "It's like crossing a bridge": complexities preventing physicians from discussing deactivation of implantable defibrillators at the end of life. *J Gen Intern Med.* 2008;23(suppl 1):2–6.

54. Kelley AS, Reid MC, Miller DH, Fins JJ, Lachs MS. Implantable cardioverter-defibrillator deactivation at the end of life: a physician survey. *Am Heart J.* 2009;157(4):702–708 e701.

55. Matlock DD, Nowels CT, Masoudi FA, et al. Patient and cardiologist perceptions on decision making for implantable cardioverter-defibrillators: a qualitative study. *Pacing Clin Electrophysiol.* 2011;34(12):1634–1644.

56. Swetz KM, Freeman MR, AbouEzzeddine OF, et al. Palliative medicine consultation for preparedness planning in patients receiving left ventricular assist devices as destination therapy. *Mayo Clin Proc.* 2011;86(6):493–500.

CHRONIC CRITICAL ILLNESS

Chapter 58
What Is Chronic Critical Illness and What Outcomes Can Be Expected?

CHRISTOPHER E. COX AND J. RANDALL CURTIS

INTRODUCTION AND SCOPE OF THE PROBLEM

Since the evolution of the modern intensive care unit in the 1940s,[1] clinicians have recognized that a group of patients survives the acute phase of their critical illness yet is unable to be liberated completely from life support in a timely manner. During the past few years, evolving trends in clinical care and health policy have brought this group under increasing scrutiny. First, the number of patients with chronic critical illness is increasing markedly—a finding that temporally is associated with expected age-related population trends. Second, the health care resources that chronic critically ill patients use exceed that of nearly every other patient group and are drawing increased attention in the current era of health care cost scrutiny. Third, the outcomes of chronic critical illness are disappointing for patients and represent an intense caregiving burden for patients' loved ones. Finally, decision making for the chronically critically ill can be extremely challenging for both providers and loved ones. For all these reasons, palliative care practitioners should familiarize themselves with this important group of patients.

How Do You Define Chronic Critical Illness?

Chronic critical illness is a syndrome of prolonged mechanical ventilator use typically accompanied by signs of multisystem organ dysfunction.[2] Accompanying features of chronic critical illness include ventilator dependence, delirium and coma, neuromuscular weakness, and malnutrition. Historically, the term prolonged mechanical ventilation was used to describe this patient group as categorized by a specific number of ventilator days, placement of tracheotomy for prolonged respiratory failure, or both. Such a definition was popular because of the relative simplicity of case identification and its facilitation of administrative database-driven research such as using the International Classification of Disease (ICD) and Diagnosis Related Group (DRG) systems.[3] However, various authors have defined prolonged mechanical ventilation as ranging from 2 days to a month, although not all have incorporated the placement of a tracheotomy in their research populations. This has led to confusion for practitioners, who have rightly questioned the relevance of these varying definitions to clinical practice. Additionally, researchers have increasingly thought that defining a patient group by a procedure such as tracheotomy likely represents an overspecification. For example, is the outcome significantly different between a patient ventilated for 2 weeks with a tracheotomy and one patient without? Also, tracheotomy practices are significantly different between and even within hospitals. Although the indication for early tracheotomy is unclear,[4] it is being performed earlier over time.[5] In an effort to promote clarity in clinical and research settings, Nelson and colleagues proposed a case definition of chronic critical illness as a requirement of 10 or more days of ventilation—a definition that captures 10% to 20% of all patients receiving ventilation.[2] Further efforts to better define this population are underway by the Centers for Medicare and Medicaid Services (CMS). Specifically, CMS is currently seeking to redefine chronic critical illness beyond just patients receiving ventilation by soliciting input from researchers and policymakers.

RELEVANT CONSIDERATIONS

What Is the Clinician Thinking in the Case of Chronic Critical Illness?

Although an operational definition is necessary for clinicians and researchers to be able to communicate effectively about a patient group, it is instructive to consider how clinicians intuitively approach the chronically critically ill patient—that is, the patient who has received life support from advanced technologies for much longer than average. In general, patients with chronic critical illness, more specifically those who undergo tracheotomy, are thought by clinicians to have a reasonable likelihood of short-term survival. From clinicians' decision-making perspective, proceeding with tracheotomy may represent their sense that an investment in continuing ventilatory support is likely to result in improved survival. That is, although a patient may have had an acute critical illness such as sepsis or pneumonia, the patient survived the initial insult and may have in fact stabilized (Figure 58-1).

Because of this relative stability—or perhaps a lack of deterioration—clinicians may feel uncomfortable deviating from the current course of care toward an emphasis on palliation. It may also reflect a clinician's sense that some processes such as intracerebral hemorrhage or trauma may have trajectories of recovery that sometimes necessitate prolonged ventilatory support.

What Are Family Members and Other Loved Ones of These Patients Thinking?

The critically ill patient is often bewilderingly complex for clinicians. In our experience, it is often difficult for many family members to conceive of an illness of such severity, complexity, and requiring such intense decision making. It is no surprise that family members and loved ones, patients' informal caregivers, and surrogate decision makers are often overwhelmed in the case of chronic critical illness. This affects the communication and decision-making process and is important for the practitioner to consider when working with these individuals.

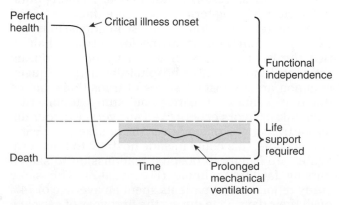

FIGURE 58-1. Health status, critical illness, and the development of chronic critical illness.

Family members often have poor comprehension of basic medical facts that are important to decision making. One study showed that over half of families did not comprehend the diagnosis, prognosis, or treatment of their critically ill loved one—even after a clinician–family meeting.[6] Over two thirds of families suffer from significant symptoms of depression or anxiety during the period in which their loved one is hospitalized.[7] Other stresses exist as well. Many families must travel from out of town to be with their loved one, leaving work and families. Past authors reported that nearly one third of families lost most of their life's savings as a result of a family member's serious illness.[8] Taken together, families suffer an enormous emotional and financial burden during the hospitalization, leading some authors to question the appropriate role of these surrogate decision makers in making decisions about the goals of treatment.[7]

Who Is the Typical Patient With Chronic Critical Illness?

Chronic critical illness is predominantly a syndrome of the elderly, with the notable exception of younger parents who are injured in trauma. Most of the medical literature addressing this patient group has reported remarkably similar age (average approximately 65) and gender (roughly 50% female) across studies. Although relatively little comparative study of the chronically critically ill to other critically ill patients has been done, some studies suggest that no significant differences exist in either baseline functional status limitations or chronic medical comorbidities between those with acute versus those who progress to chronic critical illness.[9]

Why Is Chronic Critical Illness Important to Health Care Systems and Policymakers?

Chronic critical illness has a significant effect on the U.S. health care system, including acute care hospitals and postacute care facilities. As noted earlier, the number of patients with chronic critical illness is increasing markedly. In 2003, it was estimated that there were 300,000 annual cases, with an acute care hospital cost of approximately $16 to 20 billion.[10,11] To contextualize these costs, this represents nearly two thirds of all costs associated with mechanical ventilation and more than one third of all critical illness–associated resource usage.[12,13] Some researchers have reported that prolonged mechanical ventilation has poor value in general societal perspective terms compared to palliative care, finding that costs per quality adjusted life-year gained with this treatment exceeded $100,000 for those 65 and older.[10] Using population-based data tables and forecasts, the number of annual cases of chronic critical illness is expected to reach 600,000 per year by 2020, largely because of the aging of the U.S. population.[14]

Sociodemographic trends behind these data are useful to understand. The incidence of acute respiratory failure increases substantially after 65 years of age,[15] as does the incidence of chronic critical illness—peaking among those 75 and older.[5] Many hospitals struggle with these patients, particularly the uninsured and those with long stays. In addition, because of high costs for this group of patients, difficulties in postdischarge placement, the requirement for high-intensity staffing related to patients' residual need for life support, and diminishing reimbursement to cost ratios, these patients may have unique financial implications for hospitals. In fact, only about half of acute care hospitals cover their costs for Medicare-paid chronically critically ill patients.[16]

Over the past two decades, the care of chronically critically ill patients has shifted in part from the acute care hospital to other specialized centers.[12] Because fewer than 10% on average are able to be discharged from the acute care hospital to home,[9,17-20] postacute care facilities are a common reality for these patients, and these settings of care have received an increasing level of scrutiny in both the medical literature and lay press.[21] Skilled nursing facilities, inpatient rehabilitation facilities, chronic ventilator facilities, and long-term acute care facilities routinely provide extended care for these patients.

Long-term acute care facilities in particular have been most prominent in the health care policy discussions surrounding chronic critical illness.[22] They typically offer mechanical ventilator weaning, physical therapy, speech therapy, wound care, and other services. Long-term acute care facilities have the unique distinction of being the only Medicare providers that are defined by an average length of stay (25 days) rather than specific services provided or a patient population served. Their number more than doubled between 1996 and 2007,[23] expanding more rapidly than any other segment of acute care in the United States, driven in part by the desire of acute care hospitals to offload costly long-stay outliers and generous reimbursement for long-term acute care facilities from health care payers.[24] Coincident with these trends has been a tripling of both post–critical care patient volume and costs, to totals of 43,000 and $1.3 billion in 2007.[23] During this time period, long-term acute care facility mortality remained flat at 50%, whereas the number of comorbidities rose slightly. Long-term acute care facilities have consistently had higher operating margins than any other facility type, likely because of generous base payment rates from Medicare as well as bias in DRG-based payment weighting.[25] As an example, in 2004 the median margin for ventilator support provided at a long-term acute care facility was 23.1% in contrast to the Medicare margin in acute care hospitals of essentially zero.[26] Although long-term acute care facilities offer services that could be uniquely beneficial to the chronically critically ill, little evidence exists that survival is improved by transfer from an acute care hospital.[12] Because of perceived payment inequities, unclear patient referral criteria,

and unsubstantiated clinical benefits, the Deficit Reduction Act of 2005 has directed CMS to reevaluate postacute care facility payment systems.

Little research has been done describing the entire trajectory of acute and postacute care for the chronically critically ill. However, one study of 126 such patients enrolled at a single center found that costs of health care for the entire first year inclusive of postacute care averaged over $300,000 per patient.[20] Because most research has focused on acute care costs alone, it is likely that the overall health care cost burden associated with the care of these patients has been dramatically underestimated.

SUMMARY OF EVIDENCE REGARDING OUTCOMES AND RECOMMENDATIONS

What Are the Outcomes of Chronic Critical Illness?

Understanding the outcomes of chronic critical illness is important to the palliative care practitioner, both to anticipate questions from families and to offer the best support possible during decision making.

Patients. In general, the chronically critically ill have high mortality, substantial persistent physical and cognitive disability, and continued requirement for either hospital readmission or postacute care facility use after discharge.

Acute care hospital mortality for these patients varies by study, ranging from 20% to 50%, with more recent studies consistently reporting mortality in the 20% to 25% range. Although these data reflect lower hospital mortality than other conditions such as septic shock or acute respiratory distress syndrome, it is important to remember that the data reflect a selected population who has survived the acute phase of critical illness. Patient length of stay ranges from 30 to 50 days in most studies, with intensive care accounting for most of this time. About half of patients are liberated from mechanical ventilation during the acute hospital admission, with an average ventilator requirement of around 1 month.[19-20,27]

On average, fewer than 10% of patients with chronic critical illness are discharged home; most require postacute care facility transfer, and the distribution of this care is divided equally among nursing facilities, long-term acute care facilities, and inpatient rehabilitation facilities. Readmissions are extremely common, occurring for between half to two thirds of patients; this usually occurs during the first 3 months after hospital discharge. Equally common are a constant series of transitions among different venues of care. One study found that hospital survivors experienced an average of four different transitions of care over the course of 1 year.[20] For example, this could include hospital to long-term acute care facility to hospital readmission to skilled nursing facility to home (Figure 58-2). The same study reported that patients spent an average of 74% of all their days alive during the first year of care in a hospital, in a postacute care facility, or as dependent at home receiving care.[20] By 1 year, several findings are clear. First, in keeping with a mortality risk that

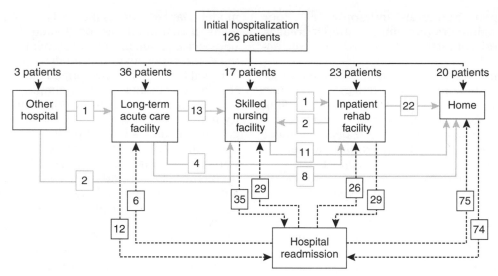

FIGURE 58-2. One-year trajectories of the chronic critical illness experience. *(From Unroe M, Kahn JM, Carson SS, et al. One-year trajectories of care and resource utilization for recipients of prolonged mechanical ventilation: a cohort study.* Ann Intern Med. *2010;153[3]:167-175.)*

remains constant even after discharge, fewer than half of patients are still alive. Of those who survive, only 10% to 15% have no major limitations in basic activities of daily living 1 year after intensive care unit (ICU) admission.[17,20,28,29] Many have persistent cognitive deficits, as well.[28] Few are able to return to work. Finally, long-term quality of life is much worse than population averages, but similar to that of other survivors of critical illness.[9,18,19,30]

Family Members. The experience of family members of a chronically critically ill patient is difficult. Up to 75% of family members of ICU patients experience psychological distress during the patient's hospitalization,[7] which can persist thereafter for years.[31] Patients' newly acquired disability also presents a persistent informal caregiving burden, even when institutional or home care is being provided.[32-34] One study reported that at 1 year after discharge, more than 60% of survivors still required daily informal caregiving assistance, whereas over 80% of family members had to either alter job schedules or stop working altogether.[35] The cumulative stress of patients' intense care needs, frequent readmissions and medical needs, and financial strain are remarkable.[8] Unfortunately, evidence suggests that these commonly reported findings are rarely discussed during the decision-making process surrounding the provision of prolonged life support.[35]

Prognosis and Decision Making in Chronic Critical Illness

Problems With Communication, Prognosis, and Decision Making. What may be concerning for the reader is exactly what has challenged clinicians and researchers alike for years—survival and weaning likelihood is approximately 50% for these patients as a group. Therefore, on the surface, great uncertainty exists—in fact, maximal uncertainty—associated with chronic critical illness decision making in the absence of further individualization. Further, past work has shown that the most commonly used ICU-based prognostic models become (predictably) less accurate over time and are unreliable to use during the most common period of chronic critical illness decision making occurring during the second week of ventilation.[36] Also, until recently, few studies had reported patient-centered outcomes that could be used in decision making, such as postdischarge quality of life and functional status limitations. Finally, because it is rare that these patients are able to participate in decision making because of their severe illness, surrogate decision makers must typically consider this information on their behalf when considering whether to proceed with a course of prolonged life support. These are all formidable challenges to the palliative care provider.

In addition to this prognostic uncertainty, even more basic problems exist with the clinician–patient–family or surrogate decision-maker interaction. First, studies have shown that clinicians do not meet family members' informational needs,[6,37-40] notably for prognosis—the information surrogates cite as most valued in their decisional role.[41,42] Physicians are underprepared to provide prognosis,[43] which leads to infrequent and inaccurate prognostication, as well as excessive optimism—particularly in chronic critical illness.[35,44] Indeed, surrogate decision makers have reported that only 33% of physicians discussed prognosis for survival, functional limitations, quality of life, or expected caregiving needs with them.[35] Another study found that clinicians discussed future cognitive status and financial implications less than 25% of the time.[45] It is concerning that 31% of surrogates recently reported feeling that physicians made the decision to proceed with tracheotomy and 28% believed that the physician wanted surrogates to agree to prolonged life support.[35] Even if families receive medical information, they are often ill equipped to integrate and apply it.[35,46] Poor comprehension impairs communication, increases discordance and conflict,[35,47–49] and reduces consensus building.[6,50–53]

Clinicians also have an incomplete understanding of patients' life support preferences[54–56] because they either fail to elicit surrogates' understanding or they inaccurately interpret them.[45,57–58] This is a key barrier to patient-centered care because most deaths among patients receiving ventilation therapy follow a decision to withdraw life support.[59–60] Also, physicians commonly do not explore a surrogate decision-maker's preferences for involvement in decision making. This is important because surrogates have varied preferences for their decisional role[61] and commonly use nonconventional information sources in deliberation beyond just the prognosis given by clinicians.[62]

The ICU family conference is an important opportunity for improving communication with family members. These conferences have been associated with improved patient and family outcomes, yet frequently do not occur for many patients and families.[63,64] Importantly, staffing and reimbursement limitations are perceived to be challenges by some.[65] The lack of good communication with family members can delay decision making, which may in turn increase length of stay and resource utilization.[66–69] Communication interventions described by Lautrette and colleagues[63] and Lilly[64] and associates are important for health systems to consider to address these problems, although the most effective and cost-effective way to implement such interventions has not been determined. Furthermore, growing clinician shortages in ICUs that are increasingly staffed by multiple shifts represent a serious challenge to good communication and continuity.[70–73]

What Are the Decision Points—and When and How Is Ongoing Life-Sustaining Treatment Best Considered?

An important consideration in the discussion of chronic critical illness is defining the decision points. In the authors' experience, medical disciplines often use a discussion about tracheotomy as a convenient conversation point around which to discuss the provision of prolonged life support. Surgical teams often view tracheotomy less symbolically. Many patients who received tracheotomies have in fact stated that although not pleasant, it was not one of their main memories of critical care.[74,75] This is notable, given an average length of stay of nearly 1 month, because chronically critically ill patients may undergo surgical procedures; multiple venous, arterial, and bladder catheterizations; scores of radiological procedures; and weeks of ventilation with frequent deep suctioning.

One way to have conversations with families is instead of focusing on specific procedures (e.g., tracheotomy, hemodialysis), explore the decision at hand with families as a range of goals of treatment—a model adapted from Gillick.[76] These patient-centered goals of treatment can be depicted as a continuum between maximizing life prolongation and maximizing comfort, with an intermediary area of aiming for survival but avoiding prolonged life support. Framing the decision in this way may simplify the process and help to set up a structure within which more specificity may be introduced as necessary. Early, proactive communication is important.[77]

Because these patients are too cognitively impaired to participate in decision making,[78] family members or friends must act on their behalf as surrogate decision makers.[28] Instead of focusing on a particular medical procedure when communicating with family members, it may be more effective to promote the practice of shared decision making.[44,77] Shared decision making is a collaborative communication process that involves the exchange of information, elicitation of patient preferences and participants' preferred role in decision making, and achievement of consensus about the treatment that is most consistent with patient values.[44,79] Shared decision making lies between the model of parentalism and complete patient autonomy.[77] A decision about chronic critical illness provision meets the requirements for the shared decision-making model because it is often a serious condition with no "right" decision. Treatment options with different risks and benefits exist, and outcomes are often perceived to be uncertain. Although shared decision making is endorsed by all major critical care professional societies,[44,80] its effective use in the ICU is incomplete and infrequent, with only 2% of ICU family conferences meeting all major shared decision-making criteria.[44]

What Can Help in Prognostication?

In general, it is both intuitive and correct that elderly patients with multiple medical comorbidities have high mortality and poor recovery of function.[2] Similarly, younger patients, particularly trauma victims, do comparatively well. As we mentioned earlier, few methodologically sound models have been developed to guide decision making when undertaken later in the ICU course. However, a prediction model for 1-year mortality among a cohort of patients receiving ventilation for 21 or more days was recently developed.[27] This simple model includes four variables (age, platelet count, requirement for dialysis, and need for vasopressors) and demonstrates good calibration and discrimination. A model for day 14 of ventilation is being validated in a larger multicenter cohort study.[81]

Although prognosis is not the sole factor that drives decision making, currently a notable discordance exists between surrogate decision makers and physicians. Both groups greatly overestimate survival, surrogates more so, and neither is particularly accurate in their predictions. The agreement between surrogates and clinicians for

1-year survival, functional disability, and quality of life is no better than a coin toss in current clinical care.[35] It is important that clinicians consider how the gap between expectations and the actual likely outcomes can be bridged. Perhaps as important to families as understanding mortality is appreciating the reality of what may be a dramatically changed life for the patient—a requirement for prolonged facility-based care and the likelihood that full recovery may be unachievable.

What Can Palliative Care Clinicians Do for These Patients and Their Loved Ones?

As noted, the term chronic critical illness describes an important and challenging patient group. The palliative care clinician can provide valuable assistance in their care in several important ways. First, working with ICU clinicians to promote good, early, and effective communication is an important goal that can be facilitated by the involvement of palliative care specialists.[77] Building rapport and building or repairing trust can be an important and time-consuming goal in the care of these patients. Some general communication elements that have demonstrated increased quality of care, decreased family member distress, or improved ratings of communication itself include conducting a family meeting within 72 hours of ICU admission, increasing the amount of time spent listening to family members rather than speaking, providing printed information, and providing palliative care consultation.[59,77] Second, continuity of care and consistency of communication are key elements of high-quality care and can be very challenging in the care of the chronically critically ill. Palliative care specialists can help improve continuity of care and consistency of communication about the goals of care. Finally, because the symptom burden among the chronically critically ill is considerable, this is another important area in which palliative care specialists may be able to offer additional expertise.

KEY MESSAGES TO PATIENTS AND FAMILIES

Clinicians should help patients and families understand that chronic critical illness is a unique syndrome seen in patients who need prolonged mechanical ventilation and it is associated with poor functional outcomes and a high rate of mortality. Families should understand that the likelihood their loved one will return to the previous state of functioning is low, and clinicians should assist with decision making to determine the overall goals of care when patients are unable to speak for themselves. Likewise clinicians should help patients and families understand the inherent uncertainties in the illness and that the course is often marked by the need for prolonged stays in care facilities with multiple transfers between them.

CONCLUSION AND SUMMARY

Chronically critically ill patients and their family members are an important and challenging group that frequently prompts the involvement of palliative care providers. In general, patients' outcomes are poor and the burden on their families is substantial. Because there is a great need in current practice to improve the decision making process surrounding the provision of prolonged life support, we believe this represents an ideal opportunity for palliative care clinicians to advance the overall care of these patients. In doing so, it is important for palliative care professionals to understand the definitions, clinical trends, outcomes, and complexities of prognostication, as well as to help encourage a sound conceptual approach to the decision making process.

SUMMARY RECOMMENDATIONS

- When working with patients with chronic critical illness, providers should remember that there is also a significant burden on the patients' families.
- The decision making process surrounding the provision of prolonged mechanical ventilation is currently inadequate. However, palliative care professionals can facilitate communication and assist in promoting shared decision making.
- For palliative care clinicians to best support patients and their families, it is important that the clinicians understand the definitions, clinical trends, outcomes, and complexities of prognostication in chronic critical illness.

REFERENCES

1. Weil MH, Tang W. From intensive care to critical care medicine: a historical perspective. *Am J Respir Crit Care Med.* 2011;183(11):1451–1453.
2. Nelson JE, Cox CE, Hope AA, Carson SS. Chronic critical illness. *Am J Respir Crit Care Med.* 2010;182(4):446–454.
3. Kahn JM, Carson SS, Angus DC, Linde-Zwirble WT, Iwashyna TJ. Development and validation of an algorithm for identifying prolonged mechanical ventilation in administrative data. *Health Serv Outcomes Res Methodol.* 2009;9:117–132.
4. Terragni PP, Antonelli M, Fumagalli R, et al. Early vs late tracheotomy for prevention of pneumonia in mechanically ventilated adult ICU patients: a randomized controlled trial. *JAMA.* 2010;303(15):1483–1489.
5. Cox CE, Carson SS, Holmes GM, Howard A, Carey TS. Increase in tracheostomy for prolonged mechanical ventilation in North Carolina, 1993–2002. *Crit Care Med.* 2004;32(11):2219–2226.
6. Azoulay E, Chevret S, Leleu G, et al. Half the families of intensive care unit patients experience inadequate communication with physicians. *Crit Care Med.* 2000;28(8):3044–3049.
7. Pochard F, Azoulay E, Chevret S, et al. Symptoms of anxiety and depression in family members of intensive care unit patients: ethical hypothesis regarding decision making capacity. *Crit Care Med.* 2001;29(10):1893–1897.
8. Covinsky KE, Goldman L, Cook EF, et al. The impact of serious illness on patients' families. *JAMA.* 1994;272(23):1839–1844.
9. Cox CE, Carson SS, Hoff-Linquist JA, Olsen MA, Govert JA, Chelluri L. Differences in one-year health outcomes and resource utilization by definition of prolonged mechanical ventilation. *Crit Care.* 2007;11:R9.

10. Cox CE, Carson SS, Govert JA, Chelluri L, Sanders GD. An economic evaluation of prolonged mechanical ventilation. *Crit Care Med.* 2007;35(8):1918–1927.

11. Zilberberg MD, Luippold RS, Sulsky S, Shorr AF. Prolonged acute mechanical ventilation, hospital resource utilization, and mortality in the United States. *Crit Care Med.* 2008;36(3):724–730.

12. Kahn JM. The evolving role of dedicated weaning facilities in critical care. *Intensive Care Med.* 2010;36(1):8–10.

13. Wagner DP. Economics of prolonged mechanical ventilation. *Am Rev Respir Dis.* 1989;140(2 Pt 2):S14–S18.

14. Zilberberg MD, de Wit M, Pirone JR, Shorr AF. Growth in adult prolonged acute mechanical ventilation: implications for healthcare delivery. *Crit Care Med.* 2008;36(5):1451–1455.

15. Behrendt CE. Acute respiratory failure in the United States: incidence and 31-day survival. *Chest.* 2000;118(4):1100–1105.

16. Cooper LM, Linde-Zwirble WT. Medicare intensive care unit use: analysis of incidence, cost, and payment. *Crit Care Med.* 2004;32(11):2247–2253.

17. Carson SS, Bach PB, Brzozowski L, Leff A. Outcomes after long-term acute care: an analysis of 133 mechanically ventilated patients. *Am J Respir Crit Care Med.* 1999;159(5 Pt 1):1568–1573.

18. Combes A, Costa MA, Trouillet JL, et al. Morbidity, mortality, and quality-of-life outcomes of patients requiring > or=14 days of mechanical ventilation. *Crit Care Med.* 2003;31(5):1373–1381.

19. Engoren M, Arslanian-Engoren C, Fenn-Buderer N. Hospital and long-term outcome after tracheostomy for respiratory failure. *Chest.* 2004;125(1):220–227.

20. Unroe M, Kahn JM, Carson SS, et al. One-year trajectories of care and resource utilization for recipients of prolonged mechanical ventilation: a cohort study. *Ann Intern Med.* 2010;153(3):167–175.

21. Berenson A. Long-term care hospitals face little scrutiny. *New York Times.* February 9, 2010.

22. Research Triangle International. *Post-acute care payment reform demonstration.* http://www.pacdemo.rti.org/; 2009 Accessed September 24, 2012.

23. Kahn JM, Benson NM, Appleby D, Carson SS, Iwashyna TJ. Long-term acute care hospital utilization after critical illness. *JAMA.* 2010;303(22):2253–2259.

24. MedPAC. *Defining long-term care hospitals. Report to Congress: New approaches in Medicare.* Washington, DC: MedPAC; 2004.

25. Gage B, Pilkauskas N, Dalton K, et al. *Long-Term Care Hospital Payment System Monitoring and Evaluation: A Phase II Report.* Durham, NC: Research Triangle Institute; 2007.

26. MedPAC. *Healthcare spending and the Medicare program.* Washington, DC: MedPAC; 2010.

27. Carson SS, Garrett J, Hanson LC, et al. A prognostic model for one-year mortality in patients requiring prolonged mechanical ventilation. *Crit Care Med.* 2008;36(7):2061–2069.

28. Nelson JE, Tandon N, Mercado AF, Camhi SL, Ely EW, Morrison RS. Brain dysfunction: another burden for the chronically critically ill. *Arch Intern Med.* 2006;166(18):1993–1999.

29. Stoller JK, Xu M, Mascha E, Rice R. Long-term outcomes for patients discharged from a long-term hospital-based weaning unit. *Chest.* 2003;124(5):1892–1899.

30. Chelluri L, Im KA, Belle SH, et al. Long-term mortality and quality of life after prolonged mechanical ventilation. *Crit Care Med.* 2004;32(1):61–69.

31. Jones C, Skirrow P, Griffiths RD, et al. Post-traumatic stress disorder-related symptoms in relatives of patients following intensive care. *Intensive Care Med.* 2004;30(3):456–460.

32. Douglas SL, Daly BJ. Caregivers of long-term ventilator patients: physical and psychological outcomes. *Chest.* 2003;123(4):1073–1081.

33. Douglas SL, Daly BJ. Caregiving and long-term mechanical ventilation. *Chest.* 2004;126(4):1387; author reply 1387–1388.

34. Van Pelt DC, Milbrandt EB, Qin L, et al. Informal caregiver burden among survivors of prolonged mechanical ventilation. *Am J Respir Crit Care Med.* 2007;175(2):167–173.

35. Cox CE, Martinu T, Sathy SJ, et al. Expectations and outcomes of prolonged mechanical ventilation. *Crit Care Med.* 2009;37:2888–2894.

36. Carson SS, Bach PB. Predicting mortality in patients suffering from prolonged critical illness: an assessment of four severity-of-illness measures. *Chest.* 2001;120(3):928–933.

37. Azoulay E, Pochard F, Chevret S, et al. Meeting the needs of intensive care unit patient families: a multicenter study. *Am J Respir Crit Care Med.* 2001;163(1):135–139.

38. Curtis JR, Engelberg RA, Wenrich MD, Shannon SE, Treece PD, Rubenfeld GD. Missed opportunities during family conferences about end-of-life care in the intensive care unit. *Am J Respir Crit Care Med.* 2005;171(8):844–849.

39. Davis-Martin S. Perceived needs of families of long-term critical care patients: a brief report. *Heart Lung.* 1994;23(6):515–518.

40. Nelson JE, Kinjo K, Meier DE, Ahmad K, Morrison RS. When critical illness becomes chronic: informational needs of patients and families. *J Crit Care.* 2005;20(1):79–89.

41. Evans LR, Boyd EA, Malvar G, et al. Surrogate decision-makers' perspectives on discussing prognosis in the face of uncertainty. *Am J Respir Crit Care Med.* 2009;179(1):48–53.

42. White DB, Engelberg RA, Wenrich MD, Lo B, Curtis JR. Prognostication during physician-family discussions about limiting life support in intensive care units. *Crit Care Med.* 2007;35(2):442–448.

43. Christakis NA, Iwashyna TJ. Attitude and self-reported practice regarding prognostication in a national sample of internists. *Arch Intern Med.* 1998;158(21):2389–2395.

44. White DB, Braddock 3rd CH, Bereknyei S, Curtis JR. Toward shared decision making at the end of life in intensive care units: opportunities for improvement. *Arch Intern Med.* 2007;167(5):461–467.

45. Nelson JE, Mercado AF, Camhi SL, et al. Communication about chronic critical illness. *Arch Intern Med.* 2007;167(22):2509–2515.

46. Rodriguez RM, Navarrete E, Schwaber J, et al. A prospective study of primary surrogate decision makers' knowledge of intensive care. *Crit Care Med.* 2008;36(5):1633–1636.

47. Baggs JG, Schmitt MH, Mushlin AI, et al. Association between nurse-physician collaboration and patient outcomes in three intensive care units. *Crit Care Med.* 1999;27(9):1991–1998.

48. Zwarenstein M, Bryant W. Interventions to promote collaboration between nurses and doctors. *Cochrane Database Syst Rev.* 2000;(2): CD000072.

49. Azoulay E, Timsit JF, Sprung CL, et al. Prevalence and factors of intensive care unit conflicts: the conflicus study. *Am J Respir Crit Care Med.* 2009;180(9):853–860.

50. Heyland DK, Tranmer JE, Kingston General Hospital ICURWG. Measuring family satisfaction with care in the intensive care unit: the development of a questionnaire and preliminary results. *J Crit Care* 2001;16(4):142–149.

51. Maillet RJ, Pata I, Grossman S. A strategy for decreasing anxiety of ICU transfer patients and their families. *Nursingconnections.* 1993;6(4):5–8.

52. Azoulay E, Pochard F, Chevret S, et al. Impact of a family information leaflet on effectiveness of information provided to family members of intensive care unit patients: a multicenter, prospective, randomized, controlled trial. *Am J Respir Crit Care Med.* 2002;165(4):438–442.

53. Larson CO, Nelson EC, Gustafson D, Batalden PB. The relationship between meeting patients' information needs and their satisfaction with hospital care and general health status outcomes. *Int J Qual Health Care.* 1996;8(5):447–456.

54. Uhlmann RF, Pearlman RA, Cain KC. Physicians' and spouses' predictions of elderly patients' resuscitation preferences. *J Gerontol.* 1988;43(5):M115–M121.

55. Wenger NS, Phillips RS, Teno JM, et al. Physician understanding of patient resuscitation preferences: insights and clinical implications. *J Am Geriatr Soc.* 2000;48(5 suppl):S44–S51.

56. Hofmann JC, Wenger NS, Davis RB, et al. Patient preferences for communication with physicians about end-of-life decisions. SUPPORT Investigators: Study to Understand Prognoses and Preference for Outcomes and Risks of Treatment. *Ann Intern Med.* 1997;127(1):1–12.

57. Davidson JE, Powers K, Hedayat KM, et al. Clinical practice guidelines for support of the family in the patient-centered intensive care unit: American College of Critical Care Medicine Task Force 2004–2005. *Crit Care Med.* 2007;35(2):605–622.

58. The Support Investigators. The Study to Understand Prognoses and Preferences for Outcomes and Risks of Treatments (SUPPORT) Investigators: a controlled trial to improve care for seriously ill hospitalized patients. *JAMA.* 1995;274(20):1591–1598.

59. Scheunemann LP, McDevitt M, Carson SS, Hanson LC. Randomized, controlled trials of interventions to improve communication in intensive care: a systematic review. *Chest.* 2011;139(3):543–554.

60. Cook D, Rocker G, Marshall J, et al. Withdrawal of mechanical ventilation in anticipation of death in the intensive care unit. *N Engl J Med.* 2003;349(12):1123–1132.

61. White DB, Malvar G, Karr J, Lo B, Curtis JR. Expanding the paradigm of the physician's role in surrogate decision-making: an empirically derived framework. *Crit Care Med.* 2010;38(3):743–750.

62. Boyd EA, Lo B, Evans LR, et al. "It's not just what the doctor tells me:" factors that influence surrogate decision-makers' perceptions of prognosis. *Crit Care Med.* 2010;38(5):1270–1275.

63. Lautrette A, Darmon M, Megarbane B, et al. A communication strategy and brochure for relatives of patients dying in the ICU. *N Engl J Med.* 2007;356(5):469–478.

64. Lilly CM, De Meo DL, Sonna LA, et al. An intensive communication intervention for the critically ill. *Am J Med.* 2000;109(6):469–475.

65. Lilly CM, Daly BJ. The healing power of listening in the ICU. *N Engl J Med.* 2007;356(5):513–515.

66. Fried TR, Bradley EH, Towle VR, Allore H. Understanding the treatment preferences of seriously ill patients. *N Engl J Med.* 2002;346(14):1061–1066.

67. Gilmer T, Schneiderman LJ, Teetzel H, et al. The costs of non-beneficial treatment in the intensive care setting. *Health Aff (Millwood).* 2005;24(4):961–971.

68. Lloyd CB, Nietert PJ, Silvestri GA. Intensive care decision making in the seriously ill and elderly. *Crit Care Med.* 2004;32(3):649–654.

69. Siegel MD. Do you see what I see? Families, physicians, and prognostic dissonance in the intensive care unit. *Crit Care Med.* 2010;38(5):1381–1382.

70. Angus DC, Kelley MA, Schmitz RJ, White A, Popovich Jr J. Current and projected workforce requirements for care of the critically ill and patients with pulmonary disease: can we meet the requirements of an aging population? *JAMA.* 2000;284(21):2762–2770.

71. Embriaco N, Azoulay E, Barrau K, et al. High level of burnout in intensivists: prevalence and associated factors. *Am J Respir Crit Care Med.* 2007;175(7):686–692.

72. Meier DE, Back AL, Morrison RS. The inner life of physicians and care of the seriously ill. *JAMA.* 2001;286(23):3007–3014.

73. US Department of Health and Human Services. *Projected Supply, Demand, and Shortages of Registered Nurses: 2000–2020.* Washington, D.C: US Department of Health and Human Services; 2002.

74. Cox CE, Docherty S, Brandon D, et al. Surviving critical illness: the experience of acute respiratory distress syndrome patients and their caregivers. *Crit Care Med.* 2009;37(4):2702–2708.

75. Jones C, Griffiths RD, Humphris G, Skirrow PM. Memory, delusions, and the development of acute posttraumatic stress disorder-related symptoms after intensive care. *Crit Care Med.* 2001;29(3):573–580.

76. Gillick MR. Choosing appropriate medical care for the elderly. *J Am Med Dir Assoc.* 2001;2(6):305–309.

77. Curtis JR, White DB. Practical guidance for evidence-based ICU family conferences. *Chest.* 2008;134(4):835–843.

78. Prendergast TJ, Luce JM. Increasing incidence of withholding and withdrawal of life support from the critically ill. *Am J Respir Crit Care Med.* 1997;155(1):15–20.

79. Braddock 3rd CH, Edwards KA, Hasenberg NM, Laidley TL, Levinson W. Informed decision making in outpatient practice: time to get back to basics. *JAMA.* 1999;282(24):2313–2320.

80. Carlet J, Thijs LG, Antonelli M, et al. Challenges in end-of-life care in the ICU. Statement of the 5th International Consensus Conference in Critical Care: Brussels, Belgium, April 2003. *Intensive Care Med.* 2004;30(5):770–784.

81. Carson SS, Kahn JM, Hough CL, et al. Development and validation of a mortality prediction model for patients receiving at least 14 days of mechanical ventilation. Poster presentation at the annual International Conference of the American Thoracic Society. Denver, CO. May 13–18, 2011.

HEAD AND NECK CANCER

Chapter 59

What Special Considerations Are Needed in Patients With Head and Neck Cancer?

NATHAN E. GOLDSTEIN AND ERIC M. GENDEN

INTRODUCTION AND SCOPE OF THE PROBLEM
RELEVANT PATHOPHYSIOLOGY
SUMMARY OF EVIDENCE REGARDING TREATMENT
RECOMMENDATIONS
Physical Symptoms and Mechanisms of Treatment
Psychological Symptoms and Mechanisms of Treatment
Concerns in Late-Stage Disease
Unique Nature of the Interdisciplinary Team
KEY MESSAGES TO FAMILY
CONCLUSION AND SUMMARY

INTRODUCTION AND SCOPE OF THE PROBLEM

Although the term *head and neck cancer* is often used somewhat generically, these cancers are actually a diverse group that includes cancers of the skin, oral cavity, larynx, skull base, trachea, jaw, thyroid, and sinuses. Recent data demonstrate that the median age at diagnosis is 62 years and the incident rate is 15 cases per 100,000 men and 6 cases per 100,000 women.[1] Overall 5-year survival rates for head and neck cancer from 2001 to 2007 from the national Surveillance Epidemiology and End Results (SEER) dataset were 60.8%, with better survival for whites and men as compared to blacks and women.[1]

What these statistics do not reveal, however is the unique challenges faced by patients with head and neck cancer. The nature of this group of cancers is that patients have relapsing and remitting disease; they will have periods during which they are relatively symptom free and have no evidence of disease (including no pathological evidence of cancer) interspersed with bouts of serious illness, debility, and numerous physical and psychological symptoms during periods when the disease is active or they are receiving treatments. Indeed, because disease relapses occur, during even those periods when patients are "cured," they may still continue to have lingering feelings of anxiety and concern that the disease will reoccur. In addition, head and neck cancers also may interfere with patients' ability to express themselves. Because of the cancer itself or the treatments used, these patients may have difficulty speaking, eating, and drinking and also may be disfigured. Given that these diseases affect the face, this disfigurement can be particularly disturbing and emotionally destabilizing. Unlike other cancers that may result in body alterations that can be hidden (such as amputation or colostomy), changes to the face are apparent to the public and thus often interfere with ability and desire to socialize with others. For all of these reasons, patients with head and neck cancer may benefit from having palliative care as a core element of the interdisciplinary team caring for them.[2,3]

RELEVANT PATHOPHYSIOLOGY

The tumors tend to be primarily squamous cell carcinomas[4] and affect men more than women. There is a strong relationship with both alcohol and tobacco consumption,[5,6] and in recent years the evidence that this link is causal has been reinforced by recent data demonstrating an increased incidence of mutations in the *p53* gene in patients with head and neck cancer who have a history of either smoking or alcohol use.[7] Likewise, a large percentage of patients with head and neck cancer test positive for human papillomavirus (HPV), and it is thought that these patients may have a distinct clinical course different than those who have not been exposed to oncogenic strains of HPV.[7-9] It also has been proposed that alcohol and tobacco use and HPV may have a synergistic relationship in the development of head and neck cancers.[10] In terms of variations related to patient age, an increasing number of cases are being seen in younger adults, presumably because of the link with sexual transmission of HPV.[10] Likewise, an increasingly large number of cases are also being seen in older patients, related to mucosal irritation from ill-fitting dentures.

In terms of treatment for the disease, surgical resection, followed by concomitant use of both chemotherapy and radiation remain the mainstays of treatment for these diseases. However, as the genetic and subcellular mechanisms relating to the causal pathway of the disease are becoming further elucidated, advances in the development of targeted therapies such as monoclonal antibodies to control the disease (especially in terms of distant metastases) continue to be promising.[11-14] Specific techniques and the indications for chemotherapy and radiation depend on the origin of the tumor and thus are difficult to summarize because staging and appropriate therapies differ for each tumor type.[15]

SUMMARY OF EVIDENCE REGARDING TREATMENT RECOMMENDATIONS

Physical Symptoms and Mechanisms of Treatment

Numerous physical symptoms occur in patients with head and neck cancer, including pain, mucositis, dysphagia and odynophagia, sialorrhea (overproduction or inability to control saliva), xerostomia (dry mouth from reduced production of saliva), and difficulty with speech. (For a summary of these symptoms and techniques used to treat them see Table 59-1.)

Pain in patients with head and neck cancer often consists of both nociceptive and neuropathic components. Nociceptive pain may result from the cancer itself or from surgical treatments used to alter its course. Although treatment of the nociceptive elements of cancer pain in this group is not different from that for other types of cancer (see Chapters 1 and 2), these patients may have difficulty taking medications. Some formulations can be crushed and swallowed, and use of alternative formulations and delivery methods often may be of benefit to these patients. For example, for patients with both constant and episodic pain, an appropriate regimen might include a transdermal opioid delivery system (e.g., fentanyl patch) along with the use of liquid morphine that can be administered via a gastrostomy or jejunostomy tube. Also in this group, neuropathic pain can occur as a result of the invasion of nerves by tumor and sequelae of surgical or radiation therapy. As for nociceptive pain the treatment for neuropathic pain in this group should involve the use of medications that can be administered via alternative routes (e.g., topical lidocaine patches or medications that can be crushed and administered via gastrostomy tube).

Mucositis may occur as a result of radiation therapy and is often worsened with concomitant chemotherapy. It is one of the most frequent side effects of radiation in this patient group, occurring in almost all patients undergoing radiation treatment, and is the most significant dose-limiting aspect of treatment.[16,17] It is related to destruction of mucosal cells in the field of radiation, and its onset and duration are related to the turnover of these cells. That is, it usually starts about 10 to 14 days after treatment begins (corresponding with loss of regenerative capabilities of the cells exposed to radiation) and abates between 4 and 6 weeks after treatment ends.[4] A recent Cochrane review demonstrated that effective agents for prevention include amifostine, Chinese herbs, ice chips, and hydrolytic enzymes, although the effect size for many of these agents was relatively small.[18] A separate Cochrane review showed that agents that are effective for treatment of mucositis include allopurinol mouthwash, granulocyte-macrophage colony-stimulating factor (GM-CSF) mouthwash, immunoglobulins, human placental extract, with similarly small effect sizes.[19] These studies both found that "magic mouthwash"—often a mixture of oral topical agents used to treat the pain—is not effective in either prevention or treatment. Systemic analgesia

TABLE 59-1. Common Symptoms Encountered in Patients With Head and Neck Cancer and Suggested Treatments

SYMPTOM	TREATMENT*	NOTES
Pain	Opioids	May need to be given by alternative route (e.g., transdermal fentanyl patches, morphine elixir by gastrostomy tube).
Mucositis	Opioids Multiple other medications	Evidence supporting use of many commonly used agents is poor.
Dysphagia	Consultation with speech-language therapists Artificial hydration and nutrition	Degree of dysphagia depends on origin of tumor and types of treatments. May be transient or permanent. May be severe and lead to dehydration or malnutrition.
Xerostomia	Frequent intake of water, ice chips Use of sugarless candy, gum Artificial saliva Pilocarpine (starting dose 2.5 mg enterally q8h)	Should be left to patient preference within boundaries of what is deemed medically indicated (e.g., avoid water if significant aspiration risk). Pilocarpine has multiple side effects that may limit its use, particularly in the elderly.
Change in speech	Consultation with speech-language pathologist Adaptive devices (e.g., amplifier)	Many patients can relearn speech, so this symptom does not always interfere with long-term function, but speech may not return to baseline patterns.
Decreased quality of life	Supportive treatments, including counseling and psychotherapy	In many patients, quality of life will return to baseline level over the long term.
Depression	Emotional support Referral to psychotherapy, counseling Antidepressant medications	May be transient or prolonged. Antidepressants are associated with side effects and interactions with other medications.
Anxiety	Emotional support Referral to psychotherapy, counseling Anxiolytics	Anxiolytics can be associated with fatigue, delirium.

From McPhee SJ, Winker MA, Rabow MW, et al (eds): *Care at the Close of Life: Evidence and Experience.* New York: McGraw-Hill; 2010; 233.
*Consultation with speech and language therapists is useful for many of these conditions as well.

with nonsteroidal agents and opioids has been shown to be effective in symptom control, especially when the opioids are given via patient-controlled analgesia (PCA). Superinfection of oral mucosa by candida can worsen the pain of mucositis and should be treated with appropriate antifungals. Special care must be taken to ensure appropriate intake of hydration and nutrition in patients with mucositis, and these individuals may often require a gastrostomy tube or parenteral nutrition to ensure they do not become dehydrated or malnourished.

Dysphagia (difficulty swallowing) and odynophagia (painful swallowing) in patients with head and neck cancer may result from the tumor or from surgical interventions, chemotherapy, or radiation (including mucositis). For this reason, placement of a gastrostomy tube often occurs as a prophylactic measure in patients before treatment begins so it may be used as needed. It may be used for all nutrition or to supplement oral intake. Used in this manner, its purpose is short term, with clear benefits, unlike when it may be used in patients near the end of life (see later discussion). Consultation with a nutritionist is essential for patients who develop these symptoms to ensure adequate intake of fluids and calories. In addition nutritionists can teach techniques such as bolus feedings that may be helpful to ensure that artificial hydration and nutrition does not interfere with quality of life and lifestyle.

Sialorrhea and xerostomia may not be as common as other physical symptoms in patients with head and neck cancer, but for those patients who do have these side effects, they can be severe and permanent. Although most patients do not routinely give much thought to the importance of saliva, it is essential for speech, eating, and swallowing and it reduces dental caries.[20,21] Sialorrhea and xerostomia are caused by the cancer destroying salivary glands and may be worsened by radiation and chemotherapy. Major avenues of treatment include (1) increasing saliva production through activities such as chewing gum, sucking on hard candies, or using pharmacological stimulation with agents such as pilocarpine; (2) using saliva substitutes, ice chips, or sips of water; and (3) meticulous mouth care.[22] Sialorrhea may result from changes in the architecture of the oral cavity as a result of surgery. Referral to a speech pathologist is often useful so that patients can be taught techniques to better manage oral secretions. Likewise, anticholinergic medications such as glycopyrrolate or hyoscamine are beneficial for reducing secretions, although their side effects (constipation, urinary retention, orthostatic hypotension, delirium) may limit use in older patients.[23,24]

Changes in speech result from alterations to the tongue, teeth, palate, and larynx.[4] Referral to speech-language pathologists should occur *before* surgical intervention, so patients and their families can be educated on the changes to come and so they can learn adaptive techniques early. The use of assistive speaking devices (e.g., electric larynx) may be beneficial in this population, as are additional speech techniques such as tracheoesophageal speech.

Psychological Symptoms and Mechanisms of Treatment

Because of the unique nature of head and neck cancer, these patients are particularly susceptible to psychological conditions related to the disease. The inability to eat and speak related to the disease creates social isolation, and disfigurement from the disease may make it upsetting for patients to leave the house. These may lead to patients being less able to participate in social, religious, and cultural rituals that add meaning to their life. Because the disease is often related to factors such as alcohol and tobacco consumption, patients with head and neck cancer may feel guilt and blame themselves for their disease. This may be compounded by the fact that the disease may place restrictions on the family and the patient may be unable to join them in traditional social situations (e.g., dining out in restaurants), thus only adding to these feelings of guilt and self-blame.

The severity of psychological symptoms is related to tumor type, stage, and therapies received. Approximately 20% to 50% of patients may develop depression at some point in their illness, and the high recurrence rate may result in constant anxiety about relapse.[25–28] Benzodiazepines and selective serotonin reuptake inhibitors (SSRIs) are medications traditionally used in this population.[29] Likewise, pretreatment counseling may help to educate patients and reduce psychological symptoms during the course of their disease. Support groups may also be useful for these patients and their families.[28,30] Clinicians should ask about the impact of the disease on patients and their families during routine office visits to assess the need for additional supportive counseling and referral to psychiatric support when needed. Studies on quality of life in this patient group demonstrate decreases near the start of treatment, but after 12 to 36 months it may return to near baseline levels.[31–33]

Changes in body image and body appearance are almost universal.[34] This is particularly challenging given that the treatments used for the disease may be curative or life-prolonging, but also worsen ability to function.[35] This paradox means that these patients and their families may be particularly amenable to the additional support provided by the palliative care team. Recent changes to treatment regimens have dramatically changed the course of this disease and patients' ability to adapt to it. For example, techniques such as microvascular free tissue transfer allows for resection of diseased tissue with reconstruction using bone, muscle, arteries, nerves, and other tissues harvested from the patient and transferred to another locations. Developed in the last decade, these techniques allow for reconstruction of tongue, jaw, and facial elements that often result in excellent cosmetic outcomes with little to no long-lasting disfigurement.[36] The use of new robotic techniques allows for minimally invasive surgery for lesions that were once associated with significant postoperative morbidity, especially in terms of excision of oropharyngeal lesions and reconstruction during surgery.[37–40]

Concerns in Late-Stage Disease

Given the relapsing nature of head and neck cancer, it can sometimes be difficult to determine when patients are near the end of life; thus focus should be on continual evaluation of goals of care and the benefits and burdens of treatments. Like with other cancers, however, factors associated with late-stage disease include cachexia, fatigue, decreased oral intake, and increasing time spent in bed.[22,41] However, the majority of deaths from head and neck cancer are a result of distant metastases and not local disease. Simultaneously, patients may have continued growth of regional disease resulting in continued disfigurement and nonhealing ulcers and wounds.[42] Control of these lesions may be particularly difficult, and wound care becomes palliative, focusing on ensuring comfort and decreasing odor. A concern for patients being cared for at home includes "carotid blowout" syndrome—a condition related to the disease eroding into the carotid artery (or other large vessel in the neck) that may be a slow process of bleeding or result in rapid exsanguination. This complication is now much less common because of current palliative surgical techniques.[43] If this condition is expected, patients should be cared for in an inpatient palliative care setting whenever possible.

Although artificial hydration and nutrition is often beneficial earlier in the disease course when it can supplement caloric intake as patients are recovering from surgery or radiation therapy, the benefit to burden ratio for this treatment changes in late-stage disease. The changing nature of this treatment, especially as patients are no longer able to control their secretions, should be clearly explained to the family so they can understand that a once beneficial treatment may no longer be indicated. In some cases, either for uncontrolled physical symptoms or existential suffering relating to disfigurement, palliative sedation may be necessary. This consists of sedating patients so they are kept asleep in their final hours or days of life using a combination of opioids, benzodiazepines, or barbiturates. These techniques often require careful explanation for all members of the team caring for the patient and the patient's family.

Unique Nature of the Interdisciplinary Team

As shown in Table 59-2, the interdisciplinary team for patients with head and neck cancer includes many clinicians not normally considered part of the palliative care team. The team is headed and coordinated

TABLE 59-2. Roles of Members of Interdisciplinary Team in Caring for Patients With Malignancies of the Head and Neck*

CLINICIAN	ROLE IN TEAM
Otolaryngologist/head and neck surgeon	Given the chronic and complex nature of illness in patients with head and neck cancer, the head and neck surgeon not only coordinates the interdisciplinary team but in many cases becomes the primary care physician who refers the patient to other specialist and oversees the plan of care.
Radiation oncologist	Charged with creating the plan for radiotherapy. Must be familiar with various options for treatment (e.g., brachytherapy, fractionated) to allow for maximal effectiveness while minimizing side effects.
Medical oncologist	Works with team to provide chemotherapeutic agents—both in terms of antineoplasitc agents and radiosensitizers to improve effectiveness of radiotherapy.
Plastic and reconstructive surgeon	Assists head and neck surgeon in planning surgical resection but may work side-by-side in operating room to ensure best possible cosmetic outcomes.
Dentist/prosthodontics providers	Ensures adequate dental health before, during, and after interventions. May be called on to create prosthetics for patients undergoing resection of teeth or jaw.
Psychiatrist/psychologist	Provides emotional and psychological support for patients and families, either individually or in a group setting. May prescribe antidepressants or anxiolytics.
Neurosurgeon	Consults with head and neck surgeon in cases in which resection or treatment plan involves major structures of the nervous system.
Ophthalmologist	Consults with head and neck surgeon in cases in which malignancy involves eyes or orbits.
Palliative care providers	Physicians, nurses, social workers, and chaplains with expertise in palliative care are necessary to provide relief of pain and other symptoms, assistance with decision making, and supportive care for these patients and their families.
Specialized nursing care	Nurses with expertise in care of patients with head and neck cancer are necessary because of specialized interventions such as tracheostomy and gastrostomy tubes. May also provide specialized wound care. Also play a role in educating patient and caregiver in the use of these interventions.
Speech-language pathologists	Provide assistance, therapies, and education for patients with difficulty swallowing or speaking. May also educate family in terms of techniques for meal preparation, etc.
Physical and occupational therapists	Provide care for patients with general debility or who have undergone resection or reconstructive procedures that interfere with daily function and ability to care for themselves.
Clinical social worker	Provides care coordination across settings and assists with discharge planning. Depending on background and training, may provide supportive care and counseling for patient and family.
Clinical nutritionist	Ensures patients receive adequate hydration and nutrition, especially in cases in which patients have gastrostomy tubes, debility, or hypermetabolic states.

From McPhee SJ, Winker MA, Rabow MW, et al (eds): *Care at the Close of Life: Evidence and Experience.* New York: McGraw-Hill; 2010; 237.
*Because the management of patients with head and neck cancers is complex, patients may need access to the services of the range of clinicians shown here. The order in which clinicians are listed is chosen for clarity and is not meant to imply that any one role is more important than others in the care of these patients. For more information see reference 46.

by the otolaryngologist or head and neck surgeon and includes the radiation oncologist, medical oncologist, speech-language pathologist, social worker, and nutritionist. Depending on the nature of the disease and the complexity of the surgical techniques employed, the team may also include dentist or prosthodontics providers, neurosurgeons, plastic and reconstructive surgeons, and ophthalmologists. For patients undergoing free tissue transfer, physical and occupational therapists may be added to the team. Patients may need specialized nursing care, whether it is for teaching related to the gastric tube or specialized wound care. The role of palliative care in this team is to ensure expert relief of pain and other symptoms, assist with decision making, and continue to provide supportive care for these patients and their families throughout the complex course of the disease. Like other forms of cancer, involvement of the palliative care team or hospice for patients with head and neck cancers may improve outcomes for patients and their families.[44,45]

KEY MESSAGES TO FAMILY

One of the core elements for patients with head and neck cancer and their families to understand relates to the relapsing and recurring nature of head and neck cancer. Patients and families should understand that although cure is a real potential for many individuals, recurrence of disease is common even if prophylactic chemotherapy or radiation is given. Likewise, it is important that the head and neck surgeon honestly discuss the incurable nature of the disease with the patient and family as appropriate based on the stage and nature of the disease.[22] The role of the palliative care provider can be to facilitate these conversations with the family and ensure understanding while also providing emotional and psychological support. Helping the family to understand the role of each member of the interdisciplinary team and how they contribute to the overall care of the patient can be beneficial given the large number of clinicians involved and the need for coordination of care among all of these individuals.

CONCLUSION AND SUMMARY

Head and neck cancers are a diverse group of diseases, and patients with these cancers have a complex set of physical and psychological symptoms regardless of the tumor type and treatments administered. Numerous domains of both physical and psychological suffering are experienced by these patients, and thus a large and comprehensive multidisciplinary team can provide the wide range of expertise to best address the needs of the patient and the family. The role of palliative care is to ensure that symptoms are controlled and coordinate care among this diverse group. Finally, unique challenges exist related to late-stage disease, and expert communication is essential to ensure that patients and their families understand the circumstances and appropriate therapeutic options.

SUMMARY RECOMMENDATIONS

- Head and neck cancers are a diverse group of diseases, and the overall course is often characterized by relapse. Clinicians should help patients and families understand this unusual and complex trajectory, so that relapse is expected.
- Physical and psychological symptoms are numerous and relate to both the disease itself and the treatments provided. Palliative care clinicians should be familiar with these symptoms, because many can be explained and even treated in a proactive manner.
- Because artificial hydration and nutrition can be beneficial early in the disease course but then later may become burdensome, clinicians should discuss its use over time and explain when the benefit/burden ratio shifts.
- The interdisciplinary team required to treat head and neck cancers is large and may be particularly beneficial in this disease, so palliative care practitioners need to explain why so many clinicians are involved and the role of each member of the team.

REFERENCES

1. Howlader N, Noone AM, Krapcho M, et al. *SEER Cancer Statistics Review, 1975–2008.* Bethesda, MD: National Cancer Institute; http://seer.cancer.gov/statfacts/html/oralcav.html. Based on November 2010 SEER data submission, posted to the SEER website, 2011. Accessed September 14, 2012.
2. Davies L, Rhodes LA, Grossman DC, Rosenberg MC, Stevens DP. Decision making in head and neck cancer care. *Laryngoscope.* 2010;120(12):2434–2445.
3. Goldstein NE, Genden E, Morrison RS. Palliative care for patients with head and neck cancer: "I would like a quick return to a normal lifestyle". *JAMA.* 2008;299(15):1818–1825.
4. Murphy BA, Cmelak A, Bayles S, Dowling E, Billante CR. Head and neck cancer. In: Doyle D, Hanks G, Cherny NI, Calman K, eds. *Oxford Textbook of Palliative Medicine.* 3rd ed. New York: Oxford University Press; 2005:658–673.
5. Dikshit RP, Boffetta P, Bouchardy C, et al. Lifestyle habits as prognostic factors in survival of laryngeal and hypopharyngeal cancer: a multicentric European study. *Int J Cancer.* 2005;117(6):992–995.
6. Boffetta P, Merletti F, Faggiano F, et al. Prognostic factors and survival of laryngeal cancer patients from Turin, Italy: a population-based study. *Am J Epidemiol.* 1997;145(12):1100–1105.
7. Forastiere A, Koch W, Trotti A, Sidransky D. Head and neck cancer. *N Engl J Med.* 2001;345(26):1890–1900.
8. Gillison ML, Koch WM, Capone RB, et al. Evidence for a causal association between human papillomavirus and a subset of head and neck cancers. *J Natl Cancer Inst.* 2000;92(9):709–720.
9. Kreimer AR, Clifford GM, Boyle P, Franceschi S. Human papillomavirus types in head and neck squamous cell carcinomas worldwide: a systematic review. *Cancer Epidemiol Biomarkers Prev.* 2005;14(2):467–475.
10. Pannone G, Santoro A, Papagerakis S, Lo Muzio L, De Rosa G, Bufo P. The role of human papillomavirus in the pathogenesis of head & neck squamous cell carcinoma: an overview. *Infect Agent Cancer.* 2011;6:4.
11. Burgos-Tiburcio A, Santos ES, Arango BA, Raez LE. Development of targeted therapy for squamous cell carcinomas of the head and neck. *Expert Rev Anticancer Ther.* 2011;11(3):373–386.
12. Licitra L, Bergamini C, Mirabile A, Granata R. Targeted therapy in head and neck cancer. *Curr Opin Otolaryngol Head Neck Surg.* 2011;19(2):132–137.

13. Ma BB, Hui EP, Chan AT. Systemic approach to improving treatment outcome in nasopharyngeal carcinoma: current and future directions. *Cancer Sci.* 2008;99(7):1311–1318.

14. Goerner M, Seiwert TY, Sudhoff H. Molecular targeted therapies in head and neck cancer: an update of recent developments. *Head Neck Oncol.* 2010;2:8.

15. Pfister DG, Ang K, Brizel D, et al. *NCCN Clinical Practice Guidelines in Oncology for Head and Neck Cancers.* http://www.nccn.org/professionals/physician_gls/pdf/head-and-neck.pdf; 2011 Accessed September 14, 2012.

16. Scully C, Epstein J, Sonis S. Oral mucositis: a challenging complication of radiotherapy, chemotherapy, and radiochemotherapy. II. Diagnosis and management of mucositis. *Head Neck.* 2004;26(1):77–84.

17. Elting LS, Keefe DM, Sonis ST, et al. Patient-reported measurements of oral mucositis in head and neck cancer patients treated with radiotherapy with or without chemotherapy: demonstration of increased frequency, severity, resistance to palliation, and impact on quality of life. *Cancer.* 2008;113(10):2704–2713.

18. Worthington HV, Clarkson JE, Eden OB. Interventions for preventing oral mucositis for patients with cancer receiving treatment. *Cochrane Database Syst Rev.* 2007;(4): CD000978.

19. Clarkson JE, Worthington HV, Eden OB. Interventions for treating oral mucositis for patients with cancer receiving treatment. *Cochrane Database Syst Rev.* 2007;(2): CD001973.

20. Dirix P, Nuyts S, Van den Bogaert W. Radiation-induced xerostomia in patients with head and neck cancer: a literature review. *Cancer.* 2006;107(11):2525–2534.

21. Brosky ME. The role of saliva in oral health: strategies for prevention and management of xerostomia. *J Support Oncol.* 2007;5(5):215–225.

22. Elackattu A, Jalisi S. Living with head and neck cancer and coping with dying when treatments fail. *Otolaryngol Clin North Am.* 2009;42(1):171–184, xi.

23. Agostini JV, Leo-Summers LS, Inouye SK. Cognitive and other adverse effects of diphenhydramine use in hospitalized older patients. *Arch Intern Med.* 2001;161(17):2091–2097.

24. Agostini JV, Tinetti ME. Drugs and falls: rethinking the approach to medication risk in older adults. *J Am Geriatr Soc.* 2002;50(10):1744–1745.

25. Pandey M, Devi N, Thomas BC, Kumar SV, Krishnan R, Ramdas K. Distress overlaps with anxiety and depression in patients with head and neck cancer. *Psychooncology.* 2007;16(6):582–586.

26. Duffy SA, Ronis DL, Valenstein M, et al. Depressive symptoms, smoking, drinking, and quality of life among head and neck cancer patients. *Psychosomatics.* 2007;48(2):142–148.

27. Birkhaug EJ, Aarstad HJ, Aarstad AK, Olofsson J. Relation between mood, social support and the quality of life in patients with laryngectomies. *Eur Arch Otorhinolaryngol.* 2002;259(4):197–204.

28. Vakharia KT, Ali MJ, Wang SJ. Quality-of-life impact of participation in a head and neck cancer support group. *Otolaryngol Head Neck Surg.* 2007;136(3):405–410.

29. Block SD. Assessing and managing depression in the terminally ill patient. ACP-ASIM End-of-Life Care Consensus Panel. American College of Physician–American Society of Internal Medicine. *Ann Intern Med.* 2000;132(3):209–218.

30. Luckett T, Britton B, Clover K, Rankin NM. Evidence for interventions to improve psychological outcomes in people with head and neck cancer: a systematic review of the literature. *Support Care Cancer.* 2011;19(7):871–881.

31. Hammerlid E, Taft C. Health-related quality of life in long-term head and neck cancer survivors: a comparison with general population norms. *Br J Cancer.* 2001;84(2):149–156.

32. Murphy BA, Ridner S, Wells N, Dietrich M. Quality of life research in head and neck cancer: a review of the current state of the science. *Crit Rev Oncol Hematol.* 2007;62(3):251–267.

33. Babin E, Sigston E, Hitier M, Dehesdin D, Marie JP, Choussy O. Quality of life in head and neck cancers patients: predictive factors, functional and psychosocial outcome. *Eur Arch Otorhinolaryngol.* 2008;265(3):265–270.

34. Dropkin MJ. Coping with disfigurement and dysfunction after head and neck cancer surgery: a conceptual framework. *Semin Oncol Nurs.* 1989;5(3):213–219.

35. Callahan C. Facial disfigurement and sense of self in head and neck cancer. *Soc Work Health Care.* 2004;40(2):73–87.

36. de Bree R, Rinaldo A, Genden EM, et al. Modern reconstruction techniques for oral and pharyngeal defects after tumor resection. *Eur Arch Otorhinolaryngol.* 2008;265(1):1–9.

37. Genden EM, Park R, Smith C, Kotz T. The role of reconstruction for transoral robotic pharyngectomy and concomitant neck dissection. *Arch Otolaryngol Head Neck Surg.* 2011;137(2): 151–156.

38. Mukhija VK, Sung CK, Desai SC, Wanna G, Genden EM. Transoral robotic assisted free flap reconstruction. *Otolaryngol Head Neck Surg.* 2009;140(1):124–125.

39. Iseli TA, Kulbersh BD, Iseli CE, Carroll WR, Rosenthal EL, Magnuson JS. Functional outcomes after transoral robotic surgery for head and neck cancer. *Otolaryngol Head Neck Surg.* 2009;141(2):166–171.

40. Weinstein GS, O'Malley Jr BW, Cohen MA, Quon H. Transoral robotic surgery for advanced oropharyngeal carcinoma. *Arch Otolaryngol Head Neck Surg.* 2010;136(11):1079–1085.

41. Ellershaw J, Ward C. Care of the dying patient: the last hours or days of life. *BMJ.* 2003;326(7379):30–34.

42. Sesterhenn AM, Folz BJ, Bieker M, Teymoortash A, Werner JA. End-of-life care for terminal head and neck cancer patients. *Cancer Nurs.* 2008;31(2):E40–E46.

43. Cohen J, Rad I. Contemporary management of carotid blowout. *Curr Opin Otolaryngol Head Neck Surg.* 2004;12(2):110–115.

44. Shuman AG, Yang Y, Taylor JM, Prince ME. End-of-life care among head and neck cancer patients. *Otolaryngol Head Neck Surg.* 2011;144(5):733–739.

45. Lin YL, Lin IC, Liou JC. Symptom patterns of patients with head and neck cancer in a palliative care unit. *J Palliat Med.* 2011;14(5):556–559.

46. Pfister DG, Ang K, Brockstein B, et al. NCCN practice guidelines for head and neck cancers. *Oncology (Williston Park).* 2000;14(11A):163–194.

END-STAGE RENAL DISEASE

Chapter 60

What Special Considerations Are Needed in Treating Symptoms in Patients With End-Stage Renal Disease?

ALVIN H. MOSS

INTRODUCTION AND SCOPE OF THE PROBLEM

Patients on dialysis have tremendous symptom burden. Indeed, they are just as symptomatically sick as patients with cancer, but their survival rate is only 60% of that of patients with cancer. Patients with cancer have been found to have an average of nine symptoms,[1] and those on dialysis have been found to have a comparable number of symptoms when tested with a validated symptom instrument for patients on dialysis.[2] Patients who have cancer have on average a 5-year survival of 67%,[3] whereas patients with end-stage renal disease (ESRD) have a 5-year survival of only 40%.[4] In a more recent study using a modified version of the Patient Outcome Scale-Symptom Module, British researchers noticed that patients with stage 4 chronic kidney disease before dialysis and managed without dialysis at stage 5 had a median of seven symptoms.[5] In a recent study of patients with stage 5 chronic kidney disease treated without dialysis, British researchers used a patient-completed Memorial Symptoms Assessment Scale-Short Form and found that in the month before death the median number of symptoms reported by these patients was 16.6.[6] In surveys of patients on dialysis in one study the most commonly reported symptoms were dry skin, fatigue, itching, and bone and joint pain,[2] and in a second study of Canadian dialysis patients using the Modified Edmonton Symptom Assessment Scale (ESAS), the most common symptoms were essentially the same—tiredness, decreased well-being, itching, and pain.[7]

Of particular concern, especially in light of the high symptom burden of patients on dialysis, is the fact that renal providers (nephrologists, nephrology nurse practitioners, nephrology physician assistants) are largely unaware of the presence and severity of symptoms in patients on maintenance hemodialysis. In one study, renal providers underestimated the presence of 27 of 30 symptoms and underestimated the severity of 19 of 30 symptoms.[8] Perhaps this failure to recognize symptoms in patients on dialysis patients should not be a surprise, because only one third of nephrology fellows report that they were taught to assess pain during their nephrology fellowship training.[9]

Because symptoms of patients on dialysis are underrecognized, and pain is one of the most common and severe symptoms of these patients, it is not unexpected that three studies document that pain is undertreated in 75% of patients on dialysis with pain.[10–12] The underrecognition and undertreatment of pain in patients on hemodialysis is particularly noteworthy in the Dialysis Outcomes and Practice Patterns Study (DOPPS) of 3749 patients in 142 U.S. dialysis units between May 1996 and September 2001. Although moderate to severe pain is known to be present in approximately 50% of patients on dialysis, only 18% of the DOPPS study population were prescribed pain medications. Three quarters of patients reporting moderate to very severe pain were not prescribed any analgesics. Worse yet, the most commonly prescribed opioid medication (47% of patients) was a combination of propoxyphene and acetaminophen. This is an older study, but it is alarming because propoxyphene is one of the pain medications that is specifically recommended to be used with caution or not at all in patients on dialysis because of the accumulation of a renally excreted toxic metabolite, norpropoxyphene.[13]

The underrecognition and undertreatment of symptoms in patients on dialysis is a particular concern because researchers have found an inverse correlation between the number of troublesome symptoms experienced by a patient on dialysis and the patient's reported quality of life.[2,14,15] Therefore, if they want to promote an excellent quality of life for patients on dialysis, those treating these patients need to understand the importance of systematic pain and symptom assessment and treatment. Nephrologists who are not expert in these areas may want to consult palliative care clinicians for assistance in this aspect of care for patients on dialysis.

RELEVANT PATHOPHYSIOLOGY

The kidney is responsible for homeostasis and excretion of sodium, potassium, calcium, phosphorous, magnesium, water, acids, metabolic end-products such as urea, and some toxins and drugs. It also produces and secretes hormones: (1) renin, which is part of the renin–angiotensin system, which is involved in salt balance and blood pressure regulation; (2) erythropoietin, which stimulates the maturation of erythrocytes in the bone marrow; and (3) 1,25-dihydroxyvitamin D_3, which regulates calcium and phosphate balance.[16] Consequently, kidney failure results in many disorders that can cause symptoms such as hyperkalemia (weakness), calcium-phosphorous deposition in the skin (pruritus), fluid overload (swelling, shortness of breath), metabolic acidosis (shortness of breath, anorexia), uremia (nausea, vomiting, hiccups, chest pain from pericarditis, daytime somnolence, insomnia, confusion, weakness, myoclonic jerking, seizures), hypertension (which may or may not be symptomatic), anemia (weakness, shortness of breath), hyperphospatemia, hypocalcemia, and secondary hyperparathyroidism (pruritus, bone and joint pain).

Many drugs are excreted by the kidney, and dose adjustments are necessary to avoid drug toxicity in patients with chronic kidney disease, especially in patients on dialysis who within 6 months of starting dialysis usually have less than 5% of the normal glomerular filtration rate. To avoid toxicity, dosages must be decreased or alternative drugs must be used. Consideration also needs to be given to whether a substantial amount of the drug or its metabolites are removed by dialysis and whether a supplemental dose is needed after dialysis. It is best to refer to dosing guidelines for patients with renal dysfunction, including dialysis, before prescribing medications eliminated by the kidneys.[17]

SUMMARY OF EVIDENCE REGARDING TREATMENT RECOMMENDATIONS

Pain is one of the most common and most severe of the symptoms reported by patients on dialysis.[2,7,8,15] For most patients undergoing dialysis, pain is musculoskeletal in origin. Smaller numbers of patients have pain related to the dialysis procedure, peripheral neuropathy, peripheral vascular disease, or carpal tunnel syndrome. Less common causes of pain include that from polycystic kidney disease, malignant disease, or calciphylaxis (calcification of cutaneous blood vessels associated with skin necrosis).[10] Several studies have shown that nociceptive and neuropathic pain are equal in severity in patients on dialysis and can both be effectively treated.[10,11]

The Mid-Atlantic Renal Coalition and the Kidney End-of-Life Coalition assembled a panel of nephrologists and palliative care physicians who were international experts on pain management in chronic kidney disease and developed an evidence-based brochure for treating pain in patients on dialysis, "Clinical Algorithm and Preferred Medication to Treat Pain in Dialysis Patients," which is accessible on the Internet (http://www.kidneyeol.org).[18] This brochure recommends fentanyl and methadone as the safest opioids to use in chronic kidney disease and patients on dialysis because of their lack of active renally excreted metabolites (Figure 60-1). It also provides recommendations for initiation and titration of medications to treat nociceptive and neuropathic pain in patients on dialysis using the World Health Organization (WHO) Three-Step Analgesic Ladder (Figures 60-2 and 60-3). Use of the WHO Three-Step Analgesic Ladder has been found to be effective in the treatment of pain in patients

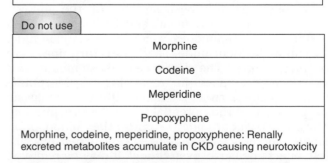

Preferred opioid medications in chroinc kidney disease

Recommended
Fentanyl
Methadone
Hydromorphone
Acetaminophen
Gabapentin
Doses up to 300 mg/d generally considered safe in ESRD, but doses up to 600 mg should be used with caution; note that gabapentin use for neuropathic pain is off-label but effectiveness has been documented
Pregabalin
Doses up to 100 mg/d are generally considered safe in ESRD

Use with caution
Tramadol
Limit dose to 50 mg BID. Higher doses have been used but caution needs to be taken since pharmacokinetics are not well established.
Hydrocodone/Oxycodone
Insufficient pharmacokinetic evidence to establish safety in CKD, but literature reports use without major adverse effects
Desipramine/Nortriptyline
Alternative to treat neuropathic pain, but more adverse effects than gabapentin and pregabalin

Do not use
Morphine
Codeine
Meperidine
Propoxyphene
Morphine, codeine, meperidine, propoxyphene: Renally excreted metabolites accumulate in CKD causing neurotoxicity

FIGURE 60-1. Preferred opioid medications in chronic kidney disease. (*CKD,* Chronic kidney disease; *ESRD,* end-stage renal disease.) (*Mid-Altlantic Renal Coalition and Kidney End-of-Life Coalition:* Clinical Algorithm & Preferred Medications to Treat Pain in Dialysis Patients. *Richmond, Virginia, 2009.*)

Approaches to pain management in chronic kidney disease

NOCICEPTIVE PAIN TREATMENT

Note: Monitor for opioid toxicity (sedation, hallucinations, myoclonus, and/or asterixis) and opioid adverse effects (constipation, nausea, and vomiting).

- Confirm patient is able to swallow oral medications.
- Long-acting opioids should be started after the needed dosage to control pain is established with short-acting opioids.
- A rescue dose equivalent to 10% of the 24-hour dose of opioid should be available to be taken every 1–2 hours prn for breakthrough pain. Remember to recalculate the rescue dose when increasing the base dose (long-acting dose).
- If the patient is experiencing pain when he/she takes the long-acting opioid, he/she should take a rescue dose at the same time and not expect the long-acting opioid to relieve the breakthrough pain.

NEUROPATHIC PAIN TREATMENT

First

Gabapentin:
- Start 100 mg po qhs and increase weekly by 100 mg per night to a maxiumum of 300 mg qhs. Occasionally doses up to 600 mg a day can be safely used.
- If effective at maximum tolerated dose, discontinue and start Pregabalin.

Second

Pregabalin:
- 25 mg qhs and increase every few days to 100 mg a day.
- If pain control is inadequate at target dose for 2 to 4 weeks, or intolerable adverse effects, discontinue and start Desipramine.

Third

Desipramine:
- 10 mg po qhs. Titrate to adequate pain control or maximum dose of 150 mg qhs.
- If pain control still remains inadequate, institute WHO 3 step analgesic ladder (see Fig. 60-3).

FIGURE 60-2. Approaches to pain management in chronic kidney disease. *(Mid-Altlantic Renal Coalition and Kidney End-of-Life Coalition. Clinical Algorithm & Preferred Medications to Treat Pain in Dialysis Patients. Richmond, Virginia, 2009.)*

World Health Organization 3-step analgesic ladder

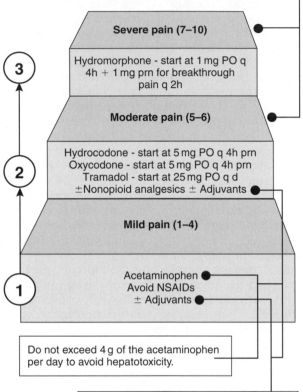

Titrate upwards, increasing the dose until either analgesia or intolerable side effects occur. For mild-moderate pain, increase dose by 25%–50%; for severe pain, increase dose by 50%–100%.

3

Severe pain (7–10)

Hydromorphone - start at 1 mg PO q 4h + 1 mg prn for breakthrough pain q 2h

2

Moderate pain (5–6)

Hydrocodone - start at 5 mg PO q 4h prn
Oxycodone - start at 5 mg PO q 4h prn
Tramadol - start at 25 mg PO q d
±Nonopioid analgesics ± Adjuvants

Mild pain (1–4)

1

Acetaminophen
Avoid NSAIDs
± Adjuvants

Do not exceed 4 g of the acetaminophen per day to avoid hepatotoxicity.

Adjuvants include medications such as anticonvulsants for neuropathic pain. It may also refer to medications that are administered to manage an adverse effect of an opioid, or to enhance analgesia, such as steroids for pain from bone metastases.

FIGURE 60-3. Nociceptive pain management in chronic kidney disease. (CKD, Chronic kidney disease; *ESRD*, end-stage renal disease.) *(Mid-Altlantic Renal Coalition and Kidney End-of-Life Coalition: Clinical Algorithm & Preferred Medications to Treat Pain in Dialysis Patients. Richmond, Virginia, 2009.)*

on dialysis.[11] Other clinical experience also suggests that application of the WHO analgesic ladder results in effective pain relief for patients undergoing dialysis, and the panel recommended its use to nephrologists treating patients with ESRD; however, because morphine, codeine, meperidine, and propoxyphene metabolites are renally excreted and active, the panel did *not* recommend the use of these drugs for pain in patients on dialysis.[18]

Morphine is the best studied of the opioids used for pain management, and its most common metabolites (including morphine-3-glucuronide, morphine-6-glucuronide, and normorphine) are excreted renally. The clearance of these metabolites therefore decreases in renal failure. Morphine-6-glucuronide is an active metabolite with analgesic properties and the potential to depress respiration. Morphine-6-glucuronide crosses the blood–brain barrier and may have prolonged central nervous system effects because, even though it may be removed by dialysis, it diffuses slowly out of the central nervous system. Morphine-3-glucuronide does not have analgesic activity, but it may cause neurotoxicity manifested by agitation, myoclonus, or confusion. Morphine is 35% protein bound, and it has

intermediate water solubility. Studies suggest that morphine is dialyzable to a limited degree. Some clinicians recommend the use of morphine for patients undergoing dialysis but with a decreased dose or an increased dosing interval. A comprehensive review of the use of opioids in renal failure recommended that morphine not be used in patients with kidney disease because it is so difficult to manage the complicated adverse effects of the morphine metabolites.[19]

Codeine is metabolized to codeine-6-glucuronide, norcodeine, morphine, morphine-3-glucuronide, morphine-6-glucuronide, and normorphine. Studies of codeine pharmacokinetics suggest that codeine metabolites would accumulate to toxic levels in a majority of patients undergoing hemodialysis. It is recommended that codeine not be used in patients with kidney failure because of the accumulation of active metabolites and because serious adverse effects have been reported from codeine use in patients with chronic kidney disease.[19]

Hydromorphone is metabolized in the liver to hydromorphone-3-glucuronide as well as to dihydromorphine and dihydroisomorphine. Small quantities of additional metabolites are also formed. All metabolites are excreted renally. The hydromorphone-3-glucuronide metabolite does not have analgesic activity, but it is neuroexcitatory in rats. This metabolite also accumulates in patients with kidney disease. Some studies suggest that hydromorphone is removed with dialysis or is rapidly converted to hydromorphone-3-glucuronide which is removed by dialysis. It is recommended that hydromorphone be used cautiously in patients stopping dialysis because hydromorphone-3-glucuronide accumulates in between dialysis treatments and when dialysis is stopped and can cause opioid neurotoxicity.[20]

On the WHO analgesic ladder, oxycodone is recommended for treatment of both moderate and severe pain. Use of oxycodone in patients with kidney disease has not been well studied. The elimination half-life of oxycodone is lengthened in patients undergoing dialysis, and excretion of metabolites is impaired. Almost all of the oxycodone metabolites are inactive. Anecdotal reports of opioid neurotoxicity have been made when oxycodone has been used in patients with kidney disease. Oxycodone has limited water solubility and 45% plasma protein binding, both of which suggest limited dialyzability. The Mid-Atlantic Renal Coalition expert panel recommended that oxycodone be used with caution and careful monitoring in patients on dialysis.[18] Oxycodone was used effectively and without toxicity in one study of 45 patients on hemodialysis who had moderate to severe pain.[11]

The WHO analgesic ladder recommends fentanyl as one of the opioids to be used for severe pain. Fentanyl is metabolized in the liver primarily to norfentanyl. No evidence exists that any fentanyl metabolites are active. Several studies have found that fentanyl can be used safely in patients with chronic kidney disease. Because 85% of fentanyl is protein bound and fentanyl has very low water solubility, it has negligible dialyzability.[19] The Mid-Atlantic Renal Coalition expert panel deemed fentanyl to be one of the safest opioids to use in patients with chronic kidney disease.[18]

The WHO analgesic ladder recommends methadone as one of the opioids to be used for severe pain. Approximately 20% to 50% of methadone is excreted in the urine as methadone or as its metabolites, and 10% to 45% is excreted in the feces as a pyrrolidine metabolite. Studies in anuric patients found that nearly all of methadone and its metabolites doses are excreted in the feces, mainly as metabolites. Methadone metabolites are inactive. Methadone is 89% bound to plasma proteins and has moderate water solubility. These two factors suggest that it is poorly removed by dialysis. No dose adjustments are recommended for patients undergoing dialysis. The use of methadone appears safe in patients with chronic kidney disease and those undergoing dialysis.[19] The Mid-Atlantic Renal Coalition expert panel deemed methadone to be one of the safest opioids to use in patients with chronic kidney disease.[18]

In addition to their use for pain, opioids are often used to treat dyspnea at the end of life in patients regardless of whether they are continuing or stopping dialysis. In the setting of withdrawal of dialysis, the clinician may be challenged to distinguish uremic encephalopathy from opioid neurotoxicity. Both can cause metabolic encephalopathy with sedation, hallucinations, myoclonus, and asterixis. If respiratory depression with oxygen desaturation is also present and causing respiratory distress, it is advisable to stop the opioid until the respiratory depression subsides. If the patient's respiratory rate is not compromised, the opioid can usually be continued, and a benzodiazepine such as lorazepam is added as an intravenous dose of 1 mg every 6 to 8 hours to control the myoclonus. Occasionally, a lorazepam continuous intravenous infusion at 1 or 2 mg/hr is necessary to control the myoclonus. Seizures occur only 10% of the time after dialysis withdrawal as a major complication of the uremic metabolic encephalopathy. They also can be controlled with lorazepam.[21]

Although nonsteroidal antiinflammatory drugs are recommended for use in step 1 on the WHO analgesic ladder, the use of these drugs in patients with chronic kidney disease is discouraged because of their nephrotoxicity, and their use in patients undergoing dialysis is risky because of the higher frequency of upper gastrointestinal bleeding in these patients. The use of these drugs may also cause loss of residual renal function.[13]

Because of the number of disorders that occur with a uremic state, patients on dialysis develop various symptoms (Table 60-1). As noted, the greater the number of troublesome symptoms reported by patients undergoing dialysis, the lower they rate their quality of life.[2,14,15] For this reason, it is very important for clinicians who treat these patients to assess and manage symptoms aggressively. Treatment with erythropoietin therapy in patients undergoing dialysis led to a correction of the anemia with improved quality of life, decreased fatigue, increased exercise tolerance, and improved overall general well-being. It also has been shown to improve sexual desire and performance in some, but not all, patients undergoing dialysis. Pain from muscle cramps is a common symptom among patients on dialysis, especially if they undergo significant fluid removal during dialysis. Decreasing the volume of fluid removed during any given dialysis treatment may lessen cramps. For patients with chronic kidney disease who are not yet undergoing dialysis, decreasing the dose of diuretic often works to eliminate cramps. Patients need to limit their intake of fluids and salt-containing fluids to avoid worsening of edema and fluid overload if diuretic doses are decreased. Benzodiazepines may be helpful for cramps.

TABLE 60-1. Treatment of Symptoms in Chronic Kidney Disease

SYMPTOM	DISORDER	TREATMENT IF eGFR 10-60 mL/min	TREATMENT IF eGFR* <10 mL/min
Weakness	Hyperkalemia	Dietary potassium restriction, polystyrene resin	Dialysis
Shortness of breath	Fluid overload	Fluid restriction and diuretics	Dialysis
	Anemia	Erythropoietin and intravenous iron	
	Metabolic acidosis	Sodium bicarbonate by mouth to raise total CO_2 to 24	Dialysis
Itching	Hyperphosphatemia with calcium and phosphorus deposition in skin	Dietary phosphate restriction Phosphate binders with meals	Dialysis
Hypertension	Sodium and water overload	Diuretics, antihypertensive medication Salt and water restriction	Dialysis
Uremia	Pericarditis Encephalopathy Gastritis	—	Dialysis
Nausea and vomiting	Uremic gastritis		Dialysis
	Drug toxicity	Adjust dose of medication downward (e.g., digoxin) or stop medication (e.g., nitrofurantoin)	
Bone pain	Secondary hyperparathyroidism	Phosphate binder, vitamin D supplementation with active drug such as calcitriol, and calcimimetic such as cinacalcet Pain medication appropriate to severity of pain	Dialysis

*Dialysis is indicated in addition to other treatments if symptoms below an eGFR of 10 mL/min cannot be controlled with other medical treatment.
eGFR, Estimated glomerular filtration rate in mL/min.

Pruritus, or itching, is one of the most common and frustrating symptoms experienced by patients undergoing dialysis. Secondary hyperparathyroidism, increased calcium-phosphate deposition in the skin, dry skin, inadequate dialysis, anemia, iron deficiency, and low-grade hypersensitivity to products used in the dialysis procedure leading to chronic inflammation have all been identified as possible contributory factors.[22] In addition to careful management of these factors, the following interventions have been tried for pruritus with some success: emollient skin creams; phototherapy with ultraviolet B light three times weekly; intravenous lidocaine (100 mg) during dialysis for severe, refractory itching; and thalidomide (100 mg at bedtime; must not be used in pregnant women).

Insomnia is also reported by the majority of patients undergoing dialysis. In one study it was among the top five symptoms in intensity and severity.[15] In obese patients, sleep apnea should be excluded. The patient should also be evaluated for adequacy of dialysis. Avoidance of caffeinated beverages, alcoholic drinks, and naps have been recommended. If these measures are not effective in improving insomnia, anxiolytic/hypnotics (e.g., zolpidem) or benzodiazepines (e.g., triazolam) are generally safe in patients undergoing dialysis.[23]

Depression is a common symptom in patients on dialysis, with estimates of the point prevalence ranging from 20% to 30%. Diagnosis of depression with instruments such as the Beck Depression Inventory is more difficult because these patients often have somatic symptoms from their kidney disease that are typical of depressed patients.[24] The second edition of the Renal Physicians Association clinical practice guideline on shared decision-making recommended the Patient Health Questionnaire (PHQ-9) as an easy-to-use and validated instrument to screen for depression in patients on dialysis.[25,26] Depression in patients on dialysis has been associated with increased morbidity and mortality. It is estimated that only half of patients on dialysis with depression are diagnosed and that an even smaller number are given adequate doses of antidepressants.[24] Some studies have suggested promising pharmacological and nonpharmacological approaches to treat depressive symptoms in patients on dialysis, but further research is needed to determine the impact of these approaches on morbidity and mortality, hospitalizations, costs, and health-related quality-of-life measures.[24]

Patients on dialysis typically experience significant pain and other symptoms that are underrecognized and undertreated. Dialysis patient care will improve if nephrologists start using simple validated symptom assessment screening instruments such as the 10-item modified ESAS[7] and the 17-item Patient Outcome Scale-symptom (POSs) module.[5] The longer 31-item Dialysis Symptom Index is an excellent tool for research on the symptom burden of patients on dialysis.[2]

KEY MESSAGES TO PATIENTS AND FAMILIES

Patients on dialysis and their families should understand that part of the course of ESRD is a high symptom burden compared to that of most other patients with chronic diseases. They should communicate to their providers about these symptoms, because pain and other symptoms in these patients are underrecognized and undertreated. Indeed, patients and families should be encouraged to seek out nephrologists who systematically assess for pain and symptoms or who routinely consult with palliative care physicians for these aspects of dialysis treatment. It is important to emphasize that symptoms are treatable and proper management of these symptoms in patients with dialysis has been found to improve patient quality of life.

CONCLUSION AND SUMMARY

Because of their comorbid illnesses, patients undergoing dialysis are among the most symptomatic of any population with chronic disease. The greater the number of troublesome symptoms reported by patients on dialysis, the lower they rate their quality of life. For this reason, it is very important for clinicians who treat these patients to assess and manage symptoms aggressively. Treatment of pain in patients on dialysis is more difficult because many of the medications commonly used to treat pain should be avoided in patients on dialysis because they have active, renally excreted metabolites that accumulate in renal failure and can cause adverse effects. Validated instruments are available to assess and manage pain and symptoms for patients on dialysis. The nephrology literature recommends that nephrologists who do not feel prepared to assess and manage pain and symptoms should seek referrals from palliative care consultants.

SUMMARY RECOMMENDATIONS

- Because of their high symptom burden, dialysis patients should be systematically assessed using validated instruments for pain and symptoms using tools modified for dialysis patients such as the Edmonton Symptom Assessment Scale and the Patient Outcome Scale-symptom module scale.
- Pain should be treated using the World Health Organization Three-Step Analgesic Ladder with those medications preferred in chronic kidney disease because of their lack of renally excreted active metabolites (the Mid-Atlantic Renal Coalition pain algorithm is an excellent resource).
- Nephrologists and other nephrology clinicians who do not feel prepared to manage pain and symptoms in patients on dialysis should consult with palliative care specialists. The reason to consult is because the nephrology literature documents a higher patient quality of life when dialysis patients' symptoms are managed well.

REFERENCES

1. Chang VT, Hwang SS, Feuerman M, Kasimis BS. Symptom and quality of life survey of medical oncology patients at a Veterans Affairs Medical Center: a role for symptom assessment. *Cancer.* 2000;88(5):1175–1183.
2. Weisbord SD, Fried LF, Arnold RM, et al. Prevalence, severity, and importance of physical and emotional symptoms in chronic hemodialysis patients. *J Am Soc Nephrol.* 2009;16:2487–2494.
3. Surveillance, epidemiology, and end results (SEER) program 5-year relative survival rates, all sites, all ages, all races, both sexes: SEER*Stat Database: Incidence-SEER 9, (1975–2003). National Cancer Institute, DCCPS, Surveillance Research Program, Cancer Statistics Branch. http://seer.cancer.gov/faststats/selections.php?series=cancer; Accessed September 20, 2012.
4. United States Renal Data System. *USRDS 2010 Annual data report: atlas of end-stage renal disease in the United States. Patient survival; Table I.5: Five-year survival probabilities: Incident ESRD patients.* Available http://www.usrds.org/reference.htm; 2010 Accessed September 20, 2012.
5. Murphy EL, Murtagh FEM, Carey I, Sheerin NS. Understanding symptoms in patients with advanced chronic kidney disease managed without dialysis: use of a short patient-completed assessment tool. et al. Symptoms in the month before death for stage 5 chronic kidney disease patients managed without dialysis. *J Pain Symptom Manage.* 2010;40:342–352.
6. Murtagh FE, Addington-Hall J, Edmonds P, et al. Symptoms in the month before death for stage 5 chronic kidney disease patients managed without dialysis. *J Pain Symptom Manage.* 2010;40:342–352.
7. Davison SN, Jhangri GS, Johnson JA. Longitudinal validation of a modified Edmonton symptom assessment system (ESAS) in haemodialysis patients. *Nephrol Dial Transplant.* 2006;21:3189–3195.
8. Weisbord SD, Fried LF, Mor MK, et al. Renal provider recognition of symptoms in patients on maintenance hemodialysis. *Clin J Am Soc Nephrol.* 2007;2:960–967.
9. Holley JL, Carmody SS, Moss AH, et al. The need for end-of-life care training in nephrology: National survey results of nephrology fellows. *Am J Kidney Dis.* 2003;42:813–820.
10. Davison SN. Pain in hemodialysis patients: Prevalence, cause, severity, and management. *Am J Kidney Dis.* 2003;42:1239–1247.
11. Barakzoy AS, Moss AH. Efficacy of the World Health Organization Analgesic Ladder to treat pain in end-stage renal disease. *J Am Soc Nephrol.* 2006;17:3198–3203.
12. Bailie GR, Mason NA, Bragg-Gresham JL, Gillespie BW, Young EW. Analgesic prescription patterns among hemodialysis patients in the DOPPS: potential for underprescription. *Kidney Int.* 2004;65:2419–2425.
13. Kurella M, Bennett WM, Chertow GM. Analgesia in patients with ESRD: a review of available evidence. *Am J Kidney Dis.* 2003;42:217–228.
14. Kimmel PL, Emont SL, Newmann JM, Danko H, Moss AH. ESRD patient quality of life: symptoms, spiritual beliefs, psychosocial factors, and ethnicity. *Am J Kidney Dis.* 2003;42:713–721.
15. Yong DSP, Kwok AOL, Wong DML, Suen MHP, Chen WT, Tse DMW. Symptom burden and quality of life in end-stage renal disease: a study of 179 patients on dialysis and palliative care. *Palliat Med.* 2009;23(2):111–119.
16. Briggs JP, Kriz W, Schnermann JB. Overview of renal function and structure. In: Greenberg A, ed. *Primer on Kidney Diseases.* 3rd ed. New York: National Kidney Foundation; 2001.
17. Brater DC. Drug dosing in renal failure. In: Wilcox CS, ed. *Therapy in Nephrology & Hypertension: A Companion to Brenner & Rector's The Kidney.* 3rd ed. Philadelphia: Saunders; 2008:1049–1072.
18. Kidney End-of-Life Coalition. *Clinical Algorithm & Preferred Medications to Treat Pain in Dialysis Patients.* http://www.kidneyeol.org; 2009 Accessed September 20, 2012.
19. Dean M. Opioids in renal failure and dialysis patients. *J Pain Symptom Manage.* 2004;28(5):497–504.
20. Davison SN, Mayo PR. Pain management in chronic kidney disease: the pharmacokinetics and pharmacodynamics of hydromorphone and hydromorphone-3-glucuronide in hemodialysis patients. *J Opioid Manage.* 2008;4(6):339–344.

21. Keely KJ, Roxe DM. Palliative care/hospice and the withdrawal of dialysis. *J Palliat Med.* 2000;3(1):57–67.
22. Lugon JR. Uremic pruritus: a review. *Hemodial Int.* 2005;9(2):180–188.
23. Murtagh F, Weisbord SD. Symptoms in renal disease; their epidemiology, assessment, and management. In: Chambers EJ, Brown EA, Germain MJ, eds. *Supportive Care for the Renal Patient.* 2nd ed. New York: Oxford University Press; 2010:103–132.
24. Hedayati SS, Finkelstein FO. Epidemiology, diagnosis, and management of depression in patients with CKD. *Am J Kidney Dis.* 2009;54:741–752.
25. Renal Physicians Association. *Shared Decision-Making in the Appropriate Initiation of and Withdrawal from Dialysis.* 2nd ed. Rockville, MD: Renal Physicians Association; 2010:123–124.
26. Abdel-Kaher K, Unruh ML, Weisbord SD. Symptom burden, depression, and quality of life in chronic and end-stage kidney disease. *Clin J Am Soc Nephrol.* 2009;4:1057–1064.

How Is the Patient Who Stops Dialysis Best Managed?

Alvin H. Moss

INTRODUCTION AND SCOPE OF THE PROBLEM

United States Renal Data System (USRDS) annual reports have consistently shown that stopping dialysis is the third most common cause of dialysis patient death after cardiovascular diseases and infections.[1] In the earliest major study calling attention to the frequency of dialysis withdrawal, researchers in one large dialysis program noted that stopping dialysis (or what has also been termed dialysis withdrawal or discontinuation) accounted for 22% of deaths.[2] In 2009 the 18 End-Stage Renal Disease (ESRD) Networks in the country reported 20,854 deaths from stopping dialysis, which constituted 26% of the 79,886 dialysis patient deaths that year.[3] Patients on dialysis who stop dialysis die on average 8 days later[4] and 96% die within a month.[5] The two most common reasons for patients to stop dialysis are progressive physical deterioration (called failure to thrive in the USRDS reports) and an acute intercurrent disorder (called a medical complication in the USRDS reports) such as a stroke.[4,6]

Death after dialysis withdrawal is much more predictable than death of a patient with cancer. Because of the short timeframe between dialysis withdrawal and death, it would be expected that most patients on dialysis are referred to hospice for terminal care. The first study to examine hospice use by patients on dialysis covered the period 2001 to 2002 and found that fewer than half (41.5%) of patients stopping dialysis were referred for hospice. In this study, overall only 13.5% of patients on dialysis in the United States used hospice before death, a usage roughly half that of the general population (25%). This same study also found that withdrawal from dialysis and hospice use both rose steadily with older age.

Because of the recognition that there was a need to improve palliative care and hospice care for patients on dialysis, the Robert Wood Johnson Foundation national program, Promoting Excellence in End-of-Life Care, convened an ESRD workgroup in 2000 that met for an 18-month period and released a report in 2002 that made 46 recommendations to improve end-of-life care for patients on dialysis.[7] The report recommended that dialysis units incorporate palliative care into their treatment of patients on dialysis and refer dying patients on dialysis to hospice. Numerous articles were subsequently published based on the findings of the workgroup, and the Kidney End-of-Life Care Coalition (www.kidneyeol. org) was formed.[8] Participants in the workgroup and Coalition published a core curriculum in palliative care for nephrology fellowship programs that included a discussion of the medical, ethical, and legal considerations in stopping dialysis.[9] One result of these efforts was increased attention to the palliative care needs of patients on dialysis, including the appropriateness of referring patients who stop dialysis to hospice. There was a 50% increase in the hospice referral of patients who stopped dialysis in 2009 compared to 2002 (65% versus 41.5%).[3]

RELEVANT PATHOPHYSIOLOGY

Patients who stop dialysis die a "uremic death." Stopping dialysis is usually associated with an accumulation of uremic toxins, electrolyte imbalance, metabolic acidosis, and fluid excess because patients with ESRD continue to drink but have little or no urine output.[10] Despite years of research, these uremic toxins have not been well characterized, but it is well known that their buildup results in a metabolic encephalopathy progressively characterized by somnolence, confusion, hallucinations, myoclonus, asterixis, and ultimately coma. Seizures occur in about 10% of patients who stop dialysis.[10] The metabolic acidosis worsens over time, and patients hyperventilate and become dyspneic to compensate for it.

SUMMARY OF EVIDENCE REGARDING TREATMENT RECOMMENDATIONS

In one study, 79 patients on dialysis were followed prospectively until death after stopping dialysis. Twenty-five percent or more of patients had pain, agitation, myoclonus, and dyspnea in the last 24 hours of life.[4] For years, death from uremia was considered "painless" because patients eventually become comatose.[10] The prospective study of dialysis withdrawal indicates that pain is the most common symptom of dying patients after stopping dialysis and that it is the most severe.[4] Because they do not have active renally excreted metabolites, fentanyl and methadone are the preferred medications to treat pain and dyspnea in dying patients who have stopped dialysis.[8] Benzodiazepines are the drugs of choice for myoclonus and seizures in renal failure, and no dosage adjustment is necessary.[10] Haloperidol can be safely used in renal failure for agitation and delirium and requires no dosage adjustment.[10]

Other opioids commonly used in dying patients are not safe for long-term use in dying patients who are on dialysis because of the accumulation of active renally excreted metabolites. Included in this list of drugs to be avoided in patients stopping dialysis are morphine, hydromorphone, codeine, meperidine, and propoxyphene.[8,11]

No randomized, controlled trials have been conducted on the use of hospice versus standard care for patients who have stopped dialysis, but some early evidence suggests that the complex needs of these patients are best addressed through the collaboration of nephrology professionals with family, community-based professionals, and hospice or palliative care providers.[12,13] The actual care provider may be determined by the strengths of local service programs, but the approach is characterized by the following:
- Holistic and patient-centered care
- Multidisciplinary professional collaboration to provide this care
- High-quality, skilled communication and sensitive advance care planning
- Attention to needs across the physical, psychological, social, and spiritual domains of care
- Consideration of family needs, including bereavement support

In addition, based on the experience of hospice personnel in managing pain, symptoms, and psychosocial and spiritual issues at the end of life, the ESRD Peer Workgroup[7] and the *Shared Decision-Making in the Appropriate Initiation of and Withdrawal from Dialysis* clinical practice guideline[14] both recommend hospice for dying patients who are on dialysis. Table 61-1 presents the recommendation of the clinical practice guideline.

Almost all patients die within a month of stopping dialysis; therefore it is important that patients and families be prepared for imminent death. Part of this preparation is for clinicians involved in the patient's care to explain that cardiac arrest from uremia will occur and that a do-not-resuscitate order is necessary to prevent the patient from being traumatized at the time of death. A "Preparation for Dying Checklist" is included in the toolkit for the Shared Decision-making clinical practice guideline[14] to ensure that pertinent medical, financial, spiritual, and legal matters are considered in advance of death when a patient with ESRD decides not to start dialysis or before a patient stops dialysis (Table 61-2).

KEY MESSAGES TO PATIENTS AND FAMILIES

Death from stopping dialysis is not uncommon. Every year, thousands of patients on dialysis (or their family members) make the decision to stop dialysis because of a medical complication or a progressive deterioration in the patient's condition so that life is no longer satisfactory. Because death occurs on average 8 days after stopping dialysis, it is necessary for patients and families to take care of medical, financial, spiritual, and legal matters before stopping dialysis to avoid stress and difficulties at or after the patient's death. Nephrologists recommend referral to hospice for patients stopping dialysis so that the patient receives careful attention to pain and symptom management, and the patient and family receive psychosocial and spiritual support. Hospice continues to provide bereavement support to the family after the patient's death.

CONCLUSION AND SUMMARY

Because patients die on average 8 days after stopping dialysis, clinicians caring for them need to take a proactive approach to ensure that patients are comfortable and the needs of the families are met.

TABLE 61-1. Clinical Practice Guideline Recommendation for Palliative Care and Hospice for Patients Stopping Dialysis

Providing Effective Palliative Care
Recommendation No. 9
To improve patient-centered outcomes, offer palliative care services and interventions to all acute kidney injury, chronic kidney disease, and ESRD patients who suffer from burdens of their disease.
Palliative care services are appropriate for people who chose to undergo or remain on dialysis and for those who choose not to start or to discontinue dialysis. With the patient's consent, a multi-professional team with expertise in renal palliative care, including nephrology professionals, family or community-based professionals, and specialist hospice or palliative care providers, should be involved in managing the physical, psychological, social, and spiritual aspects of treatment for these patients, including end-of-life care. Physical and psychological symptoms should be routinely and regularly assessed and actively managed. The professionals providing treatment should be trained in assessing and managing symptoms and in advanced communication skills. Patients should be offered the option of dying where they prefer, including at home with hospice care, provided there is sufficient and appropriate support to enable this option. Support also should be offered to patients' families, including bereavement support where appropriate. Dialysis patients for whom the goals of care are primarily comfort should have quality measures distinct from patients for whom the goals are aggressive therapy with optimization of functional capacity.

Data from the Renal Physicians Association. *Shared Decision-Making in the Appropriate Initiation of and Withdrawal from Dialysis,* 2nd ed. Rockville, MD: Renal Physicians Association; 2010: 65–66.
ESRD, End-stage renal disease.

TABLE 61-2. A Preparation for Dying Checklist

A patient who has decided not to initiate or to withdraw dialysis should have or consider preparing the following documents:

A will

Signed advance directive (living will, durable health care power of attorney or health care proxy) complying with applicable state law

A durable power of attorney complying with applicable state law designating someone to act on the patient's behalf on all matters other than medical, including legal, financial, banking, and business transactions. (A power of attorney must be "durable" if it is to remain in effect even if the individual becomes unable to make his or her own decisions or dies.)

Medical orders specifying treatment the patient is to receive at the end of life, including a do-not-resuscitate order and a physician order for life-sustaining treatment (POLST) or comparable form if available in the state in which the patient dies[15]

An inventory, including the location of her/his bank, brokerage and other financial accounts, stock and bond holdings not in brokerage accounts, real estate and business records and documents, medical and other insurance policies, pension plans, and other legal documents.

Names, addresses, and telephone numbers of attorney, accountant, family members/significant other, friends, and business associates who should be notified of the death or may have information that will be helpful in dealing with estate affairs

Documentation concerning preferences for funeral/memorial services, burial or cremation instructions, and decisions about organ, tissue, or body donation

Written or videotaped or audiotaped message to family/significant other, business associates, and friends

Modified from Renal Physicians *Association. Shared Decision-Making in the Appropriate Initiation of and Withdrawal from Dialysis*, 2nd ed. Rockville, MD: Renal Physicians Association; 2010: 148.

In most circumstances, patients should be referred to hospice before dialysis is stopped so that hospices become familiar with the patients and families and are prepared to manage patients' pain and symptoms and provide support to patients and families during patients' brief life after dialysis is stopped.

SUMMARY RECOMMENDATIONS

- Patients who stop dialysis require active medical management of their pain and symptoms.
- Fentanyl and methadone are the preferred drugs to treat pain and dyspnea in patients who have stopped dialysis.
- Myoclonus is best managed with benzodiazepines.
- Advance preparation for death is necessary, with attention to medical orders and financial, legal, and spiritual matters.
- Nephrologists recommend referral to hospice before stopping dialysis so that the hospice becomes familiar with the patient's and family's needs during the patient's brief life after stopping dialysis.

REFERENCES

1. USRDS Annual Data Report Reference Tables. *Mortality and causes of death: table H.12*. http://www.usrds.org/reference.htm; 2010 Accessed September 20, 2012.

2. Neu S, Kjellstrand CM. Stopping long-term dialysis: an empirical study of withdrawal of life-supporting treatment. *N Engl J Med.* 1986;314(1):14–20.

3. *Standard Information Management System [ESRD Network database]*. Midlothian, VA: Mid-Atlantic Renal Coalition: 2010.

4. Cohen LM, Germain M, Poppel DM, Woods A, Kjellstrand CM. Dialysis discontinuation and palliative care. *Am J Kidney Dis.* 2000;36(1):140–144.

5. Murray AM, Arko C, Chen S-C, Gilbertson DT, Moss AH. Utilization of hospice in the United States dialysis population. *Clinical J Am Soc Nephrol.* 2006;1(6):1248–1255.

6. USRDS Annual Data Report Reference Tables. *Mortality and causes of death: table H.11*. http://www.usrds.org/reference.htm; 2010 Accessed September 20, 2012.

7. Robert Wood Johnson Foundation ESRD Peer Workgroup. *Completing the continuum of quality ESRD patient care: recommendations to the field*. http://www.promotingexcellence.org/downloads/esrd_report_summary.pdf; 2002 Accessed September 20, 2012.

8. Mid-Atlantic Renal Coalition and Kidney End-of-Life Coalition. *Clinical algorithm and preferred medications to treat pain in dialysis patients*. http://www.kidneyeol.org; Accessed September 20, 2012.

9. Moss AH, Holley JL, Davison SN, et al. Core curriculum in nephrology: palliative care. *Am J Kidney Dis.* 2004;43(1):172–185.

10. Keely KJ, Roxe DM. Palliative care/hospice and the withdrawal of dialysis. *J Palliat Med.* 2000;3(1):57–67.

11. Dean M. Opioids in renal failure and dialysis patients. *J Pain Symptom Manage.* 2004;28(5):497–504.

12. Poppel DM, Cohen LM, Germain MJ. The Renal Palliative Care Initiative. *J Palliat Med.* 2003;6(2):321–326.

13. Noble H, Kelly D, Rawlings-Anderson K, Meyer J. A concept analysis of renal supportive care: the changing world of nephrology. *J Adv Nurs.* 2007;59(6):644–653.

14. Renal Physicians Association. *Shared Decision-Making in the Appropriate Initiation of and Withdrawal from Dialysis*. 2nd ed. Rockville, MD: Renal Physicians Association; 2010:7.

15. Citko J, Moss AH, Carley M, Tolle S. *The National POLST Paradigm Initiative*. 2nd ed. http://www.eperc.mcw.edu/fastFact/ff_178.htm; Accessed September 20, 2012.

Chapter 62

Which Patients With End-Stage Renal Disease Should Not Be Started on Dialysis?

ALVIN H. MOSS

INTRODUCTION AND SCOPE OF THE PROBLEM
SUMMARY OF EVIDENCE REGARDING TREATMENT
  RECOMMENDATIONS
KEY MESSAGES TO PATIENTS AND FAMILIES
CONCLUSION AND SUMMARY

INTRODUCTION AND SCOPE OF THE PROBLEM

The history of the ethical question of which patients with end-stage renal disease should not be started on dialysis dates back to the early 1960s, when the technique of chronic dialysis was developed. In 1962 the Seattle Artificial Kidney Center, the first dialysis center in the country, opened; they faced the unprecedented ethical problem of determining which patients should be given access to chronic hemodialysis in their nine-bed-capacity dialysis center. Many more patients were seeking treatment than there were trained staff and machines available to provide dialysis to them. Journalist Shana Alexander called national attention to this ethical problem in her *Life* magazine article, "They Decide Who Lives, Who Dies: Medical Miracles Puts Moral Burden on Small Committee."[1] The King County Medical Society solved the question in part by instructing the Seattle Artificial Kidney Center Admissions Committee that children and patients over the age of 45 years were not to be started on dialysis. Furthermore, patients who were not otherwise healthy with the exception of kidney disease were not to be started.

In 1972 the passage of the end-stage renal disease (ESRD) Amendment to H.R. 1 virtually eliminated the need to ration dialysis. This legislation classified patients with a diagnosis of ESRD as disabled, authorized Medicare entitlement for them, and provided the financial resources to pay for their dialysis. The only requirement for this entitlement was that the patients or their spouses or (if dependent children) parents were insured or entitled to monthly benefits under Social Security. When Congress passed this legislation, its members believed that money should not be an obstacle to providing life-saving therapy.[2] Although the legislation stated that patients should be screened for "appropriateness" for dialysis and transplantation, the primary concern was to make dialysis available to those who needed it. Neither Congress nor physicians thought it necessary or proper for the government to determine patient-selection criteria.

By 1978 many patients with ESRD who would not previously have been accepted as dialysis candidates were started on treatment.[3] A decade later, the first report of the U.S. Renal Data System documented the progressively greater acceptance rate of patients onto dialysis,[4] and subsequent reports showed that the sharp rise in the number of patients on dialysis could be explained in part by the inclusion of patients who had poor prognoses, especially the elderly and those with diabetic nephropathy.[5]

In its 1991 report the Institute of Medicine (IOM) Committee for the Study of the Medicare End-Stage Renal Disease Program raised concerns about the appropriateness of treating many patients with ESRD with dialysis.[6] Specifically, questions were raised about the appropriateness of providing dialysis to those with a limited life expectancy despite the use of dialysis and those with severe neurological disease. The first group included patients with kidney failure and other life-threatening illnesses, such as atherosclerotic cardiovascular disease, cancer, chronic pulmonary disease, and acquired immunodeficiency syndrome (AIDS). The second group included patients whose neurological disease rendered them unable to relate to others, such as those in a persistent vegetative state or with severe dementia. The IOM committee acknowledged that the existence of the public entitlement for treatment of ESRD did not obligate physicians to treat all patients who have kidney failure with dialysis. The committee recommended that guidelines be developed for who should receive dialysis and that the guidelines allow physician discretion in assessing individual patients. The committee thought that such guidelines might help nephrologists make dialysis decisions more uniformly, with greater ease, and in a way that promoted patient benefit and the appropriate use of dialysis resources. Subsequent studies confirmed the committee's concerns and demonstrated that nephrologists differed on how they made decisions to start or stop dialysis for patients.[7,8]

In 2000, following the recommendation of the IOM committee, the Renal Physicians Association and the American Society of Nephrology published a clinical practice guideline that included recommendations about which patients should not be started on dialysis.[9] This guideline was based on a systematic review of the medical literature and included more than 300 citations. It marked a turning point in how nephrologists familiar with this guideline made decisions about not starting dialysis.[10,11]

SUMMARY OF EVIDENCE REGARDING TREATMENT RECOMMENDATIONS

The Renal Physicians Association and American Society of Nephrology working group, who wrote the clinical practice guideline "Shared Decision-Making in the Appropriate Initiation of and Withdrawal from Dialysis," used the research evidence, case and statutory law, ethical principles, and expert consensus opinion to formulate two separate recommendations with regard to patients with ESRD for whom dialysis should not be started. The first identified patients for whom it was appropriate not to start dialysis (Table 62-1). The second was not as strong and noted patients for whom it was reasonable to consider not starting dialysis, such as those with a terminal illness from a nonrenal cause or those whose medical condition makes the technical process of dialysis particularly challenging.

In 2010, prompted by a substantial body of new research evidence on dialysis decision-making and poor outcomes with dialysis in increasingly older patients with significant comorbid conditions, the Renal Physicians Association published a second edition of the clinical practice guideline "Shared Decision-Making in the Appropriate Initiation of and Withdrawal from Dialysis."[12] In particular, the second edition is noteworthy for an extensive discussion of the poor prognosis of many elderly patients with stage 4 (estimated glomerular filtration rate 15-29 mL/min) and stage 5 (estimated glomerular filtration rate <15 mL/min) chronic kidney disease who are not likely to benefit from dialysis and for whom it would be appropriate not to start dialysis.

The guideline reviewed several studies that showed that patients 75 years of age and older with stage 4 or 5 chronic kidney disease are far more likely to die than to live to start dialysis, because of increasing cardiovascular mortality with higher stages of chronic kidney disease.[13] Furthermore, the guideline found that patients 75 years of age and older with

---

TABLE 62-1. Patients for Whom It Is Appropriate NOT to Start Dialysis

It is appropriate to withhold dialysis from patients with ESRD in the following situations:

Patients with decision-making capacity, who being fully informed and making voluntary choices, refuse dialysis or request dialysis be discontinued

Patients who no longer possess decision-making capacity who have previously indicated refusal of dialysis in an oral or written advance directive

Patients who no longer possess decision-making capacity and whose properly appointed legal agents refuse dialysis or request that it be discontinued

Patients with irreversible, profound neurological impairment such that they lack signs of thought, sensation, purposeful behavior, and awareness of self and environment

---

TABLE 62-2. Patients for Whom It Is Reasonable to Consider NOT Starting Dialysis

Those whose medical condition precludes the technical process of dialysis because the patient is unable to cooperate (e.g., advanced dementia patient who pulls out dialysis needles) or because the patient's condition is too unstable (e.g., profound hypotension).

Those who have a terminal illness from nonrenal causes (acknowledging that some in this condition may perceive benefit from and choose to undergo dialysis)

Those with stage 5 chronic kidney disease older than age 75 years who meet two or more of the following statistically significant very poor prognosis criteria: (1) clinicians' response of "No, I would not be surprised" to the surprise question, "Would I be surprised if this patient died in the next year?"; (2) high comorbidity score; (3) significantly impaired functional status (e.g., Karnofsky Performance Status score less than 40); and (4) severe chronic malnutrition (i.e., serum albumin <2.5 g/dL using the bromcresol green method).

---

stage 4 or 5 chronic kidney disease with ischemic heart disease, more than one significant comorbidity, or poor functional status had no survival advantage with dialysis. Accordingly, the second edition of the guideline revised and expanded its recommendation for patients for whom it is reasonable to consider not starting dialysis (Table 62-2). Because of the severe comorbidities, functional impairment, and malnutrition of some elderly patients with chronic kidney disease, the guideline recommended that nephrologists should not take an "age neutral" approach to the management of patients with chronic kidney disease. On the other hand, age alone should not constitute a contraindication to starting dialysis, because comorbidity is the single most important determinant of outcome in patients receiving dialysis.

KEY MESSAGES TO PATIENTS AND FAMILIES

The key message to patients and families is that dialysis does not benefit every patient. Factors that have been found to be independently statistically significant predictors of early mortality in patients on dialysis are age, nutritional status, functional status, and comorbidities.[12] Therefore it is important for patients and families to engage in an extended discussion with the patient's nephrologist about the patient's overall condition considering these factors and the likelihood of benefit of dialysis for the patient. As part of the discussion, nephrologists need to estimate each patient's prognosis. Elderly patients with severe comorbidities need to be apprised of potential burdens of dialysis for them (Table 62-3).

CONCLUSION AND SUMMARY

In the 1960s, when dialysis first was developed as a therapy for ESRD, the vast majority of patients were not started on it. It was thought that adults below the age of 45 who were otherwise healthy were the only appropriate candidates. When federal funding through

TABLE 62-3. Particular Informed Consent Considerations for Elderly Patients With Chronic Kidney Disease With Comorbidities

Dialysis may not confer a survival advantage.

Patients with their level of illness are more likely to die than live long enough to progress to ESRD.

Life on dialysis entails significant burdens that may detract from patient quality of life.

Patients may not experience functional improvement with dialysis and may undergo significant functional decline during the first year after dialysis initiation.

The burdens of dialysis include surgery for vascular or peritoneal access placement and complications from the vascular access or peritoneal dialysis catheter.

Patients may experience adverse physical symptoms on dialysis such as dizziness, fatigue, and cramping, and a feeling of "unwellness" after dialysis.

Life on dialysis requires travel time and expense to and from dialysis and long hours spent on dialysis and reduces time available for physical activity.

Dialysis may entail an "unnecessary medicalization of death" resulting in invasive tests, procedures, and hospitalizations.

Medicare became available, slowly over the last few decades of the late twentieth century, virtually all selection criteria for patients on dialysis were abandoned and patients with increasingly poor prognoses were started on dialysis. In 2000 the Renal Physicians Association and American Society of Nephrology published a clinical practice guideline that recommended which patients should not be started on dialysis. In 2010 this guideline was updated based on a considerable body of new research evidence pointing to poor outcomes for dialysis in elderly patients with multiple comorbidities and poor functional status. Because of this new evidence, the guideline recommends that nephrologists engage in informed consent discussions with patients and families in which the patient's prognosis is estimated. For patients who choose not to start dialysis, the guideline recommends palliative care and referral to hospice.

SUMMARY RECOMMENDATIONS

- Patients who have indicated through oral or written advance directives that they do not want dialysis should not be started on dialysis.
- Patients whose families think that dialysis would not be in the patient's best interest and refuse dialysis should not be started on dialysis.

- Patients with profound neurological disease such that they lack awareness of self and others should not be started on dialysis.
- Patients age 75 and older with severe comorbidities should be informed about the benefits and burdens of dialysis based on their overall condition, and nephrologists should recommend to such patients that they not be started on dialysis if they do not believe that dialysis will confer a survival advantage over active medical management without dialysis.

REFERENCES

1. Alexander S. They decide who lives, who dies: medical miracles puts moral burden on small committee. *Life.* 1963;53:102–125.
2. Rettig RA. Origins of the Medicare Kidney Disease Entitlement: The Social Security Amendments of 1972. In: Hanna KE, eds. *Biomedical Politics.* Washington, DC: National Academies Press; 1991:176–208.
3. Fox RC, Swazey JP. *The Courage to Fail: A Social View of Organ Transplants and Dialysis.* 2nd ed, rev. Chicago: University of Chicago Press; 1978:367–371.
4. U.S. Renal Data System. *Annual Data Report.* Bethesda, MD: National Institutes of Health, National Institute of Diabetes and Digestive and Kidney Diseases, Division of Kidney, Urologic, and Hematologic Diseases; 1989.
5. Rosansky SJ, Jackson K. Rate of change of end-stage renal disease treatment incidence 1978–1987: has there been selection? *J Am Soc Nephrol.* 1992;2(10):1502–1506.
6. Rettig RA, Levinsky NG. *Kidney Failure and the Federal Government.* Washington, DC: National Academies Press; 1991:51–61.
7. Moss AH, Stocking CB, Sachs GA, et al. Variation in the attitudes of dialysis unit medical directors toward reported decisions to withhold and withdraw dialysis. *J Am Soc Nephrol.* 1993;4(2):229–234.
8. Singer PA. Nephrologists' experience with and attitudes towards decisions to forego dialysis. The End-Stage Renal Disease Network of New England. *J Am Soc Nephrol* 1992;2(7):1235–1240.
9. Renal Physicians Association and the American Society of Nephrology. *Shared Decision-Making in the Appropriate Initiation of and Withdrawal from Dialysis.* Rockville, MD: Renal Physicians Association; 2000.
10. Davison SN, Jhangri GS, Holley JL, Moss AH. Nephrologists' reported preparedness for end-of-life decision-making. *Clin J Am Soc Nephrol.* 2006;1(6):1256–1262.
11. Holley JL, Davison SN, Moss AH. Nephrologists' changing practices in reported end-of-life decision-making. *Clin J Am Soc Nephrol.* 2007;2(1):107–111.
12. Renal Physicians Association. *Shared Decision-Making in the Appropriate Initiation of and Withdrawal from Dialysis.* 2nd ed. Rockville, MD: Renal Physicians Association; 2010:39–92.
13. O'Hare AM, Choy AI, Bertenthal D, et al. Age affects outcomes in chronic kidney disease. *J Am Soc Nephrol.* 2007;18(10):2758–2765.

FRAILTY

Chapter 63

What Is Frailty?

FRED C. KO AND JEREMY D. WALSTON

INTRODUCTION AND SCOPE OF THE PROBLEM

Frailty Syndrome: Conceptualization and Definitions

Frailty syndrome describes a clinical state of increased vulnerability that is recognized by progressive multisystemic decline, reduced physiological reserve and ability to cope with acute stress, and increased adverse health outcomes.[1] Poor clinical events such as recurrent falls and injuries, frequent hospitalization, or progressive disability often provide clinicians with evidence that a patient is afflicted with frailty.[2] In contrast to these late manifestations, frailty in its earliest stage is often not clinically apparent. Although various frailty screening tools have been developed and validated, and several have been studied in multiple population and biological studies, no single definition of frailty has been widely accepted and incorporated into clinical practice.[2] This is in part due to differences in the conceptualization of frailty—some have considered it a physiological condition related to multisystemic declines that are age-related, and others have conceptualized frailty as an accumulation of functional deficits, disease states, and cognitive decline.

Given this difference in conceptualization, definitions of frailty can be divided into two major categories: one category that primarily focuses on compromised energetics, muscle weakness, and physiological decline[1,3,4] and one category that is based on an accumulation of deficits and clinical conditions.[5] In the former category, frailty is usually characterized by physical decline in strength, balance, mobility, endurance, activity, and weight.[1,4] The most widely used definition of this category was operationalized by Fried and colleagues[1] as a syndrome meeting three of the following five criteria: (1) low grip strength, (2) slowed walking speed, (3) low physical activity, (4) self-reported exhaustion, and (5) unintentional weight loss (Table 63-1). Those with profound cognitive deficits and medical conditions that would greatly affect the physical measurements were not included in the original validation studies. This is assessed by a series of questions about activity and energy levels and with measurements of walking speed and grip strength. Robust individuals meet none of the criteria, a prefrail state is present when one or two criteria are met, and frailty is present when three to five of the criteria are met. Importantly, the prefrail state predicts a higher risk for progression to frailty. The Fried criteria attempt to capture the idea of a cumulative multisystem physiological decline that underlies frailty, with this accumulation of defects in phenotypes ultimately influencing vulnerability to adverse health outcomes of all kinds, including mortality. This definition was validated in community-dwelling men and women 65 years or older of the Cardiovascular Health Study (CHS)[1] and the Women's Health and Aging Studies (WHAS).[3] In these population studies, older adults with the frailty phenotype had significantly worsened mobility and activities of daily living (ADLs) disability, increased falls, hospitalization, and mortality, even after adjustment for medical comorbidities, socioeconomic status, and disability. This phenotype of frailty has also been widely used to study biological underpinnings of frailty and in the development of a frail mouse model, as detailed later.[6-10]

Other investigators built on this concept and operationalized alternative definitions in large population cohort studies. The Study of Osteoporotic Fracture (SOF) research group developed a frailty index in a prospective cohort of 6701 women over the age 69 years that used unintentional weight loss, poor ability to stand from chair, and reduced energy level to calculate frailty.[11] The tool was effective at

TABLE 63-1. Frailty Phenotype Defined as per the Cardiovascular Health Study

FRAILTY CHARACTERISTICS*	ASSESSMENT	
Unintentional weight loss	*Baseline:* Lost >4.5 kg in the last year *Follow-up:* ([Weight in previous year − Current weight]/[Weight in previous year]) ≥0.05	
Weakness (loss of strength)	Grip strength *Women:* ≤17 kg for BMI ≤23 ≤17.3 kg for BMI 23.1-26 ≤18 kg for BMI 26.1-29 ≤21 kg for BMI >29	*Men:* ≤29 kg for BMI ≤24 ≤30 kg for BMI 24.1-26 ≤30 kg for BMI 26.1-28 ≤32 kg for BMI >28
Exhaustion	Self-report of either: Feeling that everything the person did was an effort in the last week or inability to get going in the last week	
Slowness	Observed walking for 4.57 m at usual pace *Women:* Time ≥7 sec for height ≤159 cm Time ≥6 sec for height >159 cm	*Men:* Time ≥7 s for height ≤173 cm Time ≥6 s for height >173 cm
Low physical activity	*Women:* Energy <270 kcal on activity scale (18 items) *Men:* Energy <383 kcal on activity scale (18 items)	

Data from Fried LP, Tangen CM, Walston J, et al. Frailty in older adults: evidence for a phenotype. *J Gerontol A Biol Sci Med Sci.* 2001;56(3):M146-M156; and Xue QL. The frailty syndrome: definition and natural history. *Clin Geriatr Med.* 2011;27(1):1–15.
*Frail if ≥3 criteria present; prefrail if 1 or 2 criteria present.

predicting adverse health outcomes of falls, disability, fracture, and mortality in this cohort, and the authors suggest that it may be simpler to use and calculate a frailty score compared to the Fried frailty criteria. The Survey of Health, Ageing, and Retirement in Europe (SHARE) investigators developed a tool they claim is easier and faster to use for calculations of frailty, particularly in the community or primary care setting.[12] This tool was developed from questions that approximated the Hopkins frailty tool (Fried frailty criteria) that were included in the SHARE survey of over 21,000 Europeans over age 65. Frailty as measured by this tool was also found to be highly predictive of mortality compared to nonfrail individuals, with an odds ratio of 4.8, similar to that seen in the Hopkins frailty tool. Other tools that used measures of physical decline to operationalize frailty syndrome included lower extremity performance battery of gait speed, chair stand, tandem balance,[13] and inactivity plus weight loss,[4] both of which accurately predicted hospitalization, health and functional decline, and mortality in frail older adults.

Another frequently used definition of frailty, developed by Mitnitski and colleagues,[14] conceptualizes frailty as an at-risk state caused by the age-associated accumulation of deficits. This frailty index (FI) accounts for deficits across the range of health problems to include signs and symptoms, laboratory abnormalities, ADLs, and instrumental ADLs (IADLs) disabilities, diseases, physical and psychosocial risk factors, and geriatric syndromes, identified through a routine comprehensive geriatric assessment (FI-CGA) (Table 63-2).[5,15] The FI and similar tools with smaller numbers of measures have been demonstrated to be predictive of adverse health outcomes, with increasing values of FI corresponding with increased deficits and frailty.[5,15]

TABLE 63-2. Summary of Deficits Assessed by Frailty Index–Comprehensive Geriatric Assessment

CATEGORY	DEFICITS
Cognitive status	MCI, dementia, delirium
Emotional	Depression, anxiety, fatigue
Motivation	Degree, health attitude
Communication	Speech, hearing, vision
Strength	Proximal and distal upper and lower extremities
Mobility	Level of dependence on transfer, walking
Balance	Balance, falls
Elimination	Bowel and bladder incontinence
Nutrition	Weight, appetite
ADLs	Feeding, bathing, dressing, toileting
IADLs	Cooking, cleaning, shopping, medications, driving, banking
Sleep	Disrupted sleep, daytime drowsiness
Socially engaged	Frequency of social interaction
Social and home environment	Marital status, living arrangement, support system, caregiver relationship, caregiver stress
Medications	Type and indication

Data from Jones DM, Song X, Rockwood K. Operationalizing a frailty index from a standardized comprehensive geriatric assessment. *J Am Geriatr Soc.* 2004;52(11):1929-1933; and Jones D, Song X, Mitnitski A, Rockwood K. Evaluation of a frailty index based on a comprehensive geriatric assessment in a population based study of elderly Canadians. *Aging Clin Exp Res.* 2005;17(6):465-471.
ADLs, Activities of daily living; *IADLs,* instrumental activities of daily living; *MCI,* mild cognitive impairment.

Prevalence

Because the Fried criteria of frailty developed in the CHS has been widely used in clinical investigation, epidemiological data on frailty in older adults is now available from various regions across the globe.[16] In the United States, the overall prevalence of frailty in community-dwelling adults older than 65 years and recruited as part of CHS ranged from 7% to 12%.[1] This prevalence increased with age from 3.9% in 65 to 74 years to 25% in those older 85 years, and older women (8%) were more likely to be frail than older men (5%). Frailty was less common in white Americans (6%) than African Americans (13%),[1] but similar to that in Hispanic Americans.[17] In the WHAS, a study of community-dwelling older women that were recruited to span the spectrum of disability, the prevalence of frailty was 11%.[3] In a survey of community-dwelling older adults in 10 European countries, the overall prevalence of frailty is 17%, with a geographical variation that is higher in southern Europe (e.g., 27% in Spain, 23% in Italy) than in northern Europe (e.g., 5.8% in Switzerland, 8.6% in Sweden).[18] Similarly, in Central and South America, geographical variation of frailty prevalence is also present and ranges from 30% to 48% in women and from 22% to 35% in men, with values that are higher than the American and European cohorts.[19] In all of these studies, the prevalence of frailty demonstrates similar age trends and gender differences.

Clinical Course and Natural History

The cycle of frailty theoretical framework helps explain the natural history of frailty.[16,20] Based on this hypothesis, the clinical manifestations of frailty result from a cycle of dysregulated energetics (e.g., decreased total energy expenditure, resting metabolic rate), poor nutrition, and loss of muscle mass that contributes to the five core clinical features in the Fried criteria: (1) loss of strength (weakness), (2) decreased exercise tolerance (fatigue and exhaustion), (3) slowed motor performance (decreased walking speed), (4) reduced physical activity, and (5) poor nutritional intake (unintentional weight loss).[1,20] According to this theory, any of these five clinical features could initiate the cycle of frailty, resulting in the culmination of an aggregate syndrome.[16] However, a partial hierarchical order in the onset of frailty indicates that weakness is the most common initial manifestation and that the occurrence of weakness, slowness, and low physical activity precede exhaustion and weight loss in 76% of community-dwelling women in the WHAS.[20] The notion that muscle weakness precedes frailty has significant implications because sarcopenia, defined as the loss of muscle mass and strength, is a well-characterized phenomenon in aging muscle, associates strongly with poor clinical outcomes, and develops secondary to dysregulation in aging-related biological pathways.[21,22] Moreover, in the same WHAS cohort, women with initial presentation of exhaustion and weight loss were 3 to 5 times more likely to become frail and 80% of transitions to frailty involved adding exhaustion or weight loss.[20] These findings suggest that wasting conditions characterized by significantly decreased energy production or increased utilization may be a critical step in the final progression toward frailty.

In clinical practice, the clinical description of frailty often implies an irreversible premorbid state that precedes the end of life. However, recent epidemiological data suggest that older community-dwelling adults could in fact transition among the stages of frailty (nonfrail, prefrail, and frail).[16,23] Gill and colleagues[23] demonstrated that in a cohort of 754 participants age 70 years or older, 57.6% had at least one transition between any two of the three frailty states during 54 months of follow-up, and 36.8%, 21.5%, and 9.2% had rates of one, two, and three transitions, respectively. Moreover, transitions to states of greater frailty were more common (up to 43.3%) than transitions to states of lesser frailty (rates up to 23.0%). However, the probability of transitioning from being frail to nonfrail was rare (0%-0.9%).[23] Similar rates of transition between stages of frailty were identified in WHAS, although the rate of transition from frail to nonfrail was higher (17%).[16] Thus the trajectory and rate of progression of frailty in older adults are variable and therefore present opportunities for its prevention and treatment.

RELEVANT PATHOPHYSIOLOGY

The biological cause that underlies frailty is an active area of research. Although incompletely determined, causal mechanisms underlying frailty are likely to be many and likely to be age related, thus reflecting a multisystemic and cyclical physiological decline. Therefore the dysregulation of aging-related physiological and homeostatic pathways have been hypothesized to contribute to this decline.[24] The operationalization of the Fried frailty phenotype in population studies and the development of a frail mouse model have provided opportunities to explore alterations in homeostatic pathways hypothesized to underlie frailty, that is, inflammation, neuroendocrine, and sympathetic nervous system pathways. Furthermore, aging biology–related hypotheses and emerging molecular evidence from the frail mouse model and from pilot genetic studies suggest that cellular senescence, oxidative stress, and apoptosis may also be operant in frailty and ultimately contribute to the impaired systems in frailty.[6,7,24] This section summarizes evidence that supports inflammation, the endocrine system, and sarcopenia and their interactions as likely etiological causes of frailty.

Inflammation

Inflammation is in general an essential systemic response of the innate and adaptive immune system to stressors such as infections, injuries, and disease states.[25] As humans age, adaptive immunity declines because immunosenescence and innate immune systems become chronically activated in a subset of older individuals. This in turn leads to a state of persistent, low-grade inflammation as measured by increased levels of serum inflammatory mediators such as white blood cells, the cytokine interleukin-6 (IL-6) and C-reactive protein (CRP).[24] This proinflammatory state has been associated with various diseases of aging, including cancer, diabetes, cardiovascular diseases, and Alzheimer disease.[24] Similarly, frailty in older adults in large cohort studies, including CHS, WHAS, and the Longitudinal Aging Study Amsterdam (LASA), is associated with markers of low-level inflammation and innate immune system activation. These measurable changes include increased serum CRP and IL-6,[8,10,26,27] elevated neutrophils and macrophages,[28,29] and activation of the molecular inflammatory pathway via monocytic gene expression of C-X-C motif chemokine 10 (CXCL10).[30]

Of the inflammatory changes associated with frailty, IL-6 is the most predictive of poor clinical outcomes in older adults. For example, chronically elevated serum IL-6 level is associated with atherosclerosis, heart failure, osteoporosis, sarcopenia, diabetes, disability, and all-cause mortality.[31–34] In addition, IL-6 inhibits erythropoiesis and iron metabolism and activates clotting factors; therefore it has significant hematological effects in older adults.[10,35] The mechanism by which IL-6 affects multiple physiological systems and influences the pathogenesis of chronic diseases and frailty remains unknown. Although IL-6 stimulates skeletal muscle growth and development after exercise,[36] many other studies suggest that IL-6 plays a key role in mediating muscle atrophy.[37,38] It is possible that the chronic elevation of inflammatory mediators contributes to frailty development by (1) directly causing the phenotypic changes described by the Fried criteria, (2) causing widespread tissue changes and therefore indirectly increasing susceptibility to chronic disease development, or (3) interacting with other intermediate homeostatic pathways.[39]

Endocrine System

The hypothalamic-pituitary-testicular and growth hormone–insulin-like growth factor–1 (GH-IGF-1) axes are key regulators in energetics. Sex hormones (e.g., dehydroepiandrosterone sulfate [DHEA-S]) and growth factors (e.g., IGF-1, transforming growth factor–β [TGF-β]) in particular, are essential to skeletal muscle metabolism. Thus alterations in bioavailability and activity of these hormones may contribute to frailty development in older adults.[40,41] The development of sarcopenia in older men and women with decreasing serum testosterone and estrogen, respectively, is well established.[41,42] More recently, frailty-associated alterations in anabolic hormones have been described in WHAS. In these community-dwelling older adults, frailty is associated with decreased serum DHEA-S and IGF-1, a downstream target of pituitary GH.[9] In addition, low IGF-1 is independently associated with progressive disability, poor strength, slow walking speed, and increased mortality.[43,44] Moreover, the likelihood of being frail is increased when two or three hormonal deficiencies in DHEA-S, free testosterone, and IGF-1 are simultaneously present.[45] Given the multiple endocrine derangements associated with frailty, the overall burden of anabolic hormonal deficiencies is a strong predictor of frailty status.[46]

25-Hydroxyvitamin D is an important hormone that is crucial to bone, muscle, and nervous tissue health in older adults.[47] Numerous epidemiological studies suggest that vitamin D deficiency impairs muscle function and therefore increases risks for falls, sarcopenia, poor physical function, and disability.[27,48,49] Recent findings from large cohorts in Invecchiare in Chianti (InCHIANTI), LASA, Osteoporotic Fractures in Men Study (MrOS), and Third National Health and Nutrition Survey (NHANES III) clearly demonstrate that vitamin D insufficiency is also associated with several-fold increase in prevalent and incident frailty in noninstitutionalized older men and women.[27,48,50–52] Finally, age-related cortisol increase secondary to the loss of stringent hypothalamic-pituitary-adrenal (HPA) regulation likely contributes to decreased skeletal muscle mass and strength.[53] In WHAS, frailty in older women is associated with elevated evening and 24-hour mean cortisol level and its blunted diurnal variation, suggesting that HPA dysregulation may play a role in frailty pathogenesis.[54]

Sarcopenia

Sarcopenia, defined as age-related loss of muscle mass and strength, may be a key physiological component of frailty.[22] In humans, peak muscle mass and strength occur in early adulthood between ages 20 and 30 years. This is followed by the gradual loss of muscle mass and strength until age 50 years and accelerated decline (e.g., 12%-15% per decade in strength) after age 50.[55,56] The rate and extent of sarcopenia in patients with chronic illnesses are accelerated.[22] Some candidate mechanisms leading to sarcopenia include age-related decline in α-motor neurons, IGF-1, and DHEA-S and increase in catabolic cytokines (e.g., IL-6).[22,57] Recent evidence from an aging animal model strongly suggests that increased levels of TGF-β play an important role in fibrotic replacement of skeletal muscle and perhaps in the development of disuse atrophy.[58] Importantly, this pathway appeared to be disrupted by the angiotensin receptor type 1–blocker losartan, effectively decreasing both the amount of skeletal muscle fibrosis and the amount of disuse atrophy.

Despite these findings, the relative contribution of these factors to the development of sarcopenia is not completely understood.[22,59] Because muscle weakness, loss of strength, and poor physical function are central features in frailty syndrome, sarcopenia likely has an etiological role in frailty.[22] Moreover, overlapping hormonal and inflammatory changes in IGF-1, DHEA-S, and IL-6 in sarcopenia and frailty further support the presence of a shared pathophysiology.[8,9,60,61]

Molecular Changes

Some aging-related molecular changes, including increased apoptosis, cellular senescence, increased oxidative stress, and altered mitochondrial function, have all been hypothesized to underlie some of the physiological changes and the vulnerability to disease observed in frail older adults.[62] Gene expression data from the skeletal muscle of a frail mouse model in part supports this hypothesis.[6] Genetic evidence in human population studies support the role of cellular senescence in frailty with associations between specific loci in the $p16^{(INK4a)}$ gene and frailty.[63] Furthermore, associations between frailty status and single-nucleotide polymorphism (SNPs) in genes related to apoptosis, senescence, and mitochondrial function have been identified.[7,64] These findings suggest that these aging-related processes may be operant in triggering the syndrome of frailty and certainly warrant further investigation.

Multisystemic Disease

The hypothesis that frailty results from alterations in multiple molecular, cellular, and physiological systems is gaining evidence. Although inflammatory, neuroendocrine, and neuromuscular dysregulation are independently associated with frailty in older adults, several studies suggest that aggregate alterations in these systems may be synergistic in frailty development and frailty-associated adverse outcomes.[9,44,65-67] For instance, progressive disability and mortality were increased in participants in WHAS when high levels of serum IL-6 and low IGF-1 were simultaneously present compared with either changes alone.[9,44] In the same population, the likelihood of frailty increased nonlinearly in relationship to the number of abnormal physiological systems, and the number of abnormal systems is more predictive of frailty than any individual abnormal system.[67] Similarly, Gruenewald and colleagues[65] showed that greater levels of multisystem physiological dysregulation, or allostatic load, were associated with greater risk for frailty in a longitudinal cohort study of community-dwelling older adults. Allostatic load in this study was determined by 13 biomarkers of endocrine (DHEA-S, epinephrine), immune (CRP, IL-6), and metabolic (cortisol) functions, with each 1-unit increase in allostatic load at baseline associating with a 10% greater likelihood of frailty at the 3-year follow-up.[65] Together, these findings support the hypothesis that aggregate loss of aging-associated complexity in physiological systems is an important cause of frailty.

SUMMARY OF EVIDENCE REGARDING TREATMENT RECOMMENDATIONS

Exercise intervention and patient-centered interdisciplinary geriatric care models are beneficial on various characteristics and adverse outcomes of frailty. However, whether these interventions favorably modify the frailty phenotype remains unknown. This section discusses the clinical care of frail older adults, centering on evidence-based exercise interventions

and interdisciplinary geriatric care models. Despite the association between inflammation and neuroendocrine dysregulation and frailty, the use of pharmacological intervention targeting these physiological systems is currently not recommended.[68] Discussions on the goals of care, symptom management, and palliative and hospice care—as they relate to frailty—will be presented in Chapter 64.

Exercise Intervention

A considerable amount of evidence indicates that aerobic and resistance exercise interventions improve strength, endurance, balance, mobility, and ADLs and reduces falls and chronically elevated inflammatory mediators in older adults.[69,70] For instance, a 9-month program of strength training and walking and a 3-month program of cycle ergometer training improved oxygen uptake by 14% and aerobic capacity by 30%, respectively.[71,72] In a systematic review of 121 randomized, controlled trials in adults 60 years or older, progressive resistance training performed 2 or 3 times per week as the primary intervention showed improvement in gait speed, muscle strength, and physical ability.[73] In this review, pain reduction was observed in older adults with baseline osteoarthritis and no serious events directly related to the exercise programs were reported. The beneficial effects of progressive resistance training extends to nursing home residents, a subset of the frailest older adults.[74] In this study, participants showed significant increases in muscle strength (113%), gait velocity (12%), and cross-sectional thigh muscle area (3%) after 10 weeks of training.

Although the relative efficacy of a unique exercise regimen (aerobic versus progressive resistance training; duration, frequency; facility versus group versus home based) in frail older adults are not known, most exercise training programs appear to be beneficial. Chin and colleagues[75] evaluated the effects of 23 exercise programs from 20 randomized, controlled trials on physical performance in older adults with varying degrees of frailty. These interventions were mostly facility-based, group exercise programs that comprised progressive resistance training (n = 9), Tai Chi (n = 2), or multicomponent training including resistance, endurance, balance, and flexibility exercises (n = 12) performed in 45- to 60-minute sessions three times per week. Most of these exercise regimens improved functional performance in frail older adults. However, several of these exercise interventions showed few benefits in performance measures in the frailest subset, suggesting that severity of frailty may influence effectiveness of exercise therapy.[75] Moreover, Gill and colleagues[76] showed that home-based resistance, flexibility, and balance exercises and home safety and assistive device evaluations administered over 6 months improved disability score based on ADLs in moderately frail community-dwelling older adults, thus demonstrating that home exercise intervention could be beneficial in treating physical frailty. Finally, exercise intervention in older adults may improve domains other than physical function. For example, exercise intervention in the Frailty and Injuries: Cooperative Studies of Intervention Techniques (FICSIT) trials was associated with improved quality of life and emotional health in older adults.[77]

Exercise is well tolerated and has positive effects on physical and functional performance, fall reduction, and quality of life in frail older adults. To date, specific exercise intervention guidelines targeting the treatment of frailty have not been published. Although much more research is needed, the 2008 U.S. Department of Health and Human Services Physical Activity Guidelines could be used in caring for frail older adults.[69] Specifically, adults older than 65 years should participate in at least 150 minutes per week of moderate-intensity aerobic physical activity; aerobic activity should be performed in episodes of at least 10 minutes and spread throughout the week; and muscle strengthening resistance training involving all major muscle groups should be incorporated 2 or more days per week as their abilities and conditions tolerate.[78] In more frail patients, structured and supervised exercise training could be administered with assistance by caretakers and therapists for community-dwelling patients or incorporated into restorative therapy programs for residents in long-term care facilities.

Interdisciplinary Geriatric Care

Patient-centered, comprehensive geriatric assessment implemented by an interdisciplinary treatment team improves the clinical outcome and quality of life of frail elderly.[53,68,79] Interdisciplinary geriatric care is administered across outpatient (Geriatric Evaluation and Management [GEM], Comprehensive Geriatric Assessment [CGA], Program for All-Inclusive Care of the Elderly [PACE]) and inpatient (Acute Care for Elderly [ACE]) settings and tailored for older adults with varying degrees of frailty. These studies general define an interdisciplinary team as consisting of a geriatrics-trained physician or practitioner, nurse, social worker, occupational or physical therapist, and nutritionist. Through a team approach, each patient is assessed with a detailed medical history and physical examination. This is followed by thorough analyses of relevant medical, psychosocial, and environmental data, and the formulation of patient-centered treatment goals and care plans. The objectives of intervention often include setting goals of care, improving or maintaining physical and psychological function, reducing frequent hospitalizations, and improving quality of life.[68]

GEM, in which the interdisciplinary team directs medical care, and CGA, a consultative service, both improve clinical outcomes in frail older adults.[80–82] In a randomized controlled trial of GEM intervention, participants of GEM had fewer health-related restrictions in daily activities, lost less physical function, and used fewer home health care services for 12 to 18 months after randomization.[80] Rueben and colleagues[81] showed that a single outpatient CGA prevented decline in function and quality of life in community-dwelling older adults with a history of falls, urinary incontinence, depressive symptoms, or functional impairments. The improvement in survival and function in older adults participating in CGA were also demonstrated in a meta-analysis of 28 controlled trials.[82] Moreover, GEM and CGA were most effective when patients and caregivers actively participated in formulating and implementing treatment plans.[80,82]

PACE is an alternative model to deliver care for frail older adults who are nursing home eligible but choose to live in the community. In this capitated program reimbursed by Medicare and Medicaid, modest medical intervention and palliative care are provided by an interdisciplinary team through adult day care centers and home services.[83] Palliative care is a mainstay of PACE, aiming to improve participants' function, independence, and quality of life. For frail older adults who are acutely hospitalized, the patient-centered interdisciplinary geriatric approach has been demonstrated by randomized controlled trials to be effective in improving functions and reducing hospital length of stay, readmission, and mortality.[84,85] The most widely adopted model, ACE incorporates geriatric principles of care; frequently creates a home-like, elderly friendly physical environment that facilitates patient participation; includes nurse-initiated clinical protocols of care; and ensures comprehensive discharge planning and management

KEY MESSAGES TO PATIENTS AND FAMILIES

Because frailty syndrome is associated with increased morbidity and mortality, older patients and their caregivers should be mindful of its presenting symptoms of exhaustion, weakness, and declines in activity. Early diagnosis of frailty may help to facilitate the implementation of exercise interventions and patient-centered interdisciplinary care. This in turn may decrease the vulnerability of frail, older adults to illness, disability, and complications from medical procedures.

CONCLUSION AND SUMMARY

Frailty is a common geriatric syndrome. Clinicians need to be familiar with the range of defining characteristics of frailty to make early diagnosis and hence deliver evidence-based care. As researchers further refine the phenotypes of frailty and gain more understanding of its molecular, cellular, and physiological bases, more effective and targeted interventions will likely be developed.

SUMMARY RECOMMENDATIONS

- Numerous definitions of frailty exist; however, the two most common are those that primarily focus on declines in energetics, muscle strength, and activity and those that are based on an accumulation of deficits and detrimental clinical conditions. Clinicians should be familiar with these definitions, as they are used throughout the medical literature.
- Frailty is a unique physiological syndrome that is associated with progressive decline in physiological reserve, increased vulnerability to stressors, and poor clinical outcomes, including recurrent falls and injuries, hospitalization, and progressive disability. As such, clinicians should consider frailty as a potential diagnosis when working with older adults with serious illness.
- Exercise and participation in interdisciplinary geriatric care teams have both been shown to improve health outcomes in frail older adults. Patients with frailty should be referred to these interventions whenever feasible.

REFERENCES

1. Fried LP, Tangen CM, Walston J, et al. Frailty in older adults: evidence for a phenotype. *J Gerontol A Biol Sci Med Sci.* 2001;56(3):M146–M156.
2. Hamerman D. Toward an understanding of frailty. *Ann Intern Med.* 1999;130(11):945–950.
3. Bandeen-Roche K, Xue QL, Ferrucci L, et al. Phenotype of frailty: characterization in the women's health and aging studies. *J Gerontol A Biol Sci Med Sci.* 2006;61(3):262–266.
4. Chin A.P.M.J., Dekker JM, Feskens EJ, Schouten EG, Kromhout D. How to select a frail elderly population? A comparison of three working definitions. *J Clin Epidemiol.* 1999;52(11):1015–1021.
5. Jones DM, Song X, Rockwood K. Operationalizing a frailty index from a standardized comprehensive geriatric assessment. *J Am Geriatr Soc.* 2004;52(11):1929–1933.
6. Walston J, Fedarko N, Yang H, et al. The physical and biological characterization of a frail mouse model. *J Gerontol A Biol Sci Med Sci.* 2008;63(4):391–398.
7. Ho YY, Matteini AM, Beamer B, et al. Exploring biologically relevant pathways in frailty. *J Gerontol A Biol Sci Med Sci.* 2011;66(9):975–979.
8. Leng S, Chaves P, Koenig K, Walston J. Serum interleukin-6 and hemoglobin as physiological correlates in the geriatric syndrome of frailty: a pilot study. *J Am Geriatr Soc.* 2002;50(7):1268–1271.
9. Leng SX, Cappola AR, Andersen RE, et al. Serum levels of insulin-like growth factor-I (IGF-I) and dehydroepiandrosterone sulfate (DHEA-S), and their relationships with serum interleukin-6, in the geriatric syndrome of frailty. *Aging Clin Exp Res.* 2004;16(2):153–157.
10. Walston J, McBurnie MA, Newman A, et al. Frailty and activation of the inflammation and coagulation systems with and without clinical comorbidities: results from the Cardiovascular Health Study. *Arch Intern Med.* 2002;162(20):2333–2341.
11. Ensrud KE, Ewing SK, Taylor BC, et al. Comparison of 2 frailty indexes for prediction of falls, disability, fractures, and death in older women. *Arch Intern Med.* 2008;168(4):382–389.
12. Romero-Ortuno R, Walsh CD, Lawlor BA, Kenny RA. A frailty instrument for primary care: findings from the Survey of Health, Ageing and Retirement in Europe (SHARE). *BMC Geriatr.* 2010;10:57.
13. Studenski S, Perera S, Wallace D, et al. Physical performance measures in the clinical setting. *J Am Geriatr Soc.* 2003;51(3):314–322.
14. Mitnitski AB, Mogilner AJ, Rockwood K. Accumulation of deficits as a proxy measure of aging. *ScientificWorldJournal.* 2001;1:323–336.
15. Jones D, Song X, Mitnitski A, Rockwood K. Evaluation of a frailty index based on a comprehensive geriatric assessment in a population based study of elderly Canadians. *Aging Clin Exp Res.* 2005;17(6):465–471.
16. Xue QL. The frailty syndrome: definition and natural history. *Clin Geriatr Med.* 2011;27(1):1–15.
17. Graham JE, Snih SA, Berges IM, Ray LA, Markides KS, Ottenbacher KJ. Frailty and 10-year mortality in community-living Mexican American older adults. *Gerontology.* 2009;55(6):644–651.
18. Santos-Eggimann B, Cuenoud P, Spagnoli J, Junod J. Prevalence of frailty in middle-aged and older community-dwelling Europeans living in 10 countries. *J Gerontol A Biol Sci Med Sci.* 2009;64(6):675–681.
19. Alvarado BE, Zunzunegui MV, Beland F, Bamvita JM. Life course social and health conditions linked to frailty in Latin American older men and women. *J Gerontol A Biol Sci Med Sci.* 2008;63(12):1399–1406.
20. Xue QL, Bandeen-Roche K, Varadhan R, Zhou J, Fried LP. Initial manifestations of frailty criteria and the development of frailty phenotype in the Women's Health and Aging Study II. *J Gerontol A Biol Sci Med Sci.* 2008;63(9):984–990.
21. Fried LP, Hadley EC, Walston JD, et al. From bedside to bench: research agenda for frailty. *Sci Aging Knowledge Environ.* 2005;2005(31):pe24.
22. Roubenoff R. Sarcopenia: a major modifiable cause of frailty in the elderly. *J Nutr Health Aging.* 2000;4(3):140–142.
23. Gill TM, Gahbauer EA, Allore HG, Han L. Transitions between frailty states among community-living older persons. *Arch Intern Med.* 2006;166(4):418–423.
24. Fedarko NS. The biology of aging and frailty. *Clin Geriatr Med.* 2011;27(1):27–37.
25. Stout RD, Suttles J. Immunosenescence and macrophage functional plasticity: dysregulation of macrophage function by age-associated microenvironmental changes. *Immunol Rev.* 2005;205:60–71.
26. Leng SX, Yang H, Walston JD. Decreased cell proliferation and altered cytokine production in frail older adults. *Aging Clin Exp Res.* 2004;16(3):249–252.
27. Puts MT, Visser M, Twisk JW, Deeg DJ, Lips P. Endocrine and inflammatory markers as predictors of frailty. *Clin Endocrinol (Oxf).* 2005;63(4):403–411.
28. Leng SX, Xue QL, Tian J, Huang Y, Yeh SH, Fried LP. Associations of neutrophil and monocyte counts with frailty in community-dwelling disabled older women: results from the Women's Health and Aging Studies I. *Exp Gerontol.* 2009;44(8):511–516.
29. Leng SX, Xue QL, Tian J, Walston JD, Fried LP. Inflammation and frailty in older women. *J Am Geriatr Soc.* 2007;55(6):864–871.
30. Qu T, Yang H, Walston JD, Fedarko NS, Leng SX. Upregulated monocytic expression of CXC chemokine ligand 10 (CXCL-10) and its relationship with serum interleukin-6 levels in the syndrome of frailty. *Cytokine.* 2009;46(3):319–324.
31. Cesari M, Penninx BW, Newman AB, et al. Inflammatory markers and cardiovascular disease (The Health, Aging and Body Composition [Health ABC] Study). *Am J Cardiol.* 2003;92(5):522–528.
32. Cohen HJ, Harris T, Pieper CF. Coagulation and activation of inflammatory pathways in the development of functional decline and mortality in the elderly. *Am J Med.* 2003;114(3):180–187.
33. Ershler WB, Keller ET. Age-associated increased interleukin-6 gene expression, late-life diseases, and frailty. *Annu Rev Med.* 2000;51:245–270.
34. Harris TB, Ferrucci L, Tracy RP, et al. Associations of elevated interleukin-6 and C-reactive protein levels with mortality in the elderly. *Am J Med.* 1999;106(5):506–512.
35. Ershler WB. Biological interactions of aging and anemia: a focus on cytokines. *J Am Geriatr Soc.* 2003;51(3 suppl):S18–S21.
36. Toth KG, McKay BR, De Lisio M, Little JP, Tarnopolsky MA, Parise G. IL-6 induced STAT3 signalling is associated with the proliferation of human muscle satellite cells following acute muscle damage. *PLoS One.* 2011;6(3):e17392.

37. Haddad F, Zaldivar F, Cooper DM, Adams GR. IL-6-induced skeletal muscle atrophy. *J Appl Physiol.* 2005;98(3):911–917.
38. Tsirpanlis G. Cellular senescence and inflammation: a noteworthy link. *Blood Purif.* 2009;28(1):12–14.
39. Yao X, Li H, Leng SX. Inflammation and immune system alterations in frailty. *Clin Geriatr Med.* 2011;27(1):79–87.
40. Morley JE, Baumgartner RN, Roubenoff R, Mayer J, Nair KS. Sarcopenia. *J Lab Clin Med.* 2001;137(4):231–243.
41. Morley JE, Kaiser FE, Sih R, Hajjar R, Perry 3rd HM. Testosterone and frailty. *Clin Geriatr Med.* 1997;13(4):685–695.
42. Poehlman ET, Toth MJ, Fishman PS, et al. Sarcopenia in aging humans: the impact of menopause and disease. *J Gerontol A Biol Sci Med Sci.* 1995;50(Spec No):73–77.
43. Cappola AR, Bandeen-Roche K, Wand GS, Volpato S, Fried LP. Association of IGF-I levels with muscle strength and mobility in older women. *J Clin Endocrinol Metab.* 2001;86(9):4139–4146.
44. Cappola AR, Xue QL, Ferrucci L, Guralnik JM, Volpato S, Fried LP. Insulin-like growth factor I and interleukin-6 contribute synergistically to disability and mortality in older women. *J Clin Endocrinol Metab.* 2003;88(5):2019–2025.
45. Cappola AR, Xue QL, Fried LP. Multiple hormonal deficiencies in anabolic hormones are found in frail older women: the Women's Health and Aging studies. *J Gerontol A Biol Sci Med Sci.* 2009;64(2):243–248.
46. Maggio M, Cappola AR, Ceda GP, et al. The hormonal pathway to frailty in older men. *J Endocrinol Invest.* 2005;28(11 Suppl Proceedings):15–19.
47. Zhang R, Naughton DP. Vitamin D in health and disease: current perspectives. *Nutr J.* 2010;9:65.
48. Shardell M, Hicks GE, Miller RR, et al. Association of low vitamin D levels with the frailty syndrome in men and women. *J Gerontol A Biol Sci Med Sci.* 2009;64(1):69–75.
49. Visser M, Deeg DJ, Lips P. Low vitamin D and high parathyroid hormone levels as determinants of loss of muscle strength and muscle mass (sarcopenia): the Longitudinal Aging Study Amsterdam. *J Clin Endocrinol Metab.* 2003;88(12):5766–5772.
50. Ensrud KE, Blackwell TL, Cauley JA, et al. Circulating 25-hydroxyvitamin D levels and frailty in older men: the osteoporotic fractures in men study. *J Am Geriatr Soc.* 2011;59(1):101–106.
51. Ensrud KE, Ewing SK, Fredman L, et al. Circulating 25-hydroxyvitamin D levels and frailty status in older women. *J Clin Endocrinol Metab.* 2010;95(12):5266–5273.
52. Wilhelm-Leen ER, Hall YN, Deboer IH, Chertow GM. Vitamin D deficiency and frailty in older Americans. *J Intern Med.* 2010;268(2):171–180.
53. Walston JD, Fried LP. Frailty and its implications for care. In: Morrison RS, Meir DE, eds. Geriatric Palliative Care. New York: Oxford University Press; 2003:93–109.
54. Varadhan R, Walston J, Cappola AR, Carlson MC, Wand GS, Fried LP. Higher levels and blunted diurnal variation of cortisol in frail older women. *J Gerontol A Biol Sci Med Sci.* 2008;63(2):190–195.
55. Metter EJ, Conwit R, Tobin J, Fozard JL. Age-associated loss of power and strength in the upper extremities in women and men. *J Gerontol A Biol Sci Med Sci.* 1997;52(5):B267–B276.
56. Rice CL, Cunningham DA, Paterson DH, Lefcoe MS. Arm and leg composition determined by computed tomography in young and elderly men. *Clin Physiol.* 1989;9(3):207–220.
57. Larsson L, Ramamurthy B. Aging-related changes in skeletal muscle: mechanisms and interventions. *Drugs Aging.* 2000;17(4):303–316.
58. Burks TN, Andres-Mateos E, Marx R, et al. Losartan restores skeletal muscle remodeling and protects against disuse atrophy in sarcopenia. *Sci Transl Med.* 2011;3(82):82ra37.
59. Rolland Y, Czerwinski S, Abellan Van Kan G, et al. Sarcopenia: its assessment, etiology, pathogenesis, consequences and future perspectives. *J Nutr Health Aging.* 2008;12(7):433–450.
60. Schaap LA, Pluijm SM, Deeg DJ, et al. Higher inflammatory marker levels in older persons: associations with 5-year change in muscle mass and muscle strength. *J Gerontol A Biol Sci Med Sci.* 2009;64(11):1183–1189.
61. Valenti G, Denti L, Maggio M, et al. Effect of DHEAS on skeletal muscle over the life span: the InCHIANTI study. *J Gerontol A Biol Sci Med Sci.* 2004;59(5):466–472.
62. Walston J, Hadley EC, Ferrucci L, et al. Research agenda for frailty in older adults: toward a better understanding of physiology and etiology: summary from the American Geriatrics Society/ National Institute on Aging Research Conference on Frailty in Older Adults. *J Am Geriatr Soc.* 2006;54(6):991–1001.
63. Popov N, Gil J. Epigenetic regulation of the INK4b-ARF-INK4a locus: in sickness and in health. *Epigenetics.* 2010;5(8):685–690.
64. Moore AZ, Biggs ML, Matteini A, et al. Polymorphisms in the mitochondrial DNA control region and frailty in older adults. *PLoS One.* 2010;5(6):e11069.
65. Gruenewald TL, Seeman TE, Karlamangla AS, Sarkisian CA. Allostatic load and frailty in older adults. *J Am Geriatr Soc.* 2009;57(9):1525–1531.
66. Roubenoff R, Parise H, Payette HA, et al. Cytokines, insulin-like growth factor 1, sarcopenia, and mortality in very old community-dwelling men and women: the Framingham Heart Study. *Am J Med.* 2003;115(6):429–435.
67. Fried LP, Xue QL, Cappola AR, et al. Nonlinear multisystem physiological dysregulation associated with frailty in older women: implications for etiology and treatment. *J Gerontol A Biol Sci Med Sci.* 2009;64(10):1049–1057.
68. Ko FC. The clinical care of frail, older adults. *Clin Geriatr Med.* 2011;27(1):89–100.
69. Liu CK, Fielding RA. Exercise as an intervention for frailty. *Clin Geriatr Med.* 2011;27(1):101–110.
70. Nicklas BJ, Brinkley TE. Exercise training as a treatment for chronic inflammation in the elderly. *Exerc Sport Sci Rev.* 2009;37(4):165–170.
71. Ehsani AA, Spina RJ, Peterson LR, et al. Attenuation of cardiovascular adaptations to exercise in frail octogenarians. *J Appl Physiol.* 2003;95(5):1781–1788.
72. Harber MP, Konopka AR, Douglass MD, et al. Aerobic exercise training improves whole muscle and single myofiber size and function in older women. *Am J Physiol Regul Integr Comp Physiol.* 2009;297(5):R1452–R1459.
73. Liu CJ, Latham NK. Progressive resistance strength training for improving physical function in older adults. *Cochrane Database Syst Rev.* 2009;(3):CD002759.
74. Fiatarone MA, O'Neill EF, Ryan ND, et al. Exercise training and nutritional supplementation for physical frailty in very elderly people. *N Engl J Med.* 1994;330(25):1769–1775.
75. Chin A.P.MJ, van Uffelen JG, Riphagen I, van Mechelen W. The functional effects of physical exercise training in frail older people: a systematic review. *Sports Med.* 2008;38(9):781–793.
76. Gill TM, Baker DI, Gottschalk M, Peduzzi PN, Allore H, Byers A. A program to prevent functional decline in physically frail, elderly persons who live at home. *N Engl J Med.* 2002;347(14):1068–1074.
77. Schechtman KB, Ory MG. The effects of exercise on the quality of life of frail older adults: a preplanned meta-analysis of the FICSIT trials. *Ann Behav Med. Summer.* 2001;23(3):186–197.
78. US Department of Health and Human Services. *2008 Physical activity guidelines.* http://www.health.gov/paguidelines/ guidelines/summary.aspx; Accessed September 21, 2012.
79. Espinoza S, Walston JD. Frailty in older adults: insights and interventions. *Cleve Clin J Med.* 2005;72(12):1105–1112.
80. Boult C, Boult LB, Morishita L, Dowd B, Kane RL, Urdangarin CF. A randomized clinical trial of outpatient geriatric evaluation and management. *J Am Geriatr Soc.* 2001;49(4): 351–359.
81. Reuben DB, Frank JC, Hirsch SH, McGuigan KA, Maly RC. A randomized clinical trial of outpatient comprehensive geriatric assessment coupled with an intervention to increase adherence to recommendations. *J Am Geriatr Soc.* 1999;47(3): 269–276.
82. Stuck AE, Siu AL, Wieland GD, Adams J, Rubenstein LZ. Comprehensive geriatric assessment: a meta-analysis of controlled trials. *Lancet.* 1993;342(8878):1032–1036.
83. Eng C, Pedulla J, Eleazer GP, McCann R, Fox N. Program of All-inclusive Care for the Elderly (PACE): an innovative model of integrated geriatric care and financing. *J Am Geriatr Soc.* 1997;45(2):223–232.
84. Landefeld CS, Palmer RM, Kresevic DM, Fortinsky RH, Kowal J. A randomized trial of care in a hospital medical unit especially designed to improve the functional outcomes of acutely ill older patients. *N Engl J Med.* 1995;332(20):1338–1344.
85. Rubenstein LZ, Josephson KR, Wieland GD, English PA, Sayre JA, Kane RL. Effectiveness of a geriatric evaluation unit: a randomized clinical trial. *N Engl J Med.* 1984;311(26):1664–1670.

What Are the Special Needs of Patients With Frailty?

Fred C. Ko and Jeremy D. Walston

INTRODUCTION AND SCOPE OF THE PROBLEM

Overview of Frailty Syndrome

Frailty syndrome in older adults is characterized by progressive decline in physiological reserve, increased vulnerability to stressors, and poor clinical outcomes, including recurrent falls and injuries, hospitalization, or progressive disability.[1] Although definitions vary, several operational definitions of frailty have become widely accepted and validated in population studies in older adults.[2,3] The frailty phenotype described by Fried and colleagues[2] characterizes frailty as a syndrome of compromised energetics with five core clinical features: (1) low grip strength, (2) slowed walking speed, (3) low physical activity, (4) self-reported exhaustion, and (5) unintentional weight loss. A frail state is present when three or more of these clinical characteristics are met, and a prefrail state is present when one or two criteria are met. The frailty index (FI) developed by Mitnitski and colleagues[3] is another commonly used tool to assess frailty and conceptualizes frailty as an at-risk state characterized by the age-associated accumulation of deficits. The FI calculates risks for frailty in older adults by accounting for deficits across a range of health problems, including signs and symptoms, activities of daily living (ADLs) and instrumental ADLs (IADLs) disabilities, diseases, physical and psychosocial risk factors, and geriatric syndromes identified through a routine Comprehensive Geriatric Assessment (FI-CGA).[4,5] Embedded in both of these definitions is the concept that age-related multisystemic accumulation of physiological decline underlies frailty and that the sum of these deficits contributes to the development of adverse clinical outcomes. Moreover, frail older adults identified by these definitions have increased adverse clinical outcomes, including worsened mobility, ADL disability, increased falls, hospitalization, and mortality, reflecting a loss of physiological reserve.[2,4,6,7]

Frailty in older adults demonstrates an age trend and gender differences in multiple cohort studies from North, Central, and South America and Europe.[8] For example, in the United States, community-dwelling adults 65 years or older have an overall frailty prevalence of 7% to 12%. This prevalence is lower in individuals 65 to 74 years old (4%) compared to those older than 85 years (25%).[2] In addition, frailty is more common in older women (8%) than men (5%) and in African Americans (13%) than white Americans (6%).[2] In terms of clinical course, epidemiological studies that used the Fried frailty phenotype as its operational definition suggest that the physiology that underlies the development of any of its five core clinical features (low grip strength, slowed walking speed, low physical activity, self-reported exhaustion, and unintentional weight loss) may be a first step in a cycle of decline that culminates in an aggregate syndrome of frailty and its related adverse health outcomes.[8] Of these clinical features, weakness is the most common initial manifestation, whereas exhaustion and weight loss, which reflect wasting conditions, are most highly associated with transitions to a more severe frailty state.[9] In two population studies, transition to states of greater frailty is more common (up to 43.3%); nevertheless, transition to states of lesser frailty (up to 23.0%) also occurs.[8,10] In contrast, the probability of transitioning from being frail to nonfrail is less frequent (0%-17%).[8,10]

Exercise intervention and patient-centered interdisciplinary care models have been demonstrated to be beneficial in the clinical care of frail, older adults.[11,12] Aerobic or progressive resistance training exercise performed 2 or 3 times per week, in particular, improves muscle strength, gait velocity, aerobic capacity, endurance, balance, mobility, and functional performance and reduce falls in older adults.[13,18] Moreover, the beneficial effects of exercise regimen extend to the frailest subset of older adults, including those who are home bound or institutionalized.[17,19] Implementation of patient-centered, geriatrics-focused comprehensive assessment and management improves the clinical outcome and quality of life in frail older adults.[11,12,20] Through a team approach, an interdisciplinary team consisting of a geriatrics-trained physician, nurse, social worker, occupational or physical therapist, and others provides comprehensive care with particular emphasis on setting goals of care, improving or maintaining functional status, and improving quality of life.[11] Both outpatient (Geriatric Evaluation and Management [GEM], Comprehensive Geriatric Assessment [CGA], Program for All-Inclusive Care of the Elderly [PACE]) and inpatient (Acute Care for Elderly [ACE]) interventions have been shown to reduce functional decline, home health care usage, hospital length of stay and readmission, and mortality in frail older adults.[21-25]

Challenges in Caring for Patients With Frailty. Frailty syndrome and chronic diseases share many characteristics, including a higher prevalence in older adults,[2,8] associated multimorbidities and disabilities,[2] and general progression toward more severe disease states over the course of the illness.[8,10] Moreover, frailty and chronic diseases present a common set of challenges to patients and their caretakers, namely, dealing with persistent symptoms, emotional distress, disability and functional loss, complex medical regimens, difficult lifestyle adjustment, and obtaining helpful medical care.[26] Therefore the clinical management of frailty in older adults should incorporate unique and effective features of chronic illness care.

The clinical care of patients with frailty is challenging for patients, their caretakers, and clinicians. Because frail older adults often have medically and psychosocially complex issues and frailty exists across a spectrum that is often not obvious clinically until a very late stage, every stage of frailty presents a unique opportunity for interventions tailored to meet the specific needs of these patients. The following section highlights some of the challenges in the care of frail older adults and addresses associated management principles.

RELEVANT PATHOPHYSIOLOGY

Screening and Timely Recognition

Frailty in older adults exists across a broad spectrum. When severe, frailty is often recognizable because of the poor tolerance to medical, social, and psychological stressors and the development of adverse health outcomes.[1] In contrast, frailty in its early clinical stage may lack readily recognizable connections to adverse outcomes and therefore may be unrecognized by patients and undiagnosed by clinicians.[11] Several factors may present a diagnostic challenge in frailty in older adults. First, unlike organ-specific diseases such as heart failure and diabetes, frailty does not fit into a classic disease model.[27] For example, the Fried frailty phenotype uses five clinical features to capture compromised energetics, the likely cause of frailty; none of these features are organ-specific.[2] The FI developed by Mitnitski and colleagues[3] diagnoses frailty by the summation of age-associated deficit accumulation that accounts for some organ-specific diseases

as well as ADLs and IADLs disabilities, physical and psychosocial risk factors, and geriatric syndromes. Therefore this "organless" diagnostic approach to frailty may pose a challenge to those who are accustomed to the conventional organ-specific model of disease. Second, clinical features of frailty such as loss of strength and weight, slowed walking speed, decreased physical activity, and exhaustion can occur gradually and therefore may be incorrectly attributed to aging-related decline. This in turn may delay or prevent a patient with early-stage frailty, a family member, or a health care provider from recognizing increased risks for adverse health outcomes associated with frailty.[27,28] Finally, although frailty has long been recognized by clinicians and is a well-established entity in research, no single clinical definition of frailty has been adopted into clinical practice, therefore limiting its diagnosis and management in vulnerable older adults.

Frailty screening may enable the timely diagnosis of frailty in older adults and facilitate the implementation of appropriate care and risk assessment.[11,27] Although a gold standard definition and diagnostic criteria for frailty are not available, the use of validated assessment tools predicative of functional decline, disability, and frailty that can be administered across sites of care may be used for diagnostic purposes.[11,29] For patients who receive CGA, the use of FI-CGA, a validated tool for frailty risk assessment, could be administered (see Table 63-2).[4,5] The Fried criteria of frailty validated in the Cardiovascular Health Study (CHS) could be administered in patients who do not receive CGA (see Table 63-1).[2] Because some of the criteria used in CHS cannot be readily assessed in the nonresearch setting, the Study of Osteoporotic Fractures (SOF) index, a more easily determined index, could be used instead. The SOF index has three criteria: (1) weight loss of 5% in the past year, (2) inability to rise from a chair five times without use of arms, and (3) a "no" response to the question "Do you feel full of energy?" with frailty defined to be present when two or three of these criteria are met.[30] The SOF and CHS indices have been shown to be comparable in predicting risks for falls, disability, fracture, hospitalization, and death.[31,32]

SUMMARY OF EVIDENCE REGARDING TREATMENT RECOMMENDATIONS

When frailty is recognized in older adults, a care plan should be tailored and quickly implemented to meet the specific needs presented by varying degrees of frailty. Because overlapping clinical features may be present in frailty, occult malignancy, rheumatological disease, major depression, chronic infection, heart failure, and other medical conditions that are potentially treatable should be optimally managed.[11,20,27] Appropriate exercise intervention and patient-centered interdisciplinary care that have been shown to improve clinical outcomes in these vulnerable patients should be prescribed and introduced depending on the patient's level of frailty.[11,12,20] For those in the frailest category, hospice care may be appropriate.[11,20,27] Finally, symptom management and setting goals of care should remain essential aspects of management in all patients with frailty.[27]

Interdisciplinary Care: Communication and Collaboration

In 2001 the Institute of Medicine report *Crossing the Quality Chasm: A New Health System for the 21st Century* made specific recommendations toward creating a high-quality health care delivery system.[33] Several of these recommendations are highly relevant to the care of patients with chronic illness and frailty. These include (1) continuous healing relationship with the treatment team, (2) individualized and customized care according to patient needs and values, (3) evidence-based decision making, (4) anticipation of patient needs and services, and (5) cooperation among clinicians to optimize coordination of care. Where the recommendations in the Chronic Care Model (CCM) described by Wagner and colleagues[26] are effectively implemented, productive interactions could be anticipated among the patient, patient's caretakers, and management team to (1) elicit relevant patient-centered clinical, psychosocial, and environmental data; (2) clarify and set goals of care; (3) enact clinical, behavioral, and environment interventions to minimize complications and optimize disease management and personal well-being; and (4) ensure continuous follow-up.

The patient-centered interdisciplinary geriatric and palliative models of care have many overlapping features with CCM. The outpatient care delivery models (GEM, CGA, PACE) and the inpatient model (ACE) are designed to optimize a healing and collaborative relationship between the frail patient and the interdisciplinary team. The plans of care are patient-centered geriatrics and palliative care focused and therefore enable the treatment team to provide services that meet the unique medical and psychosocial needs of these vulnerable patients.[11] Also, the comprehensive approach of interdisciplinary models ensures coordination of care. Thus these interventions may be effective in reducing functional decline, home health usage, hospital length of stay and readmission, and mortality in frail older adults.[21–25]

Effective communication and collaboration between frail patients and the management team play a role in increasing the effectiveness of interdisciplinary care.[23,25] In the chronic disease literature, these productive interactions achieve better disease control, higher patient satisfaction, and better adherence to management.[26] Similarly, frail patients and their family members who are empowered to be active and informed participants in care become effective collaborators in health management.[34] Several studies have shown that GEM and CGA are most effective when patients and caregivers actively participate in formulating and implementing treatment plans.[23,25] Moreover, a collaborative relationship between the

patient and the patient's primary care physician has been shown to be a strong predictor of both physician implementation and patient adherence to CGA recommendations made by a consultative interdisciplinary team.[34]

Establishing Goals of Care

Given the high prevalence of frailty in older adults, the likely progression toward more severe disease, and the absence of curative interventions, goals of care conversations are indicated at the time a patient is identified to be frail.[27] A benefit–burden assessment could be used to guide patient-centered discussions in setting management goals. Although frailty tends to transition toward more rather than less severe states and complete reversal to robustness is rare,[8,10] its time course of progression is not well defined. Therefore discussions on goals of care in older adults with primary physical frailty should focus on maintenance or improvement of function, relief of symptoms and pain, optimization of quality of life, maintenance of control and autonomy, and support for family and loved ones.[35] Furthermore, although those who are frail are at higher risk for all causes of mortality than age- and gender-matched robust older adults, little information is available that can help predict life expectancy. However, conversations around that topic may be relevant and important for advance planning purposes.

In frail patients with other comorbid conditions and significant pain and discomfort, procedures intended to diagnose and treat specific medical conditions and to prolong life may be too burdensome and risky to undertake.[20,27] Conversations around these issues with patients, their families, and health care providers may help control the risk related to adverse outcomes. Severely frail patients should be offered palliative care, similar to patients with other serious illness. Thus early and systematic initiation of goals of care discussions in these patients could allow them to make more informed decisions, achieve better palliation of symptoms, and have more opportunity to attend to issues of life closure.[36] On the other hand, the benefit of diagnostic workup and treatment for occult conditions may outweigh its burden in patients who are less frail.[11,20] Thus clearly setting goals of care, constructing advance directives, and appointing a health care proxy are necessary actions that should benefit all patients along the spectrum of frailty.

Symptom Management

Although specific guidelines targeting frailty and its symptomatic management are not available, a growing number of studies suggest exercise interventions are beneficial. Variations of aerobic and progressive resistance training exercises performed several times per week, approximately 30 to 45 minutes per session, may improve muscle strength, gait velocity, endurance, balance, mobility, and functional performance and reduce falls in frail older adults.[13–18] Some of these beneficial effects extend to home bound or institutionalized patients, a subset of the frailest patients.[17,19] Hence, weakness (low grip strength), slowness (reduced walking speed), low physical activity, and exhaustion, four core clinical features of the Fried frailty phenotype, are likely to improve from regular, increased physical activity.[2] Thus all patients along the entire spectrum of frailty could potentially benefit from some form of exercise regimen that is safely tolerated if symptom management is a part their care goals[11,12,27]

Adherence to exercise intervention in frail older adults may be challenging because of limitations in their functional ability and social support. Thus exercise prescription should be crafted to suit the physical capacity of the patients and interfaced with their available environmental resources. In less frail patients, the U.S. Department of Health and Human Services Physical Activity Guidelines recommendation of participation in 150 minutes per week of moderate-intensity aerobic physical activity plus muscle-strengthening resistance training 2 or more days per week may be appropriate[13,37] In more frail patients, the duration, intensity, and frequency of an exercise regimen should be modified to ensure safe participation. Center- or facility-based group exercise programs are generally effective in improving physical performance in older adults.[18] This is likely in part due to the increased exercise training stimuli provided in a structured and supervised setting.[38] Therefore center- or facility-based group exercise programs, including those at senior centers, adult day care facilities, or PACE, may be a reasonable option for early- to moderate-stage frail older adults who can financially and physically access these resources. However, in more frail patients who are home bound, home exercise interventions may be safely and effectively implemented.[19,38] The home-based exercise program offers several advantages over facility-based programs. For instance, evaluation in the home setting allows direct observation and modification of home environment to optimize safe and effective mobility-related activities and exercise regimen.[38,39] Moreover, it provides therapy to frail older adults who have limited access to transportation or are unwilling to leave their homes. On the other hand, home-based exercise intervention likely requires assistance by caretakers and provides a lower training stimulus because of the lack of direct supervision.[38] In the frailest patients who are institutionalized, physical activities incorporated into restorative therapy programs also should be implemented.[11]

Insufficient data exist to recommend the use of pharmacological intervention and supplemental nutrition for the treatment of frailty and its symptoms.[11,12,27] Although more research is needed, non-pharmacological interventions commonly used in the treatment of fatigue, failure to thrive, and the anorexia and cachexia syndrome may be useful in the symptomatic management of frailty. For example, liberalizing diet, providing favorite foods, varying texture and flavor of foods, and assisting with feeding and oral care may improve oral intake.[27,40,41] In patients who are severely frail, modifications to the environment and daily procedures to reduce energy expenditure may be beneficial for treating exhaustion.[27] Specific helpful tasks include placing the phone within closer reach, using a bedside commode, adjusting room temperature, and reordering the sequence of daily tasks, such as eating, followed by resting, then bathing.[42]

Palliative Care

The referral to palliative care in managing frail older adults is highly appropriate in many cases.[11,20,27] Palliative care programs provide patient-centered comprehensive interdisciplinary care for frail patients and their families, with particular focus on effective communication; symptom management; advance care planning; psychosocial, spiritual, and bereavement support; and coordination of care.[43] Multiple studies have demonstrated that palliative care has beneficial effects on symptom relief, patient and family satisfaction, increased likelihood of dying at home, and decreased hospital costs.[44] Hospice care should be provided to severely frail patients who are likely to die within 6 months. Because the prognostication of life expectancy in frail older patients is difficult, the National Hospice and Palliative Care Organization guidelines for determining prognosis for noncancer disease can be applied.[27,45] Specific guideline criteria include (1) multiple emergency department visits or inpatient hospitalizations over the prior 6 months, (2) a recent decline in functional status, and (3) unintentional progressive weight loss of more than 10% over the prior 6 months.[46]

Caring for the Caretaker

Caring for a family member with chronic physical illness results in increased financial, physical, and emotional responsibilities for the caregiver.[47] Tasks such as extensive coordination of care, managing symptoms, disability and mobility deficits, and others can lead to caregiver isolation, burnout, stress, anxiety, and depression.[48] Thus caring for a chronically ill family member can have a considerable negative impact on the physical and psychosocial health and quality of life of the caretaker.[49] Because the clinical management of frailty and chronic disease share many similarities, caregiver stress and its associated negative consequences are likely to be experienced by family members who provide care to frail older adults. Therefore caretakers and the primary management team should be highly cognizant of the signs and symptoms of caregiver stress and burnout. Appropriate coping strategies and interventions, including individual therapy, family therapy, education, and problem-solving programs should be implemented when indicated.[48]

Improving Access to Geriatric Care: Modification of Primary Care Practice

The patient-centered interdisciplinary geriatric and palliative models address several key processes of care for vulnerable older adults—communication, developing a personal care plan, and care coordination.[50] Thus the interdisciplinary team–based approach to care used by GEM, CGA, PACE, ACE, patient-centered medical homes, palliative care, and hospice fulfills these needs. However, with a limited number of programs that deliver high-quality interdisciplinary care and an aging population, primary care physicians will need to take an increasing role in managing frail older patients. Ganz and colleagues[50] described two models of care delivery, through reorganizing traditional primary care practice, to address the specific needs of vulnerable older adults.[50] In the comanagement model, a nurse practitioner or physician assistant comanages serious and chronic conditions common in frail older adults with a primary care physician. Nurses, social workers, or psychologists with specialized geriatrics or palliative care training provide support to treating practitioners by assessing patient and caregiver needs, coordinating care, and counseling on chronic diseases. In the augmented primary care model, trained office staff perform screening and basic assessment for chronic conditions common in frail older adults and therefore lend enhanced support for clinicians. Other essential practice modifications include (1) facilities making accommodations for frail patients with adjustable-height tables, clearance for wheelchair maneuvering, and adaptive equipment for the hearing impaired; (2) staff education to improve communication with frail older adults; (3) team meetings to discuss management of complicated patients; (4) integration of electronic communications and health records; and (5) partnership with community resources for housing, health promotion, and caregiver support. These modifications may be creative solutions to improve access and quality of primary care for frail older adults in the community.

KEY MESSAGES TO PATIENTS AND FAMILIES

Patients and family members should be familiar with the special needs in patients who are frail. This knowledge will facilitate the appropriate implementation of care plans that most benefit the frail patient. Patients and families should be proactive and collaborative with the interdisciplinary management team in establishing goals of care, partaking in exercise intervention, managing symptoms, and initiating palliative and hospice care when appropriate. Caretakers of a frail patient must recognize signs and symptoms of caregiver stress to cope successfully.

CONCLUSION AND SUMMARY

The management of frail older adults presents many challenges because of a broad frailty spectrum, lack of definitive therapy, and high medical and psychosocial complexity of these patients. Therefore clinical care of this vulnerable population must be tailored individually to meet their special needs. Interventions that address these specific needs and have beneficial effects in frail older patients include (1) screening and timely recognition; (2) implementing interdisciplinary care that focuses on effective communication, personalized care plans, and care coordination; (3) establishing goals of care; (4) managing symptoms; (5) initiating palliative and hospice care; and (6) caring for the caregivers.

SUMMARY RECOMMENDATIONS

- Screening patients for frailty is a key first step in caring care for older patients who may be frail and therefore at higher risk for adverse health outcomes.
- Care plans for frail older adults should be interdisciplinary and include appropriate symptom management, establishing goals of care, and making referrals to palliative care and hospice as appropriate.
- Given the multiple stressors placed on family members caring for frail patients, clinicians should be aware of caregiver burden and refer caregivers to supportive services as appropriate.
- Improving delivery models for patients with frailty can streamline care and create environments that are adapted specifically to the needs of frail older adults.

REFERENCES

1. Hamerman D. Toward an understanding of frailty. *Ann Intern Med.* 1999;130(11):945–950.
2. Fried LP, Tangen CM, Walston J, et al. Frailty in older adults: evidence for a phenotype. *J Gerontol A Biol Sci Med Sci.* 2001;56(3):M146–M156.
3. Mitnitski AB, Mogilner AJ, Rockwood K. Accumulation of deficits as a proxy measure of aging. *ScientificWorldJournal.* 2001;1:323–336.
4. Jones DM, Song X, Rockwood K. Operationalizing a frailty index from a standardized comprehensive geriatric assessment. *J Am Geriatr Soc.* 2004;52(11):1929–1933.
5. Jones D, Song X, Mitnitski A, Rockwood K. Evaluation of a frailty index based on a comprehensive geriatric assessment in a population based study of elderly Canadians. *Aging Clin Exp Res.* 2005;17(6):465–471.
6. Bandeen-Roche K, Xue QL, Ferrucci L, et al. Phenotype of frailty: characterization in the women's health and aging studies. *J Gerontol A Biol Sci Med Sci.* 2006;61(3):262–266.
7. Rockwood K, Andrew M, Mitnitski A. A comparison of two approaches to measuring frailty in elderly people. *J Gerontol A Biol Sci Med Sci.* 2007;62(7):738–743.
8. Xue QL. The frailty syndrome: definition and natural history. *Clin Geriatr Med.* 2011;27(1):1–15.

9. Xue QL, Bandeen-Roche K, Varadhan R, Zhou J, Fried LP. Initial manifestations of frailty criteria and the development of frailty phenotype in the Women's Health and Aging Study II. *J Gerontol A Biol Sci Med Sci.* 2008;63(9):984–990.

10. Gill TM, Gahbauer EA, Allore HG, Han L. Transitions between frailty states among community-living older persons. *Arch Intern Med.* 2006;166(4):418–423.

11. Ko FC. The clinical care of frail, older adults. *Clin Geriatr Med.* 2011;27(1):89–100.

12. Espinoza S, Walston JD. Frailty in older adults: insights and interventions. *Cleve Clin J Med.* 2005;72(12):1105–1112.

13. Liu CK, Fielding RA. Exercise as an intervention for frailty. *Clin Geriatr Med.* 2011;27(1):101–110.

14. Ehsani AA, Spina RJ, Peterson LR, et al. Attenuation of cardiovascular adaptations to exercise in frail octogenarians. *J Appl Physiol.* 2003;95(5):1781–1788.

15. Harber MP, Konopka AR, Douglass MD, et al. Aerobic exercise training improves whole muscle and single myofiber size and function in older women. *Am J Physiol Regul Integr Comp Physiol.* 2009;297(5):R1452–R1459.

16. Liu CJ, Latham NK. Progressive resistance strength training for improving physical function in older adults. *Cochrane Database Syst Rev.* 2009;(3):CD002759.

17. Fiatarone MA, O'Neill EF, Ryan ND, et al. Exercise training and nutritional supplementation for physical frailty in very elderly people. *N Engl J Med.* 1994;330(25):1769–1775.

18. Chin A.P.M.J., van Uffelen JG, Riphagen I, van Mechelen W. The functional effects of physical exercise training in frail older people: a systematic review. *Sports Med.* 2008;38(9):781–793.

19. Gill TM, Baker DI, Gottschalk M, Peduzzi PN, Allore H, Byers A. A program to prevent functional decline in physically frail, elderly persons who live at home. *N Engl J Med.* 2002;347(14):1068–1074.

20. Walston JD, Fried LP. Frailty and its implications for care. In: Morrison RS, Meier DE, eds. *Geriatric Palliative Care*. New York: Oxford University Press; 2003:93–109.

21. Landefeld CS, Palmer RM, Kresevic DM, Fortinsky RH, Kowal J. A randomized trial of care in a hospital medical unit especially designed to improve the functional outcomes of acutely ill older patients. *N Engl J Med.* 1995;332(20):1338–1344.

22. Rubenstein LZ, Josephson KR, Wieland GD, English PA, Sayre JA, Kane RL. Effectiveness of a geriatric evaluation unit: a randomized clinical trial. *N Engl J Med.* 1984;311(26):1664–1670.

23. Boult C, Boult LB, Morishita L, Dowd B, Kane RL, Urdangarin CF. A randomized clinical trial of outpatient geriatric evaluation and management. *J Am Geriatr Soc.* 2001;49(4):351–359.

24. Reuben DB, Frank JC, Hirsch SH, McGuigan KA, Maly RC. A randomized clinical trial of outpatient comprehensive geriatric assessment coupled with an intervention to increase adherence to recommendations. *J Am Geriatr Soc.* 1999;47(3):269–276.

25. Stuck AE, Siu AL, Wieland GD, Adams J, Rubenstein LZ. Comprehensive geriatric assessment: a meta-analysis of controlled trials. *Lancet.* 1993;342(8878):1032–1036.

26. Wagner EH, Austin BT, Davis C, Hindmarsh M, Schaefer J, Bonomi A. Improving chronic illness care: translating evidence into action. *Health Aff (Millwood).* 2001;20(6):64–78.

27. Boockvar KS, Meier DE, Boockvar KS, Meier DE. Palliative care for frail older adults: "there are things I can't do anymore that I wish I could . . .". *JAMA.* 2006;296(18):2245–2253.

28. Williamson JD, Fried LP. Characterization of older adults who attribute functional decrements to "old age". *J Am Geriatr Soc.* 1996;44(12):1429–1434.

29. Corapi KM, McGee HM, Barker M. Screening for frailty among seniors in clinical practice. *Nat Clin Pract Rheumatol.* 2006;2(9):476–480.

30. Ensrud KE, Ewing SK, Taylor BC, et al. Comparison of 2 frailty indexes for prediction of falls, disability, fractures, and death in older women. *Arch Intern Med.* 2008;168(4):382–389.

31. Ensrud KE, Ewing SK, Cawthon PM, et al. A comparison of frailty indexes for the prediction of falls, disability, fractures, and mortality in older men. *J Am Geriatr Soc.* 2009;57(3):492–498.

32. Kiely DK, Cupples LA, Lipsitz LA. Validation and comparison of two frailty indexes: the MOBILIZE Boston Study. *J Am Geriatr Soc.* 2009;57(9):1532–1539.

33. Institute of Medicine. *Crossing the Quality Chasm: A New Health System for the 21st Century*. Washington, DC: The National Academies Press; 2001:65–94.

34. Maly RC, Leake B, Frank JC, DiMatteo MR, Reuben DB. Implementation of consultative geriatric recommendations: the role of patient-primary care physician concordance. *J Am Geriatr Soc.* 2002;50(8):1372–1380.

35. Singer PA, Martin DK, Kelner M. Quality end-of-life care: patients' perspectives. *JAMA.* 1999;281(2):163–168.

36. Quill TE. Perspectives on care at the close of life: initiating end-of-life discussions with seriously ill patients: addressing the "elephant in the room". *JAMA.* 2000;284(19):2502–2507.

37. US Department of Health and Human Services. *2008 physical activity guidelines*. http://www.health.gov/paguidelines/guidelines/summary.aspx; Accessed September 22, 2012.

38. Gill TM, Baker DI, Gottschalk M, et al. A prehabilitation program for physically frail community-living older persons. *Arch Phys Med Rehabil.* 2003;84(3):394–404.

39. Gill TM. Preventing falls: to modify the environment or the individual? *J Am Geriatr Soc.* 1999;47(12):1471–1472.

40. Fabiny AR, Kiel DP. Assessing and treating weight loss in nursing home patients. *Clin Geriatr Med.* 1997;13(4):737–751.

41. Alibhai SM, Greenwood C, Payette H. An approach to the management of unintentional weight loss in elderly people. *CMAJ.* 2005;172(6):773–780.

42. Reuben DB, Herr KA, Pacala JT, et al. *Geriatrics at Your Fingertips: 2010*. New York: The American Geriatrics Society; 2010.

43. Morrison RS, Meier DE. Clinical practice: palliative care. *N Engl J Med.* 2004;350(25):2582–2590.

44. Finlay IG, Higginson IJ, Goodwin DM, et al. Palliative care in hospital, hospice, at home: results from a systematic review. *Ann Oncol.* 2002;13(suppl 4):257–264.

45. Lunney JR, Lynn J, Foley DJ, Lipson S, Guralnik JM. Patterns of functional decline at the end of life. *JAMA.* 2003;289(18):2387–2392.

46. National Hospice Organization. Medical guidelines for determining prognosis in selected non-cancer diseases. *Hosp J.* 1996;11(2):47–63.

47. Rees J, O'Boyle C, MacDonagh R. Quality of life: impact of chronic illness on the partner. *J R Soc Med.* 2001;94(11):563–566.

48. Lim JW, Zebrack B. Caring for family members with chronic physical illness: a critical review of caregiver literature. *Health Qual Life Outcomes.* 2004;2:50.

49. Jones DA, Peters TJ. Caring for elderly dependents: effects on the carers' quality of life. *Age Ageing.* 1992;21(6):421–428.

50. Ganz DA, Fung CH, Sinsky CA, Wu S, Reuben DB. Key elements of high-quality primary care for vulnerable elders. *J Gen Intern Med.* 2008;23(12):2018–2023.

Chapter

65

What Are Special Considerations for Treating Pediatric Patients and Their Families?

RICK GOLDSTEIN AND JOANNE WOLFE

INTRODUCTION AND SCOPE OF THE PROBLEM
  Epidemiology
RELEVANT PATHOPHYSIOLOGY
  Developmental Physiology: Pain, Symptoms, and Their
   Treatment
  Developmental Psychology
  Cosmology
  Bereavement
KEY MESSAGES TO PATIENTS AND FAMILIES
CONCLUSION AND SUMMARY

INTRODUCTION AND SCOPE OF THE PROBLEM

The prospect of managing the palliative care needs of seriously ill children can be intimidating to many. Children with complex chronic conditions and those facing the end of life experience a spectrum of disease outside the practice of most health practitioners. Not only are deaths in pediatric patients relatively infrequent, but many children receiving palliative care suffer from rare and complex conditions. In addition, they have complicated treatment plans that involve a broad array of health care providers. The research on which to base medical decisions is substantially thinner than in adult medicine, and many decisions involve extrapolations from research on adults. Yet, despite the unique aspects of pediatric care, the principles and core set of skills remains the same as in palliative care of adults. This chapter reviews the evidence to provide an understanding of the epidemiology, developmental physiology, developmental psychology, cosmology, and bereavement issues specific to the palliative care of children.

Epidemiology

Deaths in newborns, infants, children, and adolescents under 20 years of age number about 53,000 each year in the United States.[1] This represents less than 1% of total U.S. mortality figures[2] and only 0.4% of all U.S. pediatric hospital stays.[3] It is estimated that 500,000 children cope with life-threatening conditions.[4]

Generally speaking, child deaths in the United States are dominated by newborns and infants. In 2008, 55% of deaths in children occurred in those under 1 year of age, with 20.1% of those infant deaths attributed to congenital malformations, deformations, and chromosomal abnormalities; 16.9% to short gestation and low birth weight; 8.2% to sudden infant death syndrome; 6.2% to newborns affected by maternal complications of pregnancy; and 4.6% to unintentional injuries. For older children, 1 to 19 years of age, the leading causes of death were unintentional injuries (38.8%), homicide (12.4%), malignant neoplasms (8.6%), suicide (8.0%), and congenital malformations, deformations, and chromosomal abnormalities (4.7%). However, palliative care for children is not only end-of-life care. Although the potential certainly exists for a helpful role for pediatric palliative care specialists in the deaths of all children, the focus of the field does not follow that of child death overall.

The population who will benefit from pediatric palliative care may be described as children suffering from a wide array of life-threatening conditions. Although not necessarily beyond cure, these children tend to have courses marked by prognostic uncertainty and diminished expectations for health and longevity. Their care often involves medical decision making balancing quality of life with the risks and burdens of life-sustaining interventions.[5] Pediatric palliative care principally addresses four categories of illness (Table 65-1): (1) conditions for which curative treatment is possible but may fail (e.g., cancer with a poor prognosis); (2) conditions requiring intensive long-term treatment aimed at maintaining the quality of life (e.g., cystic fibrosis, advanced muscular dystrophy); (3) progressive conditions in which treatment is exclusively palliative after diagnosis (e.g., progressive metabolic disorders, spinal muscular atrophy type 1); and (4) conditions involving severe, nonprogressive disability, causing extreme vulnerability to health complications (e.g., holoprosencephaly or other severe brain malformations).

It is difficult to make general statements about a young, evolving field such as pediatric palliative care, but some conclusions may be reached based on two studies describing cohorts of the patients cared for in pediatric palliative care programs.[6,7]

TABLE 65-1. Conditions Appropriate for Pediatric Palliative Care*

Conditions for Which Curative Treatment Is Possible but May Fail
    Advanced or progressive cancer or cancer with a poor prognosis
    Complex and severe congenital or acquired heart disease

Conditions Requiring Intensive Long-Term Treatment Aimed at Maintaining the Quality of Life
    Human immunodeficiency virus infection
    Cystic fibrosis
    Severe gastrointestinal disorders or malformations such as gastroschisis
    Severe epidermolysis bullosa
    Severe immunodeficiencies
    Renal failure in cases in which dialysis, transplantation, or both are not available or indicated
    Chronic or severe respiratory failure
    Muscular dystrophy

Progressive Conditions in Which Treatment Is Exclusively Palliative After Diagnosis
    Progressive metabolic disorders
    Certain chromosomal abnormalities such as trisomy 13 or trisomy 18
    Severe forms of osteogenesis imperfecta

Conditions Involving Severe, Nonprogressive Disability, Causing Extreme Vulnerability to Health Complications
    Severe cerebral palsy with recurrent infection or difficult-to-control symptoms
    Extreme prematurity
    Severe neurological sequelae of infectious disease
    Hypoxic or anoxic brain injury
    Holoprosencephaly or other severe brain malformations

From Himelstein BP, Hilden JM, Boldt AM, et al. Pediatric palliative care. *N Engl J Med.* 2004;350:1753.
*Premature death is likely or expected with many of these conditions.

In contrast to adults, patients with cancer do not make up a majority but rather constitute only about one fifth of the patients. In fact, the leading diagnoses of children enrolled in these studies were genetic and congenital conditions (40.8%), followed by neuromuscular conditions (39.2%). These are populations of children marked by medical complexity. More than half of the children had more than one principle diagnosis, and the mean number of medications received was more than 9. Only 20.4% did not have some element of medical technology in their care, and 67.3% had gastronomy or jejunostomy tubes, 6.7% had a tracheostomy, and 8.5% were ventilator dependent. In addition to illustrating the importance of complex chronic conditions (CCCs) in pediatric palliative care in the United States, prolonged survivorship is also noted, with more than two thirds of the patients in pediatric palliative care programs surviving beyond 1 year from enrollment. The studies also conclude that pediatric palliative care is relatively underused, particularly in the care of neonates, with an estimate that only 5% to 12% of children who might benefit from pediatric palliative care actually receiving those services.

The concept of CCCs is important in understanding the epidemiology of pediatric palliative care. CCCs have been defined as (1) medical conditions in which the child can reasonably be expected to survive for at least 12 months (unless death intervenes) and (2) that involves either several different organ systems or one organ system severely enough to require specialty pediatric care and probably some period of hospitalization in a tertiary center.[8] Children with CCCs constitute more than 22% of all pediatric deaths. Overall, the main categories of CCCs leading to death are cardiovascular (22.2%), malignancy (21.4%), congenital or genetic (19.4%), neuromuscular (18.1%), and respiratory (9.3%).

Socially determined risk and disparities fill the place that lifestyle choices hold in adults, and understanding this is an essential factor to consider when examining the epidemiology of child mortality. Disparities research has shown that the risk for child death is not randomly or homogeneously shared; the suffering of many children facing death is a medical consequence of socially determined risk. Race has been shown to be a factor in disparities in mortality as varied as diabetes, fatal injuries, congenital heart defects, asthma, and Down syndrome,[9] whereas socioeconomic status is an independent and contributory factor in differential health outcomes in a similarly broad number of diseases.[10-12] Uninsured children are 60% more likely to die during a hospitalization compared with insured children (0.75% versus 0.47%), independent of their medical condition.[13] Even in the case of children with CCCs, in which the illnesses may themselves be a risk factor for poorer results, outcomes are affected by race and socioeconomic status.[14-16]

As in adults, the location of death is an important consideration in end-of-life care. Overall, slightly more than 40% of U.S. children die in the hospital setting. Among children with CCCs, more than 80% die in a hospital and half of them on a ventilator. However, studies of bereaved parents have found that, in retrospect, 88% would choose home as the most appropriate location of death.[17] Trends indicate that children with CCCs are increasingly dying at home, perhaps because of factors such as longer survival, the migration of advanced medical technology into the home, and shifting attitudes about what is better care—with a greater focus on quality of life among children with life-threatening conditions.[8] However, this trend toward home as a setting of death is not seen in black or Hispanic children.

The integration of hospice and palliative care for children has been endorsed by the Institute of Medicine[18] and the American Academy of Pediatrics,[19] but it is difficult to get a clear picture of hospice enrollment in U.S. children. A study of Florida children enrolled in Medicaid[20] found that 11% used hospice care in their last year of life. Of hospice-enrolled children, 55% died at home and 90% had a chronic condition. Research on pediatric providers has found they think that hospice's clearest advantages are in location of death and the provision of nonmedical services; these data also suggest that hospice affords better psychosocial services, better anticipatory grief support, better care coordination, and better symptom management, with less chaos, fewer interventions, and more dignity.[21]

Nonetheless, a survey of the Children's Oncology Group institutions found that only 60% have hospice programs available for referrals.[22]

RELEVANT PATHOPHYSIOLOGY

Developmental Physiology: Pain, Symptoms, and Their Treatment

After centuries of scientific opinion stating otherwise, it is now thought that children, even premature newborns, experience pain. The view that children cannot experience pain because of immature myelination, propagated until the 1980s, is no longer accepted.[23] Research has found that, in fact, nociceptive impulses are carried through unmyelinated and thinly myelinated nerve fibers and that although this conduction is slower, the shorter interneuron and neuromuscular distances in newborns compensate. Another view, that young children cannot experience pain because they lack the painful memories to provide the emotional context for the painful stimulus, has also been countered by a body of research, and the inadequate prevention and treatment of pain in young children has been found to have an enduring impact on the future experience of a child's pain.[24]

The current view of developing pain perception in fetuses and infants is fairly nuanced though hardly definitive. It involves an understanding of the role of spinal reflexes, thalamic afferents, and cortical function in the experience of pain.[25] In developmental terms, nociception precedes the experience of pain. Cutaneous nociceptors are developed between 7.5 and 15 weeks postconceptional age, and very strong reflexes to tactile and noxious stimuli can be seen from the first trimester because of the established circuitry of nociceptor–spinal reflexes.[26] These sensory signals, however, do not ascend to the cortical level until 25 weeks postconceptional age.[27] Even then, the cortical activity has not been shown to be discriminant, that is, not only able to register input but also to discriminate whether the input is noxious or not, until 35 weeks postconceptional age.[28] At issue is when thalamocortical pathways, necessary to the experience of pain as the affective psychological experience it is understood to be, become functional in humans. There have been no human studies to directly demonstrate the establishment of the pathways, but they begin to appear between 23 to 30 weeks postconceptional age and functionality occurs in the third trimester, at 29 to 30 weeks postconceptional age. An understanding of these

issues becomes especially important in the neonatal intensive care unit and in areas of prenatal palliative care consultation, including novel in utero interventions.

Developmental physiology aside, the assessment of pain in young children can be difficult. Objective assessment tools can be very helpful when caring for preverbal children or children with developmental disabilities affecting expression and cognition. These scales can assess the presence and severity of pain and are also helpful in understanding the symptom of pain over time. Analog pain scales (Figure 65-1), generally scales of 1 to 10 for pain intensity, have some reliability when used in the same patient over time. However, their use in younger children is limited by the child's difficulty with the concept of quantity or the meaning of greater intensity. Children's reports of pain over time tend to be greatly influenced by their pain at the moment they are asked, which typically obscures the perspective necessary for a general assessment. Children with severe cognitive impairments experience frequent pain that is often unrecognized and untreated.[29]

For children older than of 3 years, the Wong-Baker FACES Pain Rating Scale[30] (Figure 65-2) is often used. After showing the child the faces, it is explained that Face 0 is happy because he has no pain but Face 5 is sad because he has a lot of pain. The child is then asked to choose the face that best describes how he is feeling. An important modification of the analog scale for children with impaired communication skills or cognition is an Individualized Numeric Rating Scale[31] (Figure 65-3), in which parents' observations of their child's facial expression, body movements, activity and interaction, cry, and ability to be consoled as the child experiences worsening pain are used to label the points of the scale. The perspective of parents and others familiar with the child is crucial to any assessment of a child's pain. More comprehensive pain assessment tools that incorporate function and mood are available but infrequently used.

The World Health Organization Three-Step Pain Ladder (Figure 65-4) is the basic approach to pain management in children with life-threatening illness, as in adults. Important issues specific to the care of children are noted at each step.[32] Step 1 involves the use of nonopioid analgesics and possibly an adjuvant. Relevant considerations are (1) analgesia from acetaminophen and ibuprofen has only been established from roughly 3 to 6 months of age, and newborn efficacy trials found them no different from placebo; (2) aspirin is a critical agent in

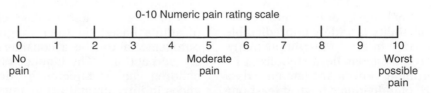

FIGURE 65-1. Visual analog scale.

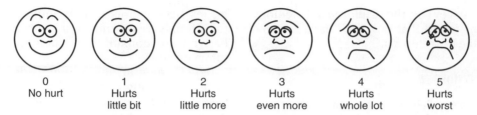

0
No hurt

1
Hurts
little bit

2
Hurts
little more

3
Hurts
even more

4
Hurts
whole lot

5
Hurts
worst

Figure 65-2. Wong-Baker FACES Pain Scale. *(From Wong DL, Hockenberry-Eaton M, Wilson D, et al (eds).* Wong's Essentials of Pediatric Nursing. *6th ed. St Louis: Mosby; 2001:1301.)*

The following scale will help us assess and manage your child's pain.

Directions:
1. Think about your child's past painful events. How does your child act when in mild pain, moderate pain, or severe pain?
2. In the diagram below, write your child's typical pain behaviors on that line that corresponds to its pain intensity where 0=no pain and 10=worst possible pain.
3. When describing your child's pain, think about changes in:
   1. Facial expression
      Squinting eyes, frowning, distorted face, grinds teeth, thrusts tongue
   2. Leg or general body movements
      Tenses, gestures (more or less), or touches part of body that hurts
   3. Activity, or social interaction
      Not cooperative, cranky, irritable, unhappy; not moving, less active, quiet or more active, fidgety
   4. Cry or vocalization
      Moaning, whimpering, crying, yelling
   5. Consolability
      Less interaction, seeks comfort or physical closeness, difficult to distract/satisfy
   6. Other changes: Tears, sweating, holds breath, gasping

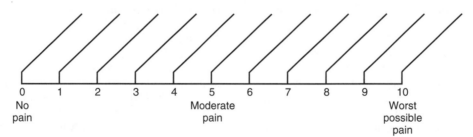

0   1   2   3   4   5   6   7   8   9   10
No   Moderate   Worst
pain   pain   possible
                                                              pain

Figure 65-3. Parent instructions for the Individualized Numeric Rating Scale (INRS). *(From Solodiuk J, Curley M. Pain assessment in nonverbal children with severe cognitive impairments: the Individualized Numeric Rating Scale (INRS),* J Pediatr Nurs. *2003;18:295-299.)*

the cause of Reye syndrome, and its use is avoided in pediatrics; (3) inadvertent or excess amounts of acetaminophen, with particular risk from combined acetaminophen–opioid combinations (step 2), is a major cause of pediatric overdoses and causes 16% of pediatric liver failure.

Issues also exist that are specific to step 2, which calls for weak opioids and combined opioid–nonsteroidal anti-inflammatory drug (NSAID) use. The use of codeine in children is problematic; pediatric research has shown that codeine may be a weaker analgesic than a standard dose of many NSAIDs, and it has a ceiling effect. Its oral bioavailability is widely unpredictable and may range from 15% to 80%. Most importantly, codeine is a prodrug that must be metabolized by the liver into morphine. Pharmacogenomic data show that nearly 50% of individuals have at least one reduced functioning allele resulting in suboptimal

conversion of codeine to active analgesic, and it is estimated that 35% of children do not metabolize codeine in the anticipated way.[33] Another consideration for step 2 is that combination acetaminophen–opioid products have little clear advantage and the decided disadvantage of inadvertent overdose in children. Studies show that their efficacy in somatic pain is comparable to that of ibuprofen.

Step 3 of the pain ladder illustrates important considerations in pediatrics because of the child's physical and physiological development. Although it is usually sufficient to dose children as fractions of adults based on their weight, an awareness of ontogenic factors is a consideration in drug delivery and action.[34] The kinetics of drug absorption in children can be affected by developmental differences in intraluminal pH in segments of the gastrointestinal tract, biliary function, gastric emptying

WHO's Pain Relief Ladder

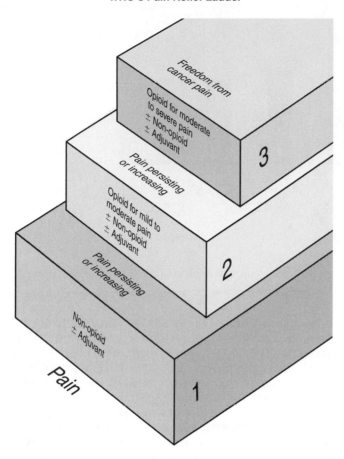

Freedom from
cancer pain

3
Opioid for moderate
to severe pain
± Non-opioid
± Adjuvant

Pain persisting
or increasing

2
Opioid for mild to
moderate pain
± Non-opioid
± Adjuvant

Pain persisting
or increasing

1
Non-opioid
± Adjuvant

Pain

Figure 65-4. World Health Organization Three-Step Pain Ladder. *(From the World Health Organization. http://www.who.int/cancer/palliative/painladder/en/. Accessed September 24, 2012.)*

and intestinal motility, passive and active translumenal transport, intestinal surface area, splanchnic blood flow, activity of drug-metabolizing enzymes and efflux transporters, intestinal microflora, percutaneous absorption, and intramuscular absorption because of skeletal muscle blood flow and capillary density. For example, phenobarbital, which is a weak acid, must be given in much higher doses in neonates because of their relatively elevated gastric pH. Drug distribution is affected by changes in extracellular and total body water distribution, the quantity and composition of circulating binding proteins, and differences in the rate of diffusion of drugs across the blood–brain barrier. For example, highly lipid-soluble psychoactive medications have shorter half-lives and require more frequent dosing in school-aged children with less body fat than adults.[35] Although all of this detail may not be used on a day-to-day basis, its impact is that pediatric drugs must be prescribed in a manner that accounts not only for children's size but also their development as it is relevant to the drug in question. Perhaps the most important developmental factor for pain management is the maturation of drug metabolizing enzymes. The delayed maturation of hepatic cytochromes limits the clearance of

midazolam in the neonate. Conjugation reactions involving phase II enzymes affect the metabolism of acetaminophen and morphine. Whereas neonates have less clearance of many drugs because of immature hepatic enzyme systems, children 2 to 6 years of age have a greater relative liver mass, which leads, for example, to three times daily rather than twice daily dosing of long-acting opioid preparations.[36] Overall, an age-dependent increase in the plasma clearance of drugs metabolized in the liver occurs in the first 10 years of life. An additional factor related to clearance is renal development, because the glomerular filtration rate (GFR) approaches adult values by 1 year of age and continues to increase for the first decade. For all practical purposes, equianalgesic opioid conversion ratios are the same for children as for adults.

Studies of dying children have found that many are troubled by distressing symptoms. Wolfe and colleagues[37] investigated the symptoms and suffering of children dying from cancer and found that the majority of the children experienced fatigue, pain, dyspnea, anorexia, nausea and vomiting, and constipation in the last month of their life (Figure 65-5). Findings consistent with this work have been found in other populations of seriously ill children. This burden in neurologically impaired children is difficult to assess but is likely even more significant. Research on parents has found that their greatest concerns are not specific to the type of symptoms the child experiences so much as the distress caused when those symptoms cannot be satisfactorily controlled. In those children unable to reliably report symptoms it becomes crucial to partner with parents or other family members who may be expert interpreters of the child's expression of symptoms.

It is also essential to remember that children carry a different risk for secondary effects than adults, complicated by the fact that most medications in pediatrics are used off-label and there is little available study of side effects. The risk for extrapyramidal side effects is greater in children. Metoclopramide or the phenothiazines carry a heightened risk for acute dystonic reactions. A study of clonazepam in children 7 to 13 years of age found irritability in two thirds of children treated.[38] Rapid administration of fentanyl can cause chest wall rigidity in infants. High accumulated levels of diphenhydramine causes hallucinations. The risk for suicidality is elevated in adolescents using selective serotonin reuptake inhibitors (SSRIs). Infants treated with opioids are more susceptible to respiratory failure given the immaturity of receptors to hypoxia and hypercarbia found in the first year of life. Table 65-2 lists commonly used medications in palliative care, their age-dependent dosing where necessary, and comments on metabolism and side effects. Importantly, although it is necessary to be aware of the risks, all of these medications can be safely and effectively used to relieve distress in children.

Although the research base is of variable quality and results have been inconsistent,[39] the use of hypnosis for analgesia has shown promise in pain management

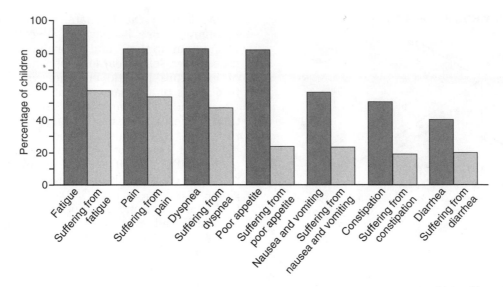

Figure 65-5. The presence and degree of suffering from specific symptoms in the last month of life. *(From Wolfe, Grier HE, Klar N, et al. Symptoms and suffering at the end of life.* N Engl J Med. *2000;342:326-333.)*

during bone marrow aspirations, lumbar punctures, and procedure-related pain and anxiety.[40] The analgesic effect of hypnosis depends most importantly on the hypnotic susceptibility of the patient, and children are more susceptible than adults. The potential for hypnosis is limited for those children younger than 3 years old, with a peak in those between the ages 7 and 14 years. Hypnosis seems a promising nonpharmacological adjunct in the care of seriously ill children, but its contribution needs to be clarified by further research.

The role of distraction can be overrated by some parents and providers. Distraction may be thought of as an assessment tool, and maybe as an adjunct, but not as treatment. Although a child who can be substantially distracted from pain for a considerable period need not be treated with medication, if the child's distress is apparent once the cajoling stops, the pain needs pharmacological management. What is to be avoided is the distressed child dutifully engaging in the distraction to please adults while the pain goes unabated. Similarly, there is no place for the use of placebos in the treatment of pain in children.

Developmental Psychology

An appreciation of the developmental aspects of what death is in the eyes of children is central to their care. Parents want to know what their children can understand as they go through the process of difficult illness or dying. Caregivers, too, wonder what children can understand or express as they try to assess their needs or reckon with enigmatic statements from them. Most would agree that children's suffering because of avoidance of discussions of their fears about their condition and death is especially tragic. Children's cognitive limitations will obviously have an impact on their understanding, as will the effects of illness on a child's development. On the

other hand, it has been noted that chronically ill children may possess a precocious and advanced understanding of certain things, for instance, the details of their illness or the way to address their symptoms, while being quite immature in other developmental areas at the same time.[41]

Much of the central work on loss in children has been conducted with bereaved child survivors. The use of these observations in ill and dying children, though borne out by experience, is nonetheless limited by the assumption that personal mortality is understood similarly to the loss of cherished others. The child's concept of death reflected in the medical literature has changed very little from that extrapolated from Jean Piaget's work in cognitive development[42] and is based on the developmental stages of sensorimotor, preoperational, concrete operations, and formal operations.

Children up to 2 years of age (sensorimotor stage) probably have no concept of death. Death is a separation. Grief stems from the loss of an attachment figure and is expressed through protesting and difficulties in attaching to other adults. The child's difficulty depends on the availability of other nurturing people who have been primary caretakers and with whom the child has had a good previous attachment.

When they are 3 years of age, children recognize death as a changed state. In the preoperational stage (3 to 5 years of age), however, they cannot understand the meaning of a severe illness or the finality and universality of death. Limited language abilities can give the appearance of little insight, and moods and behavior can provide evidence of distress. Children this age think that bad things happen for an immediately identifiable reason, and because of their egocentric perspective, death may be viewed as punishment. They may need concrete reassurance that they are not at fault for the gravity of their illness. Their understanding of what happens to people when they die is that life continues under changed

TABLE 65-2.   Commonly Used Medications and Dosing in Pediatric Palliative Care

MEDICATION	NEONATAL DOSE	INFANT	CHILD	DETERMINANTS OF DIFFERENCES/SIDE EFFECTS
Morphine	*IV:* 0.05 mg/kg/ dose q4-6 hr	*PO:* 0.2-0.5 mg/kg/dose q4-6 hr (half-life goes from 0.2 hr in 1-3 mo to 1-2 hr at age 4-6 yr)	*PO:* 0.2-0.5 mg/kg/dose q4-6 hr (half-life goes from 0.2 hours in 1-3 mo to 1-2 hr at age 4-6 yr)	Glucuronide conjugation in liver, excreted in urine; Under 3 mo old more susceptible to respiratory depression
Hydromorphone	Not studied in neonates	*PO: <50 kg:* 0.03-0.08 mg/kg/dose (max dose 5 mg)	*PO: <50 kg:* 0.03-0.08 mg/kg/dose (max dose 5 mg); *>50 kg:* 1-2 mg/kg/dose q2-4 hr	Potential CNS effects in neonates
Fentanyl	*IV:* 0.5-3 mcg/kg/ dose q2-4 hr; Slow push to prevent chest wall rigidity	*IV:* 1-4 mcg/kg/dose q2-4 hr; Slow push to prevent chest wall rigidity	*IV:* 1-2 mcg/kg/dose q2-4 hr	90% hepatic cytochrome; Highly lipophilic; Nearly 4 times greater volume of distribution in children under 14 yr
Oxycodone	Not studied in neonates	*PO: <50 kg:* 0.1- 0.2 mg/kg/dose q3-4 hr	*PO: <50 kg:* 0.1- 0.2 mg/kg/dose q3-4 hr; *>50 kg:* 10 mg q3-4 hr	Hepatic cytochrome
Methadone	*PO:* 0.05 mg/kg q12-24 hr	*PO:* 0.1 mg/kg/dose q4 hr for 2-3 doses, then q6-12 hr as needed, or 0.7 mg/kg/day divided q4-6 hr	*PO:* 0.1 mg/kg/dose q4 hr for 2-3 doses, then q6-12 hr as needed, or 0.7 mg/kg/day divided q4-6 hr	N-demethylated in liver; Shorter half-life in children
Phenobarbital (hypnotic)	*PO:* 3-5 mg/kg/day divided qd-bid	*PO:* 5-6 mg/kg/day divided qd-bid	*PO: 1-5 yr:* 6-8 mg/kg/d divided qd-bid; *6-12 yr:* 4-6 mg/kg/day divided qd-bid	Hydroxylation and glucuronide conjugation in liver; Absorption affected by gastric pH
Gabapentin (neuropathic pain)	Not studied in neonates	*PO:* 5 mg/kg/dose qhs day 1, then bid day 2 then tid day 3; titrate to effect	*PO: <12 yr:* 5 mg/kg/dose qhs day 1, then bid day 2 then tid day 3; titrate to effect; *>12 yr:* begin 100 mg tid and titrate to effect	Not metabolized; Excreted unchanged in urine and feces
Lorazepam (anxiety)	*PO/IV:* 0.05 mg/kg/ dose q4-8 hr; Reports of neurotoxicity and myoclonus in neonates	*PO/IV:* 0.05 mg/kg/dose q4-8 hr	*PO/IV:* 0.05 mg/kg/dose q4-8 hr	Glucuronide conjugation in liver
Clonazepam	*PO/IV:* 0.01-0.03 mg/ kg/day in 2-3 divided doses, then titrate q3 days	*PO/IV: <30 kg:* 0.01- 0.03 mg/kg/day in 2-3 divided doses, then titrate q3 days	*PO/IV: <30 kg:* 0.01-0.03 mg/kg/ day in 2-3 divided doses, then titrate q3 days; *>30 kg:* 1.5 mg in 3 divided doses, then titrate q3 days	Extensive liver metabolism
Ondansetron	*PO:* guidelines based on body surface area	*PO:* guidelines based on body surface area	*PO: <4 yrs:* guidelines based on body surface area; *4-11 yr:* 4 mg tid; *>11 yr:* 8 mg tid	Hepatic hydroxylation and glucuronide conjugation; Data limited for children under 3 yr
Haloperidol (agitation)	Not used in neonates	Not used in infants	*PO: 3-12 yr:* 0.25-0.5 mg/kg/day divided bid-tid; *>12 yr:* 2-5 mg q1 hr	Hydroxylated in liver
Melatonin (insomnia)	Unstudied	*PO: <40 kg:* 3 mg	*PO: <40 kg:* 3 mg; *>40 kg:* 6 mg	Limited information
Glycopyrrolate (secretions)	*PO:* 40-100 mcg/kg/ dose 3-4 times/day	*PO:* 40-100 mcg/kg/dose 3-4 times/day	1-2 mg/dose tid-qid	Biliary elimination

CNS, Central nervous system; *IV,* intravenous; *PO,* by mouth.

circumstances, and they may, for example, worry about how the dead are able to breath underground or wonder whether not coming back after death is the fault of the person who has died.[43] Children this age can feel overwhelmed when confronted with the strong emotional reactions of their parents to the stresses and disappointments of a difficult medical course or to loss. As with pain assessment, at this age children typically lack the ability to understand their symptoms over time; their perspective is overshadowed by their immediate experience, and trying to understand whether they feel better or worse can be complicated.

School-aged children, 6 to 11 years of age, are considered to be in the late preoperational to concrete operational stages of cognitive development. In this age range, children can understand the seriousness of their illness and the finality of death comes to be understood. Eight-year-olds are aware of personal mortality, and work by Hinds and colleagues[44] has found that children as young as 10 years of age are able to speak about their experiences and decisions at the end of life. Magical thinking gives way to a need for detailed information to gain a sense of control. The development of identity at this age requires experiences in which competence, empathy, and autonomy can be explored and assumed, something considerably challenged by their illness. Children this age develop a separateness and internal world, which may lead to minimizing or amplifying their reactions out of concern for the effect on others. Older children in this range will often feel a need to control their emotions by compartmentalizing and intellectualizing.

Adolescents (>12 years of age) are considered to be in the developmental stage of formal operations. Their concept of death includes universality and finality, and they can understand personal mortality. Adolescents handle death issues at an abstract or philosophical level and can be realistic. They may seem closed off to information and resist present, frank discussion with undercurrents of deep emotion. They may instead rely on anger or disdain. Communication with peers, perhaps involving social networking technologies, can be less limited. However, critically ill children seem sensitive to not burden their friends and they often feel their friends are unable to fully comprehend their situation. They may also feel the need to protect family members and parents, and attention should be placed on helping them understand their preferences independent of the views of caring family members. Adolescents can discuss withholding of treatments. Their goals should be understood, respected, and discussed on their own terms.

Parents can struggle with whether they should talk with their children about their imminent death. Although research supports the bias to speak frankly to dying children, each individual case presents its own complexities based on the child's age, cognitive development, disease, timeline of disease, and parental psychological state. Cultural considerations often have great influence on how the child's voice is elicited, validated, or reinforced. In the study by Kreicsberg and colleagues[45] of parental disclosure to children with impending cancer death, no parent who had talked with their children about their death regretted doing so, and, of those parents who did not speak frankly about imminent death, 27% regretted not having done so. Among those who did not talk with their children about death, 47% of parents who sensed their child was aware of imminent death felt regret.

Most initial disclosures to children about their prognosis come from their parents. For parents who seek advice about how to speak with their children, they may be encouraged to use language that is developmentally appropriate and familiar to the child, to be as honest as the child can bear, in their judgment, and rather than failing to address central issues that the child is likely to be thinking about already, to "scaffold" the information by titrating disclosure and contextualizing it with an emphasis on how they will confront it together. They should be reminded that listening to their child and responding with words as well as physical comforting is a critical part of the disclosure, and, although compassion often tints honesty, they should be discouraged from falsely reassuring. It can sometimes be helpful for the parents to know that terminally ill children may be grieving the loss of their abilities or their future and may worry about being forgotten, experiencing pain, or causing distress in those they will leave behind.[46]

Cosmology

One of the great difficulties in caring for children with life-threatening illnesses is confronting the particular suffering and burden of the family. Much of this suffering feels worse as a result of the unsettling challenge to cosmological order that is presented by pediatric illness. Most people find it more difficult to see children confronting death or impaired by illness to the point that quality of life is in question than confronting the same in people who have lived longer lives. Parents experience an almost primal distress when they are unable to protect their child and can find little comfort in a life lived but cut short. There is a feeling that what is occurring is against nature, out of the proper order. And in an important sense, it is.

When families find themselves in such challenging situations, the work of the palliative care practitioner is to practice compassionate care for the complete child—care that is responsive to both perceived and unrecognized needs. It requires sensitivity to the precarious spiritual state of the families, and to their vulnerability to worry that a focus on comfort may lead to the abandonment of their child by the team or feel to them as "giving up." It requires an appreciation for the need to facilitate meaning making, finding how their child's life is of meaning and value in spite of the circumstances.

Parents are unable to help their child if they have not confronted their child's problems and reconciled themselves enough to participate in decision making. Research has found that the most influential factor in decision making is the ability of parents to confront the impending loss of their child.[47] This requires the careful disclosure of prognosis but does not imply that they need to be directly confronted with blunt facts. Honest, sensitive communication with parents, titrated to their tolerance, allows them to understand their child's situation and its risks and is prerequisite to the restoration of their equipoise. It is very diffi-cult for them to make positive decisions from a posi-tion of fear, mistrust, or misinformation. Research on peace of mind, which is a more positive state than equipoise, finds that peace of mind is not determined by parental or clinical characteristics. It suggests, rather, that parents are more likely to find peace of mind when they have discussed prognosis with the child's physician.[48] Moreover, more detailed prognos-tic disclosure has been found to support hope[49] and earlier recognition of prognosis promises a stronger emphasis on lessening suffering and a greater inte-gration of palliative care.[50]

Parents are likely to consider their core obligation to be protecting their child from harm by making ben-eficial medical decisions and remaining at their child's side despite difficult medical circumstances.[51] Parents need to know that everything is being done to prevent pain and suffering. This is done by scrupulous atten-tion to the management of pain and symptoms, often the "foot in the door" for the palliative care team. Once a relationship is formed with the patient and family, listening becomes essential and can lead to the impor-tant work of promoting a continued sense of valued living and clarification of the goals of care.

Parents often focus on understanding what their children want, even in cases of extraordinary impair-ment. They search for signs of their child's character and strive to find meaning in their life and its course. A focus on their child's development and personality can become an important, positive alternative to the disease and disability they otherwise face. There is an important role for functional-based services (e.g., child life, occupational therapy, physical therapy, educational services) in child treatment and paren-tal coping. Response shift, that is, changes in what is considered to be quality of life because of changes in internal standards, values, or conceptualization, can often be seen in this focus on development in parents.[52] Thresholds for meaningful existence may change. Although finding more meaning in the rip-tide between development and disease progression should be understood sympathetically, it also under-scores the importance of helping families articulate their goals of care and then documenting them, par-ticularly in severely affected children with long ill-ness trajectories. The documentation has a unique potential to remind parents what their perspective was previously, once the illness has evolved.

Clinicians tend to focus on the biomedical aspects of care. However, research on parents finds that they consider communication to be the principle determinant of quality of care regardless of symptom control.[53] In the charged environment of protracted or severe illness, parental fatigue, helplessness, changing medical teams, and the lonely injustice of their child's illness can strain communication. Most conflicts at end of life between parents and the care team are due to parents having a more positive view of prognosis or religious objections to treatment discontinuation.[54]

Bereavement

In the contemporary United States, experiencing the death of a child is a rare and abnormal event. Classic research investigating upsetting life events found that the death of a child rated the most stressful with great consistency across sociodemographic groups.[55] Bereavement research shows parental bereavement to be more intense, complicated, and long-lasting, with huge fluctuations over time.[56] This bereave-ment seems intensified because the loss is hostile to the feelings, hopes, and meanings projected onto the child by the parents; the assumed and socially assigned responsibilities of parents and their incor-poration into their identity; and the closeness and intensity of the parent–child relationship. In keep-ing with this, however, more recent work on parental bereavement stresses the importance of continuing bonds between the bereaved parent and the child[57,58] through memories, rituals, recollections, and saved objects, rather than focusing solely on the separation tasks of grief. Parents may appreciate being unbur-dened by the unrealistic expectation that they will "get over" their loss. Parents who share their prob-lems with others during the child's illness, who have had access to psychological support during the last month of their child's life, and who have had closure sessions with the attending staff, are less likely to experience prolonged grief.

The loss of a child has been shown to dramatically affect the health of a bereaved parent and under-scores the critical importance of bereavement care. Although levels of prolonged grief have not been consistently found to be elevated among bereaved parents, 41% have been shown to expe-rience heightened amounts of grief-related separa-tion distress[59] and 26% of parents continue to report difficulties working through grief 4 to 9 years after their loss, with clear negative health and functional outcomes.[60] Hospitalizations for mental illness are elevated for 5 years after the loss of a child, espe-cially among mothers.[61] Mortality from both natu-ral and unnatural causes remains elevated for up to 18 years in mothers and by unnatural causes for 3 years among fathers.[62] Bereaved parents with unre-solved grief have more physician visits, more missed work, and more sleep difficulties. In fact, a sample of bereaved parents in the United States and Australia showed work disruption in excess of 80%, with 60% losing more than 10% of their annual income. Also, 16% of U.S. families and 22% of Australian families in the sample fell below the poverty line during bereavement.[63]

Siblings have a distinct experience as their brother or sister struggles with complex illness and death. They have a different sort of empathy, identification, and sense of responsibility for the predicament of their ill sibling, sometimes feeling they need to vocal-ize what the patient will not or cannot say. Attempts by parents and the health care team to protect and shield siblings from difficult developments can create a space that becomes filled with misunderstanding or misinterpretation. The same cognitive development issues that complicate the ill or dying child's experience also complicate theirs, and they may feel burdened that angry wishes or ambivalent feelings toward their sibling have caused the illness or complicated its outcome. They must deal with their grief for their loss of a brother or sister in a home compromised by parental mourning, withdrawal, and, not uncommonly, marital discord.

Research on bereaved siblings is limited, but there does not appear to be an elevated risk for depression, anxiety, or behavioral problems rising to the pathological level.[64] However, research suggests that their coping is markedly strained, with observations of diminished quality of life, negative mood states, survivor guilt, and conversion symptoms.[65] Of bereaved siblings with conversion symptoms, 58% have unresolved grief. One third of bereaved siblings have the presence of adjustment problems that impede their health and relationships.[66] The way they are parented may be affected by the idealization of the lost sibling or overprotection by their parents.[67] Primary pediatricians and school-based services can be very helpful to these children, and they may benefit from communication that alerts them to concerns.

KEY MESSAGES TO PATIENTS AND FAMILIES

Complex illness and the loss of a child is a profound and complicated experience. Having a seriously ill child should not undermine a parent's sense of being the parent and having the responsibility to make the decisions that determine the course of their child's life. They need to be supported through this process. As in the care of adults, good communication and support between the medical team and the patient and family during the process has a meaningful, positive impact. Although differences exist in how symptoms are treated, parents should be reassured that every effort will be made to address the child's symptoms safely and effectively. Overall, children with serious illness and their families should understand that high-quality palliative care will focus on the entire family, through the child's illness and beyond the child's death.

CONCLUSION AND SUMMARY

The treatment of children with life-threatening illness is challenging. Although the basic skills involved in the care of children with complex illness or facing death are universal to the practice of palliative care, specific considerations are necessary in the care of children, often related to developmental aspects of their care. Developmental considerations are important to understanding the presence of symptoms and treating them; developmental aspects of understanding death and illness are also important in advising parents or approaching the child. Family bereavement carries its own unique and important considerations.

SUMMARY RECOMMENDATIONS

- Pediatric palliative care should encompass not only end-of-life care but also the care of children with life-threatening conditions and courses marked by prognostic uncertainty and diminished expectations for health and longevity.
- The approach to care must consider a child's physiological development influences pain, symptoms, and potential treatments.
- Recommendations and interactions should be influenced by how a child's cognitive development affects symptom expression and the child's understanding of illness and death.
- The bereavement needs of parents and siblings are significant, and addressing them is critical to high-quality pediatric palliative care.

REFERENCES

1. Mathews TJA, Minino M, Osterman MJ, et al. Annual summary of vital statistics: 2008. *Pediatrics.* 2011;127(1):146–157.
2. Kochanek KD, Xu J, Murphy SL, et al. Deaths: preliminary data for 2009. *Nat Vital Stat Rep.* 2011;59(4). http://www.cdc.gov/nchs/data/nvsr/nvsr59/nvsr59_04.pdf. Accessed September 24, 2012.
3. Healthcare Cost and Utilization Project (HCUP). HCUP *Kids' Inpatient Database (KID)*. Rockville, MD: Agency for Healthcare Research and Quality; 2006.
4. Himelstein BP, Hilden JM, Boldt AM, et al. Pediatric palliative care. *N Engl J Med.* 2004;350(17):1752–1762.
5. Liben S, Papadatou D, Wolfe J. Paediatric palliative care: challenges and emerging ideas. *Lancet.* 2008;371(9615):852–864.
6. Widger K, Davies D, Drouin DJ, et al. Pediatric patients receiving palliative care in Canada: results of a multicenter review. *Arch Pediatr Adolesc Med.* 2007;161(6):597–602.
7. Feudtner C, Kang TI, Hexem KR, et al. Pediatric palliative care patients: a prospective multicenter cohort study. *Pediatrics.* 2011;127(6):1094–1101.
8. Feudtner C, Feinstein JA, Satchell M, et al. Shifting place of death among children with complex chronic conditions in the United States, 1989–2003. *JAMA.* 2007;297(24):2725–2732.
9. Wise PH. The transformation of child health in the United States. *Health Aff (Millwood).* 2004;23(5):9–25.
10. Todd J, Armon C, Griggs A, et al. Increased rates of morbidity, mortality, and charges for hospitalized children with public or no health insurance as compared with children with private insurance in Colorado and the United States. *Pediatrics.* 2006;118(2):577–585.
11. Pressley JC, Barlow B, Kendig T, et al. Twenty-year trends in fatal injuries to very young children: the persistence of racial disparities. *Pediatrics.* 2007;119(4):e875–e884.
12. Brooks-Gunn J, Duncan GJ. The effects of poverty on children. *Future Child.* 1997;7(2):55–71.
13. Abdullah F, Zhang Y, Lardaro T, et al. Analysis of 23 million US hospitalizations: uninsured children have higher all-cause in-hospital mortality. *J Public Health (Oxf).* 2010;32(2):236–244.
14. Newacheck PW. Poverty and childhood chronic illness. *Arch Pediatr Adolesc Med.* 1994;148(11):1143–1149.
15. Newacheck PW, Hung YY, Wright KK. Racial and ethnic disparities in access to care for children with special health care needs. *Ambul Pediatr.* 2002;2(4):247–254.
16. Wang C, Guttmann A, To T, et al. Neighborhood income and health outcomes in infants: how do those with complex chronic conditions fare? *Arch Pediatr Adolesc Med.* 2009;163(7):608–615.
17. Hechler T, Blankenburg M, Friedrichsdorf SJ, et al. Parents' perspective on symptoms, quality of life, characteristics of death and end-of-life decisions for children dying from cancer. *Klin Padiatr.* 2008;220(3):166–174.

18. Field MJ, Behrman RE, Institute of Medicine (US) Committee on Palliative Care for Children and Their Families. *When Children Die: Improving Palliative and End-of-Life Care for Children and Their Families.* Washington, DC: National Academies Press; 2003.

19. American Academy of Pediatrics, Committee on Bioethics and Committee on Hospital Care. Palliative care for children. *Pediatrics.* 2000;106(2 Pt 1):51–357.

20. Knapp CA, Shenkman EA, Marcu Mi, et al. Pediatric palliative care: describing hospice users and identifying factors that affect hospice expenditures. *J Palliat Med.* 2009;12(3):223–229.

21. Dickens DS. Comparing pediatric deaths with and without hospice support. *Pediatr Blood Cancer.* 2010;54(5):746–750.

22. Johnston DL, Nagel K, Friedman DL, et al. Availability and use of palliative care and end-of-life services for pediatric oncology patients. *J Clin Oncol.* 2008;26(28):4646–4650.

23. Anand KJ, Hickey PR. Pain and its effects in the human neonate and fetus. *N Engl J Med.* 1987;317(21):1321–1329.

24. Weisman SJ, Bernstein B. Schechter. Consequences of inadequate analgesia during painful procedures in children. *Arch Pediatr Adolesc Med.* 1998;152(2):147–149.

25. Lee SJ, Ralston HJ, Drey EA, et al. Fetal pain: a systematic multidisciplinary review of the evidence. *JAMA.* 2005;294(8):947–954.

26. Fitzgerald M. The development of nociceptive circuits. *Nat Rev Neurosci.* 2005;6(7):507–520.

27. Slater R, Cantarella A, Gallella S, et al. Cortical pain responses in human infants. *J Neurosci.* 2006;26(14):3662–3666.

28. Slater R, Worley A, Fabrizi L, et al. Evoked potentials generated by noxious stimulation in the human infant brain. *Eur J Pain.* 2010;14(3):321–326.

29. Breau LM, Camfield CS, McGrath PJ, et al. The incidence of pain in children with severe cognitive impairments. *Arch Pediatr Adolesc Med.* 2003;157(12):1219–1226.

30. Wong DL, Hockenberry-Eaton M, Wilson D, et al., eds. *Wong's Essentials of Pediatric Nursing.* 6th ed. St Louis: Mosby; 2001:1301.

31. Solodiuk J, Curley MA. Pain assessment in nonverbal children with severe cognitive impairments: the Individualized Numeric Rating Scale (INRS). *J Pediatr Nurs.* 2003;18(4):295–299.

32. Berde CB, Sethna NF. Analgesics for the treatment of pain in children. *N Engl J Med.* 2002;347(14):1094–1103.

33. Williams DG, Hatch DJ, Howard RF. Codeine phosphate in paediatric medicine. *Br J Anaesth.* 2001;86(3):413–421.

34. Kearns GL, Abdel-Rahman SM, Alander SW, et al. Developmental pharmacology: drug disposition, action, and therapy in infants and children. *N Engl J Med.* 2003;349(12):1157–1167.

35. Tosyali MC, Greenhill LL. Child and adolescent psychopharmacology: important developmental issues. *Pediatr Clin North Am.* 1998;45(5):1021–1035, vii.

36. Blanco JG, Harrison PL, Evans WE, et al. Human cytochrome P450 maximal activities in pediatric versus adult liver. *Drug Metab Dispos.* 2000;28(4):379–382.

37. Wolfe J, Grier HE, Klar N, et al. Symptoms and suffering at the end of life in children with cancer. *N Engl J Med.* 2000;342(5):326–333.

38. Graae F, Milner J, Rizzotto L, et al. Clonazepam in childhood anxiety disorders. *J Am Acad Child Adolesc Psychiatry.* 1994;33(3):372–376.

39. Wild MR, Espie CA. The efficacy of hypnosis in the reduction of procedural pain and distress in pediatric oncology: a systematic review. *J Dev Behav Pediatr.* 2004;25(3):207–213.

40. Richardson J, Smith JE, McCall G, et al. Hypnosis for procedure-related pain and distress in pediatric cancer patients: a systematic review of effectiveness and methodology related to hypnosis interventions. *J Pain Symptom Manage.* 2006;31(1):70–84.

41. Bluebond-Langner M. *The Private Worlds of Dying Children.* Princeton, NJ: Princeton University Press; 1978:210–230.

42. Piaget J. *The Child's Conception of the World.* Savage, MD: Littlefield Adams; 1951:37–60.

43. Nagy M. The child's view of death. In: Feifel H, ed. *The Meaning of Death.* New York: Blakiston Division, McGraw-Hill; 1959.

44. Hinds PS, Drew D, Oakes LL, et al. End-of-life care preferences of pediatric patients with cancer. *J Clin Oncol.* 2005;23(36):9146–9154.

45. Kreicbergs U, Valdimarsdottir U, Onelöv E, et al. Talking about death with children who have severe malignant disease. *N Engl J Med.* 2004;351(12):1175–1186.

46. Hinds PS, Schum L, Baker JN, et al. Key factors affecting dying children and their families. *J Palliat Med.* 2005;8(suppl 1):S70–S78.

47. Kars MC, Grypdonck MH, Beishuizen A, et al. Factors influencing parental readiness to let their child with cancer die. *Pediatr Blood Cancer.* 2010;54(7):1000–1008.

48. Mack JW, Wolfe J, et al. Peace of mind and sense of purpose as core existential issues among parents of children with cancer. *Arch Pediatr Adolesc Med.* 2009;163(6):519–524.

49. Mack JW, Wolfe J, Cook EF, et al. Hope and prognostic disclosure. *J Clin Oncol.* 2007;25(35):5636–5642.

50. Wolfe J, Klar N, Grier HE, et al. Understanding of prognosis among parents of children who died of cancer: impact on treatment goals and integration of palliative care. *JAMA.* 2000;284(19):2469–2475.

51. Hinds PS, Oakes LL, Hicks J, et al. "Trying to be a good parent" as defined by interviews with parents who made phase I, terminal care, and resuscitation decisions for their children. *J Clin Oncol.* 2009;27(35):5979–5985.

52. Sprangers MA, Schwartz CE. Integrating response shift into health-related quality of life research: a theoretical model. *Soc Sci Med.* 1999;48(11):1507–1515.

53. Mack JW, Hilden JM, Watterson J, et al. Parent and physician perspectives on quality of care at the end of life in children with cancer. *J Clin Oncol.* 2005;23(36):9155–9161.

54. de Vos MA, van der Heide A, Maurice-Stam H, et al. The process of end-of-life decision-making in pediatrics: a national survey in the Netherlands. *Pediatrics.* 2011;127(4):e1004–e1012.

55. Paykel ES, Prusoff BA, Uhlenhuth EH. Scaling of life events. *Arch Gen Psychiatry.* 1971;25(4):340–347.

56. Rando TA. *Parental Loss of a Child.* Champaign, IL: Research Press; 1986:45–58.

57. Klass D. Solace and immortality: bereaved parents' continuing bond with their children. *Death Studies.* 1993;17:343–368.

58. Talbot K. *What Forever Means After the Death of a Child: Transcending the Trauma, Living with the Loss.* New York: Brunner-Routledge; 2002:195–210.

59. McCarthy MC, Clarke NE, Ting CL, et al. Prevalence and predictors of parental grief and depression after the death of a child from cancer. *J Palliat Med.* 2010;13(11):1321–1326.

60. Lannen PK, Wolfe J, Prigerson HG, et al. Unresolved grief in a national sample of bereaved parents: impaired mental and physical health 4 to 9 years later. *J Clin Oncol.* 2008;26(36):5870–5876.

61. Li J, Laursen TM, Olsen J, et al. for mental illness among parents after the death of a child. *N Engl J Med.* 2005;352(12):1190–1196.

62. Li J, Precht DH, Mortensen PB, et al. Mortality in parents after death of a child in Denmark: a nationwide follow-up study. *Lancet.* 2003;361(9355):363–367.

63. Dussel V, Bona K, Heath JA, et al. Unmeasured costs of a child's death: perceived financial burden, work disruptions, and economic coping strategies used by American and Australian families who lost children to cancer. *J Clin Oncol.* 2011;29(8):1007–1013.

64. Alderfer MA, Long KA, Lown EA, et al. Psychosocial adjustment of siblings of children with cancer: a systematic review. *Psychooncology.* 2010;19(8):789–805.

65. Sood AB, Razdan A, Weller EB, et al. Children's reactions to parental and sibling death. *Curr Psychiatry Rep.* 2006;8(2):115–120.

66. Fujii Y, Watanabe C, Okada S, et al. Analysis of the circumstances at the end of life in children with cancer: a single institution's experience in Japan. *Pediatr Int.* 2003;45(1):54–59.

67. Brent DA. A death in the family: the pediatrician's role. *Pediatrics.* 1983;72(5):645–651.

SPECIAL TOPICS

PALLIATIVE CARE EMERGENCIES

Chapter 66 — What Are the Signs and Symptoms of Spinal Cord Compression?

Ryan R. Nash and Christine S. Ritchie

INTRODUCTION AND SCOPE OF THE PROBLEM

Malignant spinal cord compression occurs in 2.5% to 5% of patients with cancer in the last 5 years of life. The cumulative incidence varies by cancer type, with 7.9% of patients with myeloma experiencing spinal cord compression and 0.2% with pancreatic cancer experiencing spinal cord compression before death. Systemic cancers more likely to lead to spinal cord compression include prostate, breast, renal, and lung cancer; lymphoma; sarcoma; and multiple myeloma (Table 66-1).[2–4] The thoracic spine is the most common site for spinal cord metastases (70%), with the lumbar spine being second (20%); multiple levels are involved about one third of the time.[5]

Although in most instances spinal cord compression occurs in cancer as a result of metastatic spread to the spinal cord, it can also occur as a result of ischemic or hemorrhagic insults to the circulation involving the spinal cord, complications of radiation or chemotherapy, infections, or paraneoplastic syndromes. Occasionally, spinal cord compression occurs in the setting of primary spinal cord tumors such as astrocytomas and ependymomas. The focus of this chapter will be on metastatic spread to the spinal cord or malignant spinal cord compression (MSCC). Note that treatment of spinal cord compression is considered a medical emergency and is covered in Chapter 67.

The diagnosis of MSCC generally bodes a poor prognosis. In a prospective study of 142 consecutive patients with MSCC referred for potential surgical treatment, median survival was 5 months and 1-year mortality was 50%. Prognosis was influenced by tumor type, functional status, American Society of Anesthesiologists (ASA) score and pain.[6] In a larger, population-based study of Ontario's cancer registry, median survival after diagnosis of MSCC was 2.9 months.[1] Eastern Cooperative Oncology Group (ECOG) performance status and Karnofsky scores are shown to be predictive of survival and ambulation.[7,8]

Patients' overall prognoses and health status play a key role in clinical suspicion, evaluation, diagnosis, and treatment. Those with higher functional status levels at baseline are more likely to notice new neurological deficits and have them addressed promptly; conversely, those with poor functional status to begin with may be less likely to notice subtle changes in strength and neurological function. Likewise, those who are ambulatory at baseline are more likely to benefit from treatment.[4] Rapidity of onset also influences survival and ambulation, with rapid onset of hours to days having worse prognosis than more gradual onset. This difference in onset is usually due to tumor type and aggressiveness (e.g., rapid onset is more common in lung cancer, and gradual onset is more common in breast cancer). Cancer specific median survival after diagnosis of MSCC from the Ontario Cancer Registry was 5 months for breast cancer, 4 months for prostate cancer, 6.4 months for myeloma, 6.7 months for lymphoma, and 1.5 months for lung cancer.[1]

TABLE 66-1. Cancers Commonly Associated With Spinal Cord Compression

Account for 15%-25% of those presenting with MSCC	Carcinoma of the prostate Carcinoma of the lung Breast cancer
Account for 5%-10% of those presenting with MSCC	Kidney or renal cancer (5%-10%) Lymphoma (5%-10%) Myeloma (5%-10%)
Account for <5% of those presenting with MSCC	Colorectal cancer Tumors of unknown primary Melanoma Sarcoma

MSCC, Malignant spinal cord compression.

RELEVANT PATHOPHYSIOLOGY

MSCC usually occurs by hematogenous spread of malignant cells through the vertebral bodies, with subsequent expansion into the epidural space. Spread into the epidural space can occur through extension of the tumor or can occur hematogenously by Batson's venous plexus. Other, less common modes of spread into the spinal cord are through leptomeningeal and intramedullary spread. Leptomeningeal spread can take place through seeding of the meninges by the primary tumor (as can be seen in lung and breast cancer, melanoma, and lymphoma). Signs and symptoms are similar to those seen with epidural spread (see later discussion); however, lower extremity weakness and paresthesias may be more pronounced. Intramedullary spread is relatively rare; in this instance, the primary tumor metastasizes into the spinal cord itself. Signs and symptoms are similar to those in other types of MSCC; however, weakness may be unilateral.[9]

Symptoms

Back pain is the most common symptom seen in MSCC and occurs in 69% to 90% of cases.[4,10] At presentation, many patients have already had pain for weeks to months. Pain may be initially localized and then become more diffuse and radicular in nature. Pain may also be more intense after lying down because of the expansion of the venous plexus with recumbency.[11]

Because early detection of MSCC is key to regaining mobility after treatment, MSCC must constantly be kept in the differential diagnoses of patients presenting with back pain, especially if the symptom is new, has changed in character, or involves the thoracic portion of the spine (because thoracic pain is relatively uncommon in typical osteoarthritis involving the spine). It is also important to keep in mind that in a meaningful percentage of cases, MSCC may be the initial presenting condition of a previously undiagnosed malignancy. However, pain is not as helpful in distinguishing MSCC from other conditions as other signs and symptoms. In a retrospective study of 342 episodes of suspected MSCC evaluated by computed tomography (CT), the presence of pain did not differentiate between those with and without MSCC.[12] Instead, the symptom of weakness (inability to walk) and increased deep tendon reflexes are more predictive of MSCC.

Signs

Weakness is a tell-tale sign in MSCC. It is present in 35% to 75% of patients at diagnosis; half are too weak to walk.[10,13] Thoracic spine involvement is associated with the greatest amount of weakness. Motor deficits at diagnosis influence response to treatment and survival. Patients often do not complain of sensory deficits; these deficits, however, are usually present on careful examination.[4,14] Work by Helwig-Larsen and colleagues[15] suggests that sensory deficits are more common with lumbar spine metastases and motor deficits seen more in thoracic MSCC. Lhermitte sign, which is characterized by a shock-like sensation in the back, arms, and legs when the neck is flexed, can be seen both with cervical and thoracic MSCC. Changes in bowel and bladder function tend to occur late in MSCC. At diagnosis, up to half of patients have bladder dysfunction and are catheter dependent. Patients with cauda equina syndrome predictably present with decreased sensation in a saddle distribution, urinary retention, and lax anal sphincter tone. This presentation is sensitive and specific for the diagnosis, although confirmation imaging is needed if the diagnosis is suspected.[16]

SUMMARY OF EVIDENCE REGARDING DIAGNOSTIC WORKUP

Whether to evaluate or confirm the diagnosis of MSCC is the often the first diagnostic decision confronting a clinician. Although imaging and treatment are often well tolerated, the burden of imaging in the setting of a frail patient with advanced cancer can be significant. Magnetic resonance imaging (MRI) sequencing for the complete spine requires imaging time of well over an hour and necessitates sedation in some patients. The determination of whether to pursue confirmatory imaging should be made after clear dialogue with the patient and family. The decision should be based on the likelihood that the patient will benefit from treatment, that the burden of evaluation is acceptable, that significant pretest probability for MSCC exists, and that further evaluation and potential treatment are consistent with the patient's goals. Pretest probability can be estimated with four factors on history and physical examination: an abnormal neurologic examination, a known cancer diagnosis, a known vertebral metastasis at presentation, and new mid-to upper back pain. Patients with none of these four factors had a spinal cord compression incidence of 8% (notably not an insignificant percentage), and patients with three or four of these risk factors had an 81% likelihood of spinal cord compression.[17]

Imaging

Although plain radiographs often can detect the level of abnormality in spinal cord compression, they lack the desired anatomical detail and sensitivity to be a lone test for diagnosis. Bone scintigraphy is sensitive in identifying the level of spinal cord compression, except in the case of multiple myeloma because of the lytic nature of its bony involvement. However, the bone scintigram lacks specificity and anatomical detail sufficient to direct therapy. X-ray CT allows good visualization of bony structures but is not as detailed as MRI in visualizing adjacent structures. CT with myelography is an option for patients who cannot have MRI because of hardware or other contraindications. Myelography requires a lumbar puncture and may require an additional cervical puncture. In the setting of spinal cord compression, lumbar puncture can result in worsening neurological deficits, with a risk reported as high as 15%.[18] However, one study did not detect any such cases of worsening neurological deficit following myelography.[19]

These imaging modalities have some ability to aid in the diagnosis of spinal cord compression, but they generally do not abrogate the need for MRI. Thus MRI usually should be the first imaging study performed when MSCC is suspected. It is broadly considered the current gold standard.[20-22] In addition to excellent visualization of bony structures, MRI affords detection of intraforaminal and leptomeningeal disease. MRI of the complete spine is recommended because 30% of MSCC cases may involve noncontiguous spinal levels.

Other Diagnostic Considerations

In patients with spinal cord compression as the first manifestation of malignancy, CT-guided needle biopsy has been shown to be safe and effective. Biopsy of the spinal lesion in many of these cases is preferred because the tumor is often of unknown, lung, or hematological origin.[7] Cerebrospinal fluid studies are of limited value in diagnosis of MSCC. Even in the often overlooked leptomeningeal variant of spinal cord compression, the initial cerebrospinal fluid sample fails to yield cells in 10% to 40% of cases.[23] In most instances, further diagnostic evaluation beyond MRI is not needed to confirm the diagnosis of MSCC. Additional testing may be helpful to better define the extent of disease, which might have an impact on treatment choices and prognosis.

KEY MESSAGES TO PATIENTS AND FAMILIES

MSCC is a terrifying diagnosis with the potential for invasive treatment, limited prognosis, paralysis, and radical change in quality of life and caregiver burden. Patients and families should receive clear communication and guided decision support that is informed by prognosis and benefits and burdens of evaluation and treatment. Psychological and spiritual care should be encouraged. Outcomes of MSCC are affected by delays in diagnosis; therefore patients with cancer should be encouraged to report new or changing pain or other symptoms. Further, treating physicians should routinely ask for details regarding the character and location of pain on regular visits.

CONCLUSION AND SUMMARY

MSCC is a relatively common complication of advanced cancer. Patients often present with new or changing pain, which is especially worrisome if it is in the mid to upper back. Patients may also have motor and sensory deficits. The rapidity of onset of these symptoms, the underlying malignancy, and patient's functional status all affect mortality and ambulation outcomes. History and physical examination are usually adequate to inform pretest probability; MRI of the complete spine is currently the accepted gold standard for diagnosis confirmation.

SUMMARY RECOMMENDATIONS

- Metastatic spinal cord compression is a relatively common complication of advanced cancer and should be evaluated when suspected. When present, it portends a poor prognosis.
- For patients with cancer who present with new or changed back pain with or without sensory deficits, MRI of the spine should be performed if the patient's overall prognosis and goals are consistent with evaluation and treatment. It is the gold standard for diagnosing spinal cord compression.

REFERENCES

1. Loblaw DA, Laperriere NJ, Mackillop WJ. A population-based study of malignant spinal cord compression in Ontario. *Clin Oncol.* 2003;15(4):211–217.
2. Bach F, Larsen BH, Rohde K, et al. Metastatic spinal cord compression: occurrence, symptoms, clinical presentations and prognosis in 398 patients with spinal cord compression. *Acta Neurochir (Wien).* 1990;107(1–2):37–43.
3. Schiff D, O'Neill BP, Suman VJ. Spinal epidural metastasis as the initial manifestation of malignancy: clinical features and diagnostic approach. *Neurology.* 1997;49(2):452–456.
4. Mak KS, Lee LK, Mak RH, et al. Incidence and treatment patterns in hospitalizations for malignant spinal cord compression in the United States, 1998–2006. *Int J Radiat Oncol Biol Phys.* 2011;80(3):824–831.
5. Spinazze S, Caraceni A, Schrijvers D. Epidural spinal cord compression. *Crit Rev Oncol Hematol.* 2005;56(3):397–406.
6. Pointillart V, Vital JM, Salmi R, Diallo A, Quan GM. Survival prognostic factors and clinical outcomes in patients with spinal metastases. *J Cancer Res Clin Oncol.* 2011;137(5):849–856.
7. Moon KY, Chung CK, Jahng TA, Kim HJ, Kim CH. Postoperative survival and ambulatory outcome in metastatic spinal tumors: prognostic factor analysis. *J Korean Neurosurg Soc.* 2011;50:216–223.
8. Chataigner H, Onimus M. Surgery in spinal metastasis without spinal cord compression: indications and strategy related to the risk of recurrence. *Eur Spine J.* 2000;9(6):523–527.
9. Schiff D, O'Neill BP. Intramedullary spinal cord metastases: clinical features and treatment outcome. *Neurology.* 1996;47(4):906–912.
10. Stark RJ, Henson RA, Evans SJ. Spinal metastases: a retrospective survey from a general hospital. *Brain.* 1982;105 (Pt 1):189–213.
11. Prasad D, Schiff D. Malignant spinal-cord compression. *Lancet Oncol.* 2005;6(1):15–24.
12. Talcott JA, Stomper PC, Drislane FW, et al. Assessing suspected spinal cord compression: a multidisciplinary outcomes analysis of 342 episodes. *Support Care Cancer.* 1999;7(1):31–38.
13. Husband DJ. Malignant spinal cord compression: prospective study of delays in referral and treatment. *BMJ.* 1998;317(7150):18–21.
14. Gilbert H, Apuzzo M, Marshall L, et al. Neoplastic epidural spinal cord compression: a current perspective. *JAMA.* 1978;240(25):2771–2773.

15. Helweg-Larsen S, Sorensen PS, Kreiner S. Prognostic factors in metastatic spinal cord compression: a prospective study using multivariate analysis of variables influencing survival and gait function in 153 patients. *Int J Radiat Oncol Biol Phys.* 2000;46(5):1163–1169.

16. Deyo RA, Rainville J, Kent DL. What can the history and physical examination tell us about low back pain? *JAMA.* 1992;268(6):760–765.

17. Lu C, Gonzalez RG, Jolesz FA, Wen PY, Talcott JA. Suspected spinal cord compression in cancer patients: a multidisciplinary risk assessment. *J Support Oncol.* 2005;3:305–312.

18. Posner JB. Neurologic complications of cancer. In: *Contemporary Neurology Series.* Vol 45. Philadelphia: FA Davis; 1995:112.

19. Hagenau C, Grosh W, Currie M, et al. Comparison of spinal magnetic resonance imaging and myelography in cancer patients. *J Clin Oncol.* 1987;5:1663–1669.

20. Jennelle RLS, Vijayakumar V, Vijayakumar S. A systematic and evidence-based approach to the management of vertebral metastasis. *ISRN Surg.* 2011;2011:719715.

21. Loblaw DA, Perry J, Chambers A, Laperriere NJ. Systematic review of the diagnosis and management of malignant extradural spinal cord compression: the Cancer Care Ontario Practice Guidelines Initiative's Neuro-Oncology Disease Site Group. *J Clin Oncol.* 2005;23(9):2028–2037.

22. Abrahm JL. Assessment and treatment of patients with malignant spinal cord compression. *J Support Oncol.* 2004;2(5):377–401.

23. Bach F, Bjerregard B, Soletormos G, et al. Diagnostic value of cerebrospinal fluid cytology in comparison with tumor marker activity in central nervous system metastases secondary to breast cancer. *Cancer.* 1993;72(8):2376–2382.

Chapter 67

What Are the Best Pharmacological and Surgical Treatments for Patients With Spinal Cord Compression?

RYAN R. NASH AND CHRISTINE S. RITCHIE

INTRODUCTION AND SCOPE OF THE PROBLEM

In the case of suspected or confirmed spinal cord compression, what treatments are available and which should be chosen for a specific patient? As discussed in Chapter 66, spinal cord compression is not always cancer related. Prognosis in non–cancer-related spinal cord compression is generally better than in the setting of malignancy. Surgery with another disease-targeted therapy is often the treatment of choice, if possible, in this setting. This chapter focuses on spinal cord compression as is it most commonly seen in palliative care—that caused by malignancy and often metastatic disease (metastatic spinal cord compression [MSCC]).

RELEVANT PATHOPHYSIOLOGY

A complete discussion of the pathophysiology relating to malignant spinal cord compression can be found in Chapter 66. Briefly, MSCC usually occurs via hematogenous spread of malignant cells through the vertebral bodies, with subsequent expansion into the epidural space. Spread into the epidural space can occur through extension of the tumor or can occur hematogenously through Batson's venous plexus. Other, less common modes of spread into the spinal cord can occur through leptomeningeal and intramedullary spread. Intramedullary spread is relatively rare; in this instance, the primary tumor metastasizes into the spinal cord itself.

SUMMARY OF EVIDENCE REGARDING TREATMENT RECOMMENDATIONS

Treatment

The diagnosis of spinal cord compression from metastatic cancer usually forebodes a poor prognosis. However, potentially beneficial treatments for this condition exist and are often well-tolerated by certain patients. Delay in treatment can bring further neurological complications, and time to definitive therapy has been a factor in outcomes such as ambulation.[1,2]

Immobilization

Although immobilization is de facto considered standard of care and initiated usually with any suspicion of spinal instability or cord compression, the evidence for ongoing bracing and special positioning is lacking, as is evidence for spinal stability or restriction of mobilization.[3] It is doubtful that immobilization will be put to the test of a controlled trial; however, the lack of clear data demonstrating efficacy of prolonged bracing and immobilization argues against permanent mobility restriction in cases in which definitive therapy is not possible or desired.

Pain

Pain is the most common symptom of spinal cord compression. Definitive therapy, such as radiation therapy or surgery, can help painful symptoms. However, until definitive therapy can be initiated, during treatment and often after it is completed, appropriate pain management should be provided.[4] Opioid therapy will be required in most cases, with rapid escalation to the level recommended by the World Health Organization (WHO) Three-Step Pain Ladder.[5]

Pharmacological Treatments

Steroids. Corticosteroids have long been used in the treatment of spinal cord compression. Their utility is believed to be due to anti-inflammatory and antiedema effects. For a high index of suspicion, high-dose corticosteroids have been advocated, even before confirmation of the diagnosis. However, the data are mixed on this recommendation. Three randomized, controlled trials of patients after confirmation of spinal cord compression and before x-ray therapy found no statistically significant benefit in 2-year survival, pain relief, urinary continence, and ambulation when no steroids, moderate-dose steroids (dexamethasone 10-16 mg/day), or high-dose steroids (dexamethasone 96-100 mg/day) were compared.[6] However, these studies were small and underpowered. They did show trends toward improved neurological status and ambulation with the use of high-dose steroids. These trends along with data from nonrandomized, controlled trials suggest that corticosteroids should be used if the potential untoward effects do not outweigh their benefit. High- and moderate-dose corticosteroids have been shown to significantly increase adverse effects, including psychosis and other neuropsychiatric disorders; gastrointestinal bleeding, perforation, and ulceration; and increased infection.[3,7] Current data do not clearly indicate whether moderate or high doses are preferable. One small study provides evidence that patients with preserved ambulation may not require corticosteroids.[8]

Chemotherapy. Chemotherapy does not have a clear role for most patients with MSCC. It may be considered for selected patients with hematological or germ cell malignancies or in leptomeningeal disease.[9] Hormonal therapies also may be a consideration in specific cancers such as prostate and breast cancer but do not specifically treat MSCC.

Radiation

Radiotherapy alone is the most common definitive treatment for MSCC. Radiation therapy has been shown to have benefits in terms of ambulation, neurological status, pain, quality of life, and survival. If radiotherapy alone is given, it is important to select the appropriate regimen. Similar functional outcomes can be achieved with short-course radiotherapy regimens (often 1-2 fractions) and longer-course radiotherapy regimens (i.e., >3 treatments; one randomized, controlled trial examined 8 treatments versus 2).[10] Longer-course radiotherapy is associated with better local control of MSCC and a decreased chance for recurrence than short-course radiotherapy. Patients with a more favorable survival prognosis (expected survival of ≥6 months) should receive longer-course radiotherapy (potentially with surgery), because they may live long enough to benefit from the reduced risk for MSCC recurrence. Patients with an expected survival of less than 6 months should be considered for short-course radiotherapy, because this therapy gives equal functional and symptomatic relief without the burden of repeated treatments.[2,9]

MSCC can recur after radiation in the field already radiated. Many experts consider repeat irradiation an option. One recent post hoc study analyzed a small population within a randomized, controlled trial that had recurrence in the radiation field area.[11]

It reported that approximately half received repeat irradiation. Some patients received a single fraction and others multiple fractions. Ambulation was determined by preradiation ambulatory status, and repeat irradiation did not change patients' ability to ambulate. The treatments were well tolerated, and the median response was 4.5 months. Other studies have had similar results for repeat irradiation; high-precision techniques appear to reduce the cumulative radiation dose received by the spinal cord.[7] Decompressive surgery can be considered in the previously irradiated area; however, surgery to the radiated area is associated with greater risk for complications than surgery to a nonradiated area.[10] Further prospective studies are needed to better guide individualized care for patients with MSCC.

Surgery

It has been estimated that decompressive surgery followed by radiotherapy is generally indicated in only 10% to 15% of MSCC cases.[2] However, recent data suggest a larger role for surgery in MSCC. The standard treatment for spinal cord compression caused by metastatic cancer had been corticosteroids and radiotherapy, and the role of surgery had not been clearly established until the study by Patchell and colleagues[12] was published in 2005. This study assessed the efficacy of direct decompressive surgery plus postoperative radiation therapy versus radiation therapy alone. This was a randomized, controlled multicenter trial conducted in the United States. The trial recruited participants with magnetic resonance imaging diagnosis of a single area of MSCC, a prognosis of at least 3 months, and nonradiosensitive cancers who were not paraplegic for more than 48 hours. More than one third of participants had spinal instability or pathological spine fractures. All participants received dexamethasone 100 mg initially, with a steroid taper over the course of radiation therapy. Radiation therapy consisted of 30 Gray in 10 fractions. Surgical approach was case dependent, varying from anterior approaches for vertebral body disease or spinal instability to posterior or lateral approaches for posterior or lateral disease. The study assessed ambulation, urinary continence, use of opioid analgesics and corticosteroids, change in muscle strength, change in functional and neurological status, and survival time. The study was stopped early (after 10 years) because a planned midstudy evaluation revealed that the surgical arm had significantly superior results. Significantly more patients in the surgery group (42/50, 84%) than in the radiotherapy group (29/51, 57%) were able to walk after treatment. Patients treated with surgery also retained the ability to walk significantly longer than did those with radiotherapy alone (median 122 days versus 13 days). Nonambulatory patients were more likely to regain the ability to walk if they were in the surgery group versus the radiation group (10/16 [62%] versus 3/16 [19%]). In addition, the need for corticosteroids and opioids was significantly reduced in the surgical group. Finally, there was a trend toward a survival benefit for the surgical arm (median survival 126 versus 100 days). These data were interpreted as evidence that "direct decompressive surgery plus postoperative radiotherapy is superior to treatment with radiotherapy alone for patients with spinal cord compression caused by metastatic cancer."[12] However, patient selection likely influenced findings because the study cohort had a high prevalence of spinal instability (radiation therapy is not a treatment of choice in the presence of spinal instability), and this may explain why the radiation therapy arm in this study did worse than expected compared to other radiation therapy trials.[5] Patchell and colleagues[12] unfortunately did not offer a subset analysis for the participants with spinal instability. The interpretation that seems most consistent with the results is that patients with localized cord compression (especially those with spinal instability), cancers that are not radiosensitive, and a prognosis sufficient to warrant major surgery are likely to benefit from decompressive surgery *and* radiation therapy over radiation therapy alone.[13] Ongoing trials of surgical decompression aim to clarify which patients will benefit from decompressive surgery by functional status, tumor type,[14] and presence or absence of spinal instability.

Other Procedural Treatments

Spinal radiosurgery has been shown to be a noninvasive, safe, and effective treatment method for patients with 1 or 2 small malignant spinal tumors. Patients with good to excellent clinical conditions and with considerable tumor pain receive the greatest benefit of radiosurgery. However, radiosurgery has not been studied in the setting of spinal cord compression, nor have sufficient comparative outcome studies been undertaken to warrant it being recommended for patients with MSCC outside of research protocols.[15]

Percutaneous vertebroplasty has been used for treatment of malignant compression fractures. Shimony and colleagues[16] evaluated the relative efficacy and safety of vertebroplasty in patients with malignant compression fracture and epidural involvement. In this study, 82% of patients reported improvement in pain and 52% of patients had at least temporary improvement in mobility.[16] Results were consistent whether the patient had no epidural involvement, had epidural involvement with no spinal cord or nerve root contact, or had epidural involvement with spinal cord or nerve root involvement. Of note, this study population was relatively healthy compared to those in other studies of MSCC. Vertebroplasty has been combined with radioactive seed placement in the treatment of MSCC with reported success but as of yet lacks controlled trials or comparative outcome research.[17] Although spinal augmentation with vertebroplasty or kyphoplasty has shown safety and efficacy in patients with limited disease, a risk in its use is the delay for more definitive and potentially more successful surgical or radiotherapy treatment. As of yet, spinal augmentation has not demonstrated results that are clearly equal to or better than those with surgery or radiation therapy.[18]

Rehabilitation

Rehabilitation potential for patients with spinal cord compression caused by nonmalignancy is generally better than for those with malignancy. In the population without cancer, rehabilitative prognosis is influenced by premorbid condition, overall prognosis, and initial functionality after treatment (usually surgery for nonmalignancy). However, the population most common to palliative care with spinal cord compression is patients with MSCC. Although care in MSCC has improved over the years, survival and overall rehabilitative prognosis remains very limited. With the limited prognosis for most in this group, rehabilitation must be approached with goals appropriate for the patient.[19,20] Individualized and interdisciplinary rehabilitation plans to achieve comfort and independence are essential. In cases in which ambulation and independence are not possible, rehabilitation goals may focus on training caregivers and aiding the patient in compensatory skills and adaptation to being dependent on others. Short-term rehabilitation in select patients may be appropriate, with some recommending no more than 1 month.[19,20] Given the limited prognosis in this population, any rehabilitative program must be weighed against time away from home and family. More limited home rehabilitative strategies have not been studied adequately. A main goal in rehabilitation may be to train the patient and family in adaptive strategies for managing spinal cord compression–induced mobility loss. Psychological support services should be used to help patients and families cope with the impact of disease on their lives. The added emotional burden of spinal cord compression beyond that of the serious or life-limiting illness should not be overlooked.

KEY MESSAGES FOR PATIENTS AND FAMILIES

Treatment decisions for MSCC should be met with support and guidance to ensure adequate understanding of pertinent information. Pain management can be achieved in most cases with nonopioid and opioid analgesics. Steroid use may be helpful, but the patient and especially the patient's family should be aware of the potential for psychiatric and other untoward side effects. Radiation and surgical treatments are generally well tolerated; however, the burden of treatment, including transportation (especially for patients undergoing radiation therapy), time away from home, and burdens on family need be considered. Finally, although MSCC can be treated, expectations need to be appropriate. Improvements beyond improved pain control are often not realized, and survival is often very short.

CONCLUSION AND SUMMARY

MSCC is an emergency complication of cancer. It often carries a grim prognosis; however, treatment can be effective. Initiation of pain management and corticosteroids should be prompt unless contraindicated. Radiation therapy in short courses is often sufficient in patients with limited prognosis. Long courses of radiation treatment alone are appropriate in ambulatory patients with radiosensitive cancers and stable spines. Patients with neurological impairment (short of prolonged paralysis) or a cancer that is not radiosensitive may benefit from decompressive surgery followed by radiation.

SUMMARY RECOMMENDATIONS

- Malignant spinal cord compression is a serious complication of cancer and should be treated as a medical emergency.
- Appropriate treatment regimens are dependent on the patient's prognosis, and clinicians should consult with patients and families based on the overall goals of care. Options include:
  - For patients with a prognosis of days to a few months or those with complete paraplegia, appropriate treatments should include pain management with opioids and consideration of steroids and single-fraction radiation therapy.
  - For patients with a prognosis of months or longer who have a radiosensitive tumor, management should include immediate treatment with steroids followed by radiation therapy (either a short of longer course depending on the type of cancer).
  - For patients with a prognosis of months or longer whose cancer is not radiosensitive, management should include immediate treatment with steroids followed by surgery. Radiation and/or chemotherapy may be considered after surgery if appropriate based on the type of malignancy.

REFERENCES

1. Jennelle RLS, Vijayakumar V, Vijayakumar S. A systematic and evidence-based approach to the management of vertebral metastasis. *ISRN Surg.* 2011; Epub August 2, 2011.
2. Mitera G, Loblaw A. Intervals from symptom onset to radiation treatment of malignant spinal cord compression: quantification and effect on pretreatment neurologic function. *J Support Oncol.* 2010;8:W1–W5.
3. Kilbride L, Cox M, Kennedy CM, Lee SH, Grant R. Metastatic spinal cord compression: a review of practice and care. *J Clin Nurs.* 2010;19(13–14):1767–1783.
4. Yoshioka H, Tsuneto S, Kashiwagi T. Pain control with morphine for vertebral metastases and sciatica in advanced cancer patients. *J Palliat Care.* 1994;10(1):10–13.
5. World Health Organization. *World Health Organization Pain Ladder.* Avaliable online http://www.who.int/cancer/palliative/painladder/en/; Accessed October 1, 2012.
6. George R, Jeba J, Ramkumar G, Chacko AG, Leng M, Tharyan P. Interventions for the treatment of metastatic extradural spinal cord compression in adults. *Cochrane Database of Syst Rev.* 2008;4: CD006716. DOI: 10.1002/14651858.CD006716.pub2.
7. Loblaw DA, Perry J, Chambers A, Laperriere NJ. Systematic review of the diagnosis and management of malignant extradural spinal cord compression: the Cancer Care Ontario Practice Guidelines Initiative's Neuro-Oncology Disease Site Group. *J Clin Oncol.* 2005;23:2028–2037.
8. Maranzano E, Latini P, Beneventi S, et al. Radiotherapy without steroids in selected metastatic spinal cord compression patients: a phase II trial. *Am J Clin Oncol.* 1996;19:179–183.
9. Rades D, Abrahm JL. The role of radiotherapy for metastatic epidural spinal cord compression. *Nat Rev Clin Oncol.* 2010;7(10):590–598.
10. Maranzano E, Bellavita R, Rossi R, et al. Short-course versus split-course radiotherapy in metastatic spinal cord compression: results of a phase III, randomized, multicenter trial. *J Clin Oncol.* 2005;23(15):3358–3365.
11. Maranzano E, Trippa F, Casale M, Anselmo P, Rossi R. Reirradiation of metastatic spinal cord compression: definitive results of two randomized trials. *Radiother Oncol.* 2011;98(2):234–237.
12. Patchell RA, Tibbs PA, Regine WF, et al. Direct decompressive surgical resection in the treatment of spinal cord compression caused by metastatic cancer: a randomised trial. *Lancet.* 2005;366(9486):643–648.
13. Abrahm JL. Assessment and treatment of patients with malignant spinal cord compression. *J Support Oncol.* 2004;2:377–401.
14. Chaichana KL, Pendleton C, Sciubba DM, et al. Outcome following decompressive surgery for different histological types of metastatic tumors causing epidural spinal cord compression. *J Neurosurg Spine.* 2009;11:56–63.
15. Wowra B, Zausinger S, Drexler C, et al. CyberKnife radiosurgery for malignant spinal tumors: characterization of well-suited patients. *Spine.* 2008;33(26):2929–2934.
16. Shimony JS, Gilula LA, Zeller AJ, Brown DB. Percutaneous vertebroplasty for malignant compression fractures with epidural involvement. *Radiology.* 2004;232(3):846–853.
17. Zuozhang Y, Lin X, Hongpu S, et al. A patient with T5 metastatic lung cancer and spinal cord compression treated with percutaneous vertebroplasty and iodine-125 seed implantation. *Diagn Interv Radiol.* 2011;17(4):384–387.
18. Tancioni F, Lorenzetti MA, Navarria P, et al. Percutaneous vertebral augmentation in metastatic disease: state of the art. *Arch Phys Med Rehabil.* 2011;92(1):4–10.
19. Fattal C, Fabbro M, Gelis A, Bauchet L. Metastatic paraplegia and vital prognosis: perspectives and limitations for rehabilitation care. I. *Arch Phys Med Rehabil.* 2011;92(1):125–133.
20. Fattal C, Fabbro M, Rouays-Mabit H, Verollet C, Bauchet L. Metastatic paraplegia and functional outcomes: perspectives and limitations for rehabilitation care. II. *Arch Phys Med Rehabil.* 2011;92(1):134–145.

Chapter 68

What Techniques Can Be Used in the Hospital or Home Setting to Best Manage Uncontrollable Bleeding?

ALEXANDRA E. LEIGH AND RODNEY O. TUCKER

INTRODUCTION AND SCOPE OF THE PROBLEM

Uncontrollable bleeding is a dreaded occurrence for patients, family, and providers.[1–3] Bleeding is particularly distressing if visible. The psychological distress associated with bleeding can be large, reminding patients and caregivers of the lack of control they have over the illness.

Uncontrollable bleeding can occur in seriously ill patients as rectal bleeding, melena, hematemesis, hemoptysis, vaginal bleeding, hematuria, visible vessel rupture, nasal bleeding, and as a result of fungating skin lesions. Medical devices and catheters, such as a peripherally inserted central catheter (PICC), can also serve as bleeding sources. Bleeding can be slow, such as the capillary ooze of a fungating wound, or brisk, causing an immediate change in the patient's trajectory. Terminal hemorrhage is an uncontrollable, typically arterial, bleed that within a short time ends in death.[1] The prevalence of uncontrollable bleeding at the end of life is not well established. In advanced cancer, significant bleeding is reported in 6% to 14% of patients.[1,4–6]

This chapter focuses on the care of patients who have chosen a comfort-oriented approach to care at the end of life. That is, the chapter assumes that these are patients for whom intubation, attempted cardiac resuscitation, and surgical procedures are no longer appropriate or within their goals of care. Treatment options in both the hospital and at home are reviewed.

RELEVANT PATHOPHYSIOLOGY

Control of bleeding can take the form of local or systemic measures. Pressure, such as that applied with a gloved hand or dressing, locally slows blood flow and facilitates clotting. Local agents such as epinephrine and cocaine cause vasoconstriction. Endovascular techniques are growing in number and can be used to embolize or stent bleeding arteries, stopping further flow of blood from an injured vessel or downstream tissue. Administration of blood products can provide clotting factors or platelets that may be diminished in a disease state. Fibrinolysis is the ongoing in vivo process of fibrin (clot) degradation. It may be heightened by malignancy or in disseminated intravascular coagulation (DIC).[7] Fibrinolytic inhibitors, such as the lysine analogs aminocaproic acid and tranexamic acid, counter fibrin degradation. They can be applied topically or given systemically.

SUMMARY OF EVIDENCE REGARDING TREATMENT RECOMMENDATIONS

Little research exists to guide the care of the patient receiving palliative care with uncontrollable bleeding or terminal hemorrhage when traditional approaches, such as bronchoscopy, endoscopy, radiation, and surgery are not options. Harris and Noble[1] performed a systematic review of available evidence on terminal hemorrhage in patients with advanced cancer and found only case reports and expert opinion to guide care. Less severe bleeding events among patients enrolled in palliative care programs have been examined in a case series.[8] No randomized or controlled trials exist.

Options for management include (1) resuscitative measures, including volume replacement and cardiopulmonary resuscitation; (2) specific measures to slow or halt bleeding, such as endovascular embolization or administration of antifibrinolytic medications; and (3) entirely supportive measures with a priority on preventing patient and family distress and providing patient comfort.

Identifying Patients at Risk

Before a bleeding event, whether the patient is at home or in the hospital, experts recommend that patients at risk be identified so that a plan of action is in place[1,2,4,5,9] (Table 68-1). Front-line nurses with experience managing terminal hemorrhage similarly support the need for prior training and plans of action.[10]

TABLE 68-1. Patients at High Risk for a Bleeding Event

Advanced head and neck cancer
Ulcerated lesions in areas of large vessels
Centrally located lung tumors or lung pathology
Thrombocytopenia, with platelets <10,000/mm³
Cirrhosis or severe liver disease
Acute leukemia
Blast crisis of myeloproliferative disorder
Myelodysplasia or bone marrow failure
Oral anticoagulant medication use
Patients with prior bleeding events

Data from References 1–5, 9, 16.

Management in the Home Setting

When bleeding occurs at home, management options are limited by preparedness of caregivers and availability of medical equipment and medications. For some patients, control of bleeding may be the goal; for others, the focus may be entirely supportive. Expert opinion suggests that an emergency call be made to the palliative care clinician for assistance and guidance in managing the acute episode.[1,9] Frequently, an emergent home visit by the clinician is necessary. Without prior planning, visible hemorrhage may prompt family to call emergency medical services, even if this was not the patient's desire. It is the suggestion of the authors that patients identified as at risk for an uncontrollable bleeding event have clear plans regarding resuscitation. "Do Not Resuscitate" orders should be visibly posted. Bleeding events have been noted to be a reason for emergency room visits in patients in palliative care.[11] For select patients, transfer of care to an acute facility will be appropriate.

Local Measures to Control Bleeding. If the bleeding can be localized, even if arterial, it may be possible to slow or stop it. Applying pressure with a cloth to the appropriate area using a gloved hand can slow bleeding.[1,4,9,12] Moistening the cloth with clean water or saline will ease removal.[13] Nonadherent dressings also may be used.

After the bleeding slows, compression dressing or packing may be applied. These may be soaked in hemostatic agents. Circular bandaging staunches a bleed while applying pressure; it requires the bleeding be localized to an area such as the arm. Packing is an effective way to apply pressure to a cavity, such as the nose or vagina.[5] Numerous agents are available and are discussed in detail elsewhere.[5,4,13] Topical tranexamic acid syrup–soaked pads and epinephrine-soaked pads (1:1000) have limited evidence for use in severe bleeding of surface wounds.[13] Acetone-soaked pads have slowed bleeding when used as packing.[14]

Systemic Measures to Control Bleeding at Home. Medications are available for hospital and home use in the case of a patient identified as at risk for a bleeding event. Again, placement of medications in the home requires foresight. Dean and Tuffin[8] performed a small pilot study describing the use of oral fibrinolytic inhibitors (tranexamic acid and aminocaproic acid) in 16 patients with cancer-associated bleeding problems. Types of bleeding ranged from fungating skin lesions to hematuria and hemoptysis; no major vessel bleeding was seen. The authors reported resolution of bleeding in 14 of 16 patients. The most common side effects are nausea and diarrhea; thromboembolism is rare.[7] Doses for tranexamic acid were 1.5g orally followed by 1g three times per day. The aminocaproic acid dose was 5g orally followed by 1g four times per day. At the time of printing, the cost of 6 days of therapy for aminocaproic acid at this dose is $112. The prevalence of vitamin K deficiency in advanced illness is considerable, and this deficiency may contribute to uncontrollable bleeding. However, no studies have evaluated whether reversal of deficiency provides bleeding benefit to patients receiving palliative care. Serum vitamin K levels in patients with advanced cancer receiving palliative care were found to be low in 22% of patients.[15]

Entirely Supportive Measures. When bleeding is uncontrollable despite other measures, and the goal is to keep the patient at home, focus shifts to patient comfort and covering the extent of the bleeding (Table 68-2).

Administer Crisis Medications. The available literature typically suggests that medications be given if the patient is in distress, understanding that previously used levels of medicine may need to be increased. Typically, midazolam is suggested as the drug of choice because of its fast onset in doses of 2.5 to 10mg intravenously.[1,3–5,17] It also may be given intramuscularly or subcutaneously. The presence of a subcutaneous butterfly at the bedside is suggested because it can be inserted with little prior training by caregivers.[5] How family members perform in the administration of crisis medicines when formal providers are absent has not been evaluated. The need for crisis medications in terminal, large hemorrhages in cancer was questioned in a qualitative study in which nurses reported that crisis medications had no or little role in management. "Staying with" and "supporting the patient" were reported as more helpful than the administration of medications during a typically brief event.[10]

Afterward. Often, an uncontrollable bleeding event will be heralded by a preceding, smaller bleed. An event should serve to remind providers to prepare for a larger bleed later.[1,18] Medication lists should be reviewed with consideration to stopping platelet

TABLE 68-2. Supportive Measures for Uncontrollable Bleeding in the Home or Hospital

Have equipment at the bedside in case of a bleeding event.[1]
Ensure a nurse has been called or is present.[1,9]
Continuous hospice care may be appropriate.
Place the patient in the lateral position.[1,2,4]
Consider the use of crisis medications.
Apply pressure using nonadherent dressings.[1,3,4,9]
Use suction, if available and appropriate.[1]
Use multiple dark towels to mask the blood.[1,4,13,17]

inhibitors and anticoagulants.[18] Warfarin anticoagulation can be reversed with oral vitamin K.[19] Interviews of nurses with experience caring for patients with terminal hemorrhage report the value of debriefing after an event.[10] Accepting the limits of the situation has been identified as worthwhile. In the case of terminal hemorrhage, reassuring the family that the patient likely lost consciousness quickly and did not suffer has been suggested.[17]

Management in the Hospital Setting

In the hospital, the options for therapy of uncontrollable bleeding far exceed those in the home. As with all seriously ill patients, the risks and benefits of treatment must be weighed against goals of care. For patients with relatively good performance scores, procedural options are numerous. Antifibrinolytic agents are available in intravenous formulations for patients unable to take oral medications. As described earlier, they may be helpful in patients receiving palliative care with distressing bleeding events who do not desire other interventions.[8]

Discussion of Specific Bleeding Events

The following sections discuss management for the specific conditions of carotid blowout syndrome, massive hemoptysis, upper gastrointestinal bleeds, hematuria, and patients with thrombocytopenia.

Carotid Blowout Syndrome. Carotid blowout syndrome is an arterial rupture in a patient typically with advanced head and neck cancer. Because of the size of the artery, exsanguination can occur rapidly. For patients who are hospitalized, intervention is possible. Powitzky and colleagues[20] reported on a large case series of patients with carotid blowout syndrome. Patients at risk were more likely to have had radiotherapy (89%), nodal metastasis (69%), and prior neck dissection (63%). Nearly half of patients with carotid blowout syndrome had a prior sentinel bleed that resolved initially with pressure and dressing. When intervention is desired and appropriate, endovascular therapy has become the treatment of choice, although rates of recurrence are significant. Complications are not uncommon, with postprocedure cerebral vascular attack (stroke) rates of 10%.[20,21] Options for endovascular interventions include embolization and stents.[22]

Massive Hemoptysis. Massive terminal hemoptysis is more likely in patients with bronchogenic, centrally located lung pathology. For the inpatient it is a condition that may be temporized. If the patient receiving palliative care has goals consistent with emergent therapies, including bronchoscopy and intubation, an immediate pulmonary evaluation and resuscitative efforts should be initiated; for those patients in whom these methods fail or are not appropriate, bronchial artery embolization can be considered.[23] Endobronchial stenting is a newer option.[24] Placing the patient with the diseased lung down, in the dependent position, is a temporizing measure.[25] For patients in whom intubation and procedures are not consistent with goals of care, hemoptysis has improved with use of oral antifibrinolytic agents, but the hemoptysis in these patients was not massive.[8] Supportive measures were discussed earlier; suppression of cough with opiates may additionally be helpful.

Upper Gastrointestinal Bleeds. Palliative use of aminocaproic acid to control an upper gastrointestinal bleed in a patient with gastric cancer who wished to avoid invasive procedures is described in a case report.[26] A systematic review in nonpalliative populations showed conflicting results for tranexamic acid in slowing gastrointestinal bleeding.[27] Vasopressin and octreotide are well established for slowing variceal and other upper gastrointestinal bleeds.[28,29] Endoscopy is the definitive treatment of choice.[30]

Hematuria. Ghahestani and Shalhssalim[31] performed a systematic review of the literature related to intractable bleeding in advanced bladder cancer and found no prospective or randomized trials. Based on the available case series they developed a decision tree to guide management. Embolization of renal masses causing hematuria is well established.

Thrombocytopenia. Cytopenias are common at the end-of-life. Patients with thrombocytopenia are at risk for an uncontrollable bleed when platelet levels fall below $20,000/mm^3$ or, in the absence of fever or other coagulopathy, $10,000/mm^3$.[16,18] In the United States, platelet transfusions are typically not provided by hospice agencies; they may be more readily given in other countries.[16] In the hospital, therapeutic platelet transfusion for uncontrollable bleeding from thrombocytopenia is an option. The half-life of platelets is short, and effects may be temporary.[4] Salacz and colleagues[18] examined the literature and offered palliative strategies for management.[18] Recombinant factor VIIa (NovoSeven) and cryoprecipitate have been offered as options for treatment of uncontrollable bleeding in the palliative care population. They are very expensive and currently have no evidence to guide use in the palliative care setting.

KEY MESSAGES TO PATIENTS AND FAMILIES

Patients and families should be reminded that there are options for the treatment of uncontrollable bleeding in the hospital and in the home. Treatment can focus on comfort, slowing and stopping the bleeding, or both. Families should be reminded to keep supplies near the patient and to call for assistance if a bleed becomes uncontrollable.

CONCLUSION AND SUMMARY

The interdisciplinary palliative care team should develop a plan of action for the family should a bleed develop. Such a plan, with input from the patient and family, can be made consistent with the overall goals of care.

SUMMARY RECOMMENDATIONS

- Identify patients at risk for uncontrollable bleeding before a bleeding event.
- Prepare caregivers with a plan of action that honors the patient's goals of care.
- Keep supplies near the patient. Tell the family to call for assistance if necessary when the patient is at home.
- Lysine analogs can be used orally or intravenously as a supportive measure for bleeding.
- Midazolam 2.5 mg to 10 mg may be administered for sedation during an uncontrollable bleeding event.
- Small, herald bleeds should remind the interdisciplinary team to prepare for larger bleeds later, perhaps as soon as within 24 to 48 hours.

REFERENCES

1. Harris DG, Noble S. Management of terminal hemorrhage in patients with advanced cancer: a systematic literature review. *J Pain Symptom Manage.* 2009;38(6):913–927.
2. Gagnon B, Mancini I, Pereira J, Bruera E. Palliative management of bleeding events in advanced cancer patients. *J Palliat Care.* 1998;14(4):50–54.
3. Prommer E. Management of bleeding in the terminally ill patient. *Hematology.* 2005;10(3):167–175.
4. Pereira J, Phan T. Management of bleeding in patients with advanced cancer. *Oncologist.* 2004;9(5):561–570.
5. Pereira J, Pautex S. Clinical management of bleeding complications. In: Hanks G, Cherny N, eds. *Oxford Textbook of Palliative Medicine.* New York: Oxford University Press; 2010:1093–1104.
6. Dutcher JP. Hematologic abnormalities in patients with non-hematologic malignancies. *Hematol Oncol Clin North Am.* 1987;1(2):281–289.
7. Lethaby A, Farquhar C, Cooke I. Antifibrinolytics for heavy menstrual bleeding. *Cochrane Database Syst Rev.* 2000;(4): CD000249.
8. Dean A, Tuffin P. Fibrinolytic inhibitors for cancer-associated bleeding problems. *J Pain Symptom Manage.* 1997;13(1):20–24.
9. Harris DG, Finlay I, Flowers S, Noble S. The use of crisis medication in the management of terminal haemorrhage due to incurable cancer: a qualitative study. *Palliat Med.* 2011;25(7):691–700.
10. Smith AM. Emergencies in palliative care. *Ann Acad Med.* 1992;23:186–190.
11. Barbera L, Taylor C, Dudgeon D. Why do patients with cancer visit the emergency department near the end of life? *CMAJ.* 2010;182(6):563–568.
12. Regnard C, Makin W. Management of bleeding in advanced cancer: a flow diagram. *Palliat Med.* 1992;6:74–78.
13. Alexander S. Malignant fungating wounds: managing pain, bleeding and psychosocial issues. *J Wound Care.* 2009;18(1):418–425.
14. Patsner B. Topical acetone for control of life-threatening vaginal hemorrhage from recurrent gynecologic cancer. *Eur J Gynaecol Oncol.* 1993;14(1):33–35.
15. Harrington DJ, Western H, Seton-Jones C, et al. A study of the prevalence of vitamin K deficiency in patients with cancer referred to a hospital palliative care team and its association with abnormal haemostasis. *J Clin Pathol.* 2008;61(4): 537–540.
16. Cartoni C, Niscola P, Breccia M, et al. Hemorrhagic complications in patients with advanced hematologic malignancies followed at home: an Italian experience. *Leuk Lymphoma.* 2009;50(3):313–314.
17. McGrath P, Leahy M. Catastrophic bleeds during end-of-life care in haematology: controversies from Australian research. *Support Care Cancer.* 2009;17(5):527–537.
18. Salacz ME, Lankiewicz MW, Weissman DE. Management of thrombocytopenia in bone marrow failure. *J Palliat Med.* 2007;10(1):236–244.
19. Whitling AM, Bussey HI, Lyons RM. Comparing different routes and doses of phytonadione for reversing excessive anticoagulation. *Arch Intern Med.* 1998;158(19):2136–2140.
20. Powitzky R, Vasan N, Krempl G, et al. Carotid blowout in patients with head and neck cancer. *Ann Otol Rhinol Laryngol.* 2010;119(7):476–484.
21. Desuter G, Hammer F, Gardiner Q. Carotid stenting for impending carotid blowout: suitable supportive care for head and neck cancer patients? *Palliat Med.* 2005;19(5):427–429.
22. Hague J, Tippett R. Endovascular techniques in palliative care. *Clin Oncol (R Coll Radiol).* 2010;22(9):771–780.
23. Kvale PA, Selecky PA, Prakash UBS. Palliative care in lung cancer: ACCP evidence-based clinical practice guidelines (2nd edition). *Chest.* 2007;132(3 suppl):368S–340S.
24. Brandes JC, Schmidt E, Yung R. Occlusive endobronchial stent placement as a novel management approach to massive hemoptysis from lung cancer. *J Thorac Oncol.* 2008;3(9):1071–1072.
25. Cahill BC, Ingbar DH. Massive hemoptysis: assessment and management. *Clin Chest Med.* 1994;15(1):147–167.
26. Roberts SB, Coyne PJ, Smith TJ. Palliative use of aminocaproic acid to control upper gastrointestinal bleeding [letter]. *J Pain Symptom Manage.* 2010;40(3):e1–e3.
27. Gluud LL, Klingenberg SL, Langholz SE. Systematic review: tranexamic acid for upper gastrointestinal bleeding. *Aliment Pharmacol Ther.* 2008;27(9):752–758.
28. Allum WH, Brearley S, Wheatley KE, et al. Acute haemorrhage from gastric malignancy. *Br J Surg.* 1990;77(1):19–20.
29. Lin HJ, Perng CL, Wang K, et al. Octreotide for arrest of peptic ulcer hemorrhage: a prospective, randomized controlled trial. *Heptogastroenterology.* 1995;42(6):856–860.
30. D'Amico G, Pietrosi G, Tarantino I, et al. Emergency sclerotherapy versus vasoactive drugs for variceal bleeding in cirrhosis: a Cochrane meta-analysis. *Gastroenterology.* 2003;124(5): 1277–1291.
31. Ghahestani SM, Shakhssalim N. Palliative treatment of intractable hematuria in context of advanced bladder cancer: a systematic review. *Urol J.* 2009;6(3):146–156.

What Can Be Done for Patients With Crisis Dyspnea?

ALEXANDRA E. LEIGH AND RODNEY O. TUCKER

INTRODUCTION AND SCOPE OF THE PROBLEM

Dyspnea is common and often overwhelming in the setting of serious illness, even in patients without an underlying lung or cardiovascular illness.[1-8] Seventy percent of patients with advanced cancer who are in hospice care experience dyspnea at some point in the last 6 weeks of life.[2] In patients with both malignant and nonmalignant diagnoses, moderate to extreme dyspnea was reported in more than half of patients in their last days.[1] Almost half of children with advanced cancer were reported to suffer from dyspnea.[8] Dyspnea severity increases as a patient approaches death and when uncontrolled is a top reason for admission to palliative care units.[9,10]

There is no universal definition for dyspnea. The American Thoracic Society defines dyspnea as a "subjective experience of breathing discomfort that consists of qualitatively distinct sensations that vary in intensity. The experience derives from interactions among multiple physiological, psychological, social, and environmental factors, and may induce secondary physiological and behavioral responses."[11] In this chapter, "crisis dyspnea" is defined as the subjective sensation of labored breathing or air hunger that has reached a point that the patient is in severe distress. It should be considered a palliative emergency.

RELEVANT PATHOPHYSIOLOGY

The mechanisms of dyspnea are complex and poorly understood. It is discussed in detail by many excellent sources.[4,12-14] One theory is that dyspnea results from a mismatch between central motor coordination and incoming information from central and peripheral chemoreceptors and mechanoreceptors.[4,11] However, others who study dyspnea suggest that there are different forms of dyspnea, as there are different pain syndromes.[12] For instance, descriptors of dyspnea, such as "air hunger" and "work/effort," can be induced to varying degrees through different mechanisms in normal volunteers. Research suggests that, despite the variability in symptom descriptors, the overall intensity of dyspnea can be summed on a scale.[15]

Inconsistency exists in the expression of dyspnea among patients with similar functional abnormalities.[14] It is likely that the affective dimension of the experience of dyspnea is large.[11] Many of the cortical regions activated by dyspnea are limbic or paralimbic, areas important in emotion and fear.[12] Anxiety correlates independently with the intensity of dyspnea in patients with advanced cancer.[16] A concept of "total dyspnea," echoing "total pain," has been offered.[17] Treatment for dyspnea should thus be multidimensional, focusing on the physical, physiological, social, and existential domains.

SUMMARY OF EVIDENCE REGARDING TREATMENT RECOMMENDATIONS

Figure 69-1 summarizes the authors' suggested approach to managing crisis dyspnea. Certainly, as in all palliative care, the benefits and burdens of assessment and treatment should be modified to fit patient and family goals of care. Prospective studies testing dyspnea interventions in general palliative populations are scarce; no such studies exist for the evaluation of crisis dyspnea alone.

Anticipate

It is concerning that adequate control of dyspnea at the end of life occurs less frequently than for other symptoms such as pain, even among children.[8,18] Caregivers feel ill-prepared to handle acute breathlessness at home.[19] This can contribute to fear and feelings of inadequacy. Anticipating crisis dyspnea can help to ensure that a plan of action, adjusted to the patient's disease, can be created with the interdisciplinary team. Patients who develop crisis dyspnea typically have experienced dyspnea before the event.

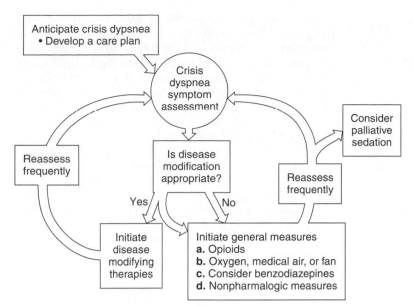

Figure 69-1. Approach to the patient with crisis dyspnea.

Thus a history of dyspnea should prompt additional preparation. An example of a shortness of breath action plan for a patient with obstructive lung disease and associated anxiety is given in Figure 69-2. Such plans may empower caregivers, especially in a home environment, although they have not been empirically evaluated. Home hospice kits, by ensuring necessary medications are in the home, may similarly aid in treatment of crisis dyspnea and avert unwanted emergency department visits.[20]

Assess

A patient experiencing crisis dyspnea is in extreme distress. Tools to assess dyspnea severity should be brief to avoid burdening the patient or delaying treatment. Validated options that can be administered quickly include the modified Borg scale (Table 69-1) and the numerical rating scale (with 0 being no shortness of breath and 10 being the most severe shortness of breath).[21-23] Functional scales or quality of

---

Shortness of breath action plan

If you get short of breath more than you normally experience, you can begin this action plan while you are calling your hospice nurse (if enrolled in hospice).

Nurse/hospice phone number: (999)–999–9999

1. Check oxygen connections to **make sure oxygen is working** correctly. Ensure the nasal cannula is positioned in your nose.
2. Make sure your room is **cool and use a fan** directed at your face to circulate air if you have one.
3. Create a **peaceful environment** using comforting music, dim lights, blankets, etc. Sit upright if you are able.
4. If it has been more than one hour since your last **breathing treatment,** you may **repeat** a breathing treatment of _albuterol and ipratropium_ .
5. You may **take a dose of your medication** such as _morphine concentrate 5mg_ or other pain med at this time to help with your shortness of breath.
6. If the above things have not helped in 30 minutes you may also now take a **dose of medication for anxiety** _Lorazepam 1mg_ .
7. Remember again to **call your hospice nurse** if you have not already done this and are enrolled in hospice.
8. If the things above have still not helped significantly after 60 minutes then your may take another dose of _morphine concentrate 5mg_ which can help with your shortness of breath.

If all of the above measures have not helped within 1–2 hours you may repeat all of the above in consultation with your hospice nurse (if enrolled in hospice).

Figure 69-2. Sample Crisis Dyspnea Plan. This plan is for a patient in hospice care with chronic obstructive pulmonary disease and an anxiety disorder.

TABLE 69-1. Modified Borg Dyspnea Scale

0	Nothing at all
0.5	Very, very slight (just noticeable)
1	Very slight
2	Slight
3	Moderate
4	Somewhat Severe
5	Severe
6	
7	Very severe
8	
9	Very, very severe (almost maximal)
10	Maximal

Patient Instructions for Borg Dyspnea Scale:
"This is a scale that asks you to rate the difficulty of your breathing. It starts at number 0, where your breathing is causing you no difficulty at all and progresses through to number 10, where your breathing difficulty is maximal. How much difficulty is your breathing causing you right now?"

Modified from Borg GA: A category scale with ratio properties for intermodal and interindividual comparisons. In Geissler HG, Petzold P (eds): *Psychophysical Judgement and the Process of Perception: Proceedings of the 22nd International Congress of Psychology.* Amsterdam: North Holland Press; 1980:25-34.

life assessments are not best suited in this time of urgency and can be administered when the patient is more comfortable.

Obtaining a brief history and performing a brief physical examination are paramount.[4,13,14] The most successful treatments require knowledge of the underlying physiology and emotional state of the patient.[24] It is important to note that assessment of the patient in a crisis should be done as preparations for relief are simultaneously being offered.

Initiate Urgent Treatment

The best approach to dyspnea is one in which disease-targeted interventions are most likely to affect symptom relief.[24,25] Many of these interventions, such as providing diuretics and nitrates for pulmonary edema, can be done rapidly. These are discussed in more detail elsewhere. However, general pharmacological and nonpharmalogical options are available that universally may offer relief in all palliative care populations (see Figure 69-1). For patients who no longer are suitable for or have maximized disease-targeted therapies, these global therapies will be their only options.

Pharmacological Options

Opioids. Opioids are the first-line treatment for dyspnea, with a good evidence base to support their use.[26–28] Opioids act through mu receptors centrally and peripherally to relieve breathlessness; they also vasodilate and sedate.[29] In the patient with crisis dyspnea, short-acting formulations can be administered immediately, with frequent reassessment of effect at the bedside.

Subcutaneous and intravenous formulations of opioids work most quickly. Dosing and choice of opioid will depend on prior or current opioid use and underlying illness, such as renal failure. In opioid-naïve patients, morphine 5 mg orally has been used as an initial treatment for dyspnea; 2 mg intravenously or subcutaneously is nearly equivalent.[30] For those on chronic opioid therapy, a supplemental dose of 50% of the equivalent 4-hour dose can be given.[31] After 10 to 20 minutes of intravenous or subcutaneous dosing, the patient should be reassessed and repeat dosing considered. Multiple doses may be needed until comfort is achieved. Respiratory depression has not been seen in studies that have evaluated oxygenation, respiration, and carbon dioxide levels in patients being treated for dyspnea.[28,32]

For patients with continued dyspnea, long-acting formulations such as sustained-release morphine may be added later and have excellent evidence to support their use.[29] Frequent dosing of oral short-acting medications, such as morphine orally every 4 hours, has proven benefit.[32] Dyspnea may be continuous or of breakthrough quality.[33] Long-acting opioids therefore may not be indicated in all patients.

The use of nebulized opioids for dyspnea has been reviewed.[28] Morphine 2.5 to 10 mg, hydromorphone 0.25 to 1 mg, and fentanyl 25 mcg are typical doses. With the exception of nebulized fentanyl,[34] randomized, controlled trials do not support either improved efficacy or reduced side effects compared to opioids delivered by conventional means. Therefore they are not routinely indicated at this time.

Oxygen and Medical Air Therapy. For patients with chronic obstructive pulmonary disease (COPD) with hypoxemia (Pao_2 <55 mm Hg), oxygen therapy has proven benefit for dyspnea and survival.[35] In palliative care, it is offered almost universally to patients with dyspnea, regardless of oxygenation.[36] This practice has increasingly been questioned in patients without hypoxia. Abernethy and colleagues[37] performed a double-blind randomized trail comparing oxygen and medical air, both delivered by nasal cannula at 2 liters per minute, to patients with life-limiting illness and Pao_2 levels greater than 55 mg Hg. No benefit was seen for oxygen therapy over medical air. Both groups, especially those with moderate to severe dyspnea, reported improvement in symptoms. A similar study in patients with COPD who did not have hypoxemia found no benefit to oxygen therapy in dyspnea, quality of life, or function.[38]

In the setting of crisis dyspnea, however, the symbol of oxygen therapy is an important one to patients.[39] Moreover, as has been suggested by numerous studies, the movement of air near the nose—whether oxygen or medical air through nasal cannula or by a portable fan—offers benefit.[37,38,40,41] At this time, it is difficult to obtain medical air in the home. Given the benefit of both medical air and oxygen in a nonhypoxemic patient, in a crisis situation it may be helpful to administer one of these by nasal cannula. If none is available, a bedside fan should be used.

Benzodiazepines. In prior published reviews, benzodiazepines are not typically recommended for first-line palliation of dyspnea in patients with advanced cancer or COPD.[42] However, more recent small studies have shown benefit. Oral midazolam improved dyspnea more than oral morphine in patients with cancer in the outpatient setting.[43] Opioids given simultaneously with lorazepam were shown to be safe and effective in a small study of patients in palliative care with moderate to severe dyspnea and concomitant anxiety.[44] In a crisis situation, there is no evidence to suggest that benzodiazepines offer inherent benefit. However, in patients with an anxiety component to their dyspnea, benzodiazepines may be helpful.

Nebulized Furosemide. There is suggestion that nebulized, inhaled furosemide may be of benefit to dyspnea in palliative populations. Patients with asthma, COPD, and even cancer may benefit through unclear mechanisms of action.[45] Larger, adequately powered, well-designed studies are needed before this promising option can be uniformly recommended.[26]

Nonpharmacological Options

General Supportive Measures. Nonpharmacological options for dyspnea have not been as well-evaluated as pharmacological options. As discussed, air delivered by fan or across the nose by nasal cannula has proven benefit, likely through trigeminal nerve stimulation.[37,41] Despite lack of evidence, it is likely that calming the patient and the environment, providing gentle and reassuring explanations, relaxation techniques, and allowing a therapeutic presence are helpful in this critical situation.[32,46] Positioning a patient in an upright manner, if appropriate, is suggested.[4] Interdisciplinary team involvement can assist in providing emotional and spiritual support, especially given the affective dimension of this symptom. Guided imagery with theta music may be helpful but may not be suited to a crisis situation.[47]

Noninvasive Ventilation. The benefit of noninvasive ventilation in patients receiving palliative care is unclear. Although some argue that a trial of noninvasive ventilation in even the sickest patients may be of benefit for dyspnea, others think the burden of treatment to patients and families is overwhelming.[48] If instituted, patients and caregivers should be educated that noninvasive ventilation is not typically a long-term option and must be discontinued if a patient deteriorates.

Palliative Sedation

In the patient for whom disease-specific and general therapies for crisis dyspnea have been given and are not effective, palliative sedation is an option. Palliative sedation is the planned sedation of a patient with intolerable suffering refractory to treatment. Refractory dyspnea is one of the most common problems requiring palliative sedation in the home. Duration is typically 1 to 3.5 days, and palliative sedation has not been statistically associated with hastened death.[49]

KEY MESSAGES TO PATIENTS AND FAMILIES

Patients and families should be told that crisis dyspnea can be anticipated and treated. It is important to explain that in addition to pursuing treatments that target the patient's underlying illness, the use of opioid medications has also been shown to offer prompt relief. Explain to families that a cool, calming environment that includes familiar sounds and sights can be comforting. They should also use oxygen by nasal cannula or a bedside fan if available. Educate families to position the patient in an upright position as appropriate. A shortness of breath action plan can be initiated if available, and the patient should be enrolled in hospice to ensure that the team can be called for additional, emergency assistance.

CONCLUSION AND SUMMARY

Dyspnea will affect a large proportion of patients receiving palliative care as they near the end of life. Although a troubling symptom for both patients and families, dyspnea can be successfully treated by incorporating an interdisciplinary multimodal plan. Disease-modifying therapies should be considered when appropriate. Anticipating dyspnea before its onset can be empowering and assist in the early management to avoid a crisis event.

SUMMARY RECOMMENDATIONS

- The clinician should recognize that dyspnea is a complex symptom with physical, psychological, spiritual, and emotional domains.
- The clinician should anticipate crisis dyspnea in patients with preexisting shortness of breath.
- Treatment of crisis dyspnea events should be disease-targeted when appropriate, and supportive in all cases.
- Opioids are a mainstay of therapy for crisis dyspnea.
- Oxygen, medical air, or even a fan blowing near the face may be beneficial.
- Palliative sedation can relieve refractory suffering from dyspnea when maximal medical therapies have failed.

REFERENCES

1. Lynn J, Teno JM, Phillips RS, et al. Perceptions by family members of the dying experience of older and seriously ill patients. SUPPORT Investigators: Study to Understand Prognoses and Preferences for Outcomes and Risks of Treatments. *Ann Intern Med.* 1997;126(2):97–106.
2. Reuben DB, Mor V. Dyspnea in terminally ill cancer patients. *Chest.* 1986;89(2):234–236.
3. Fantoni M, Ricci F, Del Borgo C, et al. *Symptom profile in terminally ill AIDS patients: AIDS Patient Care STDS.* 10(3):1996:171–173.
4. Leach RM. Palliative care in non-malignant end-stage respiratory disease. In: Hanks G, Cherny NI, Christakis NA, et al., eds.

Oxford Textbook of Palliative Medicine. 4th ed. Oxford: Oxford University Press; 2010:1231–1256.

5. Cohen LM, Germain M, Poppel DM, et al. Dialysis discontinuation and palliative care. *Am J Kidney Dis.* 2000;36(1):140–144.

6. McCarthy M, Lay M, Addington-Hall JM. Dying from heart disease. *J R Coll Physicians Lond.* 1996;30(4):325–328.

7. Lynn J, Ely EW, Zhong Z, et al. Living and dying with chronic obstructive pulmonary disease. *J Am Geriatr Soc.* 2000;48(5 suppl):S91–S100.

8. Wolfe J, Grier HE, Klar N, et al. Symptoms and suffering at the end of life in children with cancer. *N Engl J Med.* 2000;342(5): 326–331.

9. Elmqvist MA, Jodhoy MS, Bjordal K, et al. Health-related quality of life during the last three months of life in patients with advanced cancer. *Support Care Cancer.* 2009;17(2):191–198.

10. Radbruch L, Nauck F, Ostgathe C, et al. What are the problems in palliative care? Results from a representative survey. *Support Care Cancer.* 2003;11(7):442–451.

11. American Thoracic Society. Dyspnea: mechanisms, assessment, and management—a consensus statement. *Am J Respir Crit Care Med.* 1999;159(1):321–340.

12. Lansing RW, Gracely RH, Banzett RB. The multiple dimensions of dyspnea: review and hypotheses. *Respir Physiol Neurobiol.* 2009;167(1):53–60.

13. Chan K, Tse DMW, Sham MMK, et al. Palliative medicine in malignant respiratory disease. In: Hanks G, Cherny NI, Christakis NA, et al., eds. *Oxford Textbook of Palliative Medicine.* 4th ed. Oxford: Oxford University Press; 2010:587-617.

14. Dalal S, Palat G, Bruera E. Management of dypsnea. In: Berger AM, Shuster JL, Von Roenn JH, eds. *Palliative Care and Supportive Oncology.* 3rd ed.Philadelphia: Lippincott Williams & Wilkins; 2007:277–290.

15. Nishino T, Isono S, Ishikawa T, et al. An additive interaction between different qualities of dyspnea in normal human subjects. *Respir Physiol Neurobiol.* 2007;155(1):14–21.

16. Bruera E, Schmitz B, Pither J, et al. The frequency and correlates of dyspnea in patients with advanced cancer. *J Pain Symptom Manage.* 2000;19(5):357–362.

17. Abernethy AP, Wheeler JL. Total dyspnoea. *Curr Opin Support Palliat Care.* 2008;2(2):110–113.

18. Higginson I, McCarthy M. Measuring symptoms in terminal cancer: are pain and dyspnoea controlled? *J R Soc Med.* 1989;82(5):264–267.

19. Gysels MH, Higginson IJ. Caring for a person in advanced illness and suffering from breathlessness at home: threats and resources. *Palliat Support Care.* 2009;7(2):153–162.

20. Bishop MF, Stephens L, Goodrich M, et al. Medication kits for managing symptomatic emergencies in the home: a survey of common hospice practice. *J Palliat Med.* 2009;12(1):37–44.

21. Kendrick KR, Baxi SC, Smith RM. Usefulness of the modified 1-10 Borg scale in assessing the degree of dyspnea in patients with COPD and asthma. *J Emerg Nurs.* 2000;26(3):216–222.

22. Gift AG, Narsavage G. Validity of the numeric rating scale as a measure of dyspnea. *Am J Crit Care.* 1998;7(3):200–204.

23. Dorman S, Byrne A, Edwards A. Which measurement scales should we use to measure breathlessness in palliative care? A systematic review. *Palliat Med.* 2007;21(3):177–191.

24. Abernethy AP, Wheeler JL, Currow DC. Common approaches to dyspnoea management in advanced life-limiting illness. *Curr Opin Support Palliat Care.* 2010;4(3):53–55.

25. Williams M. Applicability and generalizability of palliative intervention for dyspnoea: one size fits all, some or none? *Curr Opin Support Palliat Care.* 2011;5(2):92–100.

26. Currow DC, Ward AM, Abernethy AP. Advances in the pharmacological management of breathlessness. *Curr Opin Support Palliat Care.* 2009;3(2):103–106.

27. Clemens KE, Klashik E. Symptomatic therapy of dyspnoea with strong opioids and its effect on ventilation in palliative care patients. *J Pain Symptom Manage.* 2007;33(4):473–481.

28. Jennings AL, Davies AN, Higgins JP, et al. A systematic review of the use of opioids in the management of dyspnoea. *Thorax.* 2002;57(11):939–944.

29. Abernethy AP, Currow DC, Frith P, et al. Randomised double-blind placebo-controlled crossover trial of sustained-release morphine for the management of refractory dyspnoea. *Br Med J.* 2003;327(7414):523–525.

30. Mazzocato C, Buclin T, Rapin CH. The effects of morphine on dyspnea and ventilator function in elderly patients with advanced cancer: a randomized double-blind controlled trial. *Ann Oncol.* 1999;10(12):1511–1514.

31. Allard P, Lamontagne C, Bernard P, et al. How effective are supplementary doses of opioids for dyspnea in terminally ill cancer patients? A randomized double-blind trial. *J Pain Symptom Manage.* 1999;17(4):256–265.

32. Clemens KE, Quednau I, Klashik E. Is there a higher risk of respiratory depression in opioid-naïve palliative care patients during symptomatic therapy of dyspnea with strong opioids? *J Palliat Med.* 2008;11(2):204–216.

33. Reddy SK, Parsons HA, Elsayem A, et al. Characteristics and correlates of dyspnea in patients with advanced cancer. *J Palliat Med.* 2009;12(1):29–36.

34. Coyne PJ, Viswanathan R, Smith TJ. Nebulized fentanyl citrate improves patients' perception of breathing, respiratory rate, and oxygen saturation in dyspnea. *J Pain Symptom Manage.* 2002;23(2):157–160.

35. Cranston JM, Crockett AJ, Moss JR, et al. Domiciliary oxygen for chronic obstructive pulmonary disease. *Cochrane Database Syst Rev.* 2005;19(4): CD001744.

36. Abernethy AP, Currow DC, Frith P, et al. Prescribing palliative oxygen: a clinician survey of expected benefit and patterns of use. *Palliat Med.* 2005;19(2):168–170.

37. Abernethy AP, McDonald CF, Frith PA, et al. Effect of palliative oxygen versus room air in relief of breathlessness in patients with refractory dyspnoea: a double-blind, randomized controlled trial. *Lancet.* 2010;326(9743):784–793.

38. Moore RP, Berlowitz DJ, Denegy L, et al. A randomized trial of domiciliary, ambulatory oxygen in patients with COPD and dyspnoea but without resting hypoxaemia. *Thorax.* 2011;66(1):32–37.

39. Currow DC, Fazekas B, Abernethy AP. Oxygen use: patients define symptomatic benefit discerningly. *J Pain Symptom Manage.* 2007;34(2):113–114.

40. Sin DD, McAlister FA, Man SF, et al. Contemporary management of chronic obstructive pulmonary disease: scientific review. *JAMA.* 2003;290(17):2301–2312.

41. Galbraith S, Fagan P, Perkins P, et al. Does the use of a hand held fan improve chronic dyspnea? A randomized, controlled, crossover trial. *J Pain Symptom Manage.* 2010;39(5): 831–838.

42. Simon ST, Higginson IJ, Booth S, et al. Benzodiazepines for the relief of breathlessness in advanced malignant and nonmalignant diseases in adults. *Cochrane Database Sys Rev.* 2010;(1): CD007354.

43. Navigante AH, Castro MA, Cerchietti LC. Morphine versus midazolam as upfront therapy to control dyspnea perception in cancer patients while its underlying cause is sought or treated. *J Pain Symptom Manage.* 2010;39(5):820–830.

44. Clemens KE, Klaschik E. Dyspnoea associated with anxiety-symptomatic therapy with opioids in combination with lorazepam and its effect on ventilation in palliative care patients. *Support Care Cancer.* 2010;19(12):2027–2033.

45. Newton PJ, Davidson PM, Macdonald P, et al. Nebulized furosemide for the management of dyspnea: does the evidence support its use? *J Pain Symptom Manage.* 2008;36(4):424–441.

46. Friedmann N, Alt-Eppling B. Crises in palliative care: a comprehensive approach. *Lancet Oncol.* 2008;9(11):1086–1091.

47. Lai WS, Chao CSC, Yang WP, et al. Efficacy of guided imagery with theta music for advanced cancer patients with dyspnoea: a pilot study. *Biol Res Nurs.* 2010;12(2):188–197.

48. Elliott MW. Non-invasive ventilation: establishing and expanding roles. *Clin Med.* 2011;11(2):150–153.

49. Mercadante S, Porzio G, Valle A, et al. Palliative sedation in patients with advanced cancer followed at home: a systematic review. *J Pain Symptom Manage.* 2011;41(4):754–760.

FINANCIAL ASPECTS OF PALLIATIVE CARE

Chapter 70

What Are the Arguments That Show That Palliative Care Is Beneficial to Hospitals?

Lynn Spragens

INTRODUCTION AND SCOPE OF THE PROBLEM

The case for financial support by hospitals of palliative care programs is linked to the quality of care provided, the quantity of patients receiving care, the extent to which services improve care outcomes, and the leadership relationships that confirm and reinforce these results. Cost savings emerge from "right care, right place, and right time." Cost-benefit assessment is a function of resource use (team costs minus billing) offset by cost savings or contributions to other important institutional goals. Programs that can demonstrate good stewardship of current resources are more likely to be able to leverage cost savings or other value contributions into support for wider impact.

Given the relatively small size of palliative care programs, most clinicians will need to participate in the process of resource planning and budget justification at some point in their careers. Therefore developing some awareness of the linkage between clinical impact and financial results will help plan clinical initiatives that are scalable and sustainable. Understanding some of the common linkages will also assist teams as they prioritize work, establish goals and metrics, and document activities. Many palliative care programs will need to double or triple (or more) in size over the next decade to adequately care for patients; insufficient attention to building well-aligned cases will likely result in a combination of stressed teams, clinician turnover, inadequate resource allocation, and unmet patient needs.

A succinct summary of the financial case for palliative care is as follows: palliative care teams offer customized and intensive services to a small but high-cost proportion of patients. The focus on symptom management, goals of care, and the communication necessary for the design and implementation of a plan of care that reflects the patient's goals often results in lower costs of care. Patients are more likely to be cared for outside of the intensive care unit (ICU) and are less likely to receive redundant or futile treatments.[1] Patients are more likely to enroll in hospice earlier and are less likely to be rehospitalized.

Demonstrating the value described here will require specific local work (1) demonstrating unmet patient needs and specific opportunities for improvement; (2) buy-in from leadership that closing the gap has a high value to the institution; (3) data and case stories that illustrate what the palliative care team is doing or plans to do to successfully meet patient needs and close the gap; (4) clarity about what time, skills, and resources are needed to deliver the planned services; and (5) milestones and metrics that track the team's progress and map with promises (Figure 70-1).

More than 63% of all hospitals with more than 50 beds and 85% of hospitals over 300 beds have a palliative care program[2]; however, many of these programs are underresourced and affect less than 2% of total hospital admissions. Leading programs in 2011, particularly in nonacademic settings, are serving 4% to 10% of total admissions with dedicated staffing on interdisciplinary teams (Spragens: Unpublished records from personal interviews and review of CAPC Registry detail, 2011).

The challenge for many programs will be to manage staff resources effectively and match staff growth to consult service growth as they grow from 2% to 6% or more as a percentage of total admissions. Given the scarcity of trained palliative care professionals and the need to improve the systemic capacity to identify and meet needs, the future priority is to use electronic health records to identify patients with

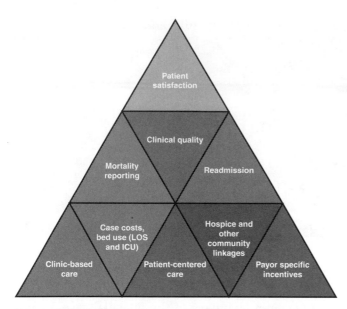

FIGURE 70-1. Palliative Care Value Pyramid. The pyramid diagrams elements that demonstrate the value of palliative care. Establishing the details of each of these elements requires specific local work. *(Reproduced with permission from the Center to Advance Palliative Care, New York, 2011.)*

potential needs and to increase the skills and awareness of other health care professionals to better care for palliative care needs directly.[3]

The challenge for the next decade is to balance palliative care's role in direct patient care (consult services, inpatient units, outpatient services) with the role of palliative care experts in systems' redesign work, mentoring, and training. For each of these activities, it is necessary to link palliative care program goals to overall hospital and system strategies and develop operational plans that meet those goals through reliable services. Concurrent with the growth and stabilization of inpatient consult services, hospitals will be expecting the extension of palliative care services into the outpatient setting (addressed in Chapter 71). In most cases the inpatient consult service will be the anchor for the outpatient service design and will be the signature service that provides a base for outreach, education, and systems' redesign work. Therefore this chapter will focus on the possible approaches to demonstrating value emphasizing the inpatient consult model.

BACKGROUND ON HOSPITAL FINANCES AND EXPECTED IMPACT OF HEALTH CARE REFORM

Since the 1980s most U.S. hospitals have been paid by Medicare through diagnosis-related groups (DRGs). The introduction of DRGs shifted payment from a "cost plus profit" structure to a fixed case rate structure. Under a case rate reimbursement, the hospital is not paid more for a patient with a longer length of stay, or with days in higher intensity units, or receiving more services. The diagnostic categorization

of the patient determines the reimbursement rate. Thus, if all other things are equal, if a patient has a shorter stay in a lower intensity bed with fewer procedures and tests, the costs to the hospital will be lower and the revenue will be unchanged, thus the contribution margin (revenue minus variable costs) will be improved. Of course, these tradeoffs will need to also result in neutral or improved quality, or the improvement will be illusory.

Under this design, in place for more than 25 years, hospitals are not at risk for costs of care outside of their doors and in fact may profit from a cycle of hospitalizations followed by extensive use of specialists and outpatient facilities (particularly affiliated outpatient surgery centers, testing and diagnostic centers, and cancer care). Costs that drive up cost per admission such as entry through the emergency department (ED), use of ICU beds, and delays in care or delays in discharge have a direct negative impact to the hospital.

All hospitals are not paid on DRGs; a small but important subset such as Veterans Administration hospitals, critical access hospitals, or "DRG exempt" hospitals have different contractual arrangements that will affect their financial case for palliative care. It is therefore important to verify how a hospital is paid based on case rates before significant financial modeling. Even in the other cases, compelling approaches may exist and many of the suggestions included in this chapter will apply, but these will need to be crafted with clarity about hospital priorities and realities.

As of 2009, national data indicated that Medicare discharges represented 37.3% of total discharges, Medicaid represented 20.4%, private insurance 32.9%, uninsured 6.1%, and other 3.2%.[4] When considering total days of care, Medicare represents a higher proportion of total care. When reviewing cases likely to have palliative care needs, Medicare often represents 60% or more of patients. Contracts with private insurance and with Medicaid often also reflect DRG case rate design, although the level of reimbursement may vary from Medicare rates. Therefore it is common for 80% or more of patients cared for by palliative care to be covered by case rate payments. However, checking payer mix and contract type through a general discussion with finance staff is advisable before building an elaborate business case. For example, a suburban hospital with a large obstetrical presence may well have needs different from those of an urban tertiary center.

In spite of the focus of hospitals on managing costs, U.S. acute-care hospital cost per case is more than double the median of 10 comparative developed countries, although median length of stay is below those of the comparison group.[5] This situation of high costs per case versus low length of stay has implications for the potential of palliative care to affect financial performance of hospitals. The high costs per day reflect high capital costs (fixed costs per bed), high intensity of care (proportion of surgical cases and ICU cases), and higher procedural activity (laboratory, radiology, other interventions) and labor costs. During the past decade the proportion of U.S. patients seeing 10 or more physicians in their last 6 months of life has grown, hitting 36.1% in 2007,[6] and the proportion of total U.S. patients being admitted through the ED has also grown from 33% to 43% as of 2010. A shortage of critical care beds is listed by hospital administrators as the top reason for ambulance diversions in 2010, accounting for 42% of diversions; 50% of urban and teaching hospitals reported ED capacity issues.[7]

The *Affordable Care Act* of 2010 has introduced significant change to the historic pattern of DRG payment for inpatient care. Changes targeted for 2012 to 2014 are expected to increase the financial risk borne by hospitals for care in and out of their doors ("bundling" for 30-day episodes of care), offer risk sharing for improved total costs of care (accountable care organizations), and introduce more penalties for gaps in quality, such as denial of payment for readmissions for certain conditions. This has accelerated the consolidation or expansion of health care delivery systems and has significantly increased interest from hospital leadership regarding continuum of care needs for patients with complex chronic illnesses.

In addition, the Hospital Consumer Assessment of Healthcare Providers and Systems (HCAHPS) survey of patient satisfaction will have a significant financial impact on the Center for Medicare and Medicaid Services (CMS) payment rates through a withholding and bonus program. The HCAHPS Survey is not specifically sensitive to palliative care activities, but includes pain management as an important component; the 2010 nationwide results show that only 64% of patients are very satisfied with pain management (this is the third lowest of all 10 satisfaction measures). Communication topics comprise five of the remaining nine measures. HCAHPS performance has the potential to affect millions of dollars of revenue per hospital and is tied to both relative performance and trended performance.[8,9]

These changes in the payment environment are collectively called value-based purchasing (VBP) and are considered very high visibility, which means that getting ready to succeed under the new rules is a top priority for most hospital senior leaders. The prospect of significant change in delivery system priorities and increased risk also increases the emphasis of hospital leadership on comprehensive change initiatives and reduces interest in small "one-off" innovations. Thus palliative care programs will need to be clearly aligned with the bigger initiatives in methodology, formal collaborations, and metrics. It is very important to note that the VBP activity is introduced by CMS for Medicare patients, with an emphasis on seniors. However, CMS payment initiatives will likely be adopted by commercial insurers, as was the trend when DRGs were introduced for case payments.

In summary, the majority of U.S. hospitals have been operating within a case rate payment system. Outpatient activities serve as independent profit centers or as feeder systems for inpatient admissions.

Expected changes in 2012 and following will significantly shift the focus to costs throughout the health care delivery system and will further highlight comparative quality results and consumer satisfaction rankings through Hospital Compare and other sources.

Palliative care has a compelling case to make about its role in improving care and reducing avoidable costs in the current system, with even more opportunity within the expanded continuum of care focus if palliative care leaders can be active in the design, delivery, and measurement of expanded services and can work in collaboration with other services.

DEMONSTRATING VALUE THROUGH PALLIATIVE CARE: MAKING THE FINANCIAL CASE

From 1995 to 2011, hundreds of palliative care programs have been effective in getting started with incremental resources and then growing gradually as they demonstrate value. Examples of results that have been used to successfully justify additional resources for growth include (1) reduction in per case costs (cost avoidance), (2) reduction in proportion of days in the ICU, and (3) improved quality and satisfaction.[1,10,11] Other benefits that matter to leadership and have been successfully leveraged (although in many cases not validated in larger studies) include earlier hospice referrals, improved discharge disposition and outpatient support, reduced conflict between nursing staff and physicians, fewer avoidable days (a case management measure), reductions in ethics consult volume, and increased satisfaction from referring physicians and from patients and families. Significant attention is being devoted to efforts to reduce readmissions and reduce length of stay of outlier patients by earlier interventions. Hopefully, future studies will show impact in these areas. Professional billing revenues (Medicare Part B) generally offset 30% to 50% of inpatient direct staff costs and are included as part of the financial justification.

Wide recognition exists within hospital senior leadership that care for patients with complex chronic illness needs improvement and that the needs of patients are not well met at the end of life. However, leadership often struggles to (1) define palliative care, (2) understand how it can be integrated into the complex delivery system without being duplicative, and (3) define the resources needed and the expected impact of the investment. Many senior leaders want to invest appropriately in palliative care. But, they need confidence that the planned services are synergistic with other initiatives and have measurable outcomes. Moving from good intent to action requires a clear and explicit linkage between specific patient population initiatives, proposed resources, and measurable outcomes.

Metrics and goals need to be customized to match local characteristics and to fill the gaps within the current medical environment; therefore a "needs assessment" is always recommended before specific financial modeling.[12] Information and examples are available on the website of the Center to Advance Palliative Care (CAPC, www.capc.org). Examples of key characteristics that vary widely and also affect the assessment of palliative care needs include (1) the relative weight of Medicare admissions, (2) presence or lack of geriatricians and nurses with geriatric training, (3) tertiary and specialty patterns, (4) ICU bed mix and percentage of inpatient deaths that occur in the ICU, (5) status of advanced care planning initiatives, (6) presence of an effective inpatient and outpatient pain service, (7) prevalence of primary care medical homes and extent of primary care provider linkages.

One strategic alignment that is obvious for palliative care programs is to seek nursing and physician leaders in geriatric care and identify points of convergence for process redesign and quality work.[13] Often initiatives arise among nursing staff to adopt geriatric models and improve skills to reduce harm and risks to geriatric patients. These initiatives can be enhanced by linkage with palliative care projects and vice-versa. For example, efforts to improve care in the ED, in the ICU, and during transitions from the hospital should engage both perspectives. Tools available from CAPC can be used to assist in building collaboration around these topics, particularly through use of the Improving Palliative Care (IPAL) series.

The strongest evidence base for direct cost savings from palliative care programs comes from the 2008 multisite cost study[1] and a 2011 study with similar structure conducted among Medicaid patients in New York.[14] These studies document consistent savings in direct costs per day for patients receiving palliative care. In the 2008 multisite study the average per case direct cost savings for live discharges was $1696 and the savings on cases ending in death versus the comparison group was $4908. The largest areas of cost savings were ICU use, laboratory costs, and pharmacy. Table 70-1 includes an overview of several important articles demonstrating the benefit of palliative care to hospital systems.

For documenting the cost savings per case impact of a program (often referred to as the cost avoidance approach), it is recommended that a program first use a proxy from the national studies and then construct the "before and after palliative care consult" portion of the study with internal data on an annual or biannual basis, if desired. It is not recommended to attempt to create a comparison group and replicate the overall study, given the difficulty of creating an appropriate comparison group of sufficient size within one hospital.

Although these studies represent the most widely replicated approach to overall cost savings impact, many programs successfully identify goals for other important areas for savings, establish a measurement plan, and report results that are credible and highly valued within their organizations. For example, targeted approaches to patients with an extended stay in the ICU, improved treatment paths for patients admitted from nursing homes through the ED, or initiatives to improve advanced care planning for patients with congestive heart failure can be used with local data support.

Another promising approach is to pursue improved payment terms from specific payers. New opportunities are emerging to achieve "pay for performance" benefits through palliative care. For example, Highmark Blue Cross Blue Shield of Pennsylvania included palliative care as a choice among quality indicators that hospitals can use to demonstrate

---

TABLE 70-1. Inventory of Articles Related to Palliative Care Financial Impact

REFERENCE	DESCRIPTION
Morrison,[1] 2008	2008 multisite large study matching palliative care patients from eight hospitals with usual care patients through propensity scores and studying costs. This is the most comprehensive study of "cost avoidance" conducted on palliative care. Study uses direct costs (vs. total costs) and demonstrates an average direct cost savings per live discharge of $1696 ($279/day) and $4908 savings for inpatient deaths. Important to be familiar with the study and also recommended that single sites not attempt to duplicate the matched study. Figure 1, page 1788 illustrates the cost pattern for palliative care patients (only) and is referred to as the "before and after" analysis. This can be replicated. See the study by Cassel[17] (below) for another example of this approach.
Morrison,[14] 2011	Similar design to the 2008 study above (matched to usual patients with propensity scores) but focused on Medicaid patients in New York State in four hospitals between 2004 and 2007 and using total costs (vs. direct costs). Savings of $6900/case (4098 for live discharges, $7563 for deaths). Per day savings were $490 for live, $3016 for deaths. Of patients receiving usual care, 58% died in the ICU vs. 34% of patients receiving palliative care. Of live discharges with palliative care, 30% were discharged to hospice vs. 1% of usual care.
Norton,[10] 2007	Study is useful in that it shows detail about a formal MICU initiative and a clear impact on the proportion of days spent in ICU vs. all days. It does not show an overall decrease in LOS. Could be used in conjunction with IPAL-ICU materials (www.capc.org) to plan an ICU initiative.
Cassel,[16] 2010	This article provides an efficient overview of 12 studies that compare patients receiving palliative care to those receiving usual care. The conclusion is that studies to date have not confirmed LOS impact beyond the reduction in the proportion of days in the ICU. The article provides a good overview of the methodology challenges to comparative analysis using LOS.
Smith and Cassel,[17] 2009	Best article presenting the results of a high-volume single site before and after palliative care consult model with inpatient unit. Clear graphics and extensive background on other studies and methodology.

ICU, Intensive care unit; *IPAL,* Improving Palliative Care; *LOS,* length of stay; *MICU,* medical intensive care unit.

quality in the Hospital Quality Blue program for 2012.[15] New York State has included palliative care in Medicaid mandates (2011). Current opportunities exist to define collaborative work with local payers toward payment innovation that will support the improvements inherent in good palliative care. These arrangements usually include outpatient activities and may be best pursued by a group of hospitals or providers in a region or state versus individually.

The other important aspect of demonstrating value is stewardship—demonstrating careful use of existing resources, primarily staff time. Palliative care programs face skepticism when describing individual and team workload. The volume of new patient consults and patient visits per day seems low compared to many other specialty areas. At least four good reasons explain the difference: (1) teams spend the time that it takes to bring diverse perspectives together to craft effective care plans, which takes a lot of time but also has a big impact; (2) care is improved through interdisciplinary involvement, which also takes time for involvement with patients and for team meetings and discussion; (3) teams maintain some open capacity so that they can respond quickly (same day) to consult requests and can adjust to the challenges of patient and family meetings (this is not work that can be prescheduled far in advance); and (4) team members consider part of their role to be reaching out and assisting other staff—helping nurses, learners, or other physicians learn palliative care skills and apply them, which is not noted in volume statistics.

However, some habits of palliative care teams are not good reasons for the difference and improvements are needed in these areas. Lack of management of these habits may reduce team credibility for future requests. Examples include (1) irregular schedules (e.g., late arrivals or early departures), (2) unreliable response times (some providers respond the same day, others let consults linger), (3) visible inefficiency in patient care (family meetings lasting 2 hours or longer, poor skills in working with discharge planning, inefficient reports to attending physicians), (4) lack of clinical schedule accountability (no definition of clinical workload, norms for leave, use of administrative time), and (5) team dysfunction and poor use of interdisciplinary team.

As teams grow, paying close attention to these possibilities and developing a culture of team accountability and transparency will help ensure that the negative attributes do not apply. Some of the dashboard metrics included under "operational," "operational-productivity," and "processes of care" measures (Table 70-2) can assist in developing this

---

TABLE 70-2. Recommended Dashboard Measures for Inpatient Consult Services

Performance dashboards should include a combination of operational, financial, and quality metrics. The quality metrics, in particular, should be updated at least annually to focus on a small number of measures of improved quality or consistent processes of care that are identified through the team's quality improvement work plan.

Recommendations for monthly measures include metrics that can support (1) overview of performance, (2) early identification of trends that may indicate bottlenecks or resource issues, and (3) comparison across sites to support exchange of best practices about processes of care. The list below is not exhaustive but is a concise summary of data that will help track performance. Detailed data capture that will support "drill down" analysis of patterns of use, patient characteristics and disease specifics, location of patients at the time of care, etc., are highly desirable.

Operational
New consults/month and trend
Follow-up visits seen, average daily census by day of month
LOS before and after consult
Discharge status (to skilled nursing facility, hospice, etc.)
Consult volume as percentage of discharges
Deaths as percentage of consults seen

Operational: Productivity
Consults and follow-up care by provider
Billed services by provider and for team as a whole
Hours of clinical time by provider (vs. budget)
Other team accomplishments for month

Processes of Care
Mean and median response time (difference between time of consult requested and consult seen)
Percentage of consults with wait time greater than target threshold (such as 24 hours)
Percentage of consulted patients with documented family meetings
Percentage of consults with documented communication with referring physician before and after consult

Financial
Monthly costs per consult (costs/volume)
Net billing revenue (overall and cumulative YTD by consult)
Percentage of patients in ICU with LOS >7 days with a palliative care consult (example of a measure that matches a quality initiative with a likely financial impact)

Quality
To be determined by team annually based on team priorities and alignment with quality initiatives such as reduced readmissions, better pain management, high reliability of handoffs and transference of care plans at discharge, implementation of advanced care plan tracking, etc.

ICU, Intensive care unit; *LOS,* length of stay; *YTD,* year to date.

culture. In addition, periodic team time tracking can be very helpful to document nondirect patient care time.

Successful documentation and collection for Part B Professional billing is also important for team reputation and stewardship. It generates revenue, and although it rarely covers team costs, it still is significant and is likely to cover 30% to 50% of costs. Teams that are reliable and thorough in their work processes to ensure credentialing of providers, collaboration with coders and billing experts, reliable and timely documentation, and reasonable coding and payment history will have more credibility when discussing future plans. Billing is a specialized topic for which there are some tools on the CAPC and American Academy of Hospice and Palliative Medicine (AAHPM) website (www.aahpm.org) and for which there are usually experts within the larger physician practices in a hospital system.

Table 70-3 illustrates an approach to net consult costs that combines four related variables in a simple relationship so that a team can track its overall costs on a per consult basis and on an aggregated basis. The four variables are (1) staff costs, (2) patient volume, (3) billing net revenue, and (4) cost savings or value estimates. This format will allow a team to see how the addition of staff, matched with volume increases and billing changes, can affect overall costs. It also puts the expected measurable value contribution (such as cost avoidance) into perspective with team costs. This simple approach may prove useful when planning team growth.

KEY MESSAGES TO THE ADMINISTRATION

Palliative care program leaders can explain to hospital administrators that the program will have an impact on health system finances in the following ways:

- Clarification of goals of care with the patient, family, and care team resulting in changes to the order sets or movement of the patient from a higher acuity bed to one more appropriate to desired care, for example from the ICU to a medical/surgical unit or from the hospital to "home with hospice."
- Use of appropriate order sets within palliative care units to meet patient needs consistently but with lower costs per day.

- Better management of acute, uncontrolled pain and symptoms enabling the patient to better tolerate treatment such as ongoing chemotherapy and to transition to other settings.
- Reducing readmissions through postdischarge follow-up, outpatient or home-based care, and communication and collaboration with primary care practices and specialty clinics as indicated.
- Working with specialists helping to manage complex patient needs, including conducting 1 hour or longer "goals of care" meetings for tightly scheduled specialists such as surgeons.
- Skill building and educational outreach to other physicians, nurses, and other care teams to improve their ability to manage these needs with a broader base of patients (15% or more of patients in the hospital are likely to have some palliative care needs).
- Enabling transfer of patients with complex issues to nursing homes and other settings by collaborative work to clarify care goals, document orders that can be implemented in the new setting, and closely adjusting medications to fit the availability in other settings.

These are statements of general characteristics. These key messages need to be tailored to reflect the needs assessment of local gaps and opportunities and must clearly describe the impact a program can have and the resources it needs to do the work in a reliable, high-quality, sustainable way.

CONCLUSION AND SUMMARY

The single most common error made by palliative care program leaders is to grow the service incrementally, without defining baseline performance, setting milestones and goals, getting buy-in up front from leadership about the linkage between growth in services and growth in resources and demonstrating value to anchor each progression. The second most frequent error is to lack clarity about program plans and the specific request to hospital administration. When seeking support for expanded team capacity, the request should include a clear and concise story of the planned future service impact, anchored by past results.

TABLE 70-3. Net Consult Costs: Sample Analysis of Net Consult Costs for Inpatient Palliative Care Service

DESCRIPTION	PER YEAR	PER CONSULT (INCLUDES ALL FOLLOW-UP)
Staffing costs for inpatient program	$850,000	$850
Expected consult volume	1,000	N/A
Expected billing revenue and other revenue	$300,000	$300
Net subsidy before cost savings or LOS	$(550,000)	$(550)
Direct cost savings (based on live patient discharge savings rate from Archives study[1] at $1,696/case)	$1,696,000	$1,696
Net Impact Including Cost Savings*	**$ 1,146,000**	**$ 1,146**

Reproduced with permission from the Center to Advance Palliative Care, New York, 2011.
*The cost savings estimate here uses the documented savings from research studies in the field. However, this is an example for illustration and does not reflect "best practices" or "benchmarks."

TABLE 70-4. Approaches to Quality Improvement Projects That Meet System Priorities and Demonstrate Palliative Care Impact

Hospitals and health systems use various terms for their high-level quality initiatives. Common characteristics are as follows: (1) focused on important system goals; (2) cross-departmental work teams; (3) professionally staffed by process/data experts; (4) methodology encourages rapid cycle improvement, small tests of change, process redesign, and clear metrics; (5) pilot results are evaluated for continuation and spread; and (6) senior executive sponsorship.

Examples of terminology: Clinical Practice Improvement Team, Six Sigma project, Process Improvement (PI), Continuous Process Improvement (CPI), Quality Improvement (QI).

Goal: Identify high-profile initiatives for which palliative care is an appropriate partner and develop collaborative work that meets organizational goals and demonstrates value for palliative care. Remember that helping others through education and design may be more feasible than implementing new services for direct patient care.

Step one: Identify the organization's respected approach, who identifies future priorities, and the current active projects.

Step two: Test some options of high-priority topics that have significant overlap with palliative care and identify which may have the strongest chance of support and success before initiating work.

Principles

Financial outcomes are a result of care quality and process improvement.

Some of the most important problems do not have to be owned by palliative care but can benefit from palliative care perspective and expertise.

Data that are gathered by a team and with formal support will be more credible than internally generated data.

Baseline data collection including case review will be useful in evaluating impact of change.

It is not necessary to get credit for all of the change. Being part of a shared initiative can be very effective in defining resource needs and getting support.

Example 1: Excellence in Pain Management

Rationale: Patients' rating of pain management is an important component of the HCAHPS Survey. Current hospital performance is ___ (national average is 69%). Improving recognition and treatment of pain is an interdepartmental initiative.

Composition might include:
  Palliative care clinician
  Geriatric resource nurse
  Surgical physician assistant
  Anesthesiologist
  Clinical pharmacist
  Psychiatry personnel
  Six Sigma coach
  Patient or family member
  Other nurses, administrator, etc.
  Community resources

Commentary: Palliative care does not want to take over this topic. Needs exist far beyond the palliative population. However, this is a good topic for palliative care to build relationships, demonstrate clinical expertise, and help build work processes and electronic monitors that will also help identify palliative care needs.

Opportunities: Working through the team to collect baseline data and identify current gaps in knowledge, process, or medication availability will identify potential focus areas for palliative care. To the extent that the interventions designed result in earlier and appropriate referrals to palliative care, outcomes will include reduced costs. Overall progress on pain will result in improvement in Hospital Consumer Assessment of Healthcare Providers and Systems (HCAHPS) score and related payments. This process might invite the introduction of palliative care triggers.

Example 2: Improving Intensive Care Unit (ICU) Capacity Through Reduction in Long Stay Cases

Rationale: A small number of cases are in the ICU for >7 days and use a disproportionate share of days. Long stays are expensive, and without reimbursement. Some of the long stay patients have unmet palliative care needs that if identified, might be managed differently.

Composition might include:
  Palliative care team members
  ICU nurses
  Intensivists, hospitalists, or pulmonologists
  Case management personnel
  Pharmacy
  Six Sigma coach
  Patient or family member
  Emergency department physician

A project such as this allows deep dive into detailed data and charts regarding a small number of patients and development of hypotheses about alternative pathways. Once again, palliative care does not take over the project but may identify a subset of patients that are well suited for an intervention.

Opportunities: The IPAL-ICU (http://www.capc.org/ipal-icu/) tools and resources on the CAPC website provide peer-reviewed tools to support the project and also reinforce the role of palliative care team as a facilitator of change and partner in care.

Both errors occur on the road paved by good intentions, and when a team gets busy solving ill-defined or unrecognized problems it is difficult to get leverage from their results. Identifying a gap, defining a pilot to test a service (with clear criteria for replication or expansion), estimating impact, and then demonstrating results is an art. One of the best ways to learn the art is to work with others on shared projects that incorporate quality planning approaches and that link you with experts. Table 70-4 provides basic orientation to quality improvement projects that may be useful to help identify activities already under way or to suggest topics with clear relevance to palliative care.

As this chapter has illustrated, palliative care has a variety of value propositions—better care, less suffering, lower hospital per case costs, fewer ICU days. The value that can be demonstrated is a function of service design, service delivery, and service volume. Figure 70-2 illustrates the building blocks of a sustainable program. Demonstrating financial impact requires local knowledge and buy-in and must reflect norms and conventions of accounting and budgeting for new programs. Value recognition depends on a clear needs assessment, good skills in defining milestones and measures, and building relationships of trust. Building strong relationships with senior leaders, with key staff such as decision support staff

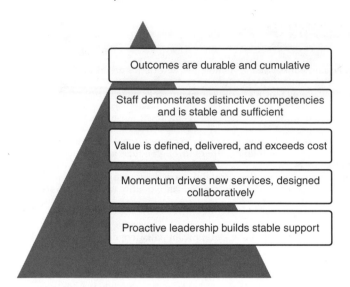

FIGURE 70-2. Characteristics of sustainability. These are the key elements required to keep a program functioning. *(Reproduced with permission from the Center to Advance Palliative Care, New York, 2011.)*

who can help with your modeling and reporting, and with collaborators such as other specialists, nursing leaders, or case managers, is critical to getting requests heard and acted upon. Simple numbers, well presented, and supported by case examples can be more effective than highly detailed projects. It is critical to remember that a team's credibility and value proposition are derived from excellent patient care and that case stories must anchor all requests.

SUMMARY RECOMMENDATIONS

- Actions are essential building blocks for the business case for a palliative care program are as follows:
  - Identify actionable quality gaps in current patient care; use basic quality improvement techniques to quantify gaps, define alternative care options, and set improvement goals. Well-defined small pilots anchored by good case examples and simple data collection are very effective in demonstrating value. Define what will be done and why it will matter, then deliver.
  - Include explicit educational initiatives to "train the trainer" or improve skills in others and show how these will increase the scale of impact. Educational efforts will not be measured in the traditional cost avoidance methodology (which looks at consulted patients) and does not create billing revenue. Therefore being more explicit about resources and goals is very important.
  - Define and then track processes of care so that resource use (team roles and time) can be accounted for. Palliative care is time consuming. However, significant variance in the effectiveness and practice patterns may exist among team members, especially in best usage of the interdisciplinary team. Demonstrating competency and accountability in resource management is important to credibility.
  - Develop dashboard metrics that include explicit performance goals defined by senior leadership and develop a reliable data tracking method. Differentiate between operational data useful to the team and summary reports for senior leadership. Show that the data can be used to identify future quality projects.
  - Collect patient case stories that illustrate the human dimension of what is done and the dramatic impact of doing it well. Use stories to connect the dots between the use of time, involvement of an interdisciplinary team, and the art of medicine. Stories are an essential part of a successful financial case because they illustrate cause and effect and increase the decision makers' confidence in the leader's ability to create changed outcomes.
  - Include measures that monitor service quality and consistency, such as time lag between consult request and consult completed. (If a good electronic health record and electronic order entry system is available, this can be done via an automated time/date stamp.) Other important measures might include "proportion of recommendations accepted." Team performance on measures such as these directly affects the extent of cost savings.
  - Set up professional billing operations. Hopefully this can be done by linking into established resources. However, it is important to pay attention to the details, meet with the billing manager, ensure useful reporting, and "own" responsibility for reviewing the coding, capture, and documentation of services so that workload is accurately captured and billable services are paid. Professionalism here is another marker of accountability.
  - Conduct retrospective financial analysis that is consistent with plans that can confirm the team's impact. This can be a combination of the "before and after cost-avoidance" methodology and customized analysis of pilots or initiatives designed based on the identified gaps. Good cases that illustrate impact are very important.

- Match growth plans with resource commitments. If gaps in care and team capacity are identified, the resources needed to take on new service commitments can be estimated. Doing this prospectively matches a future benefit (improved quality and costs) with a future resource cost. This is much more effective than incrementally overcommitting and then backtracking for resources.
- Build relationships and identify leader/sponsor/funder. The plans and offers can be effective only if they are aligned with specific priorities of someone who can approve resources. Build collaborative relationships so that requests are supported by others. Build the clinical capacity to meet patients' palliative care needs in a way that is explicitly aligned and defined.
- Take care of the team. The team is the biggest and most vulnerable asset. Self-care and professional development are essential to sustainability. Balancing operational commitments and quality goals for consistent operations with outreach efforts and educational initiatives is important. A high-functioning team that includes volunteers, partial full-time equivalent positions, and supportive interdisciplinary members who are not dedicated full time can significantly improve the capacity and effectiveness of the team and its visibility.
- Implement emerging best practices. Rapid innovation is occurring in the field and is shared through CAPC and AAHPM. Topics such as triggers (electronic screening for earlier recognition of palliative care needs),[4] IPAL-ICU, IPAL-ED, and others that will emerge provide efficient ways to add new value, be efficient, and stay fresh.
- Seek Joint Commission certification if the local hospital system values certification and external validation. This will increase the program's credibility, provide minimum requirements that support sustainable high-quality operations, and legitimize the program.
- Participate in the CAPC Registry. For more information go to www.capc.org.

REFERENCES

1. Morrison RS, Penrod JD, Cassel JB, et al. Cost savings associated with US hospital palliative care consultation programs. *Arch Intern Med.* 2008;168(16):1783–1790.
2. Morrison RS, Augustin R, Souvanna P, Meier DE. America's care of serious illness: a state-by-state report card on access to palliative care in our nation's hospitals. *J Palliat Med.* 2011;14(10):1094–1096.
3. Weissman DE, Meier DE. Identifying patients in need of a palliative care assessment in the hospital setting: a consensus report from the Center to Advance Palliative Care. *J Palliat Med.* 2011;14(1):17–23.
4. Agency for Healthcare Research and Quality. *National statistics, 1993–2009.* http://hcupnet.ahrq.gov/HCUPnet.jsp; Accessed October 1, 2012.
5. Anderson GF, Markovich P. Multinational comparisons of health systems data, 2010. www.commonwealth.org; 2011 Accessed October 1, 2012.
6. Goodman DC, Esty AR, Fisher ES, Chang C-H. *Trends and Variation in End-of-Life Care for Medicare Beneficiaries with Severe Chronic Illness.* Dartmouth Institute for Health Policy & Clinical Practice. 2011. http://www.dartmouthatlas.org/downloads/reports/EOL_Trend_Report_0411.pdf; Accessed October 6, 2012.
7. American Hospital Association. *Trendwatch Chartbook 2011: Utilization and Volume.* 2011. http://www.aha.org/research/reports/tw/chartbook/index.shtml; Accessed October 1, 2012.
8. Centers for Medicare and Medicaid Services. Summary of HCAHPS Survey Results. http://www.hcahpsonline.org; Accessed September 28, 2012.
9. Hospital Consumer Assessment of Healthcare Providers and Systems. *Fact sheet.* http://www.hcahpsonline.org/Facts.aspx; Accessed October 1, 2012.
10. Norton SA, Hogan LA, Holloway RG, Temkin-Greener H, Buckley MJ, Quill TE. Proactive palliative care in the medical intensive care unit: effects on length of stay for selected high-risk patients. *Crit Care Med.* 2007;35(6):1530–1535.
11. Temel JS, Greer JA, Muzikansky A, et al. Early palliative care for patients with metastatic non-small-cell lung cancer. *N Engl J Med.* 2010;363(8):733–742.
12. Rabow MW, Pantilat SZ, Kerr K, et al. The intersection of need and opportunity: assessing and capitalizing on opportunities to expand hospital-based palliative care services. *J Palliat Med.* 2010;13(10):1205–1210.
13. Siu AL, Spragens LH, Inouye SK, Morrison RS, Leff B. The ironic business case for chronic care in the acute care setting. *Health Aff (Millwood).* 2009;28(1):113–125.
14. Morrison RS, Dietrich J, Ladwig S, et al. Palliative care consultation teams cut hospital costs for Medicaid beneficiaries. *Health Aff (Millwood).* 2011;30(3):454–463.
15. QualityBLUE: a hospital pay-for-performance program. Level I and II program manual for fiscal year 2012. Pittsburgh: Highmark Inc; 2011. https://www.highmarkblueshield.com/health/pdfs/facility/level1-2.pdf; Accessed October 1, 2012.
16. Cassel JB, Kerr K, Pantilat S, Smith TJ. Palliative care consultation and hospital length of stay. *J Palliat Med.* 2010;13(6):761–767.
17. Smith TJ, Cassel JB. Cost and non-clinical outcomes of palliative care. *J Pain Symptom Manage.* 2009;3(1):32–44.

What Are the Arguments That Show Outpatient Palliative Care Is Beneficial to Medical Systems?

Michael W. Rabow

INTRODUCTION

Although much of the growth of palliative care in the United States has been fueled by the demonstration of cost avoidance in hospitals because of the care provided by inpatient palliative care consultation teams, the financial case for outpatient palliative care is less well developed or accepted. The evidence is preliminary, but it suggests that outpatient palliative care offers medical systems numerous potential benefits in caring efficiently for complex, seriously ill patients.

The Definition of Outpatient Palliative Care

Outpatient palliative care may be defined as palliative care services provided to patients not in hospitals. Sites of care include ambulatory practices and clinics, home, post–acute care facilities, and rehabilitation facilities. In such settings, patients typically receive palliative care *concurrently* with care intended to effect cure or management of disease. Although technically falling within the definition of outpatient palliative care, most consider hospice care separately when discussing the financial impacts of outpatient palliative care.

The Call for Outpatient Palliative Care

Although it is often noted that many patients spend some time in the hospital or the intensive care unit during the end period of their lives, the fact remains that most people spend most of their lives as outpatients. Hospital stays are typically short, and even patients with frequent hospital admissions spend the vast majority of their final years outside the hospital. It follows then from an epidemiological perspective that there is great need for palliative care to be provided outside the hospital in the outpatient setting.

The symptom burden among outpatients with serious illness is profound. Patients with cancer have been the subjects of most outpatient palliative care research, and data demonstrate that these patients suffer from numerous and distressing symptoms. Oncologists found that more than half of cancer patients need assistance with pain (81%), depression (69%), and fatigue (56%).[1] Uncontrolled symptoms result in increased health care usage.[2,3] Even symptoms that are rated mild in severity can create significant distress.[4]

Increasingly, palliative care has recognized the significant symptom burden among outpatients with non–cancer-related diagnoses. Common diseases considered are advanced heart disease (including congestive heart failure [CHF] and coronary artery disease), advanced lung disease (including chronic obstructive pulmonary disease [COPD] and pulmonary hypertension), neurological disease (including stroke and progressive diseases such as Alzheimer disease and amyotrophic lateral sclerosis), end-stage renal failure, and end-stage liver disease (including cirrhosis from alcohol and chronic hepatitis). Although much of palliative care has focused on patients with cancer, the palliative care needs of other patients may be just as significant. A 2009 study found symptom burden, depression, and spiritual distress similar among patients with symptomatic CHF and those with cancer.[5] Similarly, Fredheim and colleagues[6] demonstrated quality of life as poor for patients with chronic nonmalignant pain as for patients with cancer. Brierly and O'Brien[7] reported on the need to integrate palliative care into urological care. Harding and associates[8] reported on the benefits of palliative care in human immunodeficiency virus infection.[8]

In the setting of such significant symptom burden among outpatients, major medical organizations, including the Institute of Medicine, call for the provision of palliative care across sites of care, including in the outpatient setting, and concurrent with ongoing curative and disease-directed treatments.[9,10] The American Society of Clinical Oncology has called for concurrent oncological and palliative care, as well as comprehensive cancer care, including palliative care in multiple settings, including outpatient clinics, acute and long-term care facilities, and private homes.[11] Additionally, some professional organizations focused on non–cancer-related conditions have called for attention to palliative care among their members. The National Quality Forum emphasizes the needs for continuity of care among health care settings, for seamless follow-up, and for advance care planning in the community.[12,13]

The Growth of Outpatient Palliative Care

Outpatient palliative care appears to be a rapidly developing field.[14] Within cancer centers, Hui and colleagues[15] reported palliative care services available in 59% of National Cancer Institute (NCI) Cancer Centers but only in 22% of non–NCI-designated cancer centers. Conversely, in California, Berger[16] found only 8% of hospitals had an affiliated outpatient palliative care practice. Anecdotally, just in the last few years, outpatient practices seems to be developing quickly, either independently or as outgrowths of inpatient, oncology, or hospice-based palliative care services.

BENEFITS OF OUTPATIENT PALLIATIVE CARE TO MEDICAL SYSTEMS

Three major lines of reasoning support the presumption that outpatient palliative care is beneficial to health care systems. These include (1) the consequences of providing clinical benefit to patients and families, (2) the consequences of providing professional benefit to palliative care clinicians, and (3) improvements in efficiency of care within the medical system itself. The evidence base for many of these theoretical benefits to health care systems is limited, but is detailed in the following section.

Benefits to Patients and Families

Although gains in efficiency of care (and decreased overall costs of care) are key to medical systems, most organizations consider their financial success to be a by-product of the excellent clinical care they strive to provide. An emerging evidence base demonstrates the clinical benefits of outpatient palliative care to patients and families. Most studies show feasibility and high satisfaction with outpatient palliative care.[17,18] A few major observational trials have shown improvement in symptom burden among outpatients with cancer who are receiving palliative care. Strasser and colleagues[17] showed statistically significant improvement in pain, nausea, depression, anxiety, sleep, dyspnea, and well-being, but not in fatigue, anorexia, or drowsiness. Bruera and associates[19] showed improved symptom distress, depression, anxiety, and sensation of well-being between clinic visits in a cancer center symptom control clinic and at 2- and 4-week telephone follow-up. Follwell and colleagues[20] showed statistically significant improvements in pain, fatigue, nausea, depression, anxiety, drowsiness, appetite, dyspnea, insomnia, and constipation at 1 week and 1 month, as well as improvement in family satisfaction. Yennurajalingam and associates[21]

showed improvements in fatigue, pain, depression, anxiety, dyspnea, sleep, and well-being across an average 15-day interval between outpatient palliative care clinic visits in a large cancer center.

Among patients with non–cancer-related diagnoses as well as patients with cancer, we demonstrated improved dyspnea, insomnia, anxiety, and spiritual well-being among outpatients with advanced COPD, advanced CHF, or cancer in a primary care practice with concurrent palliative care consultation.[22]

Bakitas and colleagues[23] showed improved outcomes in a randomized trial of a psychoeducational, palliative care intervention by advanced practice nurses among patients in a rural comprehensive cancer center. The patients receiving the intervention experienced improved quality of life and depression, although not an improvement in symptom intensity, hospital length of stay, intensive care unit use, or emergency department visits.

In a widely reported and important study, Temel and associates[24] showed improved quality of life and depression, as well as 2.7 additional months of survival among patients with metastatic non–small cell lung cancer receiving early palliative care compared to those receiving usual care. Notably, the patients receiving early palliative care had prolonged survival despite less aggressive cancer-directed treatment.

With the emerging evidence and accumulating personal experience and word-of-mouth reports about the clinical benefits of outpatient palliative care, medical systems that offer palliative care may have an advantage in terms of competing for customers in the health care marketplace. The attention paid by medical systems to widely publicized surveys comparing hospitals and health systems, such as in *US News and World Report*, attests to the importance of reputation among care institutions. In competitive health care markets, patient satisfaction is paramount. Furthermore, institutions may be more competitive in these markets based on ability to provide up-to-date services such as quality outpatient palliative care. Unpublished data from the University of California, San Francisco demonstrate that patients seen in their outpatient palliative care clinic are very likely to recommend the medical center *because* of their palliative care experience.

Benefits to Palliative Care Clinicians

Many believe that palliative care work is satisfying and enlivening for clinicians.[25] Little published evidence exists, however, to support the common observation that the addition of outpatient palliative care can be a source of professional sustainability for inpatient palliative care clinicians who primarily work in the hospital. By working with outpatients, many clinicians may benefit because of the increased variety in their workday, by having more continuity in their relationships with patients, and by gaining a more complete education in the natural history of symptoms and decision making. From the perspective of medical systems, these benefits of outpatient palliative care help to sustain an effective and productive palliative care inpatient team. This allows the inpatient palliative care service to continue without interruption or degradation, thus making it more likely the inpatient team will produce the benefit of cost avoidance within the hospital.

Benefits to Medical Systems

In the current reimbursement environment, personnel and facilities costs for outpatient palliative care may increase costs for individual outpatient practices or hospices.[26] A survey of prominent, primarily academic medical center and comprehensive cancer center outpatient palliative care practices demonstrated that about half of operating revenues for these practices were supported by billing alone, with the need for institutional support for much of the rest.[27] However, a strong argument for financial benefit can be made for integrated health care systems in which the costs of care are summed across time and setting. The most direct benefits seen by medical systems from outpatient palliative care are those accrued via improvement in the efficiency of care within the system. Care integration, smoother transitions between care settings, and improved disease management are cost effective. The adage is that palliative care can help integrated systems provide *"the right care in the right place at the right time."* Within integrated systems charged with providing high-quality care for patients under a global budget, avoiding unnecessary costs while providing similar or better clinical care is a prime objective. The rise of the model of accountable care organizations (ACOs) is a tremendous opportunity for palliative care to be of service organizationally.

At least six mechanisms have been identified whereby outpatient palliative care might improve the efficiency of integrated medical systems. Primarily, these are based on an impact on health care usage resulting in decreased total costs. The published evidence to support these contentions is summarized in the following section.

Increased Hospice Use. Presuming costs for hospice care at the end of life are lower than continued attempts at cure or disease management, promoting appropriate referrals to and patient acceptance of hospice will save medical systems money while providing quality care. A 2007 study found that hospice use decreased Medicare program costs during the last year of life by $2309 on average for participants in hospice.[28]

Outpatient palliative care can increase hospice use by educating patients and families about the benefits of hospice care and by helping them choose hospice when those services are in line with the patients' goals. The advance care planning undertaken in the outpatient setting may promote hospice use among patients earlier than possible when it must wait for terminal hospitalization or catastrophic worsening of patients' well-being at the end of life. A study of Medicare decedents found that increasing length of stay in hospice would increase savings for about 70% of hospice participants.[28]

In a study analyzing the impact of comprehensive outpatient case management and enhanced hospice benefits for patients with advanced illness, one large national health plan found that patients receiving case management by nurse case managers extensively trained in palliative care had increased hospice use, increased hospice length of stay, and fewer and shorter inpatient stays compared to control patients. The study concluded that case management programs may allow insurance benefits to be liberalized without a negative impact on total costs.[29] A large health maintenance organization serving a Medicaid/Medicare population in the Midwest has unpublished data demonstrating that funding a palliative care team for patients at home to see patients for up to 9 sessions led to increased hospice admissions and an overall cost savings to the organization. The Advanced Illness Management (AIM) Program is an innovation of a large California-based health plan that provides home-based transitional and palliative care to patients with advanced illness. Participation in the AIM program was associated with an increase in hospice participation from 20% to 47%.[30]

Decreased Acute Care: Emergency Department Visits and Hospitalizations. Outpatient palliative care may be able to arm patients and families sufficiently with treatments, medications, and care plans to successfully manage symptoms at home that otherwise would prompt a visit to the emergency department for care. A significant number of hospitalizations are due to symptoms poorly managed in the outpatient setting. Ongoing symptom management as an outpatient may avoid exacerbations that might otherwise prompt an emergency room visit or hospitalizations. It is likely that provision of in-person, telephonic, or web-based supports from the palliative care team (including visiting nurses) will allow some patients to remain at home or in their nursing home. In a randomized, controlled trial of in-home palliative care for home bound, terminally ill patients, Brumley and colleagues[18] showed in-home palliative care led to fewer emergency department visits and hospitalizations, resulting in reduced costs in the intervention group. Participation in the AIM program was associated with a 68% decrease in hospitalizations for the first month in the program compared to the month before program participation, resulting in a savings of about $2000 per patient per month.[30]

Outpatient palliative care leading to earlier hospice care will typically result in fewer visits to the emergency department and fewer hospitalizations. Advance care planning accomplished in the outpatient setting may result in avoiding the hospital. There is strong evidence that outpatient advance care planning that leads to completion of the Physician Orders for Life Sustaining Treatment (POLST) form results in good comfort care and decreased transfer from nursing homes to hospitals.[31]

Decreased Hospital Length of Stay. Advance care planning accomplished in the outpatient palliative care setting may avert hospitalizations. In addition, it may have an impact on the course of hospitalizations. Outpatient advance care planning may allow hospitalizations to more closely mirror patients' goals, including avoiding lengthy stays in the intensive care unit and avoiding unwanted clinical evaluations and procedures that may delay discharge. Advance care planning conducted within the outpatient setting may lead to quicker transitions to hospice during a final hospitalization.

Importantly, many inpatient palliative care programs strive to "move upstream," seeing patients earlier in the disease process and transitioning from a service that primarily sees patients at the end of life to a palliative care program serving patients without respect to prognosis and length of life. Accordingly, as programs mature, many find the need to establish outpatient palliative care follow-up services. These outpatient services allow earlier hospital discharges because some necessary palliative care can be provided outside the hospital and more efficiently in lower-acuity settings such as home or nursing home. In the absence of robust outpatient palliative care, some patients may remain hospitalized because the inpatient palliative care service is their only source of palliative care.

Decreased Hospital Costs. Outpatient palliative care often focuses on communication about end-of-life goals. Even without affecting the *length* of hospitalization, outpatient advance care planning may improve the chance that a patient's hospital care avoids unwanted but costly interventions and workups. The impact of such advance care planning discussions has been associated with decreased health care costs generally. In particular, costs for the last week of life were $1041 lower for patients reporting end-of-life care discussions compared to similar patients who had not had such discussions.[32] This is despite the groups not differing in treatment preferences or acknowledgment of their illness. Of note as well, higher costs in this study were associated with worse quality of death. Advance care planning and end-of-life discussions in the outpatient setting may influence how patients use particularly expensive health care services, such as care in the intensive care unit, mechanical ventilation, and chemotherapy, at the end of life. Although data have not been published for outpatient palliative care consultation, inpatient palliative care has been associated in a randomized trial with decreased intensive care unit stays on readmissions (with resultant decreased costs).[33]

Decreased Hospital Readmissions. For integrated systems, the greatest cost savings may revolve around decreasing readmissions. Once patients are discharged from the hospital, outpatient palliative care may promote decreased readmissions through symptom management, continuity of care initiated in the hospital, or goal setting (including deciding on no further hospitalizations). As discussed earlier, a significant portion of rehospitalizations may be due primarily to symptoms inadequately managed in the outpatient setting. Such rehospitalizations may be averted by outpatient palliative care services.

Increased Efficiency of Specialists. Theoretically, palliative care services can save time for the referring specialist if the palliative care clinician assumes some of the work that the specialist is currently doing. For example, palliative care services can save referring clinicians time by conducting time-intense family meetings or advance care planning discussions. Another example is palliative care clinicians performing clinical tasks that limit the specialists' time to address specialty specific care (e.g., having the palliative care clinician manage pain while the oncologist manages chemotherapy). Given reimbursement structures, supporting oncologists to spend most of their time administering chemotherapy may create a financial advantage over having them spend significant time with less well-reimbursed activities. Such an arrangement can increase quality of care (through specialization of the tasks and performance of the task by an expert). Of course, if the specialist is not already performing the palliative care tasks, adding palliative care services may improve quality of care but potentially increase costs. Muir and colleagues[34] showed time saved when palliative care services were embedded in outpatient oncology practices, based on the assumption that the services provided by palliative care clinicians would otherwise have had to be performed by the oncologists.

Cautions and Limitations of the Data

Although great promise exists for realizing the potential benefits of outpatient palliative care to medical systems, the limitations of the data presented here must be recognized. Few randomized trials[24] and no multicenter trials have demonstrated support for the arguments made here. Large trials have not been conducted. Importantly, some data suggest that outpatient palliative care might be cost neutral[22] or might increase costs when added on to individual clinics or hospices. Depending on the structure of financing and reimbursement for any particular health system, decreased hospitalizations may in fact create a loss of revenue.[30]

CONCLUSION AND SUMMARY

The epidemiological and clinical benefits of outpatient palliative care are now well-established. Outpatient palliative care can improve symptoms (physical, psychological, and spiritual) for patients and thus improve the quality of health care. Paying for *quality* care may be a key mission for many medical systems, but there is an emerging *financial* argument for medical systems to promote outpatient palliative care as well. Patient satisfaction and palliative care clinician sustainability likely offer value to health systems. Through its ability to assist patients in determining and choosing the level and location of care to meet their goals, outpatient palliative care can improve the efficiency of health care, resulting in cost savings for integrated health systems. A developing evidence base supports the argument that outpatient palliative care accrues cost savings to medical systems through earlier hospice referrals; decreased frequency, length, or costs of hospitalization or readmissions; and increased efficiency of referring specialists. Outpatient palliative care offers great promise and a close alignment with the missions of developing ACOs, whose success may well hinge on scrupulous disease management, integration of care, and caring for the seriously ill patients with complex issues that palliative care serves well.

SUMMARY RECOMMENDATIONS

- Medical systems may realize benefits from providing excellent outpatient palliative care in the following ways:
  - A competitive advantage with consumers who recognize the positive clinical outcomes of outpatient palliative care
  - A workforce advantage because of sustainability for their palliative care clinicians adding variety to their inpatient work
  - A financial advantage with improved efficiency as a result of the impact of outpatient palliative care on hospice, emergency department, hospital, and specialty care.

REFERENCES

1. Whitmer KM, Pruemer JM, Nahleh ZA, Jazieh AR. Symptom management needs of oncology outpatients. *J Palliat Med.* 2006;9(3):628–630.
2. McCorkle R, Jeon S, Ercolano E, Schwartz P. Healthcare utilization in women after abdominal surgery for ovarian cancer. *Nurs Res.* 2011;60(1):47–57.
3. Burke TA, Wisniewski T, Ernst FR. Resource utilization and costs associated with chemotherapy-induced nausea and vomiting (CINV) following highly or moderately emetogenic chemotherapy administered in the US outpatient hospital setting. *Support Care Cancer.* 2011;19(1):131–140.
4. Kirkova J, Walsh D, Rybicki L, et al. Symptom severity and distress in advanced cancer. *Palliat Med.* 2010;24(3):330–339.
5. Bekelman DB, Rumsfeld JS, Havranek EP, et al. Symptom burden, depression, and spiritual well-being: a comparison of heart failure and advanced cancer patients. *J Gen Intern Med.* 2009;24(5):592–598.
6. Fredheim OM, Kaasa S, Fayers P, Saltnes T, Jordhøy M, Borchgrevink PC. Chronic non-malignant pain patients report as poor health-related quality of life as palliative cancer patients. *Acta Anaesthesiol Scand.* 2008;52(1):143–148.
7. Brierly RD, O'Brien TS. The importance of palliative care in urology. *Urol Int.* 2008;80(1):13–18.
8. Harding R, Easterbrook P, Higginson IJ, Karus D, Raveis VH, Marconi K. Access and equity in HIV/AIDS palliative care: a review of the evidence and responses. *Palliat Med.* 2005;19(3):251–258.
9. Institute of Medicine National Cancer Policy Board. *Improving Palliative Care for Cancer.* Washington, DC: Institute of Medicine; 2001:44.
10. Levy MH, Back A, Benedetti C, et al. NCCN clinical practice guidelines in oncology: palliative care. *J Natl Compr Canc Netw.* 2009;7(4):436–473.
11. Ferris FD, Bruera E, Cherny N, et al. Palliative cancer care a decade later: accomplishments, the need, next steps: from the American Society of Clinical Oncology. *J Clin Oncol.* 2009;27(18):3052–3058.
12. National Quality Forum. *A National Framework and Preferred Practices for Palliative and Hospice Care Quality: A Consensus Report.* Washington, DC: National Quality Forum; 2006. www.qualityforum.org. Accessed May 9, 2012.
13. National Consensus Project for Quality Palliative Care. Clinical practice guidelines for quality palliative care. National Consensus for Quality Palliative Care; 2004. www.nationalconsensusproject.org. Accessed May 5, 2012.
14. Meier DE, Beresford L. Outpatient clinics are a new frontier for palliative care. *J Palliat Med.* 2008;11(6):823–828.
15. Hui D, Elsayem A, De la Cruz M, et al. Availability and integration of palliative care at US cancer centers. *JAMA.* 2010;303(11):1054–1061.
16. Berger GN, O'Riordan DL, Kerr K, Pantilat SZ. Prevalence and characteristics of outpatient palliative care services in California. *Arch Intern Med.* 2011;171(22):2057–2059.
17. Strasser F, Sweeney C, Willey J, Benisch-Tolley S, Palmer JL, Bruera E. Impact of a half-day multidisciplinary symptom control and palliative care outpatient clinic in a comprehensive cancer center on recommendations, symptom intensity, and patient satisfaction: a retrospective descriptive study. *J Pain Symptom Manage.* 2004;27(6):481–491.
18. Brumley R, Enguidanos S, Jamison P, et al. Increased satisfaction with care and lower costs: results of a randomized trial of in-home palliative care. *J Am Geriatr Soc.* 2007;55(7):993–1000.
19. Bruera E, Michaud M, Vigano A, Neumann CM, Watanabe S, Hanson J. Multidisciplinary symptom control clinic in a cancer center: a retrospective study. *Support Care Cancer.* 2001;9(3):162–168.
20. Follwell M, Burman D, Le LW, et al. Phase II study of an outpatient palliative care intervention in patients with metastatic cancer. *J Clin Oncol.* 2009;27(2):206–213.
21. Yennurajalingam S, Urbauer DL, Casper KL, et al. Impact of a palliative care consultation team on cancer-related symptoms in advanced cancer patients referred to an outpatient supportive care clinic. *J Pain Symptom Manage.* 2011;41(1):49–56.
22. Rabow MW, Dibble SL, Pantilat SZ, McPhee SJ. The comprehensive care team: a controlled trial of outpatient palliative medicine consultation. *Arch Intern Med.* 2004;164(1):83–91.
23. Bakitas M, Lyons KD, Hegel MT, et al. Effects of a palliative care intervention on clinical outcomes in patients with advanced cancer: the Project ENABLE II randomized controlled trial. *JAMA.* 2009;302(7):741–749.
24. Temel JS, Greer JA, Muzikansky A, et al. Early palliative care for patients with metastatic non-small-cell lung cancer. *N Engl J Med.* 2010;363(8):733–742.
25. Sinclair S. Impact of death and dying on the personal lives and practices of palliative and hospice care professionals. *CMAJ.* 2011;183(2):180–187.
26. Passik SD, Ruggles C, Brown G, et al. Is there a model for demonstrating a beneficial financial impact of initiating a palliative care program by an existing hospice program? *Palliat Support Care.* 2004;2(4):419–423.
27. Rabow MW, Smith AK, Braun JL, Weissman DE. Outpatient palliative care practices. *Arch Intern Med.* 2010;170(7):654–655.
28. Taylor Jr. DH, Ostermann J, Van Houtven CH, Tulsky JA, Steinhauser K. What length of hospice use maximizes reduction in medical expenditures near death in the US Medicare program? *Soc Sci Med.* 2007;65(7):1466–1478.
29. Spettell CM, Rawlins WS, Krakauer R, et al. A comprehensive case management program to improve palliative care. *J Palliat Med.* 2009;12(9):827–832.
30. Meyer H. Changing the conversation in California about care near the end of life. *Health Aff (Millwood).* 2011;30(3):390–393.
31. Tolle SW, Tilden VP, Nelson CA, Dunn PM. A prospective study of the efficacy of the physician order form for life-sustaining treatment. *J Am Geriatr Soc.* 1998;46(9):1097–1102.
32. Zhang B, Wright AA, Huskamp HA, et al. Health care costs in the last week of life: associations with end-of-life conversations. *Arch Intern Med.* 2009;169(5):480–488.
33. Gade G, Venohr I, Conner D, et al. Impact of an inpatient palliative care team: a randomized control trial. *J Palliat Med.* 2008;11(2):180–190.
34. Muir JC, Daly F, Davis MS, et al. Integrating palliative care into the outpatient, private practice oncology setting. *J Pain Symptom Manage.* 2010;40(1):126–135.

Chapter 72

What Is the Effect of Serious Illness on Caregivers?

Deborah Waldrop and Jean S. Kutner

INTRODUCTION AND SCOPE OF THE PROBLEM

Demographic patterns have shifted during the past century, and life expectancy has increased such that currently most people die later in life.[1,2] In 2008, more than half of all the deaths in the world resulted from chronic illnesses. Noncommunicable diseases such as cancer, heart disease, and lung disease accounted for 36 million, or 63%, of the 57 million deaths worldwide in 2008.[1] Of every 10 deaths in the United States, 7 occur at the end of chronic illness.[3] Death from one or more comorbid chronic conditions happens slowly and over time, as physical and functional abilities dwindle and there is increased need for assistance with activities of daily living (ADLs). The Centers for Disease Control and Prevention estimate that about one quarter of people with chronic conditions need assistance with one or more daily activity,[3] and projections indicate that these numbers will continue to grow. The accompanying burden of disease has been viewed as "a slow-motion catastrophe."[4]

Families are often assumed to be readily available, willing, and able to provide care for people who are seriously ill and facing physical decline, but this is not always possible.[5] Although definitions of caregivers vary, in general, *informal* caregivers are considered to be unpaid family members and friends who assist an adult with one or more ADLs. *Formal* caregivers are considered to be paid professionals who provide health care. Currently, the number of informal family caregivers in the United States who provide personal assistance for adults with a chronic

illness is estimated to be 29.2 million. The Family Caregivers Alliance (FCA) estimates that the number of family caregivers is expected increase to 37 million by the year 2050.[6] Many family members readily assume caregiving roles as an extension of a caring relationship, but the significant physical, psychosocial, and financial burdens of caregiving for people with serious illness cannot be overstated.

Caregiving involves numerous types of care that can range in frequency from daily care (5-7 days/week), intermittent care (2-4 days/week), to rare care. Active (daily plus intermittent) caregivers, compared with nonactive (rare) caregivers, are more often women who are widowed and over age 60. Intermittent caregivers are more commonly children, other relatives, or friends and are more educated, active in paid work, and wealthier. Financial burden, the nature of the illness, the ability to adapt to loss, and the need for grief support also differ by the intensity of the caregiving experience.[6,7]

Caregiving has been conceptualized as a series of shifting configurations within relationships and a process that restructures lives. The life course perspective is a theoretical framework that views life transitions as both simultaneous and continuous in the lives of individuals and their families.[8] Considering caregiving from a life-course perspective, the sequence of transitions changes both individual and family development.[9] The transitions in a serious illness also have been viewed as the "caregiving career" which includes (1) preparation for and acquisition of the caregiver role, (2) enactment of caregiving responsibilities, and (3) disengagement from caregiving.[10] Each stage of the caregiving career generates distinct types of primary stressors that are situation-specific (e.g., learning medication management) and simultaneous secondary stressors that emerge from other life roles (e.g., work, parenting). Each caregiver brings social, personal, and material resources and coping strategies that moderate the stressors that accompany caregiving in a serious illness.[10]

The impact of caregiving on informal caregivers is complex and multifaceted. Caregivers are often referred to as "hidden patients" because they suffer from stress-induced problems that are associated with the caregiving role.[11] Informal family caregiving has significant effects on caregivers' lives in six domains: (1) physical and mental health, (2) family communication, (3) social impact, (4) work and finances, (5) social identity, and (6) positive impacts.[5] As a result, caregivers have the need for psychological and emotional support; information; help with personal, nursing, and medical care of the patient; assistance at night; respite care; and financial assistance.[12] This chapter addresses current research that illustrates the ways in which serious illness affects caregivers. Table 72-1 provides an outline of the key aspects that should be considered when working with caregivers of patients with serious illness.

RELEVANT PATHOPHYSIOLOGY

Physical and Mental Health

Caregiving for people with serious illness has potentially profound effects on the physical and mental health of caregivers. Caregiving strain has been associated with higher risk for the development of cardiovascular disease as a result of this suboptimal lifestyle and its related psychosocial stressors,[13] higher estimated stroke risk,[14] and mortality.[15,16] However, the interrelationship between providing care and the continuous exposure to a loved one with serious health problems is complex. Brown and colleagues[17] found that spending at least 14 hours per week providing

---

TABLE 72-1. Important Aspects to Consider When Working With Caregivers of Patients With Serious Illness

Elements to Assess When Taking a Comprehensive History From the Patient and Caregiver
Consider the patient and family as a unit of care
Determine the patient's level of function and associated psychosocial needs
Explore family functioning
Consider caregiver physical and mental health
Assess for family conflict
Anticipate individual and family grief

Communication Characteristics
Timely
Frequent and consistent
Congruent with the need
Clear, honest and understandable
Comprehensive when addressing prognosis and progression of the illness
Focused on the patient's desires, address aspects that require communication and planning
Encourage advance care planning
Discuss goals of care, including end-of-life care, hydration and nutrition, "Do Not Resuscitate" (DNR) order
Provide support and information
Connect patient and family to available resources
Focus on what the patient would want
Address the patient's comfort
Understand that some caregivers do not want to bother clinicians and others may reject support

Modified from Bascom PB, Tolle SW. Care of the family when the patient is dying. *West J Med.* 1995;163(3):292-266; and Hudson PL, Aranda S, Kristjanson LJ. Meeting the supportive needs of family caregivers in palliative care: challenges for health professionals. *J Palliat Med.* 2004;7(1):19-25.

---

care to a spouse actually predicted decreased mortality for the caregiver, which may suggest that in some circumstances, caregivers benefit from providing care. Moreover, although resilience is seen to be a key factor to caregivers' health and adaptation, clinical recognition of the variations in caregiver hardiness becomes central when providers are working with families who will be engaging in long-term informal caregiving.[18]

Serious illnesses have distinct trajectories with diagnosis-specific symptom clusters that present unique caregiving challenges. Caregivers must typically learn complicated and unfamiliar treatments in the home setting with only limited education and support. Difficult symptoms such as increasing pain, dysphagia, and shortness of breath can be emotionally distressing for a loved one to witness and feel responsible to manage. Caregivers must assess, report, and treat symptom exacerbations. The caregivers themselves can become stressed by providing treatments they perceive to be painful and difficult for their loved one with serious illness.

An extensive body of literature describes the unique and distinct caregiving dynamics that accompany Alzheimer disease. In fact, much of what is known about caregiving has emerged from research with caregivers of people with Alzheimer disease. Caregiving for people with dementia is time consuming and isolating. Caregivers often spend more than 40 hours per week assisting patients with ADLS and instrumental ADLs (IADLS) and report feeling that they are "on duty" 24 hours a day and ended or reduced employment to address the demands of caregiving.[19] Caregivers for people with Alzheimer disease have also been found to have a greater propensity for developing serious illness themselves; this may possibly reflect reluctance to schedule necessary medical care or attend to their own needs because caregiving requires so much time and focus.[20] Caregivers have also demonstrated high levels of depressive symptoms while caring for a relative with dementia; some express considerable relief at the death.[19] Hospice care is available for people with dementia, but the significant lack of awareness about hospice and palliative care (in both families and providers) remains a major barrier to hospice usage for people with Alzheimer disease and their caregivers.[21]

The trajectories of progressive neuromuscular diseases such as amyotrophic lateral sclerosis (ALS) and Parkinson disease involve increasing needs for physical care while observing a loved one lose all basic abilities. In addition, caregivers face difficult transitions and decisions about respiratory support and nutrition during the final stages of these diseases. Caregivers of people with ALS are faced with care for a loved one who must decide whether to choose long-term mechanical ventilation (LTMV) and a tracheostomy or death. Caregiver burden and satisfaction were assessed in a sample comparing people who chose LTMV with those who did not; burden and depressive symptoms were higher in the LTMV group[22] Similarly, there is significant physical and psychological impact of caring for someone who is in the advanced stages of Parkinson disease.[23] Observing long-term deterioration that robs the person of social and emotional coping coupled with profound deterioration and complications at the end of life creates significant emotional and psychosocial impact. Five emergent themes describe the experience of caregiving for people with Parkinson disease: (1) the emotional impact of the diagnosis with fear of the future and the unknown; (2) a need to stay connected with the ill person when speech and communication are diminished; (3) enduring financial hardships; (4) management of physical challenges such as falls, rigidity, total care; and (5) a need for help in the advanced stages, with choking and the dying process.[24]

Caregivers for people with advanced respiratory illnesses deal with unique stressors. Most people with lung disease and their caregivers fear dying, shortness of breath, and the experience of suffocation. The trajectory of end-stage lung disease typically involves a long, slow decline with increasing care needs that include at least intermittent hands-on care for an average of 41 months. Although caregivers hope for a peaceful passing, only 31.1% assessed their loved one as "comfortable" or "very comfortable" in the last stage of lung disease.[25] Caregivers for people with cystic fibrosis report that particularly distressing symptoms occur during the last week of life and include dyspnea, fatigue, anorexia, anxiety, pain, and coughing. Treatments are viewed as necessary but uncomfortable.[26] Some caregivers believe that symptoms cannot be controlled at life's end and harbor concerns that the use of opioids and anxiolytics will hasten death.

Caregivers for people with serious illnesses experience anticipatory grief in various ways and at different stages of the illness. However, disease-specific features may influence the grief process. For example, across the duration of human immunodeficiency virus infection and acquired immunodeficiency syndrome (HIV/AIDS), stigmatization and multiple losses may make it difficult for caregivers to work through grief.[27] Anticipatory loss is a common dynamic in cancer, particularly in light of the pervasive uncertainty, together with fears of recurrence and death. Recurrence increases psychosocial distress.[28]

Caregiving during the final stages of a serious illness occurs within the context of physiological and psychological changes that may not be understood or anticipated by family members. Although emotional burdens are felt by most family members, families who choose to have their loved one die at home take on enormous direct caregiving burdens. Caring for a dying relative is demanding, and often family caregivers have unmet needs for information, support, and guidance from health care professionals.[29] Anorexia and cachexia, breathlessness, the accumulation of respiratory tract secretions ("death rattle"), terminal delirium, and mottling are common in people who are dying[30] but often unfamiliar to family members. The persistence of a dying person's symptoms generates parallel distress in family members.[31]

Caregiving at the end of life has been described as "jumping into the abyss of someone else's dying." Themes developed from interviews with caregivers illustrate how caregiving is unpredictable, intense, complex, frightening, and anguishing, but also profoundly moving and affirming. Caregiving completely dissolves familiar social boundaries.[32] The powerful experiences of end-stage caregiving have been characterized as involving the comprehension of terminality (grasping the combination of prognostic information, physical and cognitive decline, personality changes, and role losses), addressing the need for near-acute care, assuming the executive functions of caregiving, and facilitating final decision making, perhaps for a person who was always in control.[33] Caregivers for people who are at the end of life report a greater sense of overload and sense of captivity than at other stages of a serious illness.[34]

Advance care planning, which involves frank and honest discussion about the dying process, advance directives, and conversations about goals of care are most effective when they occur well in advance of the terminal stage of an illness.[35,36] Although most family members feel emotional burdens, families who choose to have their loved one die at home take on enormous direct caregiving burdens. In addition to information about prognosis, disease progression, and the dying process, these caregivers need supplies, education on caregiving skills, and logistical support.[37]

Family Communication

The nature and quality of family communication significantly influences the caregiving experience. Conversations about illness and death can be painful, difficult, and laden with emotion. The level of open communication has been related to caregivers' emotional reactions (e.g., emotional exhaustion, depression), feelings of self-efficacy, and the length of time spent in the caregiving role.[38] The intense energy that is required to cope with the physical, psychological, social, and spiritual aspects of a loved one's illness also generates stress and fatigue that can cause conflict within families and with providers.[39]

Communication about serious illness can generate dissimilar responses in caregivers and care recipients. Fried and colleagues[40] found that disagreement about communication preferences is frequent in caregiver–patient pairs. In a sample of responding caregivers who desired more communication, 83.1% of the patients did not. In a sample of responding patients who desired more communication, 66.7% of the caregivers did not. More communication was desired by 39.9% of caregivers, and 37.3% reported that communication was difficult. Caregivers who wanted more communication had higher burden scores.[40] The level of openness is influenced by personality traits, the history of the relationship, the duration and intensity of caregiving, and the emotional responses to the experience.[38]

Family caregiving for people with serious illnesses occurs within the network of complex social and family relationships. Providers may encounter various patterns of care, three of which have been identified as (1) care dyads who are aging, who are chronically ill, and who compensate for each other's deficits; (2) people who are cared for by a constellation or system of multiple family members; and (3) family care chains in which one person functions as a caregiver for one but the care recipient of another (e.g., older spouses with adult children).[41] Families also respond to the advanced stages of serious illness in varied modes or styles. Family response styles can be reactive when the illness generates intense emotional responses, fused when the illness and decline are seen as shared or "we" experiences, dissonant when family members have diametrically opposed and conflicting viewpoints, resigned when death is anticipated, and assertive or advocative when the patient's vulnerability ignites responses. Providers who can recognize, acknowledge, and engage families with varying responses to serious illness can ease patients' suffering and help families manage the often unknown terrain of dying and prepare for life without the loved one.

Family–provider communication is also central to caregiver adaptation over the course of a serious illness. Cherlin and colleagues[42] investigated caregivers' perceptions of physicians' communication and found that there is little concordance between families' and providers' perceptions of their communication. Caregivers reported that physicians did not tell them the patient's illness was incurable, they were not given life expectancy information, and hospice was not introduced.[43] To ascertain patient–clinician and caregiver–clinician concurrence about prognostic discussions, Fried and colleagues[44] gathered and subsequently matched independent reports. In 46% of patient–clinician and 34% of caregiver–clinician pairs, the clinician reported saying the patient could die of the underlying disease, but the patient or caregiver said this was not discussed. In 23% of patient–clinician and 30% of patient–caregiver pairs, the clinician reported discussing an approximate life expectancy, but the patient or caregiver reported there was no discussion.[44]

Caregivers typically overestimate cancer patients' symptom burden, and accuracy does not improve over time. Improving caregiver accuracy may boost the positive effects of cognitive-behavioral interventions designed to improve cancer patients' quality of life.[45] Greater attention toward a coordinated approach to discussing options in the setting of serious illness is needed.[46] Communication about the nature of illness, symptoms, terminality, life expectancy, and prognosis is a major issue in family communication and encounters with providers. Open, honest, direct, and frank discussion of a poor prognosis, end-of-life needs, and goals of care can be difficult to initiate and to participate in, but their importance cannot be underestimated.

Social Impact

The impact of serious illness reverberates through the social context with implications for family and social support systems, communities, and the network of health care professionals. A growing societal trend toward delivering more illness-related care in the home is driven by both family preferences and reimbursement policies.[47] This pressure changes the manner of health care delivery in serious illness, placing greater responsibilities for increasingly complex caregiving on family members who are not trained health care professionals and who are simultaneously managing intense emotions as a loved one declines.

Cultural beliefs and values influence the consideration of options for health care in serious illness. Fervor about the importance of advance directive discussions and the availability of end-of-life choices has reached an all-time high, particularly after difficult cases that receive intense public attention.[48] However, such discussions are not consistent with cultural, religious, and social values in all communities. For example, after measuring levels of acculturation, Desanto-Madeya and colleagues[49] found that caregivers who were less acculturated were more likely to choose the insertion of a feeding tube, more likely to perceive that they were given too much information from their doctors, and less inclined to seek mental health care than those with higher acculturation scores. Additionally, the use of living wills or a durable power for health care is influenced by culture and sociodemographic variables.[50] Caregivers who were less acculturated felt their religious and spiritual needs were supported by both the community and the medical system, had higher degrees of self-efficacy, and had stronger more supportive family relationships.[49]

Sensitive cross-cultural and religious care can be particularly challenging at the end of life. Culturally sensitive end-of-life care involves respect, communication, and consideration of environmental desires (e.g., beliefs about the use of nursing home, hospice, hospital care).[51] Cultural differences also shape the caregiving experience. For example, cultural values of denial and secrecy about prognosis and a collective, family-centered orientation can be highly influential on decisions regarding hospice for Latinos but not non-Latinos. Discussing hospice with a patient and family who prefer not to discuss a terminal prognosis can present challenges for providers.[51]

Patients and family members sometimes express feelings of abandonment by their health care providers as they end treatments, have fewer visits to the office, and make the transition to end-of-life care. The sense of abandonment has been related to the loss of continuity between patient and physician; at the time of death or after, feelings of abandonment resulted from lack of closure for patients and families. Nonabandonment at the end of life involves bridging the gap when patients no longer come to the provider by (1) providing continuity, of both expertise and the patient–physician relationship and (2) facilitating the closure of an important relationship.[52]

Health care professionals can enhance their support for caregivers during bereavement. Bereavement care is a fundamental component of palliative care, and family caregivers identify significant benefits from receiving help from health care professionals in preparing for and responding to a loved one's dying and death.[53] Providers can assess the potential for high-risk grief responses and develop techniques to address the grief process in advance of the death.[54]

Work and Finances

The fiscal reality of prolonged caregiving is that families can experience significant financial burdens. A majority of people with serious illness who require caregiving from a family member fear leaving family members with debt.[55] Serious illness can cause economic devastation for families.[56] Burns and colleagues[57] found that nearly as many men as women balance work and caregiving (38% worked full-time). Families of younger and more functionally dependent patients with a lower annual income are most likely to report the loss of most or all of the family's savings.[58] Interviews with caregivers indicated that in 20% of cases, a family member had to leave a job to provide care for the seriously ill person. In nearly one third of these families most or all of the family's savings was used, and 29% reported the loss of the major source of income. The loss of the family's savings was more likely when the seriously ill person needed assistance with three or more ADLs, the annual family income was below $25,000, and the caregivers were younger than 45 years of age. Financial burden also differs with the intensity of need and caregiving.[6,7] The life-course impact of caregiving with forced occupational and financial strain has not been measured but most certainly also has the potential to be emotionally devastating.

Social Identity

Caregivers' social identity emerges from the family, cultural, and social context; thus, becoming a caregiver changes the preexisting relationship with a care recipient. As dependency increases care needs, issues, and concerns become the central focus replacing a focus on activities, plans, and shared mutual experiences. The need to provide intimate, personal care for a spouse, or parent (especially the opposite gender) moves people and families into an unknown realm.[32] Previous studies indicate that spouses are the most likely caregivers for all racial groups[6] except for African-American women, who identify their daughters as the most likely caregivers.[59] Caregiving is most often provided by older, close family members, but large numbers of young people (15-29 years of age) also provide hands-on care for people with advanced illness. Given the unexpected responsibility of caregiving in young adulthood and considerable influence that caregiving has on the life course, theirs may a more negative experience than for older adults.[57]

Family caregivers are often called on to take a loved one's perspective (e.g., What would she tell us if she could?) or make substituted judgments for the patient, requiring them to speak from the patient's perspective.[60] Caregivers who hold the status of Health Care Proxy (HCP) or Durable Power of Attorney for Healthcare (DPAHC) face the additional stress that accompanies substituted decision making. Pruchno and colleagues[61] found that African-American spouses were more likely than white spouses to indicate that they believed that the patient would be more inclined to continue dialysis under hypothetical conditions. However, differences in spouse substituted judgments between African-American and white spouses were found to be directly related to racial differences in perceptions about patient health and caregiver burden and indirectly related to spouses' fear of death and participation in religious services.

Positive Impacts

Caregiving has been found to be a source of positive affect, feeling useful, appreciating closeness with the person who is ill, and experiencing pride in the accomplishments of caregiving.[62] Among family members, positive effects were found for caregiving burden, depression, and anxiety; these effects were strongest for nondementing illnesses and for interventions that targeted only the family member and addressed relationship issues.[63] Caregiving interventions have been found to decrease burden and negative appraisal by increasing impact and satisfaction.[64] The term *gain* has been used to refer to positive appraisal of the caregiving experience and defined broadly as the extent to which one views the caregiver role as enhancing and enriching.[65] Other concepts used to express positive impacts of caregiving have been benefits, rewards, satisfaction, pleasure, enjoyment, uplifts, and positive aspects.[65] Recognition that a family member is dying can bring a new perspective and sense of strength to caregivers, who may need help to navigate the uncertainty of the dying process.[66] The opportunity to engage in meaningful activities that create important memories is important in the final stages and transitions before death.[33] There is a need to further explore caregiver meaning making, positive benefits, and influences on families for incorporation in palliative care.[67]

Caregivers' sense of security results from the belief that health care services will be provided by competent professionals; feeling they will have timely access to needed care, services, and information; and being secure in their own identity and self-worth as a caregiver and individual. The concept of security moves beyond description of individual satisfaction or dissatisfaction.[68]

SUMMARY OF EVIDENCE REGARDING TREATMENT RECOMMENDATIONS

The assessment of burden associated with caregiving can serve as an important intervention. First, recognition of the health and mental health effects on the caregiver can help increase awareness of the stress and the need for support and assistance. In addition, a provider's recognition of a caregivers' burden can generate important secondary effects that may go unnoticed. Second, the assessment of caregiver burden and emotional distress can lead to prevention of additional long-term health effects and mortality. Finally, assessment and intervention of caregiver burden can help families navigate the uncertainty and move toward important life closure. Numerous assessment tools are available, but individual providers will benefit from selecting tools that fit their patient population. A list of selected websites with caregiver assessment tools appears in Table 72-2.

KEY MESSAGES TO PATIENTS AND FAMILIES

Caregiving for a seriously ill loved one has considerable physical and psychological effects on the caregiver, both negative and positive. The effects of caregiving are multifactorial and depend on the nature of the patient's illness, the relationship between the patient and the caregiver, and other sociodemographic factors (e.g., age, socioeconomic status). Clinicians must not only be aware of these effects but also encourage caregivers to ask for assistance from the health care team when needed. Information about the nature of the illness and its expected trajectory is critical to the caregiver; clinicians should provide this information as well as encourage caregivers to be inquisitive about it.

TABLE 72-2. Websites With Caregiver Assessment Tools

Providers are encouraged to assess family caregivers for situation-specific stressors. Although numerous assessment tools are available, providers alone can identify those that would best serve the caregivers with whom they work. A list of sample websites with links to assessment tools is provided.

TIME: Toolkit of Instruments to Measure End-of-Life Care http://www.chcr.brown.edu/pcoc/toolkit.htm

Michigan Dementia Coalition http://www.dementiacoalition.org/resources/

International Palliative Care Family Carer Research Collaboration http://www.centreforpallcare.org/index.php/research/ipcfcrc/

Family Caregiver Alliance http://www.caregiver.org/caregiver/jsp/content_node.jsp?nodeid=1717

American Psychological Association http://www.apa.org/pi/about/publications/caregivers/practice-settings/assessment/tools/index.aspx

National Palliative Care Research Center http://www.npcrc.org/resources/resources_show.htm?doc_id=376172

CONCLUSION AND SUMMARY

Caregiving has a whole-life effect on people who provide hands-on assistance and emotional support for a loved one. Providers are encouraged to recognize that the effects of serious illness ripple through families and affect physical and mental health, family communication, financial stability, and social relationships. Providers can assist families in experiencing the positive effects of caregiving. Additional research is needed to inform evidence-based interventions and to assess caregivers who are at risk for adverse outcomes.

SUMMARY RECOMMENDATIONS

- Whole patient care should include assessment of the patient and family as a unit of care. Clinicians need to consider the following factors when working with patients with serious illness and their families: patient level of function and associated psychosocial needs, family functioning, caregiver physical and mental health, family conflict, and individual and family grief.
- Communication with patients and families should be timely; frequent and consistent; congruent with the need; clear, honest, and understandable; germane to prognosis and progression of the illness; and focused on the patient's desires.
- Clinicians should help patients and caregivers anticipate and plan for the end of the patient's life. This needs to include encouraging advance care planning; discussing the goals of care including end-stage care, hydration and nutrition, and DNR; providing support and information; connecting the patient and family to available resources; focusing on what the patient would want; and addressing the patient's comfort. It is important to remember that some caregivers do not want to feel like they are bothering clinicians and some caregivers may reject support.

REFERENCES

1. World Health Organization. *Life expectancy at birth.* http://www.who.org; 2011. Accessed October 1, 2012.
2. National Center for Health Statistics. 2010. http://www.cdc.gov/nchs/; Accessed on May 5, 2011.
3. Centers for Disease Control and Prevention. *Noncummunicable diseases.* 2011. http://www.cdc.gov; Accessed on October 1, 2012.
4. Chan M. The worldwide rise of chronic noncommunicable diseases: a slow-motion catastrophe. 2011. http://www.who.int/dg/speeches/2011/ministerial_conf_ncd_20110428/en/index.html; Accessed October 1, 2012.
5. Payne S. White Paper on improving support for family carers in palliative care I. *Eur J Palliat Care.* 2010;15(5):238–245.
6. Family Caregiver Alliance. http://www.caregiver.org; 2010. Accessed October 1, 2012.
7. Abernethy A, Burns C, Wheeler J, et al. Defining distinct caregiver subpopulations by intensity of end-of-life care provided. *Palliat Med.* 2009;23(1):66–79.
8. O'Rand AM, Campbell RT. On reestablishing the phenomenon and specifying ignorance: theory development and research design in aging. In: Bengtson VL, Schaie KW, eds. *Handbook of Theories of Aging.* Thousand Oaks, CA: Sage; 1999:59–78.
9. Pearlin LI, Skaff MM. Stress and the life course: a paradigmatic alliance. *Gerontologist.* 1996;36(2):239–247.
10. Aneshensel CS, Pearlin LI, Mullen JT, et al. *Profiles in Caregiving: The Unexpected Career.* San Diego: Academic Press; 1995.

11. Zarit SH. Caregiver assessment: voices and views from the field—a research perspective. In: *Report from a national Consensus Development Conference*. 2. Family Caregiver Alliance: National Center on Caregiving; 2006:12–37. http://www.caregiver.org/caregiver/jsp/content/pdfs/v2_consensus.pdf; Accessed October 1, 2012.

12. Payne S. White Paper on improving support for family carers in palliative care II. *Eur J Palliat Care.* 2010;17(6):286–290.

13. Aggarwal B, Liao M, Christian A, et al. Influence of caregiving on lifestyle and psychosocial risk factors among family members of patients hospitalized with cardiovascular disease. *J Gen Intern Med.* 2009;24(1):93–98.

14. Haley WE, Roth DL, Howard G, et al. Caregiving strain and estimated risk for stroke and coronary heart disease among spouse caregivers: differential effects by race and sex. *Stroke.* 2010;41(2):331–336.

15. Schulz R, Beach SR. Caregiving as a risk factor for mortality: the Caregiver Health Effects Study. *JAMA.* 1999;282(23):2215–2219.

16. O'Hara RE, Hull JG, Lyons KD, et al. Impact on caregiver burden of a patient-focused palliative care intervention for patients with advanced cancer. *Palliat Support Care.* 2010;8(4):395–404.

17. Brown SL, Smith DM, Schulz R, et al. Caregiving behavior is associated with decreased mortality risk. *Psychol Sci.* 2009;20(4):488–494.

18. Gaugler JE, Kane RL, Newcomer R. Resilience and transitions from dementia caregiving. *J Gerontol Ser B Psychol Sci Soc Sci.* 2007;62(1):P38–P44.

19. Schulz R, Belle SH, Czaja SJ, et al. Introduction to the special section on Resources for Enhancing Alzheimer's Caregiver Health (REACH). *Psychol Aging.* 2003;18(3):357–360.

20. Shaw WS, Patterson TL, Semple SJ, et al. Longitudinal analysis of multiple indicators of health decline among spousal caregivers. *Ann Behav Med.* 1997;19(2):101–109.

21. Torke AM, Holtz LR, Hui S, et al. Palliative care for patients with dementia: a national survey. *J Am Geriatr Soc.* 2010;58(11):2114–2121.

22. Albert SM, Whitaker A, Rabkin JG, et al. Medical and supportive care among people with ALS in the months before death or tracheostomy. *J Pain Symptom Manage.* 2009;38(4):546–553.

23. Hasson F, Kernohan WG, McLaughlin M, et al. An exploration into the palliative and end-of-life experiences of carers of people with Parkinson's disease. *Palliat Med.* 2010;24(7):731–736.

24. Hudson PL, Toye C, Kristjanson LJ. Would people with Parkinson's disease benefit from palliative care? *Palliat Med.* 2006;20(2):87–94.

25. Currow DC, Ward A, Clark K, et al. Caregivers for people with end-stage lung disease: characteristics and unmet needs in the whole population. *Int J COPD.* 2008;3(4):753–762.

26. Dellon EP, Shores MD, Nelson KI, et al. Family caregiver perspectives on symptoms and treatments for patients dying from complications of cystic fibrosis. *J Pain Symptom Manage.* 2010;40(6):829–837.

27. Walker RJ, Pomeroy EC, McNeil JS, et al. Anticipatory grief and AIDS: strategies for intervening with caregivers. *Health Social Work.* 1996;21(1):49–57.

28. Vivar CG, Canga N, Canga AD, et al. The psychosocial impact of recurrence on cancer survivors and family members: a narrative review. *J Adv Nurs.* 2009;65(4):724–736.

29. Hudson PL, Aranda S, Kristjanson LJ. Meeting the supportive needs of family caregivers in palliative care: challenges for health professionals. *J Palliat. Med.* 2004;7(1):19–25.

30. Plonk Jr WM, Arnold RM. Terminal care: the last weeks of life. *J Palliat Med.* 2005;8(5):1042–1054.

31. Kutner JS, Bryant LL, Beaty BL, et al. Time course and characteristics of symptom distress and quality of life at the end of life. *J Pain Symptom Manage.* 2007;34(3):227–236.

32. Phillips LR, Reed PG. Into the abyss of someone else's dying: the voice of the end-of-life caregiver. *Clin Nurs Res.* 2009;18(1):80–97.

33. Waldrop DP, Kramer BJ, Skretny JA, et al. Final transitions: family caregiving at the end of life. *J Palliat Med.* 2005;8(3):623–638.

34. Cohen CJ, Auslander G, Chen Y. Family caregiving to hospitalized end-of-life and acutely ill geriatric patients. *J Gerontol Nurs.* 2010;36(8):42–50.

35. Oliver DP, Wittenberg-Lyles E, Demiris G, et al. Barriers to pain management: caregiver perceptions and pain talk by hospice interdisciplinary teams. *J Pain Symptom Manage.* 2008;36(4):374–382.

36. Lorenz KA, Lynn J, Dy SM, et al. Evidence for improving palliative care at the end of life: a systematic review. *Ann Intern Med.* 2008;148(2):147–159.

37. Bascom PB, Tolle SW. Care of the family when the patient is dying. *West J Med.* 1995;163(3):292–296.

38. Bachner YG, Carmel S. Open communication between caregivers and terminally ill cancer patients: the role of caregivers' characteristics and situational variables. *Health Commun.* 2009;24(6):524–531.

39. Quest TE, Bone P. Caring for patients with malignancy in the emergency department: patient-provider interactions. *Emerg Med Clin North Am.* 2009;27(2):333–339.

40. Fried TR, Bradley EH, O'Leary JR, et al. Unmet desire for caregiver-patient communication and increased caregiver burden. *J Am Geriatr Soc.* 2005;53(1):59–65.

41. Lingler JH, Martire LM, Schulz R. Caregiver-specific outcomes in antidementia clinical drug trials: a systematic review and meta-analysis. *J Am Geriatr Soc.* 2005;53(6):983–990.

42. Waldrop DP, Milch RA, Skretny JA. Understanding family responses to life-limiting illness: in-depth interviews with hospice patients and their family members. *J Palliat Care.* 2005;21(2):88–96.

43. Cherlin E, Fried T, Prigerson HG, et al. Communication between physicians and family caregivers about care at the end of life: when do discussions occur and what is said? *J Palliat Med.* 2005;8(6):1176–1185.

44. Fried TR, Bradley EH, O'Leary J. Prognosis communication in serious illness: perceptions of older patients, caregivers, and clinicians. *J Am Geriatr Soc.* 2003;51(10):1398–1403.

45. Silveira MJ, Given CW, Given B, et al. Patient-caregiver concordance in symptom assessment and improvement in outcomes for patients undergoing cancer chemotherapy. *Chronic Illn.* 2010;6(1):46–56.

46. Csika EL, Martin SS. Bereaved hospice caregivers' views of the transition to hospice. *Soc Work Health Care.* 2010;49(5):387–400.

47. Wells DK, James K, Stewart JL, et al. The care of my child with cancer: a new instrument to measure caregiving demand in parents of children with cancer. *J Pediatr Nurs.* 2002;17(3):201–210.

48. Roscoe LA, Osman H, Haley WE. Implications of the Schiavo case for understanding family caregiving issues at the end of life. *Death Stud.* 2006;30(2):149–161.

49. DeSanto-Madeya S, Nilsson M, Loggers ET, et al. Associations between United States acculturation and the end-of-life experience of caregivers of patients with advanced cancer. *J Palliat Med.* 2009;12(12):1143–1149.

50. Connell CM, Janevic MR, Gallant MP. The costs of caring: impact of dementia on family caregivers. *J Geriatr Psychiatry Neurol.* 2001;14(4):179–187.

51. Kreling B, et al. "The worst thing about hospice is that they talk about death", contrasting hospice decisions and experience among immigrant Central and South American Latinos with US-born White, non-Latino cancer caregivers. *Palliat Med.* 2010;24(4):427–434.

52. Back AL, Young JP, McCown E, et al. Abandonment at the end of life from patient, caregiver, nurse, and physician perspectives: loss of continuity and lack of closure. *Arch Intern Med.* 2009;169(5):474–479.

53. Hudson PL. How well do family caregivers cope after caring for a relative with advanced disease and how can health professionals enhance their support? *J Palliat Med.* 2006;9(3):694–703.

54. Casarett D, et al. Life after death: a practical approach to grief and bereavement. *Ann Intern Med.* 2001;134(3):208–215.

55. Byock IR, Corbeil YJ, Goodrich ME. Beyond polarization, public preferences suggest policy opportunities to address aging, dying, and family caregiving. *Am J Hosp Palliat Med.* 2009;26(3):200–208.

56. Emanuel RH, Emanuel GA, Reitschuler EB, et al. Challenges faced by informal caregivers of hospice patients in Uganda. *J Palliat Med.* 2008;11(5):746–753.

57. Burns CM, LeBlanc TW, Abernethy A, et al. Young caregivers in the end-of-life setting: a population-based profile of an emerging group. *J Palliat Med.* 2010;13(10):1225–1235.

58. Covinsky KE, Cook EF, et al. The impact of serious illness on patients' families. SUPPORT Investigators: Study to Understand Prognoses and Preferences for Outcomes and Risks of Treatment. *JAMA.* 1994;272(23):1839–1844.

59. Roth DL, Haley WE, Wadley VG, et al. Race and gender differences in perceived caregiver availability for community-dwelling middle-aged and older adults. *Gerontologist.* 2007;47(6):721–729.

60. Lobchuk MM, Vorauer JD. Family caregiver perspective-taking and accuracy in estimating cancer patient symptom experiences. *Soc Sci Med.* 2003;57(12):2379–2384.

61. Pruchno R, Cartwright FP, Wilson-Genderson M. The effects of race on patient preferences and spouse substituted judgments. *Int J Aging Hum Dev.* 2009;69(1):31–54.

62. Pinquart M, Sorensen S. Associations of stressors and uplifts of caregiving with caregiver burden and depressive mood: a meta-analysis. *J Gerontol Ser B Psychol Sci Soc Sci.* 2003;58(2):P112–P128.

63. Martire LM, Lustig AP, Schulz R, et al. Is it beneficial to involve a family member? A meta-analysis of psychosocial interventions for chronic illness. *Health Psychol.* 2004;23(6):599–611.

64. Stolley JM, Reed D, Buckwalter KC. Caregiving appraisal and interventions based on the progressively lowered stress threshold model. *Am J Alzheimers Dis Other Demen.* 2002;17(2):110–120.

65. Kramer BJ. Gain in the caregiving experience: where are we? What next? *Gerontologist.* 1997;37(2):218–232.

66. Zaider T, Kissane D. The assessment and management of family distress during palliative care. *Curr Opin Support Palliat Care.* 2009;3(1):67–71.

67. Funk L, Stajduhar K, Toye C, et al. Home-based family caregiving at the end of life: a comprehensive review of published qualitative research (1998-2008). II. *Palliat Med.* 2010;24(6):594–607.

68. Funk LM, Allan DE, Stajduhar KI. Palliative family caregivers' accounts of health care experiences: the importance of "security". *Palliat Support Care.* 2009;7(4):435–447.

Chapter 73

What Can Be Done to Improve Outcomes for Caregivers of Patients With Serious Illness?

DEBORAH WALDROP AND JEAN S. KUTNER

INTRODUCTION AND SCOPE OF THE PROBLEM

Family members who become caregivers over the course of a loved one's serious illness are often deeply affected and forever changed by the experience. While providing hands-on care and emotional support they are also observing a loved one's decline and preparing for the approaching death and loss. Informal caregivers are central to the care for people who are seriously ill and dying. However, this often underappreciated care is provided at considerable personal, physical, and financial cost to the caregiver. Caregivers can experience a variety of physical, emotional, financial, and social burdens associated with caregiving. The emotional and physical impact of caregiving underscores the importance of considering caregivers "second-order patients,"[1]

The nature of the caregiving experience is influenced by numerous social factors, including (1) characteristics of the family caregiver, (2) characteristics of the patient, (3) symptoms of the illness, (4) the relational context, (5) social and professional support, and (6) circumstances surrounding the illness.[2] The relationship between caregiver and care recipient (e.g., spouse, adult child, sibling, friend) influences the perspectives, needs, issues, concerns and problems associated with the experience. Moreover, the caregiving experience is influenced by racial and cultural differences, location (rural versus urban environments), and socioeconomic status.[3,4] The negative effects of caregiving, which are commonly described as "burden" or "strain," have been extensively described. However, less is known about effective interventions to improve caregiver outcomes. The greatest number of interventions has been developed to improve the outcomes of caregivers for people with

dementia, specifically for Alzheimer disease. Fewer evidence-based interventions exist for people with serious nondementing illnesses and fewer still for caregivers whose loved ones are at the end of life. This chapter presents an overview of interventions that have been designed to ease the negative impact of caregiving for people with a serious illness.[5]

RELEVANT PATHOPHYSIOLOGY

The trajectories of functional decline that occur in serious illnesses are variable. Differentiating caregivers' needs according to the diagnosis and stage of illness can help providers tailor strategies and interventions.[6] The trajectory from diagnosis to death in the context of Alzheimer disease can range from 8 to 20 years and has been viewed as "the long goodbye."[7] This trajectory can also vary widely depending on how and when the disease is detected and on the specific nature of the cognitive decline.[8,9] The trajectory of other serious illnesses such as chronic obstructive pulmonary disease (COPD) and congestive heart failure (CHF) have been characterized as a slow decline with periodic crises and a seemingly "sudden" death.[10] People can live with cancer for years and generally experience a sharp functional decline in the last months before death.[11] Both situational- and diagnosis-specific stressors and needs occur across all stages of the trajectory of a serious illness, from diagnosis through end-stage care. Providers are urged to anticipate and assess evidence of caregiver distress at each stage of the illness trajectory.[12]

SUMMARY OF EVIDENCE REGARDING TREATMENT RECOMMENDATIONS

This section presents an overview of the importance of family–provider communication as a fundamental intervention that improves outcomes for caregivers in all situations. Next, it presents interventions that have been designed to ease the distress of caregiving. The selections of representative studies of interventions for caregivers of people with Alzheimer disease and serious nondementing illnesses are presented in Tables 73-1 and 73-2.

TABLE 73–1. Interventions That Improve Outcomes for Caregivers of People With Dementia

INTERVENTION	TARGET	COMPONENTS	OUTCOMES	SOURCE
Resources for Enhancing Alzheimer's Caregiver Health (REACH)	Caregiver burden; depression	Multisite RCT tested the feasibility, outcome in nine locations: Skills training Telephone Linked Computer (TLC) system Behavior care Enhanced care Family-based multisystem in-home intervention Computer Telephone Integration System Coping Minimal support Environmental Skill-building Program	Measures: ADLs, Revised Memory and Behavior Problems Checklist Depression–CES-D Mini-Mental State Exam Caregiver Health and Health Behaviors Anxiety Inventory Vigilance, Formal Care, and Services Positive aspects of caregiving Religiosity Social activities	See reference 30 for a full description of REACH See reference 31 for a special section of Psychology & Aging on REACH
Telephone Linked-Computer (REACH site)	Disruptive behaviors	12-month automated interactive voice response intervention Caregiver stress monitoring and counseling information Voice-mail linkage to experts Voice-mail telephone support group Distraction call to care recipient	Increased mastery and decrease bothersome nature of caregiving Decreased anxiety and depression	Reference 32
Video-Based Coping Skills Training	Caregiver distress	Controlled clinical trial Viewed two video modules weekly Completed homework in a skills workbook Received coaching phone call	Reduced bio markers of stress: average blood pressure remained steady Improved depressive, anxiety, stress symptoms	Reference 33
Comprehensive Educational Program Reinforced by an Individualized Component (CEPRIC)	Caregiver burden; behavior management	General information session Individualized educational component (with a nursing assessment) Educational booklet	Improved sleep and eating patterns Reduced trauma risk, anxiety Diminished depression, anxiety	Reference 34
Environment Skill-Building Program	Caregiver well-being, care recipient functioning	5 home sessions, 1 phone contact Education Problem-solving Adaptive equipment	Less distress with memory-related and disruptive behavior Less assistance needed Increased positive affect, well-being, mastery	Reference 35

Family Caregiver Role Training	Clinical Belief Set	14-hour training provided in 72-hour sessions for family caregiver–care receiver dyads	Beliefs about caregiving changed; Knowledge, skills improved; Depression, burden improved	Reference 36
Progressively Lowered Stress Threshold	Caregiver responses to memory and problem behaviors	Longitudinal, multisite, community-based intervention	Positive impact on the frequency of and response to problem behaviors	Reference 37
Psychoeducational Intervention Program	Problem behaviors	8 individual sessions over a 4-month period	Reduced caregiver distress; Development of caregiving strategies; Improved quality of life and perceived health	Reference 38
Psychoeducation	Understanding and acceptance; knowledge of resources; expression of concerns; emotions of caregiving in Hispanic caregivers	5-day, 20-hour training; Information about Alzheimer disease; Community resources; Legal issues; Social support; Grief	Increased willingness to attend support groups; Satisfaction with the program	Reference 39
Counseling	Depression	Enhanced counseling and support; 6 sessions of individual family counseling; Support group for 4 months; Ad hoc counseling	Reduced depression	References 40,41
Counseling	Burden and depression during the transition to institutionalization	6 sessions of individual and family counseling; Support group participation; Continuous availability of ad hoc telephone counseling	Reduced burden and depression	Reference 42

ADLs, Activities of daily living; *CES-D*, Center for Epidemiologic Studies Depression Scale; *RCT*, randomized, controlled trial.

TABLE 73-2. Interventions That Improve Outcomes for Caregivers of People With Nondementia Serious Illness

INTERVENTION	TARGET	COMPONENTS	OUTCOMES	SOURCE
Team-Managed Home-Based Primary Care	CHF and COPD patients' functional status Caregivers' health-related QoL and burden in patients with CHF, COPD	Home-based primary care 24-hour phone contact Prior approval for hospitalization HBPC team participation in discharge planning	Improved caregiver health-related QOL Improved satisfaction, decreased burden	Reference 43
The CARE Project	Identification and management of problems in rural areas	Home-based comprehensive geriatric assessment (CGA)	Identification of problems Modifications needed	Reference 44
Home-Based Palliative Care	Symptom relief, QoL reduced resource usage	Home visits by an interdisciplinary team: physician, nurse, case manager, psychologist, interpreter, volunteers	Decreased hospitalizations Discussion of end-of-life wishes Higher caregiver satisfaction	Reference 45
Partner-Guided Pain Management	Caregiver strain in managing advanced cancer care	Randomized intervention involving: 3-session intervention Systematic training of cognitive behavioral coping skills	Increased pain control in patients Self-efficacy in controlling other symptoms Decreased caregiver strain	Reference 46
Psychoeducation	Preparedness to care, self-efficacy, competence, anxiety in caregivers of patients with terminal cancer	Home-based palliative care Caregiver manual 2 home visits Follow-up telephone calls Condolence letter	More positive caregiver experience No intervention effects in preparedness, self-efficacy, competence, or anxiety	Reference 20
Living with Hope Program (LWHP)	Caregiver QoL	Hope video Activity: Stories of the present	LWHP is easy to use, flexible, and increases hope and QoL	Reference 47
Educate, Nurture, Advise Before Life Ends II (ENABLE II)	Caregiver burden	Patient-focused palliative care	Increased patient QoL Reduced symptom intensity Lowered depressed mood No reduction of caregiver burden	Reference 26

CHF, Congestive heart failure; *COPD,* chronic obstructive pulmonary disease; *QoL,* quality of life.

Family–Provider Communication

The concept of caring for the patient and family as a unit is deeply rooted in the precepts that guide the delivery of palliative care. However, family caregivers consistently report that they do not receive adequate communication, support, and information from health care providers.[13,14] Many potential barriers exist to adequate communication. Family functioning can complicate communication[15]; incongruent desires for the amount and timing of information can cause discrepancies[16]; impaired concentration can occur, with both patient and caregiver interfering with effective communication[13]; and "conspiracies of silence" can become problematic.[17] Communication can also be complicated by individual patient dynamics. Patients with a poor understanding of their prognosis are less likely to discuss care preferences with family members.[14] Moreover, patients may discuss their care preferences either with family members or with providers but not with both, which can result in incomplete communication.

Providers may lack training in communication skills or have limited resources (e.g., social work collaboration) or experience in this area. Additionally, the fragmentation of care that occurs when patients see multiple providers can become a barrier to communication.[13] Family–provider communication about a poor prognosis can be emotional and difficult, exacerbating painful family issues and dynamics.[14] Providers may focus on the medical and technical aspects of an illness rather than on the emotional, psychosocial, and quality of life issues[18] or be reluctant to discuss the terminal nature of a prognosis.[19] Functional decline often becomes the catalyst for the discussion of a poor prognosis. When patients and families have not had prior conversations about goals of care or end-of-life wishes, discussions at this time can become intense. Providers are encouraged to communicate prognostic information well in advance of the end stage of a serious illness[14] (see Chapter 43).

However, with respectful regard for these identified difficulties, the importance of open, honest and straightforward communication about the prognosis and goals of care simply cannot be overstated. The development of a mutual understanding about the patient's prognosis with the seriously ill person, the person's family caregivers, and providers, together with communication about and understanding of the patient's preferences is essential to ensure that seriously ill people will receive end-of-life care that is concordant with their wishes. Caregivers' experiences both before and after a death can be greatly enhanced by meaningful communication with providers that addresses emotional issues such as a life-limiting prognosis or an impending death.[20]

Interventions for Caregivers of People With Serious Illnesses

Intervention studies to improve outcomes for caregivers of people with serious illness have largely focused on caregiver burden that accompanies Alzheimer disease. Caregiver burden in Alzheimer disease has been associated with managing difficult behaviors in dementia, including aggression, agitation, confusion, hallucinations, repetitive behaviors, sleeplessness or sundowning, suspicion, unpredictable behaviors, and wandering.[21] Outcome measures that have been used in intervention studies include but are not limited to insufficient information about the illness, knowledge of behavioral issues, and behavior management. Emotional distress, which has been conceptualized as including some combination of anxiety, depression, grief, sleep and eating changes, and family conflict, has been an outcome measure of numerous studies. Intervention methods have included psychoeducation (including behavior management and coping skills) and counseling, and they often using a cognitive-behavioral therapy approach with an individual, family, and support group component. Notably, the pharmacological treatment of people with Alzheimer disease using acetylcholinesterase inhibitors has been found to positively affect cognition, activities of daily living (ADLs), and behavioral problems, thus rendering small decreases in burden for their caregivers.[22]

The assessment and treatment of both caregiver burden and emotional distress anxiety in caregivers of people with Alzheimer disease is important. The Caregivers for Alzheimer's disease Problems Scale (CAPS) has the sensitivity and specificity to detect caregivers who have symptoms of anxiety and depression.[23] Routine assessment and referral to mental health professionals and community resources is strongly recommended.

Caregiver burden in nondementia serious illnesses has been associated with the stress of managing symptoms such as pain, dyspnea, nausea, vomiting, functional decline, and the physical burden of assisting with ADLs. Emotional distress has been associated with the personality and relationship changes that accompany transition to the caregiver and care recipient roles, together with feelings of loss, sadness, anxiety, and depression. Group education that prepares families for the tasks accompanying caregiving in the setting of serious illness is effective.[24] Grief is pervasive in both people who have serious illnesses and their caregivers across the trajectory.

Interventions to improve outcomes for caregivers of people with serious nondementia illnesses have targeted improvements in pain and symptom management, health-related quality of life, satisfaction, self-efficacy (e.g., a sense of preparedness, competence), anxiety, depression, and hope. Routine assessment and screening of caregivers together with referrals to local community agencies with disease-specific support programs is recommended.

KEY MESSAGES TO PATIENTS AND FAMILIES

Caregiving can be hard and difficult work—emotionally, physically, socially, and spiritually—for the family members of patients with serious illness. It is important that family caregivers attend to their physical and mental health. Referrals should be made so they can seek assistance from community programs that offer information and support, and caregivers should be encouraged to ask their (or the patient's) clinician for assistance. Clinicians should encourage the caregivers to talk with their loved one about the patient's goals of care, particularly related to the patient's wishes for care at the end of life. Family caregivers should be encouraged to help their loved ones complete a written advance directive, and they should have one of their own.

CONCLUSION AND SUMMARY

Providers are encouraged to recognize the physical and psychosocial distress that the caregiving experience can cause. Routine screening of caregivers for anxiety, depression, and health-related quality of life is strongly recommended. Knowledge of the resources provided by community-based programs for specific serious illnesses can be helpful (e.g., American Cancer Society, Alzheimer's Association). Referrals for mental health support and counseling can be very helpful to family caregivers.

Existing interventions typically focus on helping caregivers cope with the physical and emotional demands of care provision. Although this focus is useful and may be helpful for providers, interventions often ignore a primary and central source of stress for family caregivers—the suffering of a loved one. Interventions that focus on the relief of patient suffering as a way to improve caregiver well-being have only rarely been tested.[25] The results are mixed; some but not all patient-focused interventions have a similar beneficial effect on caregiver burden.[26] Clearly, this is an important focus for future study.

Many intervention studies have reported small to moderate effects that are statistically significant on a range of outcomes, but only a few have demonstrated clinical significance. Caregiving intervention studies have increasingly shown promise of affecting important public health outcomes such as service usage, including delayed institutionalization, diminished psychiatric symptoms, and the linkage of caregivers to helpful community services. The assessment of clinical significance is needed in this research area.[27] The evaluation of intervention studies has been limited to only a few randomized controlled trials and a predominance of small sample sizes. Finally, many interventions do not actually have a focus on caregivers, which further limits the likelihood of demonstrating their impact.[28]

SUMMARY RECOMMENDATIONS

- Clinicians should conduct meetings with patients and families that address prognosis and goals of care; they also should ask about the patient's wishes during the late and end stages of the illness and ascertain congruence (or lack thereof) between patient and caregiver.
- Clinicians should ensure that advance care planning conversations occur between patients and their family caregivers and that these conversations include health care professionals (e.g., nurse and/or social work case manager, clinicians). Patient wishes should be documented, and family needs should be clarified and addressed.
- It is important for clinicians to screen patients' caregivers for emotional distress (including anxiety, depression, and anticipatory grief) and determine their needs for information and strategies to manage illness-specific problems (e.g., behavioral manifestations, symptom management).
- Clinicians can help caregivers and patients prioritize emotional and quality of life issues.
- When communicating with caregivers about caregiver stress, clinicians should enlist the help of other professionals; speak less, listen more; and offer support and emotional validation.[18] Recognize that silence is a form of expression that conveys powerful emotions.[29]
- Clinicians should refer caregivers for supportive interventions to help manage caregiver burden, emotional distress, and symptom management.
- It is important for clinicians to universalize the need for mental health care among caregivers of people with serious illness and encourage caregivers to use effective interventions (e.g., cognitive-behavioral therapy, counseling) to manage their distress.

REFERENCES

1. Kristjanson LJ, Aoun S. Palliative care for families: remembering the hidden patients. *Can J Psychiatry Rev Can Psychiatrie.* 2004;49(6):359–365.
2. Dumont I, Dumont S, Mongeau S. End-of-life care and the grieving process: family caregivers who have experienced the loss of a terminal-phase cancer patient. *Qual Health Res.* 2008;18(8):1049–1061.
3. Roth DL, Haley WE, Wadley VG, et al. Race and gender differences in perceived caregiver availability for community-dwelling middle-aged and older adults. *Gerontologist.* 2007;47(6):721–729.
4. Montoro-Rodriguez J, Gallagher-Thompson D. The role of resources and appraisals in predicting burden among Latina and non-Hispanic white female caregivers: a test of an expanded socio-cultural model of stress and coping. *Aging Mental Health.* 2009;13(5):648–658.
5. Connell CM, Janevic MR, Gallant MP. The costs of caring: impact of dementia on family caregivers. *J Geriatr Psychiatry Neurol.* 2001;14(4):179–187.
6. Lunney JR, Lynn J, Foley DJ, et al. Patterns of functional decline at the end of life. *JAMA.* 2003;289(18):2387–2392.
7. Alzheimer's Association. 2011. *Living with Alzheimer's disease.* http://www.alz.org/living_with_alzheimers_4521.asp; Accessed October 1, 2012.
8. Wilkosz PA, Seltman HJ, Devlin B, et al. Trajectories of cognitive decline in Alzheimer's disease. *Int Psychogeriatr.* 2010;22(2):281–290.
9. Carpentier N, Bernard P, Grenier A, et al. Using the life course perspective to study the entry into the illness trajectory: the perspective of caregivers of people with Alzheimer's disease. *Soc Sci Med.* 2010;70(10):1501–1508.
10. Field MJ, Cassel CK. *Approaching Death.* eds. Washington, DC: National Academies Press; 1997:1–25.
11. Teno JM, Weitzen S, Fennell ML, et al. Dying trajectory in the last year of life: does cancer trajectory fit other diseases? *J Palliat Med.* 2001;4(4):457–464.
12. Brant JM. Palliative care for adults across the cancer trajectory: from diagnosis to end of life. *Semin Oncol Nurs.* 2010;26(4):222–230.
13. Hudson PL, Aranda S, Kristjanson LJ. Meeting the supportive needs of family caregivers in palliative care: challenges for health professionals. *J Palliat Med.* 2004;7(1):19–25.
14. Wagner GJ, Riopelle D, Steckart J, et al. Provider communication and patient understanding of life-limiting illness and their relationship to patient communication of treatment preferences. *J Pain Symptom Manage.* 2010;39(3):527–534.
15. Zaider T, Kissane D. The assessment and management of family distress during palliative care. *Curr Opin Support Palliat Care.* 2009;3(1):67–71.
16. Gardner DS, Kramer BJ. End-of-life concerns and care preferences: congruence among terminally ill elders and their family caregivers. *Omega J Death Dying.* 2009;60(3):273–297.
17. Zhang AY, Siminoff LA. Silence and cancer: why do families and patients fail to communicate? *Health Commun.* 2003;15(4):415–429.
18. Fine E, Reid MC, Shengelia R, et al. Directly observed patient-physician discussions in palliative and end-of-life care: a systematic review of the literature. *J Palliat Med.* 2010;13(5):595–603.
19. Fried TR, Bradley EH, O'Leary J. Prognosis communication in serious illness: perceptions of older patients, caregivers, and clinicians. *J Am Geriatr Soc.* 2003;51(10):1398–1403.
20. Hudson PL, Aranda S, Hayman-White K. A psycho-educational intervention for family caregivers of patients receiving palliative care: a randomized controlled trial. *J Pain Symptom Manage.* 2005;30(4):329–341.
21. Alzheimer's Association. 2010. *Caregivers for Alzheimer's and dementia face special challenges.* http://www.alz.org/care/overview.asp; Accessed October 1, 2012.
22. Farcnik K, Persyko MS. Assessment, measures and approaches to easing caregiver burden in Alzheimer's disease. *Drugs Aging.* 2002;19(3):203–215.
23. Livingston G, Mahoney R, Regan C, et al. The Caregivers for Alzheimer's disease Problems Scale (CAPS): development of a new scale within the LASER-AD study. *Age Ageing.* 2005;34(3):287–290.

24. Hudson P, Quinn K, Kristjanson L, et al. Evaluation of a psycho-educational group programme for family caregivers in home-based palliative care. *Palliat Med.* 2008;22(3):270–280.

25. Hebert RS, Arnold RM, Schulz R. Improving well-being in care-givers of terminally ill patients: making the case for patient suffering as a focus for intervention research. *J Pain Symptom Manage.* 2007;34(5):539–546.

26. O'Hara RE, Hull JG, Lyons KD, et al. Impact on caregiver burden of a patient-focused palliative care intervention for patients with advanced cancer. *Palliat Support Care.* 2010;8(4):395–404.

27. Schulz R, O'Brien A, Czaja S, et al. Dementia caregiver interven-tion research: in search of clinical significance. *Gerontologist.* 2002;42(5):589–602.

28. Grande G, Stajduhar K, Aoun S, et al. Supporting lay carers in end of life care: current gaps and future priorities. *Palliat Med.* 2009;23(4):339–344.

29. Bearden DM, Childers T, Howell S, et al. Lessons from the silence. *J Palliat Med.* 2011;14(1):105–106.

30. Wisniewski SR, Belle SH, Coon DW, et al. The Resources for Enhancing Alzheimer's Caregiver Health (REACH): proj-ect design and baseline characteristics. *Psychol Aging.* 2003;18(3):375–384.

31. Schulz R, Belle SH, Czaja SJ, et al. Introduction to the special section on Resources for Enhancing Alzheimer's Caregiver Health (REACH). *Psychol Aging.* 2003;18(3):357–360.

32. Mahoney DF, Tarlow BJ, Jones RN. Effects of an automated tele-phone support system on caregiver burden and anxiety: find-ings from the REACH for TLC intervention study. *Gerontologist.* 2003;43(4):556–567.

33. Williams VP, Bishop-Fitzpatrick L, Lane JD, et al. Video-based coping skills to reduce health risk and improve psychological and physical well-being in Alzheimer's disease family caregiv-ers. *Psychosom Med.* 2010;72(9):897–904.

34. Kuzu N, Beser N, Zencir M, et al. Effects of a comprehensive educational program on quality of life and emotional issues of dementia patient caregivers. *Geriatr Nurs.* 2005;26(6):378–386.

35. Gitlin LN, Winter L, Corcoran M, et al. Effects of the home envi-ronmental skill-building program on the caregiver-care recipi-ent dyad: 6-month outcomes from the Philadelphia REACH Initiative. *Gerontologist.* 2003;43(4):532–546.

36. Hepburn KW, Tornatore J, Center B, et al. Dementia family care-giver training: affecting beliefs about caregiving and caregiver outcomes. *J Am Geriatr Soc.* 2001;49(4):450–457.

37. Gerdner LA, Buckwalter KC, Reed D. Impact of a psychoeduca-tional intervention on caregiver response to behavioral prob-lems. *Nurs Res.* 2002;51(6):363–374.

38. Martin-Carrasco M, Martin MF, Valero CP, et al. Effectiveness of a psychoeducational intervention program in the reduction of caregiver burden in Alzheimer's disease patients' caregivers. *Int J Geriatr Psychiatry.* 2009;24(5):489–499.

39. Morano CL, Bravo M. A psychoeducational model for Hispanic Alzheimer's disease caregivers. *Gerontologist.* 2002;42(1):122–126.

40. Mittelman MS, Roth DL, Coon DW, et al. Sustained benefit of supportive intervention for depressive symptoms in care-givers of patients with Alzheimer's disease. *Am J Psychiatry.* 2004;161(5):850–856.

41. Mittelman MS, Roth DL, Haley WE, et al. Effects of a caregiver intervention on negative caregiver appraisals of behavior prob-lems in patients with Alzheimer's disease: results of a random-ized trial. *J Gerontol Ser B Psychol Sci Soc Sci.* 2004;59(1):P27–P34.

42. Gaugler JE, Roth DL, Haley WE, et al. Can counseling and sup-port reduce burden and depressive symptoms in caregivers of people with Alzheimer's disease during the transition to insti-tutionalization? Results from the New York University care-giver intervention study. *J Am Geriatr Soc.* 2008;56(3):421–428.

43. Hughes SL, Weaver FM, Giobbi-Hurder A, et al. Effectiveness of team-managed home-based primary care: a randomized multi-center trial. *JAMA.* 2000;284(22):2877–2885.

44. Cravens DD, Mehr DR, Campbell JD, et al. Home-based compre-hensive assessment of rural elderly persons: the CARE project. *J Rural Health.* 2005;21(4):322–328.

45. Fernandes R, Braun KL, Ozawa J, et al. Home-based pallia-tive care services for underserved populations. *J Palliat Med.* 2010;13(4):413–419.

46. Keefe Ahles TA, Sutton L, FJ, et al. Partner-guided cancer pain management at the end of life: a preliminary study. *J Pain Symptom Manage.* 2005;29(3):263–272.

47. Duggleby W, Wright K, Williams A, et al. Developing a living with hope program for caregivers of family members with advanced cancer. *J Palliat Care.* 2007;23(1):24–31.

Chapter 74

What Is Prolonged Grief Disorder and How Can Its Likelihood Be Reduced?

DEBORAH WALDROP AND JEAN S. KUTNER

INTRODUCTION AND SCOPE OF THE PROBLEM

Loss, in many forms, occurs across the continuum of a serious illness, beginning with the diagnosis and continuing through treatment, remission, recurrence or exacerbation, rehospitalization, terminal decline, and death. Grief is the normal and inevitable response to the losses sustained during a serious illness and for loved ones after death occurs. Although grief is most often resolved over time, in a small percentage of situations, it is acutely distressing, becomes prolonged, and causes serious health concerns.[1,2] This small minority of people experience persistent emotional and behavioral disturbances that prevent them from returning to normal functioning.[1]

Difficult grief has been recognized by mental health professionals for decades and described as "the intensification of grief to the level where the person is overwhelmed, resorts to maladaptive behavior, or remains interminably in the state of grief without progression of the mourning process towards completion...."[1] and "involves processes that do not move progressively toward assimilation or accommodation but, instead, lead to stereotyped repetitions or extensive interruptions of healing."[3] Multiple terms have been used to refer to difficult adaptation in bereavement, including "abnormal," "pathological," "atypical," "neurotic," "unresolved," "chronic," "delayed," "exaggerated," "traumatic," and "complicated."[4,5] Complicated grief was chosen initially by Prigerson and colleagues[1] because it implied that the symptoms associated with the loss are both unresolved and combined with impaired performance in daily activities and also because the term is neither pejorative nor value-laden.[2,6]

Complicated grief is not a self-limited process that progresses from a stage of initial shock, to stages of acute somatic or emotional discomfort and social withdrawal, ending with the acceptance of the loss and restoration of preloss levels of functioning. Rather, complicated grief prevents the return to preloss levels of performance and well-being. Seven symptoms were determined to characterize complicated grief: (1) searching, (2) yearning, (3) preoccupation with thoughts of the deceased, (4) crying, (5) disbelief about the death, (6) feeling stunned by the death, and (7) a lack of acceptance of the death.[1] However, through ongoing research aimed at determining the psychometric validity of diagnostic criteria, Prigerson and colleagues[4] became dissatisfied with the term "complicated" because of its vague and nonspecific nature, potentially referring to multiple symptoms of distress.[4]

Subsequently, the term "traumatic grief" was chosen and conceptualized to include (1) symptoms of separation distress, such as preoccupation with thoughts of the deceased to the point of functional impairment, upsetting memories, longing, searching, and loneliness following the loss; and (2) symptoms of traumatic distress about the death, which included disbelief, mistrust, anger, detachment from others, shock, and experiencing somatic symptoms similar to those of the person who died. Traumatic grief was considered to accurately characterize the disorder because it included the dual elements of both traumatic and separation distress.[4] Ultimately, however, use of the term "traumatic grief" was confused with posttraumatic stress disorder (PTSD)[2] and influenced continuing work toward identifying an optimal diagnostic algorithm for prolonged grief disorder.[6]

Grief, of any type, has not previously been a diagnostic category in either the *Diagnostic and Statistical Manual of Mental Disorders* (DSM) or the International Classification of Diseases (ICD) codes. The DSM-IIIR acknowledged that protracted functional impairment could indicate that bereavement was complicated by depression. However, the DSM-IIIR also noted that substantial individual and cultural variations in adjustment to bereavement made it difficult to determine when reactions could be appropriately defined as complicated. DSM-IV criteria addressed the possible need for treatment early in the course of bereavement by specifying that the diagnosis of Major Depressive Disorder (MDD) may be given as early as 2 months after the loss of a loved one.[1] The DSM-IV did not specify clinically disabling grief symptoms as a separate disorder but listed bereavement as a "V" code condition that "may be a focus of clinical attention." Since that time, consensus has been developing that difficult grief reactions that include complicated grief,[1] complicated grief disorder,[7] traumatic grief,[8–12] and most recently prolonged grief disorder[2,13,14] are a distinct mental disorder that is experienced as clinically significant distress and substantive disability and warrants inclusion in both the DSM-V and ICD-11.[15]

RELEVANT PATHOPHYSIOLOGY

A panel of experts in bereavement, mood anxiety disorders, and psychiatric nosology was convened to consider the evidence for the development of diagnostic criteria for prolonged grief disorder (PGD).[6] A field trial was conducted to test the psychometric validity of criteria for PGD. PGD has been defined as a specific reaction to the loss of a loved one. Specific PGD symptoms, which include thoughts, feelings, and actions, must be elevated 6 months after the loss and associated with significant functional impairment. There are five specific criteria for the diagnosis of PGD, as follows[16]:

A. *Event Criterion:* The person is bereaved and has lost a loved one.

B. *Separation Distress:* The person experiences longing or yearning and intense feelings of emotional pain, sorrow, or pangs of grief related to the lost relationship at least daily.

C. *Duration Criterion:* The symptoms must be elevated 6 months after the loss.

D. *Cognitive, Emotional, and Behavioral Symptoms:* The respondent must experience 5 of 9 criteria at least once per day or quite a bit. The symptoms include (1) avoidance of reminders; (2) feeling stunned, shocked, or dazed; (3) feeling role confusion (e.g., part of self has died); (4) having trouble accepting the loss; (5) finds it hard to trust others; (6) feeling bitter over the loss; (7) feeling that moving on would be difficult; (8) feeling emotionally numb; (9) feeling that life is unfulfilling, empty, or meaningless

E. *Impairment Criterion:* The person has experienced significant reduction of social, occupational, or other important areas of functioning.

Assessment for PGD is encouraged. The criteria appear in Table 74-1, and Appendix 74-1 provides a guide to screen for PGD in clinical practice.

Grief is frequently confused and overlapped with and misdiagnosed as PTSD, MDD, and with generalized anxiety disorder (GAD). PGD is a postloss syndrome with core symptoms that is distinct from bereavement-related anxiety, depression, and the intrusion and avoidance dimensions of PTSD.[15] The course of PGD is distinctly different from that of normal grief, MDD, GAD, and PTSD. However, it can be difficult to distinguish a major depressive disorder from complicated grief, particularly in people with a history of depression. Depression tends to be more global in its impact on thoughts, feelings, and behaviors such that depressed individuals experience distorted cognitions directed at themselves, the world, and the future, whereas those suffering from complicated grief tend to report negative thoughts associated with specific aspects of their loss.[17]

Risk Factors

The identification of clinical risk factors is important for screening people who may be at high risk for developing PGD[14] and its consequent poor health, a risk that would be undetected with an exclusive focus on depression and anxiety.[13] PGD has been associated with poor quality of life and impaired physical and mental health (including increased risk for depression and suicidality).[13,18,19]

Childhood attachment issues have been found to create vulnerability for the development of PGD in adulthood. A history of childhood separation anxiety was significantly associated with PGD in bereavement.[20] Vulnerability for the development of PGD is also greater in people who experienced parental abuse or death during childhood[19] and people who perceived a high level of parental control in childhood.[21] The close relationship with someone

TABLE 74-1. Prolonged Grief Criteria Proposed for Inclusion in DSM-V and ICD-11*

CATEGORY	DEFINITION
A	*Event:* Bereavement (loss of a significant other)
B	*Separation distress:* The bereaved person experiences yearning (e.g., craving, pining, or longing for the deceased; physical or emotional suffering as a result of the desired, but unfulfilled, reunion with the deceased) daily or to a disabling degree
C	*Cognitive, emotional, and behavioral symptoms:* The bereaved person must have five (or more) of the following symptoms experienced daily or to a disabling degree: 1. Confusion about one's role in life or diminished sense of self (i.e., feeling that a part of oneself has died) 2. Difficulty accepting the loss 3. Avoidance of reminders of the reality of the loss 4. Inability to trust others since the loss 5. Bitterness or anger related to the loss 6. Difficulty moving on with life (e.g., making new friends, pursuing interests) 7. Numbness (absence of emotion) since the loss 8. Feeling that life is unfulfilling, empty, or meaningless since the loss 9. Feeling stunned, dazed, or shocked by the loss
D	*Timing:* Diagnosis should not be made until at least 6 months have elapsed since the death.
E	*Impairment:* The disturbance causes clinically significant impairment in social, occupational, or other important areas of functioning (e.g., domestic responsibilities)
F	*Relation to other mental disorders:* The disturbance is not better accounted for by major depressive disorder, generalized anxiety disorder, or posttraumatic stress disorder

From Prigerson HG, Horowitz MJ, Jacobs SC, et al. Prolonged grief disorder: psychometric validation of criteria proposed for DSM-V and ICD-11. *PLoS Med.* 2009;6(8):e1000121.
*See Appendix 74-1 for a version of this tool that can be used in clinical practice.

who commits suicide has been strongly associated with the development of complicated grief.[22] Suicidal behavior[23] and completed suicide[24] cluster in families, placing relatives of suicide victims at increased suicide risk. Risk factors for complicated grief may cluster in families who have experienced suicide.[25]

Higher risk for the development of PGD has also been associated with the circumstances of the death itself. The perception that a loved one's death was sudden and unexpected has been associated with the development of PGD.[14,26] PGD was found to be more prevalent in younger age family members of people who were in a vegetative state[27] and when death occurs in hospital or intensive care unit.[28] Finally, racial and cultural risk factors may exist for the development of PGD; higher rates were found in nonwhite, recently bereaved adults.[14] Risk factors are summarized in Table 74-2.

SUMMARY OF EVIDENCE REGARDING TREATMENT RECOMMENDATIONS

To date, relatively little evidence exists about treatment for PGD. The importance of screening for PGD cannot be underestimated. The timely identification of people who are at risk for or experiencing PGD will ensure that appropriate treatment can be initiated. Differential screening for the existence of comorbid depression, anxiety, or PTSD is also important. Use of the Prolonged Grief Disorder (PG-13) for risk assessment 6 months after the loss of a loved one is suggested (Appendix 74-1).

Cognitive-behavioral therapy has shown promise in the treatment of complicated grief. A combination of cognitive restructuring and exposure therapy produced more improvements in complicated grief than did supportive counseling.[29] Shear and colleagues[30] compared the use of Interpersonal Psychotherapy with a complicated grief treatment (CGT) intervention that integrated a focus on grief symptoms with a dual-process model of adaptive coping and addressing trauma-like symptoms by encouraging the person to retell the story. Participants who received CGT demonstrated a better response, which suggests that as a distinct diagnosis, PGD requires specific treatments. Family-based cognitive-behavioral grief therapy was used with relatives of suicide victims and demonstrated a decline in suicidality.[31] The combination of antidepressant medication and interpersonal psychotherapy was found to reduce bereavement-related major depression, but it did not impact complicated grief.[32]

KEY MESSAGES TO PATIENTS AND FAMILIES

Bereaved family members should understand that PGD is a distinct clinical entity that is concerning and can be disabling. It should not be considered "normal." They should understand that risk factors for its development include the death of a child, sudden death from a traumatic event such as violence or disaster, death from suicide, or death in a hospital, particularly in an intensive care unit. It is important that bereaved individuals understand that effective treatments are available and continue to be developed; cognitive-behavioral therapy and CGT interventions have been demonstrated to improve symptoms.

CONCLUSION AND SUMMARY

Rather than conceptualizing grief as a series of distinct, sequential stages, it might be more accurate to envision a proposed progression of multidimensional grief states that evolve and diminish in

TABLE 74-2. Association Between Clinical Risk Factors and Prolonged Grief Disorder

RISK FACTORS FOR DEVELOPING PGD	DOCUMENTED RISKS ACCOMPANYING PGD
Attachment Issues History of childhood separation anxiety[20] Childhood vulnerability as a result of parental abuse or death[19]	Significant association with comorbid major depressive disorder.
High level of perceived parental control in childhood[21]	Resolving high levels of dependency on the deceased spouse.
Relational proximity (closeness) with someone who committed suicide[22]	PGD is associated with suicide in parents, spouses, children, siblings, in-laws, and friends or co-workers in decreasing order.
Loss of a child and unresolved parental bereavement[34,35]	Long-term mental, physical morbidity; increased health service use and sick leave.
Place or Manner of Death Death in a hospital, ICU[29]	Associated with increased risk of PGD
Perceptions of "sudden" or "unexpected" death[14,26] Younger patients, younger caregivers, less time from the sudden, traumatic event (e.g., that results in a patient's vegetative state)[27]	African Americans have increased risk for PGD
Overall PGD	Predicts reduced QoL, poorer mental health (e.g., depression, suicidality)[13,18]

ICU, Intensive care unit; *PGD,* prolonged grief disorder; *QoL,* quality of life.

intensity over time. Decline in grief-related distress appears to correspond with an increase in peaceful acceptance of loss, which suggests a need for studies that advance our understanding of how grief resolution may facilitate adaptation. The potentially therapeutic role of clinicians and family members in facilitating adaptation should inform interventions that can be used to promote the mental health of those confronting particularly difficult losses through death.[2] Health and mental health providers are encouraged to understand the factors that contribute to particularly difficult grief that does not resolve with time, specifically PGD.

A better understanding of people who are at risk and of the predeath factors that contribute to the development of PGD will enhance the opportunity for the needs of survivors to become a central component of end-of-life care.[33] Studies demonstrating how the mind comprehends, copes with, and accepts death address the core psychological issues that need to be better understood before they can inform interventions to promote adjustment.

SUMMARY RECOMMENDATIONS

- Clinicians should become familiar with the criteria for prolonged grief disorder.
- Caregivers should be screened for risk factors for the development of prolonged grief disorder before the death.
- Clinicians should follow bereaved individuals, especially those at risk for the development of prolonged grief disorder.
- Caregivers who are at risk for or who develop prolonged grief disorder should be connected with appropriate mental health resources with consideration of pharmacological therapy if indicated.

REFERENCES

1. Prigerson HG, Frank E, Kasl SV, et al. Complicated grief and bereavement-related depression as distinct disorders: preliminary empirical validation in elderly bereaved spouses. *Am J Psychiatry.* 1995;152(1):22–30.
2. Prigerson HG, Vanderwerker LC, Maciejewski PK. A case for inclusion of prolonged grief disorder in DSM-V. In: Stroebe MS, Hansson RO, Schut H, et al., eds. *Handbook of Bereavement Research and Practice.* Washington, DC: American Psychological Association; 2008:165–186.
3. Horowitz MJ. Pathological grief and the activation of latent self images. *J Psychiatry.* 1980;137:1157–1162.
4. Prigerson HG, Jacobs SC. Traumatic grief as a distinct disorder: a rationale, consensus criteria, and a preliminary empirical test. In: Stroebe M, Hansson O, Schut H, et al., eds. *Handbook of Bereavement Research: Consequences, Coping and Care.* Washington, DC: American Psychological Association; 2001:613–646.
5. Worden JW. *Grief Counseling and Grief Therapy.* 4th ed. New York: Springer; 2009:127–151.
6. Prigerson HG, Horowitz MJ, Jacobs SC, et al. Prolonged grief disorder: psychometric validation of criteria proposed for DSM-V and ICD-11. *PLoS Med.* 2009;6(8) e1000121.
7. Horowitz MJ, Siegel B, Holen A, et al. Diagnostic criteria for complicated grief disorder. *Am J Psychiatry.* 1997;154(7):904–910.
8. Prigerson HG, Bierhals AJ, Kasl SV, et al. Traumatic grief as a risk factor for mental and physical morbidity. *Am J Psychiatry.* 1997;154(5):616–623.
9. Prigerson HG, Shear MK, Frank E, et al. Traumatic grief: a case of loss-induced trauma. *Am J Psychiatry.* 1997;154(7):1003–1009.
10. Boelen PA, van den Bout J, de Keijser J. Traumatic grief as a disorder distinct from bereavement-related depression and anxiety: a replication study with bereaved mental health care patients. *Am J Psychiatry.* 2003;160(7):1339–1341.
11. Prigerson HG, Shear MK, Jacobs SC, et al. Consensus criteria for traumatic grief: a preliminary empirical test. *Br J Psychiatry.* 1999;174:67–73.
12. Prigerson HG, Bridge J, Maciejewski PK, et al. Influence of traumatic grief on suicidal ideation among young adults. *Am J Psychiatry.* 1999;156(12):1994–1995.
13. Boelen PA, Prigerson HG. The influence of symptoms of prolonged grief disorder, depression, and anxiety on quality of life among bereaved adults: a prospective study. *Eur Arch Psychiatry Clin Neurosci.* 2007;257(8):444–452.
14. Goldsmith B, Morrison RS, Vanderwerker LC, et al. Elevated rates of prolonged grief disorder in African Americans. *Death Stud.* 2008;32(4):352–365.
15. Golden A-MJ, Dalgleish T. Is prolonged grief distinct from bereavement-related posttraumatic stress? *Psychiatry Res.* 2010;178(2):336–341.
16. Prigerson HG, Maciejewski PK, Center for Psychooncology & Palliative Care Research, eds. *Prolonged Grief Disorder (PG-13).* Boston: Dana-Farber Cancer Institute; 2010.
17. Kutner JS, Kilbourn KM. Bereavement: addressing challenges faced by advanced cancer patients, their caregivers, and their physicians. *Prim Care Clin Office Pract.* 2009;36(4):825–844.
18. Mitchell AM, Kim Y, Prigerson HG, et al. Complicated grief and suicidal ideation in adult survivors of suicide. *Suicide Life Threat Behav.* 2005;35(5):498–506.
19. Silverman GK, Johnson JG, Prigerson HG. Preliminary explorations of the effects of prior trauma and loss on risk for psychiatric disorders in recently widowed people. *Isr J Psychiatry Relat Sci.* 2001;38(3–4):202–215.
20. Vanderwerker LC, Jacobs SC, Parkes CM, et al. An exploration of associations between separation anxiety in childhood and complicated grief in later life. *J Nerv Ment Dis.* 2006;194(2):121–123.
21. Johnson JG, Zhang B, Greer JA, et al. Parental control, partner dependency, and complicated grief among widowed adults in the community. *J Nerv Ment Dis.* 2007;195(1):26–30.
22. Mitchell AM, Kim Y, Prigeson HG, et al. Complicated grief in survivors of suicide. *Crisis.* 2004;25(1):12–18.
23. Goodwin RD, Beautrais AL, Fergusson DM. Familial transmission of suicidal ideation and suicide attempts: evidence from a general population sample. *Psychiatry Res.* 2004;126(2):159–165.
24. Runeson B, Asberg M. Family history of suicide among suicide victims. *Am J Psychiatry.* 2003;160(8):1525–1526.
25. Zhang B, El-Jawahri A, Prigerson HG. Update on bereavement research: evidence-based guidelines for the diagnosis and treatment of complicated bereavement. *J Palliat Med.* 2006;9(5):1188–1203.
26. Kent H, McDowell J. Sudden bereavement in acute care settings. *Nurs Stand.* 2004;19(6):38–42.
27. Chiambretto P, Moroni L, Guarnerio C, et al. Prolonged grief and depression in caregivers of patients in vegetative state. *Brain Inj.* 2010;24(4):581–588.
28. Wright AA, Keating NL, Balboni TA, et al. Place of death: correlations with quality of life of patients with cancer and predictors of bereaved caregivers' mental health. *J Clin Oncol.* 2010;28(29):4457–4464.
29. Boelen PA, ed Keijser J, van den Bout J, et al. Treatment of complicated grief: a comparison between cognitive-behavioral therapy and supportive counseling. *J Consult Clin Psychol.* 2007;75(2):277–284.

30. Shear K, Frank E, Houck PR, et al. Treatment of complicated grief: a randomized controlled trial. *JAMA.* 2005;293(21):2601–2608.

31. de Groot M, de Keijser J, Neeleman J, et al. Cognitive behaviour therapy to prevent complicated grief among relatives and spouses bereaved by suicide: cluster randomised controlled trial. *BMJ* 2007;334(7601):994.

32. Reynolds 3rd CF, Miller MD, Pasternak RE. Treatment of bereavement-related major depressive episodes in later life: a controlled study of acute and continuation treatment with nortriptyline and interpersonal psychotherapy. *Am J Psychiatry.* 1999;156(2):202–208.

33. Workman S. Prolonged grief disorder: a problem for the past, the present, and the future. *PLoS Med.* 2009;6(8):e1000122.

34. Lannen PK, Wolfe J, Prigerson HG, et al. Unresolved grief in a national sample of bereaved parents: impaired mental and physical health 4 to 9 years later. *J Clin Oncol.* 2008;26:5870–5876.

35. Rowe J, Clyman R, Green C, et al. Follow-up families who experience a perinatal death. *Pediatrics.* 1978;62:166–170.

Appendix 74-1 Clinical Screening Tool for Prolonged Grief Disorder (PG-13)

Prolonged grief disorder (PGD) is a newly defined syndrome that is a specific reaction to the loss of someone loved very much. There are a particular set of PGD symptoms—feelings, thoughts, actions—that must be elevated at 6 months post-loss and that must be associated with significant functional impairment in order for a person to meet criteria for PGD.

1.1.1.1 INSTRUCTIONS

Below lie instructions for how to score (diagnose) Prolonged Grief Disorder (PGD). Each of the requirements for Criteria A-E must be met for an individual to be diagnosed with PGD.

A. EVENT CRITERION: In order to complete the PG-13, we assume the respondent has experienced bereavement (i.e., the loss of a loved person).

B. SEPARATION DISTRESS: The respondent must experience PG-13 questions #1 or 2 at least daily.

C. DURATION CRITERION: The symptoms of separation distress must be elevated at least 6 months after the loss. That is, PG-13 question #3 must be answered as "Yes".

D. COGNITIVE, EMOTIONAL, AND BEHAVIORAL SYMPTOMS: The respondent must experience 5 of the PG-13 questions #4-12 at least "once a day" or "quite a bit".

E. IMPAIRMENT CRITERION: The respondent must have significant impairment in social, occupational, or other important areas of functioning (e.g., domestic responsibilities). That is, PG-13 question #13 must be answered as "Yes".

PG-13 is a diagnostic tool. If a respondent meets criteria for PGD, this would suggest that he or she should seek a more thorough evaluation from a mental health professional. Only an in-person assessment by a mental health professional can determine for certain, the clinical significance of the reported symptoms, and provide recommendations or referrals for treatment.

Part I instructions: **For each item, place a check mark to indicate your answer.**
1. In the past month, how often have you felt yourself longing or yearning for the person you lost?
_____ 1 = Not at all
_____ 2 = At least once
_____ 3 = At least once a week
_____ 4 = At least once a day
_____ 5 = Several times a day

2. In the past month, how often have you had intense feelings of emotional pain, sorrow,
or pangs of grief related to the lost relationship?
_____ 1 = Not at all
_____ 2 = At least once
_____ 3 = At least once a week
_____ 4 = At least once a day
_____ 5 = Several times a day

3. For questions 1 or 2 above, have you experienced either of these symptoms at least daily
and after 6 months have elapsed since the loss?
_____ No
_____ Yes

4. In the past month, how often have you tried to avoid reminders that the person you lost is gone?
_____ 1 = Not at all
_____ 2 = At least once
_____ 3 = At least once a week
_____ 4 = At least once a day
_____ 5 = Several times a day

5. In the past month, how often have you felt stunned, shocked, or dazed by your loss?
_____ 1 = Not at all
_____ 2 = At least once
_____ 3 = At least once a week
_____ 4 = At least once a day
_____ 5 = Several times a day

Part II instructions: **For each item, please indicate how you currently feel. Circle the number to the right to indicate your answer.**	Not at all	Slightly	Somewhat	Quite a bit	Overwhelmingly
6. Do you feel confused about your role in life or feel like you don't know who you are (i.e., feeling that a part of yourself has died)?	1	2	3	4	5
7. Have you had trouble accepting the loss?	1	2	3	4	5
8. Has it been hard for you to trust others since your loss?	1	2	3	4	5
9. Do your feel bitter over your loss?	1	2	3	4	5
10. Do you feel that moving on (e.g., making new friends, pursuing new interests) would be difficult for you now?	1	2	3	4	5
11. Do you feel emotionally numb since your loss?	1	2	3	4	5
12. Do you feel that life is unfulfilling, empty, or meaningless since your loss?	1	2	3	4	5

Part III instructions: **For each item, place a check mark to indicate your answer.**
13. Have you experienced a significant reduction in social, occupational, or other important areas
of functioning (e.g., domestic responsibilities)?
_____ No
_____ Yes

Bibliography

Prigerson HG, Vanderwerker LC, Maciejewski PK. A Case for the Inclusion of Prolonged Grief Disorder in DSM-V. In: Stroebe M, Hansson R, Schut H, et al., eds. *Handbook of Bereavement Research and Practice: 21st Century Perspectives.* Washington DC: American Psycholo gical Association Press; 2008.

Prigerson HG, Horowitz MJ, Jacobs SC, et al. Prolonged Grief Disorder: Psychometric Validation of Criteria Proposed for DSM-V and ICD-11. *PLoS Med.* 2009;6(8):e1000121. doi:10.1371/journal.pmed.1000121.

Zhang B, El-Jawahri A, Prigerson HG. Update on bereavement research: evidence-based guidelines for the diagnosis and treatment of complicated bereavement. *J Palliat Med.* 2006;9:1188–1203.

Goldsmith B, Morrison RS, Vanderwerker LC, Prigerson HG. Elevated rates of prolonged grief disorder in African Americans. *Death Stud.* 2008;32(4):352–365.

Kiely DK, Prigerson H, Mitchell SL. Health care proxy grief symptoms before the death of nursing home residents with advanced dementia. *Am J Geriatr Psychiatry.* 2008;16(8):664–673.

Morina N, Rudari V, Bleichhardt G, et al. Prolonged grief disorder, depression, and posttraumatic stress disorder among bereaved Kosovar civilian war survivors: A preliminary investigation. *Int J Soc Psychiatry.* 2009 Jul 10. [Epub ahead of print].

Maciejewski PK, Zhang B, Block SD, et al. An Empirical Examination of the State Theory of Grief Resolution. *JAMA.* 2007;297:716–723.

Articles That Have Applied ICG-R to PGD Criteria

Boelen PA, Prigerson HG. The influence of symptoms of prolonged grief disorder, depression, and anxiety on quality of life among bereaved adults: a prospective study. *Eur Arch Psychiatry Clin Neurosci.* 2007;257(8):444–452.

MODELS FOR DELIVERING PALLIATIVE CARE

Chapter 75

What Are the Eligibility Criteria for Hospice?

MELISSA D. ALDRIDGE CARLSON AND MARTHA L. TWADDLE

INTRODUCTION AND SCOPE OF THE PROBLEM

Hospice is both a philosophy of care and a regulated insurance benefit. The Medicare Hospice Benefit (MHB) was enacted by Congress in 1982 and is the dominant source of payment for hospice care.[1] Specifically, 84% of patients who receive hospice services in the United States are covered by the MHB, with the remaining patients covered by private insurance (9%), Medicaid (5%), and other sources (2%).[1] When one reads about "eligibility criteria for hospice," what is actually meant is "eligibility criteria that insures reimbursement for hospice services under the Medicare Hospice Benefit." That is, patients may receive hospice services and pay for it themselves; however, if patients and their families want to receive hospice services as a covered insurance benefit, eligibility criteria apply.

Despite growth in the number of hospice agencies and patients receiving hospice care, the MHB remains one of Medicare's smallest programs and is used by only 39% of all deaths in the United States,[1] although the general trend is toward an increase in annual use. The extent to which this percentage reflects underuse of hospice is unknown, because low usage likely reflects a combination of barriers to hospice care and patient preferences not to receive such care before death. Potential barriers include lack of knowledge regarding hospice care,[2-5] hospice admission criteria,[6] and ineligibility for hospice care under the MHB.

RELEVANT REGULATIONS REGARDING HOSPICE

Patient Eligibility Criteria

Patients are eligible to receive hospice care reimbursed under the MHB if they meet the following criteria: (1) the individual has a life expectancy of 6 months or less if the disease follows its expected course, as certified by two physicians,[7] and (2) the individual forgoes Medicare reimbursement for ongoing therapy or curative medical treatment related to the terminal diagnosis.[8] Table 75-1 outlines the guidelines for determining whether a patient is eligible for hospice care.

Current eligibility under the MHB is consistent with hospice's origins and the goals of the hospice founders—interdisciplinary care for patients with a limited life expectancy and for whom curative treatments are no longer effective or desired. The limited life expectancy[7] and waiver of Medicare reimbursement for pursuit of curative treatment of the terminal condition for which hospice care is elected[8] are necessary and appropriate criteria for defining this target hospice population. The advantage of the MHB and its eligibility criteria is that it offers a comprehensive benefit to a defined population of patients, provided primarily in the home setting by an interdisciplinary health care team through an intermittent care model. The disadvantage of the current eligibility criteria is that it is difficult for individuals with uncertain prognosis or those who may be availed of more complex treatment options to access hospice in a timely manner. For example, although there has been significant growth in the range of diagnoses of individuals receiving hospice care,[1] prognostic difficulty (i.e., difficulty in certifying that a patient has 6 months or less to live as required by the MHB) remains a barrier to hospice referral,[9-11] particularly for individuals with non–cancer-related diagnoses. Similarly, the line between curative and palliative treatments has become increasingly less distinct, because some curative treatments simultaneously provide the benefit of symptom relief.

TABLE 75-1. Criteria for Hospice Coverage: General Guidelines for Certifying Terminal Illness

	CLINICAL STATUS	SYMPTOM BURDEN	SIGNS	LABORATORY (WHEN AVAILABLE)	FUNCTION
Progression of Disease (Decline in Clinical Status) *Note:* This top row outlines universal evidence for decline in a patient's status that makes him or her eligible for Medicare coverage for hospice. These criteria can be applied to assess eligibility regardless of underlying diagnosis.	Recurrent or intractable infection Weight loss not due to reversible or treatable causes, dysphagia leading to aspiration, or inadequate oral intake Progressive pressure ulcer despite optimal care Delirium or cognitive failure without the diagnosis of dementia	Dyspnea Intractable cough, nausea/vomiting, diarrhea Pain—increasing or progressive Fatigue/malaise Cognitive deterioration/confusion Anorexia	SBP <90, tachycardia Ascites Vascular/lymphatic obstruction Effusions Weakness Change in location of care FEV_1 <30%	Increased Pco_2 Decreased Po_2 or Sao_2 Chronic kidney disease—progressive or stage 4-5 Abnormal liver enzymes Increased tumor markers Progressive serum sodium abnormality or increased potassium Hyponatremia Anemia Hypoalbuminemia Hypercalcemia Elevated brain natriuretic peptide (BNP), troponin, cystatin C, or C-reactive protein	Decline in KPS, PPS Decline in FAST Decline in Mortality Risk Index score Increased health care usage because of chronic or progressive disease state (e.g., hospital admission, ED visit, MD office visits)
Disease-Specific Guidelines for Certifying Terminal Illness KPS, PPS <70% Dependent on >2 activities of daily living		Pulmonary	Dyspnea at rest supported by FEV_1 (after bronchodilator) is <30% ED/hospitalization for respiratory infection or respiratory failure AND oxygen saturation <88% on room air or Pco_2 >50 in last 3 months Supported by sequelae of right heart failure, weight loss >10% over last 6 months, or resting tachycardia >100/min		
		Heart	Optimally treated AND continued dyspnea at rest Supported by symptomatic arrhythmia, history of cardiac arrest or unexplained syncope, brain embolism of cardiac origin, concomitant HIV disease		
		Renal	Acute: CrCl <10mL/min or serum Cr >8mg/dL (15 or 6 for diabetic) with CHF and not seeking dialysis. Supported by mechanical ventilator support; malignancy; chronic or advanced lung, heart, liver disease; sepsis; immunosuppression; albumin <3.5; cachexia; platelets <25,000; disseminated intravascular coagulation; GI bleed Chronic: Supported by symptoms of renal failure: uremia, oliguria, intractable hyperkalemia, uremic pericarditis, hepatorenal syndrome, intractable fluid overload		

Disease	KPS	Criteria
Liver		INR >1.5, serum albumin <2.5 and ascites, SBP, hepatorenal syndrome, encephalopathy or variceal bleeding. Supported by progressive malnutrition, muscle wasting, use of alcohol, hepatocellular carcinoma, hepatitis B positive, hepatitis C refractory to interferon. May be waiting for liver transplant
Cancer		Pancreatic, small cell lung, brain, or others with distant metastases and continued decline with therapy or refusal of further therapy
HIV	KPS <50%	CD4 <25 or viral load >100,000 copies and either CNS lymphoma, wasting, *Mycobacterium avium* complex, progressive multifocal leukoencephalopathy, systemic lymphoma, visceral Kaposi sarcoma, renal failure, cryptospiridiosis, or toxoplasmosis. Supported by diarrhea >1 year, serum albumin <2.5, active substance abuse, age >50 years, not using HAART, advanced AIDS dementia, toxoplasmosis, heart failure class IV, advanced liver disease
Dementia (Alzheimer disease)		FAST 7 or greater. Assistance with ambulation, bathing, dressing. Urinary/fecal incontinence. < 6 meaningful words. Aspiration pneumonitis or fever despite antibiotics. 10% weight loss last 6 months
ALS		Vital capacity < 30%. Critical nutrition impairment. Life-threatening complications (Need 2 of 3)
Stroke	KPS or PPS <40%	Inability to maintain hydration and caloric intake, aspiration pneumonitis, dysphagia with no artificial feedings. Thrombotic/embolic event (ischemic) with poor prognosis: anterior infarct with cortical and subcortical involvement, large bi-hemispheric, basilar artery or bilateral vertebral artery occluded. Hemorrhagic with poor prognosis: midline shift (≥1.5 cm), obstructive hydrocephalus with no ventricular-peritoneal shunt, large (≥20 mL infratentorial and ≥50 mL supratentorial), extension to ventricles
Coma		Meets 3 of the following criteria: Day 3 with abnormal brainstem reflexes. Nonverbal. No withdrawal to pain. Serum Cr >1.5 mg/dL

This table represents a compilation of all of the local coverage determination (LCD) criteria from the Medicare Administrative Contractors (MAC). This table should not be considered the authority as to criteria, but presents a general overview. Medical Directors and Hospice team members should consult their assigned MAC LCDs because regional variation does exist and LCDs are updated and changed on a regular basis.

AIDS, Acquired immunodeficiency syndrome; *ALS*, amyotrophic lateral sclerosis; *CHF*, congestive heart failure; *CNS*, central nervous system; *Cr*, creatinine; *CrCl*, creatinine clearance; *ED*, emergency department; *FAST*, Functional Assessment Staging scale for dementia; *FEV₁*, forced expiratory volume in 1 second; *GI*, gastrointestinal; *HAART*, highly active antiretroviral therapy; *HIV*, human immunodeficiency virus; *INR*, international normalized ratio; *KPS*, Karnofsky Performance Score; *MD*, medical doctor; Pco_2, partial pressure of carbon dioxide; Po_2, partial pressure of oxygen; *PPS*, Palliative Performance Scale; Sao_2, oxygen saturation; *SBP*, systolic blood pressure.

Hospice Certification Requirements

To receive Medicare reimbursement for providing hospice care under the MHB, hospices must be certified by Medicare as being in compliance with the Hospice Conditions of Participation (CoP).[12] The CoPs are the federal health and safety requirements that all certified hospices are required to meet. They are a flexible framework for continuous quality improvement in hospice care and reflect the current standards of practice relating to the availability, staffing, and location of patient care. These federal regulations distinguish between core hospice services and noncore hospice services. Core services are those that must be provided by hospice staff employed by the hospice, including skilled nursing services, physician services, volunteer services, counseling services (including bereavement counseling), spiritual care, dietary counseling, and social services.[13] Noncore services, defined as services that may be outsourced by the hospice provider, include physical therapy; occupational therapy; speech-language pathology; home health care; homemaker services; administration and provision of drugs, biological agents, and medical supplies; continuous home care; respite care; and other services.[14] It is estimated that as of 2010, approximately 93% of hospices operating in the United States are certified by Medicare.[1]

KEY MESSAGES TO PATIENTS AND FAMILIES

Patients and families, and the health care professionals who care for them, need to be aware of not only the substantial benefits that hospice services may provide but also the eligibility criteria the beneficiary must meet to elect the MHB and thus receive insurance coverage for hospice services. Although dramatic growth has taken place in the number of individuals receiving hospice services, many patients and families enroll in hospice too late in the course of their disease to use the benefit fully. Almost one third of individuals who enroll with hospice die within 1 week of enrollment,[1] and the mean length of stay in hospice care in the United States still hovers around 21 days. Debate regarding whether to change hospice eligibility criteria is ongoing[15] and demonstration projects funded by the *Accountable Care Act* may shed light on the benefits and costs of expanding MHB eligibility criteria.

It is also important for patients and families to realize that if they do not meet the hospice eligibility criteria, alternative palliative care options are available. Specifically, palliative care is a service most often provided in the hospital setting and these services have been rapidly growing over the past decade.[16,17] Although the philosophy of palliative care is nearly congruent with that of hospice care, the scope of care is not identical because it differs in terms of both timing and types of patients served. No federal or commercial insurance benefits are specific to palliative care; thus there exist no formal eligibility criteria. Palliative care is available to patients who continue to benefit from life-prolonging treatments, and access to palliative care is not dependent on prognosis. Palliative care's independence from prognosis is especially important for individuals with conditions such as heart disease, stroke, or dementia, for which prognostication is particularly difficult. Ideally, individuals may receive palliative care services as indicated by objective measures of functional decline and need, independent of prognosis, and in conjunction with all other beneficial therapies. As the disease progresses and when eligible, individuals could transition to hospice care. Likewise, some patients with non–cancer-related diagnoses who are discharged from hospice with an extended prognosis prefer to continue with the support of palliative care until which time they again require (and are eligible for) hospice care.

CONCLUSION AND SUMMARY

Hospice is both a benefit and a philosophy of care aimed to ensure comfort and maximize quality of life for those patients who are coming to the end of their lives. While it continues to be underutilized, which is due in part to both patient concerns and its restrictive requirements for enrollment, hospice offers significant benefits to patients and their families. For patients not eligible or who choose to not enroll in hospice, palliative care is a viable option that can ensure adequate symptom control and continue ongoing conversations about goals of care until the time when a patient might otherwise become eligible or choose to enroll in hospice.

SUMMARY RECOMMENDATIONS

- Clinicians referring patients to hospice must be knowledgeable regarding eligibility criteria for the Medicare Hospice Benefit. Specifically, patients must have a prognosis of 6 months or less if the disease follows its natural course, and they are required to forgo Medicare reimbursement for ongoing therapy or curative medical treatment related to the terminal diagnosis
- Clinicians, patients, and families should consider the increasingly prevalent nonhospice palliative care options available in their community if patients do not meet Medicare Hospice Benefit eligibility criteria.

ACKNOWLEDGMENT

The authors wish to acknowledge Sally Kelley, MD, for her significant contributions to Table 75-1.

REFERENCES

1. National Hospice and Palliative Care Organization. *Facts and figures: hospice care in America.* http://www.nhpco.org/files/public/statistics_research/2011_facts_figures.pdf; Accessed September 24, 2012.

2. Rhodes RL, Teno JM, Welch LC. Access to hospice for African Americans: are they informed about the option of hospice? *J Palliat Med.* 2006;9:268–272.

3. Cherlin E, Fried T, Prigerson HG, Schulman-Green D, Johnson-Hurzeler R, Bradley EH. Communication between physicians and family caregivers about care at the end of life: when do discussions occur and what is said? *J Palliat Med.* 2005;8:1176–1185.

4. General Accounting Office. Medicare hospice care: modifications to payment methodology may be warranted. GAO-05-42. 2004.

5. Friedman BT, Harwood MK, Shields M. Barriers and enablers to hospice referrals: an expert overview. *J Palliat Med.* 2002;5:73–84.

6. Lorenz KA, Asch SM, Rosenfeld KE, Liu H, Ettner SL. Hospice admission practices: where does hospice fit in the continuum of care? *J Am Geriatr Soc.* 2004;52:725–730.

7. Code of Federal Regulations 42CFR418.22, Certification of Terminal Illness. 2002.

8. Code of Federal Regulations 42CFR418.24, Election of Hospice Care. 2002.

9. Brickner L, Scannell K, Marquet S, Ackerson L. Barriers to hospice care and referrals: survey of physicians' knowledge, attitudes, and perceptions in a health maintenance organization. *J Palliat Med.* 2004;7:411–418.

10. Simpson DA. Prognostic criteria for hospice eligibility. *JAMA.* 2000;283:2527.

11. Fox E, Landrum-McNiff K, Zhong Z, Dawson NV, Wu AW, Lynn J. Evaluation of prognostic criteria for determining hospice eligibility in patients with advanced lung, heart, or liver disease. SUPPORT Investigators: Study to Understand Prognoses and Preferences for Outcomes and Risks of Treatments. *JAMA.* 1999;282:1638–1645.

12. Code of Federal Regulations 42CFR418.50-100, Conditions of Participation. 2002.

13. Centers for Medicare & Medicaid Services. *Medicare and Medicaid Programs: Hospice Conditions of Participation; Final Rule,* Code of Federal Regulations 42CFR418. 64 Core Services.

14. Centers for Medicare & Medicaid Services. *Medicare and Medicaid Programs: Hospice Conditions of Participation; Final Rule,* Code of Federal Regulations 42CFR418. 70-78 Furnishing of Non-Core Services.

15. Carlson MD, Morrison RS, Bradley EH. Improving access to hospice care: informing the debate. *J Palliat Med.* 2008;11: 438–443.

16. Goldsmith B, Dietrich J, Du Q, Morrison RS. Variability in access to hospital palliative care in the United States. *J Palliat Med.* 2008;11:1094–1102.

17. Pan CX, Morrison RS, Meier DE, et al. How prevalent are hospital-based palliative care programs? Status report and future directions. *J Palliat.* 2001;4:315–324.

INTRODUCTION AND SCOPE OF THE PROBLEM
KEY MESSAGES TO PATIENTS AND FAMILIES

INTRODUCTION AND SCOPE OF THE PROBLEM

Hospice care in the United States began in the 1970s as a social movement that focused on providing a higher quality death than typically experienced in the hospital setting. Hospitalized dying patients often suffered from significant pain and discomfort, did not receive the emotional and spiritual support necessary to cope with their approaching death, and faced uncertainty as to whether the life-prolonging medical interventions to which they were subjected were consistent with their goals of care.[1] Hospice was originally provided by "charitable"[1] and "charismatic"[2] leaders working individually or through nonprofit community-based agencies, caring for patients in their own homes, and relying on charitable donations as the sole revenue source. Despite growing support in the early 1970s for the general principles embraced by hospice, the concept (comfort rather than curative care), setting (home rather than hospital care), and focus (patient and family rather than patient) of hospice care were still considered experimental. The passing of the *Tax Equity and Fiscal Responsibility Act* (TEFRA) in 1982 marked a critical turning point for the hospice movement in the United States. TEFRA authorized Medicare to reimburse for hospice services, and thus hospice care became publicly funded under the Medicare Hospice Benefit (MHB).

The MHB is currently the dominant source of payment for hospice care. Specifically, 89% of hospice patient care days annually are paid for by the MHB, with the balance paid by private insurance, managed care insurance plans, Medicaid, private pay, or charity care.[3] To receive reimbursement from Medicare, hospices must be certified by Medicare as being in compliance with the Hospice Conditions of Participation (CoP).[4] The CoPs are the federal health and safety requirements that all certified hospices are required to meet. They are a flexible framework for continuous quality improvement in hospice care and reflect the current standards of practice relating to the availability, staffing, and location of patient care.

Consistent with the hospice philosophy, the majority of hospice services are provided in a patient's home (Table 76-1). A "home" may be defined as the patient's private residence, a residential facility, or a nursing home. Residential hospices—assisted living specifically for hospice patients in a group setting—are rare in the United States given the robust presence of nursing homes. As part of the MHB, respite care is provided as needed to relieve the stress on family caregivers. It is delivered as short-term (usually ≤5 days) inpatient care for the patient to provide respite for the individual's family or other persons caring for the patient.[5] It may be provided by the agency or through other arrangements made by the hospice, and it must be provided by a hospice, hospital, skilled nursing facility, or intermediate care facility that meets the standards set forth in the MHB regulations.

If conditions warrant, a patient may also receive care in a hospice inpatient facility or in an acute-care hospital under the MHB. Medicare payment rules, however, are designed to limit the number of patient care days that occur outside of a patient's residence to ensure that hospice care under the MHB remains a home care delivery model. Specifically, federal regulations stipulate that payment for inpatient care is limited. The total payment to the hospice for inpatient care (general or respite) is subject to a limitation that total inpatient care days for Medicare patients not exceed 20% of the total days for which these patients elected hospice care.[6] These inpatient stays are typically time limited, and the hospice agency must have a contract with the hospital if that is the site of care delivery to provide care without disenrolling patients from the hospice benefit.

KEY MESSAGES TO PATIENTS AND FAMILIES

Hospice services are intended to enable patients to remain at home during the terminal stages of illness and to die at home with supportive services for both the patient and the family. Rules regarding reimbursement for hospice services under the MHB are designed to promote and maintain hospice as a home health model and to provide an alternative to hospital or other institutional death.

It is also important for patients and families to realize that if they cannot receive services at their private residence, alternative options are available. Many hospices serve patients who reside in nursing homes, group housing, or assisted living settings. Nursing homes and hospitals have hospice contracts

TABLE 76-1. Characteristics of Patients Receiving Hospice Care Services

LOCATION OF HOSPICE PATIENTS AT TIME OF DEATH	2010 (%)
Private residence	41.1
Nursing home	18.0
Residential facility	7.3
Hospice inpatient facility	21.9
Acute-care hospital	11.4

From National Hospice and Palliative Care Organization. Facts and figures: hospice care in America. Alexandria, VA; 2010. http://www.nhpco.org/files/public/Statistics_Research/2011_facts_figures.pdf; Accessed September 24, 2012.

enabling patients in these settings to receive palliative care outside of the MHB or be cared for in dedicated hospice units. In addition, palliative care programs outside of the hospice setting are more widely available than ever before, particularly hospital-based palliative care programs.[7,8]

SUMMARY RECOMMENDATIONS

- It is important for hospice users and referring clinicians to understand the historical roots of hospice as a social movement that focused on providing a higher quality death than typically experienced in the hospital setting.
- The majority of hospice services are provided in a patient's home, although clinicians should also understand that it can also be provided in nursing homes, inpatient hospice, or acute-care hospitals.
- It is essential for providers to explain to patients and families the limits of inpatient hospice or hospitalizations so families understand that these are time limited and only for management of acute symptoms or for patients who are actively dying.

REFERENCES

1. Paradis LF, Cummings SB. The evolution of hospice in America toward organizational homogeneity. *J Health Soc Behav.* 1986;27:370–386.
2. James N, Field D. The routinization of hospice: charisma and bureaucratization. *Soc Sci Med.* 1992;34:1363–1375.
3. National Hospice and Palliative Care Organization. *Facts and figures: hospice care in America.* Alexandria, VA; 2011. http://www.nhpco.org/files/public/Statistics_Research/2011_facts_figures.pdf; Accessed September 24, 2012.
4. Code of Federal Regulations 42CFR418.50-100, Conditions of Participation. 2002.
5. Code of Federal Regulations 42 CFR418.204(b), Special Coverage Requirements. 2010.
6. Code of Federal Regulations 42CFR 418.302, Payment Procedures for Hospice Care. 2002.
7. Goldsmith B, Dietrich J, Du Q, Morrison RS. Variability in access to hospital palliative care in the United States. *J Palliat Med.* 2008;11:1094–1102.
8. Pan CX, Morrison RS, Meier DE, et al. How prevalent are hospital-based palliative care programs? Status report and future directions. *J Palliat Med.* 2001;4:315–324.

Chapter 77

What Models Exist for Delivering Palliative Care and Hospice in Nursing Homes?

JUSTINE S. SEFCIK, ADITI RAO, AND MARY ERSEK

INTRODUCTION AND SCOPE OF THE PROBLEM

Between 1.5 and 1.8 million people currently live in U.S. nursing homes,[1] and by 2050 it is estimated that more than 3 million people will spend time in a nursing home. Nationwide, 25% of people die in a nursing home, and this percentage is expected to increase as the population ages.[2] Of persons with advanced dementia, 70% will die in a nursing home.[3] The vast majority of nursing home residents need assistance with activities of daily living (ADLs), and more than half are totally dependent or need extensive assistance with bathing, dressing, toileting, and transferring.[4]

State and federal governments spend billions of dollars every year for older adults and nursing home residents at the end of life. Nursing home care costs between $114 and $136 billion per year.[1] Medicaid pays for the majority of nursing home costs for long-term care, although Medicare covers payments for almost 18% of costs and is the major payer for the first 90 days of a nursing home stay.[1] Health care costs are particularly high for older adults, including frail nursing home residents, in the last months to year of life.[5,6]

Despite the billions of dollars spent for end-of-life care in nursing homes, the quality of care in this setting is lower than the care delivered in other health care settings, resulting in unnecessary suffering for residents and considerable distress for their families. End-of-life care in nursing homes has long been associated with poor symptom control, burdensome transitions, and decreased family satisfaction with care.[7,8]

Palliative care is one approach to care delivery that can enhance outcomes and decrease costs. Compared to usual care, palliative care is associated with improved quality and satisfaction[9,10] and decreased costs.[11] However, comprehensive palliative care has not yet been routinely integrated into the nursing home setting, where its effectiveness can be thoroughly evaluated. Reports are anecdotal, and no rigorously evaluated cost or resident outcomes have been published.[2]

This chapter describes the nursing home as a setting for palliative care. It begins by describing the social, regulatory, and financial factors that affect nursing home care and reviews the challenges and the advantages of providing palliative care in this setting. It then reviews various models for palliative care delivery. The chapter ends with important issues to discuss with residents and families about palliative care.

SPECIAL CONSIDERATIONS IN DELIVERING PALLIATIVE CARE IN NURSING HOMES

Description of the Setting

Nursing homes are complex environments in which a disparate group of caregivers attempts to form a community to care for residents who may be frail, elderly, sick, or dying.[12] The number of vulnerable residents requiring complex care is growing rapidly. Long-term care residents often have multiple chronic conditions; short-term residents are often very ill, but expected to recover and go home.[13] More than 45% of nursing home residents have dementia, and an additional 23% have various other psychological disorders. Sixty-five percent of residents are prescribed psychoactive medications, including antidepressants, anxiolytics, antipsychotics, sedatives, and hypnotics. Roughly 60% of residents are bedridden or chairfast. Many require extensive assistance by nursing staff with their ADLs, and 25% receive therapy services by physical, occupational, and speech therapists.[14] Despite these demands for care, the nursing home industry's ability to meet the public need is threatened by issues of workforce capacity and care quality.

For decades, activists, researchers, and policymakers have voiced concerns regarding the quality of care in nursing homes. To address these concerns, in

1987 the federal government implemented a stringent set of regulations with which all Medicare-certified nursing homes were required to comply. These regulations, intended to improve oversight of care quality, made the nursing home industry one of the most heavily regulated industries in the country. Since the implementation of these regulations, nursing homes have been mandated to undergo comprehensive annual inspections by state surveyors who assess the processes and outcomes of the nursing care provided. Failure to meet regulatory standards results in deficiency citations.[4,14] Although care quality has arguably improved since these regulations were put into place, they are also criticized for being burdensome and restrictive.[2,12] Directors of nursing report that much of their time is spent addressing regulatory standards, rather than working with staff or caring for residents.[15] Additionally, because of the pressure to focus on compliance, caregivers, particularly registered nurses, are often forced to spend a great deal of their time documenting care rather than directly providing it.[12]

Unlicensed nursing assistants provide the majority of direct care in nursing homes. Licensed practical nurses (LPNs) are typically the largest group of licensed caregivers and registered nurses (RNs) the smallest. Numerous studies have demonstrated that adequate staffing and greater RN presence is associated with improved quality of care. Nonetheless, staffing represents a major challenge for nursing homes.[14] Turnover rates for all nursing staff members are staggeringly high. In 2008 the American Health Care Association reported that annual turnover among nursing assistants was 53%, that of LPNs and RNs was 43%, and for directors of nursing, 18%. Making matters worse, nursing homes frequently operate under slim profit margins. Reliant on Medicare and Medicaid reimbursement rates that have not adjusted to support increased staffing, nursing homes can rarely afford to staff according to recommendations. Instead, to remain financially viable, facilities staff according to the minimum standards.[14] Therefore, despite residents' complex care needs, RNs, the most skilled caregivers, are the least utilized because they are the most expensive.

Negative reports in the popular press have given nursing homes a poor reputation. Although legitimate deficiencies do exist, nursing homes today rarely resemble the stereotypes they have been assigned.[16] Nursing staff typically care very deeply for their residents and form strong relationships with the residents and their family members.[12] Additionally, although nursing home staff have less formal education than their colleagues in acute care, nurses and nursing assistants are frequently eager to receive continuing education to support them in their practice.[2] Caregivers in nursing homes, by and large, aim to provide the best care to their frail and elderly residents. Yet, they often struggle to do so amidst a variety of financial, regulatory, and workforce issues.

Given the growing numbers of residents who die in nursing homes each year, establishing strong palliative care programs within this setting is important for enhancing the quality of life these residents experience and the quality of care they receive. Many attributes of nursing homes make them ideal settings in which to deliver these services. Given the complexities surrounding care delivery in this setting, however, challenges exist that limit progress toward this goal.

Challenges to Delivering Palliative Care in Nursing Homes

Current reimbursement patterns, regulatory structures, workforce capacity issues, and resident characteristics hamper efforts to expand the delivery of palliative care services within nursing homes. For example, payer systems favor restorative care. Efforts to administer palliative care are misinterpreted by facilities and regulators as a lack of intervention congruent with poor care quality and potentially resulting in deficiency citations for facilities. In addition, nursing home staff have limited formal educational preparation and little knowledge regarding palliative care, and this area experiences a high level of employee turnover. To increase residents' access to palliative care, these contextual challenges must be addressed.[2]

Long-term care residents in nursing homes are typically frail and elderly, suffering from cognitive impairments and multiple comorbidities. They are relatively dependent and require a great deal of care. For 64% of these residents, Medicaid is their primary insurer, and Medicaid reimburses at a lower rate than either Medicare or private payers.[14] Therefore, to stay solvent, nursing homes attempt to provide care that will maximize their reimbursement. Restorative care, rather than palliative care, is financially favorable.[2]

Primarily, Medicaid and Medicare pay nursing homes a set amount of money per day for the care they provide rather than for specific care provided. Specifics of care are instead accounted for in the facility's case mix index, a composite score reflecting the complexity of care delivered to residents in the facility. In facilities providing more medical interventions, therapy services, and assistance with ADLs, the case mix index and the reimbursement rates are higher. Therefore facilities are financially incentivized to accept residents requiring "skilled" treatments. Intravenous therapies and tube feedings, for example, are reimbursed at a higher rate than alternative, less invasive therapies. These policies disincentivize nursing homes, already operating under slim profit margins, to provide palliative care services despite the fact that palliative services may improve the overall quality of care and the residents' quality of life.[2]

Additionally, regulators have been slow to adapt to palliative, rather than restorative, care. Nursing home regulations prescribe that nursing homes must "provide services and activities to attain or maintain the highest practicable physical, mental, and psychosocial well-being of each resident."[17] Therefore surveyors and caregivers alike frequently struggle to reconcile these standards with palliative care practices. Although for many frail, elderly, long-term residents, functional decline is inevitable and likely to be marked by weight loss, eating disturbances, and decreased mobility, facilities may be reluctant to use palliative care approaches because these expected changes are misperceived as a failure to meet regulatory standards. Instead of implementing care plans that account for declines and focus on symptom management and advanced care planning, facilities may transfer residents to the hospital or attempt interventions intended to rehabilitate these residents.[2]

Workforce issues in this setting present additional challenges. Nursing home staff tend to lack training in palliative care approaches and therefore have difficulties recognizing and implementing palliative treatments as appropriate. Unlicensed nursing assistants and LPNs provide the bulk of direct care to residents, and their skills related to symptom assessment and treatment, communication, and decision-making are limited. Clinical decision making is also somewhat fragmented because LPNs and nursing assistants are only minimally involved in developing care plans despite the fact that they spend the most time at the bedside.[2] This means that valuable and nuanced resident information may not be accounted for in the care planning process. As a result, nursing homes struggle to deliver quality end-of-life care—symptoms are poorly managed, families are dissatisfied, and residents are frequently subjected to unnecessary and distressing medical interventions and hospitalizations.[7,18] Pain, for example, occurs in as many as 45% to 83% of residents but often is inappropriately assessed and undertreated or untreated, resulting in unnecessary suffering, depression, and sleep disturbances.[19] To meet the needs of residents at the end of life more completely, all nursing staff members, particularly nursing assistants, need training that will enhance their abilities to recognize, communicate, and address symptoms and participate in advanced care planning.

Finally, the substantial medical and psychosocial issues that characterize the nursing home population create challenges for achieving palliative care goals. Cognitive impairment interferes with residents' abilities to provide reliable self-report, thereby hindering symptom assessment and management. For example, the gold standard for pain assessment—self-report— must be substituted with careful observation and surrogate estimates. Many observation tools are available to assess pain in nonverbal persons, but there is a dearth of systematic psychometric testing that establishes their reliability, validity, and clinical usefulness.[20] Tools to assess symptoms other than pain are even more limited.[20] When pain and other symptoms are identified, multiple comorbidities and polypharmacy are factors that complicate effective treatment of these problems.[21]

Advantages of Nursing Homes as Sites of Palliative Care

Despite the many challenges in delivering palliative care to persons in nursing homes, this setting can be an ideal place for elders to receive end-of-life care. Most nursing homes strive to create a homelike atmosphere. Rooms are modified to include personal items such as photographs and furniture. Staff often do not wear uniforms, and many facilities have resident pets, including birds, cats, and dogs. A growing number of facilities are built or remodeled to create smaller units, often referred to as "neighborhoods," with central, shared living spaces that include eating areas. These neighborhoods are no longer dominated by the nurses' station, which in turn creates a more relaxed and comforting environment for residents and their families. Therapeutic gardens and secure outdoor spaces also are becoming commonplace.[22]

In addition to changing their physical design, many facilities have embraced the "culture-change" model in which residents' needs and preferences come first and the facilities' operations adapt to meet this priority. In this model, residents decide for themselves when to get up, eat, and bathe, and the nursing assistants are given greater autonomy in their care for residents. Although this approach to care is not pervasive, about half of nursing homes have taken steps to transform the way that they provide care.[22]

Nursing home staff who routinely care for the same residents often develop long-term relationships with them. This familiarity can promote enhanced ability to interpret resident behaviors as their communication abilities diminish. Moreover, staff become emotionally invested in residents and describe themselves as part of the resident's family.[18,23] When coupled with appropriate palliative care training and staff support, these attachments create an atmosphere that promotes the dignity and comfort of residents at the end of life.

STRATEGIES FOR ENHANCING PALLIATIVE CARE IN NURSING HOMES

Several initiatives and strategies have been implemented to enhance palliative care in nursing homes. First, training programs to teach staff about palliative care have been shown to increase knowledge and skills,[24] and a comprehensive palliative care curriculum for staff is widely available.[25] Second, programs to enhance advance care planning in nursing homes can improve completion of advance directives and ensure a delivery of care that matches residents' preferences.[26–28] Strategies to identify residents who are most likely to benefit from hospice and palliative care also can enhance end-of-life care in nursing homes.[29,30]

Descriptive studies have illuminated ways to enhance the care of nursing home residents and their families at the end of life. Families' perspectives are particularly important. For example, Thompson and colleagues[31] reported that when family members of loved ones who have died in nursing homes have been asked to reflect on their experience, they commonly reported that they had limited interaction with physicians. In addition to the lack of communication and contact with physicians and staff, family members' discontent also stemmed from a perception that their loved one was suffering and staff did not deliver care that relieved suffering.[31,32] Furthermore, the respondents with negative experiences felt that the care delivered failed to meet their expectations and that their loved ones had unmet needs.[31] When families felt that basic needs were not being met, this resulted in a loss of trust in care providers.[32]

In contrast, satisfied family members felt they were witnessing excellent care when staff members gave them attention and provided information about what to expect during the last stage of the resident's life.[31] These family members believed that when the staff members acknowledged that the resident was dying, the staff expressed concern for the resident and became more attentive to both the resident and the family's needs.[31]

Practitioners in nursing homes have the opportunity to provide not only quality end-of-life care to residents but also support to family members during a potentially difficult time. Family members' satisfaction with their loved one's end-of-life care has been linked to the nursing home staff's ability to identify and effectively communicate when a resident is nearing death.[31] This evidence suggests that palliative care practitioners should be actively involved in staff education. In-service programs can be provided to nurses and nursing assistants on symptoms related to the end of life and evidence-based care for symptom management.

Additionally, open communication with family members and efforts to provide family education on symptoms and symptom management are also extremely important. It has been found that family members and caregivers do not often agree on the symptoms that residents with dementia experience when they are dying.[33] A lack of consensus on symptom identification and care provided can create conflict between staff and family members. Practitioners should be aware that dissatisfied family members can have a negative emotional response to the particular situation of the resident and experience feelings of guilt and regret for the placement of their loved one, as well as anger and frustration over the belief that the resident did not have a good death.[31]

For some family members, relinquishing their caregiving role is difficult.[32] This should be kept in mind, and nursing home staff should strive to direct family members to continue to contribute to an aspect of care that is still meaningful for them, such as providing massages, reading to their loved one, or playing the residents' preferred music for them.

Nursing homes have the ability to provide a consistent quality of care to residents; however, this can be disrupted by the movement of a resident to a hospital or another facility. During end-of-life care, nursing homes can keep residents comfortable

and strive to meet the residents' needs and wishes. A contributor to poorer quality of end-of-life care is transferring a resident, especially one with cognitive impairment, to any other facility during the last 3 days of life.[34] Furthermore, multiple transfers to a hospital or to other facilities in the last 90 days of life has the potential to be a burdensome transition for the resident.[34] Nursing homes have the opportunity to reduce potential burdens to residents and to maintain resident comfort by providing continuous care within the facility and avoiding any type of transfer.[34] Transfers interfere with the consistency of care delivered and can expose elders to potential medical errors. Moreover, transfers can be disruptive and disorienting.[2]

EVIDENCE FOR DIFFERENT DELIVERY MODELS FOR HOSPICE AND PALLIATIVE CARE IN NURSING HOMES

Several models for incorporating palliative care into nursing homes have been described and range from hospice–nursing home partnerships, to consultations from palliative care teams that are external to the facility, to in-house teams and specialized palliative care units.[2,35] The body of scientific evidence documenting the effectiveness of these various models is limited. The following section describes each model (Table 77-1).

Hospice Care

Hospice care is the most common and well-established program for delivering palliative care in U.S. nursing homes. The Medicare Hospice Benefit (MHB) was extended to nursing homes in 1989, and by 2004, 78% of U.S. nursing homes contracted with at least one hospice agency for services.[4] Miller and colleagues[36] reported that the percentage of nursing home residents receiving hospice services rose from 14% in 1999 to 33% in 2006.

When a nursing home resident is enrolled in hospice, the hospice agency is responsible for providing all care that is related to the resident's terminal illness. These services include nursing visits, additional personal care, spiritual counseling and social work services, medications that are related to the terminal illness, and medical supplies. The nursing home continues to provide room and board and long-term care services. This shared responsibility and additional resources potentially benefit both the nursing home and the hospice agency. However, barriers do exist to adoption of hospice care in nursing homes. First, administrators and staff may believe that acceptance of hospice services is an admission that nursing home care is inadequate.[37] Further, poor communication and lack of collegial relationships can compromise care and engender ill will between nursing home and hospice staff.[2] Additionally, financial disincentives exist for nursing homes to transfer patients who were admitted under the Medicare

TABLE 77-1. Models of Hospice and Palliative Care Delivery in Nursing Homes

MODEL	DESCRIPTION	PAYMENT MODEL	COMMENTS
Hospice care delivered by hospice agency in collaboration with nursing home staff	Interdisciplinary team provides end-of-life care to residents who are eligible and consent (or whose surrogate decision-maker consents) to hospice care. Health care team members from hospice provide care within the nursing home.	Medicare Hospice Benefit	Oldest (i.e., from 1989) model of formal end-of-life care Established funding mechanism Limited to residents with ≤6 month prognosis Requires contract between hospice agency and nursing home Requires collaboration between hospice agency and nursing home Financial disincentive for nursing home to enroll short-term patients Model with strongest empirical base for effectiveness (though evidence base is modest)
External palliative care consultation team	MDs and NPs employed by a hospice/palliative care organization provide palliative care consultations to nonhospice nursing home residents.	Palliative care consultant (MD or NP) bills Medicare Part B	Does not require financial investment from nursing home or specialized training for staff Similar to existing models for delivery of specialized (e.g., mental health) services in nursing homes Consultation model does not ensure adherence to palliative care standards or recommendations Model is not widely available or financially viable for many palliative care organizations or services
Internal palliative care team and/or unit	Nursing home employs or trains an internal palliative care NP or team (NP, SW, chaplain, MD).	Nursing home absorbs costs related to hiring or training team and establishing specialized unit	Nursing home oversees entire program and is accountable for the care and outcomes Model is consistent with other "culture change" initiatives Model can empower nursing home staff and increase job satisfaction May be difficult to implement and sustain because of the necessary resources to train staff and deliver care

Modified from Hanson L, Ersek M. Meeting palliative care needs in post-acute care settings: "to help them live until they die." In: McPhee S, Winker M, Rabow M, Pantilat S, Markowitz A (eds). *Care at the Close of Life: Evidence and Experience*. New York: McGraw Hill; 2010:513-521; and Carlson MD, Lim B, Meier DE. Strategies and innovative models for delivering palliative care in nursing homes. *J Am Med Dir Assoc*. 2011;12:91-98.
MD, Medical doctor; *NP*, nurse practitioner; *SW*, social worker.

skilled nursing facility (SNF) benefit to the MHB because the reimbursement to the nursing home for patients on the MHB is much lower than reimbursement for the SNF benefit.[30]

Despite the challenges of delivering hospice care in nursing homes, many hospice agencies successfully collaborate with nursing facilities to deliver high-quality end-of-life care.[38] Several studies have documented that the addition of hospice to usual nursing home care improves the quality of end-of-life care. Specifically, family satisfaction with end-of-life care increases, pain and symptom management is enhanced, and use of invasive therapies and hospitalization is decreased.[30,39-41]

External Consultation Teams

External palliative care consultation teams typically are based at a community hospice or palliative care organization or occasionally are associated with a hospital palliative care program. In this model, an administrator from the nursing home (most commonly the medical director or director of nursing services) or a resident's primary care provider requests a consultation. Residents may or may not be hospice-eligible. The consultant (either a physician or nurse practitioner) bills under Medicare part B, and thus the costs for these services are not incurred by the nursing home. One group, Evercare Hospice and Palliative Care, is a Medicare Advantage plan that operates in a full-risk capitation model, again without cost to the nursing home.[42] Empirical evidence for the effectiveness of this model on the quality of end-of-life care is scant, although one large provider reported high patient satisfaction, fewer emergency department visits, higher staff retention, and improved symptom management.[2] In a Centers for Medicare and Medicaid Services (CMS) demonstration project, the general Evercare model, which provides nurse practitioner primary care services in nursing homes, was associated with lower hospitalizations and costs compared to usual nursing home care.[43]

This model involves several challenges. First, palliative care consultation teams are not available in every location. Also, it is difficult to staff these teams with clinicians who have expertise in palliative care and an understanding and appreciation of the nursing home setting, a characteristic that one provider of this service considers critical to its success.[2] To ensure financial viability, consultation services must be able to access large numbers of patients in one facility to maximize efficiency.[42] Because reimbursement typically is through Medicare part B, it is focused on physician and nurse practitioner visits, which hinders more comprehensive interdisciplinary care. Finally, because the service is consultative, nursing home staff and primary care providers may be inconsistent in following the recommendations made by the palliative care team.

Internal Palliative Care Teams and Units

A recent study showed that 27% of U.S. nursing homes report that they have implemented specialized programs or staff trained in hospice or palliative care. After controlling for covariates, nonprofit status, location in the southern part of the United States, having hospice contracts and other specialty programs, and employing an American College of Health Care Administrators (ACHCA) certified administrator were associated with having a specialized palliative care program.[44] There are no standard elements across these programs, although they generally encompass staff training, advance care planning, and symptom management.[42]

Several authors have described the benefits of nursing home–based palliative care services. Suhrie and associates[45] reported a decrease in the use of unnecessary medications following admission of residents to a nursing home–based palliative care unit. Specialized dementia "comfort care" units were found to be associated with higher staff satisfaction, less observed resident discomfort, and lower costs than standard nursing home care.[46]

An additional advantage to internal programs includes the ability to infuse palliative care principles into daily nursing home care. Moreover, clinicians' daily interaction with residents may facilitate timely detection of clinical changes and promote understanding of resident and family values, personal goals, and care preferences.[42] Internal programs also place the expertise and authority with the entity—that is, the nursing home itself—that is ultimately responsible and held accountable for the residents' quality of care.[47] Empowering nursing home staff to provide high-quality palliative care may also enhance staff satisfaction and decrease turnover.[2] The biggest hindrances to the growth of internal nursing home palliative care services are the lack of resources and financial disincentives for nursing homes to invest in this type of care. The need to train staff and the additional time necessary to deliver high-quality palliative care are additional barriers.

KEY INFORMATION FOR RESIDENTS AND FAMILIES

Different models of palliative care exist within nursing homes; therefore practitioners need to ensure that residents and their family members understand the model that is available to them. It is not uncommon for people to be unclear about the differences and similarities between palliative care and hospice services. Furthermore, details on how the particular program will work for the resident within a facility should be carefully explained. Educating residents and their family members about existing models before nursing home placement is a proactive method to make sure that a facility is selected for placement that will meet expectations and needs at the end of the resident's life.

The different palliative care models discussed all embrace the concept of person-centered care. Person-centered care is an approach that honors and values residents' preferences. The goal of care is not completing a task, but meeting the residents' needs and ensuring their well-being.[48-50] This approach takes the whole individual into account and is concerned with the residents' goals for their end-of-life care and their individualized wishes on how they want to live out their daily life.[51] The focus of person-centered care is getting to know the individual and honoring his or her specific wishes[52]; therefore practitioners should provide opportunities for residents and their family members to make their wishes known. Through open verbal communication, providers can offer information about treatment options and support residents and their family members during their decision-making process. Topics regarding pain management strategies, artificial nutrition and hydration, antibiotic use, and future hospitalizations versus "do not hospitalize" status should be openly discussed if they have not already been addressed.[53] By establishing and documenting a resident's end-of-life wishes, making incorrect assumptions about the kind of care the resident wants to receive can be avoided. This can also facilitate person-centered care within nursing home facilities.

CONCLUSIONS AND SUMMARY

Many clinicians have an incomplete picture of nursing homes, relying on stereotypes and exposés in the media that do not reflect the reality of care in many long-term care facilities. Although there are challenges to delivering palliative care in nursing homes, several distinct advantages to promoting palliative care practices in these facilities do exist. Nursing homes are more homelike than many other settings, and residents and families often form meaningful relationships with the nursing home staff. Furthermore, as efforts to implement culture change programs and enhance person-centered care grow, there is an expanded focus on considering resident and family needs and preferences, making the setting ripe for discussions regarding end-of-life preferences and advanced care planning.

Nursing homes do not strive to deliver curative care. Their goal, instead, is to maximize residents' functional capabilities and autonomy along with their quality of life. Therefore understanding residents' preferences regarding the degree to which they desire to participate in restorative treatments is critical. Rather than allow residents to experience disruptive, costly, and unnecessary medical interventions and transfers to the hospital, practitioners working in nursing homes should understand and address the residents' individual needs. If restorative care and medical intervention is warranted, it should be delivered. If not, it should be avoided.

Residents and families should understand their end-of-life options and have an opportunity to clarify their preferences. At the end of life, residents' symptoms, particularly pain, must be managed. With increased education, nursing home staff will be better able to incorporate palliative care into their practices. With increased awareness among regulators and payers, external challenges to palliative care can be mitigated. For the frail and elderly residents who die each year in nursing homes and their families, palliative care can make their experiences less physically and emotionally painful. To deliver this care and meet the needs of millions of residents and families, nursing homes must capitalize on their strengths and find ways to overcome their weaknesses.

SUMMARY RECOMMENDATIONS

- Changes should be made in regulation, reimbursement, and training processes within nursing homes to foster establishment of palliative care programs in nursing homes.
- Treatment goals should be matched with resident needs, and promotion of potentially inappropriate restorative therapies should be avoided.
- Weight loss, functional declines, infections, and eating disturbances should be viewed as indicators of poor prognosis meriting the use of palliative care rather than indicators of poor quality of care in nursing homes.
- Issues of turnover and training among nursing home staff must be addressed to ensure the workforce has the capacity to care for growing numbers of residents who will die in nursing homes.
- As standard of care shifts from restorative to palliative care, staff education should address potential misconceptions that may devalue residents' lives. Staff should not hold the overarching perception that medical intervention is unnecessary or unwarranted for nursing home residents.[7]
- Open communication about palliative care services and end-of-life care with residents and their families is necessary for overall satisfaction with the care delivered within a nursing home.

REFERENCES

1. Kaye HS, Harrington C, LaPlante MP. Long-term care: who gets it, who provides it, who pays, and how much? *Health Aff (Millwood)*. 2010;29(1):11–21.
2. *Improving palliative care in nursing homes*. New York: Center to Advance Palliative Care; 2008.
3. Mitchell SL, Teno JM, Miller SC, Mor V. A national study of the location of death for older persons with dementia. *J Am Geriatr Soc*. 2005;53(2):299–305.
4. Jones A, Dwyer L, Bercovitz A, Strahan G. *The National Nursing Home Survey: 2004—overview*. Hyattesville, MD: National Center for Health Statistics; 2009.
5. Goldfeld KS, Stevenson DG, Hamel MB, Mitchell SL. Medicare expenditures among nursing home residents with advanced dementia. *Arch Intern Med*. 2011;171(9):824–830.
6. Barnato AE, McClellan MB, Kagay CR, Garber AM. Trends in inpatient treatment intensity among Medicare beneficiaries at the end of life. *Health Serv Res*. 2004;39(2):363–375.
7. Meier DE, Lim B, Carlson MD. Raising the standard: palliative care in nursing homes. *Health Aff (Millwood)*. 2010;29(1):136–140.
8. Teno JM, Clarridge BR, Casey V, et al. Family perspectives on end-of-life care at the last place of care. *JAMA*. 2004;291(1):88–93.
9. Casarett D, Pickard A, Bailey FA, et al. Do palliative consultations improve patient outcomes? *J Am Geriatr Soc*. 2008;56(4):593–599.
10. Finlay IG, Higginson IJ, Goodwin DM, et al. Palliative care in hospital, hospice, at home: results from a systematic review. *Ann Oncol*. 2002;13(suppl 4):257–264.
11. Morrison RS, Penrod JD, Cassel JB, et al. Cost savings associated with US hospital palliative care consultation programs. *Arch Intern Med*. 2008;168(16):1783–1790.
12. Farrel D, Brady C, Frank B. *Meeting the Leadership Challenge in Long-term Care: What You Do Matters*. Baltimore, MD: Health Professions Press; 2011:xv–xxiv.
13. Dumas LG, Blanks C, Palmer-Erbs V, Portnoy FL. Leadership in nursing homes: 2009— challenges for change in difficult times. *Nurs Clin North Am*. 2009;44(2):169–178.
14. Harrington C, Carrillo H, Woleslagle B, O'Brian T. *Nursing facilities, staffing, residents and facility deficiencies, 2004 through 2009*. http://74.53.52.239/sites/default/files/advocate/action-center/OSCAR-2010.pdf; 2010; Accessed September 5, 2012.
15. Aroian JF, Patsdaughter CA, Wyszynski ME. DONs in long-term care facilities: contemporary roles, current credentials, and educational needs. *Nursing Econ*. 2000;18(3):149–156.
16. Collopy B, Boyle P, Jennings B. New directions in nursing home ethics. *Hastings Cent Rep*. 1991;21(2):S1–S15.
17. *Compilation of the Social Security Laws*. http://www.ssa.gov/OP_Home/ssact/title19/1919.htm; 2011 Accessed September 29, 2012.
18. Ersek M, Wilson SA. The challenges and opportunities in providing end-of-life care in nursing homes. *J Palliative Med*. 2003;6(1):45–57.
19. American Medical Directors Association. *Pain Management in the Long-Term Care Setting: Clinical Practice Guideline*. Columbia, MD: American Medical Directors Association; 2009.
20. Herr KA, Ersek M. Measurement of pain and other symptoms in the cognitively impaired. In: Hanks G, Cherny N, Christakis N, et al., eds. *Oxford Textbook of Palliative Medicine*. 4th ed. New York: Oxford University Press; 2009:466–479.
21. American Geriatrics Society Panel. Pharmacological management of persistent pain in older persons. *J Am Geriatr Soc*. 2009;57(8):1331–1346.
22. Doty M, Koren M, Sturla E. *Culture change in nursing homes: how far have we come? Findings from the Commonwealth Fund 2007 National Survey of Nursing Homes*. New York: The Commonwealth Fund; 2008.
23. Ersek M, Kraybill BM, Hansberry J. Assessing the educational needs and concerns of nursing home staff regarding end-of-life care. *J Gerontol Nurs*. 2000;26(10):16–26.
24. Ersek M, Kraybill B, Hansen N. Evaluation of a train-the-trainer program to enhance hospice and palliative care in nursing homes. *J Hosp Palliat Nurs*. 2006;8:42–49.

25. Kelly K, Ersek M, Virani R, Malloy P, Ferrell B. End-of-Life Nursing Education Consortium. Geriatric Training Program: improving palliative care in community geriatric care settings. *J Gerontol Nurs.* 2008;34(5):28–35.
26. Hickman SE, Tolle SW, Brummel-Smith K, Carley MM. Use of the Physician Orders for Life-Sustaining Treatment program in Oregon nursing facilities: beyond resuscitation status. *J Am Geriatr Soc.* 2004;52(9):1424–1429.
27. Molloy DW, Guyatt GH, Russo R, et al. Systematic implementation of an advance directive program in nursing homes: a randomized controlled trial. *JAMA.* 2000;283(11):1437–1444.
28. Morrison RS, Chichin E, Carter J, Burack O, Lantz M, Meier DE. The effect of a social work intervention to enhance advance care planning documentation in the nursing home. *J Am Geriatr Soc.* 2005;53(2):290–294.
29. Casarett D, Karlawish J, Morales K, Crowley R, Mirsch T, Asch DA. Improving the use of hospice services in nursing homes: a randomized controlled trial. *JAMA.* 2005;294(2):211–217.
30. Hanson L, Ersek M. Meeting palliative care needs in post-acute care settings: "To help them live until they die". In: McPhee S, Winker M, Rabow M, Pantilat S, Markowitz A, eds. *Care at the Close of Life: Evidence and Experience.* New York: McGraw Hill; 2010:513–521.
31. Thompson GN, Menec VH, Chochinov HM, McClement SE. Family satisfaction with care of a dying loved one in nursing homes: what makes the difference? *J Gerontol Nurs.* 2008;34(12):37–44.
32. Kehl K, Kirchhoff K, Kramer B, Hovland-Scafe C. Challenges facing families at the end of life in three settings. *J Soc Work End-of-Life Palliat Care.* 2009;5:144–168.
33. Hanson LC, Eckert JK, Dobbs D, et al. Symptom experience of dying long-term care residents. *J Am Geriatr Soc.* 2008;56(1):91–98.
34. Gozalo P, Teno JM, Mitchell SL, et al. End-of-life transitions among nursing home residents with cognitive issues. *N Engl J Med.* 2011;365(13):1212–1221.
35. Hanson LC, Ersek M. Meeting palliative care needs in post-acute care settings: "to help them live until they die". *JAMA.* 2006;295(6):681–686.
36. Miller SC, Lima J, Gozalo PL, Mor V. The growth of hospice care in U.S. nursing homes. *J Am Geriatr Soc.* 2010;58(8):1481–1488.
37. Stevenson DG, Bramson JS. Hospice care in the nursing home setting: a review of the literature. *J Pain Symptom Manage.* 2009;38(3):440–451.
38. Miller SC. A model for successful nursing home-hospice partnerships. *J Palliat Med.* 2010;13(5):525–533.
39. Miller SC, Gozalo P, Mor V. Hospice enrollment and hospitalization of dying nursing home patients. *Am J Med.* 2001;111(1):38–44.
40. Miller SC, Mor V, Teno J. Hospice enrollment and pain assessment and management in nursing homes. *J Pain Symptom Manage.* 2003;26(3):791–799.
41. Baer WM, Hanson LC. Families' perception of the added value of hospice in the nursing home. *J Am Geriatr Soc.* 2000;48(8):879–882.
42. Carlson MD, Lim B, Meier DE. Strategies and innovative models for delivering palliative care in nursing homes. *J Am Med Dir Assoc.* 2011;12(2):91–98.
43. Kane RL, Keckhafer G, Flood S, Bershadsky B, Siadaty MS. The effect of Evercare on hospital use. *J Am Geriatr Soc.* 2003;51(10):1427–1434.
44. Miller SC, Han B. End-of-life care in U.S. nursing homes: nursing homes with special programs and trained staff for hospice or palliative/end-of-life care. *J Palliat Med.* 2008;11(6):866–877.
45. Suhrie EM, Hanlon JT, Jaffe EJ, Sevick MA, Ruby CM, Aspinall SL. Impact of a geriatric nursing home palliative care service on unnecessary medication prescribing. *Am J Geriatr Pharmacother.* 2009;7(1):20–25.
46. Kovach C, Wilson S, Noonan P. The effects of hospice interventions on behaviors, discomfort, and physical complications of end stage dementia nursing home residents. *Am J Alzheimers Dis Other Demen.* 1996;11:7–15.
47. Huskamp HA, Stevenson DG, Chernew ME, Newhouse JP. A new medicare end-of-life benefit for nursing home residents. *Health Aff (Millwood).* 2010;29(1):130–135.
48. Crandall LG, White DL, Schuldheis S, Talerico KA. Initiating person-centered care practices in long-term care facilities. *J Gerontol Nurs.* 2007;33(11):47–56.
49. Fazio S. *The Enduring Self in People with Alzheimer's: Getting to the Heart of Individualized Care.* Baltimore, MD: Health Professions Press; 2008:5-31.
50. Tellis-Nayak V. A person-centered workplace: the foundation for person-centered caregiving in long-term care. *J Am Med Dir Assoc.* 2007;8(1):46–54.
51. Ragsdale V, McDougall Jr. GJ. The changing face of long-term care: looking at the past decade. *Issues Ment Health Nurs.* 2008;29(9):992–1001.
52. Jones CS. Person-centered care: the heart of culture change. *J Gerontol Nurs.* 2011;37(6):18–23.
53. Wilson S. Long-term care. In: Ferrell B, Coyle N, eds. *Oxford Textbook of Palliative Nursing.* 3rd ed. New York: Oxford University Press; 2010:879–890.

Chapter 78

How Can Palliative Care Be Integrated Into Home-Based Primary Care Programs?

Meng Zhang, Kristofer L. Smith, Jessica Cook-Mack, Ania Wajnberg, Linda V. DeCherrie, and Theresa A. Soriano

INTRODUCTION AND SCOPE OF THE PROBLEM

The number of patients living with multiple chronic medical conditions continues to rise and place a growing burden on the U.S. health care system.[1] By 2030, almost 20% of the U.S. population will be older than 65 years, with the greatest increase in those over 85.[2] A portion of these elderly, chronically ill patients suffer from functional and cognitive impairment, making them unable to leave their homes to access routine medical care. The number of these homebound seniors will grow to over 3 million in the coming decade.[3]

Before the mid-twentieth century, physician home visits were a common practice. In 1930, 40% of all physician visits took place in the home; by 1980 less than 1% did, leaving many homebound patients without regular medical care.[4,5] Recent increases in Medicare reimbursement for home care visits, coupled with the growing need, have contributed to a slow increase in the number of home care providers and practices over the last decade.[6,7] Home-based primary care (HBPC) programs are structured in a variety of ways; some are physician led and others are led by nurse practitioners. Also providing home-based care are private individual and group practices, Veterans Affairs Medical Center programs, and initiatives affiliated with health systems or academic medical centers. Some programs provide urgent medical care, others focus on transitional care, and others consist of multidisciplinary teams with community partners providing longitudinal, primary care. Common to all programs, however, is the fact that patients receiving HBPC meet the following Medicare "homebound" definition:

a patient will be considered to be homebound if they have a condition due to an illness or injury that restricts their ability to leave their place of residence except with the aid of: supportive devices such as crutches, canes, wheelchairs, and walkers; the use of special transportation; or the assistance of another person; or if leaving home is medically contraindicated.[8]

Despite the recent growth of outpatient palliative care specialty clinics, a large gap still exists in the access to palliative care for community-dwelling elderly, particularly the homebound. As noted earlier, homebound patients often have multiple chronic medical conditions, such as dementia, congestive heart failure, depression, and cancer, many of which are associated with substantial symptom burden.[9] Short-term mortality rates in this population are high; nearly one in five die each year. Many have unpredictable prognoses, and the majority have life expectancies of more than 6 months, making them ineligible for home hospice.[10] Issues such as poverty, isolation, and poor health literacy complicate the delivery of care.[11] As the chronically ill homebound population grows, the need for assessment and treatment of symptom burden concurrent to complex primary and specialty care will become increasingly necessary. Because HBPC programs provide continuity and longitudinal care for patients throughout their illnesses, integration of palliative care into HBPC can allow for earlier identification of symptom burden (physical, psychosocial, or spiritual), aggressive treatment of symptoms, better coordination of care, and continuous reevaluation of goals of care as diseases progress. However, little study has been done on these potential benefits.[12]

Given the lack of data regarding integration of palliative care into HBPC, this discussion is based on best practices and extensive experience integrating palliative and primary care in one HBPC program. The benefits and challenges of symptom management, care coordination, and communication in the home environment are discussed here, as well as a brief review of particular ethical and safety concerns specific to medical care in the patient's home.

SYMPTOM MANAGEMENT

General Considerations

Unlike in the institutional setting, monitoring of symptoms in the home is performed primarily by family members and home care workers. Although this is often ideal—who knows a patient better than his or her family?—it can also be challenging. For example, sorting out whether agitation is secondary to pain, shortness of breath, or delirium can be difficult for skilled practitioners, let alone worried family members. Furthermore, the emergence of new symptoms or a change in symptom severity can be frightening, particularly when appropriate intervention is not expeditious. HBPC providers, with the assistance of home nursing services and hospice nursing, can help provide ongoing, in-person symptom assessment and management. Ultimately, however, if symptoms are too severe or unanticipated, hospitalization for a brief period may be the most appropriate response.

Although relying on family members sometimes can be challenging, even more difficult are the cases in which informal caregivers (family members or friends) are not available. Most home health workers are not permitted to administer medications. Legally they can only assist by responding to a specific request for medication made by the patient or informal caregiver. This presents a barrier to the administration of any medication, particularly to the use of medications on an as-needed basis. If the patient is unable to express his or her need because of illness such as dementia or aphasia and the family is unavailable, the medication cannot be given. Symptom management in such patients is extremely limited, and institutionalization may become necessary.

Pain

When treating pain at home, many difficulties may arise. Opioids, a mainstay in the treatment of moderate to severe pain, are controlled substances. Neighborhood pharmacies frequently do not carry the full variety of medications and preparations.[13] Chain-store pharmacies, which are most likely to be open at night and on weekends, can be particularly restrictive in their formulary. Fortunately, advance planning can ameliorate some of these difficulties. It can be useful to forge a relationship with a particular neighborhood pharmacy that is willing to deliver. Because of the regularity and volume of orders resulting from a partnership with an HBPC program, the pharmacy is often willing to have more opioids in stock. Having medications stored in the home for "emergency use only" also can help to circumvent availability problems. However, the storage of controlled substances within a patient's home raises other problems, such as the potential for intentional misuse or overdose by the patient or others. The use of a lockbox, careful record keeping, pill counts, and the election of one responsible family member can all help to alleviate, though not eliminate, these concerns.

Another challenge associated with opioid medications used for pain is family reluctance to administer a "dangerous" medication. In these situations, it can be helpful to explore the roots of such reluctance. If the cause is misconception about a particular medication (usually morphine), caregiver education is often enough, although the switch to another opioid may be needed. Another frequent concern is that the caregiver will hasten the loved one's death by accidentally administering an overdose. Again, education and support can help. It also can be useful to place as-needed medications in a separate pre-pour box with instructions to give that dose only if the patient is experiencing pain. Similarly, prefilled syringes for liquid preparations can be reassuring to family members because they do not need to be prepared by inexperienced hands and help alleviate fears of accidental overdose.

Constipation

Constipation is a frequent symptom in the homebound. Patients take constipating medications, have limited mobility, and suffer from diseases in which constipation is a known complication (e.g., diabetes, parkinsonism). Despite its prevalence, caregivers often do not identify constipation as a concerning symptom. In addition, the unpleasantness and difficulty of turning, cleaning, and changing an incontinent loved one can lead to "convenient ignoring." Furthermore, the costs and limited insurance coverage for medical supplies (diapers, liners, gloves, etc.) can be a hindrance as families and patients try to conserve limited supplies.

Treating homebound patients with constipation requires the involvement of the entire multidisciplinary team. Providers must help families understand the ramifications of constipation (e.g., delirium, pain, perforation, overflow diarrhea). Having caregivers record each bowel movement on a calendar provides concrete, visual feedback about the problem and the effectiveness of treatment. Pre-pour monitoring and pill counts can reveal skipped laxative doses. By anticipating constipation and providing early treatment, providers underscore its seriousness and can help prevent unnecessary suffering. Nurses in the home can also teach caregivers how to administer suppositories and enemas and can demonstrate proper techniques for maintaining hygiene. Social workers can help address problems resulting from limited resources, and nutritionists can provide recommendations for diet changes that might relieve constipation.

Nausea and Vomiting

Use of oral medications, the mainstay of home-based symptom management, can become challenging when the patient suffers from nausea or vomiting. In the home, intravenous antiemetics are usually not available or require a delay while the service is arranged. In addition, many homebound are confined

TABLE 78-1. Useful Nonoral Medication Delivery Modalities in the Home Setting

INDICATION	MODALITY	EXAMPLES
Agitation/anxiety	Topical/transdermal	Transdermal compounding gel with haloperidol, lorazepam
	Sublingual	Liquid benzodiazepines (lorazepam, diazepam), quick-dissolve olanzapine
	Rectal	Clonazepam, diazepam
	Subcutaneous infusion	Haloperidol
Dyspnea	Topical/transdermal	Transdermal fentanyl patch
	Sublingual	Liquid morphine
	Rectal	Morphine, fentanyl, hydromorphone
	Subcutaneous infusion	Morphine, fentanyl, hydromorphone
Nausea	Topical/transdermal	Granisetron, scopolamine patch, transdermal compounding gel with haloperidol, lorazepam, diphenhydramine, or metoclopramide
	Sublingual	Liquid lorazepam or diazepam
	Rectal	Chlorpromazine, dexamethasone, clonazepam, diazepam, metoclopramide
	Subcutaneous infusion	Dexamethasone, haloperidol, metoclopramide
Pain (nociceptive or generalized)	Topical/transdermal	Fentanyl patch, scopolamine patch
	Sublingual	Liquid morphine
	Rectal	Acetaminophen, morphine, fentanyl, hydromorphone, dexamethasone
	Subcutaneous infusion	Morphine, fentanyl, hydromorphone, dexamethasone, octreotide
	Thermal	Heat (spasm), cold (inflammation)
Pain (neuropathic)	Topical/transdermal	Lidocaine patch or gel, capsaicin
	Rectal	Gabapentin, carbamazepine
Secretions	Topical/transdermal	Scopolamine patch
	Subcutaneous infusion	Glycopyrrolate
Seizures	Sublingual	Liquid benzodiazepines (lorazepam, diazepam)
	Rectal	Chlorpromazine, gabapentin, carbamazepine, clonazepam, diazepam

Modified from Mittelman MS, Haley WE, Clay OJ, et al. Improving caregiver well-being delays nursing home placement of patients with Alzheimer disease. *Neurology.* 2006;67(9):1592-1599; Naylor MD, Brooten D, Campbell R, et al. Comprehensive discharge planning and home follow-up of hospitalized elders: a randomized clinical trial. *JAMA.* 1999;281(7):613-620; and Meier DE, Beresford L. Outpatient clinics are a new frontier for palliative care. *J Palliat Med.* 2008;11(6):823-828.

to a single room that can be less than ideal—space is limited, ventilation is often poor, and smells that exacerbate symptoms are more difficult to control. Although some of these issues are immutable, placing the patient near a window or vent and the use of fans or an air conditioner can be helpful. Alternative routes of medication administration also can be employed. The use of suppositories can provide relief (e.g., chlorpromazine and dexamethasone are available for rectal administration). Concentrated liquid preparations (haloperidol, benzodiazepines) may be more easily tolerated. Transdermal preparations can be employed depending on the mechanism of nausea (scopolamine is readily available, and granisetron has been found to help in some cases).[14] Some practitioners with access to a compounding pharmacy may be able to use pluronic lecithin organogel (PLO gel) to deliver a variety of medications either transdermally or rectally. Finally, subcutaneous administration of antiemetics with the use of a syringe driver can be attempted if the family and practitioner are willing. See Table 78-1 for medications with alternative routes of administration useful in home-based practice.

Shortness of Breath

Shortness of breath is a particularly challenging symptom to treat in the home. The causes—some of which are immediately life threatening—are myriad, and phone evaluation is complex. Sometimes the only safe answer for diagnosis and symptom relief is referral to an emergency department. When the acuity is lower, shortness of breath can be treated at home. Disease-specific treatments (e.g., nebulizers for chronic obstructive pulmonary disease, diuresis for congestive heart failure) are the mainstay of therapy. Patients may qualify for home oxygen if criteria are met.

Treatments to palliate dyspnea include oxygen, benzodiazepines, and opioids. Difficulties associated with home-based use of opioids are discussed in the section on pain. It may be more difficult to encourage families to use opioids for shortness of breath because of lack of understanding of its utility. Oxygen also can be challenging to use at home. Family members and even patients may want to continue smoking, a dangerous combination with oxygen. Furthermore, whereas oxygen in the hospital can be used for almost anyone, home use of oxygen is limited by strict Medicare reimbursement guidelines. Although patients on hospice are not subject to these requirements, many home-based patients do not qualify for, or refuse, hospice services. Studies also suggest that oxygen does not reduce dyspnea for patients without significant hypoxia and that the use of fans, air conditioners, and proper positioning can, in combination with disease-specific treatments and the judicious use of opioids, usually relieve most dyspnea.[15–17]

Depression

Assessment and treatment of depression can be both aided and hindered by caring for patients in their home. On the one hand, HBPC providers potentially have the advantage of knowing their patients over an extended period, so changes in mood are more likely to be noted. Caregivers also are frequently very sensitive to their loved one's moods and able to report on changes. On the other hand, patients may be reluctant to express their feelings to providers in front of their loved ones. Finally, depression in patients with dementia can be particularly challenging to disentangle from other behavior changes, sometimes even requiring the evaluation of a specialist in geriatric psychiatry. Maintaining a high level of suspicion is essential, as is incorporating depression screening tools validated in those with cognitive impairment.

When the diagnosis of depression is made, treatment includes both medications and psychotherapy. As in the outpatient setting, the primary care physician can generally initiate medication treatment. Complex medication management, however, may require specialized evaluation; a challenging situation given the paucity of home-based psychiatry services. Although some patients can go to an occasional outpatient psychiatry appointment for medication management, others may require hospitalization for stabilization and initiation of treatment. Psychotherapy can be even more difficult to provide in the home, although some community mental health workers are willing to do house calls. Many HBPC programs and community organizations employ social workers who can fill this role when psychiatrists are not available. Social workers may also be able to identify community mental health resources. In addition, some nursing agencies have behavioral health teams that can be used. Depending on the situation, involving the patient's spiritual community may also be helpful.

Anorexia

Anorexia is a challenging symptom regardless of the locus of care. At home, the lack of a desire to eat can be taken as a personal rejection, because food and feeding are common ways of expressing love. Helping family members understand anorexia as part of a disease process can ameliorate some of this burden. Patients may also be embarrassed by, or in the case of dementia, unaware of, their inability to perform basic self-care and may not report that they are no longer able to prepare or consume a nutritious meal. Several screening tools are available that can help in the evaluation of anorexia and weight loss.[18,19]

When possible, a workup consistent with the patient's goals of care and illness trajectory should be undertaken. General treatment of anorexia includes offering small, frequent meals, making snacks and finger foods readily available, and providing a variety of choices. In addition, lifting dietary restrictions and stopping unnecessary medications that may be contributing to anorexia can be helpful. Supplements may prevent further weight loss. Proteins such as milk powder, tofu, or whey can be added, and fat content can be increased by adding olive oil or butter. (More information on diagnosing and treating anorexia can be found in Chapters 28 and 29.)

Agitation

Infection, dementia, delirium, pain, constipation, and many other disease states can result in agitation. In addition to being a diagnostic challenge, agitation can be extremely difficult for caregivers. Witnessing a loved one act out of character can be frightening and frustrating. Caregivers may feel that their loved one is acting volitionally and, as a result, become angry with the patient for being difficult or not responding to "reason." Furthermore, when not handled appropriately, agitated patients can be dangerous to both themselves and their caregivers.`

Treatment of the underlying cause of agitation is essential, but agitation often takes time to resolve, as with delirium, or is part of a disease process that lacks curative treatment, as in dementia. When agitation persists, caregivers are at risk for burnout. Although pharmacological intervention may become necessary, nonpharmacological interventions such as aromatherapy, thermal bath, calming music, and hand massage should be attempted first. Using social work and community supports are essential to help support the family and mobilize resources. Referral to a caregiver support group, such as those found through the Alzheimer's Association, can be a great source of relief and assistance.[20] Additionally, night-care programs can provide the caregiver much needed respite. The use of medications is controversial because often the behaviors are not bothersome to the patient, but these drugs pose definite risks to patient health and well-being. Some providers find it helpful to consider whether the behaviors are threatening the patient's overall goals. If the patient's ultimate goal was to remain at home, medication may be indicated to allow caregivers to cope and continue providing home-based care.

COMMUNICATION WITH PATIENTS AND CAREGIVER

Effective and compassionate communication is an integral part of palliative medicine in any setting and is even more essential in home-based primary and palliative care. Although the same barriers and challenges described previously exist, HBPC provides some unique opportunities, particularly in regard to sharing medical information, engaging patients and families in therapeutic dialogue, managing expectations, providing caregiver support, and establishing goals of care. The intimacy and privacy of one's own home and the shift in power dynamics when a physician visits a patient promotes and encourages meaningful communication.

A large percentage of the homebound elderly population has impaired cognition and decision-making capacity. This makes development and execution of the care plan difficult and often places this responsibility in the hands of surrogates (family or caregivers). Because these agents often have different levels of health literacy, may be cognitively impaired themselves, and may speak languages different from the patient's physician, effective communication becomes vitally important. Home visits from the multidisciplinary care team can help clarify medication use and compliance, assess understanding, and identify misunderstandings in a treatment plan. The team can also demonstrate instructions and techniques in wound care, ambulation, feeding techniques, and medication administration in person to different caregivers.

In the United States, approximately 21 million patients have limited English-language skills.[21] Although it is often convenient for providers to rely on patients' caregivers, friends, or neighbors to assist in interpretation, especially in the home setting, this can lead to inaccurate and distorted information. It can also undermine patient confidentiality or embarrass and inhibit patients in fully sharing personal information or psychosocial and spiritual concerns. This may compromise effective communication, leading to incomplete histories and ineffective assessments and treatment plans.[22] Language barriers are also associated with less health education, worse interpersonal care, and lower patient satisfaction.[23] Thus the medical team should make every effort to use a trained medical interpreter (either by phone or in person) during their encounters.

GOALS OF CARE DISCUSSIONS

Clarifying a patient's goals of care is arguably one of the most important component in providing quality palliative care. It is even more critical in providing good medical care to the homebound elderly population because they have high rates of morbidity and mortality. To best understand a patient's goals and preferences regarding medical and end-of-life care requires ongoing conversation and trust. To meaningfully participate in this conversation and to help a patient articulate his or her goals requires appreciation of the patient as a whole person. As a patient's primary care physician with an established and trusting relationship, HBPC providers are in a unique position to initiate these conversations early in the disease spectrum, before a time of medical crisis. By entering a patient's home, a physician has the rare opportunity to get to know a patient on a more personal level, learning the patient's dreams, hopes, and fears, in the context of family, culture, and religious beliefs. It is important to remember that advance care planning is a process and goals should be reassessed as a patient progresses through different stages of illness. By maintaining an ongoing relationship with the patient and actively participating in the patient's care at every stage, a home care physician can appropriately match treatment plans to evolving treatment goals. A dynamic strategy such as this can help a patient avoid unnecessary tests, emergency room visits and hospitalizations.

When the patient is no longer able to participate in goals of care conversations, surrogates often turn to the physician for guidance. Home-based care not only fosters strong bonds between the patient and the physician but also with surrogates. Within these complex relationships, it is imperative for the physician to support and encourage the surrogate decision maker to respect a patient's previously established advanced directives and stated wishes. When advanced directives are not known, a home care physician is in a unique position to help guide the surrogate decision maker through end-of-life care issues, because the physician knows the patient and has gained the trust of family and caregivers. In these cases, it is recommended to encourage the surrogate decision maker to use "substituted judgment." In this process the clinician helps the family attempt to (hypothetically) determine what the patient would decide if able to participate in the discussion about end-of-life decisions.[24,25] This approach can help unite family members with differing agendas and may alleviate family guilt after a patient's death. With goals of care in place, a physician can then recommend appropriate treatment plans to match these goals and to help the patient and family members make advance directive decisions.

All of these conversations and decisions need to be well-documented both in the medical record and at the patient's home. The medical record must have an easy way to locate code status and hospitalization and treatment preferences. If others caring for the patient cannot access this information quickly, care plans inconsistent with the wishes of the family and patient may be initiated. In the home, forms such as the health care proxy or the "do not resuscitate" (DNR) order must be readily accessible. Often this means posting them on a wall next to the patient's bed or putting them on the refrigerator. This avoids the potentially catastrophic event of having emergency responders initiate resuscitation because of lack of available documentation.

CAREGIVER EDUCATION AND BURDEN ASSESSMENT

Most homebound patients have significant functional and cognitive impairment and are able to remain home only because of dedicated formal and informal caregivers. For many, caring for the homebound can be isolating, anxiety-provoking, and stressful. This is especially true in diseases such as dementia. Whatever the underlying cause, dementia is often associated with a protracted course, high variability in disease progression, and difficult-to-manage behavioral symptoms. It almost always poses significant caregiver burden physically, emotionally, and financially. HBPC can bring an interdisciplinary team to provide ongoing in-person caregiver education and practical and emotional support. For HBPC programs that do not have a multidisciplinary staff, it is important to refer to other disciplines and make use of community resources. Frequent discussions with caregivers regarding topics such as disease progression, symptom assessment and management, aspiration and pressure ulcer prevention, and nonpharmacological interventions for behavior problems can be reassuring to the caregivers, debunk misconceptions, and help to set realistic goals and expectations. Although many patients have diseases that can be difficult to prognosticate, early introduction to the concept and benefit of hospice can help ensure timely referral and acceptance.

Caregiver burnout is associated with increased likelihood of patient nursing home placement.[26,27] Assessing caregiver burden and burnout, as well as compassionately validating the difficulties and challenges of caregiving, should be a part of every home visit. Evaluation of proper care of the patient, observation of caregiver and patient relationship dynamics, and assessment of home safety can help the care team identify early signs of caregiver burnout. Timely recognition of caregiver burnout allows early interventions to prevent crises. Interventions can include ongoing social worker involvement and referral to community agencies and programs, including respite care and support groups.

TAILORING CARE PLANS; ENSURING CONTINUITY AND COORDINATION

A great benefit of HBPC is the ability of providers to continue the care that was provided in the acute or subacute setting and adapt that plan seamlessly to meet a patient's or family's changing medical, social, and spiritual needs as they reacclimatize to the home. Despite the best assessment of home care needs while in the hospital, when the patient arrives home, additional needs are often realized and must be coordinated to prevent rehospitalization or reinstitutionalization. Patients' symptoms often change when at home: pain can be better or worse; shortness of breath can be exacerbated by dust or poor ventilation; and constipation symptoms can improve when patients return to their usual diet. Similarly, as patients and caregivers experience progression of disease or have increased acceptance of a diagnosis, their stated goals of care may change. Home care providers are able to discuss these changes to best implement appropriate interventions and services.

Ensuring seamless transitions and coordination across care providers and settings is essential to high-quality care of the homebound elderly. These patients with complex medical issues have lengthy medication regimens and multiple specialties involved in their care, putting them at high risk for errors related to poor transitions and coordination. Because of the growing division in physician responsibility between inpatient and outpatient care, many HBPC providers no longer care for their own patients in the hospital. This development makes communication between providers increasingly vital to convey and carry out often unique care plans negotiated with families and patients receiving palliative care.

A timely home visit soon after returning home from an institutional setting is beneficial for a homebound patient with medically complex issues. Providers can assess for symptom changes, review discharge medications and services, appropriately address questions and discrepancies, and adjust care plans and coordinate services. Although the optimum timing of this postdischarge assessment has not been clearly defined in the literature, it should take place within a week of discharge.[28] When a timely postdischarge visit from the provider is not possible, a visit from home nurse services can be helpful.

To ensure that home care workers, nurses, patients, or family members can receive medical guidance and care after hours, 24-hour provider availability and timely response is a necessary feature of home-based care. This is especially true for patients receiving palliative care in the home who are not enrolled in hospice, because management of urgent symptoms may require immediate attention and instructions to nurses or family caregivers. To provide this coverage and access in a feasible way, single HBPC providers may partner with other colleagues or outpatient practices to share after-hours coverage. Group practices often have a rotating after-hours coverage schedule or have providers "cover" their own primary patients at all times. Regardless of how after-hours coverage is arranged, the persons addressing calls, if not HBPC providers themselves, must be clinicians familiar with HBPC principles and patient needs. These include the ability to guide caregivers about medication administration, arrange for nursing or hospice services to make an urgent home visit, order delivery of medical equipment, coordinate radiology and phlebotomy services, and follow local rules and regulations for nonhospice patients who may die at home. After-hours coverage should never consist of an answering machine instructing patients or families to call 911 or emergency services.

As with patients receiving hospice, chronically ill patients with complex medical issues receiving home-based primary and palliative care require a care plan that is interdisciplinary, coordinated, and patient-centered. Symptoms such as pain or dyspnea often require continuous monitoring and medication adjustment even after periods of stability. A provider caring for a nonhospice patient will need to collaborate with multiple home care professionals to provide optimum care at home. For example, a provider may get a call from a family member about worsening of a patient's chronic hip pain from severe osteoarthritis and metastatic prostate cancer. After eliciting some history from the family member over the phone, the provider calls the home care nurse to make a visit to assess the pain. After the nurse's report, the provider orders a home radiograph to rule out a new fracture and arranges pharmacy delivery of liquid morphine to augment the current pain regimen. Over the following days, the provider works with the nurse and family over the phone to titrate the opioids to adequately control pain. Having ruled out an acute fracture, the provider concludes the pain crisis was precipitated by worsening of the patient's underlying disease and orders a hospital bed and patient lift, physical therapy to instruct the family how to use this new equipment, and social work services for referral to an area volunteer program to help the isolated and overwhelmed spouse. The provider will also make a medical home visit the following week to readdress hospice referral, which the patient had been declining. Much of this coordination can be managed by a provider over the telephone, and through careful documentation, some of this coordination time can be reimbursed (using codes related to home care certification and care plan oversight).

As illustrated, successful palliative, patient-centered care in the home depends on facilitating strong partnerships among many different home-based providers. Understanding the requirements for referral to a certified home health care agency is important and useful, because knowledge of what services are considered skilled (e.g., nursing for wound care, symptom monitoring, education, physical therapy for deconditioning, home safety assessment) can provide opportunity for the patient to make use of other services offered by that same agency (e.g., social work, speech therapy, nutrition). Similarly, knowledge of the criteria and appropriate diagnoses for home hospice can facilitate timely referral, allowing eligible patients and their caregivers to derive the most benefit from such services. Collaboration between HBPC providers and area home hospice programs also can benefit patients, because HBPC can institute palliative care for patients not eligible for home hospice or continue a palliative care plan if patients stabilize while on hospice and no longer meet criteria or are discharged.

For HBPC programs without internal social work services, it becomes essential for the provider to possess adequate knowledge about area resources (e.g., case management, meal services, volunteer programs, community and faith-based organizations, funeral homes) to coordinate assistance and support for the patient's and family's quality of life and ability to remain at home. Related to this, providers should familiarize themselves with local and state regulations about death reporting and certification so families and caregivers can be appropriately counseled during these situations. Contacting the local medical examiner's office is a useful resource to clarify rules and regulations about managing a death at home.

It must be noted that limitations exist in a provider's ability to coordinate optimal palliative and related care services in the home setting. The availability of home health services, such as pharmacies and specialists in wound care, psychiatry, palliative medicine, mobile radiology, phlebotomy services, and adjunct community resources, can vary widely between among communities. Rural areas or municipalities with less generous benefits programs may lack many services or the services may take longer to arrange, placing greater burden on family for symptom assessment and on the medical provider to arrange for needed medications and supplies well in advance of crises at home. Despite these variations in home-based resources, an HBPC provider can coordinate available services to provide the medical and psychosocial care important to maintain patients with complex illnesses at home.

ETHICAL DILEMMAS AND PROVIDER SAFETY

Although the intimacy of caring for patents in their homes offers countless benefits in the physician–patient relationship, this same familiarity can result in ethical dilemmas and concerns for provider safety not usually encountered by a traditional office-based practitioner. The following four clinical vignettes represent challenging moments found in delivering care to homebound patients with palliative care needs.

Case 1: Autonomy Versus Beneficence. An 89-year-old woman had debility and failure to thrive. She had few friends and no family. As she aged she had gradually withdrawn into her apartment, relying on deliveries for food and other goods. She regularly refused visits by her primary care doctor, visiting nurse services, and home care, as well as the suggestion of moving to a nursing home. In the last few weeks before her death she stopped eating and although she had substantial pain, she refused medications. She was found dead by the building utility man.

When caring for patients in the home at the end of life, beneficence and autonomy often conflict. Patients regularly make choices that, in a physician's experience, will lead to greater suffering; whether this is a patient with breast cancer refusing opioids for treatment of metastatic bone pain despite repeated education, a frugal widower who will not pay an aide to shop for food, or a bedbound patient with personality disorders refusing visits to assess pressure ulcers.

In dealing with such cases it may be useful to begin by investigating whether there is an underlying disorder that can be treated. This can range from the common, depression or a grief reaction, to the more unusual, schizoaffective disorder or brain metastases. When these problems are ruled out or treated, providers should reach out to others on the care team because they might be able to develop an alternative plan to relieve the patient's suffering. Psychiatrists or social workers can reach out to the patient to better understand the nonmedical barriers to adopting the proposed treatment plan. Family members should be contacted (after obtaining the patient's permission) to discuss the plan of care, to obtain better insights into the patient's explanatory model, and sometimes to help provide the support the patient is initially rejecting. Attempts can be made to find alternative strategies to meet the patient's need. For example, if patients will not accept a home attendant, perhaps they will agree to meal delivery services. However, in cases in which patients remain steadfast to a suboptimal plan, providers should make the best effort to respect patients' wishes. In cases in which home situations are truly unsafe and an illness precludes the patient making reasoned and internally consistent decisions, providers may have to consider adult protective services referral, guardianship, hospitalization, or nursing home placement.

Case 2: A Request to Hasten Patient Death. A 98-year-old man had end-stage dementia and metastatic prostate cancer. Long before his final weeks, he had clearly stated his hope to remain at home and be treated for discomfort. He had experienced numerous episodes of acute deterioration over the last 2 years, always recovering despite foregoing aggressive treatments. Whenever his condition worsened, his family came to say their goodbyes. Despite dire predictions by his primary care physician this time, the patient again stabilized, though he never regained consciousness. Five days later, after other family members had left, the grandson who was the primary caregiver asked if there is any way to help "speed his grandfather along."

Occasionally, the dying process extends longer than originally expected or a patient has high symptom burden despite appropriate medical treatment. In these cases, physicians may be approached by family members to assist in the dying process. These requests range from the subtle, "Is there anything we can do to stop the suffering?" to the aggressive, "Can't you help him stop breathing?" These moments bring the dilemma of the double effect to the fore.

During these difficult cases, providers must determine the root cause of the question. Family members may simply be asking for relief for their loved ones' suboptimal symptom management. Providers can reassure family of their efforts to maximize the patient's comfort, aggressively treating physical symptoms and addressing psychosocial and spiritual suffering. In these cases, it is essential to make sure that the necessary medications can be delivered to the house such as high-potency liquid opioids, antipsychotic suppositories, or quickly dissolving benzodiazepines. Caregivers may also be asking because they are experiencing caregiver burnout, which can be addressed by offering to increase home support or to enroll the patient in community respite care.

However, in rare cases one may suspect that a family member is not acting in the best interest of the patient. The provider has a responsibility to make sure the patient is not being harmed. When in doubt, involving a provider or agency with elder abuse expertise may be necessary. Referral to such a provider may help to disentangle whether malfeasance is present without starting a formal investigation that can damage the therapeutic relationship. Without this option, there may be no choice but to involve adult protective services or even the police. Careful documentation of conversations with the suspect party must be kept, and all care team members should be aware of the concerns.

Case 3: Overwhelmed Caregiver. A 71-year-old woman had New York Heart Association class IV heart failure. She lived with her daughter, a woman who had multiple medical problems. As the patient's functional status declined and the demands on the daughter increased, the daughter began to become very emotionally and physically distressed. She eventually became unable to supervise the patient's medications or coordinate her complex medical care. Moreover, as the caregiver's distress increased, she began calling the physician's office multiple times per day.

The strain inherent in caring for chronically ill patients leads many loving caregivers to become dysfunctional, incapable of providing for the patient or abiding by the patient's prior wishes. This can be particularly problematic at home because patients often have no other support and require the caregiver's assistance with many daily functions, including medication administration needed to ensure palliation of symptoms. These situations leave the primary care physician with the difficulty of deciding if and how to treat the caregiver. As they advocate on behalf of patients' prior wishes, physicians may find themselves in conflict with the caregivers. Further still, caregivers may develop disruptive communication patterns as the situation becomes more desperate. Caregivers may begin calling providers multiple times a day, rarely because the patient's condition warrants it, but instead as a result of overwhelming anxiety and the need for constant reassurance.

Often, social work visits, community resources, and support groups may help mitigate the physical and emotional toll for stressed caregivers. When appropriate, other options include hospice referrals with crisis care, increasing aide hours, respite care, or day programs for the patient. Social workers can set up regularly scheduled visits or phone calls to counsel the caregiver and provide support. When disagreements arise regarding executing the patient's wishes, providers must encourage and support the caregiver to respect the patient's chosen care plan. Ultimately, however, unless the caregiver is making decisions that will clearly harm the patient, the authority of the surrogate should be respected. When patient or family member demands on a medical practice become too heavy, a provider must set limits. It can be helpful to limit the number of phone calls allowed per week, and it is important to remind caregivers that no matter the reason for their call they must be polite and respectful to all office staff. As with any ethical dilemma arising in the home all providers should be encouraged to share the experiences with the group practice in an effort to find alternative solutions and to prevent provider burnout.

Case 4: Duty Versus Safety. A 76-year-old man with end-stage chronic obstructive pulmonary disease was on home oxygen. The past 6 months have been difficult, with multiple hospitalizations, increased breathlessness, and functional decline. More recently, his son, fired from his job, has moved home. The son shows no interest in providing help and now has increasingly erratic behavior. Drug paraphernalia has been occasionally visible during recent visits, and the provider suspects the son is using and selling drugs out of the patient's home.

Although remarkably rare, entering a patient's home can leave providers vulnerable. Often, these concerns arise from the behaviors of someone in or near the home, creating a situation in which the provider has to weigh personal safety concerns against the needs of the homebound patient. As with many dilemmas, the first step is to engage the patient about the concerns. Often, however, the patient is either unable or unwilling to deal with the issue or person in question. Attempts can be made to directly engage the third party to refrain from the risky activity. However, when the safety concern arises from illegal or violent activity, this may create antagonism and worsen safety concerns. If the provider feels sufficiently safe, then completing the visit while accompanied by a colleague or escort is recommended. When the safety risk becomes too high, the provider must acknowledge the risk to himself or herself, as well as to the program, and attempt to secure alternative outpatient care for the patient. This can often be difficult because homebound patients struggle to access care in traditional ambulatory clinics. If no suitable arrangements can be made, the provider does not have an obligation to treat the patient and the patient can be counseled to use emergency medical services to meet ongoing care needs. Finally, whenever any type of safety concern arises, it is important for the primary provider to document the issue in the medical chart in such a manner that other members of the care team can be made aware of the situation.

KEY MESSAGES TO PATIENTS AND FAMILIES

HBPC provides a unique model of care that integrates medical care in the home with simultaneous delivery of palliative care. Providers are often skilled in both disciplines and understand that the goal is to keep the patient at home as long as possible. The goal of an interdisciplinary HBPC is to ensure that the care the homebound patient receives is in line with his or her overall goals while at the same time supporting the caregivers. With appropriate support, planning, and education, many of the needs of a seriously ill patient can be met in the home environment.

CONCLUSION AND SUMMARY

Clinical experience guides many of the recommendations and tips outlined in this chapter. As the literature regarding outpatient palliative care grows, more research is necessary to evaluate and examine the effects of home-based interventions. The number of chronically ill older adults is rising, and the U.S. medical system will have to adjust to help maintain functionally and cognitively impaired patients with substantial symptom burden in the community. There is a growing need for palliative care in community-dwelling chronically ill population not eligible for or agreeable to hospice care. HBPC palliative care is one model that can bridge this gap.[29] Combining home-based primary and palliative care allows for aggressive treatment of chronic diseases alongside identification and management of symptom burden concurrent with longitudinal coordination of care and goals of care communication.

By nature of the patient population and site of care, many HPBC programs are intrinsically providing palliative care. To formalize this, providers need to obtain the medical knowledge and experience in caring for these patients. Some programs hire palliative care trained physicians or nurse practitioners into their practice. Other may use palliative care specialists on a consultative basis. Palliative care is multidisciplinary; therefore using and partnering with community health agencies and services is imperative to best provide this type of care, particularly for HPBC programs without internal social work support. Finally, providers must be able to provide around-the-clock phone access and be knowledgeable about pharmacies and other services that can provide diagnostic tests, supplies, and medications to optimally assess, treat, and manage patients' symptoms at home.

HBPC presents unique care challenges because it blurs physician–patient boundaries, requires intensive communication and care coordination by the provider, and often necessitates implementing alternative methods of symptom management that may otherwise be easier in the hospital or institutional setting. However, integrating palliative care into HBPC allows health care providers to maintain patients in their home environment with their loved ones; identify and treat symptoms tailored to the patient's abilities, preferences, and values; and promote ongoing communication about illness, prognosis, and goals of care. Together these elements ensure that the care received is truly patient and family centered.

SUMMARY RECOMMENDATIONS

- Home-based palliative should be considered for chronically ill older adults who are homebound and medically frail but are not appropriate for hospice.
- Although many home-based programs are providing care that is consistent with palliative care, providers in the home setting still need to obtain formal training in palliative care because home-based palliative care presents unique care challenges. In particular, caring for patients at home blurs physician–patient boundaries, requires intensive communication and care coordination by the provider, and often necessitates implementing alternative methods of symptom management that may otherwise be easier in the hospital or institutional setting.

REFERENCES

1. Wolff JL, Starfield B, Anderson G. Prevalence, expenditures, and complications of multiple chronic conditions in the elderly. *Arch Intern Med.* 2002;162(20):2269–2276.
2. Census Bureau *U.S. Interim projections by age, sex, race, and hispanic origin.* http://www.census.gov/popest/data/index.html; Accessed September 28, 2012.
3. Qiu WQ, Dean M, Liu T, et al. Physical and mental health of homebound older adults: an overlooked population. *J Am Geriatr Soc.* 2010;58(12):2423–2428.

4. Palfrey JS, Sofis LA, Davidson EJ, Liu J, Freeman L, Ganz ML. The pediatric alliance for coordinated care: evaluation of a medical home model. *Pediatrics.* 2004;113(5 suppl):1507–1516.

5. Goldman DP, Shang B, Bhattacharya J, et al. Consequences of health trends and medical innovation for the future elderly. *Health Aff (Millwood).* 2005;24(suppl 2):W5R5–W5R17.

6. Ornstein K, Smith KL, Boal JB. Understanding and improving the burden of unmet needs of informal caregivers of homebound patients enrolled in a home-based primary care program. *J Appl Gerontol.* 2009;28(4):482–503.

7. Smith KL, Soriano TA, Boal JB. Brief communication: national quality-of-care standards in home-based primary care. *Ann Intern Med.* 2007;146(3):188.

8. Centers for Medicare and Medicaid Services. *Medicare Benefit Policy Manual.* CMS Pub. 100-02, Chapter. 7 (Rev. 142, April 15, 2011); https://www.cms.gov/manuals/Downloads/bp102c07.pdf; Accessed September 28, 2012.

9. Kellogg FR, Brickner PW. Long-term home healthcare for the impoverished frail homebound aged: a twenty-seven-year experience. *J Am Geriatr Soc.* 2000;48(8):1002–1011.

10. Gammel JD. Medical house call program: extending frail elderly medical care into the home. *J Oncol Manag.* 2005;14(2):39–46.

11. Mor V, Zinn J, Gozalo P, Feng Z, Intrator O, Grabowski DC. Prospects for transferring nursing home residents to the community. *Health Aff (Millwood).* 2007;26(6):1762–1771.

12. Meier DE, Beresford L. Outpatient clinics are a new frontier for palliative care. *J Palliat Med.* 2008;11(6):823–828.

13. Morrison RS, Wallenstein S, Natale DK, Senzel RS, Huang LL. "We don't carry that": failure of pharmacies in predominantly nonwhite neighborhoods to stock opioid analgesics. *N Engl J Med.* 2000;342(14):1023–1026.

14. Boccia RV, Gordan LN, Clark G, et al. Efficacy and tolerability of transdermal granisetron for the control of chemotherapy-induced nausea and vomiting associated with moderately and highly emetogenic multi-day chemotherapy: a randomized, double-blind, phase III study. *Support Care Cancer.* PMID: 20835873.

15. Galbraith S, Fagan P, Perkins P, et al. Does the use of a hand-held fan improve chronic dyspnea? A randomized, controlled, crossover trial. *J Pain Symptom Manage.* 2010;39(5):831–838.

16. Bruera E, Sweeney C, Willey J, et al. A randomized controlled trial of supplemental oxygen versus air in cancer patients with dyspnea. *Palliat Med.* 2003;17(8):659–663.

17. Abernethy AP, McDonald CF, Frith PA, et al. Effect of palliative oxygen versus room air in relief of breathlessness in patients with refractory dyspnoea: a double-blind, randomised controlled trial. *Lancet.* 2010;376(9743):784–793.

18. Wilson MM, Thomas DR, Rubenstein LZ, et al. Appetite assessment: simple appetite questionnaire predicts weight loss in community-dwelling adults and nursing home residents. *Am J Clin Nutr.* 2005;82(5):1074–1081.

19. Keller HH, Goy R, Kane SL. Validity and reliability of SCREEN II (Seniors in the community: risk evaluation for eating and nutrition, Version II). *Eur J Clin Nutr.* 2005;59(10):1149–1157.

20. Belle SH, Burgio L, Burns R, et al. Enhancing the quality of life of dementia caregivers from different ethnic or racial groups: a randomized, controlled trial. *Ann Intern Med.* 2006;145(10):727–738.

21. Kao H, Conant R, Soriano T, et al. The past, present and future of house calls. *Clin Geriatr Med.* 2009;25(1):19.

22. Lanarkshire Palliative Care Guidelines. 2011. *Guidelines for the use of Subcutaneous Medicine in Palliative Care.* www.nhslanarkshire.org.uk/Services/PalliativeCare; Accessed October 5, 2012.

23. Warren DE. Practical use of rectal medicines in palliative care. *J Pain Symptom Manage.* 1996;11(6):378–387.

24. Flores G. The impact of medical interpreter services on the quality of health care: a systematic review. *Med Care Res Rev.* 2005;62(3):255–299.

25. Woloshin S, Bickell NA, Schwartz LM, Gany F, Welch HG. Language barriers in medicine in the United States. *JAMA.* 1995;273(9):724–728.

26. Ngo-Metzger Q, Sorkin DH, Phillips RS, et al. Providing high-quality care for limited English proficient patients: the importance of language concordance and interpreter use. *J Gen Intern Med.* 2007;22(suppl 2):324–330.

27. Lang F, Quill T. Making decisions with families at the end of life. *Am Fam Physician.* 2004;70(4):719–723.

28. Rabow MW, Hauser JM, Adams J. Supporting family caregivers at the end of life: "they don't know what they don't know". *JAMA.* 2004;291(4):483–491.

29. McFall S, Miller BH. Caregiver burden and nursing home admission of frail elderly persons. *J Gerontol.* 1992;47(2):S73–S79.

Chapter 79

What New Models Exist for Ambulatory Palliative Care?

MICHAEL W. RABOW

INTRODUCTION

In 2008, Meier and Beresford[1] called outpatient clinics "a new frontier in palliative care" that were filling a gap in access to palliative care. However, this new frontier remains relatively uncharted, with many in the field referring to the current environment of outpatient palliative care as the "wild west." Nevertheless, gathering and summarizing the models currently being used to provide outpatient palliative care services may be useful to clinicians and health care administrators. Beyond the academic interest of understanding how outpatient palliative care services are organized and run in the United States, a description of the elements of outpatient practices may be of benefit to new and developing programs in helping identify the advantages and disadvantages of various elements and to use this knowledge in building effective practice structures suited to their own context.[2]

Definition

Ambulatory palliative care is provided to outpatients in practices and clinics. In these models of care, patients come to the palliative care teams' facility to be seen. Although fairly well-established structures exist for inpatient palliative care consultation teams, much of ambulatory palliative care is still early in its development and a wide variety of structures and processes are used nationally.

The Growth of Ambulatory Palliative Care

The prevalence and penetration of ambulatory palliative care nationally is unknown. Clearly, palliative care clinics are sprouting up in many settings, but relatively little is known about the structure, staffing, financing, or efficacy of these services. A few studies provide the foundation of our understanding. Within cancer centers, Hui and colleagues[3] reported palliative care services available in 59% of National Cancer Institute (NCI) Cancer Centers, but in only 22% of non–NCI-designated cancer centers. This survey found great variation in the types and comprehensiveness of palliative care services. In California, Berger and colleagues found only 8% of hospitals had an affiliated outpatient palliative care practice.[4] This survey is being repeated, and it is expected that a larger percentage of outpatient practices will be found. Although outpatient services may develop de novo, many appear to grow out of maturing inpatients services, a "second wave" following the establishment of inpatient services. In addition to well-established academic outpatient services, tremendous growth has occurred in small, ambulatory palliative care services across the country, operating independently or in affiliation with hospitals.

Common Elements in Ambulatory Palliative Care Practices

A survey of 11 prominent, primarily academic medical center and comprehensive cancer center outpatient palliative care practices described common elements (Table 79-1).[5] Among these leading academic programs, most patients had cancer and were seen about three times. The practices saw an average of 250 new patients annually, operating out of an average of two rooms, during 3 days per week. Most practices included a physician, with an average of 0.6 full time equivalent (FTE). Just over half of the practices had a nurse practitioner working on average 0.9 FTE. Slightly fewer than half of the programs had a social worker, with 0.7 FTE on average. About one third of programs had nursing staff, with 1.6 FTE. About half of operating revenues for these practices was supported by billing alone, with the need for institutional support for much of the rest.

STUCTURE AND PROCESSES OF CARE

Ambulatory palliative care practice models are quite varied. Generally, services develop to address a

TABLE 79-1. Characteristics of Ambulatory Palliative Care Comparison Practices (n = 11)

PRACTICE CHARACTERISTICS	VALUE	
	MEAN (RANGE)	NO. PROGRAMS (%)
Usage and Size		
Total patients annually	501 (90-1400)	
New patients annually	250 (48-840)	
Percentage of patients with cancer	80 (20-100)	
Number of visits per patient	3 (2-4)	
Days of clinical operation per week	3 (1-5)	
Number of examination rooms available each clinical session	2 (1-8)	
Referral Sources		
Oncologists (%)	76 (0-95)	
Inpatient palliative care consult service (%)	23 (0-56)	
Primary care physicians (%)	10 (0-44)	
Funding Source		
Billing (%)	49 (0-100)	
Institutional support (%)	45 (0-100)	
Philanthropy (%)	6 (0-67)	
Affiliation		
Hospital-based		10 (91)
Within an oncology division/cancer center		10 (91)
Hospice-based		1 (9)
Staffing		
Physician		10 (91)
Mean physician FTE among programs with physician staffing	0.6 (0.1-2)	
APN/NP		6 (55)
Mean APN FTE among programs with APN staffing	0.9 (0.2-2)	
Social Worker		5 (45)
Mean social worker FTE among programs with social worker staffing	0.7 (0.25-1)	
RN		4 (36)
Mean RN FTE among programs with RN staffing	1.6 (0.2-4.6)	
Patient Data Collected Routinely		
Demographics		10 (91)
Symptoms		8 (73)
Hospital admissions		5 (45)

Reprinted from Rabow MW, Smith AK, Braun JL, Weissman DE. Outpatient palliative care practices. *Arch Intern Med.* 2010;170(7):654-655.
APN, Advanced practice nurse; *FTE,* full-time equivalent; *NP,* nurse practitioner; *RN,* registered nurse.

particular need of the inpatient palliative care service, the hospital, a cancer center, or a specific specialty service. Most recently, some health systems have begun to mandate the development of outpatient palliative care services system-wide, often leaving local administrations to develop (and pay) for the service. Despite the variety of models, certain elements can be assessed to describe the structure and processes of ambulatory palliative care services (Table 79-2).

Site of Care

Ambulatory palliative care takes place in an outpatient clinic or practice. Common models for this include being a free-standing practice, being nested within an existing, non–palliative care practice (e.g., an oncology office, primary care practice, or pain clinic), or having a roving palliative care team who travel to the clinic where a referred patient is being seen by the referring physician. A free-standing practice has the ability to define their space, environment, mood, and flow but must take on all of the tasks and financial costs of running a practice. In particular, the palliative care practice will be solely responsible for the costs of rent, electricity,

maintenance, computer systems and internet access, staffing (clerical, scheduling, and clinical), record keeping, and so forth. Nesting within another practice often allows a palliative care practice to use many of the resources of the hosting practice (rooms, lights, computers, schedulers, check-in staff). Importantly, presence in the referring clinic (e.g., co-located within an oncology clinic) is a huge opportunity to develop a close relationship with potential referrers and improve and refine the stream of patient referrals. The hosting practice typically is the source of the palliative care group's referrals (or a large portion of them). However, as a guest or even renter in a host's practice, the palliative care practice may be constrained by the skills or attitudes of the existing staff and structures. A roving team is of great convenience to patients and referring physicians but generally presents significant logistical and efficiency challenges to the palliative care team.

Type of Clinical Care

Ambulatory palliative care practices need to determine the level and scope of responsibility they will take for patients. In a pure consultation model, the

TABLE 79-2. Operational and Logistical Considerations in Ambulatory Palliative Care Services

OPERATIONAL ISSUE	POSSIBLE OPTIONS
Site of care	Freestanding Within an existing non–palliative care practice
Type of care	Consultation Co-management
Duration of care	Single visit/short term Ongoing/long term
Relationship to inpatient palliative care	Pre Post Unrelated
Referral process	Referral Automatic/triggered/via protocol
Patient population	Disease-specific Symptom-specific Task-specific Time-specific
Care process and logistics	Clinic hours and days Around-the-clock coverage or backup Length of sessions for new and follow-up patients Scheduled visits versus open access Which team members are in the room How the team communicates with the referring team Structures for processing/collecting co-payments and billing
Staffing	Choice of which disciplines on the team Choice of which disciplines in the room with a patient
Finances	Billing Institutional support Philanthropy Research support
Evaluation	Clinical outcomes Patient, family, referring clinician satisfaction Palliative care clinician satisfaction Resource usage Clinic and medical system costs

palliative care team assesses the patient and then offers recommendations to the referring physician. Patients are seen once (or perhaps a few additional times); then implementation of the longer-term plan is left to other clinicians (e.g., primary care physician, oncologist). Although this model clearly constrains the clinical responsibility that must be assumed by the palliative care team, there is no way to guarantee that the patient will receive the care recommended. Referring clinicians may not attempt to implement or successfully implement the recommendations of the palliative care team. This may be especially true around complex pain management issues (because of lack of knowledge, discomfort with or bias against opioids), time-consuming psychosocial care, or care from disciplines not commonly used by or available to the referring physician (such as chaplaincy).

Consequently, many ambulatory palliative care practices have a co-management model in which the palliative care team assumes responsibility for some clinical issues (e.g., pain management) while the referring physician simultaneously manages other relevant issues (e.g., cancer). Co-management is a higher level of responsibility and requires that the palliative care team can offer options for around-the-clock care of the issues for which they are responsible. Co-management means that the ambulatory palliative care practice assumes more responsibility, including longitudinally, which may create a burgeoning practice census. The patient care benefits in co-management are clear—the palliative care team retains the power to implement their plans, can write prescriptions, and provides follow-up assessments, monitoring, and readjustment.

Duration of Care

Closely related to the type of care is the question of the duration of care. Once the service assumes responsibility, the length of time the palliative care team will be involved should be made clear to the patient. Setting expectations appropriately with patients, families, and referring physicians is key, especially if the palliative care service plans to see the patient just once (as may be the case in a consultation), a few times (short-term co-management), or in an ongoing way (continuity, long-term co-management). Depending on the life expectancy of the patient population, assuming ongoing care can quickly create a heavy patient burden for an ambulatory palliative care service, making it difficult to maintain capacity to see new patients in the setting of a growing and long-term follow-up population.

Relationship to Inpatient Palliative Care

Given the close relationship within many institutions between inpatient and ambulatory palliative care services, another way to describe ambulatory practices is by their relationship to inpatient services. Some ambulatory practices serve as a follow-up to the inpatient service. The ambulatory practice helps patients transition back to their primary care physician or completes the plans (including medication adjustment) established by the inpatient service. The ambulatory practice might allow the inpatient service more flexibility in discharge planning, knowing that the outpatient service can help maintain good symptom control or even continue goals of care discussions. With close links to the inpatient palliative care services, the ambulatory service can enjoy the advantages of administrative efficiency, sharing of expertise and staffing, and participation in the cost-avoidance model of the inpatient service. However, disadvantages include difficulty with staff moving back and forth between the drama and acuity of the hospital and the very different outpatient palliative care culture. Additionally, the ambulatory practice ties itself to the inpatient practice reputation and patient population.

Alternatively, the ambulatory practice may not have a formal relationship with an inpatient service. Such a practice could provide hospital palliative care follow-up but would not be limited to this type of referral. Such models of practice may offer "primary palliative care," seeing patients early in the course of disease, perhaps even from diagnosis, and following patients over time and providing longitudinal management of chronic symptoms. Theoretically, an ambulatory palliative care practice can be the first to introduce patients to the concepts and practice of palliative care and can increase patient interest in subsequent inpatient palliative care.

Referral Process

Although some ambulatory palliative care practices only see patients in follow-up from an inpatient palliative care consultation, most practices are dependent on referrals from non–palliative care providers. Referrals can be ad hoc, based on the referring clinician's estimation of the need for the palliative care consultation or co-management. Such a system may be perceived as supportive of the referring clinicians, who have access to palliative care as they see the need. The challenges with such a system of referral is that, even with careful marketing, the referring physicians may not be referring the patients that the palliative care service believes need to be seen or the patient population the palliative care service is most interested in seeing.

Alternatively, "automatic," "triggered," or "protocolized" referrals can be generated based on prespecified criteria. For example, given the randomized trial data for the benefits of early ambulatory palliative care for patients with metastatic non–small cell lung cancer,[6] patients who receive this diagnosis might be referred automatically to the palliative care clinic. Almost any criteria can be used to develop a trigger for referral, including diagnoses or symptoms, number of emergency department visits or hospitalizations, clinical conditions (e.g., newly metastatic disease, consideration of feeding tube placement), or need for specific services (e.g., advance care planning discussions, completing Physician Orders for Life Sustaining Treatment [POLST] forms). Such a referral system allows the palliative care team to develop deep expertise in a particular area, to coordinate closely with referring clinicians, and to have a steady and more reliable sense of the referral stream. Uniform patient populations have advantages for conducting palliative care research. Disadvantages include a limited referral base and less variety for the interdisciplinary palliative care team.

Patient Population

A key consideration, and related to the referral process described, is the target patient population to be served in the ambulatory clinic. Practices can be open to referrals of any patient with serious illness suffering burdensome morbidities or impaired quality of life. Or, the patient population can be limited. A common limit is to focus on patients with a particular disease. Usually this is cancer, although clinics focused on a particular serious chronic illness are increasingly common. Illnesses that can be the focus of an ambulatory palliative care practice are myriad but often include congestive heart failure, chronic obstructive pulmonary disease, dementia, human immunodeficiency virus infection, or primary pulmonary hypertension. Finally, some cancer centers are developing services focused on providing care and guidance to cancer survivors.

The ambulatory palliative care practice can focus on patients with a specific disease, or with specific symptoms, such as pain or cachexia. The focus can be on a specific task or intervention, such as an advance care planning clinic or a bereavement service. Finally, the service may be specific for patients at a particular time of care, such as after hospitalization or before hospice.

Practices must decide if certain patients will be excluded from the clinic. Many outpatient palliative care practices find that referring physicians enjoy help managing their most difficult or demanding patients. Palliative care practices must prospectively decide their capacity to participate in the care of these patients. For example, patients with chronic, nonmalignant pain may have palliative care needs as great as those of patients at the end of life but may be outside the scope of practice the clinic is able to serve adequately.[7] Patients with serious mental illness (especially psychotic disorders) may be a difficult but typically underserved population who often have profound palliative care issues but may require particular expertise and staffing to manage appropriately.

Care Process and Logistics

Ambulatory palliative care practices assume some or all of the logistical and administrative challenges of running an outpatient medical practice. The site of care heavily influences these considerations, and numerous questions must be considered when designing such a practice. Practices need adequate clinical, administrative, and waiting room space. Nursing, authorization, copayment processing, and billing services are necessary. The scheduling procedures are key: scheduled visit versus open access versus a combination. On which days of the week will the practice operate? How much time will be scheduled for new patient and follow-up patient appointments? Who will provide clinical coverage on clinic off days or nights and weekends if the clinic's palliative care team is unable to cover themselves? Which clinicians on the team will actually be in the room with the patient at any one time? How will communication between the team and the referring physician be accomplished?

Staffing

Key to the ambulatory effort is the composition of the palliative care team. Most practices have some supported time for a physician or a nurse practitioner.[5] Social workers and registered nurses are also common. Other members of interdisciplinary palliative care teams can include chaplains, pharmacists, nutritionists, physical and rehabilitation therapists, psychologists, and music and art therapists. Staffing is often shared between inpatient and outpatient palliative care. The logistics of protecting time for inpatient clinicians "to run over" and staff the ambulatory clinic are complex.

Clinics must decide who is on the team and also who will be in the room with patients. It is clearly expensive to have multiple professionals seeing the patient simultaneously. Additionally, although physicians and nurse practitioners can bill for their services, the other members of the team typically cannot.

Finally, practices must develop systems to help sustain clinical and administrative staff. The clinical work of outpatient palliative care is rewarding but also difficult.[8] Each member of the palliative care team needs the ability to recover, rejuvenate, and recommit. Mourning or remembrance rituals for patients who have died, team retreats, professional psychological support, and social events are just some methods used for this purpose.

Financing

Billing for ambulatory palliative care service is relatively straightforward (billing for physician and nurse practitioner visits, typically based on symptom codes). However, the survey of prominent palliative care programs showed that billing revenue is typically insufficient to support all of the costs of running an ambulatory palliative care clinic.[5] Reimbursement is typically low despite the time-intensive nature of palliative care. Additionally, ambulatory palliative care practices must support salaries of nonbilling staff, including administrative staff, registered nurses, social workers, and chaplains. (Although the potential exists for social workers to bill for psychotherapeutic services, in most settings this is not common practice). With just half of revenues coming from billing, services need a combination of institutional support, philanthropy, and research funding to cover costs. Chapter 71 discusses some of the arguments for why outpatient palliative care is beneficial to medical systems. These arguments may help convince medical systems to support the ambulatory palliative care. Obtaining research funding to support routine clinical operational costs is difficult, and increasingly so if the clinical operations are not involved in innovative services. Philanthropy, too, may be difficult for the ambulatory palliative care practice. This is especially true given that the clinicians who refer many of the patients to the palliative care practice may be competing for donations.

A referring physician may stop referring to the clinic if the palliative care clinic is seen as a competitor for philanthropic donors.

Evaluation

To support continuous quality improvement and to justify initial, ongoing, or expanding support from the larger medical system, the ambulatory palliative care practice must collect data to demonstrate that it is achieving its goals or that the unmet need justifies expanding its services. Typically, evaluation targets include clinical outcomes such as pain, completion of advance directives, and mortality; satisfaction of patients, families, and referring physicians; satisfaction and sustainability of palliative care clinicians; resource usage, including emergency department visits, hospitalizations and readmissions, use of the intensive care unit, and hospice use; and palliative care clinic and overall medical system costs.

SUMMARY OF EVIDENCE FOR THE EFFECTIVENESS OF MODELS OF AMBULATORY PALLIATIVE CARE

Although evidence of clinical efficacy and financial success is limited, some ambulatory palliative care programs have published data on their outcomes, including patient, family, and referring physician satisfaction; feasibility; clinical efficacy; and financial data. The evidence for clinical efficacy is detailed in Chapter 71.[6,9-16] Most of the best-evaluated practices are a part of a cancer center and cater to that population. Effective practices have been physician-based or nurse practitioner–based. Common elements of successful practices include the presence of an interdisciplinary team and a close relationship with referring physicians. In the early palliative care intervention shown to improve mortality in non–small cell lung cancer, the initial palliative care intervention lasted about an hour and typically addressed symptom management, coping, illness understanding, and education.[17]

KEY MESSAGES TO PATIENTS AND FAMILIES

Outpatient palliative care helps to round out the panoply of services available to patients with serious illness and their families. Depending on the nature of the practice and the relationship to the referring physician, clinicians in the palliative care ambulatory setting must explain to patients and families the goals of the appointment(s), the expected duration of the relationship (e.g., one or several visits versus a longer-term relationship in which the patient is comanaged with the referring team), and when and how to contact the palliative care team with questions. Clinicians should explain to patients and their families the interdisciplinary nature of the team, because the models of care used in palliative care outpatient settings may be new to them.

CONCLUSION AND SUMMARY

Ambulatory palliative care is a new frontier in palliative care, filling a key gap in continuity of palliative care for patients with serious illness, most of whom spend the majority of their time outside of hospitals. The number of ambulatory care practices appears to be growing rapidly, but there is little formal evaluation of the prevalence of programs nationally. The structure of ambulatory palliative care practices nationally is varied. However, all models of ambulatory palliative care must determine solutions to a series of operational considerations that are suited to local needs and opportunities. Specifically, practices must determine the site, type and duration of care to be provided, the relationship to inpatient palliative care services, the process for referrals, the patient population to be served, the logistics of the care process, staffing, financing, and how to evaluate the program. Although some practices have demonstrated improved patient outcomes, including improved mortality in one randomized trial of early ambulatory palliative care, the elements of practice structure and process that contribute to these positive outcomes have not yet been elucidated.

SUMMARY RECOMMENDATIONS

- Ambulatory palliative care practices must determine the site, type, and duration of care to be provided.
- Relationships to inpatient palliative care services must be considered.
- Practices must provide a process for patient referrals.
- The patient population to be served must be identified.
- The logistics of the care process, staffing, financing, and how to evaluate the program must be examined.

REFERENCES

1. Meier DE, Beresford L. Outpatient clinics are a new frontier for palliative care. *J Palliat Med.* 2008;11(6):823–828.
2. Rabow MW, Pantilat SZ, Kerr K, et al. The intersection of need and opportunity: assessing and capitalizing on opportunities to expand hospital-based palliative care services. *J Palliat Med.* 2010;13(10):1205–1210.
3. Hui D, Elsayem A, De la Cruz M, et al. Availability and integration of palliative care at US cancer centers. *JAMA.* 2010;303(11):1054–1061.
4. Berger GN, O'Riordan DL, Kerr K, Pantilat SZ. Prevalence and characteristics of outpatient palliative care services in California. *Arch Intern Med.* 2011;171(22):2057–2059.
5. Rabow MW, Smith AK, Braun JL, Weissman DE. Outpatient palliative care practices. *Arch Intern Med.* 2010;170(7):654–655.
6. Temel JS, Greer JA, Muzikansky A, et al. Early palliative care for patients with metastatic non-small-cell lung cancer. *N Engl J Med.* 2010;363(8):733–742.
7. Fredheim OM, Kaasa S, Fayers P, Saltnes T, Jordhøy M, Borchgrevink PC. Chronic non-malignant pain patients report as poor health-related quality of life as palliative cancer patients. *Acta Anaesthesiol Scand.* 2008;52(1):143–148.
8. Sinclair S. Impact of death and dying on the personal lives and practices of palliative and hospice care professionals. *CMAJ.* 2011;183(2):180–187.
9. Rabow MW, Dibble SL, Pantilat SZ, McPhee SJ. The comprehensive care team: a controlled trial of outpatient palliative medicine consultation. *Arch Intern Med.* 2004;164(1):83–91.
10. Strasser F, Sweeney C, Willey J, et al. Impact of a half-day multidisciplinary symptom control and palliative care outpatient clinic in a comprehensive cancer center on recommendations, symptom intensity, and patient satisfaction: a retrospective descriptive study. *J Pain Symptom Manage.* 2004;27(6):481–491.
11. Bruera E, Michaud M, Vigano A, Neumann CM, Watanabe S, Hanson J. Multidisciplinary symptom control clinic in a cancer center: a retrospective study. *Support Care Cancer.* 2001;9(3):162–168.
12. Yennurajalingam S, Urbauer DL, Casper KL, et al. Impact of a palliative care consultation team on cancer-related symptoms in advanced cancer patients referred to an outpatient supportive care clinic. *J Pain Symptom Manage.* 2011;41(1):49–56.
13. Follwell M, Burman D, Le LW, et al. Phase II study of an outpatient palliative care intervention in patients with metastatic cancer. *J Clin Oncol.* 2009;27(2):206–213.
14. Muir JC, Daly F, Davis MS, et al. Integrating palliative care into the outpatient, private practice oncology setting. *J Pain Symptom Manage.* 2010;40(1):126–135.
15. Bakitas M, Lyons KD, Hegel MT, et al. Effects of a palliative care intervention on clinical outcomes in patients with advanced cancer: the Project ENABLE II randomized controlled trial. *JAMA.* 2009;302(7):741–749.
16. Temel JS, Jackson VA, Billings JA, et al. Phase II study: integrated palliative care in newly diagnosed advanced non-small-cell lung cancer patients. *J Clin Oncol.* 2007;25(17):2377–2382.
17. Jacobsen J, Jackson V, Dahlin C, et al. Components of early outpatient palliative care consultation in patients with metastatic nonsmall cell lung cancer. *J Palliat Med.* 2011;14(4):459–464.

Chapter 80

What New Models Exist for Palliative Care in the Emergency Department?

CORITA R. GRUDZEN AND LYNNE D. RICHARDSON

INTRODUCTION AND SCOPE OF THE PROBLEM

Patients come to emergency departments (EDs) seeking relief from pain and other burdensome symptoms. Increasingly, these patients are older and have more medically complex problems, necessitating greater skill in the delivery of palliative care services. Patients with cancer may fail outpatient management of pain or treatment of other symptoms, residents of skilled nursing facilities need evaluation of fever and respiratory distress, and older adults with multiple chronic diseases have acute decompensations that need emergent treatment. Some problems are solved by simple titration of opioids or review of an advance directive, whereas others require more complex palliative care skills, such as lengthy discussions about goals of care.

As the population ages, the number of ED visits in the United States will continue to rise. Adults 75 years and older use the ED at nearly twice the rate (62 annual ED visits/100 persons) of those 45 to 64 year old (32.2 annual ED visits/100 persons) and are more likely to have one or more chronic conditions.[1] Although Emergency Medicine developed as a specialty to provide life-sustaining treatments to patients with acute injury or illness, many ED visits are made by patients with exacerbations of chronic conditions. Recognition has been increasing of the importance of addressing the palliative care needs for these patients in the ED. For those with advanced or end-stage disease, traditional life-prolonging treatments offered by emergency providers may not be concordant with patients' goals, may have greater likelihood of harm than benefit, and may not even address the symptoms for which they sought emergency care.

Chronic diseases are now the leading causes of death, and a high prevalence is seen of physical, psychosocial, spiritual, and financial suffering associated with serious and complex illness across many systems of care, including EDs.[2] Whether because of limited access to primary care or the need for interventions or testing that exceed the resources of most outpatient settings, seriously ill patients with advanced disease are frequently cared for by emergency providers. Patients who have pain, vomiting, or other burdensome symptoms that cannot be controlled at home, in a nursing facility, or in a provider's office, often visit EDs because of their around-the-clock access and ability to deal with such crises. Such patients may have multiple palliative care needs, and it is unlikely these are all addressed, given the other pressures on emergency providers. In a cohort of older adults with functional impairment and chronic disease who visited one urban ED, the majority had physical symptoms (severe fatigue, pain, dyspnea, or depression), unmet mental health and financial needs, and trouble accessing care.[3]

Palliative medicine, with its mission to relieve pain and other burdensome symptoms and to match goals of care to treatments, could help address some of these patients' reasons for seeking emergency care. The goal of palliative medicine is to achieve the best possible quality of life, including physical, psychological, social, and spiritual aspects, for patients and families through specific knowledge and skills.[4] These include assessment and treatment of pain and other burdensome symptoms; aid with complex medical decision-making; mobilization of practical, spiritual, and psychosocial support; care coordination (especially during transitions of care); and bereavement services.[4-7]

Large gaps in the delivery of palliative care services exist in the outpatient setting, in which failure to address goals of care and to plan for and prevent predictable crises often occurs.[2] Emergency Medicine and the palliative care community have increasingly acknowledged the need to deliver palliative care services in the ED.[8] In 2008 the American Board of Emergency Medicine became a sponsoring board for the subspecialty of Hospice and Palliative Medicine. Emergency providers can work in concert with primary care providers, palliative care teams, and other specialty providers (e.g., oncology), to deliver comprehensive palliative care to patients in the ED (Figure 80-1).

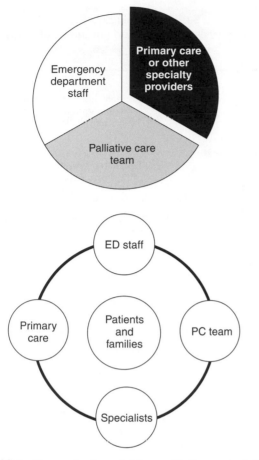

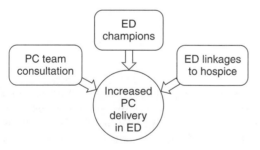

FIGURE 80-1. Conceptual model for palliative care delivery in the emergency department.

FIGURE 80-2. Current models for palliative care service delivery for patients in the emergency department.

Although more than 70% of hospitals with more than 250 beds now have palliative care services,[9–12] hospital-based consultation typically occurs more than a week into a patient's hospital stay[13,14] rather than in the first critical days of admission, when major treatment decisions are made. Preliminary data suggest that moving palliative care consultation upstream to the ED, as opposed to later during a hospital stay, can decrease hospital length of stay and reduce costs per day. A retrospective chart review of patients admitted to a community hospital in Detroit demonstrated that palliative care consultation in the ED, as opposed to after hospital admission, was associated with shorter mean hospital length of stay (6.5 days versus 11.5 days, $p = .005$).[15] A review of billing and administrative data from Virginia Commonwealth University showed that a partnership between the ED and palliative care can help identify ED patients for admission to a dedicated palliative care unit, which is associated with decreased costs per day and reduced days in the intensive care unit.[16]

CURRENT MODELS FOR PALLIATIVE CARE DELIVERY IN THE EMERGENCY DEPARTMENT

Optimal models for the delivery of ED-based palliative care services have yet to be determined. Current ED-based programs are reflective of the palliative care champions and services available at each particular hospital; these include ED-based initiatives by nursing staff, physician consultation with potential for admission, and a dedicated palliative care unit. In response to the growing numbers of patients with advanced illness cared for in the ED, several medical centers have recently initiated pilot programs to deliver ED-based palliative care consultation. These programs, as described in detail later, are of three types: ED-based consultation by an inpatient palliative care team, services or training initiated by palliative care champions in the ED, and ED partnerships with hospice providers (Fig. 80-2).

Programs Initiated by Palliative Care Teams

A select number of well-established palliative care programs have reached out to the ED to encourage consultations, including Virginia Commonwealth University, Montefiore Medical Center, and the Mount Carmel Health System. Although considerable staff and resources are often needed to begin such programs, preliminary data show that ED–palliative care partnerships can help identify patients with palliative care needs and provide needed services. Billing and administrative data from Virginia Commonwealth University Medical Center showed that ED-based consultation decreased hospital length of stay and costs for those who are admitted to and die in the hospital.[17] In addition, the ED is now the source for a significant proportion of their palliative care unit's admissions. The palliative care service at Montefiore Medical Center was able to identify chronically ill older adult patients in the ED in need of palliative care, home care, and hospice services and to link such patients with these services.[18] At three hospitals within the Mount Carmel Health System in Columbus, Ohio, the palliative care team developed training and screening tools specific to the ED, participated in ED staff meetings, and made regular ED visits, resulting in a highly successful partnership in which 9.2% of all admissions and 66.7% of all direct admissions to the palliative care unit come from the ED.[19]

Emergency Department Champions in Palliative Care

Now that palliative care is a subspecialty of Emergency Medicine, an increasing number of emergency physicians will be board-certified in both disciplines, and can serve as champions in the ED. At Scripps Mercy Hospital in San Diego, an emergency physician trained in palliative medicine began a pilot program to increase ED-based palliative care consultations. Of the 78 patients in the ED who were seen during the first 4 months, 29 were admitted to hospice agencies, suggesting that direct transfer to hospice care is feasible for patients in emergency care.[20] Not all palliative care–ED partnerships have been started at hospitals with well-established palliative care consultation services. At Los Angeles County–University of Southern California Medical Center, a physician board-certified in both emergency medicine and palliative care began the first palliative care consult team at this large, urban county hospital. With funding from the Archstone Foundation, a prospective, randomized trial of an ED-based palliative care intervention called ED-HELP showed the challenges in recruiting patients with advanced illness in the ED for research studies.[21] Even with bilingual research staff, many patients could not participate because of cognitive deficits or high symptom burden.

Linkage to Hospice Services

A subset of patients in emergency care may benefit from active partnerships between EDs and hospice providers, especially those patients at the end of life with clear goals of care and a high burden of symptoms. The ED at Stands Hospital in Jacksonville, Florida works closely with a community hospice to identify patients with end-stage illness whose pain and symptoms can be managed in the outpatient setting. The hospice provides two full-time nurses from 7 AM to 11 PM to assist the ED in identifying eligible patients and reviewing hospice benefits. While data are preliminary, the program is considered highly successful by hospital administrators and ED staff, and an increasing number of patients are discharged with hospice services in place.[22]

BARRIERS AND OPPORTUNITIES FOR EMERGENCY DEPARTMENT AND PALLIATIVE CARE PARTNERSHIPS

Although some data on pilot programs are available, optimal models of delivery of ED-based palliative care have not been rigorously studied. Research is needed to determine how these services are best organized, what effect they have on patients and caregivers, and whether they can decrease symptom burden and health care usage.

Although pilot programs such as those described earlier have demonstrated some early successes, real barriers exist to the expansion of ED-based palliative care services. Attitudes of emergency providers, attitudes of patients' other treating physicians, and limited staffing resources of palliative care teams

TABLE 80-1. Barriers to Palliative Care in the Emergency Department and Potential Solutions

BARRIER	SOLUTION
Logistical	
Limited availability	Increase hours and improve response time
	Dedicate palliative care staff to ED
Environmental	
Crowding	Dedicated private space
Lack of privacy	Sound proof curtains or door, chairs for family
Culture	
Fast-paced	Creation of observation units
Interventional/ procedural	Physician champions/key opinion leaders
Knowledge	
Emergency providers	Education in palliative care
Patients and families	Triggered consultation based on set criteria

Modified from Grudzen CR, Richardson LD, Ortiz JM, et al. Does palliative care have a future in the emergency department? Discussions with attending emergency physicians. *J Pain Symptom Manage.* 2012;43(1):1-9.

all serve to constrain their proliferation. Despite these barriers, many opportunities exist to expand palliative care services into the ED. Examples include increasing knowledge among emergency care providers, developing triggers for palliative care consultations among patients in emergency care, and continually monitoring the benefits of moving palliative care consultation upstream. Table 80-1 provides a more detailed description of the barriers to delivering palliative care in the ED and potential solutions.[23]

Attitudinal Barriers Among Emergency Providers

Emergency providers, compared to primary care providers, are at some obvious disadvantages when trying to deliver goal-directed care that is consistent with patient preferences. Emergency physicians may be meeting patients and families for the first time and may not be able to access patients' medical records or advance care planning documents. Patients are often brought to the closest appropriate facility during an emergency, which may or may not be their preferred site of care or medical home. Depending on the time of day, the emergency provider may not be able to speak with the patient's primary provider and a covering provider may not know the patient or have access to the patient's medical records. Unaccompanied patients may present in extremis, making it difficult or impossible to identify family or the primary provider before beginning potentially life-saving therapies. In addition, emergency providers may think it is not their role to discuss goals of care and that primary care providers should address these predictable crises in advance. Emergency physicians who have a more rigid view of their role may view palliative care as outside their scope of practice. Initial exploratory research in this area endorses these themes.[23,24]

In addition, fear of litigation or misunderstanding of state-specific end-of-life statutes may cause providers to think that legal issues impair their ability to forgo certain treatments, even when the potential for harm outweighs the potential for benefit.[23] Fear of litigation has been shown to influence medical decision making among emergency providers. In one study, a majority of emergency physicians admitted to ordering more tests than medically indicated because of fear of liability[25]; in another study, emergency physicians with greater fear of litigation were less likely to discharge patients with low-risk chest pain.[26]

Nursing staff is typically supportive of palliative care and may be an important source of support. In some settings, ED nurses can initiate palliative care consultation themselves or can contact social work or chaplaincy services for patients and families. At some institutions, social workers can consult one another, and an ED social worker could engage the palliative care social worker, who might have access to special resources specific to palliative care.

The Primary Care Provider

Barriers to palliative care consultation exist not only among emergency providers, but also among other physicians caring for the patient—primary care providers, hospitalists, or any of a number of specialists, such as oncologists. Although primary providers could provide background on patients' goals of care, prognosis, and trajectory of illness, they may not be immediately available during a crisis and delays in reaching them may result in the initiation of unwanted interventions. Some of these providers may equate palliative care with "giving up" and so be reluctant to ever have such services initiated on their patients. Others may not trust the emergency physician to make this judgment and may insist that they be consulted before a palliative medicine consult is called. Nevertheless, in a crisis, it may be appropriate and necessary for the emergency physician to consult palliative care without the primary provider's assent, just as the emergency physician would do for any other emergent consultation.

Staffing

In an ideal world, an interdisciplinary palliative care team would be available for immediate consultation 24 hours a day, 365 days a year. In reality, EDs will need to make plans to provide some palliative care services themselves or arrange for delayed consultation. In situations in which the team is not immediately available, ED observation units may be a useful setting to deliver symptomatic care or hold the patient until the palliative care team can get to the bedside. This allows a reevaluation regarding the need for admission after symptoms have been aggressively treated, as well as time for social work or other staff to help arrange hospice, visiting nurse, or home care services before discharge. However, patients receiving palliative care who have severe symptoms or complex needs may be too ill for discharge within 24 hours.

Training of Emergency Providers

One way to promote access to palliative care services in the ED is to train emergency providers in palliative care delivery. The Education in Palliative and End-of-life Care for Emergency Medicine (EPEC-EM) curriculum, for instance, educates emergency clinicians on the essentials of emergency palliative care, including rapid assessment of palliative care needs and appropriate referral to hospice (http://www.epec.net). All health care providers should be able to provide a minimal level of palliative care[27]; for emergency providers this should include prompt treatment of pain, nausea, and vomiting and addressing goals of care before initiating aggressive interventions for patients with advanced illness who are unlikely to benefit. Emergency medicine providers should also understand the vital role they often play as the first contact for patients requiring palliative care, because the trajectory of an inpatient hospitalization is often set in the ED.

Triggered Consultation

Triggers for palliative care consultation based on preset criteria are one way to overcome lack of knowledge and attitudinal barriers to palliative care consultation.[28] Patient-specific triggers have been developed for the surgical and medical intensive care units and can help providers recognize appropriate patients for referral.[29-31] ED criteria could be built into electronic medical records, which would generate a recommendation to the provider to refer to palliative care. The emergency provider could "opt-out" (i.e., decline consultation), or the patient or surrogate could decline services once the consult arrives. Defining criteria for consultation should involve key stakeholders, including emergency and palliative care providers, hospital administration, and other inpatient hospital providers who commonly care for such patients, such as internists and oncologists.

KEY MESSAGES TO PATIENTS AND FAMILIES

Although the ED may often seem like a chaotic environment to ill patients and their families, new models are being created to improve care for patients with serious and life-threatening illness who go to the ED. Palliative care services—whether delivered by a separate team or by the providers in the ED—can assist with management of complex symptoms or clarifying goals of care. When introducing palliative care services to patients and families in the ED setting, it should be stressed that the goal is to improve symptoms and clarify understanding, not to talk patients and families out of desired treatments. When appropriate, the patient's primary care or specialist physician should be included in conversations.

CONCLUSION AND SUMMARY

Emergency Medicine developed as a specialty to treat and stabilize patients with acute illness or injury for definitive care, but providers are increasingly providing care for acute exacerbations of chronic illness. Although not at odds with palliative care, whose mission is to relieve pain and other burdensome symptoms, Emergency Medicine has traditionally been viewed as a rescue-oriented, procedural specialty. Nonetheless, emergency visits provide a unique opportunity to relieve especially burdensome symptoms and provide goal-directed care early in a patient's hospital course. Even if patients have expressed prior preferences for treatment, these can change over time and with changes in clinical status.[32–34] Patients often visit the ED because of new or worsening symptoms, and thus it is especially vital that pain and other symptoms are promptly addressed. It also may be appropriate to readdress their goals of care during an ED visit.

In their report, the Institute of Medicine delineated many of the barriers to improving care at the end of life, including the historical separation of palliative and hospice care from potentially life-prolonging therapies.[35] Bringing palliative care into the ED, a place designed more to intervene than to comfort, is one important place to begin to break down these barriers. In fact, the integration of palliative care into Emergency Medicine is already occurring, with palliative care now an official subspecialty of Emergency Medicine. The number of ED-based pilot programs in the United States continues to rise, and preliminary data show associated reductions in hospital length of stay and costs per day. From a quality and cost-benefit perspective, offering palliative care services in the ED, at the beginning of the hospital course, might provide even greater benefit to patients, families, and hospitals than inpatient consultation, which often occurs late in a patient's hospital course.

SUMMARY RECOMMENDATIONS

- The integration of emergency medicine and palliative medicine should improve to meet the needs of the increasing number of patients with serious illness who receive care in the ED.
- Palliative care consultation for ED patients, delivery of services and promotion by ED palliative care champions, and ED linkages with local hospices are all valid models that can be implemented to integrate palliative care into the ED.
- Training of emergency medicine providers in primary palliative care skills is necessary and should become universal.

REFERENCES

1. Pitts SR, Niska RW, Xu J, Burt CW. National Hospital Ambulatory Medical Care Survey: 2006 emergency department summary. *Natl Health Stat Rep.* 2008;6(7):1–38.
2. Field MJ, Cassel CK, Institute of Medicine (U.S.) Committee on Care at the End of Life. *Approaching Death: Improving Care at the End of Life.* Washington, DC: National Academies Press; 1997.
3. Grudzen CR, Richardson LD, Morrison M, Cho E, Morrison RS. Palliative care needs of seriously ill, older adults presenting to the emergency department. *Acad Emerg Med.* 2010;17(11): 1253–1257.
4. *Clinical practice guidelines for quality palliative care.* www. nationalconsensusproject.org; 2009 Accessed September 25, 2012.
5. Billings JA. What is palliative care? *J Palliat Med.* 1998;1(1):73–81.
6. Meier DE, Morrison RS, Cassel CK. Improving palliative care. *Ann Intern Med.* 1997;127(3):225–230.
7. Morrison RS, Meier DE. Clinical practice: palliative care. *N Engl J Med.* 2004;350(25):2582–2590.
8. Quest TE, Marco CA, Derse AR. Hospice and palliative medicine: new subspecialty, new opportunities. *Ann Emerg Med.* 2009;54(1):94–102.
9. Pantilat SZ, Billings JA. Prevalence and structure of palliative care services in California hospitals. *Arch Intern Med.* 2003;163(9):1084–1088.
10. Billings JA, Pantilat S. Survey of palliative care programs in United States teaching hospitals. *J Palliat Med.* 2001;4(3):309–314.
11. Pan CX, Morrison RS, Meier DE, et al. How prevalent are hospital-based palliative care programs? Status report and future directions. *J Palliat Med.* 2001;4(3):315–324.
12. Morrison RS, Maroney-Galin C, Kralovec PD, Meier DE. The growth of palliative care programs in United States hospitals. *J Palliat Med.* 2005;8(6):1127–1134.
13. Morrison RS, Penrod JD, Cassel JB, et al. Cost savings associated with US hospital palliative care consultation programs. *Arch Intern Med.* 2008;168(16):1783–1790.
14. Osta BE, Palmer JL, Paraskevopoulos T, et al. Interval between first palliative care consult and death in patients diagnosed with advanced cancer at a comprehensive cancer center. *J Palliat Med.* 2008;11(1):51–57.
15. Waselewsky D, Zalenski R, Burn J, Hong Y. *Palliative care consultation Initiated in ED is associated with significant reductions in hospital length of stay.* New Orleans, LA: Society of Academy Emergency Medicine; 2009.
16. Cassel JB, Lyckholm LJ. *Identifying palliative care needs in the emergency department: better care, lower cost.* San Francisco, CA: Society of Academic Emergency Medicine; 2006.
17. Meier DE, Beresford L. Palliative care in inpatient units. *J Palliat Med.* 2006;9(6):1244–1249.
18. Mahony SO, Blank A, Simpson J, et al. Preliminary report of a palliative care and case management project in an emergency department for chronically ill elderly patients. *J Urban Health.* 2008;85(3):443–451.
19. Meier DE, Beresford L. Fast response is key to partnering with the emergency department. *J Palliat Med.* 2007;10(3):641–645.
20. Waugh DG. Palliative care project in the emergency department. *J Palliat Med.* 2010;13(8):936.
21. Stone SC, Mohanty SA, Gruzden C, Lorenz KA, Asch SM. Emergency department research in palliative care: challenges in recruitment. *J Palliat Med.* 2009;12:867–868.
22. Hendry H, McIntosh M, Borgman P, Belena A. *Integrating Hospice and Palliative Care Services in the ED: Effects on Resident and Faculty Education and ED Overcrowding.* New Orleans, LA: Society of Academy Emergency Medicine; 2009.
23. Grudzen CR, Richardson LD, Ortiz JM, Whang C, Hopper S, Morrison RS. Does palliative care have a future in the emergency department? Discussions with attending emergency physicians. *J Pain Symptom Manage.* 2012;43(1):1–9.
24. Smith AK, Fisher J, Schonberg MA, et al. Am I doing the right thing? Provider perspectives on improving palliative care in the emergency department. *Ann Emerg Med.* 2009;54(1): 86–93, e1.

25. Studdert DM, Mello MM, Sage WM, et al. Defensive medicine among high-risk specialist physicians in a volatile malpractice environment. *JAMA.* 2005;293(21):2609–2617.

26. Katz DA, Williams GC, Brown RL, et al. Emergency physicians' fear of malpractice in evaluating patients with possible acute cardiac ischemia. *Ann Emerg Med.* 2005;46(6):525–533.

27. von Gunten CF. Secondary and tertiary palliative care in US hospitals. *JAMA.* 2002;287(7):875–881.

28. Wood GJ, Arnold RM. How can we be helpful? Triggers for palliative care consultation in the surgical intensive care unit. *Crit Care Med.* 2009;37(3):1147–1148.

29. Norton SA, Hogan LA, Holloway RG, et al. Proactive palliative care in the medical intensive care unit: effects on length of stay for selected high-risk patients. *Crit Care Med.* 2007;35(6):1530–1535.

30. Mosenthal AC, Lee KF, Huffman J. Palliative care in the surgical intensive care unit. *J Am Coll Surg* 2002;194(1):75–83; discussion 83–85.

31. Campbell ML, Guzman JA. Impact of a proactive approach to improve end-of-life care in a medical ICU. *Chest.* 2003;123(1):266–271.

32. Wittink MN, Morales KH, Meoni LA, et al. Stability of preferences for end-of-life treatment after 3 years of follow-up: the Johns Hopkins Precursors Study. *Arch Intern Med.* 2008;168(19):2125–2130.

33. Straton JB, Wang NY, Meoni LA, et al. Physical functioning, depression, and preferences for treatment at the end of life: the Johns Hopkins Precursors Study. *J Am Geriatr Soc.* 2004;52(4):577–582.

34. Gallo JJ, Straton JB, Klag MJ, et al. Life-sustaining treatments: what do physicians want and do they express their wishes to others? *J Am Geriatr Soc.* 2003;51(7):961–969.

35. *Improving Palliative Care for Cancer.* Washington, DC: Institute of Medicine and National Research Council; National Academies Press; 2001.

Chapter 81

What Are Sources of Spiritual and Existential Suffering for Patients With Advanced Disease?

THE REVEREND GEORGE HANDZO AND RABBI EDITH M. MEYERSON

INTRODUCTION AND SCOPE OF THE PROBLEM

For all of the rightful concern in health care about the lack of attention to physical and emotional pain, spiritual and existential suffering may be the most universal and underrecognized component of the disease process. Sociologist Arthur Frank writes about his experience with heart disease and cancer, "From the perspective of the ill person, the root issue is suffering."[1] Dr. Daniel Sulmasy reminds us that "patient" comes originally from *"patiens,"* which means "one who suffers."[2]

Certainly, physical and emotional pain contribute to suffering. However, this distress alone does not necessarily produce suffering. For example, one may be familiar with the small minority of patients who welcome their physical pain because they believe it is given to them by their God as a way of wiping out some amount of sin they have committed in their lives. This expiation, they believe, increases their chances of going to heaven. These patients are not suffering. Other patients suffer greatly with the same pain because they believe the pain indicates that their God has abandoned them. The difference is the meaning the person gives to the pain rather than in the intensity of the pain itself. Some patients suffer because they are disconnected from that which is important to them—family, job, or even themselves. Other people with the same amount of pain maintain connections and so do not suffer.

This chapter outlines ways that members of the team caring for patients with advanced disease can participate in the assessment, diagnosis, and treatment of patients' suffering.

DEFINITIONS

The first step in understanding suffering is to be familiar with the definition of the key terms of "spirituality," "existential," and "suffering."

Spirituality

At a 2008 national consensus conference on spirituality in palliative care, a 50-member multidisciplinary group including physicians, chaplains, nurses, social workers, psychiatrists, clergy, and others developed the following consensus definition of spirituality:

Spirituality is the aspect of humanity that refers to the way individuals seek and express meaning and purpose and the way they experience their connectedness to the moment, to self, to others, to nature and to the significant or sacred.[3]

Although this is a consensus definition and thus subject to the limitations of that process, it is notable in that this very diverse group focused their definition on two characteristics common to many other definitions of both spirituality and existentialism—the search for meaning and purpose, and connectedness. The definition also anchors spirituality in basic humanity. Sulmasy, although not using the word, also focuses his definition on the aspect of connectedness. He writes, "Spirituality is 'an experience of something other than themselves', outside them or inside them but not equivalent to them."[4]

Existential

Dr. William Breitbart writes,

Existential issues deal with the examination of our existence acknowledging that we are grounded in the human condition. Yearning to seek what lies beyond our limitations is where the existential and the spiritual perhaps meet...[it has been suggested] that what is quintessentially a 'spiritual' pursuit of human beings is 'the search each human being undertakes to find a sense of peace in one's relationship to the universe'.[5]

This human pursuit is universal, related to but distinct from ... a search for meaning, and is perhaps at its most intense when we as human beings are confronting our mortality in the context of a life-threatening illness such as cancer.[6]

In many contexts, the distinction between "spiritual" and "existential" is important. For instance, chaplains would probably identify their skill set and primary task as focused on the realm of the spiritual and the religious within that, whereas psychotherapists might be more likely to claim the existential as their realm of practice. However, the consensus definition of spirituality and the definition of existentialism seem to share a focus on meaning making and connectedness. Although this characterization may be simplistic, that overlap may be more useful for the purposes of this chapter than any distinctions. Thus we will use "E/S" to describe the joint concept of existential and spiritual.

Suffering

If E/S points to connectedness and meaning making, suffering is what separates one from those connections (e.g., our spirituality), including the ability to make meaning. Suffering is part of the universal human condition. It is a core element of humanity, whether we are currently suffering or not. It is part of being human.

Cassell[7] writes that "Suffering can occur in relation to any aspect of the person, whether it is in the realm of social roles; group identification; the relation with self, body, or family; or the relation with a transpersonal, transcendent source of meaning." For some, as Arthur Frank[8] suggests, "suffering is the unspeakable, as opposed to what can be spoken; it is what remains concealed... beyond what is tangible even hurtful." Our role as clinicians is to create space for the suffering to be "speakable" should that be helpful for the patient or family.

SOURCES OF SUFFERING

Sources of suffering can be thought of as either a lack of connectedness to that which is essential inside and outside us and/or a lack of ability to make satisfactory meaning of our situation.

E/S encompasses a sense of wholeness and connectedness in any form of relationship, whether it be a relationship with oneself, community, nature, higher being, or so forth. E/S suffering can arise from a sense of disconnection from any of those relationships. These relationships provide a sense of wholeness in one's life; when one of those connective relationships feels fractured, a feeling of brokenness can occur and E/S suffering may be present. Cassell[7] notes, "Suffering occurs when an impending destruction of the person is perceived." Again, because spirituality is reliant on one's sense of self within relationship, when that sense of self feels compromised or threatened, suffering is present. Cassell[7] continues using the word

"intactness," meaning that it is the various relationships in one's life that can help one feel intact with a sense of foundation and grounding. When this intactness feels threatened, E/S suffering presents itself. Bruce and colleagues[9] describe spiritual suffering as a sense of groundlessness. Many find this groundlessness scary, unnerving, and difficult to navigate alone. This groundlessness is another form of disconnection.

Hindshaw[10] notes that although meaning and purpose are the essence of E/S, "it is only at the threat of a terminal diagnosis that awakens spiritual awareness within persons." Therefore all human beings carry elements of E/S. How E/S is engaged varies from person to person and on diagnosis of serious illness is when many realize, acknowledge, engage, or question E/S issues.

Park and Folkman[11] in their seminal work on meaning making posit two kinds of meaning—global meaning and situational meaning. Everyone has a system of global meaning that describes their presumptions about the world. This system can consist of beliefs such as "the world is fair" or "bad things don't happen to good people" or "if I eat the right foods, I won't get sick." For many people, their global meaning system derives partly or completely from religious belief. Situational meaning is the meaning given to a particular event such as an illness or trauma (e.g., I had a car accident because I'm a bad driver). Suffering occurs when the two kinds of meaning are incongruous. The first strategy for people in this situation is to change what they perceive to be the situational meaning to match their global system and thus reduce incongruity. For example, it is more comforting for patients to think that God is punishing them and they deserve to be punished (situational) because it fits with their global sense that God is good and just. Attribution (meaning) of an event that fits with the person's global meaning system leads to good adjustment. Most people adjust or accommodate if given time and space to process their situation.

ASSESSMENT AND DIAGNOSIS OF SUFFERING

As Bruce and colleagues[12] state, "existential concerns are inherent in being human." The question for clinicians is how to engage these concerns when patients and their families find themselves in E/S struggle. The first task is knowing how to assess and diagnose whether these concerns constitute suffering.

As Cassell[13] offers, "Suffering involves some symptom or process that threatens the patient because of fear, the meaning of the symptom, and concerns about the future. The meanings and the fear are personal and individual, so that even if two patients have the same symptoms, their suffering would be different." Because of the personal and individual nature of this suffering, assessment is necessarily subjective. However, the patient's and family's self-assessment are key components to making a diagnosis of suffering and determining its severity.

As alluded to earlier, suffering is self-defined in the same way as physical pain. There are no tests that examine the degree of one's own suffering. It is a comparison between how the person has experienced his or her own sense of wholeness and grounding up to this point and how that compares to his or her current sense of wholeness and grounding.

Because E/S is about creating, building, developing, and nourishing relationship and meaning, assessment begins by asking certain questions about an individual's E/S world. This assessment of E/S suffering should be incorporated into history taking in a routine manner. For example, pain may not simply be physical, and incorporating a few E/S questions into the process of obtaining a history will allow for a deepened connection with the patient. By asking these questions, the clinician is tapping the patient's E/S world and offering E/S care. Some of these questions might be as follows:

- How are your spirits?
- Are you suffering?
- Are you at peace?
- Are you frightened by all this?
- What are you most frightened of?
- What do you worry (are afraid) is going to happen to you?
- What is the worst thing about all this?
- What keeps you strong?
- What gives your life meaning and purpose?
- What do you value?
- How would you answer the question, Why am I here?
- What do you see as your identity? How would you answer the question, Who am I?
- What are you most proud of? What are your regrets?
- What do you think this illness is about?
- Are there questions or conversations you wish people (e.g., family, friends, clinicians) were asking or talking with you about, but they have not?

It is not necessary to ask *all* of these questions while taking a patient's history. Clinicians should choose questions with which they are comfortable and incorporate them into routine practice. The goal is simply to open the conversation. The questions also suggest themes clinicians can watch for in conversations with patients or family members. Asking these types of questions lets patients or family members know that the clinician cares about the patient and is willing to engage in these important conversations related to the patient's situation, which may in turn ultimately address the patient's suffering and potentially open up conversations about goals of care. Often though, clinicians do not ask these questions for fear of not knowing how to respond to the patient's answers. This will be addressed in the next section.

TREATMENT OF SUFFERING

E/S care fits within the generalist-specialist frame in the same way as other domains of health care.[14] Just as it is the responsibility of all members of the team to be attuned to the patient's physical pain and emotional state, all members of the team have a role in care that deals with E/S suffering. As with all other domains of care, this element of clinical practice has four major components: assessment, diagnosis, treatment, and referral. (The assessment and diagnostic phases have been discussed earlier.) Several published models now address this continuum for spiritual care.[15–17]

To treat E/S suffering, it is first necessary to see the task at hand as "healing" as opposed to "curing." Sulmasy[18] says, "Healing is a 'deeply human process.' True healing takes place only when the healer is related to the one who is healed - through, in, and with a relationship to the transcendent."

The healer needs to bring concentration, compassion, and perspective. Healing requires relationship. Indeed, healing may be accomplished by nothing more than being in relationship. Relationships built with patients and family members can restore lost connections and thus reduce the person's suffering. The clinician must be willing to hear the person's story without judgment or the intention of finding a solution; the conversation itself will form healing connections and allow the person to explore other lost connections. Creating this space for exploration, the clinician gives the patient or family member permission to give voice to suffering within a relational context with another human being. Sometimes, it is just in the asking that can provide a sense of healing for one's E/S pain.

Park and Folkman[11] claim that most people who are suffering because of incongruities in their ability to make meaning are able to solve the incongruity on their own if given the space and opportunity. Thus, again, the clinician may only have to listen and communicate willingness to journey with patients as they explore the meaning of their situation. To echo Dr. Sulmasy, what may be required is concentration and compassion rather than any particular skill or technique.[18] However, clinicians need to make it clear to patients that they are willing to give patients their undivided attention and a nonjudgmental presence. Patients need to be certain that their struggles will not be met with any kind of judgment or disapproval. For some clinicians, being in this role may raise anxieties related to the clinician's own E/S beliefs or concerns. The anxieties that a particular patient, family, or situation may invoke in the clinician should at some point be addressed by that clinician in his or her own way. Professional chaplains can be helpful in working through these situations.

Although these conversations will likely be the only E/S interventions the clinician generally engages in, structured interventions are available. Dignity Therapy, created by Dr. Harvey Chochinov,[19] engages the patient in creating a legacy document that is put in written form to preserve the patient's connections with family, friends, and others. Logotherapy, which has arisen from existentialism, is founded on the belief that it is the striving to find a meaning in one's life that is the primary, most powerful motivating and driving force in humans. This theory postulates that when it comes to decision making in a medical context, this drive to find meaning is the essence of what should guide conversations with patients and their loved ones. Logotherapy has been successfully tested with both groups and individuals by Dr. William Brietbart and colleagues.[20]

The clinician may also want to consider a referral to the professional chaplain if one is available. The professional chaplain is trained and tasked to engage the patient's "groundlessness" and their difficulties finding meaning, to help patients and their loved ones discover and use their spiritual and religious resources in the service of their healing.

SUMMARY RECOMMENDATIONS

- Primary clinicians should include in their routine history taking questions to assess E/S suffering, especially in regard to connectedness to what is important to the patient and the ability to make meaning in the current situation.
- Clinicians should encourage patients and family members to talk about their E/S struggles by making it clear that they are willing to give the patient or family member undivided attention and nonjudgmental presence.
- Patients or family members with complex E/S issues that do not seem to be resolving with routine conversation should be referred to the professional chaplain.

REFERENCES

1. Frank A. *At the Will of the Body: Reflections on Illness.* Boston, MA: Houghton Mifflin; 1991:115.
2. Sulmasy D. *The Healer's Calling: A Spirituality for Physicians and Other HealthCare Professionals.* New York: Paulist Press; 1997:101.
3. Puchalski C, Ferrell B. *Making Health Care Whole: Integrating Spirituality into Patient Care.* West Conshohocken, PA: Templeton Press; 2010:25.
4. Sulmasy D. *The Healer's Calling: A Spirituality for Physicians and Other HealthCare Professionals.* New York: Paulist Press; 1997:11.
5. Sagan C. The God hypothesis. In: Druyan A, ed. *The Varieties of Scientific Experience: A Personal View of the Search for God.* New York: Penguin Press; 2006:147–168.
6. Brietbart W. Who needs the concept of spirituality? Human beings seem to!. *Palliat Support Care.* 2007;5(2):105–106.
7. Cassell EJ. Nature of suffering and the goals of medicine. In: Henderson GE, King NM, Strauss RP, Estroff SE, Churchill LR, eds. *The Social Medicine Reader.* Durham, NC: Duke University Press; 2000.
8. Frank A. Can we research suffering? *Qual Health Res.* 2011;11(3):353–362.
9. Bruce A, Schreiber R, Petrovskaya O, Boston P. Longing for ground in a ground(less) world: a qualitative inquiry of existential suffering. *BMC Nurs.* 2011;27(10):3.
10. Hindshaw DB. Spiritual issues in surgical palliative care. *Surg Clin N Am.* 2005;85(2):257–272.
11. Park C, Folkman S. Meaning in the context of stress and coping. *Rev Gen Psychol.* 1997;1(2):115–144.
12. Bruce A, Schreiber R, Petrovskaya O, Boston P. Longing for ground in a ground(less) world: a qualitative inquiry of existential suffering. *BMC Nurs.* 2011;27(10):7.
13. Cassell EJ. Diagnosing suffering: a perspective. *Ann Intern Med.* 1999;131(7):531–544.
14. Handzo G, Koenig H. Spiritual care: Whose job is it anyway? *South Med J.* 2004;97(12):1242–1244.
15. National Comprehensive Cancer Network. *NCCN clinical practical guidelines in oncology.* http://www.nccn.org/professionals/physician_gls/f_guidelines.asp; Accessed September 24, 2012.
16. Fitchett G, Canada AL. The role of religion/spirituality in coping with cancer: evidence, assessment, and intervention. In: Holland JC, Breitbart WS, Jacobson PB, Lederberg MS, Loscalzo MJ, McCorkle R, eds. *Psycho-Oncology.* 2nd ed. New York: Oxford University Press; 2010:440–446.
17. Puchalski C, Ferrell B. *Making Health Care Whole: Integrating Spirituality into Patient Care.* West Conshohocken, PA: Templeton Press; 2010:71.
18. Sulmasy D. *The Healer's Calling: A Spirituality for Physicians and Other HealthCare Professionals.* New York: Paulist Press; 1997:14.
19. Chochinov HM, Haak T, Hassard T, Kristjanson LJ, McClement S, Harlos M. Dignity Therapy: a novel psychotherapeutic intervention for patients near the end of life. *J Clin Oncol.* 2005;23(24):5520–5525.
20. Breitbart W. Spirituality and meaning in supportive care: spirituality and meaning-centered group psychotherapy interventions in advanced cancer. *Support Care Cancer.* 2002;10(4):272–280.

Index

Note: Page numbers followed by "b" indicate boxes; "f" figures; "t" tables.